drug information

A GUIDE FOR PHARMACISTS

drug information

A GUIDE FOR PHARMACISTS

fifth edition

Editors

Patrick M. Malone, PharmD, FASHP
Associate Dean of Internal Affairs and
  Professor of Pharmacy Practice
College of Pharmacy
The University of Findlay
Findlay, Ohio

Karen L. Kier, PhD, MSc, RPh,
BCPS, BCACP
Professor of Clinical Pharmacy
Director of Assessment
Raabe College of Pharmacy
Ohio Northern University
Ada, Ohio

John E. Stanovich, RPh
Assistant Professor of Pharmacy Practice
Assistant Dean for External Programs
College of Pharmacy
The University of Findlay
Findlay, Ohio

Meghan J. Malone, PharmD, BCPS,
CACP
Clinical Pharmacist
Geisinger Health System
Danville, Pennsylvania

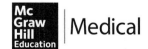

Mc Graw Hill Education | Medical

New York • Chicago • San Francisco • Athens • London • Madrid • Mexico City • Milan
New Delhi • Singapore • Sydney • Toronto

Drug Information: A Guide for Pharmacists, Fifth Edition

1 2 3 4 5 6 7 8 9 0   DOC/DOC   18 17 16 15 14

ISBN   978-0-07-180434-9
MHID   0-07-180434-X

This book was set in Century Old Style by MPS Limited.
The editors were Michael Weitz and Robert Pancotti.
The production supervisor was Catherine H. Saggese.
Project management was provided by Charu Khanna, MPS Limited.
The cover designer was Chris Bogie.
RR Donnelley was the printer and binder.

This book is printed on acid-free paper.

Library of Congress Cataloging-in-Publication Data

Drug information (Malone)
Drug information : a guide for pharmacists/editors, Patrick M. Malone, Karen L. Kier, John E. Stanovich, Meghan J. Malone.—Fifth edition.
     p. ; cm.
   Includes bibliographical references and index.
   ISBN 978-0-07-180434-9 (soft cover : alk. paper)—ISBN 0-07-180434-X
 I. Malone, Patrick M., 1954- editor.   II. Kier, Karen L., editor.   III. Stanovich, John E., editor.   IV. Malone, Meghan J., editor.   V. Title.
   [DNLM: 1. Drug Information Services. 2. Pharmacy   Administration—methods. QV 737.1]
   RS56.2
   615′.1—dc23   2014014804

International Edition ISBN 978-1-25-925555-7; MHID 1-25-925555-7. Copyright © 2014. Exclusive rights by McGraw-Hill Education, for manufacture and export. This book cannot be re-exported from the country to which it is consigned by McGraw-Hill Education. The International Edition is not available in North America.

McGraw-Hill Education books are available at special quantity discounts to use as premiums and sales promotions or for use in corporate training programs. To contact a representative, please visit the Contact Us pages at www.mhprofessional.com.

Contents

Chapter Twelve. Pharmacy and Therapeutics Committee 607
Patrick M. Malone, Nancy L. Fagan, Mark A. Malesker, and Paul J. Nelson

Chapter Thirteen. Drug Evaluation Monographs 669
Patrick M. Malone, Nancy L. Fagan, Mark A. Malesker, and Paul J. Nelson

Contributors

Robert D. Beckett, PharmD, BCPS
Assistant Professor of Pharmacy Practice
Director, Drug Information Center
College of Pharmacy
Manchester University
Fort Wayne, Indiana
Chapter 23

Elaine Blythe, PharmD
Associate Professor of Veterinary Medicine
School of Veterinary Medicine
St. Matthew's University
Omaha, Nebraska
Chapter 3

Patrick J. Bryant, PharmD, FSCIP
Director, Drug Information Center
Clinical Professor, Pharmacy Practice and
    Administration
School of Pharmacy
University of Missouri—Kansas City
Kansas City, Missouri
Chapter 5

**Karim Anton Calis, PharmD, MPH,
FASHP, FCCP**
Adjunct Clinical Investigator
Office of the Clinical Director

Eunice Kennedy Shriver National Institute of
    Child Health and Human Development
National Institutes of Health
Bethesda, Maryland
Clinical Professor
University of Maryland
Baltimore, Maryland
Clinical Professor
Virginia Commonwealth University
Richmond, Virginia
Chapter 2

**Zara Risoldi Cochrane, PharmD,
MS, FASCP**
Assistant Professor of Pharmacy Practice
Creighton University
School of Pharmacy and Health Professions
Omaha, Nebraska
Chapter 15

Sabrina W. Cole, PharmD, BCPS
Director of Biomedical Informatics
Assistant Professor of Pharmacy
School of Pharmacy
Wingate University
Wingate, North Carolina
Chapter 18

Kathryn A. Crea, PharmD, BCPS, CPPS
Director of Accreditation and Patient Safety
 Officer
OhioHealth—Riverside Methodist Hospital
Columbus, Ohio
Chapter 16

Jean E. Cunningham, PharmD, BCPS
Clinical Content Specialist
Truven Health Analytics
Greenwood Village, Colorado
Chapter 22

Lindsay E. Davison, PharmD
Silver Spring, Maryland
Chapter 22

Elizabeth A. Van Dyke, PharmD
Drug Information Consultant
Saint Clairsville, Ohio
(independent consulting)
Chapter 5

Stacie Krick Evans, PharmD
Pharmacy Implementation Manager
Central Atlantic Region
Performance Services
VHA, Waxhaw
Chapter 18

Nancy L. Fagan, PharmD
Assistant Professor of Pharmacy Practice
Creighton University
School of Pharmacy and Health Professions
Omaha, Nebraska
Chapters 12 and 13

Brent I. Fox, PharmD, PhD
Associate Professor, Department of Health
 Outcomes Research & Policy
Harrison School of Pharmacy
Auburn University
Auburn, Alabama
Chapter 24

**Maisha Kelly Freeman, PharmD, MS,
BCPS, FASCP**
Associate Professor of Pharmacy Practice
Director, Samford University Global Drug
 Information Service
Birmingham, Alabama
Chapter 4

Mary Lea Gora-Harper, PharmD
Clinical Pharmacist
University of Kentucky
Lexington, Kentucky
Chapter 1

Philip J. Gregory, PharmD, FACN
Associate Professor of Pharmacy Practice
Creighton University
School of Pharmacy and Health Professions
Omaha, Nebraska
Chapter 15

**Bambi Grilley, RPh, RAC, CCRA,
CCRC, CIP**
Assistant Professor, Pediatrics
Director, Clinical Research and Early Product
 Development
Center for Cell and Gene Therapy
Baylor College of Medicine
Houston, Texas
Chapter 17

Darren Hein, PharmD
Fellow, Drug Information & Evidence-Based
    Practice
Creighton University
School of Pharmacy and Health Professions
Omaha, Nebraska
Chapter 15

Joshua C. Hollingsworth, PharmD
Doctoral Student, Department of Health
    Outcomes Research & Policy
Harrison School of Pharmacy
Auburn University
Auburn, Alabama
Chapter 24

Peter J. Hughes, PharmD
Assistant Professor
McWhorter School of Pharmacy
Samford University
Birmingham, Alabama
Chapter 4

Vicki R. Kee, PharmD
Assistant Professor (Clinical)
Drug Information Pharmacist
The University of Iowa
Iowa Drug Information Service
Iowa City, Iowa
Chapter 7

Michael G. Kendrach, PharmD, FASHP
Professor and Associate Dean of Academic
    Affairs
McWhorter School of Pharmacy
Samford University
Birmingham, Alabama
Chapter 4

Mark A. Malesker, PharmD, FCCP,
FASHP, BCPS
Professor of Pharmacy Practice and Medicine
Creighton University
School of Pharmacy and Health Professions
Omaha, Nebraska
Chapters 12 and 13

J. Russell May, PharmD, FASHP
Clinical Professor
College of Pharmacy
University of Georgia
Augusta, Georgia
Chapter 1

Michelle W. McCarthy, PharmD, FASHP
Director, PGY1-Pharmacy and PGY2-Drug
    Information Residency Programs
Director, Medication Use Policy and
    Compliance
University of Virginia Health System
Department of Pharmacy Services
Charlottesville, Virginia
Chapter 21

Cydney E. McQueen, PharmD
Clinical Associate Professor, Pharmacy
    Practice and Administration
University of Missouri–Kansas City School
    of Pharmacy
Kansas City, Missouri
Chapter 5

Kevin G. Moores, PharmD
Associate Professor (Clinical)
Director, Division of Drug Information
    Service
College of Pharmacy
The University of Iowa
Iowa City, Iowa
Chapter 7

David P. Nau, PhD, RPh, CPHQ, FAPhA
President
Pharmacy Quality Solutions, Inc.
Springfield, Virginia
Chapter 14

Paul J. Nelson, MD
Primary Physician
Family Health Care, P.C.
Adjunct Assistant Professor—Clinician of
  Pediatrics
University of Nebraska Medical Center
College of Medicine
Omaha, Nebraska
Chapters 12 and 13

Genevieve Lynn Ness, PharmD
Director, Christy Houston Foundation
  Drug Information Center
Assistant Professor in Pharmaceutical,
  Social and Administrative Science
College of Pharmacy
Belmont University
Nashville, Tennessee
Chapter 23

Linda K. Ohri, PharmD, MPH
Associate Professor of Pharmacy Practice
Creighton University
School of Pharmacy and Health Professions
Omaha, Nebraska
Chapter 11

Heather A. Pace, PharmD
Assistant Director, Drug Information Center
Clinical Associate Professor
University of Missouri–Kansas City School
  of Pharmacy
Kansas City, Missouri
Chapter 20

Debra L. Parker, PharmD
Chair and Associate Professor
Department of Pharmacy Practice
The University of Findlay
College of Pharmacy
Findlay, Ohio
Chapter 19

Karen L. Rascati, PhD
Professor, Health Outcomes and Pharmacy
  Practice
College of Pharmacy
University of Texas
Health Outcomes and Pharmacy Practice
  Division
Austin, Texas
Chapter 6

**Martha M. Rumore, PharmD, JD LLM,
FAPhA**
Assistant Director, Pharmacy Clinical &
  Educational Services
Director, Pediatric Medication Resource
  Center
Cohen Children's Medical Center
Professor, Pharmacy & Health Outcomes
Touro College of Pharmacy
Sorrell, Lenna & Schmidt, LLP
New York, New York
Chapter 10

Amy Heck Sheehan, PharmD
Drug Information Specialist
Indiana University Health
Associate Professor of Pharmacy Practice
Purdue University College of Pharmacy
Indianapolis, Indiana
Chapter 2

Kelly M. Shields, PharmD
Assistant Dean and Associate Professor of
   Pharmacy Practice
Raabe College of Pharmacy
Ohio Northern University
Ada, Ohio
Chapter 3

Morgan L. Sperry, PharmD
Clinical Assistant Professor
Assistant Director, Drug Information Center
University of Missouri–Kansas City School
   of Pharmacy
Kansas City, Missouri
Chapter 20

Ryan W. Walters, MS
Research Analyst and Instructor
Division of Clinical Research and Evaluative
   Sciences
Department of Medicine
Creighton University Medical Center
Omaha, Nebraska
Chapter 8

James P. Wilson, PharmD, PhD
Associate Professor of Health Outcomes and
   Pharmacy Practice
College of Pharmacy
University of Texas
Health Outcomes and Pharmacy Practice
   Division
Austin, Texas
Chapter 6

Preface

Ever since the publication of the first edition of this book in 1996, there has been increasing realization of the importance of drug information. Much of this can be related to Internet information sources, along with the ever-increasing ease by which material can be located and used. This increased emphasis on information has had an effect on both the health care professional, who uses the material, and the patient, who may look up material directly and even bring it in to talk about with a health care professional. The ability to obtain, manage, evaluate, and use information has become an important core skill for the professional.

This book was originally written to provide training in drug information management. It has been tested and refined continuously, based on experience in both practice and the classroom. In this fifth edition, the goal of this book continues to be to educate both students and practitioners on how to efficiently research, interpret, evaluate, collate, and disseminate information in the most usable form. While there is no one right method to perform these professional responsibilities, proven methods are presented and demonstrated. Also, seldom-addressed issues are covered, such as the legal and ethical considerations of providing information.

The fifth edition continues to expand, updating information from previous editions and going into new areas. This includes a new chapter on assessing drug promotions by pharmaceutical representatives and the need for counterdetailing. Another new chapter is on pharmacy informatics. It always seemed that there should be a connection between pharmacy informatics and drug information—after all, both make extensive use of computer systems to manage information. However, they often seem to be treated as separate subjects. This new chapter bridges that gap.

SPECIAL TEXT FEATURES

In addition, we continue to include features that will assist the reader in learning the material:

- A series of Key Concepts at the beginning of each chapter are then identified throughout the chapter using circled numbers placed within the text.
- The main areas outlined in the Learning Objectives have been highlighted throughout the chapter using vertical rules placed in the margins alongside the relevant passages of text.
- Most chapters have cases, where a situation that might be faced by a practitioner is described, with a series of discussion points presented.
- A series of multiple-choice questions are included and many chapters provide suggested readings for further information on topics.

As in previous editions, the book begins by introducing the concept of drug information, including its history, and providing information on various places in which drug information specialists may be employed. This is followed by information on how to answer a question, from the process of gathering necessary background information, through determining the actual information need, to answering the question. The chapter on drug information resources includes descriptions of the most commonly used references and contains information on apps available for practitioners. The drug literature evaluation chapters have been updated and expanded to cover newer concepts, such as adaptive clinical trials. Chapters from the previous edition have been updated. As always, numerous practical examples are provided through the chapters and in the appendices.

With the veritable Niagara Falls of drug, medical, and pharmacy information available, much of which is complex, health care professionals have an increasing need for information management skills. This book will assist health care professionals and students with improvement in drug information skills and will allow individuals to evolve into new roles for the advancement of the profession and patient care. The authors and editors of this book hope the readers enjoy their journey toward expertise in information management.

1

Chapter One

Introduction to the Concept of Drug Information

Mary Lea Gora-Harper • J. Russell May

Learning Objectives

● *After completing this chapter, the reader will be able to*

- Define the term *drug information*, used in different contexts, and relate it to the term *medication information*.
- Identify the services provided by drug information centers.
- Describe the skills needed to perform medication information functions.
- Identify major factors that have influenced the ability to provide medication information.
- Describe how the expanding integration of information technology has changed the methods of searching, analyzing, and providing medication information to patients and health care professionals.
- Describe how the increase in cost of health care has expanded the role of medication information specialists.
- Describe practice opportunities for a medication information specialist.

Key Concepts

❶ Medication information may be patient-specific or developed for a given patient population.

❷ Medication information provision has evolved in the last 50 years as focus has shifted to medication safety, advances in informatics, evidence-based medicine, and new environments of care.

❸ With computerized medical records and order entry systems, medication information specialists can take a leadership role in incorporating automated interventions that improve safety and provide education at the point of prescribing.

❹ Medication information specialists must keep abreast of advances in information technology.

❺ Medication literature evaluation skills are essential.

❻ Leadership and career opportunities exist in a variety of settings for medication information specialists.

Introduction

The United States (U.S.) health care system is undergoing important changes, which is offering challenges and opportunities for health care providers, insurers, caregivers, and consumers. Several factors are driving these changes including new regulations in health care (e.g., expanded coverage for preventive care for patients of all ages, coverage regardless of preexisting conditions, the mandate for all Americans to acquire health insurance, expansion of Medicaid), the continued pressure to reduce health care costs, and the need to improve efficiency, quality, and safety of care.[1-3] The appropriate use of pharmaceuticals continues to be an essential element in this process because drugs represent a significant portion of the health care dollars spent in the United States. Total health care system spending on medication reached $320 billion in 2011, an increase of about $50 billion since 2006 and $125 billion since 2002.[2] The availability of patient-, disease-, and medication-specific information, and a knowledgeable decision maker are integral components of providing a system that supports the safe and appropriate use of medications.

The provision of **medication information** is among the most fundamental responsibilities of pharmacists. ❶ *Medication information may be patient-specific, or developed for a given patient population,* such as therapeutic guidelines, communication of a national quality initiative, coordination of an adverse drug event reporting and analysis program, publication of an electronic newsletter, or updating a Web site. The pharmacist can serve as a resource for issues regarding cost-effective medication selection and use, medication policy decisions (drug benefits), medication information resource selection, or practice-related issues. Medication information opportunities are developing and expanding with changes in the health care environment, national efforts to expand access to care while reducing health care costs, the rise in the self-care movement, and the integration of new health information technologies (e.g., electronic health record [EHR], telemedicine, social media, computerized physician order entry [CPOE], communication across settings of care). Medication information opportunities are growing in several areas within the health care environment including managed care organizations, the pharmaceutical industry, medical and specialty care clinics, scientific writing and medical communication companies, and the insurance industry.

The term **drug information** may have different meanings to different people depending on the context in which it is used. If asked to define this term, one could describe it as information found in a reference or verbalized by an individual that pertains to medications. In many cases, individuals put this term in different contexts by associating it with other words which include:

1. Specialist/practitioner/pharmacist/provider
2. Center/service/practice
3. Functions/skills

The first group of words implies a specific individual, the second group implies a place, and the third implies activities and abilities of individuals. The term drug information will be used in these different contexts to describe the beginnings and evolution of this area of practice. Relative to current practice, the term medication information is used in place of drug information to convey the management and use of information on medication therapy and to signify the broader role that all pharmacists take in information provision. These terms may refer to either the provision of information for a specific patient or in the context of addressing medication use issues for a population (i.e., a group of individuals defined by a set of common characteristics, such as in a set of policies and procedures on medication use developed by health professional working in the emergency department of a hospital).

Drug informatics refers to the electronic management of drug information. It emphasizes the use of technology as an integral tool in effectively organizing, analyzing, managing, and communicating information on medication use in patients. With the growing integration of EHRs and CPOE, there is greater opportunity to provide information on medications for individual patients at the point of care, and be able to assess outcomes more readily on a population of patients.[4] The impact of new technologies and opportunities in drug informatics in current and future practice is discussed later in this chapter and Chapter 24.

The goals of this chapter are to describe how the role of the pharmacist has evolved in providing medication information, to discuss factors contributing to that evolution, and to describe opportunities for use of medication information skills, either as a generalist or in a specialty practice. This chapter provides the foundation for understanding the pharmacist's need to have proficiency in the knowledge and skills discussed in this book.

The Beginning

The term *drug information* developed in the early 1960s when used in conjunction with the words *center* and *specialist*. In 1962, the first drug information center was opened at the University of Kentucky Medical Center.[5] This center desired to be a source of comprehensive drug information for staff physicians, dentists, and nurses. Another goal was to take an active role in the education of health professional students including medicine, dentistry, and nursing and specifically influence pharmacy students in developing their role as drug consultants. Several other drug information centers were established shortly thereafter. The first formal survey, conducted in 1983, identified 54 pharmacist-operated centers in the United States.[6]

The individual responsible for operation of the center was called the drug information specialist. The expectation was that drug information would be stored in the center and retrieved, selected, evaluated, and disseminated by the specialist. As practice progressed, some drug information centers evolved to drug information services where drug information activities were provided outside of a formalized center. In addition, other specific functions evolved over time, as listed in Table 1–1. A drug information center or specialist may be involved in one or all of these functions. Detailed information regarding these activities is provided in subsequent chapters.

In the 1960s, the availability of new drugs (e.g., neuromuscular blockers, first-generation cephalosporins) provided challenges for practitioners to keep abreast and make appropriate decisions for their patients. Part of the problem was finding a way to

TABLE 1–1. MEDICATION INFORMATION SERVICES

- Supporting clinical services with medication information
- Answering questions regarding medications
- Coordinating pharmacy and therapeutics committee activity
- Developing medication use policies
- Publishing or editing information on appropriate medication use through newsletters, journal columns, Web sites, e-mail, social media, etc.
- Managing investigational medication use (e.g., Institutional Review Board activities, information for practitioners—see Chapter 17)
- Providing poison information

- Coordinating formulary management initiatives
- Developing criteria/guidelines for medication use
- Analyzing the clinical and economic impact of drug policy decisions
- Managing medication usage evaluation/medication use evaluation and other quality assurance/improvement activities
- Providing education (e.g., in-services, classes, experiential education) for health professionals, students, and consumers
- Coordinating of adverse drug event reporting and analysis programs, e.g., adverse medication reactions
- Consulting on the development of informatics in the health system setting

effectively communicate the wealth of information to those needing it. The information environment relied heavily on the print medium for storage, retrieval, and dissemination of information. MEDLARS® (Medical Literature Retrieval and Analysis System) was developed by the National Library of Medicine in the early 1960s.[7] While it provided a computerized form of searching, requests for searches were submitted by mail and results returned by mail. The ability to transmit such information over telephone lines (online technology) was not available until 1971 when MEDLINE® was introduced and was limited to libraries. During this time, the drug information specialist was viewed as a person who could bridge the gap and effectively communicate drug information.[8] Of course, methods for accessing information have evolved tremendously with the creation of the Internet and the integration of EHR.

Early reports that examine the requirements for training of a drug information specialist recommended the following courses be added or strengthened in the pharmacy school curricula: biochemistry, anatomy, physiology, pathology, and biostatistics and experimental design (with some histology, embryology, and endocrinology incorporated into other courses).[9] Such topics were either not incorporated or not emphasized in curricula of the 1960s. In today's pharmacy curricula, most of these topics receive considerable emphasis. In addition to these subjects, progress has been made to incorporate evidence-based practice and patient-centered care into curricula.[10] Pharmacists today use knowledge and skills to make clinical decisions about medication use in specific patients or a group of patients in conjunction with other health care professionals. This fits nicely with providing patient- and family-centered care, known as patient-centered medical home (PCMH). Training and expertise in evidence-based practice have led pharmacists to take a leadership role in publishing in the area of therapeutic guidelines, drug policy initiatives, or outcome analyses, sometimes with support of the pharmacy professional organizations. These activities illustrate how pharmacists play a major role in meeting the needs of individual patients and large patient groups.

The Evolution

It is useful to look at the evolution of drug information practice from the perspective of drug information centers and practicing pharmacists. Calculating accurate numbers of drug information centers nationally or internationally (e.g., Puerto Rico, Japan, Saudi Arabia, Africa) is difficult, because no agency or organization is responsible for maintaining a list. Well-defined criteria are not established for using the titles of drug information centers/services. Some centers specialize in a particular area of drug information, and their name may reflect that specific function (e.g., center of drug policy and drug information, drug and poison information center, and drug information and wellness center). Some centers limit their practice to a subset of clients (e.g., pharmacists, physicians, nurses, other health professionals, attorneys, faculty, consumers) based on their source of funding (e.g., pharmaceutical manufacturer, government, college of pharmacy, managed care organization, law firm, law enforcement agencies), and some drug information centers are available for all consumers, 7 days a week, 24 hours a day, as is the case for a drug and poison information center. The center may provide services via telephone, through a Web site, face-to-face with their clients, or other methods.

One study conducted in 2008 and published in 2009 examined 89 drug information centers to test if there were changes in number or type of questions, and time spent on activities compared to 5 years earlier.[11] Eighty-four percent of the drug information centers were still in existence. There was an increase in time spent educating students (53%) and supporting adverse drug reaction reporting initiatives (44%). Seventy-six reported an increase in the number of complex questions, with 53% documenting an increase in the time required to answer questions.

When examining the availability of a drug information center specifically in the hospital setting, a 2010 survey that examined over 1950 U.S. hospitals, found that 5% had a formal drug information center as their source to provide objective drug information.[12] In an earlier survey,[13] it was found that the availability of a formal drug information center was more prevalent in larger hospitals. For instance, when examining a subset of the hospitals with more than 400 beds, 28.2% of hospitals reported that they had a formal drug information center.

A few studies have described the economic benefit of maintaining a drug information center or related activity in an academic institution or hospital. One such study examined the economic impact of drug information services responding to patient-specific requests.[14] The resultant cost-benefit ratio was found to be 2.9:1 to 13.2:1. Most of the cost savings resulted from a decreased need for monitoring (e.g., laboratory tests) or a decreased need for additional treatment related to an adverse effect. Another study examined the drug cost avoidance and revenue associated with the provision of investigational drug services, which was not part of drug information center in this study, but may be the responsibility of a drug information center.[15] The annualized drug cost avoidance plus revenue was $2.6 million. Studies of this nature are becoming increasingly important in an era of cost containment. Although these studies were completed several years ago, the basic premise of the design and results are applicable today and can be used to provide a foundation for assessment of the value of a particular center based on location, clientele, and funding. Other literature also exists that evaluates the economic return on investment for clinical services, which can help provide a framework for how to assess the value of a drug information center.[16]

DRUG INFORMATION—FROM CENTERS TO PRACTITIONERS

The responsibilities of individual pharmacists regarding the provision of medication information have changed substantially over the years. The impetus for this change was provided not only by the development of drug information centers and the clinical pharmacy concept, but also by the Study Commission on Pharmacy.[17] This external group was established to review the state of the practice and education of pharmacists and report its findings. One of the findings and recommendations stated that

> "... among deficiencies in the health care system, one is the unavailability of adequate information for those who consume, prescribe, dispense and administer drugs. This deficiency has resulted in inappropriate drug use and an unacceptable frequency of drug-induced disease. Pharmacists are seen as health professionals who could make an important contribution to the health care system of the future by providing information about drugs to consumers and health professionals. Education and training of pharmacists now and in the future must be developed to meet these important responsibilities."

The report of the Commission was issued in 1975, and since that time drug information practice has changed for both drug information centers and individual pharmacists. The development of clinical pharmacy has helped move pharmacy forward in recognizing its capabilities to contribute to the care of patients. Clinical pharmacy was thought of primarily as an institutional patient care process and did not gain widespread acceptance outside of hospitals. Over time, the activity of the pharmacist as a medication expert for patients has gained acceptance in a variety of practice settings including community pharmacies, nursing homes, and primary and specialty clinics. Pharmacists who provide patient-specific information with a goal of improving patient outcomes use the medical literature to support their choices.[18]

Pharmacists involved in patient care areas (e.g., hospitals, clinics, long-term care, home health care) now frequently answer medication information questions, participate in evaluating a patient's drug therapy, and conduct medication usage evaluation activities. In one survey of more than 1960 hospitals, approximately 97% have staff pharmacists routinely answer drug information questions.[12] The provision of medication information may be on a one-on-one basis or may occur using a more structured approach, such as a presentation to a class of patients with diabetes or a group of nurses in the practice facility. In either case, the pharmacist educates those who are the beneficiaries of the medication information. Pharmacists may also participate in precepting students in patient care or pharmacy environments. In any of these roles, the pharmacist must use appropriate information retrieval and evaluation skills to make sure that the most current and accurate information is provided to make decisions about medication use for those they are serving. This role of the pharmacist as a

TABLE 1–2. MEDICATION INFORMATION SKILLS

1. Assess available information and gather situational data needed to characterize question or issue.
2. Formulate appropriate question(s).
3. Use a systematic approach to find needed information.
4. Evaluate information critically for validity and applicability.
5. Develop, organize, and summarize response for question or issue.
6. Communicate clearly when speaking or writing, at an appropriate level of understanding.
7. Anticipate other information needs.

provider of medication information continues to be an important component of the educational outcomes developed by the Center for the Advancement of Pharmaceutical Education (CAPE). These outcomes are initiated and maintained by the American Association of Colleges of Pharmacy (AACP) to help transform the pharmacy curriculum to support education of the future.[10,19] There is a well-described systematic approach to answering drug information questions (see Chapter 2). It is important to obtain the necessary background information including pertinent patient factors, disease factors, and medication-related factors to determine the true question. Good problem-solving skills are required to fully assess the situation, develop a search strategy (see Chapter 3), evaluate the information (see Chapters 4 and 5), and then formulate and communicate a response. Good communication skills are essential to respond in a clear and concise manner, using terminology that is consistent with the patients', caregivers', or health professionals' level of understanding. Table 1–2 lists the medication information skills a pharmacist should possess when confronted with a medication information need.

Opportunities continue to grow for pharmacist participation in the continuum of care including home health care and long-term care that require a solid therapeutic knowledge base, an understanding of the medical literature, and the ability to communicate the information through either verbal or written consultation. Pharmacists in community settings counsel patients, answer medication information questions, review patient medication regimens for potential problems (medication therapy management), and participate in helping patients manage chronic diseases. The PCMH philosophy has become a widely accepted model for how primary care should be organized and delivered throughout the health care system. Patient care is considered to be comprehensive, team-based, coordinated, and accessible. As a component, the health care team helps improve the quality of care through access to information technology and other tools, to help make sure that both patients and families are making informed choices about their health. Medication information should be administered when they need it, and in a culturally and linguistically appropriate manner.

Opportunities for pharmacists are also available in the area of veterinary pharmacy practice. Information is needed by both the animal owner and the veterinarian. A pharmacist may need to practically apply information from veterinary resources (e.g., *Veterinary Drug Handbook, Textbook of Veterinary Internal Medicine, National Animal Poison Control Center*) for the benefit of an animal (see Chapter 3).

FACTORS INFLUENCING THE EVOLUTION OF THE PHARMACIST'S ROLE AS A MEDICATION INFORMATION PROVIDER

❷ *Medication information provision has evolved in the last 50 years as focus has shifted to medication safety, advances in informatics, evidence-based medicine, and new environments of care.* Other factors include new regulations in health care, the changing philosophy of practice (e.g., patient-focused medical home programs), the evaluation of outcomes, the sophistication of medication therapy, and the self-care movement.

Adverse Drug Events

As mentioned earlier in this chapter, one of the primary roles for drug information specialists in the beginning was collecting and evaluating adverse drug reactions.[5] This role will continue to expand because it is anticipated that the number of adverse drug events (ADEs) will increase in the near future for several reasons: (1) the availability of new medications and new indications with conventional medications, (2) the growing elderly population, (3) the increased use of medications for disease prevention, and (4) the improved insurance coverage for medications.[20] Pharmacists perform this function in institutional health systems, managed care, or the pharmaceutical industry. To illustrate how a central area for reporting ADEs, such as a drug information center in an institutional health system, can be beneficial, consider the following unpublished example from an academic medical center. The drug information center received three reports of patients developing methemoglobinemia within a 2-week period. The offending agent was suspected to be benzocaine spray. Upon investigation, the drug information pharmacist recognized that all reports had one thing in common: the administering nurse. The pharmacist witnessed the administration of the drug by the nurse the next time it was ordered for a patient. Instead of a single brief spray as directed by the prescribing information, several sprays were used resulting in a potentially toxic dose of drug. The drug information pharmacist developed a series of in-services for nurses. No reports of benzocaine-induced methemoglobinemia have occurred since. In managed care settings, the same benefit could be achieved on an even larger scale.

The role of the drug information specialist in the pharmaceutical industry as it relates to reporting ADEs is especially important in postmarketing surveillance activities. Because of the specific definition of a study population using inclusion and exclusion criteria in a new drug trial, many ADEs go undetected until the agent is commercially available and used in a broader population. By quickly identifying potential problems and communicating them to health care professionals, patient safety may be improved. The training and expertise of the drug information specialist qualifies them to play a major role in this process.

The importance of maintaining a comprehensive, multidisciplinary, ongoing program for monitoring, reporting, and resolving drug-related problems, and developing mechanisms to prevent future ADEs will continue to be an important element of managing medication use, with the drug information specialist providing leadership, as well as every clinical practitioner (e.g., pharmacists, nurses, physicians) contributing to the overall program. There is an estimated 700,000 emergency room visits and 120,000 hospitalizations annually attributed to ADEs, with an annual extra cost of $3.5 billion to the health care system.[21,22] Forty percent of these events are considered to be preventable.[22] These numbers are probably even higher in the elderly population because of age-related physiological changes, co-existing conditions, and polypharmacy.[23] The prevention of ADEs is important today, and will continue to be a significant health care issue in the future.[24]

Integration of New Health Information Technologies

Computer technology has drastically changed the ability to store and access information. The focus in medication information is driven toward the use and integration of data, information, knowledge, and technology involved in the medication use process to improve outcomes for patients. Even though the amount of literature is much larger today than in the past, it is more manageable. The Internet allows the user to easily access the scientific literature, government publications, news reports, and many other items, frequently without cost to the clinician or the consumer, and handheld devices (e.g., smartphones, tablets) have allowed practitioners to have a full range of applications (e.g., decision-support tools, medical references) that can be available at the point of care.[25] These devices offer the convenience of collecting and accessing information from a unit that can be carried in a user's pocket. In certain situations, these systems can be used more conveniently than a desktop computer for online searching, calculations, patient tracking, laboratory order entry, and results, to provide medication profiles, to set appointments, as a time-management tool, and to search drug information databases (e.g., general drug information text, medical specialty reference books, drug interaction resources). Patients and health care practitioners can find information on nearly every disease and treatment, and virtual health communities and forums provide a mutually supportive environment for patients and their families, and friends. The use of social media (e.g., Twitter®, Facebook®, LinkedIn), e-mail, Web forums, and blogs has simplified the way in which peers can exchange news and share opinions. Several professional organizations (e.g., American Society of Health-System Pharmacists [ASHP]; http://www.ashp.org)

have used technology to maintain awareness of important news affecting pharmacy and the health care environment (e.g., regulatory and health policy issues), drug shortages, and awareness of their meetings. Live continuing education is offered at a clinician's computer desktop through Webinars.

There is an increasing need by health professionals, as well as consumers, to get more information about medications sooner. Information is needed quickly when a new medication becomes commercially available because of the potential for health and cost implications, when a product is withdrawn from the market for safety reasons, or when data from a new study is released that could have an impact on how common ailments are treated. The lag time that occurs with the print format may not be acceptable for many direct patient care issues. The Internet allows medical information to be available sooner to both health care professionals and the public. The availability of electronic journals and texts has minimized the need to travel to a library. Online repositories for articles, such as BioMed Central (http://www.biomedcentral.com) and PubMed® (http://www.pubmedcentral.nih.gov), have allowed individuals to access millions of articles quickly, easily, and free of charge. The majority of printed medical textbooks with an online version require a subscription; however, there are exceptions (e.g., http://www.merck.com, where eight editions of Merck Manuals can be viewed and searched for free). Registries of ongoing clinical trials, such as ClinicalTrials.gov (http://www.ClinicalTrials.gov), provide information on the purpose and criteria for participation in an ongoing clinical trial. This has allowed pharmacists to anticipate new therapies, and perhaps help their patients receive medications not yet approved by the Food and Drug Administration (FDA) through enrollment in a clinical trial.

In addition to health professionals, patients are also accessing information from the Web, using sites that are sponsored by a variety of companies and individuals with diverse interests. In a recent survey, 85% of physician respondents had experienced a patient bringing Internet information to a visit.[26] Information that is either incomplete or inaccurate may result in harmful behavior, such as discontinuing medication or increasing the doses.[27] In one study,[28] information on medications on Wikipedia was found to be more narrow in scope, and had more errors of omission than the comparator database on the Web (i.e., Medscape Drug Reference, which is a free, online, evidence-based, peer-reviewed database).

There is some effort toward helping consumers accurately assess the quality of information on the Internet. Health on the Net (http://www.hon.ch) is a nonprofit, non-government organization that uses criteria to assess the quality of a Web site. The organization will give a seal of approval to those sites that apply and meet the quality criteria. If misinformation or inaccurate information is found on the Web, organizations exist to monitor fraud (e.g., Quackwatch®; http://www.quackwatch.com). One site that may be helpful in providing patients with information on a range of medical conditions and management is healthfinder (http://www.healthfinder.gov). See Chapters 19 and 20 for more information.

Drug information centers have created their own Web sites to post information about their centers and services, to provide links to related sites considered to be of acceptable quality, to accept adverse drug reaction reports, to receive and answer medication information questions conveniently, and to provide information regarding formulary changes, institution-specific therapeutic guidelines, and drug policy initiatives.[29] The advantage of having a request form for answering medication information questions or reporting adverse drug reactions on the Web is that physicians, pharmacists, or other health professionals can access computers at their practice site. This information is typically accessible only through an institution's **intranet**.[30] An intranet is a network that belongs to an organization and is designed to be accessible only by the organization's members, employees, or others with authorization. The Web site looks and acts just like other Web sites, but has a firewall surrounding it; therefore the center can provide easy access to their primary patrons, without receiving extraneous questions from outside their defined clientele.[31-33]

There is a massive effort nationally to modernize health care by making all medical records standardized and electronic.[34] This is considered to be the cornerstone for improvements in quality of care, patient safety, and efficiencies, all leading to an economic benefit.[35,36]

A properly configured medical record provides decision support, facilitates workflow, and enables the routine collection of data for performance feedback in an effort to help improve efficiency and quality of care, including patient safety.[37-40] ❸ *With computerized medical records and order entry systems, medication information specialists can take a leadership role in incorporating automated interventions that improve safety and provide education at the point of prescribing.* The use of **computer-based clinical decision support systems** (CDSS) (see Chapter 24) that provide patient information with recommendations based on the best evidence is shown to be valuable in the patient care setting, including a reported decrease in length of hospital stay.[41,42] In one study that examined the value of using a decision support program to assist physicians in using anti-infective agents, the length of hospital stay of patients who used the recommendations was compared with a group of patients who did not always use the recommendations, and compared against a group of patients who were admitted to the unit 2 years before the intervention program.[41] The length of hospital stay was statistically different with an average of 10 days, 16.7 days, and 12.9 days.

Although technology affords remote-site access to medication information sources, it is critical that pharmacists have the skills to perceive, assess, and evaluate the information, and apply the information to the situation. One of the most rapidly changing technologies in health care is information technology. ❹ *Medication information specialists must keep abreast of advances in information technology* in an effort to integrate new and

| valuable systems in a timely and efficient manner. The need for this type of training is emphasized in an Institute of Medicine (IOM) report.[43]

FOCUS ON EVIDENCE-BASED MEDICINE AND DRUG POLICY DEVELOPMENT

The pharmacist's ability to apply their medication information skills to drug policy decisions will be of growing importance in this changing health care environment. This can be done by identifying trends of inappropriate medication use in a group of patients and providing supporting scientific evidence to help change behavior. Continued growth in national health expenditures has raised the concern of government, insurance agencies, health care providers, and the public in identifying strategies to control spending while maintaining access to quality health care. The United States spent more than $307.5 billion on prescription drugs in 2010.[2] In 2014, national health spending is projected to raise to 7.4% (approximately 2 percentage points faster than without reform), with the policy changes from the Affordable Care Act (ACA) expecting to result in 22 million fewer uninsured people. There is also an anticipated increase in Medicaid spending of 18% and private health insurance growth of approximately 8%.[44] Because drug expenditures are the largest component of the pharmacy operating budget, and a significant portion of the entire health system budget, the pharmacy budget frequently attracts significant attention from leadership. In recent years, there has been a shift from a fee-for-service, inpatient focus, to a capitated, managed care, ambulatory focus.[45] Managed care, a process seeking to manage the delivery of high-quality health care in order to improve cost-effectiveness, is consuming an ever-increasing portion of health care delivery. Today, providers are relying less on impressions of what may be happening in a practice setting, and more on data that are actually being collected in that same group of patients (e.g., number of patients receiving appropriate dose of drugs). Goals are set for a particular group of patients (e.g., all patients receive beta-blocker therapy after a myocardial infarction) based on evidence found in the scientific literature. This connection of applying the scientific information to the patient care setting is made through evidence-based medicine. Evidence-based medicine (see Chapter 7) is an approach to practice and teaching that integrates current clinical research evidence with pathophysiological rationale, professional expertise, and patient preferences to make decisions for a population.[46] ❺ *Medication literature evaluation skills are essential.* Pharmacists need to have a solid understanding of medication information concepts and skills, be able to evaluate the medication use issues for a group of patients, be able to search, retrieve, and critically evaluate the scientific literature, and apply the information to the targeted group of patients.

Evidence-based medicine techniques are used in health care organizations in the development and implementation of a variety of quality assurance tools (e.g., therapeutic guidelines, clinical pathways, medication use evaluations, and disease state management) in an effort to improve patient outcomes and decrease costs across the health care system. The goal is to support the appropriate use of medications including correcting the overuse, underuse, or misuse of medicines. In the United States, the IOM designated evidence-based patient-centered health care delivery as a key feature of high-quality medical care.[47] All of these situations require pharmacists to use drug information skills and to have various kinds of medication information support at the practice site or easily accessible at a remote site. The process of evidence-based medicine requires that systems be developed to measure and report processes and outcomes that can be used to drive quality improvement efforts. Data can be collected and analyzed by a medication information specialist using scientific methods to support the decision-making process in a managed care organization.[48]

Outcomes research is a type of investigation that uses scientific rigor to determine which interventions are best for certain types of patients and under certain circumstances. This contrasts with traditional randomized controlled studies to determine *efficacy*, which examines the success of treatments in controlled environments. Outcomes research, taking place in real-life settings, is called *effectiveness* research. The branch of outcomes research, pharmacoeconomics, provides tools to assess cost, consequences (e.g., quality of life, patient functionality, patient preferences), and efficiency (see Chapter 6).[49,50] These types of publications can help guide the practitioner in developing guidelines on appropriate medication use in their practice settings. This will be discussed more fully in Chapter 7.

Sophistication of Medication Therapy

The sophisticated level of medication therapy that occurs today provides pharmacists much more opportunity to lend their expertise in assessing medication information needs of professionals, patients, or family members, and providing literature to help choose the best medication to use within a class, to convey the appropriate information to help patients correctly and safely use the more potent medications, and to address administration and delivery problems. It is increasingly difficult for health professionals to keep up with all of the developments in medication therapy, as well as keep abreast of the other information required for their practice. It is estimated that over 5400 compounds are in various stages of clinical drug development.[51] Nearly 78% of the projects in the pipeline study medications that attack a disease in a way that is unique to any other existing medicine. Several of the drugs in the different stages of development could have a substantial impact on clinical practice and drug expenditures once they are commercially available. For instance, it is anticipated that at least 3400 of these medications are anticancer agents, which could have an impact on life expectancy, quality of life, and the related expenses associated with the potential need for increased ancillary care, additional physician office visits, or hospitalization.[51] It is important that drugs in the pipeline be monitored by pharmacists to provide adequate time to identify the patient population that will most benefit from the new drug and to help anticipate the cost of treating these patients compared to traditional therapy.[2] See Chapter 17 for more information.

There is also a trend toward individualization of health care using pharmacogenomic profiling to determine potential drug effectiveness.[52] Patients may be tested for genomic patterns, and their drug therapy will be altered accordingly. There are several potential benefits of using this pharmacogenomic technique: new effective treatments for a variety of medical conditions could be identified faster and in smaller samples, computer modeling can help eliminate the medications that do not work, and, because this technique can help identify the best candidates for a particular drug, it can help patients sooner.[53] Over 155 trials are studying personalized medicine, which uses an individual's genetic profile to guide decisions on the diagnosis and treatment of disease.[51] There are medications that use cell therapy, antisense RNA interference therapy, monoclonal antibodies joined to cytotoxic agents to help target tumor cells, and gene therapy. As the types and sophistication of medication therapy continue to evolve, this will provide challenges in the future for patients, family members, and practitioners who want information on viable candidates for medication therapy, to address administration and delivery issues, and assess outcomes in real-life settings. The ability to assess information needs; search, analyze, and retrieve appropriate literature; and apply the information to patients will be important.

Rise in the Self-Care Movement

Finally, consumers have a continually growing desire for information about their medications (see Chapter 20). The growth of the self-care movement, the increase in focus on health care costs, and the improved accessibility of health information are some of the factors that have influenced patients to participate more fully in health care decisions, including the selection and use of medications. Based on these needs, direct-to-consumer advertising (DTCA) campaigns have appeared in virtually all mediums including magazines, television ads, Web-based ads (e.g., through e-mail, search engine marketing, or banner style ads on specific Web sites), and radio reports (see Chapter 23). There may be some benefits to DTCA for the patient and overall health care system.[54,55] The ads could serve to inform patients on the management of a particular disease or condition, or the appropriate use of a medication being marketed. These advertisements can also be viewed as empowering patients to have a more active role in their own health care, and for patients already taking a certain drug, the advertisement could serve as a reminder to take the medication, ultimately improving patient compliance.[54]

There are also clearly negative aspects of DTCA. There is potential for this information to result in the increased use of the advertised drugs when less expensive alternatives may be more appropriate, resulting in increases in drug spending and utilization. Patients may also lack the skills needed to evaluate comprehensive medical information, even if it has been provided.[55,56] This is because the content in DTCA often exceeds the eighth-grade reading level, which is typically recommended for information distributed to the general public. Paradoxically, the inclusion of information about risks and adverse events in DTCA may also promote an unnecessary fear of side effects, which may result in nonadherence. In general, information provided with at least some prescription drugs is not adequately understood by less-informed consumers and does not effectively communicate critical safety messages or directions.[56]

Health information is one of the most frequently searched topics on the Internet. In 2012, a study conducted by the Pew Research Center examined the use of the Internet for health information online.[57] Interestingly, 35% of U.S. adults have used the Internet to research a medical condition, and of these, half have followed up with a medical professional. Eighty-five percent of U.S. adults own a cell phone, and of those 31% say they have used their phones to look for health information online.

Because a single individual is able to serve as an author, editor, and publisher of a Web site, there is no safeguard on the quality of information available on the Internet (see Chapter 3). The end result may be a highly informed or perhaps misinformed consumer.[58-60] When a patient finds information about medications that they are either considering to start taking or are currently taking, from the Internet, through the lay press, or by DTCA, a pharmacist can help consumers critically assess the medication information that they find and add to the information based on specific patient-related needs. See Chapter 23 for more information.

The need to critically assess information regarding **complementary and alternative medicine** (CAM) has become increasingly important, with approximately 38% of U.S. adults aged 18 years and over and approximately 12% of children use some form of CAM.[61] The use of CAM (e.g., herbal or dietary supplements, meditation, chiropractic care, and acupuncture) is widespread. The 2007 National Health Interview Survey (NHIS), a nationwide government survey, found that 38% of U.S. adults reported using CAM in the previous 12 months, with the highest rates among people aged 50 to 59 (44%).[62] The NHIS data also revealed that approximately 42% of adults who used CAM in the past 12 months disclosed their use of CAM to a physician (MD) or osteopathic physician (DO).[63] Because many adults also use nonprescription medications, prescription drugs, or other conventional medical approaches to manage their health, communication between patients and health care providers about CAM and conventional therapies is vital to ensuring safe, integrated use of all health care approaches.

There is a trend toward integrating CAM with conventional medicine. In a survey of over 6400 U.S. hospitals, approximately 37% offered some sort of CAM options. This is increased from 26.5% in 2005.[64,65] Eighty-four percent and 67% of respondents claimed that patient demand and clinical effectiveness, respectively, were the primary rationale for offering CAM services. This area presents a challenging situation for pharmacists because of the need to assess relevant outcomes from well-designed clinical trials. Consumers are increasingly interested in finding reliable information regarding these products. Pharmacists are in an excellent position to help provide such information. One drug information center describes its experience with a devoted telephone line to provide information regarding herbal supplements.[66] There was an increased demand for the service over time based on a higher call volume. This is consistent with the growing use of CAM nationally. They also described the challenges and limitations of finding reliable information on herbal products. Several resources are available that have information on herbal products.[67] It is just as important that the pharmacist provide information from reliable sources, as well as identify information that is lacking in regard to a particular product (see Chapter 5).

Groups like the National Council on Patient Information and Education (NCPIE) encourage patients to seek information when they have questions. The experiences with some public access medication information hotlines have indicated the public desire and need for information.[68] Such hotlines, often established by pharmacists, are intended to enhance the relationships between health care professionals and patients.

The changing environment affords the pharmacist many opportunities to use the full spectrum of medication information skills. Factors such as the integration of new technologies, the focus on evidence-based medicine and drug policy development, the sophistication of medication therapy, and the rise in self-care movement require that all pharmacists have a strong foundation in medication information concepts.

EDUCATING STUDENTS ON MEDICATION INFORMATION CONCEPTS

The education of pharmacists continues to evolve in scope and depth. Many of the areas identified earlier as needed by the drug (medication) information specialist are now incorporated into pharmacy curricula and taught to all student pharmacists. In 1991, a consensus conference in New Mexico was held to define a set of objectives for didactic and experiential training in drug information for the year 2000.[69] Twenty-three educators and practitioners participated in the conference. There were several key concepts that were developed including: (1) drug information should be a required component of the pharmacy curriculum and include both didactic and competency-based experiential components, (2) drug information concepts and skills should be spread throughout the curriculum, beginning the day the students enter pharmacy school, and (3) problem solving should be a major technique in drug information education, with the goal of developing self-directed learners. Developing these skills should provide the foundation for the pharmacist to be a life-long learner and problem solver. Based upon the work of this conference, as well as changes in the health care system, and the movement toward outcome-based education, colleges of pharmacy are redesigning their curricula to provide a more comprehensive and integrated approach to teaching medication information concepts and skills.[70,71] The CAPE outcomes, which are guidelines used for pharmacy education, continue to include a medication information skills for all student pharmacists.[19] In a recent survey, all pharmacy schools offered didactic drug information education to first professional year students as either a stand-alone course (70%) or an integrated course throughout the professional curriculum.[72] Fifty-one of the 60 colleges offered an advanced pharmacy practice experience (APPE) in drug information, and 62% of these had it as an elective. However, 58% of respondents felt they had an inadequate number of drug information training sites. Communication skills are taught formally to facilitate the pharmacist's ability to transmit information to both health professionals and patients.

In 2009, the American College of Clinical Pharmacy (ACCP) Drug Information Practice and Research Network (DI PRN) published an opinion paper that provides recommendations regarding the curriculum and instructional methods for teaching drug information in both colleges of pharmacy and advanced training to help meet the needs of the changing health care environment and the changing culture of drug information practice.[73] In a follow-up survey examining which recommendations were included in U.S. pharmacy college curricula in the areas of drug information, literature evaluation, and biostatistics, less than half of the core concepts outlined in the opinion paper (i.e., 9 [47%]) were included in curricula of all responding institutions.[74] This supports the need to continually reevaluate and update the curriculum that focuses on medication information concepts because of changes in the health care environment. Of note, many respondents identified the areas of evidence-based medicine, medication safety, and informatics as areas of expanded focus. Technology (e.g., Twitter in a pharmacy management course, and use of e-portfolios) is also being integrated in the education process within the colleges of pharmacy.[75,76] The evolution in technology and social media has changed the way faculty teach, students learn, and faculty and students communicate in colleges of pharmacy. An academic technologist can support the college faculty and staff in the use of learning management systems, distance education programs, and classroom technology.

Upon graduation, a pharmacist can choose to enter the workforce or continue their education in a practice-based mentorship in a residency or fellowship. Postgraduate training through residencies and fellowship experiences can help prepare a pharmacist to be a skilled clinical practitioner, researcher, educator, and leader in the profession of pharmacy. Medication information and policy development are integrated throughout the three goal areas addressed in the pharmacy practice residency standards. Currently, there are 14 ASHP-accredited specialty practice (PGY-2) residencies in medication information with a total of 19 available positions (http://www.ashp.org/menu/Accreditation/ResidencyDirectory.aspx). These were designed for those who practice in health systems. Individuals who specialize in drug information can practice in a variety of different areas (e.g., scientific writing and medical communications). See Chapter 21 for more information.

Opportunities in Specialty Practice

As the role of the practicing pharmacist has changed regarding medication information activities, so has the role of the specialist. The role of the medication information specialist has changed from an individual who specifically answers questions to one who focuses on development of medication policies and provides information on complex medication information questions. ❻ *Leadership and career opportunities exist in a variety of settings for medication information specialists, including* a contract drug information center, medical informatics, managed care organizations (e.g., health maintenance organizations [HMOs]/pharmacy benefit management organizations [PBMs]), scientific writing and medical communications, poison control, pharmaceutical industry, and **academia**. A specialist in medication information can be involved in multiple activities in practice settings listed in the following.

CONTRACT DRUG INFORMATION CENTER (FEE-FOR-SERVICE)

Because of the evolution in health care and the integration of new technologies, there is an increasing demand for timely, accurate, and individualized medication information. The 34 new molecular entities launched in 2011 were the most in at least 10 years.[3] The U.S. drug expenditures were $320 billion for 2011, which is an increase of approximately $125 billion since 2002.[2] Within the next decade health care costs will increase at an alarming rate, with total expenditures reaching the $2.1 trillion mark. A majority of these costs will be shouldered by the private sector, with a significant increase in prescription drug costs. Drug information practitioners are in an enviable position to provide a service that will improve patient outcomes and decrease health care costs through the provision of unbiased information that supports rational, cost-effective, patient- and disease-specific drug therapy. One of the best ways to deliver such information is by contracting with a drug information service with formally trained health care professionals. Potential clients include managed care groups, contract pharmacy services, federal or state government, pharmacy benefits managers, buying groups, attorneys, pharmaceutical industry, small hospitals, chain pharmacies, and independent pharmacies. In one survey, 31% of managed care organizations contracted with a drug information center.[77] Several different fee structures have been used. A client may be charged a simple fee per question, or may be offered a detailed menu of services (e.g., written medication evaluations) with the final cost dependent on the number and types of services chosen by the contracting party.

Services provided within these contracts may include providing answers to medication information requests, preparation of new drug evaluation monographs, formulary drug class reviews, development of medication use evaluation criteria, pharmacoeconomic evaluations, guideline development for a particular disease, writing a pharmacotherapy publication (e.g., Web site, blog, newsletter), and providing continuing education programming.[78] Additional services the center may make available are access to in-house question files for sharing of information on commonly asked questions, and direct access to the center's Internet home page for review of medical use evaluations, formulary reviews, and newsletters. One center reports providing information on drug shortages to ASHP through a grant.[79] Frequently, the contracting drug information center also has responsibilities for pharmacy services (e.g., medication information, drug policy) as part of an entire health system, or is based in a college of pharmacy.

MEDICAL INFORMATICS IN A HEALTH SYSTEM

The majority (92%) of recently published articles on health information technology's effect on outcomes (quality, efficiency, and provider satisfaction) reached positive conclusions.[80] There are tremendous opportunities for an **informatics specialist**—an individual that has advanced medication information skills with a keen understanding of computer and information technology. This individual can help support patient care activities by improving the efficiency of workflow and increasing access to patient-specific information and the medical literature through technology by remote site availability. This individual may also be involved in the area of institutional drug policy management. As the integration of EHRs and CPOE continues to expand, data that were only accessible through a paper record will be available for those professionals who understand the type of data that are needed for quality improvement efforts, and are able to get information efficiently out of the system and into the hands of clinicians at the point of care.[81] The role of a pharmacist as an informatics specialist has been clearly described in the successful implementation of the CPOE system in an academic medical center.[82] The role goes beyond the implementation phase and includes system maintenance (e.g., formulary updates, revised clinical decision support as new guidelines and medical evidence are published, developing specialized libraries such a customized cancer chemotherapy regimen library).[83]

MANAGED CARE PHARMACY

With total U.S. drug expenditures for pharmaceuticals increasing annually (e.g., $320 billion for 2011), this offers tremendous opportunities for the medication information specialist to provide leadership in the development and implementation of mechanisms to support the cost-effective selection and use of medications managed pharmacy organizations.[2,77,84] With the appropriate training (e.g., specialized residency in drug information practice or managed care pharmacy) and expertise, opportunities are growing for the medication information specialist in the insurance industry, health maintenance organizations, PBM companies, state and national government agencies (e.g., Medicaid, Medicare) as well as other groups interested in the cost-efficient use of medications. A list of residencies in managed care pharmacy is available through the Academy of Managed Care Pharmacy (AMCP; http://www.amcp.org). A medication information specialist may be involved in several activities such as providing medication use evaluation assessments, encouraging the use of cost-effective alternatives, providing medication and practice-related information, managing formularies, providing information to support formulary guidelines (counterdetailing—see Chapter 23), and developing disease management program.[85]

Opportunities also exist to establish guidelines for selected disease states (e.g., management of patients with diabetes mellitus), or classes of drugs (e.g., selection of an appropriate antibiotic for surgical prophylaxis). Practice guidelines are becoming an increasingly important part of the biomedical literature. These clinical guidelines are systematically developed to assist practitioners and patients with decisions about health care in an effort to improve the quality and consistency of health care while minimizing costs and liability.[86] Evidence-based practice guidelines are developed through systematic reviews of the literature appropriately adapted to local circumstances and values. Key questions to consider when reviewing a practice guideline have been proposed.[86] These questions primarily rely on how accurately the guideline reflects the research used to produce it. More information on clinical practice guidelines can be found in Chapter 7.

POISON CONTROL

Poison information is a specialized area of medication information with the practitioner typically practicing in an accredited poison information center or an emergency room. Similar to the mission of traditional drug information centers, poison information centers exist to provide accurate and timely information to enhance the quality of care of patients. There are, however, several differences between a traditional drug information center and a poison control center.[87] Health professionals generate most consultations received in drug information centers, whereas, in a poison control center, most are generated from the public. Poison information centers must be prepared to provide information on management of any poison situation, including household products, poisonous plants and animals, medications, and other chemicals. Because of the type of information that the specialist provides, nearly all requests for information to a poison control center are urgent, with an average response time of 5 minutes, compared to anywhere from

30 minutes to days for drug information centers, depending on the urgency of the call and complexity of information required. A specialist in poison information requires expertise in clinical toxicology to be able to obtain a complete history that correctly assesses the potential severity of exposure. They need to know where and how to search for this type of information and be able to develop an appropriate plan for intervention. And they need to be able to communicate the plan in a comprehensive, concise, and accurate manner to a consumer at an appropriate level of understanding. A certified specialist in poison information, or a CSPI, is a registered nurse, pharmacist, or physician who has 2000 hours of experience providing telephone poison center consultations. Recertification is required every 7 years (AAPCC; http://www.aapcc.org/).

In addition to a poison control center providing patient-specific toxicology information, centers in the United States also contribute data to a larger program through the National Poison Data System (NPDS; formerly, the Toxic Exposure Surveillance System [TESS]).[88] These data can be used to compare safety profiles for similar products, to develop risk assessment guidelines for specific substances, to target national poison prevention programs, and to conduct postmarketing surveillance on products (e.g., chemicals). In 2010, poison control centers received approximately four million calls. Despite the impact that regional poison control centers have on reducing morbidity and mortality with poison exposures, they are also facing increasing emphasis on economic justification. One study used a decision analysis to compare the cost-effectiveness of treating poison exposures with the services of a regional poison control center to treatment without access to any poison control center.[89] The average cost per patient treated with the services of a poison control center was almost half of that achieved without services of a poison control center. These results were consistent regardless of exposure type, average inpatient and emergency department costs, and clinical outcome probabilities. Another study examined the public health cost savings by preventing unnecessary utilization of emergency department services by providing home management by a regional poison control center.[90] On average, 70% of requests for poison information can be managed at home, that would otherwise need to be handled in an emergency room environment. It is estimated that a median of $33 million (range $18 million to $45 million) in unnecessary health care charges were prevented by home management by a regional poison information center in 2007. A median of approximately $36 in unnecessary health care charges were prevented for each dollar of state funding the regional poison control center received. This is a large cost savings to residents compared to dollars received in state support.

PHARMACEUTICAL INDUSTRY

The pharmaceutical industry provides many career opportunities for pharmacists in a variety of areas including information technology, training and development, scientific communications, postmarketing research, regulatory affairs, professional affairs, medical information services, medical liaison, drug discovery, product development, and clinical research.[91,92] Each area requires a different skill set, which may differ between companies, depending on the infrastructure and mission of the individual companies.

A pharmacist with specialized medication information expertise or training can answer drug information questions, report and monitor adverse drug reactions, and provide information support to other departments within the pharmaceutical industry. A pharmacist, which is many times referred to as a medical liaison, can help educate health professionals about a particular group of products or provide academic support or partnership for educational initiatives. They may interact with sales and marketing, participate with regulatory affairs issues, and handle product complaints. Regulatory affairs specialists help ensure that drugs under development meet the state and federal regulations that have been developed to protect the public. Pharmacists may be called on to review adverse effects identified in clinical studies and communicate this and other information to the appropriate research and development team.

In addition to providing written information on the drug product produced by the manufacturer, there are opportunities to provide additional information at pharmacy and therapeutics committees or state drug use review (DUR) boards. Pharmaceutical companies have extensive scientific data on their products; some of which is not available through other published sources or may require a formal FOI (freedom of information) request.

Pharmacists with specialized drug information training can take a leadership role in evaluating current research, serving as an associate in managing ongoing research, or designing studies to help answer questions about new indications for future use of the product. The area of postmarketing research is a growing area that offers tremendous opportunity for pharmacists to share their knowledge of the health care environment, research design, technology, and economics from the perspective of the pharmaceutical industry. As the sophistication of drug products and information management (e.g., electronic **new drug applications** [NDAs]) has increased, so have the opportunities for pharmacists to practice in the pharmaceutical industry and focus on using the skills of a medication information specialist. Postgraduate residencies and fellowships, which are typically shared with a college of pharmacy, are available to help strengthen some of the medication information skills needed to work in the pharmaceutical industry. Other positions (e.g., in the areas of drug discovery, product development, and clinical research) require an advanced degree of study (MBA, PhD). See Chapter 22 for more information.

ACADEMIA

The medication information specialist has the opportunity to provide leadership in the pharmacy curriculum, including both didactic and experiential training.[73] In addition to teaching medication information skills that are required across practice sites, the specialist also serves as collaborator with other faculty on cases and activity designed to reinforce drug information skills for students. Approximately one-third of drug information centers are funded by a college of pharmacy.[93] This environment allows the student to be prepared to efficiently and accurately provide information to the appropriate audience, while emphasizing both didactic and competency-based experiential training. New academic opportunities for medication information training include the ACPE-required introductory pharmacy practice experiences or IPPEs (http://www.acpe-accredit.org). In this experience, students that are in their first 3 years of pharmacy school are now required to gain exposure to patient care services prior to the last year of APPEs. Answering real questions from patients and about patients may be one way to satisfy this requirement and prepare students for the more challenging mediation questions they will receive in the future.

As the prevalence of evidence-based practice increases, the importance of teaching drug literature evaluation skills increases. Courses incorporating drug literature evaluation, formulary management, and the development and management of drug use policies will be best taught by drug information specialists in academia. See Chapter 21 for more information.

SCIENTIFIC WRITING AND MEDICAL COMMUNICATION

Medical education and communications companies, separate from the pharmaceutical industry, may provide educational programming for health professionals and consumers to meet continuing education needs (e.g., symposia, workshops, monographs), or nonaccredited or promotional activities (e.g., sales training, publication planning, journal articles). These individuals may write, edit, or develop medication-related materials by gathering, organizing, interpreting, and presenting information for either medical professionals or the public. Examples of these materials include patient education materials, journal articles, regulatory documents, poster presentations, grant proposals, sales and marketing of pharmaceuticals, drug evaluation monographs for health systems.

In addition to having good writing skills, the pharmacist also needs to have scientific expertise and literature evaluation skills.[94,95] More than 77% of medical education and communication companies employ at least one licensed health care professional. These professionals may have several positions including director and scientific writer. Pharmacists in this capacity would work closely with editors, graphic designers, Web site strategists, meeting planners, and scientists. This type of information may be communicated in a variety of ways including orally, in print format, and electronically on the Web. Medical communication fellowships are available to help provide a solid foundation through experiences to various aspects of the medical communication industry.

Summary and Direction for the Future

All pharmacists must be effective medication information providers regardless of their practice site. It is one of the most fundamental responsibilities of a practitioner. Developing the skills of an effective medication information provider is the foundation for the pharmacist to be a life-long learner and problem solver. The literature is a valuable component of both of these processes and will allow the individual pharmacist to adapt to the needs of a continually changing health care system.

Opportunities abound for pharmacists to use medication information skills in all practice settings either as a generalist or as a specialist practitioner. Medication information specialists will still be needed to operate the drug information centers, to provide leadership in the area of drug informatics, managed care organizations, poison control, pharmaceutical industry, scientific writing and medical communications, and in academia.

Self-Assessment Questions

1. What percentage of adverse drug events are considered to be preventable?
   a. 1%
   b. 2%
   c. 40%
   d. 95%
   e. 99%

2. In current practice, the term medication information is used in place of drug information
   a. To convey the management and use of information on medication therapy
   b. To prevent confusion with information on drugs of abuse
   c. To signify the broader role that all pharmacists take in information provision
   d. a and b
   e. a and c

3. Which of the following is true regarding complementary and alternative medicine (CAM)?
   a. Not used in children.
   b. The use of CAM has been growing nationally.
   c. Only 5% of hospitals have some sort of CAM option for patients.
   d. It is easy to find complete and accurate information on CAM.
   e. Drug information centers do not typically answer questions regarding CAM.

4. The first drug information center was opened in 1962 at
    a. The University of Iowa
    b. The Ohio State University
    c. The University of Kentucky
    d. Misr International University in Cairo, Egypt
    e. None of the above

5. What percentage of recently published articles on health information technology's effect on outcomes (quality, efficiency, and provider satisfaction) reached positive conclusions?
    a. 15%
    b. 40%
    c. 60%
    d. 70%
    e. 92%

6. In a recent study, the cost-benefit ratio of drug information services related to patient-specific requests was found to be 2.9:1 to 13.2:1. Most savings resulted from
    a. Decreasing the books in the library by increasing the use of electronic sources
    b. Decreasing the need for drug monitoring
    c. Decreasing the need for additional treatment related to an adverse event
    d. Preventing adverse drug reactions
    e. b and c

7. Which is true regarding poison control centers?
    a. Approximately four million people contact poison information centers annually.
    b. Staff provide information only on ingestion of medications.
    c. Staff would not know how to treat snake bite.
    d. Staff do not require special training.
    e. Average response time is 30 minutes.

8. Medication information specialists' primary leadership role(s) in the move to computerized intervention programs that automatically educate at the point of prescribing should be
    a. Testing the programs once they are in place
    b. Planning and implementing the programs
    c. Providing feedback to programmers on effectiveness
    d. Developing quality improvement programs for these systems
    e. None of the above

9. For pharmacies in organized health care settings, the largest component in the pharmacy operating budget is
   a. Personnel
   b. Drug information center
   c. Clerical supplies
   d. Drugs
   e. Intravenous (IV) room equipment

10. A recent poll showed that of those who went on the Internet to find health information, what percentage of lay public followed up with a medical professional?
    a. 17%
    b. 20%
    c. 50%
    d. 5%
    e. 27%

11. What percentage of pharmacy schools offer didactic drug information education as either a stand-alone course or an integrated course throughout the curriculum?
    a. 100%
    b. 90%
    c. 80%
    d. 75%
    e. 70%

12. Which of the following changes have influenced the role of the drug information specialist?
    a. Rise in self-care movement
    b. Development of evidence-based medicine
    c. Expansion of social media
    d. Focus on medication safety
    e. All of the above

13. The number of adverse drug events will likely increase in the future because of which of the following:
    a. Ongoing availability of new medications
    b. Growing elderly population
    c. Increased use of medications for disease prevention
    d. Improved insurance coverage for medications
    e. All of the above

14. Which of the following is a registry of ongoing clinical trials?
    a. http://www.ClinicalTrials.gov
    b. http://www.newdrug.com
    c. http://www.pubmedcentral.nih.gov
    d. http://www.druginfo.com
    e. http://www.merck.com

15. Approximately how much did the United States spend on prescription drugs (2010)?
    a. $307 billion
    b. $508 million
    c. $100 billion
    d. $250 million
    e. $2 trillion

REFERENCES

1. U.S. Department of Health & Human Services. Compilation of patient protection and affordable care act [Internet]. May 2010. Available from: http://www.healthreform.gov/law/full/index.html

2. Hoffman JM, Li E, Doloresco F, Matusiak L, Hunkler RJ, Shah ND, et al. Projecting future drug expenditures—2012. Am J Health Syst Pharm. 2012;69:e5-21.

3. IMS Institute for Healthcare Informatics. The use of medicines in the United States: review of 2011 [Internet]. April 2012. Available from: http://www.imshealth.com/ims/Global/Content/Insights/IMS%20Institute%20for%20Healthcare%20Informatics/IHII_Medicines_in_U.S_Report_2011.pdf

4. Hing HS, Burt CW, Woodwell DA. Electronic health record use by office-based physicians and their practices: United States, 2006. Advanced data from vital and health statistics (DHHS Publication no. (PHS) 2008-1250). No 393. Hyattsville (MD): National Center for Health Statistics. October 26, 2007;1-7.

5. Parker PF. The University of Kentucky drug information center. Am J Hosp Pharm. 1965;22:42-7.

6. Amerson AB, Wallingford DM. Twenty years' experience with drug information centers. Am J Hosp Pharm. 1983;40:1172-8.

7. Mehnert RB. A world of knowledge for the nation's health: The U.S. National Library of Medicine. Am J Hosp Pharm. 1986;43:2991-7.

8. Walton CA. Education and training of the drug information specialist. Drug Intell Clin Pharm. 1967;1:133-7.

9. Francke DE. The role of the pharmacist as a drug information specialist. Am J Hosp Pharm. 1966;23:49.

10. Zeind CS, Blagg JD, Amato MG, Jacobson S. Incorporation of Institute of Medicine competency recommendations with doctor of pharmacy curricula. Am J Pharm Ed. 2012;76(5):article 83.

11. Rosenberg JM, Schilit S, Nathan JP, Zerilli T. Update on the status of 89 drug information centers in the United States. Am J Health Syst Pharm. 2009;66:1718-22.
12. Pedersen CA, Schneider PJ, Scheckelhoff DJ. ASHP national survey of pharmacy practice in hospital settings: prescribing and transcribing—2010. Am J Health Syst Pharm. 2011;68:669-88.
13. Pedersen CA, Schneider PJ, Scheckelhoff DJ. ASHP national survey of pharmacy practice in hospital settings: prescribing and transcribing—2007. Am J Health Syst Pharm. 2008;65;827-43.
14. Kinky DE, Erush SC, Laskin MS, Gibson GA. Economic impact of a drug information service. Ann Pharmacother. 1999;33:11-6.
15. LaFleur J, Tyler LS, Sharma RR. Economic benefits of investigational drug services at an academic institution. Am J Health Syst Pharm. 2004;61:27-32.
16. Perez A, Doloresco F, Hoffman JM, Meek PD, Touchette DR, Vermeulen LC, Schumock GT. ACCP: Economic evaluations of clinical pharmacy services: 2001–2005. Pharmacotherapy. 2009;29(1):128.
17. Study Commission on Pharmacy. Pharmacists for the future. Ann Arbor (MI): Health Administration Press; 1975. p. 139.
18. American Society of Health-System Pharmacists. ASHP Guidelines on the provision of medication information by pharmacists. Am J Health Syst Pharm. 1996;53:1843-5.
19. American Association of Colleges of Pharmacy [Internet]. Washington, DC: Center for the Advancement of Pharmaceutical Education; [updated 2004 May; cited 2009 Aug 22]. Available from: http://www.aacp.org/resources/education/Documents/CAPE2004.pdf
20. Centers for Disease Control and Prevention; National Center for Emerging and Zoonotic Infectious Diseases (NCEZID); Division of Healthcare Quality Promotion (DHQP). Medication safety basics [Internet]. August 14, 2012. Available from: http://www.cdc.gov/medicationsafety/basics.html
21. Budnitz DS, Pollock DA, Weidenbach KN, Mendelsohn AB, Schroeder TJ, Annest JL. National surveillance of emergency department visits for outpatient adverse drug events. JAMA. 2006;296:1858-66.
22. Institute of Medicine, Committee on Identifying and Preventing Medication Errors. Preventing medication errors. Washington, DC: The National Academies Press; 2006.
23. Budnitz DS, Lovegrove MC, Shehab N, Richards CL. Emergency hospitalizations for adverse drug events in older Americans. N Engl J Med. 2011;365:2002-12.
24. Wachter RM. The end of the beginning: patient safety five years after 'To err is human'. *Health Aff* [Internet]. 2004 Nov 30 [cited 2009 Aug 22]. Available from: http://content.healthaffairs.org/cgi/content/full/hlthaff.w4.534/DC1
25. Ozdalga E, Ozdalga A, Ahuja N. The smartphone in medicine: a review of current and potential use among physicians and students. J Med Internet Res. 2012;14:e128.
26. Murray E, Pollack L, Donelan K, Catania J, Lee K, Zapert K, et al. The impact of health information on the Internet on health care and the physician-patient relationship: national U.S. survey among 1,050 U.S. physicians. J Med Internet Res. 2003;5:e17.

27. Berland GK, Elliott MN, Morales LS, Algazy JI, Kravitz RL, Broder MS, et al. Health information on the Internet: accessibility, quality, and readability in English and Spanish. JAMA. 2001;285:2612-21.

28. Clauson KA, Polen HH, Boulos MN, Dzenowagis JH. Drug information: scope, completeness, and accuracy of drug information in Wikipedia. Ann Pharmacother. 2008;42:1814-21.

29. Belgado BS. Drug information centers on the Internet. J Am Pharm Assoc. 2001;41:631-2.

30. Costerison EC, Graham AS. Developing and promoting an intranet site for a drug information service. Am J Health Syst Pharm. 2008;65:639-43.

31. Dugas M, Weinzierl S, Pecar A, Hasford J. An intranet database for a university hospital drug information center. Am J Health Syst Pharm. 2001;58:799-802.

32. Ruppelt SC, Vann R. Marketing a hospital-based drug information center. Am J Health Syst Pharm. 2001; 58:1040.

33. Erbele SM, Heck AM, Blankenship CS. Survey of computerized documentation system use in drug information centers. Am J Health Syst Pharm. 2001;58:695-7.

34. Centers for Medicare and Medicaid Services. An introduction to the Medicare EHR Incentive Program for Eligible Professionals [Internet]. Available from: http://www.cms.gov/Regulations-and-Guidance/Legislation/EHRIncentivePrograms/Downloads/beginners_guide.pdf. Accessed March 20, 2013.

35. Cresswell KM, Sheikh A. Information technology-based approaches to reducing repeat drug exposure in patients with known allergies. J Allergy Clin Immunol. 2008;121:1112-7.

36. Bond CA, Raehl CL. 2006 national clinical pharmacy services survey: clinical pharmacy services, collaborative drug management, medication errors, and pharmacy technology. Pharmacotherapy. 2008;28:1-13.

37. Rind DM, Kohane IS, Szolovits P, Safran C, Chueh HC, Barnett GO, et al. Maintaining the confidentiality of medical records shared over the Internet and world wide web. Ann Intern Med. 1997;127:138-44.

38. Frisse ME. What is the Internet learning about you while you are learning about the Internet? Acad Med. 1996;71:1064-107.

39. Giacalone RP, Cacciatore GG. HIPAA and its impact on pharmacy practice. Am J Health Syst Pharm. 2003;60:433-45.

40. Elson RB, Connelly DP. Computerized medical records in primary care their role in mediating guideline-driven physician behavior change. Arch Fam Med. 1995;4:698-705.

41. Evans RS, Pestotnik SL, Classen DC, Clemmer TP, Weaver LK, Orme JF, et al. A computer-assisted management program for antibiotics and other anti-infective agents. N Engl J Med. 1998;338:232-8.

42. Hunt DL, Haynes RB, Hanna SE, Smith K. A computer-assisted management program for antibiotics and other anti-infective agents. JAMA. 1998;280:1339-46.

43. Institute of Medicine. Health professions education: a bridge to quality. Washington, DC: The National Academies Press; 2003.

44. Centers for Medicare and Medicaid Services. National Health Expenditure Projections 2011-2021. [Internet]. Available from: http://www.cms.gov/Research-Statistics-Data-and-Systems/Statistics-Trends-and-Reports/NationalHealthExpendData/Downloads/Proj2011PDF.pdf

45. Opportunities for the community pharmacist in managed care. Special Report. Washington, DC: American Pharmaceutical Association; 1994.

46. Ellrodt G, Cook DJ, Lee J, Cho M, Hunt D, Weingarten S. Evidence-based disease management. JAMA. 1997;278:1687-92.

47. Committee on Quality of Health Care in America, Institute of Medicine. Crossing the quality chasm: a new health system for the 21st century. Washington, DC: The National Academies Press; 2001.

48. Avorn J. In defense of pharmacoepidemiology—embracing the yin and yang of drug research. N Engl J Med. 2007;357(22):2219-21.

49. Vermeulen LC, Beis SJ, Cano SB. Applying outcomes research in improving the medication-use process. Am J Health Syst Pharm. 2000;57;2277-82.

50. Top 10 areas of research: report on the most popular fields of drug development. Med Ad News. 2003;137:S22.

51. Long G, Works J. Innovation in the biopharmaceutical pipeline: a multidimensional view. A report from the Analysis Group, Inc. [Internet]. January 2013. Available from: http://www.analysisgroup.com/uploadedFiles/Publishing/Articles/2012_Innovation_in_the_Biopharmaceutical_Pipeline.pdf. Accessed March 14, 2013.

52. Emilien G, Ponchon M, Caldas C, Isacson O, Maloteaux JM. Impact of genomics on drug discovery and clinical medicine. Q J Med. 2000;93:391-423.

53. Epler GR, Laskaris LL. Individualization health care and the pharmaceutical industry. Am J Health Syst Pharm. 2001;58:1042.

54. Frosch DL, Grande D, Tarn DM, Kravitz RL. A decade of controversy: balancing policy with evidence in the regulation of prescription drug advertising. Am J Public Health. 2010;100:24-32.

55. U.S. Government Accountability Office (GAO) report number GAO-07-54 entitled 'Prescription drugs: improvements needed in FDA's oversight of direct-to-consumer advertising' which was released on December 14, 2006. Available from: http://www.gao.gov/htext/d0754.html. Accessed February 15, 2010.

56. Shiffman S, Gerlach KK, Sembower MA, Rohay JM. Consumer understanding of prescription drug information: illustration using an antidepressant medication. Ann Pharmacother. 2011;45:452-8.

57. Pew Internet and American Life Project: a project of the PewResearchCenter. Health Online 2013. January 15, 2013. Available from: http://pewinternet.org/~/media/Files/Reports/2013/Pew%20Internet%20Health%20Online%20report.pdf. Accessed February 15, 2013.

58. Larner AJ. Use of internet medical websites and of NHS direct by neurology outpatients before consultation. Int J Clin Pract. 2002;56:219-21.

59. Silberg W, Lundberg GD, Musacchio RA. Assessing, controlling, and assuring the quality of medical information on the Internet. JAMA. 1997;277:1244-5.

60. Wyatt J. Measuring quality and impact on the world wide web. BMJ. 1997;314:1879-81.

61. National Institutes of Health, National Center for Complementary and Alternative Medicine.. 2007 statistics on CAM use in the United States [Internet]. Washington, DC: [updated 2008 Dec; cited 2009 Aug 22]. Available from: http://nccam.nih.gov/news/camstats/2007/camsurvey_fs1.htm

62. Barnes PM, Bloom B, Nahin R. Complementary and Alternative Medicine Use Among Adults and Children: United States, 2007. Natl Health Stat Report. 2008;10(12):1-23.

63. Complementary and alternative medicine: What people aged 50 and older discuss with their healthcare providers [Internet]. AARP and NCCAM Survey Report 2010. Available from: http://nccam.nih.gov/news/camstats/2010. Accessed March 9, 2013.

64. American Hospital Association. Latest survey shows more hospitals offering complementary and alternative medicine services [Internet].Washington, DC: cc 2006-2009. [updated 2008 Sep 15;cited 2009 Aug 22]. Available from: http://nccam.nih.gov/news/camstats.htm

65. Ananth S, Martin W. Health forum 2005 complementary and alternative medicine survey of hospitals: summary of results. Chicago (IL): Health Forum; 2006.

66. West PM, Lodolce AE, Johnston AK. Telephone service for providing consumers with information on herbal supplements. Am J Health Syst Pharm. 2001;58:1842-6.

67. Shields KM, McQueen CE, Bryant PJ. National survey of dietary supplement resources at drug information centers. J Am Pharm Assoc. 2004;44:36-40.

68. Meade V. Patient medication information hotlines multiply. Am Pharm. 1991;NS31: 569-71.

69. Troutman WG. Consensus-derived objectives for drug information education. Drug Inf J. 1994;28:791-6.

70. Ferrill MJ, Norton LL. Drug information to biomedical informatics: a three tier approach to building a university system for the twenty-first century. Am J Pharm Ed. 1997;61:81-6.

71. Gora-Harper ML, Brandt B. An educational design to teach drug information across the curriculum. Am J Pharm Ed. 1997;61:296-302.

72. Wang F, Troutman WG, Seo T, Peak A, Rosenberg JM. Drug information in doctor of pharmacy programs. Am J Pharm Ed. 2006;70:51.

73. Bernknopf AC, Karpinski JP, McKeever AL, Peak AS, Smith KM, Smith WD, et al. Drug information: from education to practice. Pharmacotherapy. 2009;29:331-46.

74. Phillips JA, Gabay MP, Ficzere C, Ward KE. Curriculum and instructional methods for drug information, literature evaluation, and biostatistics: survey of US pharmacy schools. Ann Pharmacother. 2012;46:793-801.

75. Fox BI, Varadarajan R. Use of Twitter to encourage interaction in a multi-campus pharmacy management course. Am J Pharm Ed. 2011;75:88.

76. Lopez TC, Trang DD, Farrell NC, DeLeon MA, Villarreal CC, Maize DF. Development and implementation of a curricular-wide electronic portfolio system in a school of pharmacy. Curricular-wide use of ePortfolios. Am J Pharm Ed. 2011;75:1-6.

77. McCloskey WW, Vogenberg FR. Drug Information resources in managed care organizations. Am J Health Syst Pharm. 1998;55:2007-9.
78. Foresster LP, Scoggin JA, Valle RD. Pharmacy management company-negotiated contract for drug information services. Am J Health Syst Pharm. 1995;52:1074-7.
79. Fox ER, Tyler LS. Managing drug shortages: seven years' experience at one health-system. Am J Health Syst Pharm. 2003;60:245-53.
80. Buntin BM, Burke MF, Hoaglin MC, Blumenthal D. The benefits of health information technology: a review of the recent literature shows predominately positive results. Health Affairs. 2011;30(3):464-71.
81. Woodruff AE, Hunt CA. Involvement in medical informatics may enable pharmacists to expand their consultation potential and improve the quality of healthcare. Ann Pharmacother. 1992;26:100-4.
82. Cooley TW, May D, Alwan M, Sue C. Implementation of computerized prescriber order entry in four academic medical centers. Am J Health Sys Pharm. 2012;69:2166-73.
83. Traynor K. Pharmacy informatics aids cancer center care. Am J Health Sys Pharm. 2012;69:2125.
84. Vanscoy GJ, Gajewski LK, Tyler LS, Gora-Harper ML, Grant KL, May JR. The future of medication information practices: a consensus. Ann Pharmacother. 1996;30:876-81.
85. Taniguchi R. Pharmacy benefit management companies. Am J Health Syst Pharm. 1995;52:1915-7.
86. Field JM, Lohr KN, eds. Guidelines for clinical practice: from development to use. Washington, DC: The National Academies Press; 1992.
87. AAPCC. Annual report of the NPDS. Clin Toxicol. 2012;50:911-1164.
88. Bronstein AC, Spyker DA, Cantilena LR. 2007 Annual Report of the American Association of Poison Control Centers National Poison Data System (NPDS) 25th annual report. Clin Toxicol. 2008;46:927-1057.
89. Harrison MAJ, Draugalis JR, Slack MK, Langley PC. Cost-effectiveness of regional poison control centers. Arch Intern Med. 1996;156:2601-8.
90. Lovecchio F, Curry S, Waszolek K, Klemens J, Hovseth K, Glogan D. Poison control centers decrease emergency healthcare utilization costs. J Med Toxicol. 2008;4:221-4.
91. Gong SD, Millares M, VanRiper KB. Drug information pharmacists at health-care facilities, universities, and pharmaceutical companies. Am J Hosp Pharm. 1992;49: 1121-30.
92. Riggins JL. Pharmaceutical industry as a career choice. Am J Health Syst Pharm. 2002;59:2097-8.
93. Rosenberg JM, Kournis T, Nathan JP, Cicero LA, McGuire H. Current status of pharmacist-operated drug information centers in the United States. Am J Health Syst Pharm. 2004;61:2023-32.
94. Overstreet KM. Medical education and communication companies: career options for pharmacists. Am J Health Syst Pharm. 2003;60:1896-7.
95. Moghadam RG. Scientific writing: a career for pharmacists. Am J Health Syst Pharm. 2003;60:1899-900.

SUGGESTED READINGS

1. Pedersen CA, Gumpper KF. ASHP national survey on informatics: assessment of the adoption and use of pharmacy informatics in U.S. hospitals—2007. Am J Health Syst Pharm. 2008;65(23):2244-64.

2. Hoffman JM, Shah ND, Vermeulen LC, Doloresco F, Grim P, Hunkler RJ, et al. Projecting future drug expenditures—2008. Am J Health Syst Pharm. 2008;65(3):234-53.

3. Hing HS, Burt CW, Woodwell DA. Electronic health record use by office-based physicians and their practices: United States, 2006. Advanced data from vital and health statistics (DHHS Publication no. (PHS) 2008-1250). No 393. Hyattsville (MD): National Center for Health Statistics; October 26, 2007:1-7.

4. Bernknopf AC, Karpinski JP, McKeever AL, Peak AS, Smith KM, Smith WD, et al. Drug Information: from education to practice. Pharmacotherapy. 2009;29:331-46.

5. Costerison EC, Graham AS. Developing and promoting an intranet site for a drug information service. Am J Health Syst Pharm. 2008;65:639-43.

6. Wang F, Troutman WG, Seo T, Peak A, Rosenberg JM. Drug information in doctor of pharmacy programs. Am J Pharm Ed. 2006;70:51.

7. Zeind CS, Blagg JD, Amato MG, Jacobson S. Incorporation of Institute of Medicine competency recommendations with doctor of pharmacy curricula. Am J Pharm Ed. 2012;76(5):article 83.

8. Shiffman S, Gerlach KK, Sembower MA, Rohay JM. Consumer understanding of prescription drug information: illustration using an antidepressant medication. Ann Pharmacother. 2011;45:452-8.

2

Chapter Two

Formulating Effective Responses and Recommendations: A Structured Approach

Karim Anton Calis • Amy Heck Sheehan

Learning Objectives

After completing this chapter, the reader will be able to

- Develop strategies to overcome the impediments that prevent pharmacists from providing effective responses and recommendations.
- Outline the steps that are necessary to identify the actual drug information needs of the requestor.
- List and describe the four critical factors that should be considered and systematically addressed when formulating a response.
- Define analysis and synthesis, and describe their applications in the process of formulating responses and recommendations.
- List the elements and characteristics of effective responses to medication-related queries.

Key Concepts

1. Rational pharmacotherapy can be promoted by ensuring that drug information is correctly interpreted and appropriately applied.

2. The absence of sufficient background information and pertinent patient data can greatly impair the process of information synthesis and the ability to formulate effective responses.

❸ Critical information that defines the problem and elucidates the context of the question is not readily volunteered but must be expertly elicited.

❹ Providing responses and offering recommendations without knowledge of pertinent patient information, the context of the request, or how the information will be applied can be detrimental.

❺ Formulating a response requires the use of a structured, organized approach whereby critical factors are systematically considered and thoughtfully evaluated.

❻ Approaching a question haphazardly, or prematurely fixating on isolated details, can misdirect even the most skilled clinician.

❼ Responses to drug information queries often must be synthesized by integrating data from diverse sources through the use of logic and deductive reasoning.

Introduction

Pharmacists are asked to provide responses to a variety of drug information questions every day. Although the type of requestor, query, and setting can vary, the process of formulating responses remains constant. This chapter introduces an organized, structured approach for formulating effective responses and recommendations.

As the medical literature expands, access to drug information resources by health care professionals and the public continues to grow. Yet many professionals and consumers lack the necessary skills to use this information effectively. ❶ *Rational pharmacotherapy can be promoted by ensuring that drug information is correctly interpreted and appropriately applied.* This presents an opportunity and a challenge for bona fide drug therapy experts who aspire to play a broader role in patient care.

Regardless of specialty or practice site, pharmacists with the responsibility for overseeing the safe and rational use of medications must strive to develop expertise in applied pharmacotherapy. Whether working in a community pharmacy, nursing home, outpatient clinic, hospital, or another practice site, pharmacists can apply their skills and knowledge for the optimal care of patients. Pharmacists should not be relegated to the role of information dispenser or gatekeeper, but they should instead extend their knowledge of drugs and therapeutics to the clinical management of individual patients or the care of large populations.

ACCEPTING RESPONSIBILITY AND ELIMINATING BARRIERS

Pharmacists should recognize that their responsibility extends beyond simply providing an answer to a question. Rather, it is to assist in resolving therapeutic dilemmas or managing patients' medication regimens. Knowledge of pharmacotherapy alone does not ensure success. Moreover, isolated information is not sufficient for formulating responses to questions or ensuring proper patient management. In fact, it is uncommon to find comprehensive answers in the literature that completely and effectively address specific situations or circumstances that clinicians encounter in their daily practices. Responses and recommendations must often be thoughtfully synthesized using information and knowledge gathered from a number of diverse sources. To effectively manage the care of patients and resolve complex clinical situations, added skills and competence in problem solving and direct patient care are also necessary.

In order to provide meaningful responses and effective recommendations to drug information questions, real or perceived impediments must first be overcome. One such impediment is the false perception that many drug information questions do not pertain to specific patients. Another is the perception that seemingly casual interactions with requestors and the lack of formal, written consultation somehow preclude the need for in-depth analysis and extensive involvement in patient management. Oversimplification of these interactions with requestors and failure to identify the context of the question or recognize its significance can jeopardize the clinical management of patients. ❷ *The absence of sufficient background information and pertinent patient data can greatly impair the process of information synthesis and the ability to formulate effective responses.*

IDENTIFYING THE GENUINE NEED

Historically, the approach to answering drug information queries has centered on the use of a systematic method first described by Watanabe and subsequently modified by others.[1,2] This simple approach relied on the collection of basic information to document and categorize the request and to subsequently develop an organized strategy for formulating cogent responses. Although this structure remains theoretically useful from a training standpoint, if strictly applied without proper context and guidance, it has the potential to artificially fragment the process and disrupt the natural exchange of information. A documentation form (see Appendix 2–1) may be useful to guide the process of data collection and ensure that all relevant information is considered. Ultimately success will depend largely on maintaining the flow of information with minimal distractions and unnecessary or ill-timed questions. The goal should be to remove obstacles that may obscure the actual informational needs. This is particularly relevant in clinical settings where most queries are not purely academic or general in nature. In fact, it is rational to assume that queries from health care providers will invariably involve specific patients and unique clinical circumstances. For example, a physician who asks about the association of liver toxicity with lovastatin is probably not asking this question whimsically or out of curiosity. The physician most likely is caring for a patient who has developed signs or symptoms suggestive of hepatic impairment possibly associated with the use of this medication. Although other reasonable scenarios, albeit less likely, could have prompted this question, it would be most prudent nonetheless to consider the possibility of a patient-specific drug-induced liver injury.

Even questions that are not related to patient care (refer to Case Study 2–1 as an example) must be viewed in their proper and full context. Requestors of information are typically vague in verbalizing their needs and generally provide adequate information only when specifically asked or thoughtfully prompted. Although these requestors may seem confident about their perceived needs, they may be less certain after further probing. Requestors, regardless of background, are often uncertain about the nature and extent of information that should be disclosed in order to derive the most optimal assistance. ❸ *Critical information that defines the problem and elucidates the context of the question is not readily volunteered but must be expertly elicited.* This can be accomplished through the use of effective questioning strategies (asking logical questions in a logical sequence) and other means of information gathering that are essential for formulating informed responses. Failure of the requestor to disclose critical information or clarify the question does not obviate the need for such information or relieve the pharmacist of the duty to collect it. Although it is easy to assign blame to the requestor for failing to disclose all of the necessary information, it is ultimately the responsibility of the provider of the response to obtain information completely and efficiently.

Good communication skills (both listening and questioning) are essential for gathering relevant information, discerning the real question, and identifying the genuine needs of the requestor. ❹ *Providing responses and offering recommendations without knowledge of pertinent patient information, the context of the request, or how the information will be applied can be detrimental.* Even well-equipped drug information centers with trained staff are not immune to this problem. A study of the quality of pharmacotherapy consultations provided by drug information centers in the United States found that the centers generally failed to obtain pertinent patient data, thereby risking incorrect responses and inappropriate recommendations.[3]

TABLE 2–1. QUESTIONS TO CONSIDER BEFORE FORMULATING A RESPONSE

Are the requestor's name, profession, and affiliation known?

Does the question pertain to a specific patient?

Is there a clear understanding of the question or problem?

Is the correct question being asked?

Why is the question being asked? Why now?

Are the requestor's expectations understood?

Has pertinent patient history and background information been obtained?

What are the unique circumstances that generated the query?

What information is actually needed?

When is the information needed and in what format (e.g., verbal, written)?

How will the information provided be used or applied?

How has the problem or situation been managed to date?

Are there alternative explanations or management options that should be explored?

Before attempting to formulate responses, pharmacists must consider several important questions to ensure that they understand the context of the query and the scope of the issue or problem (see Table 2–1). Without this information, pharmacists risk providing general responses that do not address the needs of the requestor. More concerning, however, is that information provided without proper context can be misinterpreted or misapplied. This not only compromises credibility of the information provider, but it also can jeopardize patient care. Pharmacists must recognize the value and potential benefits of their contributions as members of the health care team. Lack of confidence in communicating with requestors can be a limiting factor. Because a telephone call from another health care provider or even a casual face-to-face interaction may not be perceived as a formal request for a consult, the significance of such apparently informal daily interactions can easily be overlooked. Interactions with physicians and other health care providers present valuable opportunities for direct involvement in patient care. The lesson often missed is that there is a fine line between a simple, seemingly general drug information question and a meaningful pharmacotherapy consultation. Knowing the context of the question, obtaining the pertinent patient data and background information, and understanding the true needs of the requestor can often be the difference.

Some pharmacists are quick to answer questions without adequately understanding the context or unique circumstances from which they evolved. They focus exclusively on the answer and ignore or fail to obtain key information needed to establish the framework of the question. In essence, this can result in a correct response being provided to address an incorrect question. For example, in a question about the dose of an antibiotic, an incorrect response can be formulated and inappropriate recommendations made if one fails to consider such factors as the patient's age, sex, condition being treated, end-organ function, weight and body composition, concomitant diseases (e.g., cystic fibrosis), possible drug interactions, site of infection, spectrum of activity of the antimicrobial, local bacterial resistance patterns, or other factors such as pregnancy and hemodialysis or other extra-corporeal procedures.

In the absence of information that provides the proper context, a question about the half-life of a medication appears rather simple. However, if the question were posed for the purpose of assisting the requestor in determining a sufficient washout period for a cross-over study, one would be remiss if factors other than the half-life of the parent compound were not considered. Proper determination of a washout period would also necessitate consideration of other factors such as the activity and half-lives of known metabolites; the presence of potentially interacting medications; the effects of age, illness, and end-organ function; the persistence of pharmacodynamic effects of the medication beyond its detection in the plasma (e.g., omeprazole); and the effect of administration route on the apparent half-life (e.g., transdermally administered fentanyl).

The case studies in this chapter emphasize the importance of looking beyond the initial question and recognizing that the requestor's needs often go well beyond a superficial answer to the primary question. Pharmacists should always anticipate additional questions or concerns, including those that are not directly raised by the requestor. These questions nonetheless must be considered if a clinical situation is to be managed optimally. Case Study 2–4 considers a question about ranitidine as a possible cause of thrombocytopenia. Although the requestor may neglect to provide clarifying information or pose insightful questions that further inform this case, additional related issues and complementary questions should nonetheless be considered, as these will likely be critical in determining the ultimate success of the response (see Table 2–2). Failure to address such questions will undoubtedly result in an incorrect or inadequate response.

To expertly address requests for drug information, pharmacists must also depend on their patient care skills, problem-solving skills, insight, and professional judgment. Computer databases and other specialized information sources can assist in identifying critical data, but overreliance on such resources without careful attention to pertinent background information and patient data can mislead even the most experienced clinician.

FORMULATING THE RESPONSE

Building a Database and Assessing Critical Factors

Formulating optimal responses requires a series of steps that must be performed completely, objectively, and in a logical sequence. The steps in the process include assembling and organizing a database of patient-specific information, gathering information about relevant disease states, collecting medication information, obtaining pertinent background

TABLE 2–2. IMPORTANT QUESTIONS NOT POSED BY THE REQUESTOR

Initial query posed by requestor: Can ranitidine cause thrombocytopenia?
- What is the incidence of ranitidine-induced thrombocytopenia?
- Are there any known predisposing factors?
- Is the pathogenesis of this adverse effect understood?
- How does the thrombocytopenia typically present?
- Are there any characteristic subjective or objective findings?
- Does thrombocytopenia due to ranitidine differ from that caused by other histamine-2 (H_2)-receptor antagonists, other medications, or other etiologies?
- Is the thrombocytopenia dose related?
- How severe can it become?
- How soon after discontinuing the drug does it reverse (dechallenge)?
- How is it usually managed?
- What is the likelihood of cross-reactivity with other H_2-receptor antagonists?
- How risky is rechallenge with ranitidine?
- Are there treatments available that can be used in place of ranitidine?
- Are there alternative explanations for the thrombocytopenia in this patient (including other medications, medication combinations, or underlying medical conditions)?
- What complications, if any, can be expected?

information, and identifying other relevant factors and unique or special circumstances. ❺ *Formulating a response requires the use of a structured, organized approach whereby critical factors are systematically considered and thoughtfully evaluated.* Table 2–3 outlines in detail the specific types of information that may need to be considered for each factor depending on the nature of the query. A list of sample background questions is found in Appendix 2–2. It should be noted that only some of this information might be pertinent for a given query or case scenario.

For patient-related questions, development of a patient-specific database is one of the first steps in preparing a response. This requires the collection of pertinent information from the patient, caregivers, health care providers, and medical chart or other patient records. A comprehensive medication history is also essential. This database would invariably include information that overlaps with the medical and nursing databases. Because physicians, nurses, patients, and others often lack a clear understanding of the type of information needed for effective pharmacotherapy consultations, pharmacists must be able to identify and efficiently extract pivotal patient information from diverse sources.

Once these data are collected and carefully assembled, they must be critically analyzed and evaluated in the proper context before final responses and recommendations are synthesized. Background reading on topics related to the query (e.g., diseases,

TABLE 2–3. FACTORS TO BE CONSIDERED WHEN FORMULATING A RESPONSE

Patient Factors

Demographics (e.g., name, age, height, weight, gender, race/ethnic group, and setting)

Primary diagnosis and medical problem list

Allergies/intolerances

End-organ function, immune function, nutritional status

Chief complaint

History of present illness

Past medical history (including surgeries, radiation exposure, immunizations, psychiatric illnesses, and so forth)

Family history and genetic makeup

Social history (e.g., alcohol intake, smoking, substance abuse, exposure to environmental or occupational toxins, employment, income, education, religion, travel, diet, physical activity, stress, risky behavior, and compliance with treatment regimen)

Review of body systems

Medications (prescribed, nonprescription, and complementary/alternative)

Physical examination

Laboratory tests

Diagnostic studies or procedures

Disease Factors

Definition

Epidemiology (including incidence and prevalence)

Etiology

Pathophysiology (for infectious diseases consider site of infection, organism susceptibility, resistance patterns, and so forth)

Clinical findings (signs and symptoms, laboratory tests, diagnostic studies)[a]

Diagnosis

Treatment (medical, surgical, radiation, biologic and gene therapies, other)

Prevention and control

Risk factors

Complications

Prognosis

Medication Factors

Name of medication or substance (proprietary, nonproprietary, other)

Status and availability (investigational, nonprescription, prescription, orphan, foreign, complementary/alternative)

Physicochemical properties

Pharmacology and pharmacodynamics

Pharmacokinetics (liberation, absorption, distribution, metabolism, and elimination)

Pharmacogenetics

Indications (Food and Drug Administration [FDA] approved and unlabeled)

continued

TABLE 2–3. FACTORS TO BE CONSIDERED WHEN FORMULATING A RESPONSE (*CONTINUED*)

Medication Factors (*continued*)

Uses (diagnosis, prevention, replacement, or treatment)

Adverse effects

Allergy

Cross-allergenicity or cross-reactivity

Contraindications and precautions

Effects of age, organ system function, disease, pregnancy, extracorporeal circulation, or other conditions or environments

Mutagenicity and carcinogenicity

Effect on fertility, pregnancy, and lactation

Acute or chronic toxicity

Drug interactions (drug–drug or drug–food)

Laboratory test interference (analytical or physiologic effects)

Administration (routes, methods)

Dosage and schedule

Dosage forms, formulations, preservatives, excipients, product appearance, delivery systems

Monitoring parameters (therapeutic or toxic)

Product preparation (procedures, methods)

Compatibility and stability

Pertinent Background Information, Special Circumstances, and Other Factors

Setting

Context

Sequence and time frame of events

Rationale for the question

Event(s) prompting the question

Unusual or special circumstances (including medical errors)

Acuity and time constraints

Scope of question

Desired detail or depth of response

Limitations of available information or resources

Completeness, sufficiency, and quality of the information

Applicability and generalizability of the information

[a]Factors such as disease or symptom onset, duration, frequency, and severity must always be carefully assessed.

medications, and laboratory tests) is often essential (see Chapter 3). This process also often involves careful evaluation of the literature (see Chapters 4 and 5). To effectively perform the steps outlined previously, one must begin with a broad perspective (i.e., observing the big picture) to avoid losing sight of important information. ❻ *Approaching a question haphazardly, or prematurely fixating on isolated details, can misdirect even the most skilled clinician.*

Analysis and Synthesis

Analysis and synthesis of information are among the most critical steps in formulating responses and recommendations. Together they assist in forming opinions, arriving at judgments, and ultimately drawing conclusions. Analysis is the critical assessment of the nature, merit, and significance of individual elements, ideas, or factors. Functionally, it involves separating the information into its isolated parts so that each can be critically assessed. Analysis requires thoughtful review and evaluation of the quality and overall weight of available evidence. Although this process involves consideration of all relevant positive findings, pertinent negative findings should not be overlooked.

Once the information has been carefully analyzed, synthesis can begin. Synthesis is the careful, systematic, and orderly process of combining or blending varied and diverse elements, ideas, or factors into a coherent response. ❼ *Responses to drug information queries often must be synthesized by integrating data from diverse sources through the use of logic and deductive reasoning.* This process relies not only on the type and quality of the data gathered, but also on how these data are organized, viewed, and evaluated. Synthesis, as it relates to pharmacotherapy, involves the careful integration of critical information about the patient, disease, and medication along with pertinent background information to arrive at a judgment or conclusion. Synthesis can give existing information new meaning and, in effect, create new knowledge. The use of analysis and synthesis to formulate a response is akin to assembling a jigsaw puzzle. If the pieces are identified and then grouped, organized, and assembled correctly, the image will be comprehensible. However, if too many of the pieces are missing—as may be the case if patient information or supporting evidence is incomplete or absent—or are not arranged correctly (e.g., when information is not evaluated, interpreted, or applied logically), formulating a cogent response may prove to be difficult or altogether impossible.

Responses and Recommendations

An effective response obviously must adequately address and answer the question. Other characteristics of effective responses and recommendations are outlined in Table 2–4. The response to a question must include a restatement of the request and clear identification of the problems, issues, and circumstances. The response should begin with an introduction to the topic and systematically present the specific findings. Pertinent background information and patient data should be succinctly addressed. Conclusions and recommendations are also included in the response along with pertinent reference citations. The format of responses (verbal or written) is discussed in Chapter 9. In formulating responses, one should disclose the available information that is most relevant to the question and present all reasonable options and alternatives along with an explanation and evaluation of each. Specific recommendations must be scientifically sound, clearly justified, and well documented. A carefully worded record of the response must be maintained for follow-up

TABLE 2–4. DESIRED CHARACTERISTICS OF A RESPONSE

Timely
Current
Accurate
Complete
Concise
Supported by the best available evidence
Well-referenced
Clear and logical
Objective and balanced
Free of bias or flaws
Applicable and appropriate for specific circumstances
Answers important related questions
Addresses specific management of patients or situations

and for legal reasons. The records may be confidentially maintained in a patient's chart or in the provider's secure files.

Follow-Up

When recommendations are made, follow-up should always be provided in a timely manner. Follow-up is required for assessment of outcomes and, when necessary, to reevaluate the recommendations and make appropriate modifications; it is also a hallmark of a true professional and demonstrates a commitment to patient care. Furthermore, follow-up allows the provider of the information to know if their recommendations were accepted and implemented. Finally, follow-up also allows the provider to receive valuable feedback from other clinicians and to learn from the overall experience.

Conclusion

Formulating effective responses and recommendations requires the use of a structured, organized approach whereby critical factors are systematically considered and thoughtfully evaluated. The steps in this process include organizing relevant patient data, gathering information about the disease states and affected body systems, collecting medication information, obtaining pertinent background information, and identifying other relevant factors that can potentially influence outcomes. Once these data are collected and carefully assembled, they must be critically analyzed and evaluated in the proper context of each unique case. Responses and recommendations are synthesized by integrating information and evidence from diverse sources through the use of logic and deductive reasoning.

Case Study 2–1

■ INITIAL QUESTION

What is the molecular weight of enalapril?

■ POTENTIAL RESPONSE IN THE ABSENCE OF RELEVANT BACKGROUND INFORMATION

Enalapril is an oral angiotensin-converting enzyme inhibitor (ACE-I) that is indicated for the management of hypertension, symptomatic congestive heart failure, and asymptomatic left ventricular dysfunction.[4,5] The molecular weight of enalapril is 376.45.[6]

■ PERTINENT BACKGROUND INFORMATION

The requestor is a basic scientist who is conducting an *in vitro* experiment to evaluate the pharmacologic effects of enalapril. She would like to know the molecular weight of enalapril so that she can perform appropriate calculations specified for this experiment.

■ PERTINENT PATIENT FACTORS

N/A

■ PERTINENT DISEASE FACTORS

N/A

■ PERTINENT MEDICATION FACTORS

Enalapril is a prodrug that is converted *in vivo* to the pharmacologically active form, enalaprilat.[4,5] Both enalapril and enalaprilat are commercially available for use in the United States.

■ ANALYSIS AND SYNTHESIS

Considering that enalapril is a prodrug that must be converted to a pharmacologically active compound *in vivo*, and given that this researcher wishes to conduct an *in vitro* study, the researcher should use the active form of the drug in the experiment. Therefore, she should have requested the molecular weight of enalaprilat.

■ RESPONSE AND RECOMMENDATIONS

Enalapril is an oral angiotensin-converting enzyme inhibitor that is indicated for the management of hypertension, symptomatic congestive heart failure, and asymptomatic left ventricular dysfunction. Because enalapril is a prodrug that requires conversion to the active form, the requestor was advised to consider using enalaprilat in the experiment. The molecular weight of enalaprilat is 384.43.[6]

■ CASE MESSAGE

This example illustrates the importance of collecting pertinent background information, even for seemingly uncomplicated questions. Failure to understand exactly how the information that is provided will be used could result in an inaccurate or misleading response. In this case, providing the molecular weight without alerting the requestor that enalapril is pharmacologically inactive *in vitro*, would have resulted in wasted time and money, and the results of the experiment would likely have been invalid.

Case Study 2–2

■ INITIAL QUESTION

What is the maximum dose of oprelvekin?

■ POTENTIAL RESPONSE IN THE ABSENCE OF RELEVANT BACKGROUND INFORMATION

The recommended dose of oprelvekin in adult patients is 50 µg/kg given once daily.[7] Larger doses of oprelvekin (75 to 100 µg/kg/day) have been studied in patients with breast cancer.[8] Constitutional symptoms associated with oprelvekin therapy, such as myalgias, arthralgias, and fatigue, were noted to increase in a dose-dependent fashion. One patient who received 100 µg/kg/day of oprelvekin experienced a cerebrovascular event after the third dose. Dose escalation greater than 75 µg/kg/day was discontinued in this study, and the maximum tolerated dose of oprelvekin was determined to be 75 µg/kg/day.[8]

■ PERTINENT BACKGROUND INFORMATION

The requestor is a physician who is managing a patient with human T-cell leukemia/lymphoma virus Type I (HTLV-1)–associated adult T-cell leukemia. The patient received myelosuppressive chemotherapy and subsequently developed prolonged and severe thrombocytopenia. Oprelvekin was prescribed in an attempt to improve the patient's platelet count and allow continuation of therapy. After 4 days of oprelvekin therapy at a dose of 50 μg/kg/day, the patient's platelet count did not increase substantially. The physician would like to know if doses greater than 50 μg/kg/day of oprelvekin have been studied. She is planning to increase the patient's dose to achieve a better response.

■ PERTINENT PATIENT FACTORS

R.R. is a 70-year-old man with HTLV-1–associated adult T-cell leukemia who has been treated with zidovudine plus interferon α-2b and four cycles of cyclophosphamide, hydroxydaunomycin (doxorubicin), vincristine (Oncovin®), and prednisone, the combination of which is referred to as CHOP. After these treatments, R.R. developed severe and protracted thrombocytopenia, which has prevented further treatment.

Past Medical History

- HTLV-1 adult T-cell leukemia
- Cardiomegaly (ejection fraction 28%) secondary to zidovudine (AZT) and interferon α-2b treatment
- Peptic ulcer disease
- Hypertension
- Thrombocytopenia

Social History

- Ø alcohol
- Ø tobacco

Current Medications

- Oprelvekin 50 μg/kg/day subcutaneously
- Pantoprazole 40 mg orally daily
- Ramipril 5 mg orally daily
- Trimethoprim-sulfamethoxazole one double-strength tablet orally daily
- Dexamethasone 40 mg orally daily
- Loperamide 4 mg orally as needed for diarrhea
- Acetaminophen 325 mg orally as needed for headache
- Ø complementary/alternative or other nonprescription medications

Allergies/Intolerances

No known drug allergies

Laboratory Results

Sodium 135 mmol/L, potassium 4.9 mmol/L, chloride 103 mmol/L, CO_2 22 mmol/L, creatinine 1.1 mg/dL, glucose 91 mg/dL, blood urea nitrogen (BUN) 25 mg/dL, albumin 3 g/dL, calcium (total) 2.49 mmol/L, magnesium 0.75 mmol/L, phosphorus 3.4 mg/dL, liver function tests (LFTs) within normal limits, white blood cells (WBCs) 28.3×10^9/L, hemoglobin (Hgb) 10.1 g/dL, hematocrit (Hct) 28.1%

Date	Platelet Count
7/13	25 K/mm^3
7/14[a]	21 K/mm^3
7/15	26 K/mm^3
7/16	29 K/mm^3
7/17	28 K/mm^3

[a]Day 1 of oprelvekin therapy.

■ PERTINENT DISEASE FACTORS

It is not known whether patients with adult T-cell leukemia respond differently to oprelvekin than those with other types of nonmyeloid malignancies.

■ PERTINENT MEDICATION FACTORS

Oprelvekin, or recombinant interleukin-11, is indicated for the prevention of severe thrombocytopenia and the reduction of the need for platelet transfusions following myelosuppressive chemotherapy in adult patients. The U.S. Food and Drug Administration (FDA)-approved dose of oprelvekin is 50 μg/kg once daily for up to 21 days.[7] Larger doses of oprelvekin (75 to 100 μg/kg/day) have been studied in patients with breast cancer.[7,8] Constitutional symptoms associated with oprelvekin therapy, such as myalgias, arthralgias, and fatigue, were noted to increase in a dose-dependent fashion. One patient who received 100 μg/kg/day of oprelvekin experienced a cerebrovascular event after the third dose. Dose escalation greater than 75 μg/kg/day was discontinued in this study, and the maximum tolerated dose of oprelvekin was determined to be 75 μg/kg/day.[8] However, the manufacturer warns that doses greater than 50 μg/kg/day may be associated with an increased incidence of fluid retention and cardiovascular events in adult patients.[4] After initiation of therapy, platelet counts usually begin to increase between 5 and 9 days, with peak counts occurring after about 14 to 19 days of therapy.[8]

■ ANALYSIS AND SYNTHESIS

Because R.R. has only received 4 days of oprelvekin treatment and platelet counts are expected to increase between 5 and 9 days after the initiation of therapy, adequate time for an optimal response to oprelvekin therapy has not been reached. In addition, oprelvekin doses greater than 75 μg/kg/day have been associated with serious adverse effects in adult patients. Therefore, increasing the dose of oprelvekin in this patient is probably not necessary, and may increase the risk of serious adverse effects without providing additional therapeutic benefits.

■ RESPONSE AND RECOMMENDATIONS

Oprelvekin, or recombinant human interleukin-11, is a thrombopoietic growth factor that stimulates the proliferation of hematopoietic stem cells and megakaryocyte progenitor cells, resulting in increased platelet production. Oprelvekin is indicated for the prevention of severe thrombocytopenia in patients with nonmyeloid malignancies who are at high risk for severe thrombocytopenia following chemotherapy.[7] Platelet counts usually begin to increase between 5 and 9 days after initiation of oprelvekin, with peak platelet counts occurring after 14 to 19 days of therapy.[7,8] R.R. has only received 4 days of oprelvekin treatment, which is insufficient for an optimal response. In addition, the adverse effects of oprelvekin therapy (e.g., myalgias, arthralgias, fatigue, fluid retention, and cardiovascular events) are dose dependent.[7,8] Therefore, increasing the oprelvekin dose at this time is not warranted. In fact, doing so may predispose the patient to an increased risk of adverse effects without the prospect of added therapeutic benefit.

■ CASE MESSAGE

This example demonstrates the importance of understanding the proper context of the query. In this case, the physician is asking the wrong question. The pharmacist must collect critical background information to determine the actual drug information needed. Had the pharmacist failed to collect pertinent patient information, the physician may have increased the dose of the medication after being told that doses of 75 μg/kg/day of oprelvekin have been used. This would have been inappropriate, given that this patient had not received the medication for a sufficient duration to achieve optimal response. Moreover, larger doses of this medication are associated with a higher incidence of adverse effects.

Case Study 2–3

■ INITIAL QUESTION

Are there any drug interactions between labetalol, clonidine, amlodipine, lorazepam, and minoxidil?

■ POTENTIAL RESPONSE IN THE ABSENCE OF RELEVANT BACKGROUND INFORMATION

An extensive search of tertiary[4,9-12] and secondary literature sources did not reveal any significant drug–drug interactions between labetalol, clonidine, amlodipine, lorazepam, and minoxidil. However, concomitant therapy with a β-adrenergic antagonist, an α-adrenergic antagonist, a calcium channel antagonist, and a peripheral vasodilator may increase the potential for additive hypotension.

■ PERTINENT BACKGROUND INFORMATION

The requestor is a physician who is caring for a patient with severe hypertension. The physician plans to add minoxidil to the antihypertensive regimen because the patient's morning blood pressure is not optimally controlled. He would like to make sure that there are no drug interactions between minoxidil and the patient's other medications.

■ PERTINENT PATIENT FACTORS

S.L. is a 40-year-old man with severe hypertension and renal insufficiency.

Past Medical History

- HIV infection × 5 years
- Hepatitis C × 8 years
- Hypertension × 4 years
- Renal dysfunction

Social History

- 1 to 2 pints of vodka daily × 12 years
- 1 pack per day (PPD) of cigarettes × 25 years
- History of intravenous drug abuse

Current Medications

- Labetalol 400 mg orally daily (@9 AM)
- Clonidine transdermal patch 0.3 mg/day
- Amlodipine 10 mg orally daily (@9 AM)
- Lorazepam 1 mg orally as needed for anxiety
- Multiple vitamin orally daily
- Ø complementary/alternative or other nonprescription medications

Allergies/Intolerances

- Lisinopril (angioedema)

Laboratory Results

- Sodium 136 mmol/L, potassium 4.7 mmol/L, chloride 102 mmol/L, CO_2 24 mmol/L, creatinine 2.9 mg/dL, glucose 98 mg/dL, BUN 14 mg/dL
- Viral DNA <100 copies/mL
- Cluster designation 4 (CD4) count 900 cells/mm^3

Blood Pressure Measurements

4/15		4/16		4/17	
@6 AM	172/116	@6 AM	168/110	@6 AM	178/114
@noon	121/81	@noon	116/86	@noon	119/84
@8 PM	158/100	@8 PM	150/104	@8 PM	166/100

■ PERTINENT DISEASE FACTORS

It is not known whether patients with HIV infection respond differently to antihypertensive medications.

■ PERTINENT MEDICATION FACTORS

There are no primary or tertiary literature reports describing drug interactions between minoxidil and any of S.L.'s current medications.[4,9-12] A review of the patient's current antihypertensive medications suggests that the dose of each agent is appropriate for achieving adequate blood pressure control in the face of significant renal compromise.[13] However, the duration of action of labetalol is 8 to 12 hours, and this agent is typically dosed twice daily. S.L. is receiving 400 mg of labetalol daily at 9 AM.

■ ANALYSIS AND SYNTHESIS

S.L.'s blood pressure appears to be highest in the morning, just before the daily doses of labetalol and amlodipine are administered. He is receiving 400 mg of labetalol daily at 9 AM. Because the duration of action of labetalol is 8 to 12 hours, and the usual maintenance dose is 200 to 400 mg twice daily, the increase in blood pressure observed in the morning could be due, at least in part, to inappropriate dosing of labetalol. This medication should generally be administered twice daily to achieve maximal benefit. Adjustment of the labetalol dose should precede the addition of other antihypertensive agents to this patient's medication regimen. Although long-term cigarette smoking can increase the cardiovascular risk associated with hypertension, there is no indication that smoking or alcohol ingestion are contributing to this patient's present problem.

■ RESPONSE AND RECOMMENDATIONS

There do not appear to be any significant drug interactions between any of S.L.'s current medications and minoxidil.[4,9-12] Additionally, after considering the pharmacokinetics, pharmacodynamics, adverse effect profiles, and pharmaceutical properties of the patient's medications, the potential for a clinically significant drug interaction appears low. However, a review of the patient's current antihypertensive regimen suggests that the dosing of labetalol is inappropriate. The duration of action of labetalol is 8 to 12 hours, and the usual maintenance dose is 200 to 400 mg twice daily. Because S.L. is receiving 400 mg of labetalol once daily at 9 AM, the increase in blood pressure observed in the morning could be due to inappropriate labetalol dosing. The physician was directed to optimize labetalol therapy before the addition of another antihypertensive agent. If the patient's blood pressure is not controlled with proper dosing of labetalol and minoxidil therapy is required, the physician should be advised that minoxidil is usually administered with a diuretic to prevent fluid retention.

■ CASE MESSAGE

This is another example emphasizing the importance of the proper context of the question. In this case, the pharmacist was able to recommend appropriate drug therapy management, even though the initial question posed by the physician was not related to the dosage and administration of labetalol.

Case Study 2–4

■ INITIAL QUESTION

Can ranitidine cause thrombocytopenia?

■ POTENTIAL RESPONSE IN THE ABSENCE OF RELEVANT
  BACKGROUND INFORMATION

Ranitidine has been infrequently associated with thrombocytopenia.[4,14-16] This is a relatively rare but readily reversible complication of histamine-2 (H_2)-antagonist therapy.

■ PERTINENT BACKGROUND INFORMATION

The requestor is a physician who is evaluating a patient for suspected Cushing disease. The patient has been hospitalized for 8 days and has undergone extensive diagnostic tests, including serial blood sampling to establish the diagnosis. Over the last 4 days, the patient has experienced a rapid decline in her platelet count. The physician is aware that cimetidine can cause thrombocytopenia. Her patient is taking ranitidine, and she would like to know if the thrombocytopenia could be induced by this medication.

■ PERTINENT PATIENT FACTORS

L.B. is a 38-year-old obese woman with Type 2 diabetes who is being evaluated for Cushing disease.

Past Medical History

- Gastroesophageal reflux disease (GERD) × 6 years
- Type 2 diabetes × 1 year

Social History

- Ø alcohol
- Ø tobacco
- No occupational or environmental exposures

Current Medications

- Ranitidine 150 mg orally twice a day (intermittently for 6 years)
- Metformin 500 mg orally three times a day (for about 8 months)

- Heparin 100 USP units/mL (as needed for flushing heparin lock)
- Ø complementary/alternative or nonprescription medications

Allergies/Intolerances

- Penicillin (rash)

Laboratory Results

Sodium 137 mmol/L, potassium 4.9 mmol/L, chloride 102 mmol/L, CO_2 24 mmol/L, creatinine 0.9 mg/dL, glucose 133 mg/dL, BUN 12 mg/dL, albumin 3.4 g/dL, calcium 2.35 mmol/L, magnesium 0.81 mmol/L, phosphorus 3.8 mg/dL, LFTs within normal limits, WBCs 5.6×10^9/L

Date	Platelet Count
1/17	241 K/mm^3
4/20[a]	230 K/mm^3
4/24	212 K/mm^3
4/25	159 K/mm^3
4/26	114 K/mm^3
4/27	97 K/mm^3
4/28	81 K/mm^3

[a]Day of admission.

◼ PERTINENT DISEASE FACTORS

L.B.'s thrombocytopenia is of new onset and is characterized by a rapid decline in the platelet counts over a few days. This patient does not appear to have a readily identifiable medical condition as a likely cause of the thrombocytopenia. Furthermore, she does not have any clinical evidence of bleeding or thrombosis.

◼ PERTINENT MEDICATION FACTORS

A review of the literature[4,14,17] indicates that metformin has not been reported as a cause of thrombocytopenia. Ranitidine, however, has been infrequently associated with thrombocytopenia.[4,14-16] This is a relatively rare but readily reversible complication of ranitidine therapy. Ranitidine-induced thrombocytopenia usually develops within the first 30 days of therapy, but its pathogenesis remains unclear. Most hematologic toxicities reported with the H_2-receptor antagonists appear to occur in patients with serious concomitant diseases or in those receiving other treatments more commonly associated with hematologic adverse effects.[14-16] Thrombocytopenia has been reported in about 5% of patients treated with porcine heparin.[4] Heparin-induced thrombocytopenia does not appear to be dose dependent and has been reported in patients receiving less than 500 units of heparin per day. This condition typically develops within 5 to 9 days after initiation of therapy and reverses readily after discontinuation of the drug.

■ ANALYSIS AND SYNTHESIS

Although both ranitidine and heparin have been reported to cause thrombocytopenia, heparin appears to be the most likely cause in this case. L.B. has been taking ranitidine intermittently for nearly 6 years. Thrombocytopenia induced by ranitidine usually develops within the first 30 days of therapy. Moreover, heparin-induced thrombocytopenia is a more common adverse effect and has been reported in patients receiving very small daily doses of heparin (including heparin lock flush solution). It usually develops within 5 to 9 days after initiation of therapy. Based on the presentation and temporal sequence of events, heparin-induced thrombocytopenia is the most likely explanation for L.B.'s acute drop in platelet count. Assessment of causality using the Naranjo algorithm (see Chapter 15 for more information on this algorithm) implicates heparin as a probable cause of thrombocytopenia in this case, with ranitidine and metformin as possible and unlikely causes, respectively.[18]

■ RESPONSE AND RECOMMENDATIONS

A review of L.B.'s current medications reveals two agents, ranitidine and heparin, that have been reported to cause thrombocytopenia.[4,9,14] Ranitidine-induced thrombocytopenia is most likely to occur within the first 30 days of therapy.[14-16] Because L.B. has been taking ranitidine intermittently for GERD for approximately 6 years, it is unlikely that ranitidine is responsible for the acute decrement in platelet count. Ranitidine, however, cannot be immediately ruled out as a possible cause. Heparin-induced thrombocytopenia is a more common adverse effect that has been reported even with very small daily doses of heparin (e.g., heparin lock flush solution).[4] The thrombocytopenia is acute and usually develops within 5 to 9 days after initiation of therapy. Based on the presentation and temporal relationship, heparin appears to be the most likely cause of thrombocytopenia in this patient. The physician was advised to discontinue the heparin lock flush solution, closely monitor the patient's platelet count, and test for heparin antibodies in order to establish the diagnosis and guide future therapy. If the platelet counts do not begin to normalize after discontinuation of heparin, other potential causes of thrombocytopenia should be considered.

■ CASE MESSAGE

This question highlights the importance of skillful problem solving. As always, collecting appropriate background information and patient data is critical. Analyzing this information before synthesizing a logical response is paramount for effective patient management. In this case, failure to recognize that the patient was receiving heparin lock flush solution could have incorrectly excluded heparin as a possible cause of the thrombocytopenia.

Self-Assessment Questions

1. Why is it necessary to gather background information and patient data? Why do pharmacists often fail to elicit this information? Why do requestors often fail to provide this information?

2. What factors should be considered in making a recommendation regarding the dosage and administration of an antibiotic? Provide a justification for each factor you select.

3. Given the question, "Can naproxen cause nephrotoxicity?" list at least five related questions that should be considered.

4. List three patient-related factors that should be considered for a question pertaining to a potential drug interaction.

5. How can you ensure that the information you provide is correctly applied? How will you know if you were successful?

6. Can patient-specific recommendations be made in the absence of adequate background information and patient data? Elaborate.

7. What are your options in responding to patient-specific queries in cases where there is insufficient or inadequate clinical data? Elaborate.

REFERENCES
1. Watanabe AS, Conner CS. Principles of drug information services. Hamilton (IL): Drug Intelligence Publications Inc.; 1978.
2. Galt KA, Calis KA, Turcasso NM. Clinical skills program: module 3 drug information. Bethesda (MD): American Society of Health-System Pharmacists Inc.; 1995.
3. Calis KA, Anderson DW, Auth DA, Mays DA, Turcasso NM, Meyer CC, et al. Quality of pharmacotherapy consultations provided by drug information centers in the United States. Pharmacotherapy. 2000;20(7):830-6.

4. McEvoy GK, ed. AHFS drug information 2013. Bethesda (MD): American Society of Health-System Pharmacists; 2013.

5. Vasotec [package insert]. Bridgewater (NJ): Valeant Pharmaceuticals North America, LLC; 2012.

6. O'Neil MJ, Smith A, Heckelman PE, Obenchain Jr, eds. The Merck Index: an encyclopedia of chemicals, drugs, and biologicals. 14th ed. Whitehouse Station (NJ): Merck & Co; 2006.

7. Neumega [package insert]. Philadelphia (PA): Wyeth BioPharma Division of Wyeth Pharmaceuticals Inc.; 2011.

8. Gordon MS, McCaskill-Stevens WJ, Battiato LA, et al. A phase I trial of recombinant human interleukin-11 (Neumega rhIL-11 growth factor) in women with breast cancer receiving chemotherapy. Blood. 1996;87(9):3615-24.

9. DRUG-REAX System [Internet]. Greenwood Village (CO): Thomson Reuters (Healthcare) Inc.; [cited 2013 Feb 5]. Available from: http://www.micromedexsolutions.com

10. Hansten PD, Horne JR. Drug interactions: analysis and management. St. Louis (MO): Wolters Kluwer Health; 2013.

11. Tatro DS, ed. Drug interaction facts: the authority on drug interactions. St. Louis (MO): Lippincott Williams &Wilkins; 2012.

12. Zucchero FJ, Hogan MJ, Sommer CD, eds. Evaluation of drug interactions. St. Louis (MO): First Databank; 2004.

13. Aronoff GR, Bennett WM, Berns JS, Bier ME, eds. Drug prescribing in renal failure. 5th ed. Philadelphia (PA): American College of Physicians; 2007.

14. Aronson JK, Dukes MNG, Meyler L, eds. Meyler's side effects of drugs. 15th ed. Amsterdam, The Netherlands: Elsevier Science; 2006.

15. Yim JM, Frazier JL. Ranitidine and thrombocytopenia. J Pharm Technol. 1995;11:263-6.

16. Wade EE, Rebuck JA, Healey MA, Rogers FB. H_2–antagonist-induced thrombocytopenia: is this a real phenomenon? Intensive Care Med. 2002;28(4):459-65.

17. Glucophage [package insert]. Princeton (NJ): Bristol-Myers Squibb; 2011.

18. Naranjo CA, Busto U, Sellers EM, et al. A method for estimating the probability of adverse drug reactions. Clin Pharmacol Ther. 1981;30:239-45.

3

Chapter Three

Drug Information Resources

Kelly M. Shields • Elaine Blythe

Learning Objectives

After completing this chapter, the reader will be able to

- Differentiate between primary, secondary, and tertiary sources of information.
- Identify resources relevant to different pharmacy practice areas.
- Select appropriate resources for a specific information request.
- Describe the role of electronic resources in the provision of drug information.
- Evaluate resources to determine appropriateness of information.
- Describe appropriate search strategy for use with electronic databases.
- Recognize alternative resources for provision of drug information.

Key Concepts

❶ Tertiary sources provide information that has been filtered and summarized by an author or editor to provide a quick easy summary of a topic.

❷ Various systems index or abstract literature from different journals, meetings, or publications; therefore, in order to perform a comprehensive search multiple databases must be used.

❸ There are several types of publications considered primary, including controlled trials, cohort studies, case series, and case reports.

❹ At times even well-designed searches of standard medical literature do not yield sufficient information to make clinical decisions or recommendations. In these cases, alternative resources may need to be employed.

❺ Understanding where to access information is only the first step in the provision of quality drug information.

Introduction

The quantity of medical information and medical literature available is growing at an astounding rate. The technology by which this information can be accessed is also improving exponentially. The introduction of tablets, smartphones, and Internet resources has radically changed the methods and technology by which information is accessed, but not the process of providing drug information.

Pharmacists are being asked daily to provide responses to numerous drug information requests for a variety of people. It is tempting just to select the easiest, most familiar resources to find information; however, by doing that there is the possibility of missing new resources or limiting the comprehensiveness of the information found. It is for these reasons that the systematic approach discussed in Chapter 2 is helpful in order to streamline the search process.

Generally the best method to find information includes a stepwise approach moving first through tertiary (e.g., textbooks, full-text databases, review articles), then secondary (e.g., indexing or abstracting services), and finally primary (e.g., clinical studies) literature. The tertiary sources provide the practitioner with general information needed to familiarize the reader with the topic. This is also an opportunity for the practitioner to gain general information about the disease or drug in question, which ultimately results in a more structured and productive search.

If the information obtained in the tertiary resources is not recent or comprehensive enough, a secondary database may be employed to direct the reader to review primary literature articles that might provide more insight into the topic. Primary literature often provides the most recent and in-depth information about a topic and allows the reader to analyze and critique the study methodology to determine if the conclusions are valid (see Chapters 4 and 5 for more information on critiquing the primary literature).

For some requests, it may be necessary to consult news reports or Internet sites to get background information before beginning the searching process. Also, other resources, including experts or specialists in particular areas of practice, may need to be consulted. While the same general search strategy can be used for most requests, the specific resources employed vary.

Often a search for information does not employ all of these steps and does not require the use of all three types of resources. For example, a question regarding commercial availability of a product formulation, or mechanism of action, could quickly be found in a tertiary resource. The information found there may be sufficient to conclude the search and provide a response. However, a question regarding the clinical trials supporting off-label use in a specific population will likely require a search of primary literature.

The type of requestor may also substantially influence the resources used to respond to a question. Generally, a request from a consumer or patient could more appropriately be answered from available tertiary resources than from a stack of clinical trials. However, if the requestor is a prescriber requesting detailed information about the management of a specific disease state and role of investigational therapies, provision of primary literature may be appropriate.

The provision of drug information is continually expanding into new areas and technologies, which may impact selection of resources. For example, increased patient use of dietary supplements and alternative therapies has left medical professionals seeking information on these topics. Pharmacists are often expected to respond to questions about these topics and provide recommendations as to management of patients using these therapies. Also increasing interest in the practice of veterinary pharmacy underscores the need for pharmacists to be able to practically apply drug information resources for the benefit of animal patients, animal owners, and veterinary professionals. Additionally, the emergence of completely new fields of practice, such as pharmacogenomics, offer opportunities for pharmacists to apply their training in less traditional roles.

Tertiary Resources

❶ *Tertiary sources provide information that has been summarized and distilled by the author or editor to provide a quick easy summary of a topic.* Some examples of tertiary resources include textbooks, compendia, review articles in journals, and other general information, such as may be found on the Internet. These references may often serve as an initial place to identify information, due to the fact that they provide a fairly complete and concise overview of information available on a specific topic. These resources are also convenient, easy to use, and familiar to most practitioners. Most of the information needed by a practitioner can be found in these sources, making these excellent first-line resources when dealing with a drug information question.

The major drawback to print copy tertiary resources, however, is the lag time associated with publication, resulting in less current information. Medical information changes so rapidly that it is possible that information may be out of date before a text is even published. Electronically available tertiary resources have helped this situation; however, the requirement for information to be reviewed and summarized requires an inherent delay in communicating new information. It is also possible that information in a tertiary text may be incomplete, due to either space limitations of the resource or incomplete literature searches by the author. Other problems that can be seen with tertiary

TABLE 3–1. EVALUATION OF TERTIARY LITERATURE

Does the author have appropriate experience/expertise to publish in this area?
Is the information likely to be timely based on publication date?
Is information supported by appropriate citations?
Does the resource contain relevant information?
Does the resource appear free from bias and blatant errors?

information include errors in transcription, human bias, incorrect interpretation of information, or a lack of expertise by authors. For these reasons readers must judge the quality of tertiary references and may need to verify the information in multiple sources. Some types of questions that should be considered when evaluating tertiary literature are listed in Table 3–1.

It is impossible to compile a comprehensive list of tertiary resources that are useful in all areas of pharmacy practice. Differences in practice settings, available funding, patient populations seen, and types of information most commonly needed, all impact which tertiary resources should be available at a specific practice site. The legal requirements for information sources available at a practice setting vary from state to state, but rarely will the minimally required texts be sufficient to meet all information needs in a practice.

Another important factor in the selection of appropriate tertiary resources includes selecting a resource focused on the type of information needed for a specific request or situation. For example, a very well-written and comprehensive therapeutics text may have very limited use in providing information regarding pharmacokinetics of a specific drug. For this reason, it is important to consider the categories of requests received in a particular practice setting to ensure that appropriate tertiary texts are available. Table 3–2 lists resources that may be useful for specific categories of drug information requests.

A brief summary of selected tertiary resources is listed to provide examples of some resources that may be useful in the general pharmacy practice. Information is provided about the features of the resource as well as the publisher and publisher Web site. While specific electronic resources may be hosted at a different Web site, the publisher site will direct users toward the appropriate link.

This list is not comprehensive and reflects only a limited number of resources available. The Basic Resources for Pharmacy Education listing distributed by the American Association of Colleges of Pharmacy (AACP)[1] was utilized in selecting the resources described in this chapter; additional commonly used resources in drug information[2] were also included. These complete documents contain hundreds of other resources that may be useful depending on practice setting.

TABLE 3–2. USEFUL RESOURCES FOR COMMON CATEGORIES OF DRUG INFORMATION

Type of Request	Useful Tertiary Sources	Secondary Resources
General Product Information	Major compendia,* Handbook of Nonprescription Drugs,[3] product labeling	MEDLINE®, EMBASE®, IPA, IDIS
Adverse Effects	Meyler's Side Effects of Drugs,[4] Side Effects of Drugs Annual,[5] product labeling, major compendia*	Reactions Weekly, MEDLINE®, EMBASE®, IPA, IDIS
Availability of Dosage Forms	Red Book,[6] American Drug Index[7] major compendia*	IPA, IDIS, EMBASE®, MEDLINE®
Compounding/Formulations	Remington: The Science and Practice of Pharmacy,[8] Merck Index,[9] A Practical Guide to Contemporary Pharmacy Practice,[10] USP/NF,[11] Trissel's Stability of Compounded Formulations,[12] Extemporaneous Formulations,[13] Ansel's Pharmaceutical Dosage Forms and Drug Delivery Systems,[14] USP Pharmacists' Pharmacopeia[15]	
Dietary Supplements	Natural Medicine Comprehensive Database,[16] Review of Natural Products,[17] Natural Standard,[18] PDR for Herbal Medicine,[19] Trease and Evans' Pharmacognosy[20]	EMBASE®, MEDLINE®, IPA, IDIS
Dosage Recommendations (General and organ impairment)	Major compendia,* Drug Prescribing in Renal Failure[21]	MEDLINE®, IPA, IDIS, EMBASE®
Drug Interactions	Hansten and Horn's Drug Interaction Analysis and Management,[22] Drug Interaction Facts,[23] Stockley's Drug Interactions,[24] Food-Medication Interactions,[25] Drug Therapy Monitoring System,[26] major compendia*	Reactions Weekly, IPA
Drug-Laboratory Interference	Basic Skills in Interpreting Laboratory Data,[27] Laboratory Tests and Diagnostic Procedures[28]	
Geriatric Dosage Recommendations	Geriatric Dosage Handbook,[29] major compendia*	MEDLINE®, IPA, IDIS, EMBASE®
Identification of Product	Identidex,[30] Clinical Pharmacology,[31] Drugs.com, IDENT-A-DRUG,[32] Lexicomp,[33] Facts & Comparisons® eAnswers[34]	
Investigational Drug Information	FDA Web site (http://www.fda.gov),[35] Clinicaltrials.gov,[36] MedlinePlus,[37] manufacturer Web sites	Current Contents, EMBASE®, MEDLINE®, LexisNexis®, IPA, IDIS
Incompatibility/Stability	Handbook of Injectable Drugs,[38] King Guide to Parenteral Admixtures,[39] Trissel's 2 Clinical Pharmaceutics Database,[40] Extended Stability for Parenteral Drugs,[41] Trissel's Stability of Compounded Formulations,[42] Remington: The Science and Practice of Pharmacy[43]	IPA, IDIS, EMBASE®, MEDLINE®

continued

TABLE 3–2. USEFUL RESOURCES FOR COMMON CATEGORIES OF DRUG INFORMATION (*CONTINUED*)

Type of Request	Useful Tertiary Sources	Secondary Resources
International Drug Equivalency	Martindale: The Complete Drug Reference,[44] Index Nominum,[45] Internet Search Engines, Specific country resources	
Method/Rate of Administration	Major compendia*	
Pediatric Dosage Recommendations	The Harriet Lane Handbook,[46] Pediatric and Neonatal Dosage Handbook,[47] Neofax,[48] major compendia*	MEDLINE®, IPA, IDIS, EMBASE®
Pharmacokinetics	Basic Clinical Pharmacokinetics,[49] Applied Biopharmaceutics and Pharmacokinetics,[50] major compendia*	IPA, EMBASE®, MEDLINE®, IDIS
Pharmacology	Goodman & Gilman's: The Pharmacological Basis of Therapeutics,[51] Basic & Clinical Pharmacology,[52] Brody's Human Pharmacology: Molecular to Clinical,[53] Principles of Pharmacology[54]	IDIS, IPA, EMBASE®, MEDLINE®
Pharmacy Law	Pharmacy Practice and the Law,[55] Guide to Federal Pharmacy Law,[56] State Board of Pharmacy Web sites	LexisNexis®
Teratogenicity/Lactation	Drugs in Pregnancy and Lactation,[57] Medications and Mother's Milk,[58] Catalog of Teratogenic Agents,[59] Drugs during Pregnancy and Lactation,[60] REPRORISK,[61] major compendia*	Reactions Weekly, EMBASE®, MEDLINE®, IDIS, IPA
Therapy Evaluation/Drugs of Choice	Pharmacotherapy: a Pathophysiologic Approach,[62] Pharmacotherapy Principles and Practice, Applied Therapeutics: The Clinical Use of Drugs,[63] The Merck Manual of diagnosis and therapy,[64] Harrison's Principles of Internal Medicine,[65] Goldman's Cecil Medicine,[66] Textbook of Therapeutics,[67] Conn's Current Therapy,[68] Medscape	MEDLINE®, EMBASE®, IDIS, IPA
Toxicology Information	POISINDEX®[69] Goldfrank's Toxicologic Emergencies,[70] Casarett & Doull's Toxicology: The Basic Science of Poisons,[71] Poisoning & Toxicology Handbook,[72] Haddad and Winchester's Clinical Management of Drug Overdose,[73] TOXNET[74]	Reactions Weekly, EMBASE®, MEDLINE®, IPA, IDIS, BIOSIS
Veterinary Medicine	Textbook of Veterinary Internal Medicine,[75] The Merck Veterinary Manual (MVM),[76] Pet Place,[77] Pet education,[78] Pets with Diabetes[79] Plumb's Veterinary Drug Handbook,[80] Compendium of Veterinary Products (CVP),[81] Exotic Animal Formulary,[82] USP, Veterinary Medicine[83]	BIOSIS, EMBASE®, MEDLINE®

*Data from Facts & Comparisons®,[84] AHFS Drug Information®, Physicians' Desk Reference® (PDR), Micromedex,[85] Lexicomp®,[33] and Clinical Pharmacology.[31]

GENERAL PRODUCT INFORMATION

AHFS Drug Information®

American Society of Health-System Pharmacists®, http://www.ahfsdruginformation. com This drug information resource is organized by monographs containing information on both Food and Drug Administration (FDA)-approved and off-label uses of medications. This resource is designated by the U.S. Congress as an appropriate source of information for determining reimbursement of unlabeled uses of medications. Information about dosing in specific populations is also included, as is a wide variety of general information about medications. Some information is also available about compatibility and stability of injectable formulations. AHFS Drug Information is available in paper format (updated annually), an excerpted paper format (*AHFS DI® Essentials™*), and a mobile drug reference version.

Clinical Pharmacology

Gold Standard, http://www.clinicalpharmacology.com This electronic database contains monographs of prescription and nonprescription products as well as some dietary supplements. Tools within the database allow users to screen for drug interactions, create comparison tables for drug products, determine intravenous (IV) compatibility (based on Trissel's 2™ Clinical Pharmaceutics Database) and search for tablets by description or imprint codes. Patient education information is available in English and Spanish. It is available online or as a smartphone application.

Micromedex® 2.0

Truven Health Analytics, http://www.micromedexsolutions.com This electronic resource contains information about FDA-approved indications, off-label uses, pharmacokinetic data, safety information, and pharmacology. Multiple interactive tools are available to assess for drug–drug/food/supplement interactions, incompatibilities, and pharmacokinetic adjustments. There is an additional toxicology section which allows identification of drugs based on imprint codes and discussion of overdose management. Patient education materials are also included in this database. This resource is available online as well as for mobile devices. Please note that on mobile devices it is available as both a full version and an abridged application.

Facts & Comparisons®

Wolters Kluwer Health, Inc., http://www.factsandcomparisons.com This reference contains information about prescription and nonprescription drugs organized by drug class. Information is provided about specific agents, including inactive ingredients in commercial preparations. There are comparative monographs of drug classes to help discern differences between agents of the same class. This resource is available via hardcopy, online (Facts & Comparisons® eAnswers), and for mobile devices. The electronic version of this resource allows for an integrated search across a variety of Facts & Comparisons publications (depending on subscription purchased).

Drug Information Handbook

Wolters Kluwer Health, Inc., http://www.lexi.com This handbook is organized in brief product monographs, where information is presented regarding clinical use, safety, and monitoring for a variety of drugs. Data are presented about FDA-approved and off-label use of medications. There is a tablet identification section as part of the electronic format. The resource also has several helpful appendices providing treatment options and comparing agents in the same class. This resource is available via hard copy, online, and for mobile devices. The electronic versions allow for integrated searches of various Lexicomp® products (depending on subscription purchased). The online resource also includes tablet identification features as well as medication pricing information. This resource has also partnered with AHFS (described above) to offer an electronic subscription combining their two databases in a seamless search.

Handbook of Nonprescription Drugs: An Interactive Approach to Self-Care

American Pharmacists Association®, http://www.pharmacist.com This text is organized by body system, focusing on those disease states for which self-care may be appropriate. Information is provided about comparative efficacy of various over-the-counter (OTC) agents, as well as contraindications for self-treatment, drug interactions, and other safety information. The use of treatment algorithms and patient care cases make this resource especially helpful for students and new practitioners. The text is also available as an e-book.

Physicians' Desk Reference®

PDR.net®, http://www.pdr.net This resource is a compilation of prescription product package inserts. Additional information includes contact information for manufacturers, a list of poison control centers, and very limited tablet identification. The company maintains a Web site, pdrhealth.com, which contains patient appropriate information. Information from the Physicians' Desk Reference (PDR) is also available online at http://www.pdr.net or http://www.pdrhealth.com, or for mobile devices (PDRBooks®). In addition to the original PDR, there are a variety of focused editions, including the *PDR® for Herbal Medicines, PDR® for Nutritional Supplements, PDR® for Ophthalmic Medicines, PDR® for Nonprescription Drugs.*

USP Dictionary

U.S. Pharmacopeial Convention, http://www.usp.org This is the official resource for determining generic and chemical names of drugs, as well as the international nonproprietary name. Additionally, useful information such as chemical structure, molecular weight, Chemical Abstracts Services (CAS) registry number, and a pronunciation guide is provided. This resource is also available in an online format and in print.

Epocrates®

Epocrates, http://www.epocrates.com This family of electronic resources includes both mobile and online products. These resources include information about drugs (monographs, interaction checker, safety data, tablet identification) and diseases (epidemiology, prognosis, treatment).

ADVERSE EFFECTS

Meyler's Side Effects of Drugs

Elsevier Publishing, http://www.elsevier.com This reference provides a critical review of international literature in the area of adverse events. Chapters are organized by drug classification; adverse events are organized by drug name and then by organ system within each drug. Information is provided about adverse events and management.

Side Effects of Drugs Annual: A Worldwide Yearly Survey of New Data and Trends in Adverse Drug Reactions

Elsevier Publishing, http://www.elsevier.com This reference which is updated annually serves as a companion to the text Meyler's Side Effects of Drugs. A team evaluates international literature published each year identifying new information and summarizing that information in this resource.

Case Study 3-1

A 15-year-old patient has recently been started on atomoxetine for treatment of attention deficit/hyperactivity disorder. He is taking no other medications. He has noted recently that his hair is thinning and wants to know if this might be drug related.

• *What are appropriate tertiary resources to consult for a response to this request?*

AVAILABILITY OF DOSAGE FORMS

American Drug Index

Lippincott Williams & Wilkins, http://www.lww.com This reference contains brief entries, indexed by product and generic name, with information about product use, available dosage forms and sizes, and manufacturer information. Several helpful charts are also available, including look-alike/sound-alike medications, pregnancy categories, normal lab values, as well as common pharmacy calculations.

Red Book® (Red Book Drug Topics)

Truven Health Analytics, http://www.redbook.com This resource primarily contains data regarding prescription and OTC product availability and pricing. There are also a number of tables listing information such as sugar-free, lactose-free, or alcohol-free preparations. Additionally, information such as National Drug Code (NDC) numbers, routes of administration, dosage form, size, and strength are included. This resource is available in paper copy and electronically within Micromedex® 2.0.

COMPOUNDING/FORMULATIONS

Some journals are especially useful for compounding formulations, for example, the *International Journal of Pharmacy Compounding*, *U.S. Pharmacist*, or *American Druggist*.

Extemporaneous Formulations for Pediatric, Geriatric, and Special Needs Patients (Children's Hospital of Philadelphia)

American Society of Health-System Pharmacists®, http://www.ashp.org This resource is a compilation of published formulations with stability data. Most products are oral formulations to reflect the unique needs of some pediatric patients. Information is also provided about legal and technical issues in compounding practices.

Merck Index

Merck & Co., Inc., http://www.merck.com This resource provides descriptions of the chemical and pharmacological information about a variety of chemicals, drugs, and biologicals. Data include CAS number, chemical structure, molecular weight, and physical data, including solubility, which may be especially useful in compounding. This reference is available in print and online.

Remington: The Science and Practice of Pharmacy

Pharmaceutical Press, http://www.pharmpress.com This classic text contains information about all aspects of pharmacy practice. There is discussion of social issues impacting pharmacy as well as information about the basics of pharmaceutics, manufacturing, pharmacodynamics, nuclear pharmacy, and medicinal chemistry. Information is provided regarding common compounding techniques and ingredients. The paper text is divided into two volumes and also includes a companion CD-ROM.

A Practical Guide to Contemporary Pharmacy Practice

Lippincott, Williams & Wilkins, http://www.lww.com This text resource with CD-ROM is organized in an outline format to find information easily. Discussion of compounding techniques, pharmacy calculations, and explanations of additives used in compounding is very useful. Students and young practitioners may find the sample cases especially helpful.

Trissel's™ Stability of Compounded Formulations

American Pharmacists Association®, http://www.pharmacist.com This text provides information about preparation of sterile and nonsterile dosage forms. The text is organized by drugs and provides a summary of the properties of a drug, general stability considerations, and stability reports of compounded preparations. There is also extensive information provided about beyond-use dating.

USP/NF

U.S. Pharmacopeial Convention, http://www.usp.org This resource, available in print, online, and flash drive formats, contains the official substance and product standards. Also, official preparation instructions are given for a limited number of commonly compounded products.

DIETARY SUPPLEMENTS

Natural Medicine Comprehensive Database

Therapeutic Research Faculty, http://www.naturaldatabase.com This resource is available in text, online, and mobile device formats. It provides a summary of the information available for various dietary supplements and rates the relative safety and efficacy of those products. Searches can be performed by brand names of supplements or by a variety of common names. The electronic version includes an interaction checker and disease state/condition search. The electronic resource has also partnered with the USP Verified program to indicate which supplements have been certified to contain a quality product by USP Verified.

Natural Standard

Natural Standard, http://www.naturalstandard.com This resource is available in text and electronic forms. Extensive evidence-based information regarding efficacy is provided. The monographs utilize tables to quickly summarize published literature and to grade the quality of that evidence. The monographs also provide detailed dosing information reflecting the doses used in clinical studies as well as those recommended by expert opinion.

PDR® for Herbal Medicines

PDR.net®, http://www.pdr.net Products are indexed by common name and information is provided regarding action, usage, dosage, and other clinically useful information. Citations to the primary literature are also provided at the conclusion of each monograph. The focus on strictly herbal products, rather than nonbotanical dietary supplements, may limit utility in some settings.

Review of Natural Products

Wolters Kluwer Health, Inc., http://www.factsandcomparisons.com This resource provides information about the chemistry, pharmacology, and toxicology of a number of natural products, based on references to primary literature. A summary of relevant clinical trials is also available. There is also limited patient counseling information, but the strength of this resource is in the chemistry and pharmacology information. Recent revisions have dramatically increased the amount of information included in patient counseling sections. This is available in loose-leaf, bound, online, and mobile device formats.

Trease and Evans' Pharmacognosy

Saunders Ltd., http://www.elsevier.com This text offers a mixture of more classic pharmacognosy, crude plant–based drug classification and examination, and some of the more clinical applications, pharmacology, and phytochemistry. This is not a resource focused on patient care issues.

DRUG INTERACTIONS

Hansten and Horn's Drug Interactions Analysis and Management

Wolters Kluwer Health, Inc., http://www.hanstenandhorn.com This resource provides summaries of, mechanism of, and management options for reported drug interactions. The authors also provide information regarding severity of interaction and any risk factors that might predispose patients to this event. The loose-leaf version of the reference is updated quarterly while the bound is updated annually. Both provide rapid information regarding severity and likelihood of an interaction and actions needed to minimize this risk based on the case studies and primary literature available. Some of this content is integrated into other electronic Facts & Comparisons products.

Drug Interaction Facts™

Wolters Kluwer Health, Inc., http://www.factsandcomparisons.com This resource provides information about drug–drug or drug–food interactions. Discussions of significance of the interaction as well as suggestions for management are included. This resource is available in both bound and loose-leaf texts. Electronically, it is available via CD-ROM and as integrated in other electronic Facts & Comparisons products.

Food-Medication Interactions

Food-Medication Interactions™, http://www.foodmedinteractions.com This resource is available in print, online, and mobile device formats. This focuses on the impact food may have on mediations and also highlights what foods should be avoided with specific medications.

GERIATRIC DOSAGE RECOMMENDATIONS

Geriatric Dosage Handbook

Wolters Kluwer Health, Inc., http://www.lexi.com The monographs in this resource contain traditional sections of drug information, but focus on dosing recommendations for geriatric patients. There is a special section of each monograph addressing concerns specific to the geriatric population. Limited references to primary literature are provided. This reference is also available online and for mobile devices.

The Merck Manual of Geriatrics

Merck & Co., Inc., http://www.merck.com This resource available in print and online (http://www.merck.com/mkgr/mmg/home.jsp) focuses primarily on management of diseases and conditions common in geriatric patients. There is some discussion of appropriate dosing of medications in this population.

IDENTIFICATION OF PRODUCT

IDENT-A-DRUG

Therapeutic Research Faculty, http://www.indentadrug.com This resource is organized by imprint codes and provides identification of drugs based on those codes. Descriptions of medications as well as NDC and Canadian DIN numbers are provided. Electronic and text versions of this reference are available.

Drugs.com

Drugsite Trust, http://www.drugs.com This electronic resource has an easy-to-use imprint search. This is especially useful as it is available to patients and has no charge for use.

Other resources, discussed elsewhere, also have some tablet identification features including Clinical Pharmacology, Lexicomp Online, Micromedex 2.0®, and Facts & Comparisons eAnswers®.

INCOMPATIBILITY AND STABILITY

Handbook on Injectable Drugs

American Society of Health-System Pharmacists®, http://www.ashp.org This resource, commonly called Trissel's, includes information regarding the compatibility and stability of various parenteral medications. Information is primarily provided in the form of charts and tables, making finding information relatively quick. This resource also provides information about routes of administration and commercially available strengths. A pocket-sized handbook and online subscription are also available.

King® Guide to Parenteral Admixtures®

King Guide Publications, http://www.kingguide.com Over 450 IV drug monographs are provided. This resource focuses on compatibility information. Also, limited information about stability is available. This is available in loose-leaf, bound copy, online, and mobile device formats.

Trissel's™ 2 Clinical Pharmaceutics Database

TriPharma, http://trissels2.rcl.com/tsweb/. This electronic resource compiles data from other Trissel publications. Information about parenteral admixtures, compounded formulations, physical compatibility, and chemotherapy formulations is included. Extensive information describing published information is provided which can be applied to specific clinical situations. This resource is available for the intranet, as well as via CD-ROM and the Internet.

INTERNATIONAL DRUG EQUIVALENCY

Index Nominum: International Drug Directory

Medpharm Publishers, http://www.medpharm.de This drug information source contains information on drugs available in over 130 countries. Information is included regarding structure, therapeutic class, and proprietary names for single entity medications. A CD-ROM is included containing contact information for pharmaceutical manufacturers worldwide.

Martindale: The Complete Drug Reference

Pharmaceutical Press, http://www.pharmpress.com This resource includes information on a variety of domestic and international drugs. Proprietary names and manufacturer contact information are available for a variety of countries. Some information is provided about common herbal products as well as diagnostic agents, radioactive pharmaceuticals, and some veterinary products. This information is available in hardcopy, CD-ROM, via online MedicinesComplete subscription, and is also included in some Micromedex® Healthcare Series packages.

Additional resources are available that are specific to individual countries including Diccionario de Especialidases Farmaceuticas (Mexico), British Pharmacopoeia (United Kingdom), Rote Liste® (Germany), Dictionary Vidal (France), Compendium of Pharmaceuticals and Specialties (Canada), and Repertorio Farmaceutico Italiano (Italy).

PEDIATRIC DOSAGE RECOMMENDATIONS

The Harriet Lane Handbook

Mosby, http://www.us.elsevierhealth.com This resource, assembled by medical residents, contains a succinct discussion of common diseases and conditions of newborn to adolescent patients. A significant portion of the book is dedicated to medication dosing, specifically pediatrics. This section also contains information about common side effects and dosage forms available. The resource includes a variety of topic areas including palliative care and toxicology information. There is a separate publication which focuses on antimicrobial therapy. This resource is also available for mobile devices.

Pediatric Dosage Handbook

Wolters Kluwer Health, Inc., http://www.lexi.com The monographs in this resource contain traditional sections of drug information, but focus on detailed dosing recommendations for pediatrics. There is also information about common extemporaneous preparations. Limited references to primary literature are provided. This reference is also available online, on CD-ROM, and for mobile devices.

PHARMACOKINETICS

Basic Clinical Pharmacokinetics

Lippincott Williams & Wilkins, http://www.lww.com This text discusses the basic principles of pharmacokinetics especially interpretation and implications of plasma concentrations. The second section of the book provides monographs and discussions focused on drugs most commonly assessed by blood concentration levels.

Applied Biopharmaceutics and Pharmacokinetics

McGraw-Hill Professional, http://www.mcgraw-hill.com This text describes the role of pharmacokinetics as it relates to drug development and to patient care. This covers the clinical application of pharmacokinetics and also addresses the impact of pharmacogenetics on drug metabolism. This text is also included in the Access Pharmacy™ electronic subscription.

PHARMACOLOGY

Goodman & Gilman's: The Pharmacological Basis of Therapeutics

McGraw-Hill Professional, http://www.mcgraw-hill.com This classic pharmacology text also provides information about pharmacokinetics and pharmacodynamics of a number of drugs. The focus of the resource is to provide a correlation between principles of pharmacology and contemporary clinical practice. The text makes extensive use of charts and tables to convey information. This text is also included in the Access Pharmacy™ electronic subscription.

Basic & Clinical Pharmacology

McGraw-Hill Professional, http://www.mcgraw-hill.com This text, organized by therapeutic class of agents, provides general discussion of pharmacology principles as well as more detailed discussion of specific agents. Figures and tables are frequently used to illustrate difficult material. This text is also included in the Access Pharmacy™ electronic subscription.

Brody's Human Pharmacology: Molecular to Clinical

Elsevier, http://www.elsevier.com This text is designed with a student focus and emphasizes therapeutic impact of pharmacology. The text is organized by organ system impacted. The text also has accompanying mobile device downloads and Internet updates.

Modern Pharmacology with Clinical Applications

Lippincott Williams & Wilkins, http://www.lww.com This textbook is focused on the clinical application of drugs. The text has moved away from an emphasis on chemical structures to an emphasis on structure-activity relationships. This text also includes information on some common dietary supplements.

PHARMACY LAW

Information about individual state pharmacy law is best obtained through the individual state boards of pharmacy. A listing of state board Web site URLs is available at http://www.nabp.net/boards-of-pharmacy/. Often the Board will have this information available in PDF format on the Web site. The Code of Federal Regulations containing aspects of federal laws is available at http://www.gpoaccess.gov/cfr/index.html. One general text about federal law is listed below.

Pharmacy Practice and the Law

Jones and Bartlett Publishers, http://www.jblearning.com This resource contains information about federal laws and regulations impacting pharmacy practice. Additional implications for pharmacy practice are provided for some legislation. Information is provided about federal and state regulation of product development, dispensing, and development. Various summaries of case law are provided. Additionally information regarding Internet pharmacies and electronic transmission of prescriptions has been added.

TERATOGENICITY/LACTATION

Drugs in Pregnancy and Lactation

Lippincott Williams & Wilkins, http://www.lww.com As the title implies, this text (often referred to as Brigg's) focuses exclusively on information available about the use of medications in pregnant or lactating women. Summaries of the literature available regarding fetal exposure *in utero* or exposure through breast milk are provided. Animal literature is provided in cases where human literature is lacking. Additional information about recommendations by organizations such as the American Academy of Pediatrics is provided.

Catalog of Teratogenic Agents

Johns Hopkins University Press, http://www.press.jhu.edu This resource covers pharmaceuticals, chemicals, environmental pollutants, food additives, household products, and viruses and their possible teratogenicity. Special attention has been paid to including the international as well as domestic information.

Case Study 3–2

A new mother has been breast-feeding her child for 3 months. The mother has recently been prescribed levofloxacin for treatment of an infection.

- *What sources should be consulted to determine the appropriateness of this choice?*
- *Is it safe for her to continue breast-feeding during this therapy?*
- *What additional information is needed to answer this patient's question?*

THERAPY EVALUATION/DRUG OF CHOICE

Applied Therapeutics: The Clinical Use of Drugs

Lippincott Williams & Wilkins, http://www.lww.com This text includes information about disease states and treatment options. Information is presented in the form of cases with follow-up discussion. Its focus is on clinical case–based presentation of information. There is also a pocket-sized handbook designed to accompany the text. This print resource is updated every few years and comes with a CD-ROM. A version is also available for use on a mobile device.

Goldman's Cecil Medicine

Saunders, http://www.us.elsevierhealth.com This text is available in print, CD-ROM, mobile device, and Internet (http://www.cecilmedicine.com) formats. Information is organized by disease state and color-coded to speed usage. Information about etiology, manifestations, diagnosis, treatment, and prognosis is provided.

Harrison's Principles of Internal Medicine

McGraw-Hill Professional, http://www.mcgraw-hill.com This text serves as a fairly comprehensive introduction to clinical medicine. It is available in text and electronic formats. Comprehensive information is presented including pathophysiology, differential diagnosis, and disease management. This text is also included in the Access Pharmacy™ electronic subscription.

The Merck Manual of Diagnosis and Therapy

Merck & Co., Inc., http://www.merck.com This source provides a quick summary of disease state information, including pathology, symptoms, diagnosis, and treatment. This resource is also available online as a free resource at http://www.merckmanuals.com/, and mobile device version.

Medscape

Medscape, http://www.medscape.com This electronic resource provides extensive information about disease states and conditions. It includes news and updates on treatment. In addition, it includes basic monographs about prescription and OTC medications.

Pharmacotherapy: A Pathophysiological Approach

McGraw-Hill Professional, http://www.mcgraw-hill.com This text focuses on the management of a variety of disease states. Information provided about disorders include epidemiology, etiology, presentation of disease, treatment, and treatment outcomes. This is available in text and electronic formats. This resource also has accompanying texts: *Pharmacotherapy Casebook: A Patient-Focused Approach* and *Pharmacotherapy Handbook*. These texts are also included in the Access Pharmacy™ electronic subscription.

Pharmacotherapy Principles and Practice

McGraw-Hill Professional, http://www.mcgraw-hill.com This text focuses on the management of a variety of disease states, centering on the diseases most likely to be seen by pharmacists, nurse practitioners, and physician assistants. It is more concise than *Pharmacotherapy: A Pathophysiological Approach* and is focused on diseases most likely to be seen in practice, including community pharmacy; it also contains various features to help student learning. Information provided about disorders include epidemiology, etiology, presentation of disease, treatment, and treatment outcomes. This is available in text and electronic formats. This resource also has accompanying text: *Pharmacotherapy Principles and Practice Study Guide*.

Textbook of Therapeutics

Lippincott, Williams and Wilkins, http://www.lww.com PDA, CD-ROM, and print versions of this resource are available. While the resource focuses on treatment of disease states and development of a therapeutic plan, sections regarding pathophysiology and clinical presentation are also provided.

TOXICOLOGY

Casarett & Doull's Toxicology: The Basic Science of Poisons

McGraw-Hill Professional Medical Publishing, http://www.mcgraw-hill.com This resource is designed to serve as a textbook rather than a quick resource for toxicology information. Extensive information is provided regarding organ- and nonorgan-directed toxicity. This text is also included in the Access Pharmacy™ electronic subscription.

Goldfrank's Toxicologic Emergencies

McGraw-Hill Professional Medical Publishing, http://www.mcgraw-hill.com This text is designed to offer a case study approach to toxicology. Initial basic toxicology data are provided, but the majority of this text focuses on management of toxicologic emergencies with a variety of common drugs, botanicals, pesticides, and other occupational or environmental hazards.

Case Study 3–3

A pharmacy student is working on a presentation involving illicit drugs. She knows that there have been recent news stories about adolescents using Coricidin™ products for recreational use, and she is curious at what doses these products are toxic.

* *Which resources would be useful for her project?*
* *What search terms might she utilize?*

VETERINARY MEDICINE

Veterinary pharmacy as a specialty practice is a growing area in the United States, and pharmacists are interested in obtaining veterinary specific knowledge and skills. The growth in veterinary pharmacy has allowed pharmacists to apply their drug knowledge resources to veterinary situations.

Supporting the growth of veterinary pharmacy is the concept of "One Medicine," a blending of veterinary medicine and human medicine for the benefit of public health, and to better serve human and animal patients alike. From a clinical pharmacy perspective, veterinary medicine and human medicine complement each other, with the human-trained pharmacist being uniquely positioned to educate and serve veterinarians and animal owners.

Opportunities for the practical application of One Medicine can occur in community pharmacy settings as most pharmacists practicing in a community setting have been presented with prescriptions for animal patients at some time during the course of their career. Veterinarians outsource prescriptions to community pharmacists to help control inventory, high drug costs, and the need for compounded drug therapies. The use of human-labeled pharmaceuticals prescribed in an off-label manner to treat companion animal disease states is a viable option for veterinary medicine. These factors contribute to a situation where pharmacists who receive veterinary prescriptions can be challenged in their knowledge of veterinary drugs, indications, dosages, disease states, and therapeutic monitoring parameters.

Plumb's Veterinary Drug Handbook

Wiley-Blackwell Publishing, http://www.wiley.com/wiley-blackwell This resource is considered one of the most useful references for extra-label drug dosages, indications, and specific drug information on human and veterinary labeled pharmaceuticals. Monographs are listed in alphabetical order, and categorize the drugs' chemistry, pharmacology, indications, species dosing, contraindications, and interactions into an easily identifiable format. It is often referred to as "The Virus" in veterinary medicine because it is everywhere. A client information booklet is also available.

Textbook of Veterinary Internal Medicine

Saunders, http://www.us.elsevierhealth.com This is a practical, valuable, and informative two-volume resource, focusing on internal medicine topics in canines and felines. The text provides extensive coverage of pathophysiology, diagnosis, and treatment of diseases affecting dogs and cats.

Compendium of Veterinary Products (CVP)

North American Compendiums, http://naccvp.com This online reference is similar to the human PDR in terms of information provided and format. The resource contains the product monographs for over 5000 FDA-approved pharmaceuticals, USDA-approved biologicals, diagnostic, feed additive, and Environmental Protection Agency (EPA)-approved pesticide products that are currently available. The reference contains indexes of manufacturers and distributors, brand name/ingredient indexes, and product category indexes.

FDA/CVM Homepage

http://www.fda.gov/AboutFDA/CentersOffices/OfficeofFoods/CVM/default.htm This Web site provides information for pharmacists about the legal or regulatory issues that affect the practice of veterinary pharmacy or veterinary medicine. It is useful for regulatory issues pertaining to animal health. The compliance policy guide (CPG 608.400) "Compounding of Drugs for Use in Animals" and the Animal Medicinal Drug Use Clarification Act (AMDUCA) can be found at this site; these documents are considered essential reading for any pharmacist who practices veterinary pharmacy. Center for Veterinary Medicine (CVM) updates are available that detail the prohibited use of drugs in certain animal populations. Updates on the judicious use of antibiotics in food producing animals are posted at this site. A listing of all FDA-approved animal drug products, also known as the "Green Book," is available and searchable at this site. Patent information, manufacturer lists, indications, approval numbers, general drug information, code of regulations, and trade/generic names are just a few pieces of information that can be gathered from this Web site. Practitioners can also access the FDA Veterinarian Newsletter from this site.

American Veterinary Medical Association, Scientific Reference Material on Veterinary Compounding

The American Veterinary Medical Association (AVMA) has a wealth of information for pharmacists and veterinarians alike (http://www.avma.org). There is a collection of valuable veterinary compounding guidelines, brochures, federal regulations, frequently asked questions, definitions of compounding, and the AVMA compounding position statements at https://www.avma.org/KB/Resources/Reference/Pages/Compounding.aspx. This information is an excellent starting point for any health care professional wishing to prescribe, provide, or utilize compounded drug products for animal patients.

Animal Poison Control Center

The Web site, http://www.aspca.org/pet-care/poison-control/, focuses on animal toxicology and safety and is the premier resource for pharmacists in a community setting who may receive poisoning questions about animals. A toll-free number is available for immediate assistance when faced with a toxicology problem (888-426-4435), and a fee is required. The center has extensive experience in assisting veterinarians in poison management by providing immediate and specific treatment recommendations. The site also provides useful information on poison prevention, human medications that are poisonous to pets, and guidance on what to do if a pet is poisoned. References to toxicology publications and general consultation are listed in this Web site.

Veterinary Pharmacology and Therapeutics

Wiley-Blackwell, http://www.wiley.com This textbook provides comprehensive information on the basic and applied principles of veterinary pharmacology and therapeutics. Information on mechanisms of action, pharmacodynamics, and pharmacokinetics is detailed.

Small Animal Clinical Pharmacology and Therapeutics

Saunders Ltd., http://www.elseiver.com A useful pharmacology reference textbook focusing on pharmaceuticals for the prevention and treatment of small animal diseases. The book is divided into three sections detailing principles of drug therapy with special attention to clinical relevancy, the use of drugs from a categorical basis, and pharmaceutical use from a body systems approach.

The Merck Veterinary Manual (MVM)

Merck & Co., Inc., http://www.merck.com The manual has served veterinarians and other health care professionals as a concise and reliable animal health reference for over 45 years. The full-text electronic version is available for free online at http://www.merck-vetmanual.com. A guide to abbreviations used in veterinary medicine is also included.

Pet Place

The Web site, http://www.petplace.com, has pet centers focusing on different species (dog, cat, bird, horses, fish, reptiles, and small mammals) and is written for laypersons.

The database includes articles on veterinary disease states and preventative medicine. The drug library search tool allows the user to find drug information on a specific pharmaceutical. There are also text and graphics describing medication administration techniques for dogs and cats.

Pets with Diabetes

The Web site, http://www.petdiabetes.com, contains information on diabetes in small animals particularly dogs and cats. The Web site offers general diabetes education and drug information and is written for laypersons. The site also offers insight into and information on home testing and complications. There are also resources to support owners of diabetic animals.

American Veterinary Medical Association (AVMA)

From this site, http://www.avma.org/, pharmacists can read about the latest developments in One Medicine, public health issues affecting human and veterinary patients, peer-reviewed journal articles, and legal/regulatory issues and recent developments in veterinary medicine. The site provides numerous links organized by discipline for locating information. Under the scientific resources tab, there is a resource titled Veterinary Therapeutics that is valuable for educating veterinary pharmacists about current therapeutics issues in veterinary medicine.

Case Study 3–4

You have an appointment to discuss compounding services with a local veterinarian. Your pharmacy has just begun offering these services and in the dialog the veterinarian references AMDUCA. You have not heard of this.

• *What is your strategy to find the meaning and relevance of this term?*

SELECTING A FORMAT FOR TERTIARY RESOURCES

Pharmacists should also be aware that more resources are becoming available in a variety of formats. Many resources that have been traditionally available only in a paper text are now accessible via a variety of electronic formats. Electronic resources are often preferred because they may be easier to use, allow quicker access to information, allow multiple searches to be performed simultaneously, and often contain the most recent information available regarding a topic. Additionally, many electronic networked resources allow use of the same resource at more than one location. This lets many practitioners access information from a variety of physical locations rather than being restricted to only medical libraries or drug information centers.

Many texts are now being combined into electronic packages, for example, the McGraw-Hill Professional product AccessPharmacy® (http://www.accesspharmacy.com/index.aspx). The combination of multiple resources in one package may make selection of resources for a practice site much easier, but also more costly. As these combination packages increase in popularity with students and universities the expectations practitioners have for access to resources in work settings will also likely continue to increase.

REFERENCES FOR MOBILE DEVICES

The increasing incorporation of mobile devices into clinical practice settings has prompted an expanding choice of drug information databases for that medium. As described earlier in the chapter, many of the major compendia available electronically also offer a product for a mobile device. It is important to recognize that the information available in an app version of a database may differ from that available in the online or hardcopy forms.[86] One study looking specifically at dietary supplements databases highlighted some of the variations which may exist between different forms of the same resource.[87] While the specific functionality of an app and the way that one accesses information for most apps may change, the information is generally similar. Due to factors such as cost and memory requirements practitioners must be judicious in their selection of databases to purchase for a mobile device.

A limited number of critical evaluations of these databases have been performed to aid in the selection of the highest quality databases.[43,88-89] Based on the limited data available Lexicomp, ePocrates, and Clinical Pharmacology OnHand appear to be among the best quality PDA drug information databases available at the time of these studies. One additional study[90] evaluating the efficacy of PDA databases specifically for addressing drug interaction information found slightly different results from previous studies but did find Lexi-Interact to be one of the top performers, in addition to iFacts™ (http://www.skyscape.com).

Lexicomp provides access to excerpts from AHFS, the Lexicomp products, and Stedman's medical dictionary (http://www.ahfsdruginformation.com/products.aspx).

In general, it should be noted that some of the utility of mobile device apps is the ability to embed links to additional content and resources. This can be a very useful feature especially for students.

Secondary Literature

Secondary literature refers to references that either index or abstract the primary literature, with the goal of directing the user to relevant primary literature. This type of literature can be used for multiple purposes; one can be to help keep a practitioner keep abreast of recently published information[91] or to help find more recent or detailed information on a specified treatment or disease. When discussing secondary literature there are two commonly used terms, indexing and abstracting; the two terms differ slightly. Indexing consists of providing bibliographic citation information (e.g., title, author, and citation of the article), while abstracting also includes a brief description (or abstract) of the information provided by the article or resource cited. ❷ *Various systems index or abstract literature from different journals, meetings, or publications; therefore, in order to perform a comprehensive search multiple databases must be used.*

In searching most databases, a user will follow a similar search strategy, with small changes to reflect differences in database systems. There are several challenges in searching secondary database systems. Systems do not index all terms the same, so it is necessary to determine what terms a database is using in order to conduct a successful search. For example, databases through the National Library of Medicine (NLM) index terms by their Medical Subject Heading (MeSH) terms, while the Iowa Drug Information System uses the United States Adopted Name and the International Classification of Diseases. Most computerized databases also include a free-text search option, which is very useful when the defined index terms do not identify relevant data. This option may also be helpful when the term is newly emerging or before an official index term is defined.

The need to utilize a variety of terms for search strategy is illustrated in the following sample question: "Is clonidine effective in the treatment of attention deficit hyperactivity disorder (ADHD) in adolescents?" It is first important to identify the key terms. These terms might include clonidine, attention deficit hyperactivity disorder, and adolescents. However, some databases may not recognize the term adolescent and instead use the term pediatric or child. Additionally, the use of the term pediatric may just refer to the medical specialty caring for pediatric in some resources, rather than treatment of a pediatric patient population. Therefore, it is important to recognize that different databases may require different search terms to be used. Also, the name of the disease state, attention deficit/hyperactivity disorder, has changed over time, so it may be necessary to use other terms, such as attention deficit disorder.

Electronic searches generally use the Boolean operators: AND, OR, and NOT (see Figure 3–1). The operator AND will combine two terms, returning only citations containing both of those concepts or terms. Combining two terms with the operator OR will result in an equal or greater number of returns since it will include any citation where

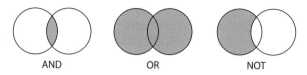

Figure 3–1. Boolean operators.

either term is used. The term NOT should be used with caution as it always decreases the number of returns. It eliminates any references having that term and may eliminate appropriate articles simply because the term happens to appear somewhere in the article.

For example, in the earlier clonidine for the treatment of ADHD question, the appropriate search terms (clonidine AND attention deficit/hyperactivity disorder) may be used with the AND operator. However, if the requestor wanted information regarding use of either clonidine or guanfacine in this disease state, then the term OR might be used. See Figure 3–2 for a graphic presentation of this search. A search using OR will return a number of results equal to or greater than a search using the term AND. The term OR might also be useful when searching for a term with synonyms, for example, attention deficit disorder OR attention deficit hyperactivity disorder. The operator NOT would be helpful if a user wants to exclude certain topics, for example, a specific disease state. In this case, a search might be performed for attention deficit hyperactivity disorder NOT Tourette's disorder. Since the use of the term NOT will exclude any article mentioning Tourette's disease, an article focused on treatment of ADHD with a small section about Tourette's disease would also be excluded. Parentheses can also be used to further streamline a search. In this example, a search may be performed for clonidine AND (attention deficit disorder OR attention deficit hyperactivity disorder), this would retrieve articles that contain the drug of interest as well as either of the two disease states of interest. An additional example of search strategy using Boolean operators is provided in Appendix 3–1.

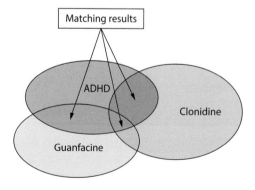

Figure 3–2. ADHD AND (clonidine OR guanfacine).

Some databases will also use the terms WITH or NEAR. These operators are similar to AND; however, they require the terms to be within a set number of words of each other. These terms may be useful when other searches are identifying a large number of articles where both terms are mentioned, but not in conjunction with each other.

Most databases allow results to be restricted via use of limit fields. For example, this may include language of publication, year of publication, type of article (e.g., human study, review, case report), or type of journal where publication is found. This is most helpful when the initial search terms return a large number of possible matches. Using too many limits with the initial search may eliminate articles or citations that would be helpful.

One additional point to bear in mind when performing electronic searches is that the same search phrase could be indexed under a variety of search terms or spellings, and in order to provide a comprehensive search it is important to address all of those. For example, if looking for information regarding the herbal product ginkgo, it may be helpful to search under the botanical name, common name(s), as well as common alternative spellings. So a possible search strategy may be to use the terms "ginkgo," "ginkgo biloba," the Latin name "Ginkgoaceae," as well as the misspelled word "gingko." This same principle holds true when considering disease states whose names may have changed over time. As databases and resources continue to modify search features, there are more Google-like search engines which allow for a natural language search.

When trying to improve the overall quality of searching secondary references, drug information specialists have looked at the use of filters to provide better searching strategies. The two most prominent types of filters are content filters and validity filters. The **content filters** are specific to the drug or disease state being searched. It helps to look at the MeSH terms to make sure that the search has the most appropriate content. It is best to use the advanced searching features in these secondary databases versus the simple searching features because advanced searching allows for filters to be utilized. The second type of filter is known as a **validity filter**, which is a way to narrow the search to only the highest quality studies. Search terminology such as randomized controlled trial or double-blind can be used to eliminate studies of weaker/poorer methodology.

Listed below are some examples of secondary databases and types of requests they are helpful in addressing.

BIOSIS PREVIEWS®

Thompson Reuters Medical, http://www.thomsonreuters.com This is a comprehensive database of biological information, covering biological and biomedical information. BIOSIS also covers abstracts from conferences relating to basic sciences. This is most helpful when seeking more basic science information about activity of compounds on a cellular level.

CANCERLIT

National Cancer Institute, http://www.cancer.gov This database is maintained by the National Cancer Institute and indexes literature from a variety of sources specific to cancer literature. This resource is most useful when looking for information about oncology therapies or quality of life issues. This resource is available electronically at http://www .cancer.gov/search/cancer_literature/.

CINAHL®

EBSCOhost, http://www.ebscohost.com This is an indexing service that covers primarily literature in the fields of nursing and allied health. This database is useful when seeking information about patient care from the perspective of allied health professionals. It is updated monthly.

COCHRANE LIBRARY

Cochrane Library, http://www.cochrane.org This database has three components: indexes of Cochrane reviews about a variety of medical treatments, conditions, and alternative therapies; abstracts of international systematic reviews; and a bibliography of systematic reviews in worldwide literature. These evidence-based medicine reviews are based on extensive analysis of current literature and provide treatment recommendations (see Chapter 7 on evidence-based medicine).

CURRENT CONTENTS CONNECT®

Thomson Reuters Medical, http://scientific.thomsonreuters.com/index.html This electronic service offers an overview of very recently published literature as it relates to scientific information. There are multiple subsets; the clinical medicine and life science subgroups are likely the most useful for practitioners and focus on useful information about recent drug research or developments.

EMBASE®

Elsevier, http://www.embase.com EMBASE® is a comprehensive abstracting service covering biomedical literature worldwide. This database covers material similar to that covered by MEDLINE®, but with greater coverage of international publications. Additionally, there is less lag time between publication and inclusion in the database. This database is useful when seeking information about dietary supplements or medications that may be available in other countries.

GOOGLE SCHOLAR

Google, http://scholar.google.com An Internet search engine that is designed to target scholarly materials available online, in a variety of professional areas including health care. Information from a variety of scholarly journals and publications is able to be searched; however, in some cases the searcher may not be able to access full-text versions of articles or works due to password restrictions.

INTERNATIONAL PHARMACEUTICAL ABSTRACTS (IPA)

Thompson Reuters Medical, http://www.thomsonreuters.com Coverage includes drug-related information, including drug use and development. This database also abstracts a variety of meeting presentations. The main focus of this database is pharmacy information, including pharmacy administration and clinical services, making it the most comprehensive global database for pharmacy specific information.

IOWA DRUG INFORMATION SYSTEM (IDIS)

Division of Drug Information Service, University of Iowa, http://itsnt14.its.uiowa.edu This is an indexing service that allows retrieval of full-text articles from a variety of biomedical publications. Indexing is done by drug- and disease-specific terms, which at times makes searching challenging. Recently an autosuggest feature has been added to this database, which provides suggested search terms that appear as the searcher begins to enter terminology. This database is useful for information about standard medications. It is unique in that it provides full-text articles, in either PDF form or, for pre-1988 articles, microfiche. There are a limited number of journals covered and not all articles from a specific journal issue are included (i.e., some articles may not be included if the editorial staff did not feel that they had sufficient focus on relevant drug or disease state information). The database has added a Comparative Effectiveness Plus tool which allows access to pivotal studies, regulatory documents, and practice guidelines to compare specific medications.

JOURNAL WATCH®

Massachusetts Medical Society, http://www.jwatch.org Journal Watch is an abstracting service including recent information, summarized by physicians, from a variety of medical literature. A general newsletter covering major medical stories of interest to generalists is published as well as additional newsletters in specific specialty areas. This is most helpful when monitoring for new clinical trials involving specific medications.

LEXISNEXIS®

LexisNexis Academic & Library Solutions, http://www.lexisnexis.com This indexing and abstracting service provides coverage of a variety of types of information, including medical, legal, and business news. Some publications are available full text through this service. This resource is helpful when attempting to locate information about recent medical news or research.

MEDLINE®

National Library of Medicine, http://www.nlm.nih.gov Coverage includes basic and clinical sciences as well as nursing, dentistry, veterinary medicine, and many other health care disciplines. Information comes from more than 5000 journals in 40 different languages. This database is available through a variety of publishers; free access to content is available via PubMed (http://www.ncbi.nlm.nih.gov/pubmed/). A sample search is provided in Appendix 3–1.

PHARMACOECONOMICS & OUTCOMES NEWS WEEKLY

Adis International, http://www.adis.com This biweekly publication covers recent publications regarding economic use of health care resources, as well as information on prescribing trends, recent health care news, and regulatory updates. The focus of this publication is the economic impact of disease states and medical interventions.

REACTIONS WEEKLY

Adis International, http://www.adis.com A weekly indexing/abstracting service summarizing literature involving adverse events, drug interactions, drug dependence, and toxicology data. This resource is especially useful when seeking case reports of adverse reactions or other information on drug safety. Also, due to the nature of this resource it has a very short lag time, so data are more timely than several other print resources.

Case Study 3–5

A physician requests information about the use of sildenafil for treatment of female sexual arousal disorder. She also requests information about use of any of the other phosphodiesterase-5 inhibitors.

- *What resources might be good places to look for this information?*
- *What search terms should be used?*
- *Should restrictors be utilized?*

In addition, there are a variety of publications targeting specific therapeutic areas that are available. For example, Adis (http://www.adisonline.com) compiles Anti-infectives Today, Cancer Today, CNS Disorders Today, and Pediatrics Today.

Primary Literature

Primary literature consists of clinical research studies and reports, both published and unpublished. Not all literature published in a journal is classified as primary literature, for example, review articles or editorials are not primary literature. ❸ *There are several types of publications considered primary, including controlled trials, cohort studies, case series, and case reports.* Additional information about study designs commonly found in medical literature and how to evaluate them is found in Chapters 4 and 5.

Advantages to the use of primary literature include access to detailed information about a topic and the ability to personally assess the validity and applicability of study results. Additionally, primary literature tends to be more recent than tertiary or secondary literature. However, there are several disadvantages to the use of primary literature alone. These disadvantages include misleading conclusions based on only one trial without the context of other research, the need to have good skills in medical literature evaluation, and the time needed to evaluate the large volume of literature available.

Due to the rapidly increasing number of specialty journals being published it is difficult to determine which journals are really most essential in a pharmacy practice setting. Appendix 3–2 provides a listing of core holdings for a college of pharmacy assembled by the AACP.[10] While this list may be more extensive than what is required in most practice settings, it does provide a core listing of journals. Each practice setting requires slightly different primary literature based on the specific areas that are of greatest importance to that facility and the patients cared for in that location.

OBTAINING THE PRIMARY LITERATURE

Once literature has been identified in a secondary searching system, the actual articles can be obtained in various ways. Many databases link users directly to the article of interest. For example, PubMed links users to open access journal publications and articles resulting from NIH-funded research through PubMed Central (http://www .pubmedcentral.nih.gov/).

However, many articles are not available via open access routes; in those cases alternative techniques may be needed. Once a citation is identified, utilizing a local library catalog is a good next step. Often a local library may carry the journal needed, or may be affiliated with other facilities that can provide that article. Articles are often available for a fee via the publisher Web site. If neither of these options are available, then the Loansome Doc ordering system might be used. This system is available through the NLM and offered for a fee to any user. Articles identified in PubMed can be easily ordered from that database through this system. Additional information about this program is available at http://www.nlm.nih.gov/pubs/factsheets/loansome_doc.html.

Alternative Resources

INTERNET SEARCHES

❹ *At times even well-designed searches of standard medical literature do not yield sufficient information to make clinical decisions or recommendations. In these cases alternative resources may need to be employed.* One such method to identify relevant resources might be a general Internet search for information. This can be especially helpful to serve as a starting point for questions about uncommon diseases, new terms, drugs in development, or marketed OTC products and combination dietary supplements. For example, if a requestor asked about use of a dietary supplement product called GABA Plus in ADHD, it would be difficult to search for information, unless the requestor was able to provide a list of ingredients contained in the product. Often requestors may not have that information; therefore, it may be necessary to search for a manufacturer Web site to identify the specific individual ingredients and then look for information on the individual components. This is also helpful in identifying information or specific product claims provided by the manufacturer. Additionally, Internet searches may be useful for topics that have recently been in the news, where information is changing more rapidly than standard paper resources can be updated.

It is important to remember that different search engines use different techniques to identify Web pages, and that no search engines identify all Web sites. Some search engines are geared toward scholarly content (such as Google Scholar, http://scholar. google.com) or scientific research, rather than general information. These might be more useful for identifying recent research about a disease or disorder, rather than the ingredients in GABA Plus. In order to efficiently perform a search, it is important to consider which search engine would most likely index the desired materials.

There are, however, several caveats to finding information on the Internet. The first is to carefully evaluate the quality of all information provided. There are millions of Web sites and there is no true quality assurance measures in place to evaluate the reliability of information available. There are some general tenets to keep in mind when evaluating this type of literature. Generally, sites maintained by educational institutions, not-for-profit medical organizations, or a division of the U.S. government are likely to contain high-quality information, whereas information maintained by a company selling a promoting a specific product may be more questionable.

In order to assess quality of online information several standards and programs now exist. These include organizations such as the Health on the Net (HON code, http://www .hon.ch), which clearly define rules to evaluate the quality of information available via a Web site. These organizations do not evaluate every Web site available, but instead only those who request evaluation. Since many Web sites do not request evaluation, the lack of an organization's quality seal does not necessarily indicate that the information is of low quality.

The following criteria should be used when determining quality of online material.

- Is the source credible, without a vested interest in promoting one particular treatment or product?
- Is the information accurate and current?
- Does the site link to other nonaffiliated sites that provide consistently good information?
- Is the information appropriately detailed and referenced?
- Is it possible to identify the author of the site to contact with additional questions or comments?

Information on evaluating Web sites is discussed further in Chapter 5. In addition, the NLM has a video and posted questions to help determine high quality sites (http:// www.nlm.nih.gov/medlineplus/evaluatinghealthinformation.html).

ALTERNATIVE INFORMATION SOURCES

Occasionally sufficient information to address a drug information request cannot be obtained from standard resources and may require the use of some alternative sources of information. If a question involves, for example, a recent news story reporting the removal of a medication from the market, a logical first place to find initial information would be to identify the original news story. This can be done by searching various newswire services such as PR Newswire or even major news network Web sites such as CNN (Table 3–3). LexisNexis, http://www.lexisnexis.com, indexes a variety of newswire stories as well as transcripts of news reports. While this news story may not provide all the information needed, it might at least serve as a point from which to search for additional information.

TABLE 3–3. MAJOR NEWS SOURCES ONLINE

News Source	URL
ABC	http://www.abcnews.go.com
AP (Associated Press)	http://www.ap.org
CBS	http://www.cbsnews.com
CNN	http://www.cnn.com
FDC Reports "The Pink Sheet"	http://www.healthnewsdaily.com/publications/the-pink-sheet
MSNBC	http://www.msnbc.msn.com
NBC	http://www.nbc.com
Reuters Health News	http://www.reutershealth.com
PR Newswire	http://www.prnewswire.com

In some cases, there may be such limited information available that it would be wise to seek out an expert in the field, for example, a question about the use of heparin in a troche dosage form. In these cases, it may be prudent to contact persons performing research in this area or practitioners who are currently using that therapy to identify information that might have been missed in an initial search or may not have been published. Some experts may be identified via medical organizations focusing on specific disease states, leadership of medical societies, or persons who have authored numerous papers on a specific medication or medical condition.

When looking for recent recommendations regarding treatment of a specific disease state, it may be helpful to identify an organization affiliated with that disease state. For example, when looking for treatment recommendations for management of irritable bowel syndrome it might be appropriate to contact the International Foundation for Functional Gastrointestinal Disorders (http://www.iffgd.org/) to obtain information about current practice standards as well as possible emerging therapies.

Additionally, when seeking information about a specific drug therapy, it may be helpful to contact the product manufacturer via their medical information department to identify information that may be available in-house. This resource could be especially helpful for obtaining difficult to access literature if a product is newly approved or for identifying a possible rare adverse drug reaction.

Case Study 3–6

A patient tells you she saw a news story on NBC that said all patients should stop taking their Coumadin™ and switch to the "new Coumadin™." She tells you she is not planning to take it anymore and wants the physician to find a different medication. She is indignant that you as a health care professional did not know this was going on.

- *Where might you find a copy of the news story that this patient saw to help her better understand what the news reporter was trying to convey?*

Consumer Health Information

As consumers become more active and educated in their health care and disease management and more computer literate, the demand for health information sources designed for consumers has been increasing. Currently there are a variety of sources where consumers obtain their health information. Since many consumers find at least some of their information online, pharmacists should be prepared to help consumers evaluate the quality of information found online as well as recommend sites where information might be found. Table 3–4 contains a listing of just a few of the sources that may be useful for consumers.

Consumers may also benefit from some text resources available at a local library. Some resources are published by organizations that produce references for health care professionals, while others are published by lay press companies. There is great variation in the quality of information provided from resource to resource. Some of the most popular resources may not be written at an appropriate level for a consumer to understand or may not provide helpful information for the patient. For this reason, it is important to discuss with patients what other resources they are using to find additional drug and medical information. Opening a dialog with patients about this topic is fairly simple and can consist open-ended questions such as "Where else have you found information on your disease state?" or "What other material have you read about your medication/disease state?"

If being asked to recommend a source of online information for a patient, one can confidently recommend health care organizations or disease societies, both of which usually provide helpful, high-quality disease-specific information geared for the average consumer. The FDA and WebMD have now launched a joint online venture (http://www.webmd.com/fda) which directs consumers to reliable information. Also, many drug companies offer Web sites with helpful disease or disease management information.

In addition to these resources aimed at consumers, there are consumer-specific sections of many tertiary resources discussed earlier. Electronic resources such as

TABLE 3–4. ONLINE CONSUMER INFORMATION SOURCES

Web Site URL	Maintained By	Information
http://www.nlm.nih.gov/medlineplus/	National Library of Medicine	Contains information about various medications as well as disease states and conditions.
http://www.fda.gov/cder	Food and Drug Administration	Contains information about new drugs as well as dietary supplements. Also contains information about recalls of drug or food.
http://www.gettingwell.com	Thomson Healthcare	Contains information about a variety of prescription drugs.
http://www.merckhomeedition.com	Merck	This is a consumer based version of the Merck Manual. It includes a variety of interactive features.
http://www.healthfinder.gov	Department of Health and Human Services	This site contains information about a variety of common medical conditions and diseases.
http://www.womenshealth.gov/www.4woman.gov	National Women's Health Information Center	This site contains information about conditions and diseases of special interest to women.
http://www.cdc.gov	Center for Disease Control and Prevention	This site has information about the treatment and prevention of infectious diseases. It also contains a listing of public health hoaxes.
http://dirline.nlm.nih.gov	National Library of Medicine and National Institute of Health	This contains a directory of health care organizations online.
http://ods.od.nih.gov	National Institute of Health	This site compiles some of the scientific information available about the efficacy and safety of dietary supplements.
http://nccam.nih.gov	National Center for Complementary and Alternative Medicine	This site is a government maintained resource describing ongoing research in the area of dietary supplements, as well as detailing efficacy information currently available.
http://www.safemedication.com	American Society of Health-System Pharmacists	This site provides a patient version of AHFS Drug Information Resource, as well as tips about medication administration and resources to empower patients to better track/manage their own health care.

Micromedex®, Lexicomp, Facts & Comparisons® eAnswers, ASHP's SafeMedication. com, or Clinical Pharmacology have subsections dedicated to consumer-level information available for a practitioner to print and provide to the patient. Specific reference recommendations for patients can be found in Chapter 20.

Conclusion

Given the rapid rate at which medical information is increasing and the amount of available technology to organize and locate this information, it is easy to become overwhelmed by the volume of data available. However, as pharmacists develop a better understanding of where to access information, provision of drug information will occur more quickly. As technological advances continue, which may change the face of physical pharmacy dispensing and compounding, reliance on pharmacists for information retrieval and interpretation will continue to grow.

Practitioners must not, however, be satisfied with merely identifying sources for drug information. ❺ *Understanding where to access information is only the first step in the provision of quality drug information.* Information must be interpreted and evaluated to become knowledge, as is described in other chapters. It is this unique knowledge that will enable practitioners to optimize patient care.

The information in this chapter helps provide guidance as to where specific types of drug information might be found and how to begin a search for drug information. The next several chapters will provide additional guidance on how to interpret and apply the information that is gathered.

Case Study 3–7

A physician is seeking information about the use of chondroitin in the management of osteoarthritis. He sees a large number of patients in his practice and is seeking information about efficacy, safety, and appropriate dosing of this product.

- *What are the advantages and disadvantages of tertiary resources in responding to this request?*
- *What are the advantages and disadvantages of primary literature in this scenario?*

Self-Assessment Questions

1. If you were looking for information on an interaction between St. John's wort and Prozac®, which source would likely provide this information?
   a. Natural Medicine Comprehensive Database
   b. Drug in Pregnancy and Lactation

    c. American Drug Index

    d. Remington: The Science and Practice of Pharmacy

    e. The Harriet Lane Handbook

2. Which of the following would be the most useful resource when determining the U.S. equivalent of an international drug?

    a. Handbook of Injectable Drugs

    b. Pharmacy Practice and the Law

    c. Index Nominum

    d. Merck Index

3. Which database would be best for finding information about a recent business merger of two large pharmaceutical manufacturers?

    a. International Pharmaceutical Abstracts (IPA)

    b. Iowa Drug Information System (IDIS)

    c. LexisNexis

    d. CINAHL

    e. Reactions Weekly

4. While searching for information on a specific medication you find an electronic document describing a clinical experience of a practitioner with a patient who had an adverse reaction to a medication. What kind of literature is this?

    a. Primary

    b. Secondary

    c. Tertiary

    d. None of the above (electronic documents are not reliable)

    e. None of the above (electronic documents do not fulfill the criteria for any type of literature)

5. Which of the following references would contain information on the normal dose of a prescription medication?

    a. Red Book

    b. AHFS

    c. American Drug Index

    d. Catalog of Teratogenic Agents

    e. Handbook of Nonprescription Drugs

6. A nurse calls you from the Intensive Care Unit and she has a patient who is receiving an intravenous solution containing amoxicillin. The doctor has now ordered morphine to be injected into the Y site of the intravenous solution every 4 hours. The nurse wants to know if these drugs will be compatible at the Y site. Which reference would provide you with this information?

a. Merck Manual
b. Review of Natural Products
c. Handbook on Injectable Drugs
d. Index Nominum
e. Red Book

7. A 75-year-old patient asks if docusate (an over-the-counter product) is safe for him to use with his other medications. Which resource would NOT be a good place to look for this information?
   a. Micromedex®
   b. Drug Information Handbook
   c. Geriatric Dosage Handbook
   d. Identidex®
   e. All of the above would be good sources for this information

8. If a pharmacist were trying to identify a tablet based on a patient description of the imprint marking, which resource might be helpful?
   a. Meyler's Side Effects of Drugs
   b. Goldfrank's Toxicologic Emergencies
   c. Clinical Pharmacology
   d. Index Nominum

9. Which of the following statements is true when considering drug information programs for mobile devices?
   a. No major drug information database companies offer mobile device apps.
   b. Mobile device versions of databases are identical to the online database.
   c. Health care professionals rarely use mobile devices for drug information.
   d. Only drug interaction checkers are available via mobile device app.
   e. None of the above are true.

10. A health care setting that wants to be able to perform comprehensive searches should make available which secondary resources to their practitioners?
    a. MEDLINE®
    b. EMBASE®
    c. Iowa Drug Information Service (IDIS)
    d. International Pharmaceutical Abstracts (IPA)
    e. All of the above

11. If a patient needed a recommendation of a nonprescription analgesic which can be safely used while breast-feeding, what resource might be useful?
    a. Brody's Human Pharmacology: Molecular to Clinical
    b. Neofax

   c. Catalog of Teratogenic Agents

   d. Drugs in Pregnancy and Lactation

12. A physician calls you to compound an ointment called Whitfield's Ointment (which his father prescribed in the early 1950s). He wants you to start compounding this for his patients. Where might you look to find the formulation?

   a. Merck Manual

   b. Index Nominum

   c. Meyler's Side Effects of Drugs

   d. Remington: The Science and Practice of Pharmacy

   e. Natural Medicine Comprehensive Database

13. If a pharmacist needed to confirm a dose of doxycycline for a dog, which resource might be useful?

   a. Pets with Diabetes

   b. Plumb's Veterinary Drug Handbook

   c. USP Veterinary Medicine

   d. Pet Place

14. Which of the following electronic databases would provide the largest international biomedical journal coverage?

   a. International Pharmaceutical Abstracts

   b. EMBASE®

   c. MEDLINE®

   d. Iowa Drug Information System

15. Which of the following publication types would be classified as primary literature?

   a. Clinical trial

   b. Textbook

   c. Case report

   d. a and b

   e. a and c

REFERENCES

1. American Association of Colleges of Pharmacy. Basic resources for pharmacy education 2008 [Internet]. Alexandria (VA): American Association of Colleges of Pharmacy ; 2013 Jan [cited 2013 Mar 1]; [54 p.]. Available from: http://www.aacp.org/governance/sections/libraryinformationscience/documents/2013janbasicresourcesforpharmacyeducation.pdf

2. Rosenberg JM, Kourmis T, Nathan JP, Cicero LA, McGuire H. Current status of pharmacist-operated drug information centers in the United States. Am J Health Syst Pharm. 2004;61(19):2023-32.

3. Krinsky DL, Berardi RR, Ferreri SP, Hume AL, Newton GD, Rollings CJ. Handbook of non-prescription drugs. 17th ed. Washington, DC: American Pharmacists Association; 2011.

4. Aronson JK. Meyler's side effects of drugs: the international encyclopedia of adverse drug reactions and interactions. 15th ed. Amsterdam, The Netherlands: Elsevier; 2006.

5. Aronson JK. Side effects of drugs annual 32: a worldwide yearly survey of new data and trends in adverse drug reactions. 32nd ed. Amsterdam, The Netherlands: Elsevier; 2010.

6. Red book: pharmacy's fundamental reference. 2013 ed. Ann Arbor (MI): Truven Health Analytics; 2013.

7. Billups NF, Billups SM. American drug index 2013. 57th ed. St. Louis (MO): Wolters Kluwer Health; 2012.

8. Allen LV, Adejare A, Desselle SP, Felton LA. Remington: the science and practice of pharmacy. 22nd ed. Philadelphia (PA): Lippincott Williams & Wilkins; 2012.

9. O'Neil MJ. Merck Index: an encyclopedia of chemicals, drugs and biologicals. 15th ed. Whitehouse Station (NJ): Royal Society of Chemistry; 2013.

10. Thompson JE. A practical guide to contemporary pharmacy practice. 3rd ed. Philadelphia (PA): Lippincott Williams & Wilkins; 2009.

11. USP 36/NF 31 2013: The official compendia of standards. Rockville (MD): United States Pharmacopeial Convention; 2012.

12. Trissel LA. Trissel's stability of compounded formulations. 5th ed. Washington, DC: American Pharmacists Association; 2012.

13. Jew RK, Soo-Hoo W, Erush SC. Extemporaneous formulations. 2nd ed. Bethesda (MD): American Society of Health-System Pharmacists; 2010.

14. Allen LV, Popovich NG, Ansel HC. Ansel's pharmaceutical dosage forms and delivery systems. 9th ed. Philadelphia (PA): Lippincott Williams & Wilkins; 2010.

15. 2008–2009 USP pharmacists' pharmacopeia. Rockville (MD): United States Pharmacopeial Convention; 2008.

16. Natural medicines comprehensive database [Internet]. Stockton (CA): Therapeutic Research Faculty; 1995 [cited 1 Mar 2013]. Available from: http://www.naturaldatabase.com

17. DerMarderosian A, Beutler JA. The review of natural products. 7th ed. St. Louis (MO): Wolters Kluwer; 2012.

18. Natural standard [Internet]. St. Louis (MO): Mosby; 2001 [cited 1 Mar 2013]. Available from: http://www.naturalstandard.com

19. PDR for herbal medicine. 4th ed. Montvale (NJ): Thomson Healthcare Inc; 2007.

20. Evans WC. Trease and Evans' pharmacognosy. 16th ed. Edinburg (TX): W. B. Saunders; 2009.

21. Aronoff GR, Bennett WM, Berns JS, Brier ME, Kasbekar N, Mueller BA, Pasko DA, Smoyer WE. Drug prescribing in renal failure. 5th ed. Philadelphia (PA): American College of Physicians; 2007.

22. Hansten PD, Horn JR. Drug interaction analysis and management 2012. St. Louis (MO): Wolters Kluwer; 2012.

23. Taro DS. Drug interaction facts 2013: the authority on drug interactions. St. Louis (MO): Facts & Comparisons; 2012.

24. Baxter K. Stockley's drug interactions. 9th ed. London: Pharmaceutical Press; 2010.

25. Pronsky ZM, Crowe JP, Elbe D, Young VSL, Epstein S, Roberts W, Ayoob TK. Food medication interactions. 17th ed. Birchrunville (PA): Food-Medication Interactions; 2012.

26. Drug therapy monitoring system v2.1 [Internet]. St. Louis (MO): Wolters Kluwer [cited 1 Jun 2010]. Available from: http://www.medispan.com

27. Lee M. Basic skills in interpreting laboratory data. 4th ed. Bethesda (MD): American Society of Health-System Pharmacists; 2009.

28. Chernecky CC, Berger BJ. Laboratory tests and diagnostic procedures. 6th ed. Philadelphia (PA): Saunders; 2012.

29. Semla TP, Beizer JL, Higbee MD. Geriatric dosage handbook. 18th ed. Hudson (NY): Lexi-Comp; 2012.

30. Identidex® [Internet]. Ann Arbor (MI): Truven Health Analytics; 2013 [cited Mar 2013]. Available from: http://www.micromedexsolutions.com

31. Clinical pharmacology [Internet]. Tampa (FL): Clinical Pharmacology; 2006 [cited 1 Mar 2013]. Available from: http://www.clinicalpharmacology.com

32. IDENT-A-DRUG reference [Internet]. Stockton (CA): Therapeutic Research Center; 1995–2013; [cited 1 Mar 2013]. Available from: http://www.indentadrug.com

33. Clinical Reference Library [Internet]. Hudson (NY): LexiComp; 1978 [cited 1 Mar 2013]. Available from: http://www.crlonline.com

34. Facts & Comparisons E Answers [Internet]. St. Louis (MO): Wolters Kluwer Health; 2003 [cited 1 Mar 2013]. Available from: online.factsandcomparisons.com

35. US Food and Drug Administration homepage [Internet]. Washington, DC: US Food and Drug Administration [cited 1 Mar 2013]. Available from: http://www.fda.gov

36. ClinicalTrials.gov [Internet]. Washington, DC: US National Institutes of Health [cited 1 Mar 2013]. Available from: http://www.clinicaltrials.gov

37. MedlinePlus® Health Information from the National Library of Medicine [Internet]. Washington, DC: National Library of Medicine; [cited 1 Mar 2013]. Available from: http://medlineplus.gov

38. Trissel LA. Handbook of injectable drugs. 17th ed. Bethesda (MD): American Society of Health-System Pharmacists; 2012.

39. King JC, Catania PN. King guide to parenteral admixtures. 35th ed. Napa (CA): King Guide Publications; 2006.

40. Trissel's 2 Clinical Pharmaceutics Database [Internet]. Cashier: TriPharma Communications; [cited 1 Mar 2013]. Available from: http://trissels2.rcl.com/tsweb/

41. Bing CM, Chamallas SN. Extended stability for parenteral drugs. 5th ed. Bethesda (MD): American Society of Health-System Pharmacists; 2013.

42. American Association of Colleges of Pharmacy. AACP core list of journals for libraries that serve schools and colleges of pharmacy 2010 [Internet]. Alexandria (VA): American Association of Colleges of Pharmacy; 2009 Jan [cited 1 Mar 2013]; [5 p.]. Available from:

http://www.aacp.org/governance/sections/libraryinformationscience/documents/2010%20core%20journals%20list.pdf

43. Lowry CM, Kostka-Rokosz MD, McClowskey WW. Evaluation of personal digital assistant drug information databases for the managed care pharmacist. J Manag Care Pharm. 2003;9(5):441-8.

44. Sweetman SC. Martindale: the complete drug reference. 37th ed. London: Pharmaceutical Press; 2011.

45. Index nominum: international drug directory. 19th ed. Stuttgart, Germany: Medpharm Scientific Publishers; 2008.

46. Tschudy MM, Arcara KM. The Harriet lane handbook. 19th ed. Philadelphia (PA): Mosby; 2011.

47. Taketomo CK, Hodding JH, Kraus DM. Pediatric and neonatal dosage handbook. 19th ed. Hudson (NY): Lexi-Comp; 2012.

48. Neofax 2011. 2011 ed. Montvale (NJ): Thomson Reuters Healthcare; 2011.

49. Winter ME. Basic clinical pharmacokinetics. 5th ed. Philadelphia (PA): Lippincott Williams & Wilkins; 2009.

50. Shargel L, Wu-Pong S, Yu AB. Applied biopharmaceutics and pharmacokinetics. 6th ed. New York: McGraw-Hill; 2012.

51. Brunton LL, Chabner B, Knollman B. Goodman & Gilman's: the pharmacological basis of therapeutics. 12th ed. New York: McGraw-Hill; 2010.

52. Katzung BG, Masters SB, Trevor AJ. Basic & clinical pharmacology. 12th ed. New York: McGraw Hill; 2012.

53. Wecker L, Crespo L, Dunaway G, Faingold C, Watts S. Brody's human pharmacology: molecular to clinical. 5th ed. Philadelphia (PA): Elsevier; 2009.

54. Golan DE. Principles of pharmacology: the pathophysiologic basis of drug therapy. 3rd ed. Philadelphia (PA): Lippincott Williams & Wilkins; 2011.

55. Abood RR. Pharmacy practice and the law. 7th ed. Sudbury (MA): Jones and Bartlett Publishers; 2012.

56. Reiss BS, Hall GD. Guide to federal pharmacy law. 7th ed. Delmar (NY): Apothecary Press; 2010.

57. Briggs GG, Freeman RK, Yaffe YJ. Drugs in pregnancy and lactation: a reference guide to fetal and neonatal risk. 9th ed. Philadelphia (PA): Lippincott Williams & Wilkins; 2011.

58. Hale TW. Medications and mother's milk 2012. 15th ed. Amarillo (TX): Hale Pub; 2012.

59. Shepard TH, Lemire RJ. Catalog of teratogenic agents. 13th ed. Baltimore (MD): Johns Hopkins University Press; 2010.

60. Schaefer C, Peters P, Miller RK. Drugs during pregnancy and lactation: treatment options and risk assessment. 2nd ed. Amsterdam, The Netherlands: Elsevier Academic Press; 2007.

61. REPOTOX [Internet]. Ann Arbor (MI): Truven Health Analytics; 2013 [cited 1 Mar 2013]. Available from: http://www.micromedexsolutions.com

62. DiPiro JT. Pharmacotherapy: a pathophysiologic approach. 8th ed. New York: McGraw-Hill; 2011.

63. Koda-Kimble M, Young LY, Kradjan WA, Guglielmo BJ, Alldredge BK. Applied therapeutics: the clinical use of drugs. 10th ed. Philadelphia (PA): Lippincott Williams & Wilkins; 2013.

64. Porter RS. The Merck manual of diagnosis and therapy. 19th ed. Whitehouse Station (NJ): Merck Research Laboratories; 2011.

65. Fauci AS, Braunwald E, Kasper DL, Hauser SL, Longo DL, Jameson JL, Loscalzo J. Harrison's principles of internal medicine. 18th ed. New York: McGraw-Hill; 2011.

66. Goldman L, Schafer AI. Goldman's cecil medicine. 24th ed. Philadelphia (PA): Saunders/Elsevier; 2011.

67. Helms RA, Quan DJ. Textbook of therapeutics: drug and disease management. 8th ed. Philadelphia (PA): Lippincott Williams & Wilkins; 2006.

68. Bope ET, Kellerman RD. Conn's current therapy 2013. Philadelphia (PA): Saunders/Elsevier; 2012.

69. Poisindex® [Internet]. Ann Arbor (MI): Truven Health Analytics; 2013 [cited 1 Mar 2013]. Available from: http://www.micromedexsolutions.com

70. Nelson LS, Lewin NA, Howland MA, Hoffman RS, Goldfrank LR, Flomenbaum NE. Goldfrank's toxicologic emergencies. 9th ed. New York: McGraw-Hill; 2010.

71. Klaassen C. Casarett & Doull's toxicology: the basic science of poisons. 7th ed. New York: McGraw-Hill; 2008.

72. Leikin JB, Paloucek FP. Poisoning and toxicology handbook. 4th ed. Boca Raton (FL): CRC; 2007.

73. Shannon MW, Borron SW, Burns MJ, Haddad LM, Winchester JF. Haddad and Winchester's clinical management of drug overdose. 4th ed. Philadelphia (PA): Saunders/Elsevier; 2007.

74. TOXNET [Internet]. Washington, DC: US National Institutes of Health; [cited 1 Mar 2013]. Available from: http://toxnet.nlm.nih.gov/.

75. Ettinger SJ, Feldman EL, eds. Textbook of veterinary internal medicine. 7th ed. Philadelphia (PA): W.B. Saunders; 2010.

76. Merck Veterinary Manual [homepage on the Internet]. Whitehouse Station (NJ): Merck & Co, Inc.; [cited 1 Mar 2013]. Available from: http://www.merckmanuals.com/vet/index.html

77. PetPlace.com [homepage on the Internet]. Weston (FL): Intelligent Content Corp; c1999; 2013 [cited 1 Mar 2013]. Available from: http://www.petplace.com

78. PetEducation.com [homepage on the Internet]. Drs. Foster & Smith Inc.; c1997–2013 [cited 1 Mar 2013]. Available from: http://www.petplace.com

79. Pets with Diabetes [homepage on the Internet]. Petdiabetes.com; c2000–2013 [cited 1 Mar 2013]. Available from: http://www.petdiabetes.com

80. Plumb DC. Plumb's veterinary drug handbook. 7th ed. Stockholm (WI): Wiley-Blackwell; 2011.

81. Compendium of veterinary products. 12th ed. Port Huron (MI): North American Compendiums; 2010.

82. Carpenter JW, Mashima TY, Rupier DJ, eds. Exotic animal formulary. 4th ed. Philadelphia (PA): W.B. Saunders; 2012.

83. USP Veterinary Medicine [homepage on the Internet]. Rockville (MD): United States Pharmacopeia; c1997–2008 [cited 1 Mar 2013]. Available from: http://www.usp.org/usp-healthcare-professionals/compounding/veterinary-compounding-monographs

84. Drug facts and comparisons 2013. St. Louis (MO): Wolters Kluwer Health; 2013.

85. *Micromedex 2.0* [Internet]. Ann Arbor (MI): Truven Health Analytics; 2013. Available from: http://www.micromedexsolutions.com

86. Clauson KA, Polen HH, Marsh WA. Clinical decision support tools: performance of personal digital assistants versus online drug information databases. Pharmacotherapy. 2007;27(12):1651-8.

87. Clauson KA, Polen HH, Peak AS, March WA, DiScala SL. Clinical decision support tools: personal digital assistant versus online dietary supplement databases. Ann Pharmacother. 2008;42:1592-9.

88. Enders SH, Enders JM, Holstad SG. Drug-information software for palm operating system personal digital assistants: breadth, clinical dependability and ease of use. Pharmacother. 2002;22:1036-40.

89. Clauson KA, Seamon MJ, Clauson AS, Van TB. Evaluation of core and supplemental drug information databases for the Palm OS and Pocket PC. Am J Health Syst Pharm. 2004;61:1015-24.

90. Barrons R. Evaluation of personal digital assistant software for drug interactions. Am J Health Syst Pharm. 2004;61:1036-40.

91. Shaughnessy AF. Keeping up with the medical literature: how to set up a system. Am Fam Physician. 2009;79(1):25-6.

4

Chapter Four

Drug Literature Evaluation I: Controlled Clinical Trial Evaluation

Michael G. Kendrach • Maisha Kelly Freeman
• Peter J. Hughes

Learning Objectives

● *After completing this chapter, the reader will be able to*

- List and explain the skills pharmacists need to locate and evaluate current information for pharmacy practice activities.
- Describe special characteristics of a controlled clinical trial that distinguish this research design as the prototype for clinical research.
- Prepare a null hypothesis (H_0) based on the clinical trial objective(s) and endpoint(s).
- Differentiate between the types of data and measures of central tendency.
- Differentiate between Type I and Type II errors; discuss methods to reduce the possibility of either of these errors occurring.
- Interpret p-values and 95% confidence intervals (CI); discuss whether to reject or fail-to-reject H_0 by using these clinical trial results.
- Calculate and interpret relative risk (RR), relative risk reduction (RRR), absolute risk reduction (ARR), and number needed to treat (NNT).
- State whether a statistical significance and clinical difference are present using the clinical trial results.
- Explain the purpose and usage of editorials, letters to the editor, and secondary journals in critiquing clinical trials and in the decision-making process of applying the results to practice.

Key Concepts

① Pharmacists need to efficiently locate, critically analyze, and effectively communicate data from the primary literature in daily activities of patient care and the medication use process.

② A controlled clinical trial is the premier study design to measure and quantify differences in effect between the intervention and control.

③ Decision making should not rely solely on reading abstracts; the entire manuscript is to be read and thoroughly evaluated.

④ The results of a controlled clinical trial should be extrapolated to the type of patient enrolled in the study, and readers should be aware of the limitations of surrogate end-points and subgroup analysis results.

⑤ Randomization is an essential component of controlled clinical trials and a significant differentiator from other study designs.

⑥ The controlled clinical trial primary endpoint should be appropriate for the study purpose and measured using valid techniques and methods.

⑦ An appropriate sample size in a controlled clinical trial is vital for the study results to have any significant meaning; conducting a power analysis is important to determine a suitable sample size.

⑧ Interpreting the p-values correctly is crucial in evaluating a controlled clinical trial; not all statistically significant p-values are clinically important. The magnitude of difference in effect between the intervention and control cannot be determined solely with the p-value.

⑨ The use of 95% CI can assist the reader in assessing the magnitude of difference in effect between the intervention and control to apply to the population.

⑩ Calculating measures of association (relative risk, absolute risk reduction, relative risk reduction, number needed to treat) for nominal data provides further information to evaluate the meaning of controlled clinical trial results.

⑪ Nonstatistically significant results do not equate to the intervention and control being the same or equal.

⑫ All controlled clinical trial results need to be assessed to determine the clinical relevance (i.e., meaningfulness) of the intervention versus control.

⑬ Controlled clinical trial investigators and authors should disclose any funding sources and potential conflicts of interest.

⑭ Editorials, letters to the editor, and commentary publications can assist in interpreting controlled clinical trial results.

Introduction

Pharmacists continuously rely on the biomedical/pharmacy literature for many day-to-day activities. The practice of medicine and pharmacy is dynamic, and drug facts acquired during formal education cannot sustain a health care provider in future practice. Changes include new medications, dosage formulations and uses approved by the Food and Drug Administration (FDA), revised drug safety information (i.e., adverse drug effects, drug interactions), and updated disease state therapeutic guidelines. During 2012, more than 35 new molecular entities/biological agents were approved by the FDA,[1] more than 115 drug safety alerts for human medical products were issued by the FDA,[2] and over 750 published articles classified as human practice guidelines were added to the National Library of Medicine database.[3] Pharmacists must employ methods to keep current with these advances in order to remain competent, trustworthy health care professionals.[4] ❶ *Pharmacists need to efficiently locate, critically analyze, and effectively communicate data from the primary literature in daily activities of patient care and the medication use process.* Therefore, skills, such as drug literature evaluation, are necessary to prepare the health care provider for practice.

Multiple resources are available for pharmacists to provide answers to questions, care for patients, make decisions, and solve problems. But pharmacists need to recognize both the advantages and limitations of the information resources to meet the challenges encountered during their daily practice activities. Advantages include ready access and electronic formats. Potential disadvantages include biases, costs, and lag time (i.e., lack of current content) that hinder the usefulness of some references. In addition, misinterpretation of the information can lead to improper patient care.

Although access to information for both health care professionals and laypersons has increased exponentially, not all information can be deemed accurate and pharmacists are repeatedly relied on to clarify, explain, defend, and/or refute information.[5] Thus, pharmacists must have skills in efficiently locating and critically analyzing drug information to appropriately formulate and effectively communicate a response. In addition, pharmacists are frequently consulted by other health care providers to assist in individual patient care regarding appropriate drug use.[6-8] Also, pharmacists are in a position to select drugs for use in a multitude of patients (e.g., third-party health care plans, drug formulary decisions).[9,10] Furthermore, pharmacists are expected to be providers of direct patient care in the new U.S. health care reform activities. All these activities require pharmacists to carefully review and critique the literature instead of accepting the authors' conclusions. Many studies have very positive conclusions, but include study design errors that limit the clinical usefulness of the results. Also, medical/pharmacy continuing education presentations may contain biases and/or inaccuracies, while textbooks/review articles may contain misinterpreted, outdated, and/or noncomprehensive information. Due to the important contribution pharmacists have in patient care, pharmacists need to have skills in identifying the strengths and limitations of the biomedical literature. This chapter is devoted to explaining and discussing core concepts for critiquing one essential type of biomedical literature, a **controlled clinical trial**.

Biomedical/Pharmacy Literature

Three types of literature serve as information resources for pharmacists: tertiary, secondary, and primary (see Table 4–1).[11] Readers are referred to Chapter 3 for more in-depth discussions of these three literature types.

Primary literature, specifically controlled clinical trials, serves as the foundation for clinical practice by providing the documentation for using therapy. Although vast numbers of primary literature articles are published every year, individuals can efficiently locate information specific and useful to their needs by incorporating appropriate search techniques.[12,13] Clinical trials are one particular type of primary literature that can be a reliable source of new information to change health care practices.[14-16] ❷ *A controlled clinical trial is the premier study design to measure and quantify differences in effect of the intervention and control.* New information may either counter or serve as the root for altering existing practice regimens; thus, pharmacists need to critique clinical trials. The special features of clinical trial design allow investigators to determine which therapeutic interventions should be used in practice.[17,18] In fact, the FDA requires clinical trials to be conducted and the results submitted before a new molecular entity (i.e., medication) can be marketed and/or receive new indications for use.[19] Proper interpretation of clinical trials is vital to providing appropriate health care. Chapter 5 reviews evaluating publications using the other types of research designs.

TABLE 4–1. THREE TYPES OF LITERATURE

Literature Type	Description	Examples
Tertiary	Established knowledge	Textbooks, review articles, Up-to-Date, WebMD, Lexicomp
Secondary	Indexing/abstracting services (i.e., databases)	PubMed® or MEDLINE® (National Library of Medicine), Embase® (Elsevier), International Pharmaceutical Abstracts (Wolters Kluwer Health)
		CINHAL (Cumulative Index to Nursing and Allied Heatlh)
		InfoTrac OneFile (Gale CENGAGE Learning), Academic LexisNexis® (Reed Elsevier)
Primary	Original research	Controlled clinical trials, case-control studies, crossover trials, case reports

In general, a controlled clinical trial consists of an investigational (intervention) group being directly compared to a control group (e.g., standard therapy, placebo).[17,18] The intervention under investigation may be a new medication, different medication dosing regimen, diet, surgery, behavioral process, exercise program, diagnostic procedure, or something else. The goal of the clinical trial is to measure and quantify the difference in effect (e.g., efficacy, safety) between the investigational and control groups. The results then can allow decisions to be made regarding proper care for patients (i.e., to use or not use the investigational therapy).[17] Although the origins of a controlled trial date back to the eighteenth century,[20] a formalized process of conducting controlled clinical trials was not implemented until the late 1940s.[21] However, poorly designed clinical trials are still published and the existence of a clinical trial may not translate into clinically useful information. Research has reported that results of well-designed clinical trials are considered to be of better quality and are usually more clinically relevant than clinical trials that are poorly designed (see Chapter 7).[22]

The published clinical trial is presented in a manner that explains the research process in an orderly format to improve the readers' comprehension of the study, results, and conclusions. Table 4–2 displays the style in which a clinical trial usually appears in printed resources.[23,24] This chapter discusses the information presented in these sections according to the CONSORT (Consolidated Standards of Reporting Trials) format. The CONSORT format was formulated to improve the quality of reporting clinical trials in the published literature, since inadequate reporting methods hinder the interpretation of results produced by clinical trials. CONSORT has been supported by an increasing number of medical and health care journals (e.g., *Journal of the American Medical Association* [*JAMA*]) and editorial groups (e.g., International Committee of Medical Journal Editors [ICMJE]).[24] Some further information about CONSORT is found in Chapter 9. Other research types (e.g., case-control study) may use a publishing style similar to a controlled clinical trial. Therefore, one should not assume all publications using this format are controlled clinical trials.

Evidence from clinical trials is used by health care providers to base their patient care decisions.[14,15,25,26] A controlled clinical trial is the most robust method to measure and quantify differences in effects between a therapy under study and the control group.[17,18] Many clinical studies are published annually, but not every study initiated is reported in the published literature.[27-29] Primary reasons for not publishing trials are lack of time, funds, or other resources.[28] In order to treat patients most appropriately, all relevant information and data, both positive and negative, are needed in the decision-making process.[28,30,31]

Readers of the biomedical literature need to consider the issues of selective reporting (i.e., publishing positive study results, but not negative studies). In addition, usually one clinical trial is not sufficient to adopt a therapy under investigation as the first choice

TABLE 4–2. FORMAT AND CONTENT OF CONTROLLED CLINICAL TRIALS

Controlled Clinical Trial Section	Type of Information Presented
Abstract	Brief overview of the research project
Introduction	Research background
	Clinical trial objective/hypotheses
Methods	Study design
	Population to be sampled
	Inclusion and exclusion criteria
	Intervention and control groups
	Randomization
	Blinding
	Endpoints
	Follow-up procedure
	Sample size calculations/power analysis
	Statistical analysis
Results	Subject characteristics
	Subject dropouts/adherence
	Endpoints quantified
	Safety assessments
Discussion	Result interpretations
	Other study results compared
	Limitations
	Conclusion/application to practice
Acknowledgments	Other contributors
	Funding source
	Peer-review dates/manuscript acceptance date (not all trials)
References/bibliography	Citations for information included from other resources (e.g., trials and reports)

to treat patients. Results of multiple trials are usually combined together to serve as the evidence for either incorporating a newly developed therapy into practice or changing the existing method of treating a disease (see Chapter 7).[32,33] Journal editors have an obligation and should publish negative studies. Results of these studies are important in formulating practice patterns based on the available evidence. Failure by investigators, authors, and journal editors to publish negative studies contributes to publication bias.[30,34,35]

The intent of this chapter is for readers not to be misled by the literature, but to correctly critique the controlled clinical trial, and then properly use the results and conclusions in health care practice settings. In addition to the discussions of critiquing clinical trials from this chapter, readers should use the principles of the evidence-based medicine (Chapter 7) in providing patient care.

Approach to Evaluating Research Studies (True Experiments)

Many different research designs are published, but the most common of these are prospective studies in which an intervention is directly compared to a control and differences between these are measured. Examples of prospective studies include clinical trials (e.g., drug A versus drug B; drug versus exercise), stability of compounded drug formulation (e.g., suspension made from drug tablets), compatibility of intravenous drug admixtures, and drug pharmacokinetic interactions. Regardless of the study design and objective, fundamental elements should be present in all studies, including appropriate qualifications of the researchers conducting the research, valid investigational methods, proper research techniques, and appropriate analysis plus interpretation of the results. A similar process is used to evaluate prospective studies. A checklist for pertinent information to be included in a clinical trial is located in Appendix 4–1. Answering the questions contained in Appendix 4–1 can allow readers to determine the strengths and limitations of a clinical trial. The remainder of this chapter discusses the questions presented in the appendix plus techniques for critiquing a clinical trial.

JOURNAL, PEER REVIEW, AND INVESTIGATORS

Numerous journals are published covering the biomedical literature, including the professions of medicine, nursing, and pharmacy. Health care practitioners need to regularly access professional journals (either print or electronic) to assist them in keeping current in their practice responsibilities.[36] Misleading information may be presented to health care providers by pharmaceutical industry representatives (see Chapter 23).[37] In addition, not all studies are published in reliable journals (i.e., in non peer-reviewed journals[38,39]). One essential journal feature is the peer-review process. Simply defined, peer-reviewed articles are evaluated by someone other than the editorial staff (i.e., evaluation by one's peers).[34,40] Most journals incorporate the peer-review process in selecting articles for publication. Briefly, manuscripts submitted to the journal for publication consideration are screened by the editor; those deemed as potential publications are sent to individuals with expertise in the appropriate area. These individuals read the manuscript and comment on the strengths and limitations, plus offer a recommendation to the journal editor regarding accepting or rejecting the manuscript for publication. The peer reviewers' comments are sent to the authors for the manuscript to be revised and, if necessary, resubmitted for publication consideration. In some cases, manuscripts may be rejected as being too flawed or inappropriate for the journal.

Although the peer-review process increases the time required before publication, the goal is to reduce the publication of manuscripts that have inappropriate methods/design, are poorly written, and/or do not meet the needs of the journal's audience.[38,40] However, the peer-review process does not always prevent publication of articles without deficiencies, and readers should assess the quality and critique each published article. Two journal sections can be checked for information addressing whether the peer-review process is used: instructions for authors and journal scope/purpose. Readers of the biomedical/pharmacy literature need to be aware of journals not incorporating a peer-review process, therefore, not having this safeguard built in. Regardless of whether a clinical trial is published in a peer-reviewed or nonpeer-reviewed journal, the article needs to be evaluated closely for biases and interpreted appropriately.

As readers become more familiar with the professional literature, they will find certain journals have a reputation for good-quality publications, such as *New England Journal of Medicine* and *Annals of Pharmacotherapy*. This too can be considered in the evaluation of literature, although poor articles can still be found in well-respected journals and excellent articles are published in other journals.

Research results can be published in other venues besides journals. A very common publication type is meeting abstracts. Research presented during a professional organization's meeting, whether as platform or poster, requires an abstract to be available for meeting attendees to review. These abstracts usually undergo the peer-review process to be selected, but readers should be cautious of the abstract content. The peer-review process may not be as thorough and the entire study details are not available to the reader. Another common publication type for research is journal supplements. The purpose of such supplements is to publish a collection of articles related to a specific topic in a separate journal issue.[34] Many, but not all supplements, are sponsored by an outside entity (i.e., pharmaceutical company), which serves as another source of revenue for the journal. The articles should undergo peer review using the same rigorous process, but readers should refer to the journal's Web site to obtain the policies regarding the peer-review process for journal supplements. However, not all articles published in journal supplements should be automatically discarded or classified as inferior information. Journal supplements can serve as a venue for organizations to publish their disease state practice guidelines. An example of a very informative journal supplement is the American College of Chest Physicians' supplement addressing antithrombotic therapy.[41] Many of the articles in this supplement are authored by recognized leaders and researchers in their field of practice.

The Internet is also a common venue to publish medical and pharmacy information. This resource is ideal for rapid communications of breaking news (i.e., contamination of drug product, study results) to better treat patients. But as many Internet users know, unreliable information is also posted and can influence some attitudes. This is especially true with Web sites posing as a legitimate health care entity, but presenting biased, unreliable, and information not supported by evidence.

Other factors to evaluate in a published study are the investigators' credentials and the practice site of these individuals. Investigators need to be properly trained and have active practice experience in the area of study. The site where the clinical trial was conducted should not immediately endorse or condemn the quality of the research, other than it should be a site that has the capability to perform the study (i.e., have the resources to properly and completely perform the necessary study methods). The quality of the research must be evaluated because even prestigious institutions can conduct poor clinical trials. Also, persons involved with the study need to be ethical and responsible to protect patients enrolled in the study.[42] Persons with specialized credentials in biostatistics need to contribute with statistical analysis of the data. Furthermore, all authors listed should have made substantial contributions to the research and/or publication. The *Uniform Requirements for Manuscripts Submitted to Biomedical Journals*, prepared by journal editors, explicitly outlines the criteria for persons to be listed as authors for a published article. According to this publication, "An author is generally considered to be someone who has made a substantive intellectual contribution to a published study...".[34] The topics of authorship and publishing are discussed in detail in Chapter 9.

Articles with authors who are employees of a pharmaceutical company should be more selectively analyzed, since there may be concern about potential bias. The pharmaceutical industry must conduct research for new therapies to be introduced to the marketplace and many companies are collaborating with academic researchers.[37,43] The concern regarding influence from the pharmaceutical industry on health care providers has not gone unnoticed, particularly involving practitioners conducting research for the pharmaceutical industry. In response, many journals now are requiring article authors to declare any conflicts of interest with the research and outside interests.[34,42] A **conflict of interest** is possible even though investigators may not consider that their relationships affect their scientific judgment.[34] Authors need to state they have received honorariums and/or research grants, and/or are members of the speaker's bureau for pharmaceutical companies. Readers should be informed of potential bias of the investigators. However, immediately discarding or discounting clinical trials in which investigators declare relationships with the pharmaceutical industry may be premature. Many investigators are required to obtain external funding for research projects and academic promotion. Clinical trials that have researchers with relationships with multiple pharmaceutical companies may not be considered to be overtly biased. Investigators have an ethical obligation to submit credible research results for publication.[34] Biases may be present, but readers having the skills of identifying study strengths and limitations can still use the clinical trial results appropriately.

TITLE

The clinical trial title is important and should be carefully evaluated by the reader. A title should be reflective of the work, unbiased, specific, and concise (i.e., usually ≤ 10 words), but not too general or detailed. Declarative sentences, which tend to overemphasize a conclusion, are not preferred for scientific articles.[44] In addition, the title should not be phrased as a question and randomized clinical trials should be identified in the title.[24] Furthermore, the title should include key words that are both sensitive (easing the task of locating the appropriate articles) and specific (excluding those not being searched for) that allow easier electronic retrieval of the article.[34]

The following is an example of a biased study title: "Improved bronchodilation with levalbuterol compared with racemic albuterol in patients with asthma."[45] The title implies levalbuterol to be better than racemic albuterol. Although the average change in lung function parameters was slightly greater with levalbuterol, no significant differences were reported.[45] Thus, one could have been misled by reading only the title, believing levalbuterol to be a superior agent. A suggested unbiased title for this trial is: "Comparison of levalbuterol and racemic albuterol bronchodilation in patients with asthma: a randomized clinical trial."

ABSTRACT

An abstract is considered to be a concise overview of the study or a synopsis of the major principles of the article. ❸ *Decision making should not rely solely on reading abstracts; the entire manuscript is to be read and thoroughly evaluated.* Abstracts include information addressing the article objective, methods, results, and conclusions. A primary use of abstracts is for readers to obtain an immediate overview of the article to determine if the entire article should be read.[46,47] Another use is publishing the abstract in secondary resources (e.g., PubMed®, International Pharmaceutical Abstracts [IPA]) for individuals conducting literature searches.

Although unique for each journal, authors are required to follow specific requirements while preparing an abstract. Many journals now require abstracts to be prepared in an organized format (i.e., structured abstract) and usually contain ≤500 words. The structured abstract includes the following sections: objective, research design, clinical setting, participants, interventions, main outcome measurements, results, and conclusions.[34,46] Structured abstracts, compared to unstructured abstracts, do have some advantages, including being more informative, easier to read, and generally preferred by readers.[48,49] However, structured abstracts usually require more journal space. Informative abstracts may entice some individuals to read the study; thus, abstracts should be thorough, complete, and unbiased in wording selection.[49]

Abstracts should be consistent with the manuscript and should not present biased and/or inaccurate information.[46,47,49] For further information regarding abstracts and preparation, refer to the appendices in Chapter 9. Regardless of the abstract presentation style, readers should not make decisions based on abstract information only. Results of three published studies illustrate the dangers of reading only the abstract.[50-52] These studies provided evidence of omissions and discrepancies between the abstract and the manuscript in medical, psychology, and pharmacy journals.

INTRODUCTION

The introduction section serves two specific purposes: discussing the study rationale and study purpose.[24,53] Usually, readers are first briefly educated on the issues that were the basis for conducting the study. The study investigators may state the reason the research was conducted was due to the lack of data to answer a question or available data are conflicting regarding an issue. Every clinical trial is designed to answer one or more primary questions. The investigators should explain how the clinical trial will overcome the shortcomings of the prior research, if applicable. The study objective is often stated within the last paragraph, if not the last sentence, of this section. Well-written studies present a clearly stated research purpose, and this statement should be understood by the reader before continuing with the remaining article content. Studies with a well-written purpose statement enable the reader to better comprehend and assess the research methods.

Once the clinical trial objective is determined, the investigators need to formulate a research and **null hypothesis** (H_0). A **research hypothesis** (also known as the alternative hypothesis) is a difference between the therapy under investigation and the control while H_0 is no difference between these two groups (see next paragraph for an example). After the study is completed, the researchers analyze the data and then the research hypothesis is either accepted (which also includes rejecting H_0) or rejected (which then means H_0 is accepted). Readers should recognize that not all clinical trials include the specific research and null hypotheses in the introduction section. While this can be considered a deficiency in the paper, it does not necessarily indicate that the paper contains incorrect information.

An example to explain some of the material thus far included in this chapter is the Celecoxib versus Omeprazole and Diclofenac in Patients with Osteoarthritis and Rheumatoid Arthritis (CONDOR) trial, which assessed gastrointestinal (GI) adverse event risk between celecoxib versus the combination of diclofenac plus omeprazole in patients with osteoarthritis (OA) or rheumatoid arthritis (RA). The CONDOR trial compared celecoxib 200 mg twice daily with diclofenac slow release 75 mg twice daily plus omeprazole 20 mg daily for 6 months.[54] The investigators expressed in the introduction section that the rationale for conducting this clinical trial was that no evidence has been published that determines whether a cyclooxygenase-2 (COX-2)-selective nonsteroidal anti-inflammatory drug (NSAID) is associated with fewer small bowel mucosal lesions compared with a nonselective NSAID plus proton pump inhibitor (PPI). The CONDOR investigators "postulated that the risk of clinical outcomes across the entire gastrointestinal tract associated with celecoxib would be lower than that associated with diclofenac plus omperazole."[54] The research hypothesis of the CONDOR trial was: "There is a difference in the incidence of clinically significant events throughout the gastrointestinal (GI) tract between celecoxib and diclofenac plus omeprazole." H_0 for this clinical trial was: "There is no difference in the incidence of clinically significant events throughout the GI tract between celecoxib versus diclofenac plus omperazole." After reading the CONDOR trial introduction, the reader has a clear understanding of the study rationale and purpose: the results of this trial should provide health care providers with evidence to prescribe either a selective NSAID or nonselective NSAID plus PPI in patients with OA or RA to reduce the risk of adverse events throughout the GI tract.

As with all sections of a clinical trial, this section needs to be carefully read. Authors may set the stage by presenting only selective (i.e., not comprehensive) information and/or weak references (which is discussed later in the chapter) to support the rationale for conducting the study. Also, the information may be presented using biased wording, which predisposes the reader to believing the prior research was insignificant in providing evidence applicable to practice.

METHODS

Following a well-designed plan is essential for the clinical trial results to be acceptable and useful to practitioners. The design of a study (i.e., methods) is important for the results to be valid, just as abiding by the blueprints is vital to building a house. The methods section of a clinical trial contains a large amount of information that includes the type of subjects enrolled, the comparative therapy description, outcome measures, and statistics. Flaws within the design of a clinical trial limit the application and significance of the results. Poor study design leads to reduced study **internal validity**, resulting in limited external study validity (see Table 4–3).[20,55] The methods section needs to be thorough in describing to the reader the process in which the study was conducted. In fact, a reader should devote the majority of time used to assess the trial in this section.

Clinical trials follow a pattern in presenting the information within the methods section.[24] This standardized format allows study details to be in an orderly fashion and quickly located. Readers of the biomedical literature should have an understanding of the overall design to appropriately critique clinical trials and use the study results for patient care activities.

TABLE 4–3. INTERNAL VERSUS EXTERNAL VALIDITY OF CLINICAL TRIALS

Term	Meaning	Application
Internal validity	Quality of the study design	Strong design should translate into reliable results
External validity	Ability to apply results to practice	Study results meaningful to practitioners and can be used for patient care

Study Design

Several study designs are available for investigators to select from when conducting research. The study questions the researchers wish to answer dictate which study design is selected to conduct the research.[56,57] Both investigators and readers of the literature need to identify the strengths and limitations of the research designs. Although many study designs are available, this chapter discusses only controlled clinical trials. For additional information on other study designs the reader is referred to Chapter 5.

A simple description of a controlled clinical trial is that it prospectively measures a difference in effect between two or more therapies. The groups are similar and treated identically with the exception of the therapies under study. The subjects in the study are assigned to one of the groups and monitored.[17,18,25,57] This study type, called parallel design, is the primary study design encountered in the literature.

Controlled clinical trials offer investigators the most rigorous method of establishing a cause-and-effect relationship between treatment and outcome.[16,18] Simply explained, the treatment under study is the cause and the result of giving the treatment is measured as the effect. The effect of the treatment under study is compared to the effect of the other group(s). Thus, investigators can use a clinical trial to claim that a treatment has some effect that may be important in modifying disease outcomes. In addition, the magnitude (i.e., size) of the difference in effect between the groups can be estimated.[16,18]

An example of a controlled clinical trial measuring a cause and effect is a study that compared atorvastatin 20 mg once daily to placebo. The study objective was to compare atorvastatin (cause) to placebo and measure the change in average LDL-cholesterol (LDL-C) levels (effect) between the two groups.[58] The study results documented atorvastatin lowered average LDL-C levels more than placebo (–33% versus –1.4%) after 4 weeks of therapy. Thus, the investigators can conclude an effect (reduction in LDL-C levels) was caused by atorvastatin, especially since placebo was used as the comparison (no minimal change in LDL-C levels anticipated with placebo). A clinical trial also quantifies the differences in the effect, such as atorvastatin compared to simvastatin in lowering LDL-C.[59] Atorvastatin 10 mg was compared to simvastatin 20 mg (both once daily) to measure how much (if any) difference the average LDL-C level was lowered by these two agents. After 6 weeks of therapy, the average LDL-C level was lowered slightly more with atorvastatin than simvastatin (−37% versus −35%). Thus, the results of this study can be used to determine the magnitude of difference in LDL-C lowering by atorvastatin 10 mg daily (compared to simvastatin) and make the decision to use, or not use, this medication instead of simvastatin 20 mg daily in practice.

Patient Inclusion/Exclusion Criteria

❹ *The results of a controlled clinical trial should be extrapolated to the patient type enrolled in the study and readers should be aware of the limitations of* **surrogate** *endpoints and subgroup analysis results.* The **inclusion criteria** lists subject demographics that must be present in order for the subject to be enrolled in the trial, while **exclusion criteria** are characteristics that prevent a subject from enrollment in the trial or necessitates withdrawal from the study, if they are later determined to be present.[24] Diagnostic criteria for conditions under study and definitions of the inclusion/exclusion criteria must be included in an article reporting study results. For instance, if subjects with hypertension are the target group to be enrolled in a trial, hypertension needs to be defined in terms of the minimal and maximum systolic blood pressure (SBP) and diastolic blood pressure (DBP). The study participant features should reflect the disease under investigation, but the existence of complex and/or extensive comorbid conditions (e.g., terminal cancer, pregnancy, numerous other disease states) in the study patients may not allow the researchers to accurately measure the differences in effect between the groups. The presence of these complex and/or extensive comorbid conditions can make for difficult decisions regarding including subjects representative of real patients versus excluding typical persons whose complicating conditions will make it impossible to accurately assess a new treatment. Whenever possible and appropriate, typical individuals with the condition being assessed, who in all probability will receive the therapy in real practice, should be represented in the trial. This includes ensuring a realistic representation of the gender, race, and other demographics. Subjects with one or more (but not numerous) other disease states and taking other medications are usually entered into the clinical trial, so the typical patients in whom the therapy under investigation is intended are represented.

The inclusion/exclusion criteria are pertinent to the extrapolation of the study results (i.e., applying the study results to practice [**external validity**]).[55] Trial results are only applicable to the type of subject included in the study. The investigators of the CONDOR trial enrolled men and women with either OA or RA who were either: at least 60 years of age; or 18 to 59 years of age with a history of gastroduodenal ulceration or GI hemorrhage.[54] Thus, the results of the CONDOR trial cannot be extrapolated to all patients less than 60 years of age since only those less than 60 years of age with a history of gastroduodenal ulceration were included in this clinical trial.

Researchers are careful in deciding which subjects to include and exclude in the clinical trial. Standard types of subjects disqualified are pregnant and lactating females or children; also, most clinical trials do not enroll subjects with severe conditions that may alter the medication's pharmacokinetics and/or pharmacodynamics (e.g., renal and/or hepatic dysfunction). Generally, the inclusion criteria attempts to include subjects who are homogeneous and are similar to the common type of patients in practice.[53]

During the process of the investigators selecting subjects to be included into a study, readers of clinical trials need to be conscious of the potential for a **selection bias** that may be present. A selection bias can occur due to various reasons, but can seriously affect the study results in a negative fashion. In general, a selection bias occurs after subjects meet the inclusion and exclusion criteria, but are not enrolled in the study.[60] The investigators may prevent a subject from being enrolled since this person may alter the results either positively or negatively.[17,25,60,61]

Although it is difficult for the reader to detect the above form of selection bias, the following paragraphs describe selection biases that can be more readily identified, but are not present in all clinical trials. One common form of a selection bias is requiring the subjects to complete a **run-in phase** (also called lead-in phase) before being officially enrolled in the study. This phase is usually short in duration (usually 2 to 4 weeks) in which the subjects may take a placebo or the therapy being investigated. The investigators should inform the reader of the intent of the run-in phase. Typical reasons include identifying subjects who may or may not adhere to the therapy regimen, experience side effects from the therapy, or did not meet prespecified criteria (e.g., blood pressure less than a set value). Afterward, these identified subjects are excluded from participating in the study even though they met the original inclusion criteria. The run-in phase produces a bias by selecting a group of subjects who do not completely represent the population, since a selected group of the subjects meeting the study inclusion criteria is not included in the study and its run-in phase results are not included in the final analysis.[62] In addition, a run-in phase can delay the time from identifying candidates to actually enrolling in the clinical trial, which can increase the chance of patients withdrawing from the study.[63]

The following examples explain a selection bias by a run-in phase. Subjects meeting the hypothetical trial inclusion criteria complete a 4-week run-in phase in which a new therapy under investigation is given to all these persons. Those persons experiencing side effects to the new therapy during the run-in phase are not allowed to be enrolled in the study. By excluding those persons eliminated after the run-in phase, the incidence and severity of the side effects of the therapy are not accurately measured during the actual study since subjects experiencing the side effects during the run-in phase were not enrolled in the study. A second example is where researchers may include a run-in phase in which only those persons achieving a preset goal are allowed to be included in the study. For instance, only subjects achieving at least a 25% reduction in LDL-C after a 4-week phase with a new therapy are enrolled in the 12-week study comparing the new therapy to placebo. By only including those with a favorable response, the final average reduction in LDL-C with the new therapy is falsely elevated since only selected subjects were allowed into the study. Those persons with less than a 25% reduction in LDL-C were excluded from the 12-week trial; if these individuals were included in the 12-week trial, the final average reduction in LDL-C most likely would have been significantly lower than actually measured.

Trials including a run-in phase are not always considered to be a study limitation.[61] The investigators may stop a therapy previously prescribed to the subjects and give a placebo during the run-in phase. This allows the effects of the prior therapy to diminish and not interfere with the effects of the therapy under study. Furthermore, a clinical trial may be designed in which the investigators enroll a very specific type of subject, which can be considered a selection bias in the inclusion criteria. The purpose of this type of selection bias is to evaluate a therapy in a very unique group of individuals, usually those who met some predetermined criteria. For instance, a trial was designed so that only subjects who experienced a GI bleed with aspirin alone were enrolled.[64] The investigators were specifically selecting a unique group of subjects (having a GI bleed due to aspirin). The combination of aspirin and esomeprazole was compared to clopidogrel to determine which therapy had a lower recurrence of GI bleeding. Even though the trial results indicated that the aspirin plus esomeprazole combination has a lower GI bleeding recurrence rate, this does not mean this drug combination should be used instead of aspirin alone in those people needing aspirin therapy. The results of this trial can only be used for selected patients; those who had a GI bleed while taking aspirin and need to continue antiplatelet therapy.

Investigators should also explain the process of recruiting subjects and define the time period of which the recruitment occurred.[24] Sponsors of clinical trials and investigators typically recruit subjects for clinical trials by four main strategies: sponsors may offer financial and other incentives to investigators to increase enrollment, investigators may target their own patients as potential subjects, investigators may seek additional subjects from other sources (e.g., physician referrals and disease registries), or sponsors and investigators may advertise and promote their studies. The most common means for advertising for recruitment to clinical trials is through newspapers, radio, Internet, television, or as posters on public transportation and in hospitals.[65] The methods in which investigators recruit subjects may have implications on the generalizability of the research results to the population (i.e., external validity). Newspaper and Internet advertisements are common; however, there are inherent problems with this form of advertisement. Survey results indicate that the majority of persons who read the newspapers are older in age, Caucasian, wealthier, more educated, and own more upscale homes than the average American. **Gender bias** can also affect recruitment rates as it has been documented that female readers consider newspaper advertising to be more important than male readers.[66]

Internet recruitment is not without similar problems. Typically, minority and elderly individuals may be less familiar and may have less access to the Internet. A study described the process of registering persons with cancer for clinical trials via the Internet and telephone call center. Most of the subjects registered via the Internet compared to the telephone call center (88% versus 12%). The majority of subjects who registered were females (73% versus 27% males; p < 0.001), Caucasian (88.9%), and received colorectal cancer screening (59%); the median age was 49 years. No differences with respect to ethnicity or gender were observed for patients registering via the Internet compared to the call center; however, subjects registering via the Internet were significantly younger than those registering through the call center. Recruitment via newspapers and the Internet may offer some benefits in terms of recruitment, although the lack of uniformity with respect to access to newspapers and the Internet for elderly and minority subjects may increase the difficulty of applying the clinical trial results to these underrepresented populations because this subject type was not included in the trials.[67]

Another important issue that affects the recruitment of patients is the increasing number of clinical studies that are outsourced to other countries due to costs associated with conducting clinical trials in the United States. Although outsourcing clinical trials to other countries may decrease the problems associated with insufficient recruitment of patients who enroll in clinical trials, other issues may occur as a result of including a large number of foreign patients in clinical trials.[68] Potential ethnic differences may affect the way drugs are handled in the body (e.g., overall response, drug distribution, metabolism, excretion). Therefore, readers of clinical studies that have included foreign patients need to ensure that the results of the study are generalizable to the patient population in which they serve. However, clinical trials including a majority of foreign patients should not be viewed with a bias. Various factors have led to more clinical research conducted in foreign countries, which include governments competing for clinical research to be conducted in their countries, increased number of health care specialists plus improving medical infrastructure in these countries, and changes in regulations.[69]

Intervention and Control Groups

Once the subjects are enrolled in the clinical trial, they will be assigned to either the intervention or control group. The intervention group consists of the therapy under investigation (e.g., medication, procedure). The intervention is compared to a control so that the fundamental principle of a controlled clinical trial can be accomplished, measuring cause and effect. The control group can consist of no therapy (e.g., placebo), another therapy (a.k.a. **active control**) (e.g., drug, exercise), or be compared to existing data (i.e., historical data). Both the intervention and control groups are to be as similar as possible in all respects (e.g., average age, number of males/females, medication use, existing disease states) other than the treatment received. Afterward, the investigators measure and quantify a difference in effect between the group assigned to the intervention with those in the control group. Thus, any identified differences in the measured effect can be attributed to intervention rather than other factors (i.e., **confounders**).[17,70,71]

A key term in the phrase controlled clinical trial is the word control, indicating another therapy is serving as the measuring point for the effect of the intervention to be assessed. Reports have been published documenting placebo effects (i.e., measured change even though no therapy was given).[72] Without a control, the effects measured by the intervention may be by chance or falsely quantified. For example, investigators of a study reported that oxandrolone caused an average increase in body weight in patients with chronic obstructive pulmonary disease (COPD).[73] However, all the subjects were treated with oxandrolone and no control group was included in the study. Although these patients gained weight, oxandrolone may not be the sole reason for this effect. Weight gain may have occurred naturally, even without the medication or by some unidentified reason. The results of this noncontrolled clinical trial may be the rationale for a clinical trial being conducted to evaluate the weight gaining effects of oxandrolone. However, they cannot be used as evidence that weight gain was solely attributed to this drug. The results of studies designed without a control can be useful, but since no control group was present, readers cannot be certain that oxandrolone caused the weight gain, even if caloric intake and exercise were held constant.

Researchers can select from a few different types of controls, including historical, placebo, or active. Historical controls are described as data that have been collected prior to the beginning of a clinical trial. Investigators conduct the study with only the intervention group and then compare the results to the existing data.[74] One advantage of using historical controls is only one group is needed to be enrolled, which may result in less time, expense, etc. Another advantage is the usefulness of studying a disease with a low occurrence or a disease with high incidence of death or other serious sequelae in which some form of therapy should not be denied.[74] Disadvantages include usually overestimating the effect of the intervention,[22] lack of homogeneity between patients in the trial and historical controls, and differences in therapeutic procedures or techniques from one study period to the next.[74]

Historical controls are not used very often in published clinical trials, but are acceptable in selected situations. For example, the use of a placebo group is not considered ethical in clinical trials evaluating new therapies in patients with epilepsy. Due to the morbidity and/or mortality associated with an uncontrolled seizure disorder, this patient type should not be denied therapy in order to investigate a new therapy. Thus, investigators may assess a new therapy in these patients and compare the research results to historical data (obtained from prior research).[75]

An intervention under investigation is compared to a placebo in many clinical trials to document and measure the pharmacological effect of the intervention. These studies are generally conducted as a requirement by the FDA to document that drug therapy is better than no therapy (placebo) for a given disease state.[72] Those trials reporting a significant difference in effect of the intervention compared to placebo could be used to support the use of the intervention in treating patients. Simvastatin was compared to placebo to determine if the incidence of death would be lower in subjects with a history of angina pectoris or myocardial infarction (MI).[76] Before this study was conducted, health care providers did not have any information indicating that simvastatin would benefit or harm this subject type. At the time this trial was designed and initiated, persons with angina pectoris or history of MI were not routinely treated with an HMG-CoA reductase inhibitor (i.e., statins); thus, a placebo was selected as the control. However, the place in therapy for the intervention may be difficult to determine when a placebo is the control, since other drugs may be found to be better than the drug in question, upon further research. For example, in this case, although simvastatin lowers LDL-C greater than placebo,[77] it is not directly known how simvastatin compares to other drugs that lower LDL-C based solely on these trial results.

Not all clinical trials will have a placebo as the control group for various valid reasons. For example, including a placebo as one of the groups in a trial may decrease the willingness of subjects to participate; some may not wish to be treated with a placebo.[78] But more importantly, denying therapy that has been documented to reduce morbidity and/or mortality to patients with selected diseases may be unethical. These studies would not include a placebo as the control, but instead may use active therapy (i.e., standard therapy).[72,79] Patients with cancer enrolled in a clinical trial are prime examples where trials do not include a placebo as the control.

Usually after the new therapy is compared to a placebo, a trial using an active therapy as the control is used to assess the difference in effect between the groups. Readers should be aware that clinical trials with a placebo as the control, particularly those funded by the pharmaceutical industry, yield a larger treatment effect than if an active therapy was selected as the control group.[80,81] For instance, the difference in the LDL-C lowering effect is expected to be significantly greater with a new statin versus placebo instead of another statin or other lipid lowering agent. Thus, the treatment effect may appear to be substantial versus placebo, but could be minimally different from another active drug that was used as the control. Also, the possibility exists that the new treatment, in fact, may be inferior in efficacy and/or safety compared to an active drug, even though the new treatment appears better in comparison to a placebo.

An appropriate control needs to be included in the study for the results to be applicable for practice. The use of historical or placebo as the control is acceptable in some clinical trials (as described above). Some studies may be designed with a control that may no longer be the preferred treatment after the trial results are published. The study may have been designed and initiated based on either recommendations of the FDA or before new therapy recommendations were available.

Also, investigators including a medication as the control need to use the dosing regimen (i.e., dose, frequency) deemed suitable.[80] Standard references should be consulted to ensure appropriate dosing regimens were included in the trial to reduce the chance of obtaining biased results. A trial concluding a new analgesic relieved pain better than morphine dosed 0.05 mg intravenously (IV) every 24 hours postsurgery in otherwise healthy adult subjects is biased because an appropriate morphine regimen was not used. However, at times investigators may not know the equivalent dosing regimen of the intervention relative to the control. Investigators directly comparing rosuvastatin to atorvastatin, both 10 mg once daily for 12 weeks, reported a greater lowering of mean LDL-C with rosuvastatin (43% versus 35%).[82] Other studies comparing these two medications have reported average LDL-C levels are similar with atorvastatin doses two times that of the rosuvastatin dose.[83] Thus, concluding rosuvastatin is a superior LDL-C lowering agent to atorvastatin based solely on the results of a single trial evaluating both agents dosed 10 mg once daily is incorrect. A more appropriate conclusion is these two agents do not have an equivalent pharmacological effect at this dose.

Institutional Review Board/Subject Consent

Research projects that use humans as study subjects must be approved before investigators begin enrolling subjects in the trial. The Institutional Review Board (IRB) is the committee charged with ensuring the subjects are protected and not exposed to unnecessary harm or unethical medical procedures,[84,85] including vulnerable populations (e.g., pediatrics, pregnant women, impaired persons[86]). The name of the actual committee may differ from place to place (e.g., local ethics committee), although the purpose of the committee remains to protect the study subjects. This committee consists of both health care and nonhealth care professionals; people specialized in ethics also need to be included.[86] The rules and regulations of human research require the study to be assessed prior to the initiation of the project.

Another primary responsibility of the IRB is to approve the informed consent form.[87,88] Before agreeing to participate in a trial, each subject is presented with an informed consent form that notifies the subjects of the study procedures, their rights and responsibilities of participating in the study, plus at least eight major points that include risks, benefits, compensation, voluntary participation, and right to withdraw from the study without any penalty. In addition to the content of the informed consent form, the IRB provides investigators with suggestions on how to write the form in language that laypersons can comprehend.[87-91] Additional information regarding the role of the IRB and investigator in clinical trial research can be obtained at http://phrp.nihtraining.com/users/login.php. Also, the reader may refer to Chapter 17. According to the Uniform Requirements, articles describing clinical trials using humans as research subjects are required to include a statement that the research was approved by the IRB (or other committee that protects subjects) and consent was obtained from the subject to partici-pate in the research project.[34] Over the past 10 years, more medical journals include IRB/ethics approval information within the published studies.[89] Trials not including the IRB/informed consent information should be questioned.

Blinding

Since clinical trials measure differences in effect between groups, outside influences (i.e., biases) should be minimized. This is especially important in studies measuring subjective outcomes (e.g., pain, depression scores). **Blinding** is a technique in which subjects and/or the investigators are unaware of who is in the intervention or control group. Blinding techniques are incorporated to reduce possible bias (defined as "differences between the true value and that actually obtained [are] due to all causes other than sampling variabil-ity").[25] Patients knowing they are taking a placebo to reduce depression symptoms are likely to report no change or worsening of the disease. The results are biased since sub-jects knowingly are taking a substance that does not reduce symptoms. Therefore, blind-ing techniques are important to reduce the influence of bias on measuring a difference in effect between the intervention and control. Four types of blinding can be used in a clini-cal trial (see Table 4–4). The specific blinding type usually is dictated by the effect being measured during the trial.

Single- and nonblinding techniques are primarily incorporated in clinical trials that have study objectives not conducible to blinding (e.g., surgery versus medication). Some trials may include a procedure that is difficult to blind (e.g., surgery) and it may not be ideal to include a placebo procedure because sham surgery is not without risks as death or infection-related complications are possible.[92] The use of placebo procedures to

TABLE 4–4. TYPES OF BLINDING

Type of Blinding	Definition
No blinding (open-label)	Investigators and subjects are aware of the assignment of subjects to the intervention or control group
Single	Either investigators or subjects, but not both, are aware of the assignment of subjects to the intervention or control group
Double	Both investigators and subjects are not aware of the assignment of subjects to the intervention or control group
Triple	In addition to both investigators and subjects not being aware of the assignment of subjects to the intervention or control group, trial personnel involved in data interpretation are not aware of subject assignment

ensure a trial remains blinded, which may increase the risk of adverse effects or other dangers, is controversial and possibly unethical if the investigators do not thoroughly discuss the rationale for including and/or not using other methods to blind the trial.[93] A clinical trial designed to compare surgery to a medication is an example of using non-blinding methods since both the investigators and subjects know which group the subjects have been assigned.

An example of single-blinding is when one group of subjects is administered a medication subcutaneously once daily versus the other group who took an oral anticoagulation medication. The subjects were not blinded since the risk of injecting a saline solution subcutaneously (i.e., bleeding complications may develop in persons taking an anticoagulant agent plus unnecessary injections) may outweigh the benefit. The investigators measured the occurrence of a blood clot, an objective outcome that cannot be biased or influenced by the subjects. Therefore, the subjects' knowledge of which therapy they were receiving cannot influence the incidence of the blood clots. Since the investigators do not know which therapy is administered, the potential for the results to be biased is minimized. There are also cases in which the subjects were blinded, but not the investigator.

Double-blinding, where neither the investigator nor the patient knows who is receiving which treatment, is considered the gold standard blinding technique and is most commonly used in clinical trials.[26] As a general rule, and regardless of whether the outcome is a subjective or objective measure, the study should be double-blinded. A clinical trial measuring an objective outcome usually assesses other study outcome measures, such as the incidence and severity of side effects, which may be biased if double-blinding was not incorporated into the trial. For instance, double-blinding was used in the CONDOR trial[54] to not only minimize biases in the objective measurements (GI tract adverse events that included hemorrhage, obstruction, perforation, anemia) but also subjective assessments (side effects) in those patients assigned to intervention or control.

In order to ensure that blinding remains intact, the therapy each group receives should be exact in frequency of administration, appearance, size, taste, smell, and other variables. Studies that compare regimens taken once daily to twice daily require the once daily group to take a placebo as the second dose (i.e., double-dummy).[17] Double-dummy methods are included in clinical trials when two therapies being compared are not the same (e.g., different routes of administration, different formulations). Patients receive two formulations, one active and one control, to ensure that blinding is maintained.[17] For example, investigators of a clinical trial evaluating the blood pressure lowering effects of amlodipine (a tablet) and the combination product of amlodipine plus benazepril (a capsule) should administer amlodipine tablets plus placebo capsules to those subjects randomized to amlodipine therapy and amlodipine/benazepril capsules plus placebo tablets to the other subjects. A similar situation may present in clinical trials in which the formulations being compared are administered via different routes. Investigators evaluating the efficacy of a once daily oral contraceptive tablet to an intramuscular contraceptive agent administered every 3 months may allocate an intramuscular placebo to those patients randomized to once daily oral contraceptives and a once daily placebo tablet to those patients randomized to the intramuscular contraceptive. Each patient receives a formulation that represents each therapy and both subjects and investigators would be less likely to determine which formulation is active.

Sometimes it is necessary to triple-blind a study. In addition to the trial investigators and subjects, other personnel involved with the trial (e.g., data collection, analysis, or monitoring; drug administration or dispensing) can have opinions regarding the outcome of the therapy being studied based on their interaction with the subjects involved in the trial or their experience with the intervention and/or control being assessed. These opinions may cause inappropriate data collection, measurement, analysis, and/or interpretation of the results by the study personnel. Also, data collection personnel having a bias for or against the intervention may not be as consistent in their data collection procedures if they know which group the subjects were assigned. This may result in an inappropriate interpretation (e.g., overestimation of the treatment effects) of the study results.[17,22,26] Therefore, it is often necessary to blind these other individuals (i.e., triple-blinding).

Randomization

Randomization is a distinguishing study attribute that separates controlled clinical trials from other study designs (e.g., case-control, cohort). ❺ *Randomization is an essential component of all controlled clinical trials and a significant differentiator from other study designs.* Randomization can be simply described as all persons in a clinical trial who have an equal chance to be in the intervention or control group.[94] Research has indicated that the results obtained from randomized trials are more dependable than nonrandomized trials. An analysis of randomized versus nonrandomized trials reported that, on average, investigators of nonrandomized trials overestimated the treatment effects of the intervention compared to the control primarily due to bias.[22] Even though including randomization in a clinical trial is important for more reliable results, it is necessary to remember not all randomized trials are without faults.

Subjects are eligible for randomization after meeting the trial inclusion criteria.[17] Subjects are randomized so the investigators cannot purposely assign selected persons to one group over another (i.e., individuals with more comorbidities in the control versus healthier individuals in the intervention group). Randomization minimizes bias by lowering the potential for an imbalance of risk factors or prognostic variations between the intervention and control groups.[25] A difference in effect measured by a clinical trial may result from many causes, and treatment may be just one of these. Disparities between the groups at baseline may cause a false result instead of measuring differences in effect between the intervention and control.[95] Therefore, to be assured that the difference is truly due to the intervention, the groups need to be as similar as possible to control for any confounding variables.[70] Besides reducing bias,[96] an additional reason to include randomization in a clinical trial is so statistical tests are valid. Most statistical tests require subjects to be randomized so that similar groups are being compared and selected statistical tests can determine whether certain subject characteristics are equivalent between groups.[25]

Measuring differences in the effect between the intervention and control group requires the groups to be as similar in as many characteristics as possible (e.g., age, gender, severity of illness) so that outside factors (i.e., confounders) do not influence the results.[96] Baseline discrepancies between the groups do not allow the true difference in effect between the intervention and group to be measured and quantified. If unbalanced factors are present between the two groups, the outcome measure is biased, and the treatment effect may be either under- or overestimated.[95]

Many randomization techniques are available and range from very simple to complex processes. The nature of the study and outcomes measured influence the randomization procedure. Various methods are available that include random number tables and computer programs. The randomization procedures should be unbiased and unpredictable by not allowing the subjects or investigators to know in advance to which group the subject will be assigned.[17,96]

Specific randomization methods include from simple (i.e., coin toss) to more advanced techniques (i.e., **stratification**). Simple randomization is an easy technique to implement and includes assigning subjects according to some criteria (e.g., day of the week, subject birthday, or subject medical record number). But this method is not considered a proper randomization method since the number of subjects in the groups can be imbalanced due to the technique. If investigators assign all subjects with an office visit on a specific day of the week to one group (i.e., control), then these subjects did not have equal opportunity to be assigned to either group. These may lead to a reduction in the ability of the investigators to detect differences in effects between the two groups. Few trials use simple randomization techniques due to the limitations of this randomization method.[25] Although the mentioned simple randomization techniques do have limitations, a random number table can be considered useful since the table allows for each study subject to have equal opportunity to be assigned to either group.

The one of the more sophisticated randomization procedures, stratification, is designed to achieve similarities in both known and unknown baseline patient characteristics between the groups. Selected factors are identified (e.g., age, smoking, presence of other disease states) and used in determining which group the subjects will be assigned so significant imbalances of these factors are not present among the groups, while all subjects with any specific factor have an equal chance of being in each group.[97] Since these patient factors can affect the outcome being measured, stratified randomization is a technique that enables these factors to be comparable between the study groups.[25] For example, the risk of developing a venous thrombosis is greater in cancer patients who are immobilized and/or receiving hormonal therapy.[41] Thus, a study comparing two agents (e.g., low-molecular weight heparin versus unfractionated heparin) to prevent a venous thrombosis in this patient type would use stratified randomization to ensure a similar number of patients with these two risk factors are assigned in each of the two study groups. If one group had significantly more patients taking hormonal therapy, this factor could be the reason more patients had a venous thrombosis instead of the drug not being effective as the other drug. Thus, a false study result could occur due to the two patient groups not being similar at the beginning of the study.

The person randomizing study participants should receive only the participant information used for the randomization process. Extra and unnecessary patient information could bias the randomization process. Unduly influencing the randomization sequence by randomizing subjects to either therapy based on some preference can occur with the extra personal information.[25] Thus, to minimize these issues, investigators should only provide the pertainent subject information that allows randomization of the subject to either the intervention or control group.

Endpoints

Clinical trials measure some effect caused by the intervention and control in order to compare these groups.[18,26,98] All trials specify one effect caused by the intervention and control as the **primary endpoint**, which can be referred to as what the investigators measured to achieve the study objective. Since significant time, money, and effort are devoted to conduct a clinical trial, researchers usually measure a primary endpoint plus **secondary endpoints**. These secondary endpoints are important, but not considered to be the primary purpose of the study. The selected primary endpoint should be a routine and useful measure.[26,98] For example, a trial evaluating the cholesterol lowering effect of an HMG coenzyme A reductase inhibitor compared to placebo selected a change in average LDL-C value, an appropriate measure, as the primary endpoint to satisfy the study objective. However, measuring a change in serum creatinine between losartan and captopril to improve heart failure (HF) symptoms[99] is not ideal, since serum creatinine is not the predominate parameter used in practice to monitor the progression or improvement in HF status.

❻ *The controlled clinical trial primary endpoint should be appropriate for the study purpose and measured using valid techniques and methods.* Investigators may combine a group of endpoint measures into one primary endpoint, referred to as a composite endpoint. The group usually consists of clinical outcomes directly related to morbidity and mortality as opposed to a pharmacological action (e.g., reduction in any incidence of stroke/MI/cardiovascular-related death versus lowering cholesterol levels). The investigators select a group of endpoints that can occur during therapy and are considered clinically important. For example, after experiencing an MI, a therapy is prescribed to reduce the occurrence of multiple adverse outcomes (e.g., reinfarction, death, chest pain), not just one clinical outcome. The rationale for measuring composite endpoints is to measure an overall effect of therapy, since one specific outcome cannot be deemed to be the most important for the study subjects.[80,100,101]

The use of composite endpoints is not without debate.[80,100-104] The results of the individual components of the composite should be reported separately and analyzed.[100,101,103] Investigators may claim the investigational therapy is better than the control based on the overall result of the composite endpoint, even though the investigational therapy was shown to significantly affect only one or a few (but not all) of the composite endpoint components. Also, the most important component of the composite may not be affected by the intervention under study. Due to the issues of using composite endpoints, researchers are in the process of designing new methods to assess the individual components of the composite endpoint (e.g., assigning weights to each endpoint) to better gauge the clinical trial results.[101,103]

The following example explains composite endpoints and issues encountered with these. The investigators of the Efficacy and Safety of Subcutaneous Enoxaparin in Non-Q-Wave Coronary Events (ESSENCE) trial used a composite primary endpoint, which consisted of death, MI (or reinfarction), or recurrent angina after 14 days of follow-up.[105] The incidence of the primary endpoint was lower with enoxaparin (intervention) than unfractionated heparin (control) (16.6% versus 19.8%, respectively; p = 0.02) in patients with angina at rest or non-Q-wave MI. However, only one of the three components of the composite endpoint was significantly different with enoxaparin, recurrent angina (12.9% versus 15.5%, respectively; p = 0.03).[105] As seen by the percentages, the majority of primary endpoint composite (~78%) consisted of this single event, which is the least robust of the three outcomes.[106] Although lowering the incidence of recurrent angina is clinically important, this outcome is not as severe as death or reinfarction. The composite endpoint effect of enoxaparin appears to be superior to heparin, even though the incidence of two of the three components of the composite endpoint indicates no difference between these two drugs. Enoxaparin was considered to be a useful therapy in this patient type, but further research was recommended to determine if the therapy reduces the occurrence of death and MI in these patients.[107]

The primary and other endpoint definitions, plus valid measuring techniques, need to be determined prior to the start of the clinical trial and incorporated in the study design.[17,26] By doing so, the investigators can be consistent throughout the trial in measuring the endpoints, thereby reducing study variances or biases. To illustrate, the CONDOR trial primary endpoint was "a composite of clinically significant events occurring throughout the gastrointestinal tract." Components of the primary endpoint were hemorrhage and/or perforation of the gastroduodenal, small bowel, or large bowel; gastric-outlet obstruction; and clinically significant anemia (decrease in hemoglobin of at least 20 g/L [2.0 g/dL] or a decrease in hematocrit of at least 10%).[54] If the reader is informed of the measurement types and methods under investigation, judgment may be made whether practical methods were used to measure the endpoints and can determine if the study can be replicated by future investigators or by individuals wanting to implement the trial results into practice to actual patients. Endpoints involving human judgment (e.g., cause of GI bleeding) also can contribute to the complexity of analyzing and interpreting the study results if strict criteria or a blinded clinical events committee designed to produce valid recommendations are not incorporated and utilized during the trial.[100]

A final type of endpoint that may be seen is a surrogate endpoint. This is discussed later in the chapter.

Follow-Up Schedule/Data Collection/Adherence

A few important issues are considered here. First, a study should be conducted for an appropriate duration; second, data need to be consistently collected throughout the entire trial. A magical number of weeks or months has not been established as a rule for all clinical trials, but the length of the study (i.e., follow-up time) should be an ideal representation to answer the question being researched.[26] Statins usually exert the maximum cholesterol lowering effect after at least 4 weeks of stable dosing.[108] Thus, the results of a study directly comparing the effects of atorvastatin 10 mg once daily to simvastatin 20 mg once daily for 6 weeks on the LDL-C level lowering differences between these two agents would be considered acceptable.[59]

A number of trials do not have an extensive follow-up time and the reader may have difficulty in interpreting the results for clinical practice. For example, in one study, the antipsychotic agent aripiprazole and placebo were administered to subjects for 4 weeks to determine the efficacy of aripiprazole in treating psychosis.[109] The investigators of the clinical trial detected a pharmacological effect of aripiprazole during this time period, but the clinical effects and tolerability of the medication beyond this time period could not be assessed due to the short duration of the trial. Considering the actual duration of aripiprazole and other antipsychotic therapy for patients with psychosis exceeds 4 weeks,[110,111] the trial should have been longer so investigators could determine the long-term clinical effects of this drug in practice.

Monitoring of the trial results at predetermined intervals is important throughout the duration of the trial. The Code of Federal Regulations and good clinical practice guidelines for clinical research state subject monitoring is required during the clinical investigation.[26] Larger trials may have a clinical trial investigator subgroup who serves as the data and safety monitoring board members. These individuals are blinded to the subject groupings and are responsible for reviewing the results obtained while the trial is ongoing. Interim analyses of the study results may indicate the intervention produces either a favorable outcome or increased risk over the control before the established duration of the study has been completed. Typically, the protocol for discontinuing the clinical trial early is established prior to enrolling study subjects.[35]

When stopping the study early due to the intervention resulting in significant harm compared to the control, subjects randomized to the intervention would not be at a greater risk for experiencing the harmful effects if a trial was allowed to continue. Conversely, if the intervention was shown to be more beneficial than the control, the investigators would be denying useful therapy to those subjects randomized to the control if the trial continued.

Prior to the start of the study, data collection methods are established. These should be reasonable in that extensive time and/or procedures are not required, so that incomplete follow-up by trial personnel and subjects at each follow-up time can be minimized. In addition, investigators should ensure trial personnel are properly trained and have sufficient resources to complete data collection.[112]

Another data collection and follow-up issue is measuring the adherence of therapy in the study participants.[26] This includes medication dosage unit counts, serum drug levels, or regular follow-up communications (i.e., telephone conversations). Subjects not complying with the therapy regimen may cause inaccuracies and less reliable data. Insufficient and/or inappropriate data collection methods and nonadherence usually lead to biased results that may make the extrapolation of results to clinical practice difficult.

Sample Size

❼ *An appropriate controlled clinical trial sample size is vital for the study results to have any significant meaning; conducting a* **power analysis** *is important to determine a suitable sample size.* Sample size (denoted by the letter n) refers to the number of subjects randomized into a study and is of considerable importance to the validity of the study results. Financial and logistical limitations prevent all subjects with the specific inclusion criteria from being enrolled in the study.[26,112] For example, investigators may want to evaluate a new drug to treat hypertension. It would be virtually impossible to enroll all people with hypertension in this clinical trial. In response, investigators will draw a representative group (i.e., sample) of individuals from all those with hypertension (i.e., population). Researchers do not wish to include too few or too many subjects in the trial. Obviously having only one subject in each group is insufficient to determine differences in effect between groups since chance alone may be the reason for a difference found (if any) between the two groups. On the other hand, having too many subjects can be excessive, costly, and may expose some subjects to unnecessary treatment. The sample size should not be determined on the basis of convenience, arbitrarily, or by the number of easily recruited subjects.[113]

The number of subjects to enroll in a clinical trial is dependent on the expected magnitude of difference in the endpoint effect between the intervention and control. The expected magnitude of difference in effect between groups is estimated based on the results of previously conducted trials or other research results assessing the intervention. In general, an inverse relationship exists between the sample size and the effect size. A large sample size is needed to detect a small difference in effect between the intervention and control outcome, while a smaller sample size is needed to detect large differences between the two groups.[21,113] A large sample size is needed to detect differences in blood pressure between two antihypertensive therapies (small difference in blood pressure reductions), while a smaller sample size is needed to measure the difference in relieving postoperative pain between morphine and placebo (large difference in pain relief).

Researchers use various procedures from table/charts to manual calculations in estimating the necessary sample size for a particular trial.[71,113] Regardless of the method selected to determine the appropriate sample size, it must be calculated prior to initiating the clinical trial. A study lacking a sample size calculation may be biased since the reader is not informed of the basis on which the investigators determined the number of subjects to enroll. Also, another important issue is that the sample size is calculated based on the guesstimated differences in the primary endpoint effect between the intervention and control groups. Investigators use existing data and information about the intervention and/or disease state to guesstimate the amount of difference between the effect in outcome by the intervention and control. The specific amount of difference in effect between the intervention and control is not known, thus the reason the study is conducted, but some estimate in the difference in effect is needed to determine a legitimate sample size. For example, the CONDOR investigators[54] used prior research results to determine an appropriate sample size for this study; they assumed the primary endpoint incidence to be 1.1% for the intervention while 2.3% for the control at month 6 of therapy in this study.

Investigators intending to measure differences in effect for other endpoints besides the primary endpoint need to include this in the process of calculating the sample size. Clinical trials consisting of larger sample sizes can be considered more reliable in measuring and detecting true difference in effect (if it exists) between the intervention and control.[114] Consequences of a clinical trial not having a sufficient sample size (i.e., too small or too large) is discussed in **Type I** and **II Errors**/Power Analysis later in this chapter and in Chapters 5 and 9.

The importance of an appropriate sample size is exemplified in the following example. Investigators conducted a small study (51 patients) to evaluate fenoldopam mesylate compared with 0.45% sodium chloride infusion in enhancing renal plasma flow in patients undergoing contrast angiography. Fewer subjects receiving fenoldopam developed a specific adverse event (radiocontrast-induced nephropathy [RCN]) at 48 hours than those treated with 0.45% sodium chloride infusion (21% versus 41%, respectively).[115] One primary contributor to the large difference in the results was the small number of sub-jects enrolled; the incidence of RCN is increased by 4% for each subject developing this outcome. Even though the percent difference was 20% (41% minus 21%), this represents a difference of only five subjects developing RCN. After the results of this large differ-ence in reducing RCN incidence were released, fenoldopam was frequently used in these patients.[116] However, the CONTRAST study (Evaluation of Corlopam in Patients at Risk for Renal Failure—A Safety and Efficacy Trial) was designed to determine if fenoldopam reduces RCN in patients after receiving iodine-based dye during cardiac angioplasty,[116] but this study had a much larger sample size (157 patients in the fenoldopam group and 158 in the placebo) than the previous study evaluating fenoldopam therapy. At 48 hours, RCN incidence was 19.9% versus 15.9% with fenoldopam and placebo, respectively. At 96 hours, incidence was 33.6% versus 30.1%, respectively. The investigators recruited slightly more than 300 subjects to accommodate potential subject discontinuation. Based on the results of this clinical trial, the incidence of RCN was actually higher with fenoldo-pam than placebo. By conducting a study with a larger sample size, the treatment effect of fenoldopam was more accurately measured compared to the study of only 51 subjects.

Statistical Analysis

Within controlled clinical trials, the use of statistics is a means to analyze sample data and apply it to the population. Many statistical tests are available and readers should be famil-iar with and have a basic understanding of the most common tests used in clinical trials. Some statistical analysis can be easily conducted using simple computer programs, while others require specialized training and extensive skills. Typically, a biostatistician is con-sulted as one of the trial investigators to perform the statistical analysis of the trial results.[117,118] However, even with biostatisticians evaluating the data, study results may be biased by using incorrect statistical analyses.[119]

The purpose of statistical analysis of the study data is to collect sufficient evidence to reject H_0 in favor of accepting the research hypothesis (H_1) (new terminology may refer to this as failure to accept H_0).[119,120] Prior to the start of the study, the appropriate tests are selected based on the type of data that will be collected and analyzed. Since the selection of statistical tests is dependent on the type of data,[94] an overview of the types of data is presented here. There are four types of data (see Table 4–5)[121]: **nominal, ordinal, interval**, and **ratio** (the latter two are usually referred collectively to as continuous). Nominal data are categorical without any sense of order; these data only can be categorized into one of the possible groups (e.g., either dead or alive, but not both). Nominal data are mutually exclusive, meaning that the data can be in only one group. Ordinal data (i.e., ranking) are categorical data with an intrinsic order, but do not have equal intervals between units. Pain severity (or other type of subjective data) measured by a scale is a typical example of ordinal data. For example, a 5-point pain scale with a score of zero indicates no pain, while

TABLE 4–5. TYPES OF DATA

Type of Data	Definition	Examples
Nominal	Categorical data; data placed in one category, but not more than one category	Yes/No; alive/dead; colors of cars in a parking lot into five categories of either red, white, blue, black, or other
Ordinal	Ranking, ordered	Likert scale; visual analog scale
Interval	Data with measurable equal distances between points, but no absolute zero	Temperature in degrees Fahrenheit
Ratio	Data with measurable equal distances between points and an absolute zero	Temperature in degrees Kelvin, blood pressure, cholesterol levels, white blood count

a score of five indicates severe pain. A 1-point change in pain intensity on this 5-point pain scale is not necessarily the same from one-to-two as from four-to-five on the scale. Interval and ratio data both have measurable equal intervals between data points, but interval data have no absolute zero (e.g., Fahrenheit temperature) while an absolute zero point (e.g., white blood cell count) is a characteristic for ratio data. Readers need to differentiate between the types of data to ensure correct statistical tests were selected in addition to the study being designed appropriately with correct data collection methods.

The type of data collected also dictates the use of inferential or descriptive statistical methods. **Inferential statistics** (e.g., Student's t-test, chi-square test) are used to draw conclusions, based on the sample, for the application of the trial results to the population.[122,123] In other words, data are analyzed to make a conclusion of the study results from the sample, which is then inferred to the population. **Descriptive statistics** describe the characteristics of the sample (e.g., average subject age, baseline endpoint values, number of subjects with another disease present) and the results in some studies (e.g., X% had an adverse effect). Descriptive data are typically presented as measures of central tendency (e.g., mean [average], median, mode) and/or measure of variability (e.g., range, standard deviation [SD], variance) (see Table 4–6).[124] Refer to Chapter 8 for further information on descriptive and inferential statistics.

TABLE 4–6. DATA PRESENTATION METHODS

Type of Data	Mode	Median	Mean	Range	Interquartile Range	Standard Deviation
Nominal	X					
Ordinal	X	X		X	X	
Interval and Ratio	X	X	X	X	X	X

NOTE: Mode: most frequently occurring data point; median: midpoint of the data (point at which the data lie 50% above and below); mean: average of the data points; range: officially the difference between the smallest and largest data point in the data set, although usually described by listing the smallest and largest data points (e.g., "the range is from 5 to 9"); interquartile range: difference between the scores at the 75th and 25th percentile; SD: degree in which individual data points deviate from the mean value of the data set.

Explaining the terms in Table 4–6 can be done best via an example of a trial in which the change in LDL-C was measured. A total of 200 subjects were enrolled in a clinical study designed to measure the reduction in LDL-C with a statin versus placebo. The LDL-C is measured in all subjects at the beginning of the trial. The values are then plotted using a histogram (see Figure 4–1). For each subject with a specific LDL-C value, a mark is placed on the graph for that value. As each subject with the same LDL-C value is plotted on the graph, an upward column for that LDL-C value forms. If the sample of subjects was randomly taken from the population, all the plotted LDL-C values would form a bell-shaped curve (also known as a normally distributed data set). After all LDL-C values are obtained, the values for the terms in Table 4–6 can be calculated. As seen from the graph, the mode (most commonly occurring LDL-C value), median (point at which 50% of the LDL-C values lie above and below), and the mean (average) LDL-C are the same. In this data set, an LDL-C of 145 mg/dL represents these three measures of central tendencies. In addition, the range for the LDL-C values can be determined by identifying the lowest and highest LDL-C values. The data can also be organized into quartiles, four groups containing 25% of the data points. The data are arranged from the lowest to highest value; afterward, the data points are divided into four groups: 25th, 50th, 75th, and 100th percentile. Therefore, an LDL-C value that corresponds to the 75th percentile would be in the upper limit of this third quartile of the distribution. In addition, the upper limit of the 50th quartile would equal the median value for the data set. The interquartile range is the difference between the scores at the 75th and 25th percentile.[124]

Since many trials present the results as an average (mean), a more detailed discussion of this measure of central tendency is warranted. Using the LDL-C example, an average

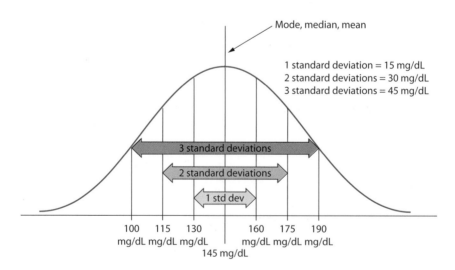

Figure 4–1. Histogram of LDL-C with standard deviation ± 15 mg/dL.

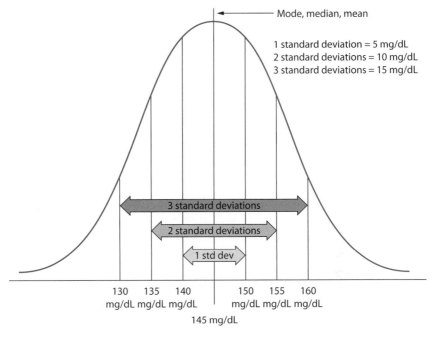

Mode, median, mean

1 standard deviation = 5 mg/dL
2 standard deviations = 10 mg/dL
3 standard deviations = 15 mg/dL

3 standard deviations

2 standard deviations

1 std dev

130   135   140   150   155   160
mg/dL   mg/dL   mg/dL   mg/dL   mg/dL   mg/dL

145 mg/dL

Figure 4–2. Histogram of LDL-C with standard deviation ± 5 mg/dL.

LDL-C value is calculated using all the measured values. However, presenting only the sample average does not inform the reader of the diversity in the set of values. Thus, SD is calculated using all of the LDL-C values. SD is presented with the mean value of the sample (e.g., 145 mg/dL ± 15, where the former number is the mean and the latter number is SD). SD is important since the average LDL-C from two distinct samples may be the same, but the dispersion of the LDL-C values may be considerably different. Figure 4–2 displays another set of LDL-C values taken from a different sample of subjects. The average LDL-C value is the same as Figure 4–1, but the spread of the values are not very dispersed away from the average.

The presentation of the average ± SD allows the readers to calculate the percentage of LDL-C values within portions of the graph. Figure 4–3 illustrates the distribution of

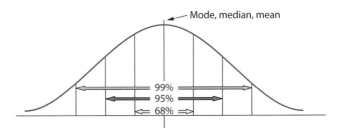

Mode, median, mean

99%
95%
68%

Figure 4–3. Histogram of LDL-C normal distribution with standard deviations +/– 15 mg/dL.

LDL-C within one, two, and three SDs from the mean in a data set that has normal distribution of the values. As a rule, ~68% of the LDL-C values would be in ±1 SD, ~95% in ±2 SDs, and ~99% in ±3 SDs. Using Figure 4–1, the average LDL-C is 145 ± 15 mg/dL. Based on these numbers, 68% of the LDL-C values are in the range of 130 to 160 mg/dL, 95% between 115 and 175 mg/dL, and 99% between 100 and 190 mg/dL. In Figure 4–2, the mean ± SD is 145 ± 5 mg/dL with corresponding values of 140 to 150 mg/dL, 135 to 155 mg/dL, and 130 to 160 mg/dL, respectively. Notice that even though the average of both LDL-C data sets is the same, 95% of the LDL-C values are in the range of 115 to 175 mg/dL in Figure 4–1, but between 135 and 155 mg/dL in Figure 4–2. SD allows for the readers to assess more than just the mean for a set of data.

Although SD is commonly used, some investigators may present the standard error of the mean (SEM), which is calculated as SD divided by the square root of the sample size (SD / $\sqrt{n}$).[123,125,126] As seen by this formula, SEM is smaller than SD, which implies a smaller dispersion of the data points away from the average. Presenting SEM instead of SD may occur when the investigators want the reader to interpret a small dispersion of the data from the mean value instead of a large variance from the mean if SD was presented. While SD measures the deviation of the individual values from the mean of the sample, SEM measures the deviation of the individual sample means from the mean of the population.[123] SEM identifies the variability in the population; 95% of the time, the true mean of the population lies within two SEMs of the sample mean.[126] At times, SEM is used appropriately, while at most times SEM is incorrectly presented.[126] Readers should be aware of these distinctions and interpret the data accordingly.

Inferential statistics are used to determine if a statistical difference is present between the intervention and control groups. A **p-value** is calculated based on trial results and statistical tests; afterward, the p-value is compared to the **alpha (α)-value** established prior to the beginning of the trial[122,124] (see Statistical Significance versus Clinical Difference later in this chapter for further discussion). The selection of the statistical test depends on the data being parametric (i.e., normal distribution) versus nonparametric. Typically, continuous data are assessed via parametric statistics; common tests are Student's t-test, analysis of variance (ANOVA), and analysis of covariance (ANCOVA). Nonparametric tests are used for nominal and ordinal data; examples are chi-square (χ^2) and Mann-Whitney U test.[94,122] A multitude of other statistical analytical procedures are available. An analysis of all research articles in six common pharmacy journals published during 2001 identified that chi-square (χ^2) test, Student's t-test, and ANOVA as the three most common statistical tests used.[127] Chapter 8 is devoted to a more in-depth discussion of statistical analyses.

Other statistical terms encountered while reading clinical trials are independent versus paired and one-tailed versus two-tailed statistical analysis. A paired analysis involves the same subject compared to themselves or to a similar matched subject.[120,128] For example, measuring the mean change in LDL-C from baseline to 12 weeks within the same subject receiving simvastatin would be a paired analysis. Analyzing the mean difference in the LDL-C reduction after 12 weeks between two independent groups, one being treated with simvastatin and the other with atorvastatin, would be considered an independent group test. Two two-tailed (also known as two-sided) statistical tests are used for trials in which investigators are not sure in which direction the primary endpoint will be affected by the intervention. These tests analyze the results in both directions, for positive or negative effects in comparison to the control.[114] Two-tailed tests are more common because the direction of change (and the degree) is not known.[30,114] For example, a two-tailed test is used for an investigational drug compared to placebo to treat elevated LDL-C. The investigators do not know the effect of the intervention on the LDL-C levels (i.e., the levels can increase or decrease relative to the placebo). A one-tailed test is primarily used in a study in which the direction of the effect of the intervention and active control (e.g., another medication, but not placebo, such as a noninferiority study) is known or can only go in one direction. The intent of this study type is to measure the difference in effect between the two groups more precisely. Some investigators have used a one-tailed test to determine differences in LDL-C changes in patients receiving statins. Prior research has documented the LDL-C lowering effects of atorvastatin and simvastatin being compared to other medications or placebo. Since these research results are available, a one-tailed test could be used to increase the statistical accuracy of detecting a difference in effect between the two statins in lowering LDL-C.

Type I and II Errors/Power Analysis

A clinical trial is conducted to test a research hypothesis that a difference in effect exists between the intervention and control treatments. Before the trial begins, the investigators develop a null hypothesis (H_0; no difference between the groups) and research hypothesis (H_1; a difference is present between the groups). The trial is conducted and the investigators measure the difference in effect between the groups (if any). If a difference is present, this could actually be due to the intervention or happen by random chance (error).[119,120] Hypothesis testing is conducted to examine how likely any observed difference between the intervention and control would be due to chance if H_0 were true. As the trial results diverge farther and farther from the finding of no difference, H_0 is rejected (i.e., failure to accept H_0) between the intervention and control groups.[120]

Two types of errors are possible in hypothesis testing (see Table 4–7). A Type I error can occur when H_0 is falsely rejected and H_1 is falsely accepted. Thus, the investigators are stating a difference in effect was measured even though there really is no difference between the intervention and control groups (also known as a false-positive finding).[96,112,114,124] On the other hand, a Type II error can occur when H_0 is falsely accepted and H_1 is falsely rejected. In this case, the investigators are stating no difference in effect is present between the intervention and control even though there really is a difference between the groups (also known as a false-negative finding).[71,114,124,129]

TABLE 4–7. TYPE I AND TYPE II ERRORS POSSIBILITIES

Error Type	Action/Decision	Interpretation
Type I	Statistical difference calculated, even though it is not really present; reject H_0	H_0 is really true, but was rejected, which leads to a false-positive result; the probability equals the α-error rate; there is one reason for a Type I error: chance
Type II	No statistical difference calculated, even though there is one; fail-to-reject ("accept") H_0	H_0 is really false, should be rejected but was accepted, which leads to a false-negative result; the probability equals the β-error rate; there are two reasons for a Type II error: chance or small sample size

Investigators attempt to control for Type I and II error occurrence by setting limits on the probability of these occurring. The only reason that a Type I error can occur is by chance. Since no research is error proof, methods are usually developed to allow up to a 5% probability that chance was the reason a difference in effect was measured between the intervention and control. The process of setting the probability of a Type I error (false-positive result) to occur no greater than 5% of the time is termed as establishing the α-value.[112,114,124] This is also referred to as setting the statistical significance to 0.05, but can also be phrased as setting the α rate at 0.05. Another phrase commonly used to state the α-value is: p-values < 0.05 are considered to be statistically significant. Most clinical trials use an α rate of 0.05; however, a few trials may use a more conservative α of 0.01. The latter rate indicates the investigators are more stringent by reducing the possibility of a Type I error to 1%. However, setting $\alpha = 0.1$ is too relaxed and permits the Type I error possibility to be very high (at 10%). The α rate is a measure of how willing the researchers are to accept the chance of making a Type I error.[119] With the α rate at 0.05, this is indicating that in one of 20 trials, a difference in effect being measured between the groups can be due to chance.[71,112] An α rate of 0.002 indicates that in two out of 1000 trials, a difference in the measured effect between groups can be due to chance. When researchers are interpreting the results of the study, they will compare the probability of making an error (p-value) to the acceptable rate of error (α). Thus, the smaller the p-values, the less likely that chance (error) was the reason for finding the differences. Also, the p-value can be expressed as the probability of rejecting a true H_0.[122] This is explained in Statistical Significance versus Clinical Difference later in the chapter.

The probability of making a Type II error is referred to as beta [β].[71,114,129] Although investigators want to avoid a Type II error, appropriately designed clinical trials allow this error (false-negative) to occur no greater than 20% of the time.[71,129] Even though investigators want to avoid making both Type I and Type II errors, they are more willing to make a Type II error than a Type I error for a few reasons. A Type II error may be easier to determine than a Type I error (specifically in studies with no power analysis and/or too small of a sample size).[119] Also, Type I errors have the potential of being more dangerous in terms of the possible direct effects on patients (see next paragraph). Therefore, this is why the α rate is set lower than the β rate. Investigators, in designing the clinical trial, aim to balance the possibility of Type I and Type II errors knowing that decreasing the probability of one error may increase the probability of the other error occurring.

Making a Type I error means a difference in effect was measured by chance but really no difference in effect exists between the two groups. The danger of using a therapy no different than the control is more serious when the control is a placebo versus an active therapy. A Type II error indicates no difference was measured between the two groups. If the control group is another therapy, then the intervention is shown to be no different. If the control is a placebo, then the intervention may not be considered a therapy to treat patients. Although the false-negative result is a concern (i.e., a useful therapy may not be used), this is less severe than a false-positive result (i.e., using a therapy that really is no difference in effect than the placebo control but was found to be by chance).

A Type II error can occur by either chance or small sample size in which the latter is usually the reason if the error occurs.[114] The ultimate goal of each clinical trial is to ensure the difference in effect size is properly measured between the intervention and control groups, which require a sufficient sample size.[71] One method for the investigators to ensure a sufficient number of subjects are enrolled in the trial is by conducting a power analysis. The **power** of a study is defined as the ability to detect a difference in the outcome between the intervention and control if a difference truly exists. Power is calculated from the β-error rate (power = $1 - \beta$).[113,129] As seen from this formula, the lower the β-error rate, the higher the power. Increasing the sample size then reduces the β-error rate, increases study power, and reduces the chance of a false-negative result.[113] In addition, the magnitude of difference in the effect that can be detected between the intervention and control groups is related to the sample size; smaller differences in the effect between the intervention and control can be detected with larger sample sizes.[21,113]

Another factor important to ensure a clinical trial has the power to detect differences in effect is estimating the absolute difference in the effect (δ) between the intervention and control groups.[25] This value is not as easily determined as the two other rates; δ is usually based on prior preliminary research results or even consensus discussion among the researchers (i.e., educated guess).[113] As an example, the CONDOR investigators[54] used prior research results to assume the primary endpoint incidence to be 1.1% for the intervention, while 2.3% for the control at month 6 of therapy. In this study, δ is calculated to be 1.2% (2.3% minus 1.1% equals 1.2%).

The sample size needed is influenced by the α-, β-, and δ-values. The purpose of the sample size calculation is to provide sufficient power to be able to reject H_0 established for the clinical trial primary endpoint if it is false and should be rejected.[71] Hopefully, a clinical trial with an appropriate sample size will not lead to erroneously detecting a difference in effect when there is no real difference (Type I error), but also have a degree of certainty that the true difference in effects was not missed (Type II error).[112] In theory, a trial having an appropriate sample size increases the precision of estimating the difference in effect (effect size) of the intervention compared to the control.[17] The total number of subjects completing the trial should be similar to the actual sample size calculation for the study to have appropriate power.[113] Normally, the investigators increase the sample size by some factor above the number calculated to be necessary (previous research can be helpful in determining that number) to account for subject attrition and therapy nonadherence. In addition, investigators can use the study results and conduct an after-the-study calculation to confirm an appropriate sample size was included.

RESULTS

After the methods section, the results of the clinical trial are presented. This section contains **primary and secondary endpoint** results and other useful information, which includes patient demographics, dropout information, and safety information. This section is to be critically appraised to verify if the study objective was met, based on the data, but also to evaluate the other types of outcomes that may have occurred. Often, data are tabulated or arranged in histogram or line graph format to provide readers with a visual interpretation of the study results that may be minimally discussed within the text of the manuscript.

Subject Demographics

The first type of information provided in the results section describes the subjects actually enrolled and randomized in the clinical trial.[24] A general overview of the average subject is described, and is usually presented in a table of demographic information.[130] Typical information in the table includes average age, gender ratio, disease states, and/or drug therapy use among the study participants at the time of enrollment that could affect the interpretation of the primary endpoint. In addition, any additional lifestyle factors that can affect the endpoint(s) or trial outcome(s) may be described, such as the number of subjects who smoke, amount of caffeine intake, etc.

The patient baseline demographic data need to be compared between treatment groups to ensure the groups are as similar as possible. The groups should not have any significant differences if proper randomization techniques are incorporated by the study investigators, but a few differences can still occur due to chance.[17] Significant dissimilarities between the groups that could contribute to differences in the outcome between the groups need to be closely scrutinized. If the patient baseline differences are substantial, a confounding variable is present and the study investigators must analyze the results to determine if these differences have affected the outcome of the study. Otherwise, the resulting interpretation of results and their subsequent applications to practice may be flawed.[114]

An example of baseline subject demographics is illustrated by select patient informa-tion from the CONDOR trial. The celecoxib and omeprazole plus diclofenac groups both had a similar number of females (83% and 81%, respectively) and subjects with OA as the primary diagnosis (84% and 84%, respectively). Average age, ethnicity, region of origin, and critical laboratory markers (e.g., hemoglobin, hematocrit) were also evenly matched.[54] The disproportion of females enrolled in the study and the abundance of OA diagnoses may be concerning to the beginning reader. However, the similar number of subjects between the two groups is more important in this study, so no differences exist between the two groups. Sometimes the disproportion of gender enrollment in a trial reflects the true prevalence in the population at large (e.g., more males with cardiovascu-lar disease). Nevertheless, for trials that involve disease states in which gender is not a prespecified risk factor, each group should consist of similar number of subjects and not be skewed in one direction for any risk factor, as this sample-based anomaly could affect interpretation and application of study results.

Subject Dropouts/Adherence

After the baseline subject information, data regarding the follow-up (i.e., subject dropout or attrition) and adherence should be presented. Not all subjects randomized in a clinical trial complete the entire duration, at which time they are then termed a study dropout or lost to follow-up.[70] Reasons vary for discontinuing study participation and include lack of desire to continue, subject relocation (e.g., moving to another city), difficulty finding transportation to clinic visits, subject protocol violation, side effects, and death. Also, not all subjects will be compliant with the therapy. Not accounting for the number of dropouts and nonadherence can have an effect on interpreting the trial results.[70,131,132] Thus, the investigators need to report the number of subjects and major reasons for discontinuing the study, adherence rates, and the techniques of assessing the data for the readers to draw appropriate conclusions about the intervention under study and subsequent trial results. All too often clinicians and industry personnel focus on the efficacy of a medica-tion, but pharmacists in particular should clearly analyze the costs of better efficacy in terms of patient safety. Dropout data can be very revealing about the overall tolerability of a medication, which can illuminate important safety risks associated with emerging thera-pies compared to conventional therapies. However, readers should be cautioned when evaluating safety data within a study that it may not be adequately powered to draw con-clusions about overall adverse effects.

The impact of attrition on the overall study results is dependent on the magnitude of subject discontinuations. A few subjects dropping out of the study may not cause a sub-stantial difference in the results, whereas a sizable percentage of attrition may alter the study results significantly. No threshold of dropout/attrition rates has been established that deems the trial results to be of no clinical value. Similar to demographic information, attrition rates should be analyzed to ensure similarity between treatment arms. Attrition rates of 60% among both groups of a clinical trial, although not ideal, is much less concerning than a study where attrition rates are 10% in one group and 50% in another. Disproportionate attrition rates can be an indicator of significant medication safety considerations for the clinician and should generate further investigation, particularly if safety endpoints were not a primary endpoint of the study.

Frequently, the study results are analyzed using data collected from all randomized subjects, regardless of whether they completed the entire study duration (i.e., results from dropouts are not discarded, but are considered to be treatment failures). This technique is referred to as the **intention-to-treat** (ITT) principle (see Chapter 5 for more on ITT and **per-protocol** [PP]). Even in cases where the subject may not have taken even one dose of the medication under investigation, these results are still included in the ITT analysis (i.e., once randomized, always analyzed). The advantage of the ITT analysis is this analysis better mimics real-life application of an intervention into practice because, similar to real life, all subjects in a clinical trial may not complete therapy as prescribed.[131] However, a concern with the ITT analysis is that data from subjects discontinuing a trial early may bias the analysis. This is of considerable importance for an endpoint measurement that worsens over time (e.g., cognitive function in subjects with dementia). The last score obtained in a subject discontinuing the trial early may suggest a better response than the last score obtained if this subject discontinued later in the trial.[133]

At times, the study results are analyzed via both ITT and the PP procedure. The latter term refers to analyzing data only from subjects completing the trial per the protocol. The advantage of this technique is for determining the effects of the intervention in subjects who followed the study protocol and completed the entire course of therapy. The ITT and PP analytical methods are simply models under which the study results are analyzed. The ITT analysis can be thought of a worst-case scenario model, whereas the PP analysis can be thought of as the best-case scenario model. The ITT analysis is typically favored by clinicians or readers of studies when analyzing results due to the desire to determine whether statistically and clinically significant differences are present between the two groups under worst-case scenario conditions. Such results are much stronger than demonstrating statistical or clinical significance under best-case scenario conditions as patients in the greater population are not completely adherent to prescriber instructions. Optimally, study investigators present both ITT and PP results; the desire is to see no significant differences between the ITT and PP results. If a significant difference exists, this can be an indirect indicator of differences in attrition rates between treatment arms that are represented in the ITT analysis. Furthermore, clinical trials including only the PP results are to be scrutinized more because results from all subjects are not assessed, which could result in an overestimation of treatment effects in favor of a treatment arm with high attrition rates.

An example of analyzing study data according to ITT and PP methods follows. The effect of caffeine therapy on the Epworth Sleepiness Scale (ESS) score in patients with Parkinson disease was assessed.[134] This scoring scheme is based on questionnaire responses to eight items and the perceived propensity of patients to fall asleep based on theoretical situations (0 = no chance of sleeping, 3 = high chance of sleeping; total score range: 0 to 24). The primary ITT analysis indicated that caffeine dosed at 200 mg twice daily (n = 30) had no significant effect on ESS scores compared to placebo (n = 31) at 6 weeks (difference of –1.71 points; 95% CI –3.57, 0.13). However, statistical significance was determined upon PP analysis for the same endpoint and treatment (difference of –1.97 points; 95% CI –3.87, –0.05), leading the investigators to conclude that caffeine therapy produces marginal but insignificant improvement in daytime sleepiness in patients with Parkinson disease. The difference in results between the ITT and PP populations is tied to the exclusion of four subjects who violated study protocol (two in each group). This example exemplifies that even very small and equal subject attrition or exclusion can significantly affect the interpretation of study results, particularly in studies with small sample sizes, and underscores the importance of analyzing both ITT and PP study results to make the most measured conclusions regarding treatment effect.[134]

Endpoints/Safety

A critical component of the results section is the primary endpoint results. These results can be displayed as tables, graphs, or other illustrations. The information should be presented clearly and completely, using transparent and unbiased methods. In addition, the investigators need to explain the results and present probability values (i.e., p-values). Results of secondary endpoints should follow and are presented in a fashion similar to the primary endpoints; however, endpoints other than the primary endpoint may not be adequately powered to detect differences between the intervention and control. Therefore, if statistically significant results occur with secondary endpoints, the results may be due to chance. Endpoints other than the primary endpoints should be adequately powered to draw meaningful conclusions regarding use in practice and are generally considered hypothesis generating.[24]

One issue to consider in evaluating the results in some clinical trials is whether medication dosing titration is allowed in the methods. The final medication dose of one group may be maximized while the other group did not require maximum doses, leading the investigators to make a conclusion based on misleading information. Thus, readers of a clinical trial should analyze the final doses in each group at the end of the trial. Ideally, both groups should have similar dose titrations at the end of the study instead of one group receiving near the maximum daily dose versus the other group not requiring much of a dose increase. Safety assessments or tolerability of all therapies should be included in the results section.[24] Investigators need to implement valid methods of defining, collecting, and analyzing these results. As with the secondary endpoints, the study may not be powered sufficiently to definitively quantify the safety/tolerability of the intervention. In addition, the frequency and severity of these results may be dissimilar to those observed in clinical practice. Investigators need to monitor the subjects closely and collect these data.[42] Other factors that need to be considered include the equipotency of doses of medications being studied, clinical trial duration, sample size, and exclusion of selected subjects from being enrolled in the trial, particularly exclusion of persons who are otherwise qualified to be part of the study according to the inclusion and exclusion criteria.

Surrogate Endpoints

Investigators of some clinical trials select a primary endpoint that can be classified as a surrogate endpoint,[135] which is described as "a measure of the efficacy of a treatment can be defined as laboratory values (e.g., HDL-C/LDL-C), symptoms (e.g., pain), or clinical parameters (e.g., blood pressure) that are employed as a substitute for a clinical endpoint (e.g., morbidity, mortality). Here it is assumed that changes in the surrogate endpoint can be directly translated into changes in the definitive clinical endpoint."[136] The primary reason surrogate endpoints are selected for clinical trials is to quickly measure an effect at a lower overall cost.[136] The established efficacy and other data collected from trials measuring the surrogate endpoint provide the rationale for larger trials with clinical endpoints (i.e., MI, stroke, death), which typically are more costly and time consuming.[26] In certain circumstances, conducting a study using surrogate endpoints versus clinical endpoints may be more ethical, particularly if a placebo is being used as the control therapy. The following conditions should be fulfilled before a surrogate endpoint is considered a valid substitute for a clinical endpoint: convenience (easily and readily assessable), well-established relationship between the surrogate and clinical outcomes (e.g., hemoglobin A_{1C} and risk/severity of diabetes), and determination of clinical benefit as a result of changes in the surrogate endpoint.[136]

The primary limitation of surrogate endpoints is illustrated by the following example. Investigators of the ILLUMINATE trial reported a significant increase in mean HDL-C with adding the investigational agent torcetrapib to atorvastatin versus atorvastatin alone (+72% versus +2%, respectively) along with change in mean LDL-C (−25% versus +3%, respectively) after 12 months of therapy. One would expect these two changes in cholesterol levels to reduce the risk of cardiovascular events (e.g., nonfatal MI, stroke). However, the incidence of a major cardiovascular event was significantly higher in patients treated with torcetrapib than atorvastatin alone (6.2% versus 5%, respectively).[137] This example illustrates that beneficial surrogate endpoint results do not always translate into positive clinical outcomes.

Subgroup Analysis

Investigators often analyze the results of subsets of the study subjects, as divided into various groups that often include gender, age, and presence of diseases or other complicating factors (i.e., diabetes versus no diabetes).[138] Reasons to analyze the results in these subgroups vary, but usually relate to providing additional information in these specific patient types as opposed to the overall trial results from all randomized subjects. For example, trial investigators may analyze the results according to various demographics that include age (i.e., <65 years and >65 years), race/ethnicity, or gender.

Although the investigators may be able to obtain more information from a trial by using subgroup analysis, limitations and other issues need to be recognized.[24,80,102,138,139] A few prerequisites should be present before subgroup analyses are conducted. The clinical trial should be well designed with sound study methods. A subgroup analysis should be defined prior to the initiation of the trial and have documented justification (e.g., past studies suggest a benefit in that patient group). Subgroup analyses should come from trials that are internally valid with well-defined study methods (e.g., ITT, randomization, blinding). For results from studies that are sufficiently flawed, there is no reason to perform subgroup analysis. Additionally, data analysis should only be conducted from those studies in which the primary endpoint was statistically significant; otherwise, investigators may be perceived to be on a fishing expedition, searching for statistically significant results.[138] Furthemore, the investigator may have conducted a multitude of subgroup analyses and reported only the statistically significant results. As the number of statistical evaluations on a data set increases, the likelihood of finding a statistical difference by chance alone increases.[138] Therefore, multiple subgroup analyses on the same data set should be avoided, unless authors can demonstrate that they have powered the endpoint for the multiple analyses *a priori* and/or have adjusted error rates statistically to control for multiple comparisons. Also, the power of the subgroup analysis is reduced, since results from a smaller number of subjects are analyzed as compared to the entire trial sample; this reduced power could lead to false positive conclusions (i.e., Type I error).[138,139] Additionally, to avoid making invalid conclusions, the ITT data set of the trial should be utilized to ensure that all dropouts are included for all treatment arms.[138] Subgroup analyses can be helpful in determining future research targets, but, unless powered appropriately, should not be used as a basis for therapeutic decision making.

Readers of clinical trials need to be aware of subgroup analyses being conducted and the potential misleading claims reported by the trial authors. For instance, an evaluation was conducted on clinical trials published during 2007 in which 41% of these trials claimed subgroup effects. However, the credibility of the claims was low. The results of this study are not to discourage conducting subgroup analyses, but authors need to be more informative and descriptive of the methods and interpretations of subgroup analyses.[140]

Overinterpretation of subgroup results can occur.[135] Reducing the sample size via a subgroup analysis can lead to a positive result that may have occurred by chance.[80,131,138,139] An illustration of this effect was documented by the African-American Antiplatelet Stroke Prevention Study (AAASPS),[141] which was conducted in response to the subgroup analysis of Ticlopidine Aspirin Stroke Study (TASS).[142] The TASS investigators documented a lower incidence of nonfatal stroke or death from any cause in subjects with recent transient or mild persistent focal cerebral or retinal ischemia taking ticlopidine compared to aspirin (17% versus 19%; p = 0.048). In addition to this overall study result, the investigators reported fewer cases of stroke and death with ticlopidine compared to aspirin in a subgroup analysis of African-Americans enrolled in this trial. The AAASPS results documented a slightly higher incidence of the composite endpoint (recurrent stroke, MI, or vascular death) in patients taking ticlopidine compared to aspirin (14.8% versus 12.4%; p = 0.12). Although the study designs of these two studies were not identical, the AAASPS results serve as an example to the limitations of selecting therapy based on subgroup analysis. Thus, practitioners should be aware that although subgroup analysis may document greater benefits in selected individuals, the differences in effect may be due to chance or other factors.

Ancillary versus Adjunctive Therapies

Clinical trials are designed to have almost identical groups with the only difference between the groups being the assignment to the intervention or control. At times, the study design may allow **ancillary therapy** to be included, in which subjects can take another therapy that can distort or confound interpretation of the results.[70] The effect of the ancillary therapy on the study results needs to be assessed and included in the study evaluation. However, readers should not confuse ancillary therapy with **adjunctive therapy**. Some studies may include, in the methods, an adjunctive therapy, which all participants receive as treatment, while ancillary therapy is not equally distributed between the intervention and control groups. Thus, any significant difference in effect between the outcomes measured between the groups should be due to the therapies under investigation. For example, a clinical trial investigated the effect of cinnamon extract on glycemic markers in patients with diabetes.[143] Study subjects received either cinnamon extract or placebo; all subjects were taking an adjunctive sulfonylurea agent each day. Although sulfonylureas can lower blood glucose levels, all subjects in the trial received this therapy. Since therapy to control blood glucose should not be withheld in patients with diabetes, the use of a sulfonylurea in this trial was appropriate and was similar between the two groups. However, ancillary therapy would occur if patients were allowed to take any other agent that could alter blood glucose levels at their own discretion, resulting in a difference between the two groups. This would create a situation where the two groups were not similar, besides one group taking the intervention and the other taking the control (i.e., would violate the principles of a controlled clinical trial).

DISCUSSION/CONCLUSION

The primary purpose of the discussion/conclusion is to evaluate and/or interpret the results of the clinical trial. Investigators should begin with a summary of the key findings of the study. Potential explanations of the study results should be addressed, in addition to discussing internal and external validity of outcomes.[24] The investigators should also interpret the trial results in comparison with results of other similarly designed studies. Also, the trial may be discussed in comparison to other trials assessing the intervention or the disease state under investigation. This is also where clinical trial limitations are identified and discussed.[24] Even though all clinical trials have limitations, these may vary from minor to those that seriously hinder the usefulness of the results, including completely invalidating the study. The discussion section should also address the clinical importance of the clinical trial results and how these results should be used in practice. All of this information should allow the reader to understand the application of the clinical trial results in practice. However, this section needs to be read just as carefully as the other sections, because it can contain biased wording. In addition, authors may only discuss selected items in relationship to the clinical trial.[80]

The investigators should ensure that strategies are included within the study design to minimize biases that may occur. Some of the strategies can include blinding, randomization, and appropriate inclusion/exclusion criteria. In addition, investigators should not be biased in interpreting the results of the trial. Readers should determine the degree that the study results compare with patients encountered in practice. One of the most commonly cited criticisms of clinical trials by clinicians is the lack of external validity of the trials and may be one explanation for the underuse of reportedly favorable treatment options in clinical trials by clinicians.[144] Although some investigators may report beneficial results of an intervention under investigation, the patient population in the clinical trial may be so dissimilar to patients encountered in practice that clinicians are not convinced that the favorable results may be beneficial in their patient population. Several issues may potentially affect the external validity of the clinical trial and should be evaluated to assess the effects of the results in practice. These include the setting of the trial, selection of patients, characteristics of randomized patients, differences between the trial protocol and routine practice, outcome measures, follow-up, and adverse effects of treatment.[144] If the characteristics of the patients and setting are very different from those encountered in practice, the clinical usefulness of the reported information may be questionable.

Study strengths and limitations should be addressed in the discussion section. All research does have inherent limitations and these usually are identified by the investigators in this section of the study. Potential limitations may include small sample size, short duration of the study, endpoint assessment techniques, or other factors that hinder the clinical usefulness of the study. The investigators should also address methods to circumvent trial limitations in subsequent clinical studies. There is no minimum or maximum number of limitations that investigators should address; a thorough discussion of the limitations should be provided so that readers can determine the applicability of the trial results to their patient population.

Comparison of the current study to previous studies should be conducted. According to the results of one study, discussion sections of trial reports were lacking complete analysis of previous clinical trial results.[145] A total of 33 randomized trials were identified in 19 issues of leading medical journals (e.g., *Annals of Internal Medicine, JAMA*). The authors of four reports claimed that their study was a first-of-a-kind study; however, reports of similar trials were located for one of these studies. In three of the reports, systematic reviews of earlier trials were mentioned; however, no attempts to incorporate the results of the new trial with the existing results were identified in the remaining 27 reports. The results of other trials should be included to allow the reader to assess the results of the current trial in context to previous trial results. The readers can determine if the study is a first-of-a-kind study that adds substantial information to a topic or is a me-too study that adds no new information to existing knowledge. The discussion section should also address future concerns and unanswered questions.

The conclusion section should provide an overall research recommendation to the readers. The investigators' conclusion should focus on the primary endpoint results, especially if no statistically significant differences between the intervention and control groups were observed, rather than favorable, secondary endpoint results. Conclusions should be limited to only that information discussed in previous sections of the trial; no new information should be discussed in this section. Also, the conclusions should be aligned with the results of the trial. Investigators should not make erroneous conclusions that are not supported by the results of the trial.

CLINICAL TRIAL RESULT INTERPRETATION

Statistical Significance versus Clinical Difference

8 *Interpreting the p-values correctly is crucial in evaluating a controlled clinical trial; not all statistically significant p-values are clinically important. The magnitude of difference in effect between the intervention and control cannot be determined solely with the p-value.* Once the clinical trial is completed, the investigators calculate a p-value for the endpoints using the collected study results and statistical tests. The p-value is an abbreviation for probability-value and is compared to the α-value established prior to the beginning of the clinical trial (*a priori*) that serves as the benchmark to which p-values are compared to determine if statistical significance is present. Also, since the entire population is not included, the investigators have to estimate the difference in effect from the sample.[119,120,146] Without statistical analysis, the likelihood of chance being the reason for any measured difference in effect is not known.[114] A p-value for the primary endpoint that is less than the α-value indicates H_0 is rejected and a statistically significant difference is declared between the intervention and control groups. This also indicates chance alone was not likely the reason that a difference in effect was measured. H_0 is accepted (failed to be rejected) with a p-value equal to or greater than the α-value and no statistically significant difference is declared.[120,146]

Statistical significance does not automatically mean a clinical difference in the effect between the intervention and control groups.[147] (See next section regarding the assessment of clinical difference.) The reader needs to make a decision in determining if the intervention is worth using instead of the control therapy, which can be dependent on the judgment and experiences of the reader (i.e., assessing both internal and external validity). Not all statistically significant studies have clinically different results (see Figure 4–4).

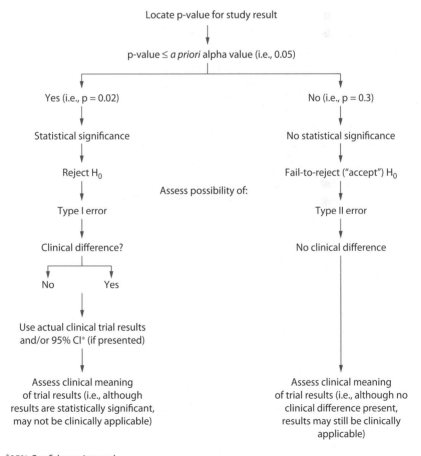

*95% Confidence interval.

Figure 4–4. Determining statistical significance, clinical difference, and clinical meaningfulness.

A p-value less than the α-value only represents the probability that a true H_0 has been rejected. In other words, the p-value can be translated into: "what is the probability of the difference in effect between the intervention and control due to chance?"[119] Lower p-values indicate a lower probability that chance alone could be the reason a difference in effect was measured between the intervention and control. Alternatively stated, what is the chance of observing this difference if there really was no difference between the two groups?[114] Recall that a Type I error is possible after rejecting H_0; the results may be statistically significant due to chance alone.

Another paramount issue in understanding clinical trials is that the p-value does not express the magnitude of difference in effect between the intervention and control.[120] Statistically significant results simply signify that the **alternative hypothesis** (H_1) is accepted. H_1 states a difference in the effect is present between the intervention and control. From this information, the reader cannot determine complex quantitative differences in effect (i.e., clinical difference between the intervention and control groups).[114,122]

In addition, specific p-values should be stated in the text of the article (i.e., $p = 0.0012$ instead of $p < 0.05$) to be more informative and helpful to the reader.[114,120] Also, all p-values should be presented in conjunction with associated endpoint results (i.e., the clinical trial concluded that drug A lowered mean DBP more than placebo, -12 versus -3 mmHg, respectively [$p = 0.001$] as opposed to the clinical trial concluded that drug A lowered mean DBP more than placebo [$p = 0.001$]). Readers should scrutinize study data that presents p-values without endpoint results (naked p-values). Such a situation should prompt the reader to ask: "Were the endpoint results not presented with the p-value because the actual difference in the effect was minimal?" Without the endpoint results being presented, statistical significance alone can be concluded with the p-value; clinical differences cannot be assessed without accompanying endpoint results. See next sections for further discussion.

Assessing Clinical Difference

Two critical items needed to assess clinical difference between the intervention and control groups of a clinical trial are the p-value and actual study results used to calculate the p-value. A fundamental first step of determining clinical difference in a given trial begins with determining if statistical significance exists (i.e., $p < a\ priori$ α-value) (see Figure 4–4). The reader must keep in mind that clinical difference is predicated on statistical significance. In other words, clinical difference between the intervention and control cannot exist with study outcome data if the results are not statistically significant. The second step in assessing clinical differences is evaluating the results used to calculate the p-value. The reader must analyze the magnitude of endpoint difference between the intervention and control results.[114,147] Once a reader determines statistical significance is present with the given study data, no magical formula is available to conclude whether clinical difference exists between the intervention and control.[120] The remainder of the process is based on clinical knowledge and experience, and may be relative in the reader's opinion to whether clinical difference is present or not. For example, an antihypertensive therapy lowers mean DBP by 14 mmHg versus 3 mmHg with placebo in subjects with a mean baseline DBP of 98 mmHg. In this case, the results are clinically different due to 11 mmHg average difference and subjects are achieving goal DBP values from baseline (< 85 mmHg). However, atorvastatin lowering mean LDL-C by 1.7% greater than simvastatin (37.1% versus 35.4%; p = 0.0097[72]) can be considered not clinically different in subjects with a mean baseline LDL-C of 181 mg/dL. The mean LDL-C was reduced by <2% with atorvastatin compared to simvastatin, a difference that most likely is not associated with producing clinical differences in effect. In addition, the actual mean LDL-C lowering was almost identical (66 mg/dL) and the mean LDL-C level at study end was <116 mg/dL in both groups.

Some readers may consider the trial results to be clinically different while others may not. In fact, two people may have different conclusions after reading the same clinical trial. This situation is very common when interpreting clinical trials in health care practice. In response, readers must justify their own conclusion regarding their decision of clinical difference. A few suggestions and examples are provided to assist in determining clinical difference.

Understanding the instrument that was used in measuring the endpoint is important in assessing clinically significant differences in trials. For example, ordinal data typically uses scales or ranking (e.g., pain, depression scales).[121] Thus, the definitions of the minimum and maximum numbers of these scales need to be known. As an example, investigators of a hypothetical clinical trial concluded that glucosamine sulfate (500 mg three times a day) reduced pain greater than placebo in men with OA of the knee. Pain intensity difference at rest was assessed by a 10-point visual analog scale (0 = no pain; 10 = severe pain). The median scores were 3.6 with placebo versus 3.3 with glucosamine (p = 0.03) at the end of the trial. Although results are statistically significant between glucosamine and placebo, the difference in scores between these two groups is minimal, only 0.3 points on a 10-point scale. Stating a clinical difference between glucosamine and placebo would be considered incorrect.

Another issue to consider is that clinical trials with too large of a sample size (i.e., overpowered) lead to smaller p-values versus those with smaller sample sizes.[113,120] The magnitude of the p-value is dependent on sample size; small differences in effect can be statistically significant with large sample size.[114] Thus, statistically significant results can occur even though a small absolute difference in effect is present. An example of this issue is a clinical trial that compared esomeprazole (n = 2624) versus lansoprazole (n = 2617). The primary endpoint, incidence of erosive esophagitis healing, was statistically significant in favor of esomeprazole (92.6% versus 88.8%; p = 0.0001).[148] The investigators (and marketing advertisements) conclude esomeprazole to be superior to lansoprazole, although the absolute difference in healing was only 4% between these two drugs. In addition, a significant number of subjects in each group (> 88%) experienced erosive esophagitis healing. Even when the results were statistically different, readers can debate whether the difference in effect is clinically different.

A data assessment technique that can be misleading is converting a continuous endpoint measure into a dichotomous value. For instance, blood pressure (continuous value) is measured after an intervention (rofecoxib—previously withdrawn from the market) and control (celecoxib) are administered. Those subjects with a blood pressure value above a predefined cut-off point are classified as being hypertensive (nominal data because subject has a blood pressure value below or above this cut-off point). Significantly more subjects taking rofecoxib versus celecoxib were diagnosed with systolic hypertension (17% versus 11%, respectively; p = 0.032). However, the change in the mean for SBP values was +2.6 versus –0.5 mmHg, respectively (p = 0.007).[149] These two data sets assessed together indicate that rofecoxib may not negatively affect SBP compared to celecoxib. The actual SBP in the subjects taking rofecoxib may have just exceeded the cut-off hypertensive value (increase >20 mmHg with absolute value >140 mmHg) while just below this value for the celecoxib (i.e., 141 versus 139 mmHg, respectively). The absolute difference between these two blood pressure values is minimal (2 mmHg), but the number of subjects counted as hypertensive is different (6%). The change in SBP between these two medications does not appear to be clinically different. Even though the measured endpoints between subjects randomized to the intervention are numerically close to the control, the subjects were categorized differently based on cut-off blood pressure values. This example illustrates the potential biases of this form of data analysis and presentation.

The foundation in determining clinical difference between an intervention and control is the p-value and actual study results. Other items can assist the reader in this endeavor and include 95% **confidence intervals** (CI) and calculating measures of association; both of these are described below. However, readers must remember that not all clinical trials may have these latter two items. Thus, the importance of analyzing and interpreting p-values and the magnitude of difference between the intervention and control cannot be overemphasized.

Confidence Intervals

Many clinical trials include 95% CI with the study results, which can assist in assessing clinical difference between the intervention and control. ❾ *The use of 95% CI can assist the reader in assessing the magnitude of difference in effect between the intervention and control to apply to the population.* CI provide data that address the size of effect (e.g., mean reduction in DBP) of the intervention under investigation in a clinical trial by presenting a range that likely covers the true but unknown value.[150,151] Although the basis of accepting or rejecting H_0 is based on the p-value, a limitation of the p-value is that the magnitude of difference in effect between the intervention and control groups of a clinical trial is not known, since it is not able to be determined based on a statistical calculation.[120,147] Because of this, the use of a CI can assist in judging the clinical usefulness of the study result.[114] Clinical trials report the effect of an intervention as a point estimate, a single value that can be considered to represent the true effect (e.g., mean reduction in DBP; incidence of MI). For instance, an angiotensin-converting enzyme (ACE) inhibitor lowered mean DBP by 8 mmHg; this value would be termed the point estimate. If the study was repeated, a similar, but not exact, reduction in mean DBP may occur (e.g., −10 mmHg, −12 mmHg). The presentation of the results only as a point estimate provides the reader with limited information. Clinical trials presenting 95% CI in conjunction with the point estimate enables the readers to further critique the study results and determine the usefulness for practice.

A CI provides an indication of the outcome within the population and is interpreted as a range of values in which the true value is included. The 95% CI for an average is calculated using the SEM from the trial sample. Recalling the formula for SEM, SD is divided by the square root of the sample size ($SD/\sqrt{n}$). A 95% CI is equivalent to approximately two SEMs from the sample mean, with an exact formula: CI = mean ±1.96 * SEM. SEM is used as opposed to SD since SEM is more reflective of the population variance, while SD is indicative of the dispersion within the sample.[120,151] A 95% CI is not the only CI reported in the literature, and readers of clinical trials need to recognize the changes in the interpretation. A 99% CI indicates more confidence that the true, but unknown, endpoint value is in this range than does a 95% CI. Thus, the 99% CI range is wider in value than a 95% CI, whereas a 90% CI range is narrower (i.e., less confident).[151,152]

A 95% CI for a point estimate is a common method of data presentation. Investigators of a clinical trial reported the mean reduction in DBP with an ACE inhibitor was −11.3 mmHg (95% CI, −8.2 to −14.4 mmHg) in subjects with a mean baseline DBP of 99 mmHg. This indicates that the investigators are 95% confident that the mean DBP reduction in the population is between −8.2 and −14.4 mmHg. An important issue to recognize in interpreting a 95% CI is a lower probability for the mean reduction in DBP at the upper and lower ends of the 95% CI range compared to numbers near the point estimate value.[123] The further away a value lies from the point estimate within the 95% CI range, the lower the probability that this value is representative of the given population. A low probability exists that the ACE inhibitor lowers mean DBP in the population by only −8.2 mmHg compared to a higher probability that mean DBP reduction is closer to the point estimate of 11.3 mmHg (the same is true with the upper end of the 95% CI).

Within this trial, the ACE inhibitor was compared to hydrochlorothiazide (HCTZ) and the mean DBP reduction with HCTZ was −9.9 mmHg (95% CI, −7.5 to −13.3 mmHg). The same principles are used to interpret this 95% CI as with the ACE inhibitor 95% CI; the investigators are 95% confident that the mean reduction of DBP in the population with HCTZ is between 7.5 and 13.3 mmHg. In addition, these two 95% CI ranges can be compared to determine any difference in effect between these two agents. Since both 95% CI ranges overlap considerably, no difference in effect is concluded.[114,120,152] However, if no overlap of the 95% CI for the two groups is present, a clinical difference can be concluded.

Another common method of data presentation is calculating a 95% CI for the difference of the point estimates between two groups. In the above trial example, the point estimate of mean DBP lowering with the ACE inhibitor was –11.3 mmHg while –9.9 mmHg for HCTZ. The difference in mean DBP between these two equals –1.4 mmHg (–11.3 minus –9.9 = –1.4). The 95% CI for the difference in the point estimates is calculated to be –3.9 to +1.1 mmHg. This is interpreted as being 95% confident that the difference in mean DBP reduction can be 1.1 mmHg greater with HCTZ (i.e., –13.1 mmHg for HCTZ versus –12 mmHg for ACE inhibitor) or 3.9 mmHg greater with the ACE inhibitor (i.e., –16.9 mmHg for ACE inhibitor versus –13 mmHg for HCTZ). Notice the upper end of the 95% CI of the difference in point estimates is a positive number (+1.1 mmHg). This does not indicate the mean DBP was increased, only that the *difference* in mean DBP lowering was 1.1 mmHg greater with HCTZ compared to ACE inhibitor (i.e., –12 minus –13.1 mmHg for ACE inhibitor and HCTZ, respectively). Also, in this 95% CI is the number zero (value of equality); this indicates with 95% confidence that there is no difference in mean DBP between these two groups (i.e., –13.2 minus –13.2 mmHg for both agents equals zero). If no zero is in the 95% CI of the difference between the two point estimates, then a clinical difference in effect between the intervention and control could be concluded.

The interpretation of clinical difference using 95% CI is dependent on clinical experience and appropriate assessment. A 95% CI without a zero in the range does not always indicate a clinical difference between the intervention and control. For example, a 95% CI for mean DBP lowering in a trial comparing an ACE inhibitor and HCTZ was –1.9 to –0.5 mmHg. Even though this 95% CI range does not contain a zero, a mean difference of only 0.5 to 1.9 mmHg greater DBP lowering effect with one agent would not be considered clinically different.

Interpreting Risks and Number Needed to Treat

Another technique to critique and interpret clinical trial results is to calculate the measures of association: relative risk (RR), relative risk reduction (RRR), absolute risk reduction (ARR), and number needed to treat (NNT). ❿ *Calculating measures of association (RR, ARR, RRR, NNT) for nominal data provides further information to evaluate the meaning of controlled clinical trial results.* However, these calculations can only be performed with clinical trials designed to determine if there is a reduction in an outcome that occurs with modification of a risk factor when comparing the intervention to the

TABLE 4–8. PRESENTING NOMINAL DATA STUDY RESULTS

Group	Adverse Event	
	Yes	No
Intervention	A	B
Control	C	D

control. Examples of outcomes could include the incidence of MI, stroke, hospitalization, or death. Since the endpoint is dichotomous (i.e., occurred or did not occur), the results can be set up in a table, as illustrated in Table 4–8. As seen from Table 4–8, the subjects randomized to the intervention are represented by either A (number of subjects experiencing the outcome) or B (those without the outcome). Subjects assigned to the control group and experiencing the outcome are designated by C while those without the outcome by D.[152,153]

Table 4–9 displays the formulas to calculate the four measure of association values plus provides a description of these measures.[152,153] A description of interpreting these values follows. RR is calculated as the proportion of the intervention group experiencing the outcome divided by the proportion of the control group with the event. RR = 1 indicates no difference between the intervention and control (i.e., the incidence of the outcome was not increased or decreased with the intervention compared to control). Anytime a numerator divided by a denominator calculates to 1, these two variables are equal. RR < 1 signifies the intervention lowered the risk of the outcome compared to the control (i.e., protective effect); a lower proportion of the intervention group compared to

TABLE 4–9. MEASURES OF ASSOCIATION DESCRIPTION AND FORMULAS

Measure of Association	Description	Formula
RR	Amount of risk removed by the intervention compared to control	[A/(A + B)]/[C/(C + D)]; in other words, (% of intervention group with primary endpoint) / (% of control group with primary endpoint)
RRR	Percent of baseline risk removed	1 − RR
ARR	Percentage of subjects treated with the intervention spared the adverse outcome compared with the control	[C/(C + D)] − [A/(A + B)]; in other words, (% of control group with primary endpoint) − (% of intervention group with primary endpoint)
NNT	Number of subjects needed to be treated to prevent one adverse event. A time course is included that represents the average (or median) duration of follow-up during the trial	1/ARR

the control experienced the outcome. RR > 1 indicates the intervention increased the risk of the outcome; a greater proportion of the intervention group had the outcome compared to control. As an example, RR of death equal to 0.70 was reported in a clinical trial in which subjects were randomized to either simvastatin (n = 2221) or placebo (n = 2223).[76] RR was calculated by dividing the proportion of the subjects who died taking simvastatin (n = 182) by the proportion of those who died taking placebo (n = 256). The calculation of RR for this trial is: (182/2221)/(256/2223). RR is < 1, which indicates simvastatin lowered the risk of death by almost one-third of the baseline risk compared to placebo. RRR indicates the relative change in the outcome rate between the intervention and control groups. RRR was calculated as 30% ((1 − 0.70)*100); Thus, the risk of experiencing death was 30% lower by treating these subjects with simvastatin instead of placebo. ARR refers to the difference in the outcome rate between the intervention and control groups. A higher proportion of subjects taking placebo died (n = 256 of 2223 or 11.5%) compared to those taking simvastatin (182 of 2221 or 8.2%). ARR for death associated with simvastatin in this trial equals 3.3% (ARR = 11.5%-8.2%); thus, 3.3% of the subjects receiving simvastatin were spared death compared to placebo. NNT of this study equals 30 (NNT = 1/0.033), meaning 30 subjects need to be treated for a median of 5.4 years with simvastatin instead of placebo to prevent one case of death. The trial had a median follow-up time period of 5.4 years.

Many clinical trials present an endpoint as a relative change, which can be a misleading value. For instance, RRR of stroke associated with atorvastatin was 48% compared to placebo in this study. Although this value appears very beneficial to subjects at risk for stroke, ARR needs to be evaluated besides just the RRR value. The actual incidence of stroke was 1.5% (21 of 1428 subjects treated with atorvastatin) versus 2.8% (39 of 1409 subjects treated with placebo), which calculates to an absolute difference of 1.3% (ARR). Even though almost 50% less subjects (a relative difference) experienced a stroke with atorvastatin, this represents only a difference of 18 in a group of just over 2800 subjects.[154]

All four measures of association can be calculated for clinical trials measuring nominal data and assessed together for the reader to determine the clinical difference in effect between the intervention and control. As seen by the simvastatin example above (in addition Table 4-9), the same study result (e.g., death) can be presented using four different methods with different meanings. However, readers should not be misled by clinical trials that only present and discuss one of these values, which usually is the most appealing value (i.e., the one that seems to show the greatest difference). In fact, studies have documented that practitioners are more inclined to select a therapy presented as RRR more often than if the same study result was presented as all four values (i.e., ARR, RR, RRR, NNT).[155] Thus, investigators may be biased and selectively present the most appealing of these four values to mislead the reader into concluding a greater difference in effect between the intervention and control, even though the difference may be minimal.

CI can also be calculated for nominal endpoints presented as RR or hazard ratio (HR). The latter is used to describe risks associated with adverse events and/or mortality data. The same formula for RR is used to calculate HR, which refers to whether the hazard of the adverse event (i.e., MI, hospitalization) is lowered or increased with the intervention compared to the control.[156] According to the formula for RR (and HR), a calculated value of 1 signifies the incidence of the adverse event is equal between the intervention and control (i.e., numerator and denominator are equal, therefore, no difference).[114,152] As previously mentioned, RR < 1 signifies the intervention lowered the risk and RR > 1 is interpreted as the intervention increasing the risk of the adverse event compared to the control. Therefore, investigators of a clinical trial presenting RR (or HR) with a 95% CI that lies entirely on one side of 1 (i.e., up to 0.99 or 1.01 and upward) indicates a difference in effect between the intervention and control. The 95% CI range for death in the simvastatin study was entirely below 1 (0.58 to 0.85)[76], which is interpreted as the investigators are 95% confident that RR associated with simvastatin is between 0.58 and 0.85 for the population. Since 1 is not in this range, the investigators are 95% confident that RR of experiencing the adverse event is reduced with simvastatin (i.e., difference in effect). Using another example, the calculated HR for the primary endpoint of CHD was 1.82 with a 95% CI of 1.49 to 2.01. This information indicates the investigators are 95% confident that the risk of CHD is increased with the intervention versus placebo in the population since HR is > 1. Also, the investigators were 95% confident that the intervention increased CHD risk in the population since the 95% CI for this endpoint did not include 1. However, a 95% CI containing the value of 1 indicates the intervention may have neither lowered nor increased the risk (or hazard) of the adverse event. For instance, HR for death due to other causes was calculated as 0.92 (95% CI, 0.74 to 1.14). The 95% CI range lies on both sides of 1 and indicates the risk of death could be lowered to 0.74 or increased to 1.14 with the intervention. Thus, the investigator (or reader) would conclude that the intervention is no different than placebo in decreasing or increasing the risk of death.

Case Study 4–1

Your uncle (67 years of age) who has nonvalvular atrial fibrillation and diabetes contacts you for your opinion on the newly approved anticoagulant medication apixaban (Eliquis®). He read an advertisement in a magazine indicating that use of apixaban led to a significant reduction in ischemic stroke, hemorrhagic stroke, and systemic embolization. He is well controlled on warfarin therapy for over 20 years with no bleeding events or other serious adverse effects and is wondering if he should switch to apixaban due to claims of being more effective than warfarin to prevent ischemic stroke secondary to systemic embolism. Other than age and medication history, he has no other risk factors for bleeding. You locate the advertisement your uncle references and determine that the data presented are extracted from the trial that is summarized below. Use the summary provided below to assist your uncle in making an informed decision before visiting his cardiologist.

A double-blind trial assessed the efficacy and safety of apixaban to warfarin in subjects with atrial fibrillation (A-fib). Individuals from 39 countries were randomized to either apixaban 5 mg twice daily (n = 9120) or adjusted-dose warfarin (target INR, 2 to 3; n = 9081). Inclusion criteria included A-fib plus one additional risk factor for stroke, age $\geq$ 75 years, previous stroke or TIA, previous systemic embolism, or symptomatic HF within 3 months or left ventricular ejection fraction of no more than 40%. Exclusion criteria included A-fib due to a reversible cause, moderate or severe mitral valve stenosis, conditions other than A-fib requiring anticoagulation, and stroke within the previous 7 days. Baseline demographics (e.g., mean age, female:male ratio) were similar in both groups with no statistical differences. The subject mean age was 70 years, approximately, 25% of the subjects resided in North America, and the mean CHADS$_2$ score was 2.1 $\pm$ 1.1 in both groups. The median follow-up duration was 1.8 years. The primary efficacy outcome was occurrence of stroke or systemic embolism, and the secondary efficacy outcome was death from any cause. The primary outcome (via ITT) occurred in 212 and 265 subjects receiving apixaban and warfarin, respectively (HR = 0.79; 95% CI, 0.66 to 0.95; p = 0.01). The study investigators concluded that apixaban is more efficacious than warfarin in this patient type.

1. Calculate the RRR for the primary endpoint and interpret this value.
2. Calculate the ARR for the primary endpoint and interpret this value.
3. Calculate the NNT for the primary endpoint and interpret this value.
4. Interpret the CI for the primary endpoint: HR = 0.79, 95% CI, 0.66 to 0.95.
5. As you read the clinical results for the different types of stroke, you locate information for ischemic stroke and systemic embolization (the events of greatest concern for your uncle):

"Ischemic stroke or uncertain type of stroke occurred in 199 and 250 subjects in the apixaban group and warfarin group, respectively (HR = 0.92, 95% CI, 0.74-1.13; p = 0.42). Furthermore, systemic embolization occurred in 15 and 17 subjects in the apixaban and warfarin groups, respectively (HR = 0.87, 95% CI, 0.44-1.75; p = 0.70)."

What would your evidence-based response to your uncle be based on the information presented?

___

No Difference Does Not Indicate Equivalency

Using the above items (e.g., 95% CI, measures of association) assists the reader in determining the clinical significance of study results with p-values less than α-values.

Remember, study results are not automatically clinically different (or significant) with p-values less than α-values. However, clinical studies reporting p-values greater than the α-value translate into no statistical significance; thus, no clinical difference in effect is declared between the intervention and control groups. H_0 is accepted (fail to be rejected) and H_1 is rejected; in response, the statement of no difference is accepted.[119,146] H_0 is not written to state the intervention and control are the same, but stated as no difference in the effect (i.e., endpoint measurement) between the intervention and control. **⑪** *Nonstatistically significant results do not equate to the intervention and control being the same or equal.* Studies accepting H_0 have the possibility of a Type II error. A difference in effect between the intervention and control groups may be present, but either by chance or a small trial sample size the difference in effect was not detected. In this latter instance, the clinical trial may not have been powered sufficiently to detect the difference. Usually (but not all of the time) clinical trials in which H_0 is accepted have too small of a sample size.[114] In fact, some studies may even be designed with an insufficient sample size so the investigators may claim equivalence between the intervention and active control after rejecting H_0 even though a trial with an appropriate sample size could detect a difference. For instance, a study comparing the blood pressure lowering effects of a new ACE inhibitor to a highly prescribed ACE inhibitor may use a small sample size to obtain study results that are not statistically different. Unfortunately, the trial results may be incorrectly interpreted by some readers as both ACE inhibitors being the same and/or the new ACE inhibitor being promoted as being equal as the comparative ACE inhibitor. This situation can occur in biased articles and/or presentations. However, the correct interpretation should be no difference detected. As one author stated, "absence of evidence is not evidence of absence."[113]

Assessing the Clinical Relevance of the Results

⑫ *All controlled clinical trial results need to be assessed to determine the clinical relevance (i.e., meaningfulness) of the intervention versus control.*[31,122,147] In other words, what do these results mean to practice? Small treatment effects and/or differences may be statistically different, but do not really mean much clinically.[61,80,114] For example, an antihypertensive medication lowered mean DBP by 5 mmHg versus 2 mmHg for placebo (p = 0.04). H_0 was rejected due to statistical difference. However, mean baseline DBP was 98 mmHg and this antihypertensive medication only lowered mean DBP to 93 mmHg, which is still classified as hypertensive.[157] Thus, practitioners would consider these results to be not clinically meaningful. In other words, these results are not useful in treating patients with hypertension.

On the other hand, a small difference in effect that is statistically different may be of clinical importance, depending on the perspective of the reader. A long-term care pharmacist who specializes in geriatrics may consider a trial reporting a reduced number of incontinence episodes, on average, by two in a 24-hour period with a new anticholinergic agent compared to placebo to be clinically meaningful compared to an infectious disease pharmacist. The new drug may reduce nursing time and improve the overall QOL in patients with incontinence.

Not all clinical trials reporting nonstatistically significant results are completely devoid of clinical importance. The overall effect of the intervention and control needs to be assessed. For example, a study compared lansoprazole (30 mg; n = 421) to omeprazole (20 mg; n = 431); each group received once daily therapy for a duration of 8 weeks. The healing rates of erosive reflux esophagitis was 87.2% versus 87%, respectively, via ITT analysis (p = nonsignificant [NS]).[158] No clinical difference is concluded from this study, but these results would be considered to be clinically meaningful (i.e., clinically relevant) since >85% of patients were healed with either therapy.

As previously mentioned, clinical trial results of the intervention may be statistically significant and clinically different than the control, but may be not clinically practical. The clinical trial methods need to be reviewed for the ability to replicate these into everyday patient care. A clinical trial may be designed that consists of technologies and/or include personnel that may not be readily accessible in patient care areas. In addition, patients may not be able to afford the new intervention. Another issue to consider is the demands on the actual patient. At times investigators offer incentives (e.g., monetary compensation, free medical care) for the subjects to strictly follow the study protocol (i.e., more motivated to be compliant). But in practice, real patients may not be as eager to follow an intricate schedule. For example, bismuth subsalicylate can be taken as a prophylaxis against traveler's diarrhea.[159] Although a clinical trial reported the suspension of subsalicylate bismuth 60 mL four times daily reduced the incidence of this unfortunate experience during travel,[160] some individuals may not be willing to adhere to this dosing schedule. Another issue to consider before applying the clinical trial results to practice is the normal care for patients with the disease/condition under study. Endpoint results of an intervention may be statistically significant and clinically different than the active control, but the control is not normally prescribed for patients with the disease/condition.[80]

BIBLIOGRAPHY

References are a very important part of the manuscript. The reference or bibliography section is at the end of the manuscript and provides documentation to support the information provided in the manuscript or acknowledgment for the work of other authors.[44] Any material that the author uses in the manuscript should be appropriately cited. References included in the manuscript should be recent (e.g., outdated articles should not be used unless the results of the article are pertinent to the manuscript) and complete. Readers should scan the references listed in the bibliography to determine if the authors used material from reputable sources. In addition, authors should refrain from extensively citing only their own work.[161] References typically should be listed in numerical order (e.g., Arabic numerals) in which these appear in the manuscript; however, several referencing styles exist and are journal dependent (refer to Appendix 9–3 for further information about referencing). At minimum, the information in the reference section should be sufficient to lead the reader to locating the same article. Some readers may wish to verify the cited information, while others search for articles in the reference section to gather additional information regarding a topic.[44]

ACKNOWLEDGMENTS

Individuals contributing to the clinical trial, but who do not meet the requirements for authorship, can be recognized in this section (see Chapter 9 for more information). Examples of persons identified are those providing manuscript preparation, technical assistance, or donors of equipment or supplies. Medical writers or editors may also be listed if their contributions were significant. A collaboration or group may receive recognition in the acknowledgment section; however, many journals have a prespecified amount of space for the acknowledgment section that must be adhered to by authors. Authors must obtain written permission from persons acknowledged before listing in this section, so the readers do not infer endorsements of the data and conclusions from these contributors.[34,44]

Other types of information may be included in this section: financial support (see below for further information) and an indication that the manuscript underwent peer review, signified by a series of dates title received/revised/accepted. Typically, at least 4 to 8 weeks are between these dates since it is necessary to allow time for the reviewers to comment, the authors to revise, and then for another review of the manuscript. Some journals present only the manuscript acceptance date, which allows readers to determine the lag time between the article being accepted in final form to publication. Hopefully, a minimal time period exists between acceptance and the publication date, which increases content currency.

FUNDING

⓭ *Controlled clinical trial investigators and authors should disclose any funding sources and potential conflicts of interest.* Due to the enormous expense often required to conduct a clinical trial, investigators may seek financial assistance to conduct the research. Various funding sources are available that include pharmaceutical companies, government agencies (e.g., National Institutes of Health [NIH]), national organizations (e.g., American Heart Association), university grants (e.g., faculty development grants), and private donations. Although financial disclosure is recommended, this may not occur. Reporting of payments by pharmaceutical companies to physicians who received greater than $100,000 has been assessed. The payments to the individuals were determined via the dollars for

Docs database during 2009 to 2010. Approximately 69% of the 103 publications evaluated did not contain disclosure of payment that was shown in the dollars for Doc database.[162]

During 2012, an estimated $48.5 billion was spent by the pharmaceutical companies for research and development (which includes clinical drug trials), but interestingly this amount has been decreasing every year since 2010.[163] The pharmaceutical industry is responsible for a significant amount of the clinical research conducted worldwide and new medications have resulted in a reduction in morbidity and mortality plus improved QOL for various disease states. Thus, readers of industry-sponsored research should not automatically disregard a clinical trial solely based on a pharmaceutical company sponsoring the research. However, readers should be cognizant of possible **conflicts of interest**, defined as "a set of conditions in which professional judgment concerning a primary interest (such as a patient's welfare of the validity of research) tends to be unduly influenced by a secondary interest (such as financial gain)"[164] that may result in potential bias. Conflicts of interest arise because the industry may be prompted to publish articles as a means of making their product appear better for a disease state in relation to the standard of care. This research may result in methods bias, premature termination of trials for nonscientific/unethical reasons, or reporting/publication bias.[165] The ICMJE has adopted a disclosure form for all their member journals to obtain financial associations of the authors submitting manuscripts. The form is posted on the ICMJE Web site (http://www. icmje.org/coi_disclosure.pdf).[166]

The study design, result presentation, data interpretations, and study conclusions should be assessed appropriately to determine if the funding source had any influences on the overall clinical trial. Pharmaceutical companies need to determine the clinical usefulness of newly developed medications. These companies are expecting to profit from the new medication being approved by the FDA and marketed to prescribers. Many organizations (e.g., government, not for profit) are not prime candidates to offer funding for these studies, which leaves the pharmaceutical company to sponsor the study. Thus, readers are going to encounter pharmaceutical companies sponsoring research and the reader is responsible to determine the quality of the research.

Not all investigator–pharmaceutical industry relationships have the potential to cause a conflict of interest, but readers should decide if a publication is biased. In fact, many well-designed, clinically important studies documenting improved patient health have been sponsored by the pharmaceutical industry and these have changed the standards of practice in treating patients.

However, there have been reports in the literature of selected pharmaceutical companies: terminating studies for various reasons unrelated to efficacy and safety,[167] employing inappropriate comparators,[168] using inappropriate study samples,[169] and suppressing the results of negative studies.[170] Also, it can be assumed that a pharmaceutical company would design studies that are most likely to show superiority of their drug in some aspect or another. Furthermore, reports have been published that indicate a favorable conclusion of studies financially supported by the pharmaceutical industry, which can be referred to as **publication bias**. This type of sponsored research usually yields larger treatment effects than not-for-profit-funded studies.[80]

Research has documented that the conclusions of some trials funded by for-profit organizations were significantly in favor of the experimental drug as the treatment of choice. But not all pharmaceutical industry–sponsored research is biased; many study results are clinically meaningful. Readers need to be aware that the pharmaceutical company has a lot at stake for an investigational drug to be approved by the FDA. In response, the pharmaceutical company attempts to design a clinical trial to meet the FDA-approval standards. However, the methods of presenting (i.e., results section), interpreting (i.e., introduction and/or discussion sections), and summarizing the data and results (i.e., conclusion) can be biased and are not governed by the regulations of the FDA. Consequently, readers need to evaluate the trial data critically to assess the appropriateness and validity of the reported conclusions based on the trial results.[171]

Furthermore, trial registration with an official governmental entity is another method for the reader to discern if publication bias exists in favor of a particular interventional therapy. Specifically, the national clinical trials registry (http://www.clinicaltrials.gov),[172] which is hosted by the NIH, is a very useful resource for the reader of biomedical literature to determine if potentially negative study results are being excluded from discussion in clinical trials or promotional materials. The Food and Drug Administration Amendments Act of 2007 (also known as FDAAA 801) mandates registration and results reporting certain clinical trials utilizing certain drugs, biologics, and devices, regardless of study outcome.[173]

ClinicalTrials.gov indexes >148,900 federally and privately funded clinical trials conducted in the United States and more than 180 countries. Furthermore, this resource provides the user details about a trial's purpose, guidelines for participation, study locations, and contact information for more details. The information contained within the national trial registry should be strictly viewed as supplementary to complement care from a health care professional. This Web site can be searched by a variety of functions, including investigational agent or disease state. With this in mind, the national clinical trials registry is also a very useful tool for the practicing pharmacist who may need to identify treatment options for a patient who cannot afford conventional intervention or who has a rare or terminal disease state and is seeking additional treatment options.[172]

COMMENTARIES/CLINICAL TRIAL CRITIQUES

Every journal should provide its readership with the opportunity for correspondence to exchange ideas about a topic or relay new information about articles published in the journal.[34,44] **⓮** *Editorials, letters to the editor, and commentary publications can assist in* *interpreting controlled clinical trial results.* Commentaries can be essential in assisting readers in interpreting and/or critiquing articles published within the journals by providing strengths and limitations of the original research, an update to published information, or questions to the authors of the original research manuscript.

Editorials, defined as, "a written expression of opinion that may reflect the official position of the publication"[44] are short essays from the editor or other experts in a particular field that are written to convey additional opinions about an article, typically, in the same issue of a journal. Not all editorials reflect the ideas/thoughts of the journal because these are opinions of the editorial author. Although editorials may contain some bias, this literature should always be considered when evaluating a clinical trial by providing additional insight into the results and aid in the comprehension of the clinical application of the trial results. For instance, an editorial in response to the CONDOR trial[54] was published in the same journal issue. The editorial authors discussed many issues ranging from the exclusion of subjects taking aspirin (a large subgroup of patients who may have OA and are at increased risk for bleeds) to the short duration of the study, and a surrogate marker of the larger composite endpoint was a significant contributor of difference between therapies. The editorial authors concluded that the novelty of the study results are a welcomed addition to existing data, however, tempered some of the investigators' conclusion regarding severity of lower GI bleeding.[174]

Several issues should be considered during the preparation or evaluation of editorials. Quality editorials are original; those editorials with nonoriginal ideas need to include a clear justification of repeating these ideas. The editorial objective should be clearly presented and reflect a complete message. The content should be significant to merit publication, along with being appliciable to practice, accurate, and thorough. The editorial points should be timely with respect to the publication in which the author is responding. Finally, the editorial author should mention the facts clearly and the material should be applicable to the readership of the publication.[175]

Not all original research reports are accompanied by an editorial. Persons seeking an editorial associated with a clinical trial can use a few methods to locate the publication. First, the journal issue that contains the clinical trial lists the editorial title in the journal issue table of contents. Another way, not always present in all clinical trials, is a notation printed on the first page of the clinical trial referring the reader to another page (i.e., "For comment, see page..."; "Commentary, page ..."). Readers not having access to the actual clinical trial or journal issue table of contents can locate the trial citation in PubMed® (using the Single Citation Matcher at http://www.pubmed.gov). Those clinical trials with an accompanying editorial will contain a notation of Comment in and an abbreviated journal citation (i.e., journal name, date, plus volume, issue, and page numbers). Another method is to search the clinical trial topic (i.e., via Medical Subject Heading [MeSH] term in PubMed®) and limit the search to the publication type of editorial.

Some journals/Web sites are published for the primary purpose of providing editorials/commentaries addressing a clinical trial. These resources are known as secondary journals and are independent of the journals that directly publish the clinical trials.[36,80,176] Secondary journals are publications that assist the busy practitioners in a few vital methods: keeping them current regarding important and relevant studies, plus presenting key study information in a concise format. Clinical trials are presented, usually in a structured abstract style, but not just copying and pasting the exact abstract prepared by the trial investigators. These prepared abstracts may present additional and/or more precise information. In addition, a commentary addressing the study strengths, limitations, and applications into practice is authored by a leading practitioner in the field of study. Readers should use these resources while critiquing the biomedical/pharmacy literature.

Examples of secondary journal Web sites include http://www.theheart.org and http://www.medscape.com. Typically, these publications provide an overview of the study followed by a commentary. Medscape is particularly useful for pharmacists since pharmacy-specific topics are addressed in a section of this Web site. *ACP Journal Club* is an online and print resource (included in *Annals of Internal Medicine* journal issues) in which biomedical literature (i.e., original research, systematic reviews) is selected, based on predefined criteria, and summarized by an expert in the field in the form of structured abstracts followed by a commentary. More than 130 journals are reviewed and are selected due to their potential impact on clinical practice.[177]

Another example is *Journal Watch,* a print and online resource that is published at least monthly in print[178] and daily on the Internet.[179] Updated information for 13 specialty areas of medical practice obtained from over 250 medical journals and other vital medical news sources is provided by physicians along with a commentary to help clinicians determine the impact or the research results on their practice.[179] Several specialty editions of *Journal Watch* are available including *Journal Watch Dermatology, Journal Watch Emergency Medicine, Journal Watch Gastroenterology,* and *Journal Watch Infectious Diseases.*[178]

Letters to the Editor

Letters to the editor can provide valuable insight into original research and can include various types of contributions. These may be in the form of comments, addenda, or updates from previously published articles, alerts regarding potential problems in practice, observations/comments on trends in medication use, opinions on trends or controversies in therapy or research, or original research. Authors of letters to the editor must adhere to strict guidelines from the journals regarding the length, number of tables, and format of the publication.[180] The primary content of letters to the editor is feedback from the journal readers regarding the published materials in the journal. Typically, these letters are published within 3 to 6 months of the original publication. The letters may disagree with the design, result interpretation, and/or conclusions of the publication. Also, the letters may ask for additional information that can be used to interpret/clarify, comprehend, and/or critique the information within the publication. Afterward, the authors of the original publication may provide a response to these published letters. The letters to the editor serve as another source of valuble information for those using and critiquing the biomedical literature.

Conclusion

Pharmacists are characterized by having the skills, ability, and knowledge to problem solve, critically think, and formulate recommendations based on the literature. All pharmacists need the skills of efficiently locating, critically evaluating, plus effectively formulating and communicating an evidence-based recommendation, regardless of the practice setting. As the role of the pharmacist in direct patient care continues to increase, incorporating these skills in daily practice is essential. A multitude of literature is published every year and the quality varies significantly. Readers of the literature should not immediately accept the authors' conclusions but assess the strengths and limitations of the source. The information within this chapter identifies and discusses many issues to consider while reading and analyzing controlled clinical trials. Although every clinical trial has limitations, those trials with appropriate design and well-presented results are still important to apply to clinical practice. Using the proper techniques in evaluating clinical trials can allow pharmacists to contribute as key stakeholders in an ever increasing interdisciplinary health care arena.

Case Study 4–2

A controlled clinical trial assessed the weight lowering effect of a new medication (lorcaserin) with a unique mechanism of action (novel selective agonist of the serotonin 2C receptor). Males and females were randomized to double-blind treatment with either lorcaserin 10 mg twice daily (n = 1561) or placebo (n = 1541) for 52 weeks. All subjects received the same specific diet and exercise routine. Overweight persons (body mass index of 30 to 45 kg/m^2) between the ages of 18 and 65 years were eligible to be enrolled in this trial. The primary endpoint was the proportion of subjects losing at least 5% of their body weight. Secondary endpoints included changes in mean body weight and cardiovascular effects (e.g., heart valve function). The investigators conducted a power analysis (>90%) to determine the appropriate sample size. Statistical tests were two sided with α-value of 5%. Study results were analyzed using intention-to-treat.

At the beginning of the trial, both groups were similar in terms of mean age (44 years), gender (females, 81%), mean body weight (100 kg), and comorbid conditions. The lorcaserin group had fewer subjects discontinued the trial as compared to the placebo group (43% versus 48%). More subjects treated with lorcaserin achieved at least a 5% body weight loss than those treated with placebo (47% versus 25%; p < 0.001). In addition, the mean body weight loss was greater with lorcaserin than with placebo (−5.8 versus −2.9 kg; p <0.001). The mean body weight loss standard deviation for both groups was ±2.4 kg. No differences in cardiovascular effects were reported between the two groups although more subjects treated with lorcaserin reported headache, nausea, and fatigue. The investigators concluded that lorcaserin therapy, in combination with diet and exercise, led to greater weight loss effects than with placebo.

1. Does this study need IRB approval?
2. Is the use of a placebo as the control group appropriate for this study?
3. Interpret the standard deviation of "± 2.4 kg" associated with the end-of-study mean change in body weight with lorcaserin.
4. Is the diet and exercise included for all subjects in this study considered adjunctive or ancillary therapy?
5. Interpret the primary endpoint p-value in terms of probability.
6. Can the primary endpoint results be interpreted as evidence that lorcaserin can reduce the risk of diabetes and cardiovascular adverse events since this agent lowered body weight?

Case Study 4–3

A pharmaceutical company representative visits you to promote an antidepressive agent to treat chemotherapy-induced peripheral neuropathy. He claims that his company's medication is very effective in reducing pain for patients with chemotherapy-induced peripheral neuropathy and this agent should be selected as first-line therapy. He presents a study to support his claim. Below is a summary of this study.

A randomized, double-blind, controlled trial was conducted to determine pain reduction with duloxetine versus placebo in persons with chemotherapy-induced peripheral neuropathy. Subjects were randomized to either duloxetine 60 mg daily (n = 115) or placebo (n = 116) for 5 weeks. Persons eligible to be enrolled in the trial were those experiencing pain for at least 3 months after completing chemotherapy. Subjects with preexisting neuropathy were excluded from the trial. Concomitant use of selected analgesics was allowed (e.g., opioids, acetaminophen, aspirin, NSAIDs), but the doses had to be stable during the 2 weeks before randomization. The primary endpoint was change in the average pain score based on the BPI-SF (Brief Pain Inventory Short Form) from start to end of the treatment period; average pain severity was measured using a pain scale (0 = no pain, 10 = worst pain). The secondary endpoints included change in chemotherapy-induced peripheral neuropathy-related quality of life (QOL) and the degree of pain-related functional interference. The study had a 90% power and α-value = 0.05.

Baseline subject demographics were similar between the two groups for age, gender, analgesic use, and cancer chemotherapy regimens. Eleven subjects never received treatment, leaving 220 being treated; the dropout rate during the study was 19%. The mean change score was greater with duloxetine (1.06; 95% CI, 0.72 to 1.40) than with placebo (0.34; 95% CI, 0.01 to 0.66) (p = 0.03). The observed mean difference in the average pain score between the two groups was 0.73 (95% CI, 0.26 to 1.20). Secondary endpoint results also indicated better results with duloxetine than placebo. The investigators concluded that duloxetine therapy resulted in significant pain reduction compared to placebo in those with chemotherapy-induced peripheral neuropathy.

1. Which type of blinding is the most appropriate for this study?
2. What is the type of data being evaluated for the primary endpoint?
3. Which measures of central tendency are appropriate to present the primary endpoint?
4. Would a larger or smaller sample size be needed with a study power of 90% versus 80%?
5. Is the pharmaceutical representative correct in his statement that duloxetine is a very effective agent to reduce chemotherapy-induced peripheral neuropathy and should be selected over other agents?

Self-Assessment Questions

Read the excerpt of the following clinical trial summary and answer the questions that follow.

A study was conducted to assess the ability of low-dose erythromycin to reduce pulmonary exacerbation in persons with frequent noncystic fibrosis (CF) bronchiectasis. Study subjects were assigned to either erythromycin 250 mg twice daily (n = 59) or placebo (n = 58); baseline demographics were factored into randomizing the subjects to the groups. Both the erythromycin and placebo tablets were similar in appearance, taste, and shape; no one knew who was in which group. Subjects were between the ages of 20 and 85 years and had to have two pulmonary exacerbations requiring systemic antibiotic treatment within the prior 12 months, daily sputum production, but stable for at least 4 weeks. Exclusion criteria included those with CF and changes in any maintenance medications in the 4 weeks prior to study entry. The primary endpoint was the mean rate of protocol-defined pulmonary exacerbations (PDPE) per patient per year (defined as subject requiring antibiotic therapy for more than 24 hours, increased sputum production, and deterioration of symptoms). The results for all subjects randomized into this study were included in the final analysis regardless of whether they completed the entire study duration (48 weeks). Other endpoints included FEV_1, change in exercise capacity, and adverse side effects. Tablet counts were used to determine adherence. Subjects returned to the clinic for follow-up 11 times over 48 weeks. Subjects also had access to contact an investigator any time of the day to report exacerbation symptoms. The investigators calculated that a total 118 subjects were needed to be enrolled in the study to have 90% ability to detect a difference between the erythromycin and placebo group for the primary endpoint. A p-value less than 0.05 was considered significant.

Baseline demographics were similar between the two groups in terms of average age (62 years), gender (60% female), and exacerbations per year. A total of 107 subjects completed the entire study duration and medication adherence was approximately 96%. Less incidences of PDPE were reported in the erythromycin group versus placebo (76 versus 114 episodes, respectively; p = 0.003). The mean PDPE was 1.29 versus 1.97 per patient per year. Less of a decrease in FEV_1 (p = 0.04) and better exercise capacity (p = 0.4) was measured with erythromycin compared to placebo. Few side effects occurred in both groups. The investigators concluded that erythromycin did provide beneficial effects versus placebo in these subjects.

1. Which of the following is a *false* statement regarding this trial?
   a. Randomization reduces bias in selecting subjects to the groups.
   b. Statistical tests are validated with randomization being included in the trial.
   c. All subjects have an equal opportunity to be assigned to either group via randomization.
   d. This study used a more advanced randomization technique (i.e., stratification).
   e. Controlled clinical trials do not require subjects to be randomized.

2. Which type of blinding is used in this study?
   a. no blinding
   b. double-blinding
   c. single-blinding
   d. open-label
   e. investigator only

3. Which of the following represents the type of data collected and evaluated for the primary endpoint in this study?
   a. nominal
   b. ordinal
   c. interval
   d. ratio
   e. continuous

4. Which of following is included in this study?
   a. Per-protocol since results from all subjects were included in the final analysis.
   b. Subgroup analysis since medication adherence was over 90%.
   c. Run-in phase since baseline demographics were similar between the two groups.
   d. Intention-to-treat since results from all subjects were included in the final analysis.
   e. Poor definition and follow-up for the primary endpoint.

5. Select the *best* written null hypothesis (H_0) for the primary endpoint.
   a. There is a difference in the mean rate of PDPE per patient per year between erythromycin and placebo.
   b. There is no difference in effect between erythromycin and placebo.
   c. There is no difference in the mean rate of PDPE per patient per year between erythromycin and placebo.
   d. There is no difference between erythromycin and placebo in persons with frequent non-CF bronchiectasis.
   e. The difference in the mean rate of PDPE per patient per year is less with erythromycin than placebo.

6. Which of the following is correct regarding the power of this study?
   a. Since at least 80% of the subjects completed the trial, the power is at least 80%.
   b. Included to estimate a sample size to reduce a Type II error.
   c. Set at 95% to reduce a Type I error.
   d. Calculated to equal 80%.
   e. No evidence of a power analysis was included in this trial.

7. Which of the following represents the statement of "A p-value less than 0.05 was considered significant"?
   a. alpha
   b. beta
   c. gamma
   d. power
   e. intention-to-treat

8. Which of the following is correct in relationship to the primary endpoint H_0?
   a. Accept H_0 since p-value is less than 0.05.
   b. Reject H_0 since p-value is greater than 0.05.
   c. Accept H_0 since p-value is less than 5%.
   d. Reject H_0 since p-value is less than 0.05.
   e. Cannot accept or reject the Ho since a specific α-value was not presented.

9. Which of the following statements should be selected based on the primary end-point p-value (p = 0.003) of this study?
   a. Statistical significance is not present and a Type I error is possible.
   b. Statistical significance is present and a Type II error is possible.
   c. Statistical significance is present and a Type I error is possible.
   d. Statistical significance is not present and a Type II error is possible.
   e. Since no study α-value was stated in the study summary, statistical difference cannot be determined.

10. Which of the following is correct to interpret the primary endpoint p-value? The probability of:
   a. accepting a false H_0 is 0.003%.
   b. rejecting a true H_0 is 0.003%.
   c. having a Type I error is 0.003%.
   d. accepting a true H_0 is 0.3%.
   e. rejecting a true H_0 is 0.3%.

11. The investigators calculated a point estimate and 95% CI difference in the effect of the primary endpoint to be 0.68 (95% CI, 0.52 to 0.84). Select the *best* interpretation of this 95% CI.
   a. A clinical difference can be present because the value of equality (zero) is not included in the 95% confidence interval range.
   b. The investigators are confident that 5% of the subjects will not experience the primary endpoint with ERY therapy.
   c. A clinician may expect that 52% to 84% of the subjects in the population will achieve a reduction in the primary endpoint with ERY therapy.
   d. If the study were repeated, 95% confident that the calculated difference in the primary endpoint would be between 52% and 84%.
   e. No clinical difference can be present because the value of equality (one) is not included in the 95% confidence interval range.

12. Which statement is the *best* in regard to whether a clinical difference between erythromycin and placebo exists?
   a. Clinical difference does not exist because the study was not appropriately powered to detect differences in the intervention and control groups.

b. Clinical difference does not exist since the results are not statistically significant.

c. Clinical difference exists because the results are statistically significant.

d. Clinical differences cannot be determined due to a placebo was used as the control.

e. Clinical difference may exist due to the p-value and 95% CI calculation.

13. Which of the following is correct for the secondary endpoint of increased exercise capacity?

a. statistically significant and accept H_0 for this endpoint

b. not statistically significant and not clinically different

c. not statistically significant and reject H_0 for this endpoint

d. not statistically significant but clinically different

e. statistically significant and reject H_0 for this endpoint

14. Which of the following patients with non-CF bronchiectasis is the *best* candidate to receive erythromycin therapy based on this study?

a. 47-year-old male with no daily sputum production

b. 55-year-old male with new hypertension therapy started last week

c. 87-year-old female with daily sputum production

d. 67-year-old female stable for prior 5 weeks

e. 16-year-old with two pulmonary exacerbations requiring systemic antibiotic treatment within the prior 12 months

15. Which of the following *best* describes a reader writing in a comment after reading this study?

a. editorial

b. acknowledgment

c. letter to the editor

d. peer review

e. readers cannot comment on published trials

REFERENCES

1. U.S. Food and Drug Administration: FDA approved drug products [Internet]. Rockville (MD): U.S. Food and Drug Administration; [updated 2013 Mar 7]. Drug approval reports; [updated 2013 Mar 7; cited 2013 Mar 22]. Available from: http://www.fda.gov/Drugs/DevelopmentApprovalProcess/HowDrugsareDevelopedandApproved/DrugandBiologicApprovalReports/default.htm

2. U.S. Food and Drug Administration: 2012 safety alerts for human medical products [Internet]. Rockville (MD): U.S. Food and Drug Administration; [updated 2013 Aug 23; cited 2013 Oct 4]. Available from: http://www.fda.gov/Safety/MedWatch/SafetyInformation/SafetyAlertsforHumanMedicalProducts/ucm285497.htm

3. PubMed homepage [Internet]. Bethesda (MD): National Library of Medicine (US). Available from: http://www.ncbi.nlm.nih.gov/pubmed/. Accessed 2013 Mar 22.

4. Gallup, Inc. Honesty/ethics in professions [Internet]. Washington, DC: Gallup, Inc. Available from: http://www.gallup.com/poll/1654/honesty-ethics-professions.aspx. Accessed 2013 October 4.

5. Calis KA, Hutchison LC, Elliott ME, Ives TJ, Zillich AJ, Poirier T, et al. Health people 2010: challenges, opportunities, and a call to action for America's pharmacists. Pharmacotherapy. 2004 Sep;24(9):1241-94.

6. Giberson S, Yoder S, Lee MP. Improving patient and health system outcomes through advanced pharmacy practice. A report to the U.S. Surgeon General [Internet]. Washington, DC: Office of the Chief Pharmacist. U.S. Public Health Service; 2011 May [updated 2011 Dec]. Available from: http://www.usphs.gov/corpslink/pharmacy/docuents/2011AdvancedPharmacyPracticeReporttotheUSSG.pdf

7. American Society of Health-System Pharmacists. ASHP statement on the role of health-system pharmacists in public health. Am J Health Syst Pharm. 2008 Mar 1;65(5):462-7.

8. American Society of Health-Systems Pharmacists. Legislative summary: Patient Protection and Affordable Care Act [Internet]. Bethesda (MD): American Society of Health-System Pharmacists; [updated 2010 Mar 22; cited 2013 Mar 22]. Available from: http://www.ashp.org/DocLibrary/AboutUs/Legislative-SummaryFinal-Reform-Bill.aspx

9. American Society of Health-Systems Pharmacists. The Patient Protection and Affordable Care Act and the Health Care and Education Reconcilation Act [Internet]. Bethesda (MD): American Society of Health-System Pharmacists; [updated 2010 May; cited 2013 Mar 22]. Available from: http://www.ashp.org/DocLibrary/SM2010/Health-Care-Reform-Reportsm2010.aspx

10. Cutler TW. The pharmacy profession and health care reform: opportunities and challenges during the next decade. J Am Pharm Assoc. 2011 Jul-Aug;51(4):477-81.

11. Wright SG, LeCroy RL, Kendrach MG. The three types of biomedical literature and systematic approach to handle a drug information request. J Pharm Pract. 1998 June;11(3): 148-62.

12. Schrimsher RS, Kendrach MG. Basic PubMed searching for pharmacists. Hosp Pharm. 2006 Sep;41(9):855-67.

13. Nelson SJ, Schulman JL. Orthopaedic literature and MeSH. Clin Orthop Relat Res. 2010 Oct;468(10):2621-26.

14. Bhandari M, Giannoudis PV. Evidence-based medicine: what it is and what it is not. Injury. 2006 Apr;37(4):302-6.

15. Hershenberg R, Drabick DA, Vivian D. An opportunity to bridge the gap between clinical research and clinical practice: implications for clinical training. Psychotherapy (Chic). 2012 Jun;49(2):123-34.

16. Whitcomb ME. Why we must teach evidence-based medicine. Acad Med. 2005 Jan;80(1): 1-2.

17. Pihlstrom BL, Curran AE, Voelker HT, Kingman A. Randomized controlled trials: what are they and who needs them? Periodontol 2000. 2012 Jun;59(1):14-31.

18. Umscheid CA, Margolis DJ, Grossman CE. Key concepts of clinical trials: a narrative review. Postgrad Med. 2011 Sep;123(5):194-204.
19. U.S. Food and Drug Administration: How drugs are developed and approved [Internet]. Rockville (MD): U.S. Food and Drug Administration; [updated 2013 Jan 3; cited 2013 Mar 22]. Available from: http://www.fda.gov/Drugs/DevelopmentApprovalProcess/How-DrugsareDevelopedandApproved/default.htm
20. Gehlbach S. Interpreting the medical literature. 5th ed. New York, NY: McGraw-Hill Company; 2006.
21. Doll R. Controlled trials: the 1948 watershed. BMJ. 1998 Oct 31;317(7167):1217-20.
22. Kunz R, Oxman AD. The unpredictability paradox: review of empirical comparisons of randomised and non-randomised clinical trials. BMJ. 1998 Oct 31;317(7167): 1185-90.
23. Kendrach MG, Anderson HG. Fundamentals of controlled clinical trials. J Pharm Pract. 1998 June;XI(3):163-80.
24. Schulz KF, Altman DG, Moher D; CONSORT Group. CONSORT 2010 Statement: updated guidelines for reporting parallel group randomised trials. Ann Int Med. 2010;152(11): 726-32.
25. Friedman L, Furberg C, DeMets D. Fundamentals of clinical trials. 4th ed. New York, NY: Springer; 2010.
26. Lader EW, Cannon CP, Ohman EM, Newby LK, Sulmasy DP, Barst RJ, et al. The clinician as investigator: participating in clinical trials in the practice setting: Appendix 1: fundamentals of study design. Circulation. 2004 Jun 1;109(21):e302-4.
27. Mathieu S, Boutron I, Moher D, Altman DG, Ravaud P. Comparison of registered and published primary outcomes in randomized controlled trials. JAMA. 2009 Sep 2;302(9): 977-84.
28. Krzyzanowska MK, Pintilie M, Tannock IF. Factors associated with failure to publish large randomized trials presented at an oncology meeting. JAMA. 2003 Jul 24;290(3): 495-501.
29. Irwin RS. The role of conflict of interest in reporting of scientific information. Chest. 2009 Jul;136(1):253-9.
30. Hayes A, Hunter J. Why is publication of negative clinical trial data important? Br J Pharmacol. 2012 Dec;167(7):1395-7.
31. Sridharan L, Greenland P. Editorial policies and publication bias: the importance of negative studies. Arch Intern Med. 2009 Jun 8;169(11):1022-3.
32. Stone GW, Pocock SJ. Randomized trials, statistics, and clinical inference. J Am Coll Cardiol. 2010 Feb 2;55(5):428-31.
33. Cook DA. Randomized controlled trials and meta-analysis in medical education: what role do they play? Med Teach. 2012;34(6):468-73.
34. International Committee of Medical Journal Editors: recommendations for the conduct, reporting, editing and publication of scholarly work in medical journals [Internet]. [place unknown]: International Committee of Medical Journal Editors; [cited 2013 Oct 4]. Available from: http://www.icmje.org. Accessed June 19, 2013.

35. Armstrong PW, Newby LK, Granger CB, et al. Lessons learned from a clinical trial. Circulation. 2004 Dec 7;110(23):3610-4.

36. Augustyn N, Welch SJ, Irwin RS. Managing information overload: the evolution of CHEST. Chest. 2012 Jul;142(1):1-5.

37. Blumenthal D. Doctors and drug companies. N Engl J Med. 2004 Oct 28;351(18):1885-90.

38. Campbell B. "Throw-away journals": tactics for dealing with office waste. CMAJ. 1990 Jan 15;142(2):100.

39. Wood BD, Ludwig RL. The difference between peer review and nonpeer review. Radiol Technol. 2012 Sep-Oct;84(1):90-2.

40. Harden RM, Lilley P. A fresh approach to publishing and reviewing papers in health professions education. Med Teach. 2013;35(1):1-3.

41. Guyatt GH, Akl EA, Crowther M, Gutterman DD, Schuünemann HJ. American College of Chest Physicians Antithrombotic Therapy and Prevention of Thrombosis Panel. Executive summary: antithrombotic therapy and prevention of thrombosis, 9th ed: American College of Chest Physicians evidence-based clinical practice guidelines. Chest. 2012 Feb;141(2 Suppl):7S-47S.

42. Lader EW, Cannon CP, Ohman EM, Newby LK, Sulmasy DP, Barst RJ, et al. The clinician as investigator: participating in clinical trials in the practice setting. Circulation. 2004 Jun 1;109(21):2672-9.

43. Studdert DM, Mello MM, Brennan TA. Financial conflicts of interest in physicians' relationships with the pharmaceutical industry—self-regulation in the shadow of federal prosecution. N Engl J Med. 2004 Oct 28;351(18):1891-900.

44. Iverson C, Christiansen S, eds. American Medical Association manual of style: a guide for authors and editors. 10th ed. New York: Oxford University Press; 2007.

45. Nelson HS, Bensch G, Pleskow WW, DiSantostefano R, DeGraw S, Reasner DS, et al. Improved bronchodilation with levalbuterol compared with racemic albuterol in patients with asthma. J Allergy Clin Immunol. 1998 Dec;102(6 Pt 1):943-52.

46. Peat J, Elliott E, Baur L, Keena V. Scientific writing: easy when you know how. London: BMJ Books; 2002.

47. Hopewell S, Clarke M, Moher D, Wager E, Middleton P, Altman DG, Schulz KF; CONSORT Group. CONSORT for reporting randomized controlled trials in journal and conference abstracts: explanation and elaboration. PLoS Med. 2008;5(1):e20.

48. Guimarães CA. Structured abstracts: narrative review. Acta Cir Bras. 2006 Jul-Aug;21(4):263-8.

49. Hartley J. Current findings from research on structured abstracts. J Med Libr Assoc. 2004 Jul-Aug;92(3):368-71.

50. Harris AH, Standard S, Brunning JL, Casey SL, Goldberg JH, Oliver L, et al. The accuracy of abstracts in psychology journals. J Psychol. 2002 Mar;136(2):141-8.

51. Pitkin RM, Branagan MA, Burmeister LF. Accuracy of data in abstracts of published research articles. JAMA. 1999 Mar 24-31;281(12):1110-1.

52. Ward LG, Kendrach MG, Price SO. Accuracy of abstracts for original research articles in pharmacy journals. Ann Pharmacother. 2004 Jul-Aug;38(7-8):1173-7.

53. Cuddy PG, Elenbaas RM, Elenbaas JK. Evaluating the medical literature. Part I: Abstract, introduction, methods. Ann Emerg Med. 1983 Sep;12(9):549-55.

54. Chan FKL, Lanas A, Scheiman J, Berger MF, Nguyen H, Goldstein, JL. Celecoxib versus omeprazole and diclofenac in patients with osteoarthritis and rheumatoid arthritis (CONDOR): a randomised trial. Lancet. 2010 Jul 17;376(9736):173-9.

55. Veith FJ. How randomized controlled trials (RCTs) can be misleading: introduction. Semin Vasc Surg. 2011 Sep;24(3):143-5.

56. Hulley SB, Cummings SR, Browner WS, Grady DG, Newman TB. Designing Clinical Research. 4th ed. Philadelphia (PA): Lippincott Williams & Wilkins; 2013.

57. Goldberg RJ, McManus DD, Allison J. Greater knowledge and appreciation of commonly-used research study designs. Am J Med. 2013 Feb;126(2):169.e1-8.

58. Bakker-Arkema RG, Davidson MH, Goldstein RJ, Davignon J, Isaacsohn JL, Weiss SR, et al. Efficacy and safety of a new HMG-CoA reductase inhibitor, atorvastatin, in patients with hypertriglyceridemia. JAMA. 1996 Jan 10;275(2):128-33.

59. Karalis DG, Ross AM, Vacari RM, Zarren H, Scott R. Comparison of efficacy and safety of atorvastatin and simvastatin in patients with dyslipidemia with and without coronary heart disease. Am J Cardiol. 2002 Mar 15;89(6):667-71.

60. Tripepi G, Jager KJ, Dekker FW, Zoccali C. Selection bias and information bias in clinical research. Nephron Clin Pract. 2010;115(2):c94-9.

61. Naylor CD, Guyatt GH. Users' guides to the medical literature. X. How to use an article reporting variations in the outcomes of health services. The Evidence-Based Medicine Working Group. JAMA. 1996 Feb 21;275(7):554-8.

62. Berger VW, Rezvani A, Makarewicz VA. Direct effect on validity of response run-in selection in clinical trials. Control Clin Trials. 2003 Apr;24(2):156-66.

63. Siddiqi AE, Sikorskii A, Given CW, Given B. Early participant attrition from clinical trials: role of trial design and logistics. Clin Trials. 2008;5(4):328-35.

64. Chan FK, Ching JY, Hung LC, Wong VW, Leung VK, Kung NN, et al. Clopidogrel versus aspirin and esomeprazole to prevent recurrent ulcer bleeding. N Engl J Med. 2005 Jan 20;352(3):238-44.

65. Department of Health and Human Services: recruiting human subjects. Pressures in industry-sponsored clinical research [internet]. Washington, DC: Department of Health and Human Services; [updated 2000 Jun; cited 2013 Jun 24]. Available from: http://oig. hhs.gov/oei/reports/oei-01-97-00195.pdf

66. Hebert R. Newspaper advertising could distort research results. Nicotine Tob Res. 2000 Nov;2(4):317-8.

67. Wei SJ, Metz JM, Coyle C, Hampshire M, Jones HA, Markowitz S, et al. Recruitment of patients into an Internet-based clinical trials database: the experience of OncoLink and the National Colorectal Cancer Research Alliance. J Clin Oncol. 2004 Dec 1;22(23):4730-6.

68. Maiti R. M R. Clinical trials in India. Pharmacol Res. 2007 Jul;56(1):1-10.

69. Nicholas J. Outsourcing clinical trials. J Natl Cancer Inst. 2012 Jul 18;104(14):1043-5.

70. Guyatt GH, Sackett DL, Cook DJ. Users' guides to the medical literature. II. How to use an article about therapy or prevention. A. Are the results of the study valid? Evidence-Based Medicine Working Group. JAMA. 1993 Dec 1;270(21):2598-601.

71. Julious SA. Sample sizes for clinical trials with normal data. Stat Med. 2004 Jun 30;23(12):1921-86.

72. Vickers AJ, de Craen AJ. Why use placebos in clinical trials? A narrative review of the methodological literature. J Clin Epidemiol. 2000 Feb;53(2):157-61.

73. Yeh SS, DeGuzman B, Kramer T. Reversal of COPD-associated weight loss using the anabolic agent oxandrolone. Chest. 2002 Aug;122(2):421-8.

74. Baker SG, Lindeman KS. Rethinking historical controls. Biostatistics. 2001 Dec;2(4):383-96.

75. Brodie MJ. Novel trial designs for monotherapy. Epileptic Disord. 2012 Jun;14(2):132-37.

76. Randomised trial of cholesterol lowering in 4444 patients with coronary heart disease: the Scandinavian Simvastatin Survival Study (4S). Lancet. 1994 Nov 19;344(8934):1383-9.

77. Simons LA, Nestel PJ, Calvert GD, Jennings GL. Effects of MK-733 on plasma lipid and lipoprotein levels in subjects with hypercholesterolaemia. Med J Aust. 1987 Jul 20;147(2):65-8.

78. Avenell A, Grant AM, McGee M, McPherson G, Campbell MK, McGee MA, et al. The effects of an open design on trial participant recruitment, adherence, and retention—a randomized controlled trial comparison with a blinded, placebo-controlled design. Clin Trials. 2004;1(6):490-8.

79. Tramer MR, Reynolds DJ, Moore RA, McQuay HJ. When placebo controlled trials are essential and equivalence trials are inadequate. BMJ. 1998 Sep 26;317(7162):875-80.

80. Montori VM, Jaeschke R, Schunemann HJ, Bhandari M, Brozek JL, Devereaux PJ, et al. Users' guide to detecting misleading claims in clinical research reports. BMJ. 2004 Nov 6;329(7474):1093-96.

81. Gluud LL. Bias in clinical intervention research. Am J Epidemiol. 2006 Mar 15;163(6):493-501.

82. Davidson M, Ma P, Stein EA, Gotto AM, Jr., Raza A, Chitra R, et al. Comparison of effects on low-density lipoprotein cholesterol and high-density lipoprotein cholesterol with rosuvastatin versus atorvastatin in patients with Type IIa or IIb hypercholesterolemia. Am J Cardiol. 2002 Feb 1;89(3):268-75.

83. Kendrach MG, Kelly-Freeman M. Approximate equivalent rosuvastatin doses for temporary statin interchange programs. Ann Pharmacother. 2004 Jul-Aug;38(7-8):1286-92.

84. Schwenzer KJ. Practical tips for working effectively with your institutional review board. Respir Care. 2008 Oct;53(10):1354-61.

85. Enfield KB, Truwit JD. The purpose, composition, and function of an institutional review board: balancing priorities. Respir Care. 2008 Oct;53(10):1330-6.

86. Schwenzer KJ. Protecting vulnerable subjects in clinical research: children, pregnant women, prisoners, and employees. Respir Care. 2008 Oct;53(10):1342-9.

87. Montori A, Onorato M. Why there is a need of an ethics committee in scientific medical societies. Dig Dis. 2008;26(1):32-5.

88. Lema VM, Mbondo M, Kamau EM. Informed consent for clinical trials: a review. East Afr Med J. 2009 Mar;86(3):133-42.

89. Freeman SR, Lundahl K, Schilling LM, Jensen JD, Dellavalle RP. Human research review committee requirements in medical journals. Clin Invest Med. 2008;31(1):E49-54.

90. Byerly WG. Working with the institutional review board. Am J Health Syst Pharm. 2009 Jan 15;66(2):176-84.

91. Mertl SL. The fundamentals of Institutional Review Board operations. J Pharm Pract. 1996;IX:437-43.

92. Macklin R. The ethical problems with sham surgery in clinical research. N Engl J Med. 1999 Sep 23;341(13):992-6.

93. Horng S, Miller FG. Is placebo surgery unethical? N Engl J Med. 2002 Jul 11;347(2): 137-9.

94. Riegelman RK. Studying a study and testing a test. Reading evidence-based health research. 6th ed. Baltimore (MD): Lippincott William & Wilkins; 2013.

95. Guyatt G, Rennie D, Meade MO, Cook DJ. User's guide to the medical literature. A manual for evidence-based clinical practice. 2nd ed. Columbus (OH): McGraw-Hill; 2008.

96. Collins R, MacMahon S. Reliable assessment of the effects of treatment on mortality and major morbidity, I: clinical trials. Lancet. 2001 Feb 3;357(9253):373-80.

97. Roberts C, Torgerson D. Randomisation methods in controlled trials. BMJ. 1998 Nov 7;317(7168):1301.

98. Slobogean GP, Sprague S, Bhandari M. The tactics of large randomized trials. J Bone Joint Surg Am. 2012 Jul 18;94(Suppl 1):19-23.

99. Pitt B, Segal R, Martinez FA, Meurers G, Cowley AJ, Thomas I, et al. Randomised trial of losartan versus captopril in patients over 65 with heart failure (Evaluation of Losartan in the Elderly Study, ELITE). Lancet. 1997 Mar 15;349(9054):747-52.

100. Freemantle N, Calvert M, Wood J, Eastaugh J, Griffin C. Composite outcomes in randomized trials: greater precision but with greater uncertainty? JAMA. 2003 May 21;289(19):2554-59.

101. Lubsen J, Kirwan BA. Combined endpoints: can we use them? Stat Med. 2002 Oct 15;21(19):2959-70.

102. Bakal JA, Westerhout CM, Armstrong PW. Impact of weighted composite compared to traditional composite endpoints for the design of randomized controlled trials. Stat Methods Med Res. 2012 Jan 24. [Epub ahead of print].

103. Kaul S, Diamond GA. Trial and error: How to avoid commonly encountered limitations of published clinical trials. J Am Coll Cardiol. 2010;55(5):415-27.

104. Pogue J, Devereaux PJ, Thabane L, Yusuf S. Designing and analyzing clinical trials with composite outcomes: consideration of possible treatment differences between the individual outcomes. PLoS One. 2012;7(4):e34785.

105. Cohen M, Demers C, Gurfinkel EP, et al. A comparison of low-molecular-weight heparin with unfractionated heparin for unstable coronary artery disease. Efficacy and Safety of Subcutaneous Enoxaparin in Non-Q-Wave Coronary Events Study Group. N Engl J Med. 1997 Aug 14;337(7):447-52.

106. Armstrong PW. Heparin in acute coronary disease—requiem for a heavyweight? N Engl J Med. 1997 Aug 14;337(7):492-94.

107. Ohman EM. Enoxaparin reduced combined coronary events in unstable angina and non-Q-wave MI at 14 and 30 days [Comment]. ACP J Club. 1998;128:34.

108. Stone NJ, Robinson J, Lichtenstein AH, Merz CN, Blum CB, Eckel RH, Goldberg AC, Gordon D, Levy D, Lloyd-Jones DM, McBride P, Schwartz JS, Shero ST, Smith SC Jr, Watson K, Wilson PW. 2013 ACC/AHA Guideline on the Treatment of Blood Cholesterol to Reduce Atherosclerotic Cardiovascular Risk in Adults: A Report of the American College of Cardiology/American Heart Association Task Force on Practice Guidelines. [Internet]. Dallas (TX). American Heart Association; 2013 Nov 12. [cited 5 March 2013]. Available from: http://circ.ahajournals.org/content/early/2013/11/11/01.cir.0000437738.63853.7a

109. Potkin SG, Saha AR, Kujawa MJ, Carson WH, Ali M, Stock E, Stringfellow J, Ingenito G, Marder SR. Aripiprazole, an antipsychotic with a novel mechanism of action, and risperidone vs placebo in patients with schizophrenia and schizoaffective disorder. Arch Gen Psychiatry. 2003 Jul;60(7):681-90.

110. American Psychiatric Association. Treatment of patients with schizophrenia [Internet]. Arlington (VA): American Psychiatric Association. [updated 2009 Nov; cited 2013 Oct 7]. Available from: http://psychiatryonline.org/guidelines.aspx

111. Woo TUW, Canuso CM, Wojcik JD, Brunette MF, Green AI. Treatment of schizophrenia. In: Schatzberg AF, Nemeroff CB, eds. Textbook of psychopharmacology. 4th ed. Washington, DC: American Psychiatric Publishing, Inc; 2009:1135-69.

112. Lader EW, Cannon CP, Ohman EM, Newby LK, Sulmasy DP, Barst RJ, Fair JM, Flather M, Freedman JE, Frye RL, Hand MM, Jesse RL, Van de Werf F, Costa F.; American Heart Association, et al. The clinician as investigator: participating in clinical trials in the practice setting: Appendix 2: statistical concepts in study design and analysis. Circulation. 2004 Jun;109:e305-7.

113. Whitley E, Ball J. Statistics review 4: sample size calculations. Crit Care. 2002 Aug;6(4):335-41.

114. Guller U, DeLong ER. Interpreting statistics in medical literature: a vade mecum for surgeons. J Am Coll Surg. 2004 Mar;198(3):441-58.

115. Tumlin JA, Wang A, Murray PT, Mathur VS. Fenoldopam mesylate blocks reductions in renal plasma flow after radiocontrast dye infusion: a pilot trial in the prevention of contrast nephropathy. Am Heart J. 2002 May;143(5):894-903.

116. Stone GW, McCullough PA, Tumlin JA, Lepor NE, Madyoon H, Murray P, Wang A, Chu AA, Schaer GL, Stevens M, Wilensky RL, O'Neill WW; CONTRAST Investigators, et al. Fenoldopam mesylate for the prevention of contrast-induced nephropathy: a randomized controlled trial. JAMA. 2003 Nov 5;290(17):2284-91.

117. Altman DG, Goodman SN, Schroter S. How statistical expertise is used in medical research. JAMA. 2002 Jun 5;287(21):2817-20.

118. Chan AW, Tetzlaff JM, Gøtzsche PC, Altman DG, Mann H, Berlin JA, et al. SPIRIT 2013 explanation and elaboration: guidance for protocols of clinical trials. BMJ. 2013 Jan 8;346:e7586.

119. Guyatt G, Jaeschke R, Heddle N, Cook D, Shannon H, Walter S. Basic statistics for clinicians: 1. Hypothesis testing. CMAJ. 1995 Jan 1;152(1):27-32.

120. Whitley E, Ball J. Statistics review 3: hypothesis testing and P values. Crit Care. 2002 Jun;6(3):222-5.

121. DeMuth JE. Overview of biostatistics used in clinical research. Am J Health Syst Pharm. 2009 Jan 1;66(1):70-81.

122. Salkind NJ. Statistics for people who (think they) hate statistics. Thousand Oaks (CA): Sage Publications, Inc; 2000.

123. Whitley E, Ball J. Statistics review 2: samples and populations. Crit Care. 2002 Apr;6(2):143-8.

124. Tu YK, Gilthorpe MS. Key statistical and analytical issues for evaluating treatment effects in periodontal research. Periodontol 2000. 2012;Jun 59(1):75-88.

125. Evans RB, O'Connor A. Statistics and evidence-based veterinary medicine: answers to 21 common statistical questions that arise from reading scientific manuscripts. Vet Clin North Am Small Anim Pract. 2007 May;37(3):477-86.

126. Glantz SA. Primer of biostatistics. 5th ed. New York (NY): McGraw-Hill; 2002.

127. Lee CM, Soin HK, Einarson TR. Statistics in the pharmacy literature. Ann Pharmacother. 2004 Sep;38(9):1412-8.

128. Swinscow TDV. Statistics at Square One. London: British Medical Association; 1983.

129. Kirby A, Gebski V, Keech AC. Determining the sample size in a clinical trial. Med J Aust. 2002 Sep 2;177(5):256-7.

130. Elenbaas JK, Cuddy PG, Elenbaas RM. Evaluating the medical literature, Part III: Results and discussion. Ann Emerg Med. 1983 Nov;12(11):679-86.

131. DeMets DL. Statistical issues in interpreting clinical trials. J Intern Med. 2004 May;255(5):529-37.

132. White IR, Carpenter J, Horton NJ. Including all individuals is not enough: lessons for intention-to-treat analysis. Clin Trials. 2012 Aug;9(4):396-407.

133. Le Bars PL, Katz MM, Berman N, Itil TM, Freedman AM, Schatzberg AF. A placebo-controlled, double-blind, randomized trial of an extract of Ginkgo biloba for dementia. North American EGb Study Group. JAMA. 1997 Oct 22-29;278(16):1327-32.

134. Postuma RB, Lang AE, Munhoz RP, et al. Caffeine for treatment of Parkinson disease: a randomized controlled trial. Neurology. 2012 Aug 14;79(7):651-8.

135. Bucher HC, Guyatt GH, Cook DJ, Holbrook A, McAlister FA. Users' guides to the medical literature: XIX. Applying clinical trial results. A. How to use an article measuring the effect of an intervention on surrogate end points. Evidence-Based Medicine Working Group. JAMA. 1999 Aug 25;282(8):771-8.

136. Weihrauch TR, Demol P. Value of surrogate endpoints for evaluation of therapeutic efficacy. Drug Inf J. 1998;32:737-43.

137. Barter PJ, Caulfield M, Eriksson M, Grundy SM, Kastelein JJ, Komajda M, et al; ILLUMINATE Investigators. Effects of torcetrapib in patients at high risk for coronary events. N Engl J Med. 2007 Nov 22;357(21):2109-22.

138. Cook DI, Gebski VJ, Keech AC. Subgroup analysis in clinical trials. Med J Aust. 2004 Mar 15;180(6):289-91.

139. Ghert M, Petrisor B. Subgroup analyses: when should we believe them? J Bone Joint Surg Am. 2012 Jul 18;94(Suppl 1):61-4.

140. Sun X, Briel M, Busse JW, You JJ, Akl EA, Mejza F, et al. Credibility of claims of subgroup effects in randomised controlled trials: systematic review. BMJ. 2012 Mar 15;344:e1553.

141. Gorelick PB, Richardson D, Kelly M, Ruland S, Hung E, Harris Y, Kittner S, Leurgans S. African American Antiplatelet Stroke Prevention Study Investigators. Aspirin and ticlopidine for prevention of recurrent stroke in black patients: a randomized trial. JAMA. 2003 Jun 11;289(22):2947-57.

142. Hass WK, Easton JD, Adams HP, Jr., Pryse-Phillips W, Molony BA, Anderson S, et al. A randomized trial comparing ticlopidine hydrochloride with aspirin for the prevention of stroke in high-risk patients. Ticlopidine Aspirin Stroke Study Group. N Engl J Med. 1989 Aug 24;321(8):501-7.

143. Lu T, Sheng H, Wu J, Cheng Y, Zhu J, Chen Y. Cinnamon extract improves fasting blood glucose and glycosylated hemoglobin level in Chinese patients with type 2 diabetes. Nutr Res. 2012 Jun;32(6):408-12.

144. Rothwell PM. External validity of randomised controlled trials: "to whom do the results of this trial apply?" Lancet. 2005 Jan 1-7;365(9453):82-93.

145. Clarke M, Alderson P, Chalmers I. Discussion sections in reports of controlled trials published in general medical journals. JAMA. 2002 Jun 5;287(21):2799-801.

146. Anderson G, Kendrach MG, Trice S. Basic biostatistics and hypothesis testing. J Pharm Pract. 1998 Jun;XI(3):181-95.

147. Pocock SJ, Ware JH. Translating statistical findings into plain English. Lancet. 2009 Jun 6;373(9679):1926-8.

148. Castell DO, Kahrilas PJ, Richter JE, Vakil NB, Johnson DA, Zuckerman S, Skammer W, Levine JG. Esomeprazole (40 mg) compared with lansoprazole (30 mg) in the treatment of erosive esophagitis. Am J Gastroenterol. 2002 Mar;97(3):575-83.

149. Whelton A, Fort JG, Puma JA, Normandin D, Bello AE, Verburg KM. Cyclooxygenase-2-specific inhibitors and cardiorenal function: a randomized, controlled trial of celecoxib and rofecoxib in older hypertensive osteoarthritis patients. Am J Ther. 2001 Mar-Apr;8(2):85-95.

150. Ranstam J. Why the P-value culture is bad and confidence intervals a better alternative. Osteoarthritis Cartilage. 2012 Aug;20(8):805-8.

151. Guyatt G, Jaeschke R, Heddle N, Cook D, Shannon H, Walter S. Basic statistics for clinicians: 2. Interpreting study results: confidence intervals. CMAJ. 1995 Jan 15;152(2):169-73.

152. Guyatt GH, Sackett DL, Cook DJ. Users' guides to the medical literature. II. How to use an article about therapy or prevention. B. What were the results and will they help me in caring for my patients? Evidence-Based Medicine Working Group. JAMA. 1994 Jan 5;271(1):59-63.

153. Jaeschke R, Guyatt G, Shannon H, Walter S, Cook D, Heddle N. Basic statistics for clinicians: 3. Assessing the effects of treatment: measures of association. CMAJ. 1995 Feb 1;152(3):351-7.

154. Colhoun HM, Betteridge DJ, Durrington PN, Hitman GA, Neil HA, Livingstone SJ, et al. Primary prevention of cardiovascular disease with atorvastatin in type 2 diabetes in the Collaborative Atorvastatin Diabetes Study (CARDS): multicentre randomised placebo-controlled trial. Lancet. 2004 Aug 21-27;364(9435):685-96.

155. Kendrach MG, Covington TR, McCarthy MW, Harris CM. Calculating risks and number-needed-to-treat: a method of data interpretation. J Managed Care Pharm. 1997 Mar/Apr;3(2):179-83.

156. Feinstein AR. Principles of medical statistics. Boca Raton (FL): Chapman & Hall/CRC Press Co; 2002.

157. James PA, Oparil S, Carter BL, Cushman WC, Dennison-Himmelfarb C, Handler J, Lackland DT, LeFevre ML, MacKenzie TD, Ogedegbe O, Smith SC Jr, Svetkey LP, Taler SJ, Townsend RR, Wright JT Jr, Narva AS, Ortiz E. 2014 evidence-based guideline for the management of high blood pressure in adults: report from the panel members appointed to the Eighth Joint National Committee (JNC 8). JAMA. 2014 Feb 5;311(5):507-520.

158. Castell DO, Richter JE, Robinson M, Sontag SJ, Haber MM. Efficacy and safety of lansoprazole in the treatment of erosive reflux esophagitis. The Lansoprazole Group. Am J Gastroenterol. 1996 Sep;91(9):1749-57.

159. Advice for travelers. Treat Guidel Med Lett. 2012 Jun;10(118):45-56.

160. DuPont HL, Sullivan P, Evans DG, Pickering LK, Evans DJ, Jr., Vollet JJ, et al. Prevention of traveler's diarrhea (emporiatric enteritis). Prophylactic administration of subsalicylate bismuth). JAMA. 1980 Jan 18;243(3):237-41.

161. Mosdell KW. Literature evaluation I: controlled clinical trials. In: Malone PM, Mosdell KW, Kier KL, Stanovich JE, eds. Drug information: a guide for pharmacists. 2nd ed. New York: McGraw-Hill;2001:160.

162. Norris SL, Holmer HK, Ogden LA, Burda BU, Fu R. Characteristics of physicians receiving large payments from pharmaceutical companies and the accuracy of their disclosures in publications: an observational study. BMC Med Ethics. 2012 Sep 26;13(1):24.

163. Pharmaceutical Research and Manufacturers of America. Biopharmaceutical Research Pharmaceutical Industry—2013 Profile [Internet]. Washington, DC: Pharmaceutical Research and Manufacturers of America; [updated July 2013; cited 2013 July 27]. Available from: http://www.phrma.org/sites/default/files/pdf/PhRMA%20Profile%202013.pdf

164. Thompson DF. Understanding financial conflicts of interest. N Engl J Med. 1993 Aug 19;329(8):573-6.

165. Wynia M, Boren D. Better regulation of industry-sponsored clinical trials is long overdue. J Law Med Ethics. 2009 Fall;37(3):395,410-9.

166. International Committee of Medical Journal Editors. ICMJE form for disclosure of potential conflicts of interest resource page [Internet]. [cited Mar 7, 2013]. Available from: http://www.icmje.org/coi_disclosure.pdf. Accessed March 7, 2013.

167. Lievre M, Menard J, Bruckert E, Cogneau J, Delahaye F, Giral P, et al. Premature discontinuation of clinical trial for reasons not related to efficacy, safety, or feasibility. BMJ. 2001 Mar 10;322(7286):603-5.

168. Gotzsche PC, Johansen HK. Meta-analysis of prophylactic or empirical antifungal treatment versus placebo or no treatment in patients with cancer complicated by neutropenia. BMJ. 1997 Apr 26;314(7089):1238-44.

169. Rochon PA, Berger PB, Gordon M. The evolution of clinical trials: inclusion and representation. CMAJ. 1998 Dec 1;159(11):1373-4.

170. Blumenthal D, Campbell EG, Anderson MS, Causino N, Louis KS. Withholding research results in academic life science. Evidence from a national survey of faculty. JAMA. 1997 Apr 16;277(15):1224-8.

171. Als-Nielsen B, Chen W, Gluud C, Kjaergard LL. Association of funding and conclusions in randomized drug trials: a reflection of treatment effect or adverse events? JAMA. 2003 Aug 20;290(7):921-8.

172. US National Institutes of Health [Internet]. Washington, DC: ClinicalTrials.gov Web page; [cited June 27, 2013]. Available from: http://www.clinicaltrials.gov/. Accessed June 27, 2013.

173. US National Institutes of Health [Internet]. Washington, DC. FDAAA 801 Requirements Web page. [reviewed 2012 Dec; cited 2013 June 27]. Available from: http://www.clinicaltrials.gov/ct2/manage-recs/fdaaa. Accessed June 27, 2013.

174. Rahme E, Bernatsky S. NSAIDs and risk of lower gastrointestinal bleeding. Lancet. 2010 Jul 17;376(9736):146-8.

175. Sage Publications. Thousands Oak (CA). Annals of Pharmacotherapy journal website. Manuscript Guidelines Web page. [cited 2013 Oct 4]. Available from: http://www.sagepub.com/journals/Journal202238/title#tabview=manuscriptSubmission.www.theannals.com/site/misc/Guidelines_Com.pdf. Accessed June 28, 2013.

176. Devereaux PJ, Manns BJ, Ghali WA, Quan H, Guyatt GH. Reviewing the reviewers: the quality of reporting in three secondary journals. CMAJ. 2001 May 29;164(11):1573-6.

177. About ACP Journal Club. Welcome! Here's what we do. ACP Journal Club [Internet]. [cited 2013 Oct 4]. Purpose and procedure. Available from: http://acpjc.acponline.org/shared/purpose_and_procedure.htm. Accessed June 28, 2013.

178. NEJM Journal Watch subscription Webpage [Internet]. [cited 2013 Oct 4]. Available from: https://secure.jwatch.org/subscribem?cpc=SMAAALLV0513A&promo=OJFLSB21&prc=OJFLSB21&step=0. Accessed June 28, 2013.

179. NEJM Journal Watch [Internet]. Waltham (MA). About Journal Watch Online. [cited 2013 Oct 4]. Available from: http://www.jwatch.org/about/journal-watch. Accessed June 28, 2013.

180. American Journal of Health-System Pharmacy website [Internet]. Columns of AJHP. [cited 2013 Oct 4]. Available from: http://www.ashp.org/DocLibrary/AJHP/AJHP-Sections-Columns.aspx. Accessed June 28, 2013.

SUGGESTED READINGS

1. Schulz KF, Altman DG, Moher D; CONSORT Group. CONSORT 2010 Statement: updated guidelines for reporting parallel group randomised trials. Ann Int Med. 2010;152(11):726-32.

2. Stone GW, Pocock SJ. Randomized trials, statistics, and clinical inference. J Am Coll Cardiol. 2010 Feb 2;55(5):428-31.

3. Guyatt G, Rennie D, Meade MO, Cook DJ. User's guide to the medical literature: a manual for evidence-based clinical practice. 2nd ed. Coulmbus (OH): McGraw-Hill; 2008.

4. Kaul S, Diamond GA. Trial and error: how to avoid commonly encountered limitations of published clinical trials. J Am Coll Cardiol. 2010 Feb 2;55(5):415-27.

5. Guller U, DeLong ER. Interpreting statistics in medical literature: a *vade mecum* for surgeons. J Am Coll Surg. 2004 Mar;198(3):441-58.

6. Pihlstrom BL, Curran AE, Voelker HT, Kingman A. Randomized controlled trials: what are they and who needs them? Periodontol 2000. 2012;59(1):14-31.

7. Tu YK, Gilthorpe MS. Key statistical and analytical issues for evaluating treatment effects in periodontal research. Periodontol 2000. 2012;59(1):75-88.

8. DeMuth JE. Overview of biostatistics used in clinical research. Am J Health Syst Pharm. 2009 Jan 1;66(1):70-81.

9. Whitley E, Ball J. Statistics review 3: hypothesis testing and P values. Crit Care. 2002 Jun;6(3):222-5.

10. Kendrach MG, Covington TR, McCarthy MW, Harris CM. Calculating risks and number-needed-to-treat: a method of data interpretation. J Managed Care Pharm. 1997 Mar/Apr;3(2):179-83.

5

Chapter Five

Literature Evaluation II: Beyond the Basics

Patrick J. Bryant • Cydney E. McQueen • Elizabeth A. Van Dyke

Learning Objectives

● *After completing this chapter, the reader will be able to*

- Describe examples of other study designs besides the basic controlled clinical trial.
- Discuss the potential utility, limitations, and questions to ask when evaluating other study designs.
- Describe the characteristics of various observational trial designs.
- Differentiate between the three types of literature reviews: narrative (nonsystematic) review, systematic review, and meta-analysis.
- Describe common quality-of-life (QOL) measures used in health outcomes research and discuss the appropriate use of these measures in the medical literature.
- Discuss common issues encountered in dietary supplement (botanical and nonbotanical) medical literature.
- Describe how to efficiently and effectively evaluate the available evidence associated with a clinical question and categorize the quality of that evidence to develop a recommendation/clinical decision.

Key Concepts

① Although the randomized controlled trial is the most frequently used study design for clinical research, several other designs are used in specific situations, such as investigating rare outcome incidences, studying equivalency/noninferiority between drugs, or minimizing patient exposure to new drugs with inadequate efficacy.

② Observational study designs offer an alternative to interventional trials and are used in specific situations, such as when large populations must be followed over extended periods of time. Results from these trials only allow associations to be formed rather than true cause-and-effect relationships.

③ Case studies, case reports, and case series are reports describing patient or patient group exposure to a drug or technology and can be valuable to record preliminary findings that lead to further study. A key characteristic to these reports is the lack of a control or comparison group.

④ Survey research is information gathered from an identified group with conclusions drawn and applied to a larger population. This gathered information is considered either descriptive (such as opinions and attitudes) or explanatory (such as explaining a cause and effect) in nature and the validity of the results depends on quality of the study's internal rigor.

⑤ Meta-analyses are the only type of review providing new quantitative data derived from combining the results of each study in the meta-analysis and performing a statistical analysis on that data set. The overall reliability of a meta-analysis is ultimately dependent on the quality of the individual studies, homogeneity between these studies, and the appropriateness of the analysis.

⑥ The value assigned to quality and quantity of life affected by many different variables including disease, injury, treatment, or policy is termed health-related quality of life (HR-QOL) and is used to assist in decision making regarding interventions such as procedures and pharmacotherapy.

⑦ The principles and criteria used to analyze the quality of drug literature are used to analyze dietary supplement (DS) literature; however, unique additional points such as standardization and purity must be considered.

⑧ An understanding of strengths and limitations inherent with each study design is essential to determine the overall quality of the evidence produced. Those trial designs with a high level of quality provide the most reliable evidence and that translates into the strongest recommendation/clinical decision.

Introduction

❶ *Although the randomized controlled trial is the most frequently used study design for clinical research, several other designs are used in specific situations, such as investigating rare outcome incidences, studying equivalency/noninferiority between drugs, or minimizing patient exposure to new drugs with inadequate efficacy.* Principles that apply to randomized controlled trials (see Chapter 4) also apply to other types of study designs. There are situations where other research designs are more effective in answering specific questions or providing the only data available to answer the questions. For example, there has been a tremendous increase in the use of noninferiority study design to establish a drug's position in therapy.[1] Typically, a superiority trial design is used in this instance. The issue arises when no statistically significant difference in efficacy between the new drug and control or reference drug (often considered to be standard treatment) is shown. The only conclusion to be made at that time is that the new drug is not superior to the reference drug. When a noninferiority trial design is used and the results confirm that the new drug is noninferior to the reference drug, a conclusion can be made that the new drug is "no worse" than the reference drug regarding efficacy. If noninferiority is established, the same data can be analyzed for superiority of the new drug over the reference drug. If no statistically significant difference in efficacy is shown from this analysis and, therefore, no superiority is established, the researchers at least know the new drug is still no worse than the reference drug. As another example, **adaptive clinical trial** design has become more common in assisting to establish efficacy for a particular drug. Adapting the number of patients, eligibility criteria, drug dose, or randomization allocation can significantly improve the efficiency of drug development and provide a more realistic clinical environment to test a new drug. Table 5–1 lists commonly encountered biomedical literature.

To effectively determine the quality of these trials, the practitioner must first evaluate major considerations that apply to the design. One approach uses a list of essential study components referred to as the **Ten Major Considerations** Checklist.[2] The Ten Major Considerations include

1. Power of the study set/met (to estimate adequate sample size that will identify a difference between groups if one truly exists)?
2. Dosage/treatment regimen appropriate?
3. Length of study appropriate to show effect?
4. Inclusion criteria adequate to identify target study population?
5. Exclusion criteria adequate to exclude patients who may be harmed in study?
6. Blinding present?
7. Randomization resulted in similar groups?
8. Biostatistical tests appropriate for type of data analyzed?
9. Measurement(s) standard/validated/accepted?
10. Author's conclusions are supported by the results?

Once this is completed, additional considerations unique to a specific study design discussed in this chapter must be evaluated. For example, it is necessary to determine the similarity of studies used to conduct a **meta-analysis** since the results of each study will be combined and new data created and analyzed.

TABLE 5–1. COMMONLY ENCOUNTERED BIOMEDICAL LITERATURE

Study Design	Study Purpose
Clinical study	Determine cause-and-effect relationships
Noninferiority study	Identify if one drug is therapeutically no worse than another drug, usually the accepted reference control drug
N-of-1 study	Compare effects of drug to control during multiple observation periods in a single patient
Adaptive clinical trial	Provides flexibility in design to incorporate continuously emerging knowledge generated as the trial progresses
Stability study	Evaluate stability of drugs in various preparations (e.g., ophthalmologic, intravenous, topical, and oral)
Bioequivalence study	Assess the bioequivalency of two or more products
Programmatic research	Determine the impact and/or economic value of clinical services
Cohort (follow-up) study	Determine association between various factors and disease state development
Case-control (trohoc) study	Determine association between disease states and exposure to various risk factors
Cross-sectional study	Identify prevalence of characteristics of diseases in populations
Case study, case report, or case series	Report observations in a single patient or series of patients
Survey research	Study the incidence, distribution, and relationships of sociologic and psychologic variables through use of questionnaires applied to various populations
Postmarketing surveillance study	Evaluate use and adverse effects associated with newly approved drug therapies
Narrative review	Nonsystematic, qualitative, subjective summary of data from multiple studies
Systematic review	Systematic, qualitative, and objective summary of data from multiple studies
Meta-analysis	Combine, statistically evaluate, and create new data from combining multiple studies in a quantitative manner
Outcomes studies (pharmacoeconomic and health-related-QOL measures)	Compare outcomes (QOL) and costs (pharmacoeconomics) of drug therapies or services

ABBREVIATION: QOL = quality of life.

The purpose of this chapter is to familiarize the health care practitioner with these unique study designs. In addition, specific considerations unique to each design and in addition to the Ten Major Considerations are identified for the practitioner to evaluate (see Appendix 5–1). Finally, a process is provided to bring all the results of trials focused on a particular clinical question together and develop a recommendation/clinical decision based on this evidence. For these reasons, this chapter can be extremely valuable and useful to anyone who depends on the medical literature to provide answers to their daily clinical challenges.

This chapter covers the variations on randomized clinical trial design (noninferiority, N-of-1, and adaptive clinical trials), observational trial design (**cohort, case-control**, and **cross-sectional**), and uncontrolled study designs (**case studies, case series**, and **case reports**). Specific types of studies such as bioequivalency, postmarketing surveillance, and programmatic research are discussed. Differences between narrative (qualitative), systematic (qualitative), and meta-analysis (quantitative) reviews are addressed. A discussion of the specialized area of health outcomes research is included to introduce concepts directly related to patient quality-of-life (QOL) trials. A section on evaluation of dietary supplement (DS) medical literature including issues specific to these trials and common methodological flaws is provided.

Good literature evaluation skills and application of a systematic evidence-based medicine (EBM) process provide the foundation that allows clinicians to make the best recommendations and decisions.[3] In light of rapidly emerging evidence and busy practitioner schedules, an understanding of inherent strengths and limitations associated with various types of clinical trial design provides a powerful clinical tool. In general, those trials with a greater number of identified strengths than limitations, especially if those limitations have a minimal effect on the study results, provides a high level of reliability. Using these high-quality trials that represent the best evidence, a stronger recommendation/clinical decision can be made. This in turn ensures the highest level of patient care, whether for one specific patient or large patient populations.

Beyond the Basic Controlled Trial

NONINFERIORITY TRIALS

Description

Randomized, controlled clinical trials are utilized to determine one of three different outcomes between comparative drugs: superiority, equivalency, or **noninferiority** (NI).[4] All three trial designs involve a new test drug compared to the accepted active control or standard of care drug. With superiority trials, the aim is to determine that one drug is superior to the other.[5] In contrast, equivalency trials are designed to determine if the new drug is therapeutically similar to the control drug. This trial design is used primarily to determine bioequivalence between two drugs. Noninferiority trials seek to show that any difference between two treatments is small enough to conclude the test drug has "an effect that is not too much smaller than the active control"[6] also referred to as the reference drug or standard treatment.[1,6-9] This section will focus on description, interpretation, and evaluation of NI trials.

There has been a dramatic increase in rate of the NI studies since 1999.[1] Along with this increase has come an understanding of several potential study design issues including choice of reference drug, at what point the test drug's **treatment effect** will be considered inferior to the reference drug, and optimal analytical approaches, therefore, requiring rigor in design and conduct of these trials.[10,11] An NI study design is often considered when superiority of a test drug over a reference drug is not anticipated.[12] In this case, the objective is showing the test drug to be statistically and clinically not inferior to the reference drug based on efficacy, yet the test drug could offer other potential advantages related to safety, tolerability, convenience, or cost.[7,8] These ancillary benefits can justify use of the test drug to replace standard treatment. NI trials are also considered when the use of a superiority trial would be considered unethical.[6] For example, it is unethical to use a placebo when there is available effective treatment that possesses an important benefit, such as preventing death or irreversible injury to the patient. For this reason, NI trials may provide an alternative method to using superiority trials for meeting United States (U.S.) Food and Drug Administration (FDA) marketing approval requirements.[6] Between 2002 and 2009, 14% of the New Drug Applications (NDAs) approved contain evidence from pivotal NI trials.[13] Rather than going through the process of showing a new drug is therapeutically superior to the reference drug treatment or a placebo, pharmaceutical companies are choosing to use an NI design. This is a developmental strategy to confirm the new drug has a valid therapeutic effect and that the drug's effect is not, at minimum, worse than the reference drug. Often the anticipated key differentiating factor for the test drug in this situation is improved safety profile. For example, a new drug for cardiac arrhythmias is anticipated to have similar efficacy but less serious side effects than the standard treatment. It should be noted that NI design is not recommended when the reference drug treatment effect is not consistently superior to placebo (both statistically and clinically).[14]

Establishing the NI Margin

The NI margin is an important component of an NI trial and is a prespecified amount used to show the test drug's treatment effect is not worse than the reference drug by more than this specific degree.[15] A combination of statistical reasoning and clinical judgment is required to best determine the NI margin.[7,8,16,17] Another way to think of the NI margin is the extent to which the test drug's effect can be worse than the reference drug, but still be considered no worse.[18] For instance, if the reference drug's minimal treatment effect is determined to be a 5 mmHg drop in diastolic blood pressure compared to placebo, then the test drug could not be worse than this 5 mmHg change to be considered noninferior to the reference drug. In other words, if the results from the NI trial showed the test drug's treatment effect to be 4 mmHg, then the test drug would be considered potentially inferior to the reference drug. The FDA draft guideline document defines the NI margin as the largest clinically acceptable difference (degree of inferiority) of the test drug compared to the reference drug.[6] Methods to determine the NI margin have been proposed; however, concern exists with the subjectivity and potential **bias** associated with any method that relies on an indirect comparison of historical data rather than a true placebo arm built into the NI study.[19-22]

A simple method to determine the NI margin is to look at the confidence interval (CI) for the reference drug treatment effect (reference drug – placebo = treatment effect). This treatment effect is best determined from examining the historical reference drug versus placebo-controlled trials. A meta-analysis of these historical placebo-controlled trials is preferred to obtain the most accurate overall treatment effect when several studies are involved.[8] The CI around the mean reference drug treatment effect is used to establish the NI margin (see Chapter 8 for an understanding of CIs). The lower bound of that CI represents the smallest expected reference drug treatment effect. For example, if the CI around the mean reference drug treatment effect is 3 to 14 mmHg diastolic blood pressure, then the lower bound of that CI would be 3 mmHg. This lower bound can be used to set the NI margin; however, a 5 mmHg change in diastolic blood pressure could be considered the smallest **clinically significant** change. Given this information, the NI margin can be set at 5 mmHg.

Interpretation of Results

The NI design focuses on the mean treatment difference between the test drug and the reference drug (see Figure 5–1). To determine NI, the CI around the mean treatment difference between the test drug and the reference drug is compared against the NI

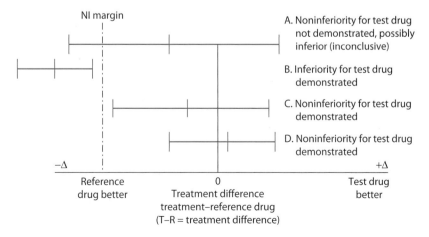

Figure 5–1. Noninferiority trial design concept.

margin. If the CI around the mean treatment difference includes (or crosses) the NI margin, then the possibility of the test drug being inferior to the reference drug exists (inconclusive), and thus, the test drug fails to exhibit noninferiority (see Scenario A in Figure 5–1). The test drug would be determined inferior if the entire CI around the mean treatment difference was located on the inferior side of the NI margin (see Scenario B in Figure 5–1). However, if the CI around the mean treatment difference does not include or cross the NI margin, then a conclusion can be made that the test drug is noninferior to the reference drug (see Scenarios C and D in Figure 5–1).

For example, an NI study of a new antihypertensive agent (test drug) compared to reference drug is published in the literature. The overall treatment effect of the reference drug compared to previous placebo-controlled studies is a reduction of 12 mmHg (CI 6 to 15 mmHg) for a sitting diastolic blood pressure. The lower bound of that CI = 6 mmHg. This lower bound or some percentage of that taking into consideration clinical significance can be used to help set the NI margin. In this case, the lower bound of the CI of 6 mmHg treatment effect is easily considered a clinically significant difference or change in sitting diastolic blood pressure. Given this, the NI margin is established as 6 mmHg sitting diastolic blood pressure. In other words, when the NI trial is completed the test drug's lower bound of the CI associated with the mean treatment difference cannot include or cross the set NI margin of 6 mmHg on the graph (see Figure 5–2). If the test drug's lower bound of the CI includes (or crosses) the NI margin, this would suggest the test drug failed to exhibit noninferiority (possibly inferiority) to the reference drug (see Scenario A in Figure 5–2). This situation would be considered an inconclusive result unless the entire CI for the mean treatment difference is located on the inferiority side of the NI margin of 6 mmHg, confirming inferiority. Upon completion of the example antihypertensive NI study, the actual results confirm noninferiority of the new antihypertensive

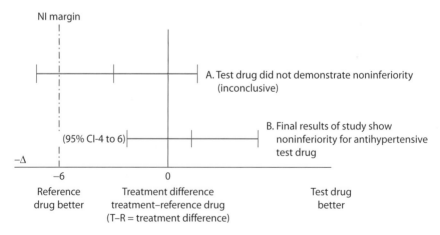

Figure 5–2. Noninferiority trial design example.

agent based on the lower bound of the CI interval for the test drug treatment effect not including (or crossing) the NI margin (see Scenario B in Figure 5–2). In the case where noninferiority is determined, three assumptions are made: (1) test drug exhibits noninferiority to the reference drug, (2) test drug performs better than placebo if placebo was included as a comparator group, and (3) test drug may offer ancillary benefits and these could include safety, tolerability, convenience, or cost.[7]

If an NI margin and/or CI are not provided, then noninferiority can still be determined if an alpha and p-value have been given. To use p-values for this purpose there must be an understanding that statistical rationale for NI trials differs from that used with superiority trials.[23,24] Specifically, defining parameters for the null and alternative hypotheses (see Chapters 4 and 8) are different from those used with superiority trials. In fact, the definitions for the two hypotheses are essentially switched or reversed and relabeled compared to superiority trial hypotheses[7,8] (see Figure 5–3). The null hypothesis for a superiority trial postulates there is no statistically significant difference between treatment groups, and the alternative hypothesis states there is a statistically significant difference between the treatment groups. With NI trials, the null hypothesis states the test drug fails to exhibit noninferiority to the reference drug or at the very least the results are inconclusive for noninferiority versus inferiority.[12] The alternative hypothesis states that the test drug is noninferior to the reference drug (not significantly worse). With NI trials, the null hypothesis must be rejected in favor of the alternative hypothesis to conclude noninferiority for the test drug. This requires a p-value less than the set alpha value. For example, an alpha of 0.05 indicating the significance level, a p-value <0.05 would indicate NI for the test drug. If the null hypothesis is not rejected, then the test drug fails to exhibit noninferiority. In this case the p-value would be equal to or greater than the set alpha value. For example, a p-value is provided rather than an NI margin and/or CI around the mean treatment difference.

Some controversy exists whether an NI trial alone can show superiority of the test drug over the reference drug.[5,23,25] Once NI is established, superiority can be tested using the results for the primary outcome measure(s).[7,8] According to guidance from the FDA, an NI study can be designed to first test for noninferiority with a predetermined NI margin, and if successful proving noninferiority, the data can be analyzed for potential

SUPERIORITY TRIAL DESIGN

Null Hypothesis	Test Drug vs Comparator Drug → NO DIFFERENCE
Alternative Hypothesis	Test Drug vs Comparator Drug → DIFFERENCE

NONINFERIORITY TRIAL DESIGN

Null Hypothesis	Test Drug vs Reference Drug → DIFFERENCE (Test Drug possibly inferior-inconclusive)
Alternative Hypothesis	Test Drug vs Reference Drug → NONINFERIOR (Test Drug possibly superior)

Figure 5–3. Differences in defining parameters for null and alternative hypotheses.

superiority of the test drug. Note the importance of the sequential process of first proving noninferiority, then analyzing for superiority. For instance, if the new antihypertensive NI trial discussed earlier provided results that showed the test drug to be noninferior, then an analysis of superiority would be appropriate and acceptable. This should be stated in the original noninferiority trial protocol. Superiority can be tested prior to NI, but the NI margin must be stated *a priori* to avoid potential manipulation of the margin. Adjusting the NI margin to avoid the CI from crossing over would give a false NI result and is unacceptable. In addition, seeking the conclusion of NI from a failed superiority trial (one that shows no statistically significant difference between treatment groups) is not acceptable.[6,26] The only conclusion that can be made from this scenario is that the test drug is not superior to the reference drug. If a noninferiority conclusion is anticipated, an NI study design should be the initial choice.

Evaluation

Several study design characteristics must be considered when evaluating the quality of an NI trial.[5] The Ten Major Considerations Checklist discussed in the Introduction section is used to identify specific major strengths and limitations.[2]

Of significant importance is how the NI margin used to determine noninferiority is defined.[23,27] Correctly determining this margin is considered the greatest challenge in the design and interpretation of NI trials.[6] If noninferiority is established for the test drug, further concluding the test drug is effective can only be made if the reference drug's efficacy has been confirmed with high-quality clinical trials against placebo. This is referred to as **assay sensitivity**.[6,21,26] The NI margin is set using historical studies to determine the actual effect of the reference drug. Two approaches to determine the NI margin are most frequently referenced: the fixed margin approach and the synthesis approach. Both these approaches use historical data. The fixed-margin approach is preferred by the FDA since that approach is more conservative than the synthesis approach.[28]

Historical evidence of sensitivity to drug effects (HESDE) is a term used to describe appropriately designed and conducted past trials using the reference drug and regularly exhibiting the reference drug to be superior to placebo. Meta-analytic methods can be used to develop more precise estimates of reference drug effect when several studies are available. When multiple studies exist, all studies should be considered to avoid overestimating the reference drug's effect.[6] Only after a determination is made that these past studies are similar in design and conduct compared to the NI trial regarding features that could alter the effect size can the HESDE be used to select the NI margin. In other words, the historical studies and new NI study should be as identical as possible regarding important characteristics. This is called the **constancy assumption**.[12,21] Note that establishing efficacy for the test drug using an NI trial design is seriously complicated by assay sensitivity and constancy assumptions that cannot be completely verified, leading to potentially inflated Type I error rate (see Chapters 4 and 8).[28] The concern is that approval of an ineffective therapy can result with inflated Type I error rates since the test drug is falsely determined to be noninferior to the reference drug.

Another concern called **biocreep** or **placebo creep** can exist that complicates using an active control to confirm efficacy as is done with an NI trial.[12,21] Biocreep is the phenomenon where a somewhat inferior test drug is chosen as the reference drug for a future generation of NI trials. When this occurs with generation after generation of NI trials, the future reference drug becomes no better than placebo.

As mentioned earlier, but important enough to reiterate, setting the NI margin *post hoc* can be interpreted as potential manipulation by investigators to show desired results. For this reason, it is critical that the NI margin be set prospectively before the beginning of the trial. This is considered acceptable practice. For all of these reasons, the investigators should provide a detailed description of how the NI margin was determined.

The type of analysis used should also be determined prospectively. For the purposes of NI study analysis, a per-protocol (PP) analysis where only the patients that completed the study are included is preferred over an intention-to-treat (ITT) analysis (see Chapters 4 and 8).[5,23] The ITT analysis includes all patients that were randomized to treatment regardless of whether they completed the study duration. With the ITT analysis, smaller observed treatment effects can result since patients may not have stayed in the study long enough to see the maximum effect of the test drug. Using an ITT analysis with an NI trial can significantly increase the risk of falsely claiming noninferiority due to the potential of smaller observed treatment effects.[8,26] For this reason, when an ITT analysis is used, a PP analysis is also used to cross-validate the ITT analysis.[8,29] Note that the PP analysis can be invalidated based on significant variation in dropout rates between treatment groups.[29] For example, a noninferiority study is completed but there is an excessively large dropout rate due to safety and lack of return to the clinic visits. This provides a much smaller PP population to be analyzed. If that PP population is less than the required number of patients to meet the set power, then questions arise if no statistical significance ($p < 0.05$ if alpha set at 0.05) is shown. This lack of statistical significance shown could be real and the test drug would fail to exhibit noninferiority (fail to reject the null hypothesis). Since power was not met the result could represent a Type II error (no statistical significance is shown when there really is one and, therefore, the test drug is noninferior to the reference drug) that invalidates the PP analysis (see Chapters 4 and 8 for explanation of Type II errors). The FDA and others suggest conducting and reporting both a PP and ITT analyses.[6,9,29,30] Any differences in results between these two separate analyses should be examined closely by the reader.

Case Study 5–1: Noninferiority Trial Design

A 14-day multicenter randomized double-blind double-dummy noninferiority (NI) trial was conducted to compare short-term efficacy of a generic alginate/antacid to omeprazole on GERD symptoms in general practice. Alginate is the salt of alginic acid and the combination of the alginic acid and bicarbonate creates a barrier which prevents stomach acid from refluxing back up into the esophagus. In addition, safety was compared between the two drugs throughout the study. The primary outcome measure was the mean time to onset of the first 24-hour heartburn-free period after initial dosing. Based on the most recent study, an NI margin was set at 0.5 days. An NI margin of 0.5 days means noninferiority of the alginate/antacid would be shown by a clinically relevant value of 0.5 days less than for omeprazole. In other words, the mean difference in onset of the first 24-hour heartburn-free period between the alginate/antacid and omeprazole with the corresponding 95% CI was used for the noninferiority test. If the lower limit of the CI was within 0.5 days and did not cross this NI margin, then the noninferiority hypothesis was confirmed for the alginate/antacid product. Intent-to-treat and per protocol analyses were used. Safety was assessed by the number of reported adverse drug reactions for each drug.

- *Identify the null hypothesis and alternative hypothesis for this noninferiority study.*
- *When setting the NI margin, what specific things did the investigators need to take into consideration?*
- *Did the investigators use the appropriate analysis type for an NI study?*
- *What is your conclusion if the 95% CI around the mean treatment difference of onset of first 24-hour heartburn-free period between alginate/antacid and omeprazole does not include or cross over the established NI margin?*
- *If the 95% CI around the mean treatment difference of onset of first 24-hour heartburn-free period between alginate/antacid and omeprazole includes or crosses over the established NI margin, what is your conclusion?*
- *After showing noninferiority for the two drugs, the investigators performed a superiority analysis on the data. What is your reaction to this second analysis?*

NI trials typically have a larger sample size compared to superiority trials since the NI margin is frequently smaller than the treatment difference anticipated with superiority trials.[26,31] Sample size determination before the study is started can be difficult since variance of the estimated treatment effect and event rate can be unknown for the test drug at this point. When this issue is present for superiority studies, an **independent data monitoring** group/committee is formed to examine the blinded information during the trial (interim analysis). This committee is looking for the occurrence of an unexpectedly low event rate so an upward adjustment in sample size can be proposed. This same approach to sample size reassessment and adjustment is applied to NI trials.[32,33] A clear explanation of how the blinded information was handled and how the **independent data monitoring committee (IDMC)** was conducted should be provided in the article for evaluation.

Reporting NI trials in the literature is still not consistent and this can often be the biggest issue to evaluating and interpreting trial results for quality.[34] The Consolidated Standards of Reporting Trials (CONSORT) statement, first published in 1996 and then updated in 2010 to improve randomized controlled trial reporting in the medical literature.[35,36] Extensions to the CONSORT statement that specifically address reporting of NI trials have been proposed.[5,8,37] Specifically, these points include:

- Rationale for conducting trial
- Research objective(s)
- Clearly defined primary and secondary outcome measures
- Statistical methods used to evaluated objective(s)
- Methods used for sample size determination
- Inclusion/exclusion criteria comparable to previous trials using the active comparator (reference drug/devise/procedure)
- Description accounting for patients that are screened, randomly allocated, violated protocol, and completing study
- Explanation of how NI margin was determined
- Rationale for choosing comparator with historical study results confirming efficacy of this comparator
- Explanation of interim analyses and study discontinuation rules
- Interpretation of the real and estimated treatment exposures
- Explanation of the impact withdrawals or crossovers could have had on length of exposure to treatment assigned
- Summary of results for each primary and secondary outcome measure providing estimated effect size and precision (e.g., 95% CI)
- Interpretation of results considering the noninferiority hypothesis, potential biases, concerns with any multiple analyses.

As mentioned previously, an attempt to rescue a failed superiority study that concludes the results really demonstrate NI should not be accepted.[23] Unfortunately, this situation is more common than would be expected.[38] The plan to determine NI of a test drug compared to the reference drug must be established prospectively utilizing the proper study design to test for NI. In other words, lack of superiority in a superiority trial design does not equal NI.

Case Study 5–2: Noninferiority Trial Design

A 2-year double-blind randomized parallel group noninferiority (NI) trial was conducted to compare the safety and efficacy of a dipeptidyl peptidase-4 inhibitor (linagliptin) to a commonly used sulfonylurea (glimepiride) in Type 2 diabetic patients inadequately controlled on metformin. Patients already on metformin, but not adequately controlled, were randomized to receive either linagliptin or glimepiride for 104 weeks. Power was set and met with a sample size of over 707 patients per treatment group. The primary efficacy endpoint was change in hemoglobin A_{1c} (HbA_{1c}) from baseline to week 104. The mean difference between treatment groups in change of HbA_{1c} from baseline to week 104 was the primary outcome for noninferiority. Even though this was an NI study, no mention of an NI margin was made throughout the study. Hypotheses based on noninferiority were established and a p-value of 0.03 was presented based on an alpha of 0.05. Safety was assessed by the number of reported adverse drug reactions for each drug.

- *Identify the null hypothesis and alternative hypotheses for this noninferiority study.*
- *Since there was no NI margin, how do you determine if noninferiority exists between these two drugs? Did the investigators use the appropriate analysis type for an NI study?*
- *Let us say the p-value for the noninferiority evaluation is p = 0.063 with alpha set at 0.05. What is your conclusion? After showing noninferiority for the two drugs, the investigators performed a superiority analysis on the data. What is your reaction to this second analysis?*

Appendix 5–1 contains a list of additional questions specific to NI studies. These specific questions are in addition to the standard questions used to evaluate other randomized clinical trials noted in Chapter 4 and using basic tools like the Ten Major Considerations Checklist discussed in the Introduction section.

N-OF-1 TRIALS

Description

The **N-of-1 trial** attempts to apply the principles of clinical trials, such as randomization and blinding, to individual patients.[39] These trials are useful when the beneficial effects of a particular treatment in an individual patient are in doubt. It is advantageous if the treatment has a short half-life (allowing multiple crossover and washout periods without carryover effects—see Chapter 8 for further explanation) and is being used for symptomatic relief of a chronic condition.[40] An N-of-1 trial can be used to determine whether a drug is effective in an individual patient. Taken as a whole, a group of N-of-1 trials can help identify characteristics that differentiate responders from nonresponders. Trials of multiple doses can identify the most effective dose and the clinical endpoints most influenced by the drug.[41]

An N-of-1 trial is similar to a crossover study conducted in a single patient who receives treatments in pairs (one period of the experimental therapy and one period of either alternative treatment or placebo) in random order.[41] As described below, the study usually consists of several treatment periods that are continued until effectiveness is proven or refuted. Randomization to active drug or placebo, and blinding of the physician and patient to the treatment being administered, helps reduce **treatment order effects** (the order in which patients receive the treatments in the trial affects the results), **placebo effects** (therapeutic activity provided by administering a placebo), and **observer bias** (person collecting the data from the trial knows or has some idea what study drug each patient is receiving and, therefore, this may have some effect on the results reported). Desired outcomes are identified prior to initiation of the study to ensure that objective criteria that are meaningful to both the prescriber and the patient are used to assess treatment efficacy.[40]

N-of-1 trials may improve appropriate prescribing of drugs in individual patients. For example, carbamazepine may be an option for relief of pain in a patient with diabetic neuropathy, but definitive information on the efficacy of such treatment is limited. Therefore, investigators may conduct an N-of-1 trial to determine whether such therapy is useful in a particular patient. N-of-1 trials are especially useful when long-term treatment with a specific drug may result in toxicity and the prescriber wishes to determine whether benefits outweigh potential risks.[40]

The effectiveness of N-of-1 trials has been evaluated in a study.[41,42] In this instance, of 57 N-of-1 trials completed, 50 (88%) provided a definite clinical or statistical answer to a clinical question, leading to the conclusion by the authors that N-of-1 trials were useful and feasible in clinical practice.[42] Simply stated, the goal of an N-of-1 trial is to clarify a therapeutic management decision.[42] Of 34 completed N-of-1 trials evaluated over a 2-year period, 17 (50%) were judged to provide definitive results (10 showed treatment to be effective, five showed treatment no better than no treatment, and two demonstrated harmful effects to the patients).[43] The remaining 17 N-of-1 trials showed trends toward equivalence to control or actually favored placebo. Overall, clinician confidence in the therapy was found to increase or decrease depending on the direction of trial results.[43]

Evaluation

General evaluation requirements have been recommended for N-of-1 trials.[43] Readers should determine whether the treatment target (or measure of effectiveness) was evaluated during each treatment period.[44] This target should be a symptom or diagnostic test result, but must be directly relevant to the patient's well-being (e.g., the visual analog scale for pain in the example of carbamazepine). Two other critical characteristics of an N-of-1 trial are that the symptom under investigation shows a rapid improvement when effective treatment is begun and that this improvement regresses quickly (but not permanently) when effective treatment is discontinued.[44] The longer it takes to see a therapeutic effect provided by a drug, the longer the testing period of the trial. This also holds true for how long it takes for the therapeutic effect to disappear after stopping the drug; a longer washout period results in an overall increase in trial duration. The length of the treatment period is important to know. For those diseases that remain constant, this treatment period is easy to establish. When dealing with a disease that is not constant, such as multiple sclerosis, the treatment period must be long enough to observe an exacerbation of the condition. A general rule is that if an event occurs an average of once every X days, then a clinician needs to observe three times X days to be 95% confident of observing at least one event. One should ask if a clinically relevant treatment target is used and can it be accurately measured? It is advisable to measure symptoms or the patient's QOL directly, with patients rating each symptom at least twice during each study period.

It is important to determine if sensible criteria for stopping the trial is established. Specification of the number of treatment pairs in advance strengthens the statistical analysis of the results and it has been advised that at least two pairs of treatment periods are conducted before the study is unblinded.[41]

N-of-1 trials provide more objective information than case reports or case studies because there is a control group, and are useful for providing definitive information for drug prescribing in individual patients. See Table 5–2 for a comparison of N-of-1 trials and case studies.

Appendix 5–1 contains a list of additional questions specific to N-of-1 studies. These specific questions are in addition to the standard questions used to evaluate other randomized clinical trials noted in Chapter 4 and using basic tools like the Ten Major Considerations Checklist discussed in the Introduction section.

TABLE 5–2. COMPARISON OF N-OF-1 TRIALS AND CASE STUDIES

	N-of-1 Trial	Case Study
Design	Prospective	Retrospective (most often)
Predefined methods	Yes	No
Clearly defined outcome measures	Yes	No
Randomization	Yes	No
Blinding	Yes	No
Multiple treatment periods	Yes	Not usually

Source: Adapted from Spilker B.[98]

ADAPTIVE CLINICAL TRIALS

Adaptive clinical trial (ACT) design has become a topic of great interest recently by both the pharmaceutical industry and the FDA.[44] In simplest form, the ACT is known as a staged protocol or group sequential trial.[45] One example of this group sequential design is called a 3+3 trial used in a Phase I trial to identify the maximum tolerated dose (MTD). Three patients start at a specific dose and if no toxicity is noted, a second group of three patients are given a higher dose. If one patient experiences a limiting toxicity, then a third group of three patients are given that same dose. From this third group, two or maybe all three patients experience toxicity, which leads to claiming that the previous lower dose is the MTD. This is one basic framework of the design that can be used for a specific purpose, dose response.

Key to this study design is that ACT provides the ability to use more adaptive sampling strategies. These strategies include response-adaptive designs for clinical trials where the emerging data or observations from the trial are used to make adjustments in the ongoing study.[46] As illustrated in this example where an ACT design is incorporated into a dose-response study, emerging patient outcomes are utilized to adjust allocation of future enrolled patients or some other study design component.

Classical clinical trial design is rigidly structured to investigate a set number of variables and prevent additional variables from being introduced that will confound the results. For instance, a traditional, randomized, controlled trial stipulates inclusion and exclusion criteria to allow only a specific population of patients entering into the trial. The benefit of these strict criteria is a well-defined population to be studied that excludes patients predicted to be potentially harmed if entered into the trial. However, the disadvantage of such rigidity is the inability to make adjustments to the inclusion and exclusion criteria as the study progresses and new information comes from those patients who have completed the trial. If the investigators discover there is a specific patient group that responds to the treatment during the trial, adjustments to include only that patient population are not allowed. For that reason, a significant number of patients who are anticipated to not respond are exposed to a treatment that may cause severe side effects. ACT design provides enough flexibility to incorporate continuously emerging knowledge generated as a trial is carried out. In essence, the ACT design provides the researcher with an opportunity to change some study methodology when they identify things that may need to be done differently, such as using a different dose, different patients, or measuring different outcomes over a different period of time. Ideas from industry, academia, and regulatory agencies, such as the FDA Critical Path Initiative (http://www.fda.gov/ScienceResearch/SpecialTopics/CriticalPathInitiative/default.htm), are leading a movement toward ACT design as a potential alternative method to gather data for use in the FDA drug approval process.

The primary benefit of ACT design is that fewer patients are allocated to a less effective therapy, a greater number of responding patients can be monitored for safety of the effective therapy, and fewer patients overall may be required to determine statistical and clinical significance of the drug.[47] Other potential benefits include a more efficient developmental pathway for the drug, patients benefit from effective therapies earlier, and prescribers have more information on patients most likely to benefit from the drug.

The majority of studies utilizing the ACT design have been dose-response trials used to identify the range of effective doses to be used in future efficacy confirmatory studies.[47] A much smaller number of pivotal, efficacy confirming studies have used this design due to company concerns about FDA's skepticism of ACT design including potential bias and increase in false-positive rates. With time, the ACT design is becoming more common in agreements made between the FDA and sponsors (also known as **Special Protocol Assessments**) for later stages of clinical development.

Higher level, more powerful, and complex ACTs require the use of Bayesian statistics that allow for much more flexibility than traditional statistical approaches can provide.[46] Traditional statistical approaches determine the likelihood that the efficacy of a specific drug could have happened by chance. On the other hand, the Bayesian approach provides a probability (or relative likelihood) that the drug is effective. This approach estimates the relative likelihood by using new data as it is created from the ongoing study. The Bayesian approach continuously updates the relative likelihood of the subject being investigated.

Pfizer's ASTIN trial (Acute Stroke Therapy by Inhibition of Neutrophils) is an example of how ACT methodology can be incorporated into a randomized, double-blind, placebo-controlled dose-response study.[48] This trial represents the first time that computer-assisted, real-time learning was successfully implemented in a large international study to look at dose response effects. In this study, ACT design methodology was used to help determine the maximum effective dose and ensure the study drug's best chance of showing efficacy. At the same time, the use of the ACT design decreased the exposure of patients to a drug that was not found to be efficacious in this particular disease state. The ACT study design is computationally and logistically complex, but today's rapid data collection methods and computing power is adequate to meet the requirements. Software programs developed in-house by pharmaceutical industry statisticians are used to handle these complexities.

Studies based on the ACT design are evaluated similar to other randomized clinical trials; however, there are some questions that are specific for assessing the ACT component. These questions are best understood using the ASTIN trial as an example.

The specific methodologies used to make adaptive changes in the trial are important. In the ASTIN trial, allocation of treatment was provided by a central location at baseline, days 7, 21, and 90, using a computer generated Bayesian design algorithm. This algorithm determined the current real-time optimal dose and provided information regarding the need to vary the number of patients required, distribute the patients differently between placebo and the study drug, and correct the optimal dose of the study drug. An automated fax system (e-mail in today's world) from other patients on the study drug provided information that was used to adjust and optimize the dose. In addition, an IDMC was established to utilize a termination rule for recommending discontinuation of the study after futility or efficacy was established. Termination for futility could be recommended only after a minimum of 500 evaluable patients had completed the study. A minimum of 250 evaluable patients were required before a recommendation could be made to terminate the study for efficacy reasons. Those patients with confirmed ischemic stroke by computerized axial tomography (CAT) scan who were still alive at study day 90 were termed evaluable patients.

Existing logistical issues and how they are being handled is important to know when evaluating an ACT study. In the ASTIN study, patient response information was transferred to a central location using an automated fax system. The adjusted dosing information was then sent back to the study site using this same fax system.

In ACTs, all proposed adaptive changes should be based on evidence and good clinical judgment. In the ASTIN study, the proposed adaptive changes were based on the dose-response information from other patients active and/or completed in the trial. The computer-generated specific adaptations that determined the current real-time optimal dose were provided by the Bayesian design algorithm. As mentioned earlier, information regarding the need to vary the number of patients required, distribute the patients differently between placebo and the study drug, and correct the optimal dose of the study drug was provided by this algorithm. A termination rule was established with specific criteria to be applied to the actual patient response information. This was developed to assist the IDMC in making a recommendation to discontinue the study after futility or efficacy was established.

It is important to know if extensive adaptation to the protocol occurred during the ACT. When adaptation is extensive in efficacy confirming trials, the key hypothesis can become unclear and protection of the study's integrity is at risk. The ASTIN study was a dose-response trial, not an efficacy-confirming trial. Adaptations of the dosing strength did occur and these were associated primarily with lack of efficacy or safety issues. The study's integrity was not jeopardized.

As with other study designs, obvious indications of bias entering the study and having effects on the results should be identified. Bias is a term used to describe a preference toward a particular result when this preference interferes with the ability to be impartial or objective. Several types of bias have been identified that can have major effects on the results of a study. See Table 5–3 for a list of biases from different causes that should be ruled out as having significant effects on the results of an ACT. Possible ways that bias could have

TABLE 5–3. TYPES OF BIAS

Category of Bias	Name of Bias	Description	Methods of Control	Cohort	Case-Control	Cross-Sectional
Selection bias	Admission rate (Berkson) bias	Admission rates of exposed and unexposed cases and controls differ, resulting in a distortion of odds of exposure in hospital-based studies	A priori define inclusion and exclusion criteria		X	
			All groups of subjects should have undergone identical diagnostic testing and there should be no difference in how exposure or disease status is determined			
	Nonresponse bias	Nonrespondents may exhibit exposures or outcomes that differ from respondents, resulting in over or under estimation of odds or risk	Match or adjust for confounding variables	X	X	X
			Use more than one control group			
	Prevalence-incidence (Neyman) bias	Timing of exposure identification causes some cases to be missed		X	X	
	Unmasking bias	An innocent exposure causes a sign or symptom that precipitates search for a disease, but does not itself cause the disease		X	X	±
Information bias	Family history bias	Family members tend to share more information with family members who have similar diseases or exposures	Establish a priori explicit criteria for data collection methods on exposures and outcomes	X	N/A	X
		Those family members without the disease or exposure may be unaware	Blinded interviewer and subject to the hypotheses investigated			
		Family historical information may vary widely depending on whether the person is a case or a control	Standardize data collection procedure, i.e., train observers, develop and refine survey questions and methods of recording answers			

	Recall bias	Difference in how data collection occurs exists between cases and controls, or the exposed and unexposed, resulting in an abnormally high rate of recall of exposure or outcome in one group	Maintain aggressive contact with subjects to limit attrition (cohort designs) For surveys, obtain response rates ≥80% Assess for effects of potential confounders	X	N/A	X
	Exposure suspicion bias	Knowledge of a subject's disease status may influence both intensity and outcome of a search for exposure		X	N/A	±
Data analysis bias	Post hoc significance bias	When decisions regarding level of significance are selected a posteriori, conclusion may be biased	Establish a priori the statistical methods to be used to evaluate data	X	X	X
	Data dredging bias	When data are reviewed for all possible associations without prior hypotheses, results are only suitable for hypothesis-forming activities	Report how missing data are handled Assess associations between confounders and exposures and outcomes	X	X	X
	Significance bias	Confusing statistical significance with clinical significance		X	X	X
	Correlation bias	Correlation do not equate with causation; concluding that correlation equates with causation can lead to serious errors		X	X	X

Source: Data from Fletcher RH et al.[75]

entered the study should be identified and confirm the effect of that bias on the results determined. In the ASTIN study, several things were instituted to minimize the chance of bias. An IDMC consisting of three stroke clinicians and a statistician was established prospectively. This group worked independent of the study investigators and would make recommendations based on the patient information to the steering committee. For instance, changing doses based on patient safety and determining if the trial should be terminated according to predetermined criteria for efficacy or futility are two types of recommendations made by this committee. The executive steering committee consisting of expert stroke physicians also worked independent of the study investigators and monitored the conduct of the study, reviewed center performance, and made study decisions based on information provided by the IDMC. In addition, the study was double-blinded so neither the patient or study investigators were aware of what treatment the patient was receiving.

If an interim analysis was conducted, exactly who had access to the information created from the interim analysis and how could this have affected any of the results are crucial to know. As mentioned previously, the ASTIN study had an IDMC formed to conduct interim analyses on the patient information received from the ongoing study. Based on the description of this group in the article, it would appear members of that committee had few, if any, interactions with Pfizer, the company sponsoring the trial.

Sometimes the ACT is stopped early based on an interim analysis. A determination should be made if stopping the trial early had any effect on the results that would prevent development of strong conclusions. If the discontinuation significantly shortens the period of treatment, evidence may be lacking for any conclusions to be made. The ASTIN study was stopped early due to lack of the test drug's dose response in efficacy. The effect on the evidence was minimal since specific numbers of patients needed to be enrolled before discontinuation could even be considered were predetermined before the study was initiated. A total of 551 evaluable patients had been enrolled (stopping rule required a minimum of 500 evaluable patients), received some dose of the study drug within the allotted range, and completed the study to day 90 before the trial was discontinued. An adequate sample size appeared to be obtained to meet the set power.

The benefits of ACT design are obvious and this encourages further exploration for appropriate application to clinical programs. Adaptations to number of patients, eligibility criteria, drug dose, and randomization allocation can significantly improve the efficiency of drug development and overall patient care. This is an area of study design research that is being implemented more frequently for specific uses. See Chapter 8 for further discussion of ACT.

Appendix 5–1 contains a list of additional questions specific to ACTs. These specific questions are in addition to the standard questions used to evaluate other randomized clinical trials noted in Chapter 4 and using basic tools like the Ten Major Considerations Checklist discussed in the Introduction section.

STABILITY STUDIES/*IN VITRO* STUDIES

Stability studies determine the stability of drugs in various preparations (e.g., ophthalmologic, intravenous, topical, and oral) under various conditions (e.g., heat, freezing, refrigeration, and room temperature). Stability of a pharmaceutical product is defined by the United States Pharmacopeia (USP) as "extent to which a product retains, within specific limits and throughout its period of storage and use (i.e., its shelf-life), the same properties and characteristics that it possessed at the time of its manufacture."[49] These studies are extremely important to the practice of pharmacy. For example, pharmacists who prepare intravenous solutions for use by patients at home often want to know how long a drug admixed in a particular solution is stable. Another stability question could be whether the length of time to maintain stability would be increased with freezing the admixture. This information helps determine how many intravenous admixtures may be dispensed at a time. It is also important for pharmacists involved with extemporaneous compounding to know the length of time a particular preparation is stable.

Stability study requirements and expiration dating are presented in the Current Good Manufacturing Practices (cGMPs),[50] the USP,[51] and the FDA and International Conference on Harmonization (ICH) guidelines. The listings for FDA Guidelines associated with various stability testing can be located at http://www.fda.gov/drugs/guidancecomplianceregulatoryinformation/default.htm. The ICH guideline Web page is located at http://www.ich.org/products/guidelines/quality/article/quality-guidelines.html. The cGMPs require a written testing program designed to assess the stability characteristics of drug products.[50] The USP contains detailed stability and expiration dating information in addition to stability considerations in dispensing practices.[51] Design of stability studies to acquire expiry and product storage, in addition to directions for submission of this information, is found in the FDA guidance documents. The ICH guidelines provide common approaches used by the pharmaceutical industry for assessing stability of drug products.

Generally, stability studies are not published but remain unpublished data on file with the pharmaceutical company or compounding pharmacy and in some cases not available to the public since they represent trade secrets. Trissel and associates have provided study guidelines for assessing the quality of stability studies that do get published.[52] These guidelines state that investigators conducting stability studies should provide:

- Complete description of study methodology and test conditions.
- Appropriate, validated assays should be used.
- Samples should include a baseline time zero measurement and an appropriate number of samples to assess stability over the time period. For example, if the goal of the study is to determine the stability of an antibiotic at room temperature, then

taking measurements at time zero and 30 days may not be adequate. Planning the study so that testing is done at multiple time points (i.e., time zero, 6 hours, 12 hours, 18 hours, and 24 hours) would yield more information about the degradation timeline of the product.

Appendix 5–1 contains a list of additional questions specific to stability studies. These specific questions are in addition to the standard questions used to evaluate other randomized clinical trials noted in Chapter 4 and using basic tools like the Ten Major Considerations Checklist discussed in the Introduction section.

BIOEQUIVALENCE TRIALS

An ever-increasing number of generic products are becoming available in the marketplace and there is a need to establish that the quality, safety, and efficacy of these generic drugs are the same as the brand name product, which is the purpose of this type of trial.[53] The health care practitioner is often placed in the position of having to select one from among several apparently equivalent products for individual patients or for use on formularies of health care organizations. The more skilled the health care practitioner is at interpreting the data, the more comfortable he or she will be in selecting the appropriate product for the specific patient or organization.

According to the Director of the FDA Office for Generic Drugs, "The standards for quality are the same for brand name and generic products."[54] Current FDA regulations require bioequivalence between each new generic product and the brand name product be demonstrated, but do not require that bioequivalence among generic copies of the same brand name drug be demonstrated.[54] This is based on the fact that if each generic copy must show bioequivalence to the brand name product, then the copies should be within the same range of bioequivalency.

Bioequivalent products are products that are equivalent in rate and extent of absorption (by definition, the rate and extent of absorption differ by –20% to +25% or less).[55] These criteria are based on an arbitrary medical decision that, for most products, a –20% to +25% difference in the concentration of the active ingredient in blood will not be clinically significant.[55] For some drugs with a **narrow therapeutic index (NTI)**, such as certain anticonvulsants and antipsychotics, there is concern this large of a margin may be unsafe. The area under the blood concentration time curve (AUC), the peak height concentration (C_{max}), and the time of the peak concentration (T_{max}) are the primary pharmacokinetic parameters used to assess the rate and extent of drug absorption. Additionally, for approval of a generic product, a manufacturer must show that a 90% CI for the ratio of the mean response of its product compared to that of the innovator product is within the limits of 0.8 to 1.25 (80% to 125%).[55,56]

Bioequivalence trials are often conducted under standardized conditions in normal healthy adult volunteers unless safety considerations prohibit administering the drug to healthy individuals. Standardized conditions and normal healthy adult volunteers are preferred because of availability and lack of confounding factors in this population.[55] This procedure has been questioned since data from healthy volunteers may not reflect the population for whom the medication is prescribed. In situations where the disease state along with comorbid diseases may have an effect on absorption, studying the bioequivalence in patients with this clinical picture would potentially yield more accurate results. Single doses of the test and control drugs are administered and blood or plasma levels of the drug are measured over time. Multidose studies are also conducted on occasion to establish bioequivalence at steady state. Often a crossover study design is used so that the subject serves as his or her own control, thus improving precision of results.

When evaluating bioequivalence trials for application in clinical practice, it is important to focus on the methods of the study. The following are specific components to look for in the methods section[57]:

- Acceptable age and weight range for the subjects are defined.
- Clinical parameters used to characterize a normal, healthy adult (e.g., physical exam observations, hematological evaluations) are described.
- Subjects should be free of all drugs, including caffeine, nicotine, alcohol, and other recreational drugs, for at least 2 weeks prior to testing, because these factors can affect pharmacokinetic parameters.
- Subjects should be free of all dietary supplements (botanical and nonbotanical), as many of these products can interact with products under bioequivalence review.
- All subjects should receive the drug under the same conditions and all blood levels should be taken at the same intervals, which should be based on the half-life of the drug.
- The assay used to determine the blood levels should be validated.
- The same assay should be used for the test and reference drugs. Multiple assays are available to measure serum levels for some products. Results from the same assay for two drugs may demonstrate equivalence. However, if one assay type is used for the reference drug and another assay type is used for the test drug, the results may not demonstrate equivalence because the sensitivity and specificity of assays may be different.
- Bioequivalence testing may be performed in both fasting and fed states to assess the impact of food on bioavailability; however, food intake should be closely monitored and controlled.

One of the most common errors in the use of bioavailability data is comparing two products based on data obtained from separate studies.[57] Different subject populations, study conditions, and assay methodologies are reasons why comparisons of data from different studies are dangerous and can lead to false conclusions.[57] For example, a pharmacy and therapeutics committee may identify two generic products that each have individually shown bioequivalence to the brand product in two separate studies. A false conclusion can be made that both generic products are bioequivalent to each other. When examining the results of bioequivalence studies, lack of statistical significance does not equate to bioequivalence.[56] The standards for a bioequivalence trial are completely different from a superiority trial. In a bioequivalence trial, a 10% difference between products would be equivalent, whereas a 10% difference between the products in a superiority trial could easily be interpreted as a difference.

For additional information, scientific and medical evaluations by the FDA are available on the FDA Web site at http://www.accessdata.fda.gov/scripts/cder/ob/default.cfm.

Appendix 5–1 contains a list of additional questions specific to bioequivalence studies. These specific questions are in addition to the standard questions used to evaluate other randomized clinical trials noted in Chapter 4 and using basic tools like the Ten Major Considerations Checklist discussed in the Introduction section.

PROGRAMMATIC RESEARCH

Programmatic research is another type of research important to overall health care is focused on the impact and economic value of programs and services provided by practitioners in community and institutional settings. This research is particularly important because limited resources and budget constraints demand that only those services that improve patient care in a cost-effective manner be implemented. As an example, the body of evidence in support of the economic benefit of pharmacists providing clinical pharmacy services has grown over the past decade, and is diverse.[58] The evidence includes contemporary practice sites and services. The study design and methodology has improved, in addition to economic, clinical, and humanistic outcomes assessed in many practice environments. Pharmacists, working in interprofessional settings with physicians and other health care providers, have demonstrated that they can improve drug therapy effectiveness and safety.[59] This study also showed that pharmacists enhanced the efficient delivery of health care in collaboration as part of an interprofessional team, applying their specific drug therapy knowledge, skills, and abilities to complement the other types of care provided by the collaborating professionals. The American College of Clinical Pharmacy (ACCP) has published a succession of position statements that review published literature regarding the value of clinical pharmacy services.[59] These position papers discuss strengths and limitations of existing literature, and include recommendations for further studies in order to facilitate continued documentation of value provided by pharmacists in progressive roles and settings, while utilizing methodology that ensures a high **level of evidence**-based rigor.

Appendix 5–1 contains a list of additional questions specific to programmatic research studies. These specific questions are in addition to the standard questions used to evaluate other randomized clinical trials noted in Chapter 4 and using basic tools like the Ten Major Considerations Checklist discussed in the Introduction section.

Observational Study Design

❷ *Observational study designs offer an alternative to interventional trials and are used in specific situations, such as when large populations of patients must be followed over extended periods of time. Results from these trials only allow associations to be formed rather than true cause-and-effect relationships.* They can be prospective, retrospective, or a single snapshot (or slice) in time. Observational study designs involve subject groups that are based on presence or absence of a disease or exposure, with observations being made and recorded regarding patient characteristics. The observational study design seeks to evaluate questions based on less rigidly controlled practice conditions than those used in experimental study designs. Research questions are addressed by comparing outcomes or experiences of patients arising from naturally occurring assignment to different treatments, subject characteristics, or exposures.[60,61] For instance, if an agent is particularly toxic and of no therapeutic value, it would be unethical to ask subjects to voluntarily expose themselves to the agent, thus an observational study would be used.[62] An example of this type of situation is the evaluation of risk factors for diseases such as cancer. An investigator wishing to evaluate the toxicity of environmental or industrial hazards or the teratogenicity of drugs administered during pregnancy would have to employ specific observational studies that will be discussed in this section to study these problems. These research techniques allow associations rather than cause-and-effect relationships to be determined. Thus, when evaluating overall results of any observational study (e.g., cohort, case-control, cross-sectional, or case study), it is important to remember that a correlation or an association between exposure and outcome does not prove causation.[63] Other factors possibly related to both the exposure and outcome must be considered.

The following discussion will present observational study designs commonly encountered within health literature: the cohort, case-control, and cross-sectional designs. Differences between these study designs will be discussed and specific uses identified for each design, see Table 5-4. In addition, evaluation techniques for each will be discussed.

TABLE 5–4. CHARACTERISTICS OF OBSERVATIONAL STUDY DESIGNS

Observational Study Design	Prospective Data Collection	Retrospective Data Collection	Exposure Known at Beginning of Study	Outcome Known at Beginning of Study	Study Determines Exposure Status	Study Determines Outcome Occurrence
Cohort	X	X	X			X
Case-control (trohoc)		X		X	X	
Cross-sectional	X				X	X

See Table 5–4 for differentiating factors between observational trial designs: cohort, case-control, and cross-sectional. In addition, see Table 5–3 for specific types of bias associated especially with observational studies. Note the suggested methods to control for bias and which types of observational studies are at the highest risk for each bias discussed.

COHORT STUDIES

Description

The term cohort is derived from the Latin word *cohors*, which means a group of soldiers.[64] In ancient Roman times, soldiers were assigned into one of 10 divisions of a legion where they remained over the duration of their service or died. This term is used today to describe a group of individuals with a common characteristic or experience.[65] That experience is often a specific exposure to a particular agent such as a vaccine, medication, procedure, or environmental toxin. Participants in a cohort study are grouped by their exposure and followed over time to determine the incidence of symptoms, disease, or death.[65] Two groups are usually compared. Generally, these two groups are made up of those participants exposed and those nonexposed. Other terms for cohort studies are follow-up, incidence, and longitudinal studies.

See Figure 5–4 for a schematic representation of this study design.

The study hypothesis for a cohort study attempts to establish a relationship between an exposure or risk factor and a subsequent outcome.[66] A measurement, such as **relative risk**, is frequently used to determine the extent of this relationship. Relative risk is the risk of developing a disease or adverse event in those participants exposed to a specific variable compared to those not exposed to that variable.[2,67]

$$\text{Relative Risk} = \frac{\text{Outcome or Adverse Event (exposure group)}}{\text{Outcome or Adverse Event (no exposure group)}}$$

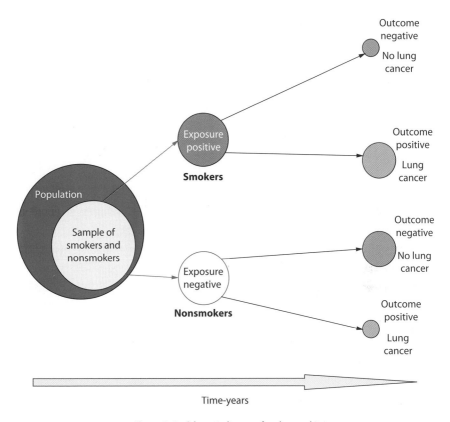

Figure 5–4. Schematic diagram of a cohort study.

The relative risk values can be greater than, less than, or equal to 1. For instance, if the relative risk calculated for a relationship between a specific drug exposure and cervical cancer is 5, this means that participants are five times more likely to contract cervical cancer when given the drug compared to those not being exposed to the drug. Other measurements such as **attributable risk, number needed to treat**, and **life table methods** can be used to analyze the data from cohort studies.[66]

Relative risk gives an idea of the magnitude of an effect, but does not provide information about precision or statistical significance of the result.[68] Alternatively, calculation of CIs (usually at a level of 95%) is utilized for evaluation of statistical significance of results. The CI provides a range in which the true value for the population lies. The concept is that the wider the CI, the greater the variability, and, therefore range that contains the true value. Because a relative risk of 1 indicates no difference exists between groups, the CI cannot include 1 and still maintain statistical significance. See Chapters 4 and 8 for further discussion on relative risk.

Categories of Cohort Studies

• There are three basic categories of cohort studies used based on timing of the events: prospective (looking forward in time), retrospective (looking backward in time), and ambidirectional (looking both forward and backward in time).[65] The prospective cohort study, also known as concurrent because participants are monitored over time, groups the participants based on current or past exposure and then follows these groups over time observing the various predetermined outcomes. In the prospective cohort design, outcomes have yet to develop and investigators are required to wait for their occurrence. For example, observing the long-term effects of lead exposure on cognitive function as children grow to be adults.

• Retrospective or historical cohort studies, also referred to as nonconcurrent since both the exposure and the outcome are already recorded in a database, uses computerized data on patients that have been recorded over the natural course of their health care.[66,69] Information regarding the treatment received by individuals in 2000 is obtained from a database in 2010. In addition, the assessment of outcomes due to this treatment is known and recorded in this database by 2010. For instance, a computer database is searched for all patients who received medication or surgical treatment for a disease in 2000. Once identified, the investigators observe the assignment to study or control groups. The database is then searched to determine the outcomes occurring for each group from 2000 to 2010.

• Finally, the ambidirectional cohort study involves both prospective and retrospective components.[65] An example of this type of cohort is the Air Force Health Study looking at men involved in aerial spraying of herbicides, including Agent Orange, during the Vietnam War.[70] The retrospective portion of the study observed the incidence of cancer and mortality from time of exposure in the war through the 1980s,[71,72] while the prospective component involves observing these men well into the future.[73]

Other terms describing cohort studies are based on the characteristics of the population that makes up the cohort, changes or no changes in the exposure over time, and existence of losses to follow-up.[65] Cohort studies where the participants may enter or leave based on changing characteristics, such as smoking, alcohol consumption, occupation, specific geographical location, are referred to as open or dynamic. For instance, a participant is a member of an open cohort group of Kansas City residents as long as they continue to live in Kansas City. A fixed cohort is identified by an unchangeable event such as having undergone a surgical procedure or been exposed to a potential toxin, such as Agent Orange, at a specific time, like the 1960s, and place, such as Vietnam. For this reason, exposures do not change or are considered fixed in this type of cohort. A third type of cohort is referred to as closed. Similar to the fixed cohort, a closed cohort involves an unchangeable event. A closed cohort also has a specific starting and ending point that involves follow-up. For example, a closed cohort may be conducted with participants attending a high school football game to determine if the nachos and spicy cheese consumed at the game provided them discomfort, such as gastritis, throughout the remainder of the evening until morning.

Uses of Cohort Studies

Cohort study designs are primarily used to explore the possible causes or risk factors, but not confirm the cause of a disease or the benefits and safety risks of both medication and procedures.[66] For instance, important information on the risk of cancer in individuals undergoing radiation therapy for noncancerous disease states has been identified. The cohort study is the simplest approach for studying disease incidence.[74] Key characteristics of each participant are determined prior to the study initiation and monitored during the follow-up period. From this information, important risk factors relating to the disease incidence are identified. In this way, risk factors are measured prospectively before the disease occurs. For example, cohort studies have been responsible for identifying the risk factors associated with cardiovascular disease such as high blood pressure, high cholesterol, physical inactivity, obesity, and smoking.

Primary disadvantages of cohort studies are expense and time consumption.[75] For example, with rare outcomes, such as the occurrence of aplastic anemia with use of clozapine, a prospective investigation may require extremely large numbers of patients, need decades of data collection, and accrue large project costs to acquire answers. It takes many years for adequate assessment of disease development or to establish disease-free status.[64] Such research questions are investigated more efficiently with the retrospective case-control design.

Evaluation of Cohort Studies

When critically evaluating a cohort study, the practitioner should be concerned with several points.[76] With a cohort study, there is no randomization process used to ensure that each participant has an equal opportunity to be in either the exposed or nonexposed group. The investigator selects the group each participant is relegated for the duration of the study. Certainly, those who have been, are, or will be exposed are assigned to that group, as are those who never have or never will be exposed assigned to the nonexposed group. Unlike a randomized controlled trial where patients are similar in their demographic characteristics between groups due to the randomization, a cohort study has no assurance of this similarity. For this reason, two concerns arise: **selection bias** and **confounders**.[25,77,78]

Selection Bias

Selection bias is a potential whenever the investigator is allowed to decide who is brought into the study and who is not selected to participate. This can result in differences within and/or between the groups that can have an impact on the final study results. For instance, an investigator either knowingly or unknowingly selects from the general population only the healthiest individuals to be assigned to the nonexposure group while at the same time a mixture of healthy and unhealthy participants are selected for the exposure group. With this scenario, there is an imbalance between groups that could set the exposed group up for an exaggerated negative effect to the exposure. When compared to the nonexposed group who were extremely healthy from the start of the study, this selection bias can produce an amplified difference that would not have been observed if both groups were balanced in regard to the initial healthiness of the participants. Simply stated, when a study starts out with dissimilar groups, the observed results at the study completion may be due to the exposure or due to the fact that the groups were different from the start.

Confounding Factor

A confounding factor or confounder is a variable related to one or more variables defined in the study.[79] These confounding factors can be known or unknown depending on whether they have been discovered. Confounding factors are common in cohort studies since they are the product of not using a randomization schedule that evenly distributes the confounding factors between the exposure and nonexposure groups. For instance, in a cohort trial that is studying the effects of sleep deprivation on pharmacy students during their schooling, sleep deprivation is a defined variable (exposure) and various outcomes associated with sleep deprivation such as grades, interaction during lectures, and volunteer time provided to student organizations are other defined variables. An example of a confounder would be age. If there were a greater number of older students in the exposure group, the outcomes could be poorer since older students have established lives with families and possibly other activities competing for their time. These confounding factors could certainly have an effect on the outcome measures, but have nothing to do with sleep deprivation. Confounding factors can mask actual associations or falsely demonstrate an apparent association that actually does not exist between variables in a study.[77] In the example of sleep-deprived pharmacy students, time taken away from studying and volunteer work that results in a negative effect on grades and volunteer time for organizations could be due to other competing activities related with older age (confounding factor) of participants. With age as a confounding factor in this example, it is possible to see how this confounder falsely demonstrates an apparent association between sleep deprivation and negative outcomes. In other words, an association between sleep deprivation and poorer grades or less volunteer time can be made when in reality the difference in age between groups is the real cause of the negative outcomes. Whether the investigators have used a systematic process to identify known confounders should be identified. In addition, careful consideration can sometimes identify confounders not mentioned by the authors. This would be considered a limitation and should raise caution with regard to reliability of the results.

There are methods and techniques that can be used to assess, correct, control, or adjust for confounding variables.[78,79] One method is putting restrictions on the selection criteria.[78] If the investigators had recognized age as a potential confounding factor prior to initiating the pharmacy student sleep deprivation study described earlier, an age range restriction such as 20 to 25 years of age could have been incorporated into the selection criteria. By restricting the age to no greater than 25 years, the confounding factor of older age and the potential effects on the results are removed from the scenario. Other analytical strategies can be used on the data to increase confidence that confounding factors had no or minimal effects on the results.[80] One analytical technique is regression that uses the data to determine if confounders are related to the outcomes. If regression analysis determines confounders have affected the results, an adjusted estimate of the actual exposure effect of interest on the outcomes is provided. For example, if age was shown by regression analysis to have affected the outcomes in the pharmacy student study, an adjusted estimate of actual sleep deprivation without the confounder effect on the outcomes would be provided. Stratification is another analytical technique that creates subgroups that are more balanced regarding baseline participant characteristics than the entire study population. Confounders such as age are balanced between subgroups. For example, applying a stratification analysis to the sleep deprivation study would result in age being more balanced between subgroups. The overall effect of sleep deprivation is calculated from the difference in average outcomes between the exposure and nonexposure groups within each stratum. The result of stratification is less confounder effect on the results of the association between sleep deprivation and measured outcomes of pharmacy student grades, lecture interaction, and volunteer time. Whether the investigators have used any of these techniques should be identified. Use of the technique can determine if confounding factors played a significant role in the final results based on what these analysis strategies reveal.

Outcome Measurement

Accurate measurement of the outcome is essential.[25] Surveillance bias is a potential problem when one group, generally the exposed group, is more intensely monitored for changes in the outcome measure than the comparison group. Blinding the investigator responsible for performing the outcome measurement is one potential way of minimizing the chances for surveillance bias. Sources for acquiring the outcome data can vary. When this happens, the different sources can affect the results since one source can be more sensitive than others. For example, the details provided regarding follow-up can be significantly different when looking at medical chart versus nursing notes versus the actual interpretation of the radiology report by an expert. Making sure that the same source is used to obtain all measurements for both groups is crucial. Furthermore, information bias can occur if the same efforts to measure outcomes are not made for both the exposed and nonexposed groups.[64,77]

Follow-Up

Adequate follow-up is important.[25,65] The practitioner must ensure that the length of follow-up was adequate for the outcome being measured. For instance, a 3-month cohort study to determine risk factors associated with long-term cardiovascular events such as myocardial infarction is inadequate. Also, dropouts should be accounted for by the authors and assessed to determine if there were factors that caused a greater number in one group compared to the other. For instance, participants who are sicker in one group might drop out of the study due to death that is not associated with the risk factor being studied, but rather because they were more prone to death due to some other cause. Studies where loss to follow-up exceeds 20% in either the exposed or nonexposed cohort should be interpreted with caution.[64]

Appendix 5–1 contains a list of additional questions specific to cohort studies. These specific questions are in addition to the standard questions used to evaluate other randomized clinical trials noted in Chapter 4 and using basic tools like the Ten Major Considerations Checklist discussed in the Introduction section.

Case Study 5–3: Cohort Study Design

A cohort study is published in *Cancer Epidemiology, Biomarkers, and Prevention*. The study is a prospective observation on the relation between coffee consumption and risk of endometrial cancer. Coffee consumption was prospectively assessed in relation to endometrial cancer risk in the Nurses' Health Study with 67,470 females aged 34 to 59. The questionnaires collected the cumulative average coffee intake over a specific time period. Cox regression models calculated incidence rate ratios. The results showed that consumption of fewer than four cups of coffee per day were not related to endometrial cancer risk. Women who consumed four or more cups of coffee had a 25% lower risk of endometrial cancer than those who consumed less than one cup of coffee per day (multivariable $RR = 0.75$, 95% $CI = 0.57$ to 0.97, $p = 0.02$). Decaffeinated coffee consumption suggested an inverse relationship. The authors concluded that these observations suggest four or more cups of coffee per day are associated with a lower risk of endometrial cancer in women.

- *What would indicate that there is some potential for selection bias in this study?*
- *What are some of the potential confounding factors associated with this study?*
- *What are some of the other characteristics of a cohort study that should be evaluated?*
- *What cause-effect relationship can be established with this study?*

CASE-CONTROL STUDIES

Case-control studies (also termed case-referent, case history, or retrospective studies) are a type of observational study that offers an epidemiologic research alternative to cohort studies. The latter requires a large number of subjects, and is often expensive and time consuming.[63] Case-control studies seek to retrospectively identify potential risk factors of diseases or outcomes. In a case-control study, subjects (cases) with a particular characteristic or outcome of interest (e.g., disease) are recruited, matched with, and compared to a similar group of subjects (controls) who have not experienced the characteristic or outcome.[63,80,81] Data regarding the history of exposures are collected via patient interviews or by reviewing subject data records, and the two groups are compared to identify possible risk factors or contributors for development of the disease or outcome of interest. Note both the exposure and the outcome are known for all subjects at the beginning of the case-control study. This is a key differentiating factor for case-control versus cohort study design. See Figure 5–5 for a schematic of the case-control study design.

Case-control studies can be more useful than cohort studies when diseases have a rare prevalence or when many years of exposure to the risk factor is required.[59,64,81]

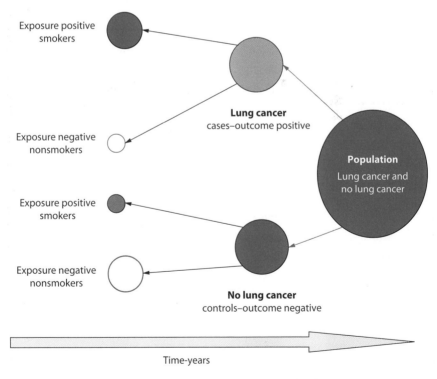

Figure 5–5. Schematic diagram of a case-control study.

Case-control studies are always conducted in a retrospective design compared to random-ized clinical trials and cohort studies, which are usually performed in a prospective man-ner and that is why case-control studies are sometimes called trohoc studies (i.e., cohort spelled in reverse).[81]

• Exposure of study subjects to the risk factor should reflect what occurs in the general population. If subjects with higher or lower exposure rates to the risk factor are excluded from the study, determination of possible associations between the exposure and a par-ticular disease may be biased and inaccurate.[81] For example, case-controls often use sub-jects drawn from hospitalized populations, whose risk factor exposure may differ from individuals in the community, a problem termed **Berkson's bias**.[81] Table 5–3 presents this and other types of bias that may be found within observational study designs, along with methods that provide control of potential biasing factors.

• Predisposition to the disease of interest should be similar in both cases and controls, except for exposure to the risk factor under investigation; however, this is extremely dif-ficult to ensure.[77,82,83] **Matching** is often used to ensure that cases and controls are simi-lar. With matching, each case has a comparable control or controls in terms of demographic and exposure characteristics. At the beginning of the study in Figure 5–5, patients with lung cancer and those without have matching demographics and exposure characteris-tics. Often it is difficult to determine which variables should be used to match cases to controls (e.g., sex, age, and date of admission). Such matching allows assessment of only the risk factor under investigation such as smoking. No other variables that may have contributed to the disease are taken into consideration.[81,82,84] Matching may even result in a negative impact on the interpretation of study results if cases and controls are matched for a factor that is itself related to the exposure.[64] Using the example, this type of situation could exist if the patients were required to have a family background of smokers. This exposure to second-hand smoke may confound the results regarding effects of direct smoking on the case group since the nonsmokers have been exposed to a factor that is itself related to the exposure. The result is both groups being exposed to indirect smok-ing in the past, which may contribute to the development of lung cancer.

• Cases and controls should undergo the same diagnostic evaluation to determine the presence or absence of the disease under investigation (e.g., chest x-ray and bronchos-copy for definitive diagnosis of lung cancer), because detection of a disease is more likely to be found in individuals who undergo extensive diagnostic testing.[83] In addition, indi-viduals administering the tests should be blinded to the presence or absence of the risk factor to eliminate **diagnostic review bias**.[81,83] This blinding can be achieved if the x-rays and bronchoscopies are reviewed and interpreted by an independent, noninvestigator who is unaware of the study protocol details. A problem is that many diagnostic tests can only be performed in individuals suspected of having a particular disease state due to risks associated with their use. This would be the situation with bronchoscopies due to the invasiveness of the test. In this situation, the independent, noninvestigator is left with only a chest x-ray and the physician's subjective final diagnosis in the medical records.

Case-control study designs have both advantages and disadvantages. These studies are relatively inexpensive and can be completed in a shorter timeframe than cohorts.[85] Both of these advantages are related to how subjects are recruited and data are acquired. When rare events are studied prospectively in a cohort design, recruitment of large numbers of patients is required due to the uncertainty of events occurring during the study period and the resulting need to ensure study power. In contrast, case-control studies reduce the need for large sample sizes, as subjects are recruited based on *a priori* knowledge of occurrence of outcomes as stated in the medical records.

Several points should be considered when evaluating these types of trials. Most limitations inherent to case-control studies are due to the retrospective design.[82] Overall, the two major methodological issues include appropriate selection of controls and accurate determination of the level of exposure.[77] Historical data used in case-control studies, which are obtained from medical records, may be inaccurate or incomplete.[81,82,84] When patients are interviewed regarding historical events, equal distribution of patients' ability to recall events that have happened in the past between the two groups may not be ensured.[83] For example, patients with lung cancer may be more likely to recall events preceding development of the disease than patients who are healthy. Patients with disease have probably contemplated factors they believe may have contributed to disease development (recall bias). For this reason, there should be some explanation in the study addressing the issue of recall bias. Unblinded investigators who collect data may also question individuals exposed to the disease more intensely than control subjects. To reduce variation in data obtained from cases and controls, trained data collectors should be blinded to the status of the subjects as cases or controls (lung cancer or no lung cancer).[81]

Another prominent disadvantage is that information about the exposure and outcome is collected simultaneously, so it is difficult to sort out the temporal relationship between the two.[77] For instance, it is often difficult to determine if the outcome preceded the exposure, a situation termed **protopathic bias**, where the disease may lead to risk factor exposure rather than vice versa.[77,83] Consider the following illustration. Abnormal vaginal bleeding may be an early sign of uterine cancer. Vaginal bleeding, however, may lead to prescribing hormonal therapies such as progesterone. An investigator may later erroneously conclude that use of progesterone was associated with development of uterine cancer, when in fact the cancer preceded use of the progesterone in this case.[83]

Some experts have suggested use of several control groups selected on the basis of different criteria in an attempt to reduce some of the biases discussed above.[81] A well-designed case-control study may have multiple controls for each case. If results of comparing cases to the various control groups are in agreement with one another, bias in the control groups is less likely to be present.[81]

Odds ratios are used to help interpret the results from case-control studies. The odds ratio is an estimate of relative risk.[63]

$$\text{Odds Ratio} = \frac{\text{\# cases with disease \& exposure} \div \text{\# cases with disease \& no exposure}}{\text{\# cases without disease \& exposure} \div \text{\# cases without disease \& no exposure}}$$

Although relative risk is preferred for prospective trials, the odds ratio is the appropriate measure for retrospective studies.[25] Consider the situation presented in Table 5–5, where industrial exposure to formaldehyde in patients with and without respiratory illness is assessed. Odds of exposure to formaldehyde is 20/180 (0.11) in the cases with respiratory illness and 5/195 (0.03) in the controls. The odds ratio is calculated as 0.11/0.03 = 3.7. Interpretation is the same as with relative risk; greater than 1 denotes increased risk, equal to 1 indicates no effect, and less than 1 indicates a protective effect. As with cohort studies, 95% CIs should be calculated.[86] CIs are preferred because they provide some indication of precision and variability of the individual participant's outcome. A narrow CI suggests precision and less variability of the individual outcome measures. The wider the CI, the more variability observed between outcome measurements that make up the mean.

Appendix 5–1 contains a list of additional questions specific to case-control studies. These specific questions are in addition to the standard questions used to evaluate other randomized clinical trials noted in Chapter 4 and using basic tools like the Ten Major Considerations Checklist discussed in the Introduction section.

CROSS-SECTIONAL STUDIES

Cross-sectional studies or prevalence surveys can be thought of as a snapshot (or slice) of time because data are collected only once on members of the study population over a period of time and evaluated as a single point in time.[87] Members of the study population do not need to all be studied at once, but each member can be studied at a different time. The key is that data are only collected once on each member. These studies differ from longitudinal studies that make a series of observations more than once on each member of the study population over a period of time. The cross-sectional study design

TABLE 5–5. **CASE-CONTROL STUDY—DETERMINATION OF ODDS RATIOS IN INDUSTRIAL FORMALDEHYDE EXPOSURE IN PATIENTS WITH RESPIRATORY ILLNESS**

Risk Factor	Respiratory Illness	No Respiratory Illness	Total
Formaldehyde exposure	20	5	25
No industrial exposure to formaldehyde	180	195	375
Total	200	200	400

is hypothesis generating as opposed to hypothesis testing, and is not suited for testing the effectiveness of interventions.[77] Only an association can be drawn from the results, not a cause-effect relationship. Typical examples of cross-sectional studies are surveys that evaluate opinions or situations at a fixed point in time. For a hypothetical situation concerning a drug, a cross-sectional study design could be developed to look into a large insurance database and determine how many people died suddenly within 5 years of receiving that drug. Cross-sectional studies are relatively quick and easy to perform and may be useful for measuring current health status or setting priorities for disease control.[77]

A study is classified as cross-sectional because measurements are taken at a single point in time, even though observations may cover a period of several months or years. For example, a survey of smokers is cross-sectional when the questionnaire is administered once, even though the questions contained in the survey may focus on smoking habits over the past 10 years.

As in other observational trial designs, the research question and the relevant inclusion and exclusion criteria must be clearly and unambiguously stated.[77] Also, selection of cases must be clearly described.[64]

Problems that may occur during cross-sectional studies include errors in data collection and transient effects that may influence observations. Because measurements occur at only one point in time, inaccuracies in data collection may go unnoticed because there are no prior data for comparison. In studies where multiple observations occur, data collection errors, seen as outlier data, may be more easily recognized. For instance, the prevalence of a disease state may be recorded as 15% of the U.S. population in 2007. However, if looking at the same statistics for 2006, 2008, and 2009, it is possible to see the prevalence was 2.1%, 2.2%, and 2.0%, respectively. Obviously, the 2007 prevalence of 15% is quite different than the prevalence 1 year before and the next 2 years after this observation. The 2007 observation would be considered a data outlier that probably represents a data collection error. The problem is, taken as a single observation without the other years, the 2007 prevalence would appear accurate and not recognized as an error in data collection. Transient effects are temporary occurrences that are found at the time a cross-sectional study is conducted, but are not identified if the study were repeated. A good example of transient effects is student evaluations of university professors. If a professor chooses to have students evaluate a course after a particularly grueling examination, chances are the evaluations would be poor based on students' response to the examination just taken. However, if the evaluations were administered after a curve had been applied for final grades, students may reflect on the course positively based on overall knowledge they received from the instructor, rather than a single negative experience. Transient effects are difficult to identify by a study evaluator. They may only be uncovered through retrospective evaluation of the study by the investigator. The investigator must perform a thorough assessment of all factors that may have impacted the results of the trial.

Appendix 5–1 contains a list of additional questions specific to cross-sectional studies. These specific questions are in addition to the standard questions used to evaluate other randomized clinical trials noted in Chapter 4 and using basic tools like the Ten Major Considerations Checklist discussed in the Introduction section.

Reports Without Control Group

CASE STUDIES, CASE REPORTS, AND CASE SERIES

❸ *Case studies, case reports, and case series are observational or interventional reports describing patient or patient group exposure to a drug or technology and can be valuable to record preliminary findings that lead to further study. A key characteristic to these reports is the lack of a control or comparison group.*

Each one is different as described below:

- Case study is a record of descriptive research that documents a practitioner's experiences, thoughts, or observations related to the care of a single patient.
- Case report is a descriptive record of a single individual (case report) in which the possibility of an association between an observed effect and a specific intervention or exposure (often an unexpected complication of treatment or procedure) based on detailed clinical evaluation and history of the individual.
- Case series is a group of records (case studies) that documents a practitioner's experiences, thoughts, or observations related to the care of multiple patients with similar medical situations.

Because these reports lack comparison to a control group, they do not take into consideration other influencing factors which may also have played a role in observed outcomes. In contrast to N-of-1 trials, a case study (either interventional or observational) does not apply clinical trial principles such as randomization and blinding to individual patients. The case study can be prospective or retrospective, whereas the N-of-1 trial design is prospective. The case study usually does not involve multiple treatment periods like that seen with N-of-1 trials. Comparisons of single patient clinical trials (N-of-1) and case studies are presented in Table 5–2.[88]

Interpretation of case studies can be difficult.[89] Design and methods describing conduct of a case study are not well defined.[90] For example, beneficial effects attributed to a drug or treatment under investigation may actually be a function of spontaneous regression of signs and symptoms of the disease, a placebo effect, and/or related to physicians' attitudes that may influence patient outcome.[90]

Case studies, however, are an integral part of the biomedical literature. They have played an important role in identifying treatments for rare disorders where large subject pools cannot be identified.[90] Case studies, reports, or series may also be useful for early recognition of drug toxicities and teratogenicity. A newly recognized value of case reports is utilization for understanding potential toxicities of DS products (botanical and nonbotanical). Because the FDA does not regulate these products and adverse event reporting is scarce, often safety information is not well defined for these products. Thus, published case reports may play a somewhat larger role for dietary supplements in suggesting potential safety problems than for traditional drug products.

When possible, results of case studies, reports, or series should be confirmed with randomized controlled clinical trials. Case studies, reports, and series serve as an important initial step in the formulation of hypotheses.[91] When case studies, reports, or series show a beneficial effect of a drug or treatment in diseases whose outcomes are consistently grim, or when all other treatments have failed, the results can be applied to patients in clinical practice.[91]

Appendix 5–1 contains a list of additional questions specific to case studies, reports, and series. These specific questions are in addition to the standard questions used to evaluate other randomized clinical trials noted in Chapter 4 and using basic tools like the Ten Major Considerations Checklist discussed in the Introduction section.

Survey Research

❹ *Survey research is information gathered from an identified group with conclusions drawn and applied to a larger population. This gathered information is considered either descriptive (such as opinions and attitudes) or explanatory (such as explaining a cause and effect) in nature and the validity of the results depends on the quality of the study's internal rigor.* Survey research is used to study the incidence, distribution, and relationships of sociologic and psychological variables.[91] It is used to collect information from a sample and generalize the findings to a larger, **target population**.[92] Data obtained from survey research have been used for many purposes including helping investigators identify, assess, and compare respondents' ideas, feelings, plans, beliefs, and demographics.[93] Surveys may be used to determine how health care programs should be implemented by utilizing the opinions of experts with experience in a particular area, to study effectiveness of a program by surveying individuals who have used its services, or to understand attitudes and behaviors of patients or members of the profession the program affects. For example, directors of pharmacy may survey other hospitals to determine salary ranges in order to decide whether salary increases are needed to remain competitive in the job market. Patient surveys are prepared and sent to postsurgical patients to document the care and satisfaction perceptions so changes can be made in the process for improvement. The ability to critically evaluate such literature has become a necessity for the practitioner due to an increased emphasis on this type of research in the medical literature.

TYPES OF SURVEYS

There are two basic types of surveys seen published in the biomedical literature. Descriptive surveys attempt to identify psychosocial variables such as attitudes, opinions, knowledge, and behaviors in a population, while explanatory surveys attempt to explain causal relationships between variables.[93] These dependent variables such as knowledge and behavior are often compared to independent variables such as age, sex, or education.[94]

TYPES OF DATA COLLECTED

Several types of data are collected in survey research and include incidence, attitudinal, knowledge, and behavior measurements. Incidence data try to determine the occurrence of events without drawing any relationships between variables.[95] An example of incidence data is the morbidity or mortality data reported weekly in the Centers for Disease Control and Prevention's *Morbidity and Mortality Weekly Report* (http://www.cdc.gov/mmwr). Manpower data are also incidence data frequently reported in pharmacy literature.[95] The number of residency-trained specialists in drug information is an example of data that might be collected in a nationwide manpower survey. Attitudinal data such as job satisfaction surveys often try to compare this dependent variable with independent variables such as age, education, or salary. Knowledge data attempt to document a person's knowledge or level of understanding about a specific topic. Examples include surveys asking physician's knowledge of retail prices of medications or pharmacist's knowledge of state pharmacy laws.[95] Behavior data documents what a person actually does in a particular situation rather than asking him or her in a survey, which may reflect an attitude, rather than the actual observed behavior. Observing the number of specific points that a pharmacist addresses during patient education sessions is an example of behavior data.[95]

DATA COLLECTION METHODS

Data collection for surveys may involve questionnaires, examination of historical records, telephone interviews, face-to-face interviews, Web-based questionnaires, focus groups, or panel interviews.[95] Well-conducted surveys have several important characteristics—they are objective and carefully planned, data are quantifiable, and subjects surveyed are representative of the target population.[96] In evaluating survey research, just like any other research, one must ask if the results are reliable and valid, and if they can be generalized.[93]

ERRORS AFFECTING PRECISION AND ACCURACY

Four sources of error have been described that can threaten the reliability of survey results and must be evaluated by readers.[93] Each source will be described and how to evaluate a survey article for these errors will be discussed in the Evaluation of Survey section.

Coverage Error

The first type of error, **coverage error**, is a bias in a statistic that occurs when the target population you want to survey does not coincide with the sample population that is actually surveyed. This type of error can compromise the ability to generalize study results.[93] Coverage error can be due to an inadequate sample frame or flaws in execution of the data collection. For example, people without telephones or those with unlisted numbers would be excluded from a **sample frame** of names from a telephone directory. In the case of a Web-based survey of a target population that includes urban and rural areas, those persons without a computer or e-mail address would be excluded from the list of e-mail addresses provided for the survey.

Sampling Error

Sampling error refers to the difference between the estimate derived from a sample survey and the true value that would result if a census of the entire target population were taken under the same conditions. This error occurs when the researcher surveys only a subset (sample) of all possible subjects within the population of interest.[93] The use of random sampling procedures and larger sample sizes can be used to minimize sampling error. This error describes variation around the true value of the population mean seen when multiple samples are pulled from the same population.[96] Sample error is reported usually as the mean ±1 **standard error of the mean (SEM)** (see Chapter 8 for more information).

Measurement Error

Measurement error occurs when the collection of data is influenced by the interviewer or when the survey item itself is unclear from the respondent's point of view. When measurement error occurs, a subject's response cannot be compared to other responses.[93] The survey method used to collect the data may be one source of measurement error. Face-to-face interviewers may influence the responses of the person being surveyed. The survey instrument itself may be ambiguous and open to interpretation. Bias can be introduced into a survey by the cover letter or sponsoring body; either may lead the respondent to one desired response rather than measuring the true response.

Lastly, measurement error can occur when a respondent replies with a preferred or more socially acceptable answer rather than the real answer. A well-designed survey instrument can minimize the chances of this type of error occurring. The well-designed survey instrument takes into account the abilities and motivation of the respondent to respond correctly (i.e., written at an appropriate educational level). **Parallel forms** (usually consisting of alternatively worded items placed throughout the survey) of either specific survey items or the entire survey instrument have been used to increase reliability of survey research. The use of such forms requires the calculation of correlation coefficients (see Chapter 8) between the parallel items and survey instruments.

Accurate assessment of measurement error relies on the availability of the questionnaire or tool used to collect data so that readers may analyze wording. Unfortunately, many articles relating results of survey research do not include the actual questionnaire used in the survey due to space and ownership issues. Lengthy questionnaires take up valuable journal space and the publisher may decide not to include them. Some authors do not want to give away the intellectual work that they invested in developing a good questionnaire and decide not to publish it. These factors make it impossible for the reader to evaluate the wording and, thus, the objectivity of questions or quality of the survey instrument. Readers need to look for author information provided on the reliability and validity of their survey instrument to ensure that quality measures were evaluated.

Nonresponse Error

Finally, **nonresponse error** occurs when a significant number of subjects in a sample do not respond to the survey. A type of bias called **nonresponse bias** can result in surveys, where the answers of respondents differ from the potential answers of those who did not answer. If the responders' demographics, characteristics, or responses differ significantly from the nonresponders in a way that influences the results, then nonresponse error would be suspect.[93] Unfortunately, this error is difficult to assess since the nonresponders' answers are never known. One way researchers attempt to minimize the chances of this error is to strive for response rates in the 80% to 90% range. This level of response rate provides some assurance that the small number of nonresponders will not alter results and, therefore, the author's conclusions.[94] Other authors argue that response rates of 80% for face-to-face interviews, 70% for telephone interviews, and 50% for mailed questionnaires are acceptable.[94]

EVALUATION OF SURVEY

In order to accurately assess the survey's validity (i.e., robustness) and evaluate these potential sources of error and bias, the methods section, which must be explicit, should be heavily scrutinized. Foremost, a description of study methodology with enough detail to replicate the study should be provided. Additionally, the methods section should relate each type of error associated with survey research and state how investigators attempted to control those errors.[97]

Factual Data and Internal Validity

Attempts to assess validity and reliability of the survey and efforts made to validate factual data should be described. For example, demographics of individual hospitals can be verified using American Hospital Association data. Asking more than one question about a concept can increase the **internal validity** of a survey.[93] For example, a respondent who answers yes to a positively worded statement would be expected to answer no to the same concept when worded in a negative fashion. A correlation analysis such as the Cronbach alpha or similar statistical test that measures correlation between items should be calculated and the coefficient factor(s) reported in the article.[93] The coefficient alpha is interpreted in the same fashion that coefficients of reliability are interpreted (i.e., 0 indicates no consistency between responses while increasing consistency is seen as you approach 0.8 to 1).

Sample Size

The methods section should report sample size, along with a description of how it was determined. The validity of both survey research and clinical trials relies on sample size. In order to have sufficient statistical power to demonstrate a difference between two groups, studies must have an adequate sample size. In designing survey research, the population of interest is first determined then subdivided into smaller groups around a variable of interest. For example, the population of interest may be all patients who attend an asthma clinic. This population could be subdivided into smaller groups based on the severity of asthma and then surveyed as to level of customer satisfaction. In establishing sample size for survey research, investigators must then determine the minimum number of subjects that must be sampled for the sample to be representative of the entire population.[97] This determination is made by consulting references that describe variability in sampling or consulting a statistician.

Sample Frame

Additionally, the reader should evaluate the comprehensiveness, probability of selection, and efficiency of the sample frame. A sample frame describes the population that will actually be drawn from to make up the survey sample. A sample is comprehensive if all members of a population had a chance to be chosen and no one was systematically excluded.[97] Determining efficiency of a sample relates to how well the sample frame excluded individuals who are not the subject of the survey. For example, to survey elderly people, it is appropriate to survey all households to determine if elderly individuals live there.[97]

In addition to providing information about the sampling frame, the methods section should provide a description of interviewers (age, sex, ethnicity, and so forth) and the effect interviewers may have had on the data.

Sampling Strategy and Response Rates

Sampling strategy and response rates should also be stated. The methods section should supply the reader with enough information to ensure that nonresponse error was assessed and measures were taken to control the error.[93] Repeated attempts to obtain completed questionnaires from initial nonrespondents will yield higher response rates and more accurate results than if no follow-ups are performed.[97] For example, attempts at other times of the day should be made for phone surveys and a second reminder postcard should be sent for mailed surveys. For Web-based surveys, e-mail reminders serve as follow-ups. Additionally, one way to minimize the problem of poor response rates is to sample (by phone) a small group of nonresponders to determine if their responses differ substantially from responders, although this may not be possible.[96] If results do not differ, the survey remains valid. Furthermore, authors should relate as much information about nonresponders as possible. Although survey result information has not been gathered, authors may have demographic and geographic data based on addresses and other information originally obtained.

Survey Instrument Reliability

The methods section should also describe techniques used to assess the reliability (i.e., can the results of the survey be repeated by another investigator) of the survey instrument and present the results of reliability estimates.[93] As discussed earlier under internal validity, a statistical test that measures correlation between items should be used as a reliability estimate. In general, the higher the reliability estimate (correlation coefficient), the more confidence the reader may place in the results published. A more complete review of correlation analysis is presented later (see Chapter 8). Additionally, any relevant elements of the survey research administration process (i.e., whether a pretest or pilot test was used) should be described. A pretest or pilot test is an assessment of a questionnaire made before full-scale implementation to identify and correct problems such as faulty questions, flawed response options, or interviewer training deficiencies.[98] Subjects administered the pretest not only answer the survey questions, but also answer questions about the clarity, length, and ease of understanding the actual instrument and may contribute other questions that should be included.[94]

Other Considerations

Of note, informed consent is generally not required in survey research as the risk is minimal and the respondent has the opportunity to withdraw from participating every time a new question is asked, although many surveys now do include an informed consent.[97] If the respondent does withdraw part way through the survey or interview, the data should not be included in the final analysis. In situations where sensitive information might potentially harm the subject, asking for a signed informed consent document allows the researchers the opportunity to reassure their commitment to confidentiality and reinforce the limits of how the data can be used.

Surveys are a commonly used research tool and are capable of providing a wealth of information on many aspects of a given target population. Ensuring validity of information gained through survey research, however, relies on critical evaluation of results through a thorough assessment of the study's internal rigor.[93] The ability to evaluate such research results is highly dependent on the amount and quality of information presented in the methods section.

Appendix 5–1 contains a list of additional questions specific to survey research studies. These specific questions are in addition to the standard questions used to evaluate other randomized clinical trials noted in Chapter 4 and using basic tools like the Ten Major Considerations Checklist discussed in the Introduction section.

Postmarketing Surveillance Studies

Prior to approval by the FDA, drugs undergo testing in a limited number of patients. Once approved, experience in patients escalates and previously unrecognized rare adverse events may be identified. The drug may also be found to be useful for conditions not described in the product labeling.

Postmarketing surveillance studies are phase IV studies that follow drug use after market approval and are sometimes referred to as **pharmacoepidemiologic studies**. See Chapter 17 for further explanation of the phases of the drug development process. The phase IV studies are useful in identifying new, potentially serious effects of drugs. A number of drugs have been removed from the market after approval following identification of such problems (e.g., fenfluramine, rofecoxib [Vioxx™], valdecoxib [Bextra®], propoxyphene (Darvon®), and hydromorphone hydrochloride extended release capsules [Palladone™ Extended-Release]). Postmarketing surveillance studies also allow assessment of drug use outside of product labeling and may identify areas for further research.

Many types of study designs are used in phase IV studies, including cross-sectional, case-control, cohort, and randomized controlled clinical trials. These studies can answer questions about drug interactions, identify potential new indications for the product, and gather information about the consequences of an overdose. In addition, the studies can provide efficacy in a larger and broader population (patients with different disease states and demographics that may not have been fully evaluated in the original clinical trials).[98]

Perhaps one of the most important functions of postmarketing surveillance is in the area of adverse event reporting. Currently, most of the information on postmarketing safety of the product comes from spontaneous adverse reaction reports. Reporting of events associated with a product by the health care practitioner to a regulatory agency or the pharmaceutical company that markets the product is the primary means for gathering this information. Each pharmaceutical company is required to maintain a database of these spontaneous reports. This database is monitored for increases in frequency of certain events or the appearance of serious unexpected events. If it is determined there is a causal relationship between the drug and the event, the product labeling may be changed to reflect either new events or events with increasing frequency. For more information about this topic, see Chapter 15.

There are several limitations to this type of data collection. The information is taken from the reporter who must make a diagnosis and assessment of causality. Data may be underreported because it is a voluntary system and this may bias the estimation of incidence. Reports may vary in quality or thoroughness and the database may not be suitable for detecting adverse reactions with high background rates in the population.[99] See Chapter 15 for additional information.

The principles of literature evaluation described in previous sections are also applicable to these studies. The method used to evaluate the study is dependent on the type of information collected. Note that when the purpose of these trials is focused on safety, they may be only powered for efficacy, which may not be sufficient. This can cause confusion when the results show "no statistically significant difference" between the drug and the comparator for various side effects. The reader is directed to the specific section of this chapter or book for the exact method to evaluate the study.

Appendix 5–1 contains a list of additional questions specific to postmarketing surveillance studies. These specific questions are in addition to the standard questions used to evaluate other randomized clinical trials noted in Chapter 4 and using basic tools like the Ten Major Considerations Checklist discussed in the Introduction section.

Review Articles

Review articles consist of three very different entities—the narrative (nonsystematic) review (qualitative review), the systematic review (qualitative review), and the meta-analysis (quantitative review). ❺ *Meta-analyses are the only type of review providing new quantitative data derived from combining the results of each study in the meta-analysis and performing a statistical analysis on that data set. The overall reliability of a meta-analysis is ultimately dependent on the quality of the individual studies,* **homogeneity** *between these studies, and appropriateness of the* *analysis.* Reviews are becoming more common in the literature and are relied on as an efficient method for keeping up with the large amount of information presented to the health care professional every day. Once a reader understands differences between individual study designs and characteristics for evaluating strengths and weaknesses within individual studies, it will become easier to analyze differences between publications that attempt to combine results from multiple studies.

Review articles, with the exception of meta-analyses that essentially consist of analysis and interpretation of previously conducted research studies, are classified as tertiary literature (see Chapter 3), although they are often used as secondary sources because they can lead readers to primary literature references. Meta-analyses are classified as primary literature since they create new data. Review articles discussing treatment of disease states or clinical aspects of drug therapy enable practitioners to gain insight into a topic or question of interest and may provide more current information than textbooks.

Although the purpose of review articles is to present the truth found among conflicting and variable primary literature, this does not always occur. Reviews may be subject to author biases or inaccuracies in the literature search.[99] Narrative (nonsystematic) literature reviews generally do not apply systematic methods, such as formal criteria for selection of studies, and they address broad rather than focused clinical questions. In addition, they provide qualitative rather than quantitative information. They often educate readers about the authors' interpretations of selected evidence, rather than using a systematic approach to evidence evaluation. Frequently, authors are experts on the topic and know the conclusions prior to conducting the review.

In contrast, systematic reviews do use formal criteria for trial selection and interpretation of study results, and authors determine the conclusions based on the data reviewed. These reviews provide qualitative information that is of a higher quality than narrative reviews based on the fact that a systematic approach was utilized. Meta-analyses (sometimes referred to as quantitative systematic reviews) differ from both narrative and systematic reviews in that they provide new data that are quantitative in nature. Due to increased emphasis on evidence-based practice, narrative reviews have largely been replaced by both systematic reviews and meta-analyses as a source of authoritative, summative information.

It is important to note that it is not uncommon to find conclusions of general overviews, systematic reviews, or meta-analyses conflict with one another.[100,101] Differences in research methodology may explain conflicting conclusions noted in selected published studies. Other explanations for conflicting conclusions include differences in study populations, type of intervention, or study endpoint, as well as chance or confounding issues.[102] In some cases, the amount of high-quality data may not be sufficient to come to a valid conclusion; in others, clinical judgment of authors may place more weight on certain findings over other results. Readers of review articles need to determine whether studies included in the review are broad enough to apply to their clinical situation.

NARRATIVE (NONSYSTEMATIC) REVIEW—QUALITATIVE

A narrative (nonsystematic) review is a summary of research that lacks a description of systematic methods. Narrative reviews are considered tertiary literature because they provide information in much the same manner as found in textbooks, but are sometimes used like secondary references because they also contain extensive and up-to-date bibliographies. Narrative reviews may pertain to one specific clinical question or disease state, or to topics related to pharmacy administration (e.g., pharmacy and therapeutics committees).

Appendix 5–1 contains a list of questions specific to narrative reviews that can be used to evaluate the quality of these reviews. These specific questions are in addition to the standard questions used to evaluate other randomized clinical trials noted in Chapter 4 and using basic tools like the Ten Major Considerations Checklist discussed in the Introduction section.

SYSTEMATIC REVIEW—QUALITATIVE

If the purpose of nonsystematic reviews is to find the truth, then the purpose of the systematic review is finding the whole truth.[103] Cook and associates describe systematic reviews as scientific investigations with predefined methods and original studies as their subjects.[104] Two general types of systematic reviews exist. The term systematic review has been applied to a summary of results of primary studies where the results are not statistically combined.[105] In contrast, a quantitative systematic review, or meta-analysis, has been described as a systematic review that uses statistical methods to combine the results of two or more studies. Perhaps, more appropriately, meta-analyses can be thought of as a specific methodological and statistical technique (or tool) for combining quantitative data that generates new data. Table 5–6 illustrates the primary differences between narrative reviews—qualitative, systematic reviews—qualitative, and meta-analyses—quantitative reviews.[105]

Systematic overviews that summarize scientific evidence (in contrast to nonsystematic narrative reviews that mix opinions and evidence) are becoming increasingly prevalent. These overviews address questions of treatment, causation, diagnosis, or prognosis and are considered superior to nonsystematic (narrative) reviews of any given topic.[101]

Systematic reviews should concentrate on a clearly defined issue that is of importance to practice.[101,102] Specific criteria should be used to select articles from the primary literature to be included in the review.[101] For valid conclusions to be derived from systematic reviews, authors must clearly define the study population or topic of interest and include only those studies using valid research methods.[101] For example, authors would have the choice of assessing women who are either pre- or postmenopausal in a systematic review focused on the utility of chemotherapy in improving survival following mastectomy in

TABLE 5-6. COMPARISON OF DIFFERENT TYPES OF REVIEWS

Feature	Narrative Review	Systematic Review	Meta-Analysis
Clinical question	Often broadly defined	Clearly defined and focused	Clearly defined and focused
Literature search	Methods not usually explicitly described	Predefined strategy, explicit, and comprehensive	Predefined strategy, explicit, and comprehensive
Studies included	Inclusion methods not usually described	Predefined inclusion and exclusion criteria	Predefined inclusion and exclusion criteria
Unpublished literature included	Not usually	Possibly	Possibly
Blinding of reviewers	No	Yes	Yes
Analysis of data—results of that analysis	Variable and subjective—no new data produced	Rigorous and objective—no new data produced	Rigorous and objective—new data produced
Results statistically evaluated	No	No	Yes
Type of results	Qualitative	Qualitative	Quantitative

SOURCE: Data from Cook DJ et al.[104] and Bryant PJ et al.[2]

breast cancer patients. Conclusions of this systematic review are likely to be very different depending on which subsets of breast cancer patients are selected. In addition, the authors' initial literature search would probably reveal a collection of studies that use a wide variety of research techniques. Only those studies meeting strict criteria for validity as discussed in Chapter 4 should be included in the review. Poorly controlled, nonrandomized, unblinded studies should be excluded to produce the most reliable results.

Authors should use a variety of resources to identify studies for the systematic review. Use of a single database is not likely to capture all relevant studies and results in reference bias. A combination of databases (such as MEDLINE®, PubMed®, Iowa Drug Information Service, International Pharmaceutical Abstracts, and Embase®, for literature published outside the United States), study bibliographies, and experts in the field should be used to identify studies for evaluation.[101,102]

Consideration should be given to inclusion of unpublished data (e.g., data on file at the manufacturer or personal communication with investigators) in addition to published studies, because it has been determined that published studies are more often of a positive nature than unpublished studies, a situation termed **publication bias**.[101] Researchers are now required to register their studies and provide data to an FDA Web site (http://www.clinicaltrials.gov), and this is a good site to find unpublished studies ongoing or completed. Unfortunately, this Web site only provides summative information, so the quality of the evidence often cannot be determined. The benefit of using unpublished studies is to include more data from which to draw a conclusion. A drawback is that unpublished studies have likely not undergone a peer-review and revision process; errors and unclearly stated conclusions may be present. **Language bias,** in which only articles published in the author's primary language are used, may also affect results. In order to reduce selection bias, review authors choosing articles should be blinded to (1) names of the study authors (to avoid political or personal issues), (2) institution of publication, and (3) results of the studies. For the initial choice of study inclusion, only the methods section should be reviewed.[105,106] In addition, because of the subjective nature of some aspects of analysis, two or more authors should critique each study under consideration and all evaluators should concur on which studies will be included in the systematic review.[101]

A systematic review article should provide a table that summarizes the results from each study included in the review.[101] Outcomes described in the systematic review article should be meaningful, and, if the trial is a clinical trial, clinically relevant.[101] For example, improved survival rate is a more desirable endpoint than reduction in total cholesterol for the hydroxymethylglutaryl-Coenzyme A (HMG-CoA) reductase inhibitors literature. Authors should also assess benefits versus risks associated with the therapy under review.[101]

Systematic reviews are retrospective observational trials and for this reason are subject to systematic and random errors.[105] Just as for nonsystematic reviews, techniques can be applied to evaluate the quality of systematic reviews.[107]

Appendix 5–1 contains a list of additional questions specific to systematic reviews. These specific questions are in addition to the standard questions used to evaluate other randomized clinical trials noted in Chapter 4 and using basic tools like the Ten Major Considerations Checklist discussed in the Introduction section.

META-ANALYSIS—QUANTITATIVE

Meta-analysis is a technique that has been developed to provide a quantitative and objective assessment.[108] This analysis is widely used to provide supporting evidence for clinical decision making. In a meta-analysis, results of previously conducted clinical trials are combined and statistically analyzed.[106,109]

Types of Meta-Analyses

Generally, a conventional **pair-wise meta-analysis** is conducted. The pair-wise approach is the traditional method to compile a meta-analysis by synthesizing the results of different trials to obtain an overall estimate of the treatment effect of one intervention relative to the control (intervention A to B). In other words, trials do exist and are used to compare intervention A to B. The alternative approach is called the **network meta-analysis** also known as the multiple treatment comparison or the mixed treatment meta-analysis. In this case, a network of randomized controlled trials is developed where all these trials have one intervention in common. This network allows an indirect estimate for comparison of interventions A and B when head-to-head trials do not exist. For example, treatment effects from trials comparing intervention A with C and other trials comparing intervention B with C can now be integrated into a network that indirectly estimates the treatment effects of interventions A compared to B.[110] All trials must have at least one intervention in common with another and this is what creates the network.

Uses for Meta-Analyses

Meta-analyses are designed to provide greater insight into clinical dilemmas than individual clinical trials. They are especially useful when previous studies have been inconclusive or contradictory, or in situations where sample size may have been too small to detect a statistically significant difference between treatment and control groups (i.e., power not met with required sample size). Meta-analyses assist in (1) supporting or refuting lesser quality evidence, (2) overcoming reduced statistical power of small studies, (3) assessing occurrence of rare events, (4) providing guidance with limited/conflicting data, (5) displaying sample sizes and treatment effects graphically, (6) assessing **heterogeneity** between studies and publication bias, (7) evaluating the natural history of disease, (8) improving estimates of effect size , and (9) answering new questions not posed at the start of individual trials.[106,109] Meta-analyses can be used to look at both clinical trials and epidemiologic research, such as cohort and case-control studies, and are particularly useful when definitive trials cannot be conducted, results of available trials are inconclusive, or while awaiting the results of definitive trials.[106,107,109] The meta-analysis study design has been used to address important clinical questions, such as whether aspirin reduces the risk of pregnancy-induced hypertension, cholesterol lowering decreases mortality, fluoxetine increases suicidal ideations, or estrogen replacement therapy increases the risk of breast cancer.[109] The thought process involved in identifying the need for this type of analysis can be presented with a hypothetical situation regarding a drug used for the treatment of myocardial infarction. Suppose this drug is shown to be related to increases in sudden death through proarrhythmic effects based on results from a number of small trials. A meta-analysis could be performed to statistically combine the results of these small trials and increase the power of the finding that there is an association or lack of association with increased sudden death for this drug.

Issues with Meta-Analyses

Methodological problems with meta-analyses have led to controversy surrounding their use in clinical decision making. Potential errors and biases to watch out for are associated with specific vulnerable steps in the meta-analysis process.[111] These vulnerable steps include study identification, study selection for inclusion, availability of information, data extraction, data analysis and synthesis, and data interpretation and reporting. When results from multiple trials are combined, biases of the individual studies are incorporated and new sources of bias arise.

A major concern with meta-analyses is the issue of publication bias found by LeLorier and associates described above.[106,108,109] Publication bias is a form of selection bias where publication of studies is based on the magnitude, direction, or statistical significance of the results.[112] It has been documented that researchers are more likely to publish studies that demonstrate positive effects of drugs. Therefore, studies that show lack of efficacy are less likely to be located than those that demonstrate beneficial effects of a drug. **Funnel plots** are used to identify the potential existence of publication bias.[113] A funnel plot is a scatterplot of treatment effect versus sample size of the studies included in the meta-analysis.[114] The treatment effect estimates should cluster around a constant value with variability in this treatment effect decreasing as size of the trial increases with a resultant funnel shape.[114] If the funnel plot shows an inverted symmetrical funnel shape, publication bias is probably not present (see Figure 5–6). However, if an asymmetrical funnel is noted, this suggests a relationship between treatment effect and study size. An asymmetrical funnel plot indicates the possibility that publication bias is present.[115]

The quality of the meta-analysis depends on the quality of the individual studies used to develop the meta-analysis.[116] Indeed, LeLorier and coworkers have compared the results of a series of large randomized controlled trials with those of previously published meta-analyses examining the same questions. They found that outcomes of 12 large randomized controlled trials studied were predicted inaccurately by previously published meta-analyses 35% of the time.[116] The randomized controlled clinical trials corresponded to meta-analyses in terms of population studied, therapeutic intervention, and at least one outcome. In this study, 46% of divergences in results involved a positive meta-analysis

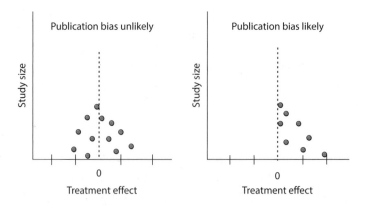

Figure 5–6. Symmetrical versus asymmetrical funnel plots.

being followed by a negative randomized controlled trial while the remaining 54% of iden-tified divergences involved a negative meta-analysis followed by a positive randomized controlled trial. Reasons for divergences, as cited by the authors, included the heteroge-neity (differences in the way the studies being included in the meta-analysis were con-ducted) of the trials included in the meta-analyses and publication bias (tendency of investigators to preferentially submit studies with positive results for publication).[116] There can be varying degrees of heterogeneity; however, if there are significant variations in true effects underlying the studies, then the meta-analysis results are in question.

Evaluation of Meta-Analyses

Several points should be considered when evaluating meta-analyses.[117] Specific stan-dards have been developed and accepted to help authors improve the reporting of meta-analyses in the literature.[118-120] These standards that consist of a 27-item checklist are referred to as the Preferred Reporting Items for Systematic Reviews and Meta-Analyses (PRISMA) statement.

A quality meta-analysis must clearly define the clinical question addressed by the anal-ysis.[106,107] Prior to conducting a meta-analysis, the hypothesis should be stated and a detailed protocol developed.[121] As with systematic reviews, details of literature searches that were conducted to locate primary research articles must be given and criteria for inclusion of studies in the meta-analysis must be determined prior to conducting the analysis.[106,107,109] Because computerized searches may not locate all of the relevant articles, other resources such as textbooks, experts in the field, and reference lists from clinical studies should also be consulted.[106] Whether to include trials from **gray literature** (i.e., documents provided in limited numbers outside the formal channels of publication and distribution) is controver-sial.[122] Access to this gray literature is not always available.[123] There are risks using data from gray literature including inaccurate information (not completely correct information), misinformation (incorrect information), and disinformation (false information deliberately provided in order to influence opinions) that can confound the meta-analysis results.

The studies should be similar enough (also referred to as homogeneity) to allow pooling of data.[106,107,124] Statistical tests that evaluate homogeneity or heterogeneity should be used to assess similarity of studies.[107,125] The more statistically significant the results of these tests, the more likely differences in study results are due to chance alone. If results of the tests of homogeneity are not significant, the studies are heterogeneous and differences in study results may be due to research design, rather than chance alone. Even heterogeneity brought into the meta-analysis by smaller sized studies should be determined.[126] Caution should be used when pooling results of heterogeneous studies. Factors that preclude pooling of results include discrepancies and poor quality of studies in general, inconsistencies in methods, improper conduct of the trial and reporting of data, and widely disparate findings.[116]

Authors should address the validity of articles used in the meta-analysis (see Chapter 4) such as randomization techniques, compliance, blinding, appropriate dosing and length of studies, and ITT analyses.[106,109] Some experts believe that studies should receive higher weight in the analysis if they are deemed to be of higher quality, but this practice is controversial because it is felt such assessments are too subjective.[109] Trials included in and excluded from the meta-analysis should be listed, along with explanation of reasons for exclusion.[123,127] Authors of meta-analyses should be blinded and choose trials to include in the meta-analysis that match prespecified criteria based solely on the methods section of studies. Strict standards should be established prior to the initiation of the meta-analysis to ensure that criteria used for inclusion of participants, administration of the principal treatment, and measurement of outcome events are similar in all trials studied.[122] Types of patients, their diagnosis, treatments, and therapeutic endpoints used in the original clinical studies should be given. The source of financial support for the original articles should be identified; however, as with analysis of individual trials, this becomes a major source of concern only when evidence of possible bias is present (e.g., strong positive conclusions, when results are inconclusive or only weakly positive).[106,107] Interpretation of meta-analyses results are limited by what studies were included or excluded, how homogeneous (or heterogeneous) the studies were, and the methodological quality of the studies.[64]

Common statistical tests used to combine the data include the **Mantel-Haenszel** test for categorical data and the **Inverse Variance** test for continuous data.[113] In addition, the probability of false-positive (e.g., Type I error) and false-negative (e.g., Type II error) results should be discussed. The 95% CIs for each study included should be calculated.[106] These CIs provide the range of values where the true value of the mean is contained 95% of the time. See Chapter 8 for more information.

The preferred method to present results obtained from meta-analyses is the **forest plot**.[122] The forest plot illustrated in Figure 5–7 describes the results of a meta-analysis conducted to determine the 1-year effectiveness of transdermal nicotine versus placebo patches for smoking cessation.[128] A closer look reveals the mean odds ratio (including the CI for nicotine patch) compared to placebo patch is plotted for each study. The odds ratio represents a ratio between two values, for instance abstinence rates from smoking between two interventions such as nicotine patch and placebo patch. The odds ratio is the preferred measurement over relative risk to be calculated for retrospective analyses. The null hypothesis value defined as no difference between treatment groups for the odds ratio (nicotine patch versus placebo patch) is one. Because of this, a statistically significant difference in favor of the nicotine patch would be illustrated as a mean odds ratio and CI greater than one (e.g., mean = 2.30 with 95% CI, 1.20 to 4.41), as noted by D'Agostino and associates in the forest plot. A statistically significant difference in favor of placebo over the nicotine patch would be represented as a mean odds ratio less than 1 (0.40 with 95% CI, 0.23 to 0.80). Note there were no studies in this meta-analysis that favored placebo over nicotine patch. At the bottom of the forest plot is the pooled odds

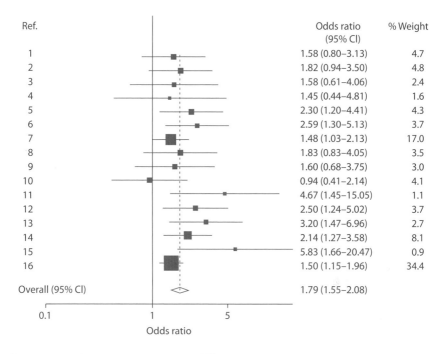

Ref.		Odds ratio (95% CI)	% Weight
1		1.58 (0.80–3.13)	4.7
2		1.82 (0.94–3.50)	4.8
3		1.58 (0.61–4.06)	2.4
4		1.45 (0.44–4.81)	1.6
5		2.30 (1.20–4.41)	4.3
6		2.59 (1.30–5.13)	3.7
7		1.48 (1.03–2.13)	17.0
8		1.83 (0.83–4.05)	3.5
9		1.60 (0.68–3.75)	3.0
10		0.94 (0.41–2.14)	4.1
11		4.67 (1.45–15.05)	1.1
12		2.50 (1.24–5.02)	3.7
13		3.20 (1.47–6.96)	2.7
14		2.14 (1.27–3.58)	8.1
15		5.83 (1.66–20.47)	0.9
16		1.50 (1.15–1.96)	34.4
Overall (95% CI)		1.79 (1.55–2.08)	

Odds ratio

Heterogeneity chi-square statistic $Q = 16.59$ (d.f. $= 15$), $p = 0.344$
Test of OR $= 1$: $z = 7.74$, $p = 0.000$

Figure 5–7. Forest plot.
SOURCE: Originally published in Myung SK, Yoo KY, Oh SW, Park SH, Seo HG, Hwang SS, Park SK. Meta-analysis of studies investigating one-year effectiveness of transdermal nicotine patches for smoking cessation. 2007;64:2471-2476 © 2007, American Society of Health-System Pharmacists, Inc. All rights reserved. Reprinted with permission. (R1301)

ratio from all the individually plotted studies included in the meta-analysis. For this meta-analysis the overall mean odds ratio was 1.79 with a 95% CI of 1.55 to 2.08. These values represent a statistically significant difference in odds ratios favoring nicotine patch compared to placebo. The advantage of illustrating the meta-analysis results using a forest plot is that each study's results are presented in a visual display. With this visual display, the practitioner can quickly interpret the overall results of the meta-analysis at the same time being able to see the contributions made to the overall result by each included study.

Sensitivity analysis is an integral part of the process and the authors should at the very least mention that this analysis has been conducted to determine how the results of the meta-analysis vary depending on use of different variables, such as assumptions, tests, and criteria.[106,107] Generally, sensitivity analysis is done among the articles included in the meta-analysis. A sensitivity analysis is done on any articles that seemed to not be as similar as the others combined. Once those articles are identified, the sensitivity analysis is done on the entire data set that makes up the meta-analysis and then repeated without each of those suspicious articles. An important difference between the outcomes of those two sensitivity analyses would be reported in the article you are evaluating. This allows a better understanding of how these different variables affect the results of the meta-analysis. Oftentimes, complete studies are removed from the analysis to improve overall homogeneity. This allows further sensitivity analyses to be completed to determine if this changes the overall results or conclusions. Sensitivity testing is essential to confirm the accuracy of the results produced by the meta-analysis. For example, in the meta-analysis for smoking cessation discussed earlier, the investigators only included studies with a follow-up of 1 year. The question that sensitivity testing answers is whether limiting the follow-up criteria to 6 months will change the overall results of the meta-analysis. In addition, the economic implications of the meta-analysis should be considered.

Overall, meta-analyses should be interpreted with caution, remembering that conclusions depend on the quality and similarity of the studies included. Findings of subsequent randomized controlled trials may differ from those of the meta-analysis.[64] This point was recently illustrated when the results of subsequent randomized controlled trials did not support previously published meta-analyses on the same subject.[121] Meta-analyses, on the surface, appear to be an extremely valuable tool allowing the practitioner to efficiently stay abreast of new information; however, oversimplification may lead to inappropriate conclusions.[121] Like all types of research evidence, meta-analyses require careful evaluation to determine their validity and applicability in practice.[112]

Appendix 5–1 contains a list of additional questions specific to meta-analyses.[129] These specific questions are in addition to the standard questions used to evaluate other randomized clinical trials noted in Chapter 4 and using basic tools like the Ten Major Considerations Checklist discussed in the Introduction section.

Case Study 5–4: Meta-Analysis

A meta-analysis was performed to determine the effect of dark chocolate and flavanol-rich cocoa products on reduction of blood pressure in hypertensive and normotensive individuals. MEDLINE®, Cochrane, and international trial registries were searched between 1995 and 2009 for randomized controlled trials investigating the effects of cocoa when consumed as food or drink compared with placebo on systolic and diastolic blood pressures. A minimum of 2 weeks consumption was required to be included in the study. A random effects meta-analysis of all studies meeting the inclusion criteria was conducted. A subgroup analysis by baseline blood pressure (hypertensive/normotensive) was included. Meta-regression analysis was used to determine the relationship, if any, between type of treatment, dosage, duration, or baseline blood pressure and blood pressure outcome. The level of significance was set at alpha = 0.05. Funnel plots of trials included were performed.

The results of the meta-analysis of all 17 trials showed a statistically significant reduction in blood pressure for cocoa/chocolate compared to control (p = 0.001). Forest plots were utilized to display the results of the meta-analysis. The results from homogeneity testing showed a low score indicating heterogeneity between the trials was high. All but 3 of the 15 trials assessed blood pressure as the primary outcome measure. In addition, participant attrition was less than 20% except for three trials where it was greater than 20%. Eight of the trials used a parallel group study design while the remaining seven trials used a crossover design. Intervention periods were at least 2 weeks in all trials (8 trials = 2 weeks; 7 trials ranged 4 to 18 weeks). Most importantly, polyphenol content (vasoactive chemical ingredient in chocolate) varied widely between trials. The authors concluded that chocolate effectively reduced blood pressure in hypertensive patients.

- *The quality of this meta-analysis depends on the quality of what component of the meta-analysis?*
- *One concern with meta-analyses is publication bias. What is publication bias and what specifically has this meta-analysis performed to correctly analyze and determine the likelihood of this bias being present?*
- *The studies included in a meta-analysis should be similar. What factors associated with these studies suggest there may be a problem with homogeneity between some of the studies?*
- *The results of this meta-analysis are provided in the text of the article. What method did the authors use to provide the results and why is this method preferred?*
- *Although the results of this study showed a statistically significant reduction in blood pressure for cocoa/chocolate compared to control (pooled mean SBP: –3.16 mmHg [p = 0.001]; pooled mean DBP: –2.02 mmHg [p = 0.003] with an alpha of 0.05), does this represent a clinically significant difference with these findings?*

Practice Guidelines

Three types of practice guidelines are published at the present time: evidence-based, formal consensus-based, and a mixture of EBM and consensus-based. These various types are differentiated by the source of information used to develop the practice guideline as well as the rigor of the process for evaluating that information. EBM practice guidelines utilize a rigorous systematic process involving review and critical evaluation of the medical literature to develop final recommendations. Formal consensus-based practice guidelines utilize experience of experts in their practice area to draw conclusions and develop recommendations. This is useful for those instances where the evidence does not exist, is not complete, or not conclusive enough to allow the development of a final recommendation. In these situations, experts are used to assist completion of practice guidelines using their expertise in those deficient areas. The mixed EBM and consensus-based practice guideline uses evidence to construct the guideline and supplements those steps without evidence with experience of the experts.

Practice guidelines are created primarily for facilitating clinical decision making, improving the quality of health care, providing consistent treatment across environments, decreasing costs, diminishing professional liability, and identifying individualized alternative treatment.[130,131] Key questions to be considered when evaluating a practice guideline are proposed.[132,133] Appendix 5–1 contains a list of these questions in addition to information presented in Chapter 7.

Useful guidelines provide information regarding therapeutic options and most appropriate choices for a specific disease and patient.[134] Important attributes for useful guidelines include validity, reproducibility/reliability, clinical applicability, clinical flexibility, accessibility, clarity, multidisciplinary development process, scheduled review, and documentation.[135] To be applicable, practice guidelines must be regularly maintained. Research has shown that within 2 years of development, a practice guideline may become outdated.[134]

Practice guidelines are becoming a common tool to use for patient population decisions. Factors are identified that influence the impact of a particular practice guideline.[76] One of the most important factors is strength of the evidence used to develop guidelines. Other factors include intensity of dissemination, follow-through of dissemination, type of problem addressed, source of guidelines, physician participation in development and adoption, format and specificity of the guideline recommendation, legal considerations, and financial/administrative issues.

Health Outcomes Research

Health outcomes research encompasses literature pertaining to discussion of pharmacoeconomic, therapeutic, and nontherapeutic outcomes (such as number of visits to the emergency room and number of hospital admissions), along with QOL outcomes. Readers are referred to Chapter 6 for information on evaluating pharmacoeconomic outcome studies. This section will focus on evaluating literature that includes QOL outcome measures.

QUALITY-OF-LIFE MEASURES

Clinical trials have traditionally focused on health outcomes related to physical or laboratory measurements of response.[136] How the patient feels and functions relative to daily activities is not always captured by these measurements. A patient's perception of well-being can be the most important outcome in specific disease states. Investigators make assumptions that changes in therapy improve the patient's QOL. These assumptions require testing. For this reason, additional health outcome measurements have been developed to address a patient's QOL.

QOL is a term that has acquired several different definitions. General agreement exists that QOL is a multidimensional concept focusing on impact of a disease and treatment relative to the well-being of a patient.[137] Physical and social environment affects QOL. Emotional and existential reactions to this physical and social environment also have an influence. ❻ *The value assigned to quality and quantity of life affected by many different variables including disease, injury, treatment, or policy is termed* **health-related quality of life (HR-QOL)** *and is used to assist in decision making regarding interventions such as procedures and pharmacotherapy.*[137] Direct measure of HR-QOL is impossible. Only inferences from patient symptoms and reported perceptions provide measurement of HR-QOL.

Two types of HR-QOL measurements exist: health status assessment and patient preference assessment.[130] Heath status assessment is a self-assessment that measures multiple aspects of a patient's perceived well-being. This assessment is primarily designed to either compare groups of patients receiving different treatments or effect of a treatment for a single group over time. Thus, health status assessments are most often used in clinical trials comparing treatment regimens. Context of questions used range from perceived impact of disease and treatments to disease frequency and severity. Examples of health status assessments include Functional Living Index-Cancer (FLIC), European Organization for Research and Treatment of Cancer (EORTC QLQ-C30), and the Functional Assessment of Cancer Therapy (FACT).[138-140] Health status assessments take approximately 5 to 10 minutes to complete.

Patient preference assessments reflect an individual's decision-making process at a time when the eventual outcome is unknown.[137] These assessments measure the patient's trade-off between quality and quantity of life. For example, a patient with a terminal illness may be assisted with decision making of treatment options based on a time trade-off instrument. This instrument is designed to assess a patient's preference with respect to their wishes regarding QOL versus quantity of life. Specifics of patient preference assessments are beyond the scope of this discussion because they are seldom used in clinical trials.

Two types of instruments are used to measure HR-QOL: generic and disease-specific.[141] Generic instruments assess HR-QOL in patients with and without active disease. An example of a generic instrument is the Sickness Impact Profile, a health profile instrument that attempts to measure multiple aspects of HR-QOL. Generic instruments are useful for comparing completely different groups or following groups after treatment is discontinued. Disease-specific instruments are narrower in scope, more sensitive, and focus on specific treatment or disease impact. A battery of several disease-specific instruments can be used to obtain a comprehensive understanding of impact associated with different interventions. For example, a variety of disease-specific instruments, including sleep, sexual dysfunction, and physical activity, can be used to demonstrate differing effects of antihypertensive therapy on HR-QOL. HR-QOL trials should use validated HR-QOL instruments.[142] Reviewers can confirm validation of HR-QOL instruments from statements, backed by citations, indicating the questionnaires have been validated. Lack of these references or some other description of a validation process should cause concern and skepticism. Similarly, use of a combination or a series of valid HR-QOL measurements as described above should also document validity for the resultant HR-QOL battery. In practice, this integrative approach may reduce validity of HR-QOL measurements due to interactions of the various instruments on one another. Investigators must document the validity of each test used in a series as well as validity of the series as a whole. Reviewers should be aware of potential bias or problems resulting from this.

When reviewing a study containing HR-QOL measurements, the reader should consider several study characteristics,[143] and a list of suggested questions to ask when reviewing these trials. Appendix 5–1 contains a list of these questions. These specific questions are in addition to the standard questions used to evaluate other randomized clinical trials noted in Chapter 4 and using basic tools like the Ten Major Considerations Checklist discussed in the Introduction section. Because there is no commonly accepted method to determine clinical significance of changes in most HR-QOL measurements, interpretation of HR-QOL results from clinical trials can be difficult.[144] A standardized method to indicate appropriate interpretation of clinically important changes and/or differences between groups in HR-QOL measurements is needed.

Trials measuring HR-QOL should be powered to detect a statistically significant difference.[137] Adequate sample size is calculated by the investigator to meet a designated level of power with a resultant number of subjects required to detect a statistically significant difference, if a difference truly exists. For example, if a study required 400 patients in each group to meet power but only 270 patients in each group were included in the final statistical analysis, power would not have been met. This is particularly important if no difference is noted between groups, in which case a difference may actually exist, but due to inadequate sample size that difference was not detected. Inadequate enrollment to allow for attrition, large patient dropout rates, and numerous protocol violators, all contribute to a reduced sample size. Often HR-QOL is designated as a secondary endpoint with study power calculated to detect differences in only primary outcome measurements. Note that is subgroups are analyzed, the sample size of those subgroups must also be determined prior to statistical analysis and the samples sizes need to be large enough to meet the designated power. Additional information

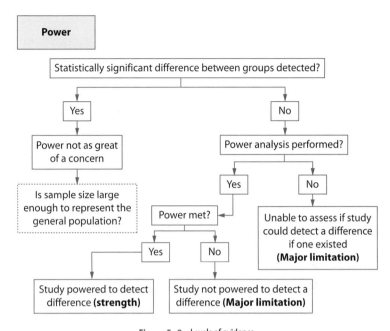

Figure 5–8. Levels of evidence.

regarding power can be found in Figure 5–8 in this chapter and in Chapter 8. Authors should document inclusion and applicability of relevant HR-QOL measurements in the assessment instrument.[145,146] For instance, if the study is evaluating a drug for treatment of a particular disease state, rheumatoid arthritis, outcome measurements should be specific to this disease (e.g., outcome measures for rheumatoid arthritis would include mobility, hand activities, personal care, home chores, and interpersonal activities). The HR-QOL measurements represent unique personal perceptions that reflect how individual patients feel about their health status and/or nonmedical aspects of their lives. These perceptions can be difficult to capture, resulting in HR-QOL measurements that inadequately reflect patient's values and preferences.[147] The reviewer should evaluate the HR-QOL measurements to determine if individual patients are given opportunities to express opinions and reactions rather than just an assessment of disease progression. For example, the HR-QOL measurement instrument for hand activities associated with rheumatoid arthritis should capture patients' perception of how well they can move their hand, not just a determination of range of hand motion. In addition, the HR-QOL instrument should be sensitive to changes in patients' status throughout the clinical trial and should measure aspects of their lives considered important by the patients.[148] Benchmarking these measures with those used in similar published studies helps identify standard or accepted measurements for a specific disease state.

These can be difficult parameters to isolate and, thus, many measurements of HR-QOL fall short of capturing this important concept.[114] Trials overlooking important issues related to patients' health status and/or nonmedical aspects of their lives can provide misleading results.

Timing of HR-QOL measurements should be appropriate to answer research questions.[137] This timing of test administration should be related to the anticipated timing of clinical effects. In some cases, outcomes may lag behind clinical effects, and in other situations, they could precede clinical effects. For instance, when evaluating a subject's perception of mood improvement following initiation of a course of antidepressant drug therapy, the measurement should not occur for several weeks to allow the medication adequate time to demonstrate efficacy. Alternatively, an HR-QOL measurement of overall QOL related to cancer therapy may include pretreatment anxiety and anticipatory nausea and vomiting preceding a chemotherapy session.

HR-QOL measurements should occupy the same timing within test sequences. For example, it is recommended that HR-QOL measurements be obtained at the beginning of clinic visits, unless there are substantial reasons provided by the authors to perform these tests at a different time. This is due to cognitively demanding assessment instruments and the fact that most subjects are fresh at the beginning of the visit. Additionally, if several measurements are obtained for each subject throughout the course of a trial, care should be taken to ensure similar timing between subjects occurs for sequential testing.

The mode of data collection is important because self-reporting is sufficient with some types of questions, while other specific types of questions are better asked by an interviewer.[137] When a trained interviewer is used, interview location is important to obtaining unbiased answers. In a case regarding a treatment for a terminal illness, the patient may be more interested in QOL, while the family member is prioritizing quantity of life. An interview conducted in the presence of that family member could affect that patient's QOL response. Thus, HR-QOL measurements are best obtained in a private setting to reduce risk of biased responses.

Results are usually reported as a composite; however, individual patient data are often reported in smaller studies, for instance, when a rare disease limits sample size. When individual patient data are reported, the reviewer should attempt to determine if patients' answers were potentially biased due to their awareness of this public disclosure.

Assessment instrument response rates are critical since nonresponse can introduce significant bias into the results.[149] In addition, data should be reasonably complete throughout the study since missing data can suggest investigator bias.[137] The reviewer should determine if data appear to be randomly missing. If a pattern of missing data is recognized (e.g., if a specific question or group has been excluded), the omission should be explained by authors. In this situation, the reviewer should determine if missing data have the potential to counter the author's hypothesis, thus identifying one explanation for incomplete data reporting. Reviewers must determine if HR-QOL measurements in a multicenter trial were performed at all sites. If HR-QOL measurements are not performed at all sites, authors should provide the reason for this methodology deviation.

Repeated use of HR-QOL measurements can lead to a training effect on the patient and/or interviewer, resulting in misleading conclusions.[147] The reviewer should determine if this effect is present and how that affects results. Showing test subjects their prior responses to HR-QOL measurement questions in an attempt to decrease variability should generally not be done unless acceptable supportive rationale for this procedure is given by the authors.

For the HR-QOL analysis, appropriate statistical tests should be used for the type of data analyzed such as use of categorical tests such as the Mann-Whitney U test for nonparametric data. All specific analytical features should be described at the time of trial design (i.e., *a priori*). A reviewer should look for an author explanation of which specific tests are used on QOL data and should not assume that the same statistical tests are used on the QOL data as are discussed for the other trial outcomes (i.e., efficacy or safety outcome data) if not directly discussed. Selective reporting of favorable or statistically significant results is also a problem. Both positive and negative findings, in addition to neutral or insignificant results, should be reported for completeness.

Several other items are worth consideration when evaluating trials with HR-QOL outcome measurements. Use of HR-QOL measurements for reporting of adverse drug events is not appropriate.[144] Trials should evaluate efficacy, safety, and HR-QOL separately and as distinctly different outcomes. An assumption that adverse events determine HR-QOL (or vice versa) can lead to erroneous results. For instance, consider a trial with breast cancer patients in whom surgery and chemotherapy is expected to eradicate all cancer cells. An appropriate assessment of HR-QOL outcomes for some patients may be positive despite troublesome adverse reactions such as low blood counts, decreased energy, and increased susceptibility to infection, based on the perception that treatment will ultimately result in a complete cure. Alternatively, other patients' HR-QOL outcomes may reflect poor QOL, even in the absence of treatment-related adverse events but instead due to an overall situational depression. Without separate assessments of adverse events experienced and HR-QOL outcomes, linking adverse events with QOL can result in inaccurate interpretations.

Finally, culturally defined factors may impact patient's QOL and assessment of HR-QOL measurements. Validity of HR-QOL measurements across different cultures or subcultures should be considered by the reviewer. For instance, an HR-QOL instrument may effectively measure outcomes for HIV-infected men living in the United States, but may be completely inadequate for measuring outcomes in HIV-infected women living in Africa. Assessment instruments must account for and reflect the variability between outcomes perceived as important to patients, considering that perceptions may be quite diverse between cultures and must be assessed accordingly.

Dietary Supplement Medical Literature

❼ *The principles and criteria used to analyze the quality of drug literature are used to analyze DS literature; however, unique additional points such as standardization and purity must be considered.* DS (botanical and nonbotanical) information is a rapidly growing body of medical literature that many health practitioners must delve into more frequently as patients continue to use herbal and nonherbal supplements. The ability to discern strong from weak clinical evidence is an important skill that enables practitioners to make solid recommendations to patients and to other health care professionals.

Provision of DS information is similar to provision of standard drug information. Evidence is described and ranked according to the quality of the literature supporting or refuting DS product claims. The same evidence-based criteria utilized for drug literature analysis apply to DS literature. Thus, large, well-designed, randomized, controlled, clinical trials or well-done meta-analyses lend stronger support versus retrospective data, case series, observational data, and experiential testimonials. However, it is not unusual to only have poorly designed published trial data to support or refute a DS product's claims. This means that, for some products, the only data available concerning theoretical actions, interactions, and side effects are animal and/or *in vitro* data.

To further compound misinformation, often trials touted as supporting claims for efficacy of a botanical DS have actually been conducted using chemical extracts or single chemical agents. Even if trials are of good quality, it is inappropriate to apply those results to the supplement. For example, if a trial of a concentrated echinacea extract from the whole plant of *Echinacea purpurea* shows positive results for shortening duration and severity of cold symptoms, that trial cannot be used to support efficacy of a product consisting of capsules of ground *Echinacea angustifolia* root.

While many evidence-based principles are easily applied to DS literature, what follows are a few issues unique to DS trials as well as the most commonly encountered methodological flaws. In addition to standard literature evaluation criteria, specifics to consider include:

- Standardization of chemical components
- International literature inclusion
- Adequate trial duration and sample size

- Limited availability of high-quality evidence-based literature
- Quality and purity of product formulations

STANDARDIZATION

One important characteristic to look for in a botanical DS study is standardization of the chemical components. Plant-derived products contain many different chemical entities that fluctuate with the growing and harvesting conditions, the plant's age, and which part of the plant is used. One or more chemical entities could be considered active constituents, i.e., responsible for desired pharmacologic action, which may or may not be accurately identified. Other components may be marker compounds that allow estimation of levels of other, less-easily assayed chemicals. Control of the amount of one chemical entity, either an active constituent (if known) or a marker compound, is used to standardize the supplement. Using a standardized chemical concentration allows for uniformity between study product and marketed product as well as between various brands of one product. For trial evaluation, it is important to assess standardization methods used by investigators. Trial investigators should discuss and document the plant or chemical substance as well as the strength or salt form utilized. This is an essential element to consider when grouping trials, so to make apples-to-apples comparisons.

Plant parts are also important to consider. If a trial evaluated use of a herb's root, but the product about which a practitioner is searching for information contains the herb's leaves and flowers, the results cannot be extrapolated. The apples-to-apples concept also applies to nonbotanical products, although often would refer to differences in salt forms. For example, glucosamine sulfate has substantial evidence documenting benefit in osteoarthritis patients, while glucosamine hydrochloride has less supportive evidence and other salt forms have almost none or even negative evidence.

Chemical constituents of botanicals, or products derived from them, can be volatile; possible degradation must be considered in interpreting results of a trial.[150] Researchers should verify that products used in studies have appropriate stability throughout the duration of a clinical trial.

INTERNATIONAL TRIALS AND INFORMATION RETRIEVAL

The majority of DS trials are conducted in Europe and Asia. Appropriateness of generalizing results to a practitioner's own patient population must always be considered, just as with prescription drug trials. This may even be of greater concern for DS trials, as many supplements are often used as food products as well, either in the United States or in other parts of the world.

Most health professionals are familiar with the MEDLINE® database, whether searched through PubMed® or another platform. Unfortunately, studies of supplements published in foreign language journals may be overlooked when doing a literature search only with one database. Embase® (http://www.embase.com) is another large, commonly used database that indexes abstracts from additional international journals (which are often published in English). It must be remembered that, while abstracts are useful to estimate the amount of potential supportive data, they do not contain enough information to properly analyze a trial's quality. Therefore, original studies must be reviewed.

Whatever databases are searched, use of adequate keywords or indexing terms is important. This is especially true for botanical supplements—plants have multiple common names and different spellings (e.g., ginkgo, gingko, ginko), different plants share common names, and official taxonomy can change frequently. This can be frustrating. A database search should include multiple search terms in order to ensure thoroughness. Additionally, searching the references of obtained articles (i.e., bibliographic searches) is useful to identify citations of trials.

TRIAL DURATION

As with drug clinical trials, duration of therapy is important for accurate assessment of efficacy and safety. Inadequate duration is a common flaw in DS trials. Dependent on the mechanism of action, some supplements may take several weeks to several months before patients experience benefit. DSs may appear less efficacious than they actually are if study duration is too short. If benefits are only small to moderate, a short trial may tend to overestimate responses as patients will often exhibit greater responses in the beginning of clinical trials, perhaps because of contributing placebo effect. That response may attenuate as the trial proceeds. And, just as with drug clinical trials, shorter study periods cannot predict outcomes or safety issues associated with long-term use.

TRIAL SIZE

Small subject population is very common flaw in DS trials. Small-sized groups may not have adequate statistical power to detect a potential difference between a DS and a placebo, if one truly exists. Adverse reactions or drug interactions can be overlooked in smaller groups versus a larger one. In addition, a small subject population can decrease trial generalizability (external validity) to broader patient populations.

MINIMAL EVIDENCE

For most DSs, few large, controlled, methodologically sound clinical trials exist. Many products have only animal, *in vitro*, or theoretical data to support their claims. Without a body of human data, practitioners must often make counseling or recommendation decisions based on safety and efficacy data that are theoretical, from case reports or flawed trials, or from animal and/or *in vitro* studies. This often entails a very patient-specific risk-benefit analysis, i.e., weighing risks of occurrence of an interaction or side effect against possible benefits of the supplement. However, more rigorous studies are underway as DS use becomes more prevalent, acceptable, and recognized by health practitioners. All DS clinical trials should be evaluated for quality with the same criteria as used for FDA-approved medications. However, additional questions do become especially important when considering both internal and external validity of the trial:

- Which plant part was utilized?
- Was a standardized botanical extract utilized?
- Was the study product standardization appropriate?
- Was a specific plant species or specific salt form utilized?

QUALITY AND PURITY

DSs can be adulterated with heavy metals or prescription medications. ConsumerLab.com, LLC (http://www.consumerlab.com) is an example of an organization that independently evaluates specific DS brands for content purity and accurate labeling and publishes results online. When a product meets the quality standard, the company may use, for a fee, a seal of approval on DS labels. Manufacturers may also voluntarily agree to have manufacturing plants and products inspected to earn approval from agencies such as the USP-Dietary Supplement Verification Program (USP-DSVP, http://www.uspverified.org/). Approved manufacturers are permitted to display a seal of approval on product labels and are listed on the USP-DSVP Web site.

Appendix 5–1 contains a list of additional questions specific to evaluation of DS studies. These are in addition to the standard questions used for evaluation of randomized clinical trials noted in Chapter 4 and using basic tools like the Ten Major Considerations Checklist discussed in the Introduction.

OTHER SPECIAL CONSIDERATIONS

Unlike prescription drugs, DSs are not legally required to be reviewed and approved by the FDA for safety and efficacy prior to marketing. The FDA can take action if problems are discovered with either, once a product is available to consumers. The bottle a consumer purchases in the health store or supermarket is not guaranteed to be labeled or dosed appropriately. Therefore, even when clinical evidence clearly supports use of an herb or supplement, the patient may not experience a benefit because the product is mislabeled, dosed subtherapeutically, or incorrectly standardized.

DS use continues to be prevalent despite fluctuations in ages or ethnicities choosing to use supplements and changes in the popularity of specific products.[151,152] Health practitioners must serve as reliable and approachable information resources for DS information just as they do for other medications. In community settings, supplements are often placed with nonprescription products near the pharmacy, making pharmacists easily accessible for consumer questions and counseling. The ability to effectively evaluate DS literature is essential to making informed recommendations and appropriately counseling patients who have DS questions.

Case Study 5–5: Trials Testing Natural Products

You are evaluating a trial comparing a natural product called *Pelargonium sidoides* (pelargonium) to placebo for treating acute bronchitis in adults. Pelargonium has been shown to stimulate the immune system and contain some minor bacteriostatic effect. The trial utilized a flavored syrup containing a standardized proprietary dose of pelargonium. The randomized, double-blind, placebo-controlled trial was conducted in multiple centers throughout Europe. Four hundred adult patients with acute bronchitis were randomized to receive either two teaspoons full of pelargonium syrup or an identical appearing placebo syrup three times daily for 7 days. The primary outcome measure to determine efficacy was a change in intensity of five typical bronchitis symptoms (Integrative Medicine Outcome Scale [IMOS]). These symptoms include coughing, wheezing/whistling on expiration, expectoration, pain in the breast during coughing, and dyspnea. The IMOS is a five-point scale (from not present to extremely pronounced) and added to produce a total score with a maximum of 20 points. The data were evaluated using both intention-to-treat and per-protocol analyses.

Power was set at 0.80 and met based on the per-protocol analysis. The results of the study showed a statistically and clinically significant reduction in the intensity of the symptoms as measured by the IMOS data ($p = 0.001$; alpha set at 0.05). No side effects that could be attributed to the treatment were noted. The investigators concluded that pelargonium was effective in treating bronchitis in adult patients.

You are evaluating this trial because you would like to have pelargonium as an option to include in the overall therapy of acute bronchitis in your patients. You have noticed several different nonprescription products containing various amounts of pelargonium.

- *How could this proprietary standardization of the product used in this study be a problem to extrapolating the results of this study to your patients?*

- *Like this trial, many natural product trials are conducted outside the United States. Why should you take this into consideration?*
- *Is there any concern with the duration of pelargonium therapy in this trial?*
- *What is your opinion regarding the patient numbers for this trial?*

Getting to a Clinical Decision

❽ *An understanding of strengths and limitations inherent with each design is essential to determine the overall quality of the evidence produced. Those trial designs with a high level of quality provide the most reliable evidence and that translates into the strongest recommendation/clinical decision.*

Once the study is evaluated, the overall quality of that trial must be determined. Categorizing the quality of the trial is the bridge from literature evaluation to developing a defensible conclusion/recommendation/clinical decision. In general, trial designs can be categorized by quality. This categorization ranks each study design from very low to high in quality. These categories of different quality are referred to as levels of evidence.[2]

Several different scales that rank the quality of evidence have been developed.[153] Although many of these levels of evidence scales follow a similar continuum of quality, labeling of each level is highly variable. For instance, one scale may use an alphabetical system (A = highest quality and D = lowest quality of evidence) while another scale uses a numerical system (1 to 5). There are even scales that combine the two systems (e.g., 1a, 1b, 1c, 2a, 2b) to rank the study design from highest to lowest quality within each level. In addition, several of these levels of evidence scales use ambiguous descriptors such as poorly designed or high-quality study. This complicates the use of the scale and adds subjectivity, which leads to variability between scales. In other words, reproducing the same ratings between scales is difficult.

A standard level of evidence scale developed by combining the best attributes from several individual scales that are currently available has been proposed.[2] Figure 5–8 illustrates this proposed level of evidence scale. Using the level of evidence scale illustrated, the level of quality can be assigned to a trial based on the specific study design characteristics. For example, a randomized, double-blind, controlled, N-of-1 trial used to test the efficacy and safety of a new antihypertensive would be assigned either a Level 1 or Level 2 ranking. On further examination of the study's methodology section, the practitioner identifies that power was set; however, an inadequate number of patients were entered into the trial to meet the set power. In this case, there is a high risk of a Type II error being present, or in other words, no difference is noted when in fact a true difference actually exists. It is unknown whether adding the additional patients needed to meet power would have resulted in actually observing the true difference between treatment groups. Using the diagram, the practitioner can identify that this study design is ranked as a Level 2 for quality of evidence. Note the one difference between the Level 1 and Level 2 categories is power being set and met. See Figure 5–9 for a better understanding of how power can affect the quality of a study design. As mentioned in the introduction section, additional study characteristics are also considered to further evaluate the strengths and limitations and how these attributes impact the results of the trial. The greater number of individual strengths identified, the greater the quality and reliability of the evidence produced by that trial. From the assigned level of evidence based on the study design and attributes, the practitioner has an understanding of the overall quality of the trial. This understanding allows the practitioner to develop a clinical decision that can be easily defended based on the evidence. Three inputs have been identified that are involved with developing an EBM recommendation/clinical decision[2]: quality of evidence, logical reasoning, and clinical judgment. Organizing the trials by the highest level of evidence, outcome of the trial, and associated limitations allows the practitioner to formulate an initial recommendation/clinical decision statement. Identifying key points associated with efficacy, safety, cost, and special considerations/special populations can help the practitioner justify and defend their recommendation/clinical decision. Note that a conservative approach is taken with population-based decisions such as drug additions to a hospital formulary. These types of decisions require a more conservative approach since a whole population is affected and little detail exists about

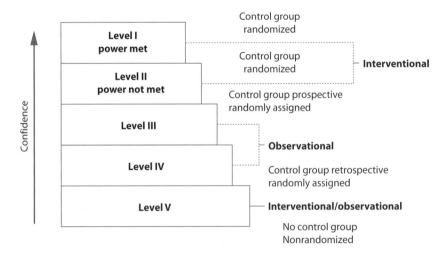

Figure 5–9. Power algorithm.
Source: Bryant PJ et al.[2] (Copyright 2009, American Society of Health-System Pharmacists.) Used with permission.

each patient in that group. This is in contrast to an individual patient therapeutic decision where a great amount of detail from the medical chart is known about that single patient, and for this reason the decision requires a less conservative approach.

Putting it all together in an EBM manner is critically important to clinical decision making. No matter what study design is used, a thorough evaluation and categorization of the quality of that evidence is necessary. Practitioners need high-quality and reliable evidence to make firm clinical recommendations/decisions. Caution should be exhibited making these decisions when lower quality or no evidence is available. In this situation the practitioner must rely on the other two components mentioned: logical reasoning and clinical judgment. Unfortunately, clinical decisions made in this manner tend to overestimate the efficacy of the intervention and underestimate the safety risk to patients.[154] For this reason, clinical decisions and recommendations should be made using the highest quality of evidence available to ensure the best patient care.

Conclusion

Although the randomized controlled trial is the most frequently used study design for clinical research, several other designs are used in specific situations. The design is chosen based on the specific clinical questions needing to be answered. In some cases, a design is used because it represents the only way a particular data set can be obtained ethically. This chapter has provided an overview of those additional types of designs. There are general questions that should be answered when evaluating any study design type. This chapter provides additional questions/points to consider that are unique for each specific design. Many clinical decisions depend on knowledge provided in the medical literature. To ensure the highest quality of care for patients, the practitioner needs to be able to determine, through efficient and effective evaluation practices, the quality and reliability of that knowledge gained from the medical literature.

Self-Assessment Questions

For questions 1 to 4, please select the *best* answer regarding which study design is presented.

1. A crossover study to prospectively evaluate the use of an anticonvulsant drug for treatment of peripheral neuropathy in an individual patient.
   a. Case study
   b. Case report
   c. N-of-1 study

2. A patient develops agranulocytosis after administration of dronedarone. The clinician writes and publishes this single patient observation.
   a. Case report
   b. Case series
   c. N-of-1 study

3. An investigator evaluates the question of whether or not different digoxin products can be used interchangeably.
   a. Case series
   b. Bioequivalence
   c. Postmarketing
   d. Stability

4. A company designs a trial to show that their new drug is therapeutically no worse than the standard of care therapy.
   a. Bioequivalence
   b. Inferiority
   c. N-of-1
   d. Noninferiority

5. When the 95% CI for a treatment difference between a test drug and reference drug crosses the NI margin, which of the following conclusions can be made?
   a. The test drug is noninferior to the reference drug.
   b. The reference drug is noninferior to the test drug.
   c. The results are inconclusive.
   d. The test drug is inferior to the reference drug.

6. Adaptive clinical trial (ACT) design provides the ability to use:
   a. Emerging data to make adjustments in the study
   b. Flexible noninterim analysis strategies
   c. Adaptive sampling designs for reallocation of patients
   d. All of the above

7. After reading the following three cases, identify the study design for each trial in the correct order.
   Trial #1: There is a concern that the use of hormone replacement therapy (HRT) in postmenopausal women may cause an increased risk of breast cancer. A study is conducted to test this hypothesis. Medical charts from a group of patients previously admitted to the hospital with the diagnosis of breast cancer is compared to medical charts from a group of patients previously admitted to the hospital without breast cancer. The groups are matched by age, sex, date of

admission, and other confounding factors such as alcohol use. Use of HRT in each group is assessed and compared. An odds ratio for the risk of breast cancer related to use of HRT is calculated.

Trial #2: An investigator identifies a study sample of women aged 20 to 45 years. During a single office visit, the investigator measures bone mass in the women. He also questions them about their past and present exercise habits. The investigator determines that women involved with rigorous exercise before the onset of menses have a greater bone mass.

Trial #3: It is hypothesized that hormone replacement therapy (HRT) in post-menopausal women may play a beneficial role in preventing osteoporosis. A group of patients receiving HRT and a group of patients not receiving HRT are followed over a 20-year period. The development of osteoporosis as assessed by bone mineral density in each group is compared, and the relative risk associated with the use of HRT and the development of osteoporosis is calculated.

a. Cohort, cross-sectional, case-control
b. Cross-sectional, case-control, cohort
c. Case-control, case series, cohort
d. Cohort, case-control, cross-sectional
e. Cohort, case-control, case series

8. Indicate which selection ranks trial designs in order of increasing rigor.
   a. Case series → Cohort → Case-control
   b. Powered randomized controlled trial → Nonpowered randomized controlled trial
   c. Case report → Case-control → Cohort
   d. Cohort → Case-control → Case series

9. Match the correct example for a prospective observational study design with control group.
   a. N-of-1 study
   b. Case-control
   c. Cohort
   d. Case series

10. Which example best matches an uncontrolled study design?
    a. Cohort
    b. Case series
    c. N-of-1 study
    d. Case-control

11. Several small studies that show no statistically significant difference between an alginate/antacid product (alginate is the salt of alginic acid and the combination

of the alginic acid and bicarbonate creates a barrier which prevents stomach acid from refluxing back up into the esophagus) and omeprazole for prevention of minor gastroesophageal reflux disease (GERD) have been published. Unfortunately, none of these studies set and met power with a large enough sample size. An investigator systematically identifies both published and unpublished studies in this area, combines the results, and performs statistical analysis to create new data. The resulting document would be classified as with of the following?

a. Narrative (nonsystematic) review—qualitative
b. Meta-analysis—quantitative
c. Systematic review—qualitative
d. Case series

12. Two types of health-related quality-of-life (HR-QOL) measurements that exist include:

a. Health status assessment and patient preference assessment
b. Functional Living Index—cancer and health status assessment
c. Generic instruments and disease-specific instruments
d. Direct measures and functional measures

13. Important characteristics to look for in a dietary supplement study include:

a. Standardization since plant-derived products can contain different chemical entities
b. Adequate size of study subject population
c. Trial duration because plant-derived product studies are often inadequate in duration for appropriate assessment
d. All of the above

14. The most reliable evidence with a high level of confidence comes from which of the following?

a. Randomized, controlled interventional trial designs conducted properly
b. Observational cohort studies
c. Observational case-controlled retrospective studies
d. Interventional studies without a comparison group

15. Key components to an evidence-based medicine process include:

a. Systematic method to evaluate the evidence
b. Method to determine the quality of evidence
c. Method to determine a defensible recommendation/clinical decision
d. All of the above

Acknowledgments

Authors wish to gratefully acknowledge Denise Woolf at the University of Missouri—Kansas City School of Pharmacy Drug Information Center—for her editing, macroformatting, and proofreading of the text and Kerry Cain for her assistance with citations. Also, the authors wish to thank and acknowledge N. Seth Berry, Pharm.D., Director, Clinical PK/PD Modeling & Simulation at Quintiles, for his assistance with the noninferiority trial and adaptive clinical trial sections, in addition to consultation on appropriate statistical methodologies. Many thanks to Timothy A. Candy, Pharm.D., M.S., BCPS, Senior Manager, Global Regulatory Affairs and Pharmacovigilance at Baxter Healthcare Corporation, for his assistance with the noninferiority trial section.

REFERENCES

1. Suda KJ, Jurley AM, McKibbin T, Motl Moroney SE. Publication of noninferiority clinical trials: changes over a 20-year interval. Pharmacotherapy. 2011;31(9):833-9.
2. Bryant PJ, Pace HA, eds. The pharmacist's guide to evidence based medicine for clinical decision making. Bethesda (MD): American Society of Health-System Pharmacists; 2009:198.
3. Fairman KA, Curtiss FR. Rethinking the "whodunnit" approach to assessing the quality of health care research—a call to focus on the evidence in evidence-based practice. JMCP. 2008;14(7):661-74.
4. De Muth JE. Basic statistics and pharmaceutical statistical applications. 2nd ed. Boca Raton (FL): Chapman & Hall/CRC; 2006:714.
5. Piaggio G, Elbourne DR, Altman DG, Pocock SJ, Evans SJ. Reporting of non-inferiority and equivalence randomized trials: an extension of the CONSORT statement. JAMA. 2006;295:1152-60.
6. U.S. Department of Health and Human Services, Food and Drug Administration, Center for Drug Evaluation and Research, and Center for Biologics Evaluation and Research. Guidance for industry non-inferiority clinical trials [Internet]. Silver Springs (MD); 2010 Mar [cited 2013 Apr 2]: [63 p.]. Available from: http://www.fda.gov/Drugs/GuidanceComplianceRegulatoryInformation/Guidances/default.htm
7. Kaul S, Diamond GA. Good enough: a primer on the analysis and interpretation of noninferiority trials. Ann Intern Med. 2006;145:62-9.
8. Dasgupta A, Lawson KA, Wilson JP. Evaluating equivalence and noninferiority trials. Am J Health Syst Pharm. 2010;67:1337-43.
9. Head SJ, Kaul S, Bogers AJ, Kappetein AP. Non-inferiority study design: lessons to be learned from cardiovascular trials. Eur Heart J. 2012;33:1318-24.
10. Durkalski V, Silbergleit R, Lowenstein D. Challenges in the design and analysis of non-inferiority trials: a case study. Clin Trials. 2011;8:601-8.
11. Schumi J, Wittes J. Through the looking glass: understanding non-inferiority. Trials. 2011;12:106.

12. D'Agostino RB Sr, Massaro JM, Sullivan LM. Non-inferiority trials: design concepts and issues—the encounters of academic consultants in statistics. Statist Med. 2003;22:169-86.
13. New Drug Approval: FDA's consideration of evidence from certain clinical trials—Report to Congressional Requesters. Washington, DC: United States Government Accountability Office; 2010 July, 33 p. Report No.: GAO-10-798.
14. Gotzsche PC. Lesson from and cautions about noninferiority and equivalence randomized trials. JAMA. 2006;295(10):1172-4.
15. Guidelines on the choice of noninferiority margin. London: European Medicines Agency (EMA); 2006.
16. Fleming TR, Odem-Davis K, Rothmann MD, Shen YL. Some essential considerations in the design and conduct of non-inferiority trials. Clin Trials. 2011;8:432-9.
17. Hung JH, Wang SJ, Tsong Y, Lawrence J, O'Neil RT. Some fundamental issues with non-inferiority testing in active controlled trials. Statist Med. 2003;22:213-25.
18. Musch DC, Gillespie BW. The state of being noninferior. Ophthalmology. 2006;113(1):1-2.
19. Hung JH, Wang SJ, O'Neil R. Challenges and regulatory experiences with non-inferiority trial design without placebo arm. Biometrical J. 2009;2:324-34.
20. Huitfeldt B, Hummel J. The draft FDA guideline on non-inferiority clinical trials: a critical review from European pharmaceutical industry statisticians. Pharmaceut Statist. 2011; 10:414-9.
21. Julious SA. The ABC of non-inferiority margin setting from indirect comparisons. Pharmaceut Statist. 2011;10:448-53.
22. Wang SJ, Blume JD. An evidential approach to non-inferiority clinical trials. Pharmaceut Statist. 2011;10:440-7.
23. Norman GR, Streiner DL, eds. Biostatistics: the bare essentials. Shelton (CT): People's Medical Publishing House; 2008:393.
24. Chiquette E, Posey LM, eds. Evidence-based pharmacotherapy. Washington, DC: American Pharmaceutical Association; 2007:211.
25. Pater C. Equivalence and noninferiority trials—are they viable alternatives for registration of new drugs? (III). Current controlled trials in cardiovascular medicine [Internet]. 2004 Aug 17 [cited 2013 Apr 2];5(8): [7 p.]. Available from: http://trialsjournal.com/content/5/1/8
26. Snapinn SM. Noninferiority trials. Curr Control Trials Cardiovasc Med. 2000;1:19-21.
27. Hung JH, Wang SJ, O'Neill R. A regulatory perspective on choice of margin and statistical inference issue in non-inferiority trials. Biometrical J. 2005;47:28-36.
28. Snapinn S, Jiang Q. Controlling the type 1 error rate in non-inferiority trials. Statist Med. 2008;27:371-81.
29. Scott IA. Non-inferiority trials: determining whether alternative treatments are good enough. MJA. 2009;190:326-30.
30. International Conference on Harmonization. Note for guidance on statistical principles for clinical trials. London: European Medicines Agency (EMA). 1998 September 37p. Report No.: CPMP/ICH/363/96 ICH Topic E9.

31. Kaul S, Diamond G. Making sense of noninferiority: a clinical and statistical perspective on its application to cardiovascular clinical trials. Prog Cardiovasc Dis. 2007;49(4):284-99.
32. Friede T, Kiser M. Blinded sample size reassessment in non-inferiority and equivalence trials. Statist Med. 2003;22:995-1007.
33. Brown D, Volkers P, Day S. An introductory note to CHMP guidelines: choice of the non-inferiority margin and data monitoring committees. Statist Med. 2006;25:1623-7.
34. Henanff AL, Giraudeau B, Baron G, Ravaud P. Quality of reporting of noninferiority and equivalence randomized trials. JAMA. 2006;295(10):1147-51.
35. Moher D, Hopewell S, Schulz KF, Montori V, Gøtzsche PC, Devereaux PJ, et al. CON-SORT 2010 explanation and elaboration: updated guidelines for reporting parallel group randomized trials. BMJ. 2010;340:c869.
36. Schulz KF, Altman DG, Moher D. CONSORT 2010 statement: updated guidelines for reporting parallel group randomized trials. Int J Surg. 2011;9:672-7.
37. Gomberg-Maitland M, Frison L, Halperin JL. Active-control clinical trials to establish equivalence or noninferiority: methodological and statistical concepts linked to quality. Am Heart J. 2003;146(3):398-403.
38. Green WL, Concato J, Feinstein AR. Claims of equivalence in medical research: are they supported by the evidence? Ann Int Med. 2000;132:715-22.
39. Larson EB, Ellsworth AJ. N-of-1 trials: increasing precision in therapeutics [editorial]. ACP J Club. 1993 July/Aug;119(1):A16-7.
40. Cook DJ. Randomized trials in single subjects: the N of 1 study. Psychopharmacol Bull. 1996;32:363-77.
41. Guyatt GH, Keller JL, Jaeschke R, Rosenbloom D, Adachi JD, Newhouse MT. The n-of-1 randomized controlled trial: clinical usefulness. Our three year experience. Ann Intern Med. 1990;112:293-9.
42. Larson EB, Ellsworth AJ, Oas J. Randomized clinical trials in single patients during a 2-year period. JAMA. 1993;270:2708-12.
43. Guyatt G, Sackett D, Taylor DW, Chong J, Roberts R, Puosley S. Determining optimal therapy-randomized trials in individual patients. N Engl J Med. 1986;314:889-92.
44. Durham TA, Turner JR, eds. Introduction to Statistics in Pharmaceutical Clinical Trials. London: Pharmaceutical Press; 2008:226.
45. Lowe D. What you need to know about adaptive trials. Pharm Exec [Internet]. 2006 Jul 1 [cited 2013 Apr 2]. Available from http://www.pharmexec.com/pharmexec/article/articleDetail.jsp?id=352793
46. Gottlieb S. Adaptive trial design. Paper presented at: Conference on Adaptive Trial Design. 2006 Jul 10; Washington, DC.
47. Adaptive designs in the real world by Deborah Borfitz [Internet]. WHERE: BioIT World. com. Despite potential advantages, pharma is taking a cautious approach to adaptive designs, resulting in a slow but sure restyling of the research enterprise; 2008 Jun 10 [cited 2013 Apr 2]: [6 p.]. Available from: http://www.bio-itworld.com/issues/2008/june/cover-story-adaptive-trial-designs.html?terms=tessella

48. Krams M, Lees KR, Hacke W, Grieve AP, Orgogozo J, Ford GA. Acute stroke therapy by inhibition of neutrophils (ASTIN): an adaptive dose-response study of UK-279,276 in acute ischemic stroke. Stroke. 2003;34:2543-8.

49. Bokser AD, O'Donnell PB. Stability of pharmaceutical products. In: Lawson LA, Adejare A, Desselle SP, Felton LA, Moffat AC, et al., eds. Remington: the science and practice of pharmacy. 22nd ed. Philadelphia (PA): Pharmaceutical Press; 2013: 335-47.

50. Current good manufacturing practice for finished pharmaceuticals [Internet]. U.S. Department of Health and Human Services, Food and Drug Administration. 2013 Jul 8 [cited 2013 Aug 15]. Available from: http://www.fda.gov/Drugs/GuidanceComplianceRegulatoryInformation/Guidances/ucm064971.htm

51. United States Pharmacopeia, Inc. United States Pharmacopeia 36–National Formulary 31. Rockville (MD): US Pharmacopeia Convention, Inc. 2012.

52. Trissel LA, Flora KP. Stability studies: five years later. Am J Hosp Pharm. 1988;45:1569-71.

53. Guidance for industry: bioavailability and bioequivalence studies for orally adminstered drug products—general considerations [Internet]. U.S. Department of Health and Human Services, Food and Drug Administration Center for Drug Evaluation and Research. 2003 Mar 1 [cited 2013 Aug 15]. Available from: http://www.fda.gov/downloads/Drugs/.../Guidances/ucm070124.pdf

54. FDA ensures equivalence of generic drugs [Internet]. U.S. Food and Drug Administration. 2002 Aug 1 [cited 2013 Aug 10]. Available from: http://www.fda.gov/Drugs/EmergencyPreparedness/BioterrorismandDrugPreparedness

55. The United States Pharmacopeial Convention, Inc. Food and Drug Administration Center for Drug Evaluation and Research approved drug products with therapeutic equivalence evaluations. USPDI. 27th ed. Vol. III, Approved drug products and legal requirements. Massachusetts; 2007:I/5-17.

56. The United States Pharmacopeial Convention, Inc. Food and Drug Administration Center for Drug Evaluation and Research approved drug products with therapeutic equivalence evaluations. USPDI. 27th ed. Vol. III, Approved drug products and legal requirements. Greenwood Village (CO): Thompson Healthcare; c2007:1700.

57. Johnson SB. Bioavailability and bioequivalency testing. In: Lawson LA, Adejare A, Desselle P, Felton LA, Moffat AC, Perrie Y, et al., eds. Remington: the science and practice of pharmacy. 22nd ed. Philadelphia (PA): Pharmaceutical Press; 2013: 349-59.

58. Willett MS, Bertch KE, Rich DS, Eveshehefsky L. Prospectus on the economic value of clinical pharmacy services. A position statement of the American College of Clinical Pharmacy. Pharmacotherapy. 1989;9:45-56.

59. Hammond RW, Schwartz AM, Campbell MJ, Remington TL, Chuck S, Blair MM, et. al. Collaborative drug therapy management by pharmacists: 2003. Pharmacotherapy. 2003;23(9):1210-25.

60. Mann CJ. Observational research methods. Research design II: cohort, cross sectional, and case-control studies. Emerg Med J. 2003;20:54-60.

61. Gottlieb M, Anderson G, Lepor H. Basic epidemiologic and statistical methods in clinical research. Urol Clin North Am. 1992;19:641-53.
62. Feinstein AR, Horwitz RI. Double standards, scientific methods, and epidemiologic research. N Engl J Med. 1982;307:1611-7.
63. Dolan MS. Interpretation of the literature. Clin Obstet Gynecol. 1998;41:307-14.
64. Aschengran A, Seage GR, eds. Essentials of epidemiology in public health. 2nd ed. Sudbury (MA): Jones and Bartlett Publishers; 2008:516.
65. Greenhalgh T. How to read a paper. 3rd ed. Malden (MA): Blackwell Publishing Ltd.; 2006:229.
66. Slaughter RL, Edwards DJ, eds. Evaluating drug literature: a statistical approach. New York: McGraw-Hill; 2001:369.
67. Matthews DE, Farewll VT, eds. Using and understanding medical statistics. 4th ed. Basel, Switzerland: Karger; 2007:322.
68. Peipert JF, Glennon Phipps M. Observational studies. Clin Obstet Gynecol. 1998;41:235-44.
69. Riegelman R. Studying a study and testing a test. 5th ed. Philadelphia (PA): Lippincott Williams & Wilkins; 2005:356.
70. Lanthrop GD, Wolfe WH, Albanese RA, Moynahan PM. An epidemiologic investigation of health effects in air force personnel following exposure to herbicides. Baseline morbidity results. Washington, DC: U.S. Air Force; 1994.
71. Wolfe WH, Michalek JE, Miner JC, Rahe A, Silva J, et al. Health status of Air Force veterans occupationally exposed to herbicides in Vietnam I. Physical health. JAMA. 1990; 264:1824-31.
72. Michalek JE, Wolfe WH, Miner JC. Health status of Air Force veterans occupationally exposed to herbicides in Vietnam II. Mortality. JAMA. 1990;264:1832-6.
73. Ketchum NS, Michalek JE. Postservice mortality in Air Force veterans occupationally exposed to herbicides during the Vietnam War: 20 year follow-up results. Mil Med. 2005;170:406-13.
74. Matthews DE, Farewell VT, eds. Using and understanding medical statistics. 4th ed. Basel, Switzerland: Karger; 2007:322.
75. Fletcher RH, Fletcher SW, Wagner EH, ed. Risk. In: Fletcher RH, Fletcher SW, Wagner EH, eds. Clinical epidemiology: the essentials. 3rd ed. Baltimore (MD): Williams & Wilkins; 1996:94-110.
76. Katz DA. Barriers between guidelines and improved patient care: an analysis of AHCPR's unstable angina clinical practice guideline. Health Serv Res. 1999;34(1): 377-89.
77. Rochon PA, Gurwitz JH, Sykora K, Mamdani M, Streiner DL, Gafinkel S, et al. Reader's guide to critical appraisal of cohort studies: 1. role and design. BMJ. 2005 Apr 16; 330:895-7.
78. Mamdani M, Sykora K, Li P, Normand ST, Austin PC, Rochon PA, et al. Reader's guide to critical appraisal of cohort studies: 2. assessing potential for confounding. BMJ. 2005 Apr 23;330:960-2.

79. Normand ST, Sykora K, Li P, Mamdani M, Rochon PA, Anderson GM. Reader's guide to critical appraisal of cohort studies: 3. analytical strategies to reduce confounding. BMJ. 2005 Apr 30;330:1021-3.

80. Hayden GF, Kramer MS, Horwitz RI. The case-control study. A practical review for the clinician. JAMA. 1982;247:326-31.

81. Niemcryk SJ, Kraus TJ, Mallory TH. Empirical considerations in orthopaedic research design and data analysis. Part I: strategies in research design. J Arthroplasty. 1990;5:97-103.

82. Horwitz RI, Feinstein AR. Methodologic standards and contradictory results in case-control research. Am J Med. 1979;66:556-64.

83. Study design: the case-control approach. In: Gehlbach SH, ed. Interpreting the medical literature. 4th ed. New York: McGraw-Hill; 2002:31-54.

84. Gullen WH. A danger in matched-control studies. JAMA. 1980;244:2279-80.

85. Kleinbaum DG, Kupper LL, Morganstern H, eds. Typology of observational study designs. In: Epidemiologic research: principles and quantitative methods. New York: John Wiley & Sons; 1982:62-95.

86. Hartzema AG. Guide to interpreting and evaluating the pharmacoepidemiologic literature. Ann Pharmacother. 1992;26:96-8.

87. Grimes DA, Schulz KF. Cohort studies: marching towards outcomes. Lancet. 2002;359:341-5.

88. Spilker B. Single patient clinical trials. Guide to clinical trials. New York: Lippincott-Raven; 1996:277-82.

89. Jaeschke R, Sackett DL. Research methods for obtaining primary evidence. Int J Technol Assess Health Care. 1989;5:503-19.

90. Lukoff D, Edwards D, Miller M. The case study as a scientific method for researching alternative therapies. Altern Ther Health Med. 1998;4:44-52.

91. Kerlinger FN. Foundations of behavioral research. 2nd ed. New York: Holt, Rinehart & Winston; 1973:401.

92. Harrison DL, Draugalis JR. Evaluating the results of mail survey research. J Am Pharm Assoc. 1997;NS37:662-6.

93. Shi L. Health services research methods. 2nd ed. Clinton Park, New York: International Thomson Publishing; 2008:481.

94. Manasse H, Lambert R. Types of research: a synopsis of the major categories and data collection methods. Am J Hosp Pharm. 1980;37:694-701.

95. Segal R. Designing a pharmacy survey. Top Hosp Pharm Manage. 1985:37-45.

96. Fowler F. Survey research methods. In: Bickman L, Rog D, eds. Applied social research methods series. Vol. 1. Newbury Park (CA): Sage; 1993.

97. Fairman K. Going to the source: a guide to using surveys in health care research. J Manag Care Pharm. 1999;5:150-9.

98. Spilker B. Classification and description of phase IV postmarketing study designs. In: Spilker B, ed. Guide to clinical trials. New York: Lippincott-Raven; 1996:44-58.

99. Mulrow CD. The medical review article. State of the science. Ann Intern Med. 1987;106:485-8.

100. Oxman AD, Cook DJ, Guyatt GH. Users' guides to the medical literature. VI. How to use an overview. JAMA. 1994;272:1367-71.

101. Oxman AD, Guyatt GH. Guidelines for reading literature reviews. CMAJ. 1988; 138:697-703.

102. Joyce J, Rabe-Hesketh S, Wessley S. Reviewing the reviews. The example of chronic fatigue syndrome. JAMA. 1998;280:264-6.

103. Mulrow CD, Cook DJ, Davidoff F. Systematic reviews: critical links in the great chain of evidence [editorial]. Ann Intern Med. 1997;126:389-91.

104. Cook DJ, Mulrow CD, Haynes RB. Systematic reviews: synthesis of best evidence for clinical decisions. Ann Intern Med. 1997;126:376-80.

105. Sacks HS, Berrier J, Reitman D, Pagano D, Chalmers TC. Meta-analyses of randomized control trials. An update of the quality and methodology. In: Bailar JC, Mosteller F, eds. Medical uses of statistics. 2nd ed. Boston, MA: NEJM Books; 1992:427-42.

106. Einarson TR, Leeder JS, Koren G. A method for meta-analysis of epidemiological studies. Drug Intell Clin Pharm. 1988;22:813-24.

107. Greenhalgh T. Papers that summarize other papers (systematic reviews and meta-analyses). BMJ. 1997;315:672-5.

108. Gibaldi M. Meta-analysis. A review of its place in therapeutic decision-making. Drugs. 1993;46:805-18.

109. Pucino F. Use of meta-analysis to support clinical decision making. Paper presented at: Meta-analysis: Principles and Practice Session. Proceedings of the 43rd American Society of Health-System Pharmacists Midyear Clinical Meeting; 2008 Dec 7-11; Orlando, Florida.

110. Li T, Phuna MA, Vedula SS, Singh S, Dickersin K. Network meta-analysis—highly attractive but more methodological research is needed. BMC Medicine. 2011;9:79.

111. Calis, KA. Pitfall and limitations of meta-analysis. Paper presented at: Meta-analysis: Principles and Practice Session. Proceedings of the 43rd American Society of Health-System Pharmacists Midyear Clinical Meeting; 2008 Dec 7-11; Orlando, Florida.

112. Guyatt G, Rennie D, eds. User's guides to the medical literature: a manual for evidence-based clinical practice. Chicago (IL): AMA Press; 2002:706.

113. Crowther M, Lim W, Crowther MA. Systematic review and meta-analysis methodology. Blood. 2010;116(17):3140-6.

114. Armitage P, Berry G, Matthews JN, eds. Statistical methods in medical research. 4th ed. Malden (MA): Blackwell Science, Inc.; 2005:817.

115. Egger M, Smith GD, Schneider M, Minder C. Bias in meta-analysis detected by a simple, graphical test. BMJ. 1997;315:629-34.

116. LeLorier J, Gregoire G, Benhaddad A, Lapierre J, Derderian F. Discrepancies between meta-analyses and subsequent large randomized, controlled trials. N Engl J Med. 1997;337:536-42.

117. Stroup DF, Berlin JA, Morton SC, Olkin I, Williamson GD, Rennie D, et al. Meta-analysis of observational studies in epidemiology: a proposal for reporting. JAMA. 2000; 283(15):2008-12.
118. Moher D, Cook DJ, Eastwood S, Olkin I, Rennie D, Stroup DF. Improving the quality of reports of meta-analyses of randomized controlled trials: the QUOROM statement. Lancet. 1999;354:1896-900.
119. Moher D, Liberati A, Tetzlaff J, Altman DG; The PRISMA Group. Preferred reporting items for systematic reviews and meta-analyses: the PRISMA Statement. PLoS Med. 2009;6(7):e1000097. Doi:10.1371/journal.pmed.1000097.
120. Liberati A, Altman DG, Tetzlaff J, Mulrow C, Gøtzsche PC, Ioannidis JP, et al. The PRISMA statement for reporting systematic reviews and meta-analyses of studies that evaluate health care interventions: explanation and elaboration. PLoS Med. 2009;6(7):e1000100. Doi:10.1371/journal.pmed.1000100.
121. Moores KG. Meta-analysis: principles and practice. Paper presented at: Meta-Analysis. Principles and Practice Session. Proceedings of the 43rd American Society of Health-System Pharmacists Midyear Clinical Meeting; 2008 Dec 7-11; Orlando, Florida.
122. Cook DJ, Guyatt GH, Ryan G, Clifton J, Buckinham L, Willan A, et al. Should unpublished data be included in meta-analyses? Current convictions and controversies. JAMA. 1993;269(21):2749-53.
123. Van Iddekinge CH, Roth PL, Raymark PH, Odle-Dusseau HN. The crucial role of the research question, inclusion criteria, and transparency in meta-analyses of integrity test research. J Appl Psychol. 2012;97:543-9.
124. DerSimoniam R, Laird N. Meta-analysis in clinical trials. Controlled Clin Trials. 1986;7:177-88.
125. Higgins JP, Thompson SG. Quantifying heterogeneity in a meta-analysis. Statist Med. 2002;21:1539-58.
126. Moreno SG, Sutton AJ, Thompson JR, Ades AE, Abrams KR, Cooper NJ. A generalized weighting regression-derived meta-analysis estimator robust to small-study effects and heterogeneity. Statist Med. 2012;31:1407-17.
127. Sackett PR, Schmitt N. On reconciling conflicting meta-analytic findings regarding integrity test validity. J Appl Psychol. 2012;97(3):550-6.
128. Myung SK, Yoo KY, Oh SW, Park SH, Seo HG, Hwang SS, et al. Meta-analysis of studies investigating one-year effectiveness of transdermal nicotine patches for smoking cessation. Am J Health Syst Pharm. 2007;64:2471-6.
129. Thacker SB, Stroup DF, Peterson HB. Meta-analysis for the practicing obstetrician gynecologist. Clin Obstet Gynecol. 1998;41:275-81.
130. Zinberg S. Practice guidelines—a continuing debate. Clin Obstet Gynecol. 1998;41:343-7.
131. Rush AJ, Crismon ML, Toprac MG, Trivedi MH, Rago WV. Consensus guidelines in the treatment of major depressive disorder. J Clin Psychiatry. 1998;59(Suppl 20):73-84.
132. Hayward RS, Wilson MC, Tunis SR, Bass EB, Guyatt G. Users' guide to the medical literature. VIII. How to use clinical practice guidelines. A. Are the recommendations valid? JAMA. 1995;274:570-4.

133. Shekelle PG, Ortiz E, Rhodes S, Morton SC, Eccles MP, Grimshaw JM, et al. Validity of the agency for health care research and quality clinical practice guidelines: how quickly do guidelines become outdated? JAMA. 2001;286(12):1461-7.

134. Wilson MC, Hayward RS, Tunis SR, Bass EB, Guyatt G. User's guide to the medical literature. VII. How to use clinical practice guidelines. B. What are the recommendations and will they help you in caring for your patients? JAMA. 1995;274:1630-2.

135. Field MJ, Lohr KN. Clinical practice guidelines: directions for a new program. US Dept. of Health and Human Services. US Institute of Medicine Committee to advise the public health service on clinical practice guidelines. Washington, DC: National Academy Press; 1990.

136. Fairclough DL. Design and analysis of quality of life studies in clinical trials. Boca Raton (FL): Chapman & Hall; 2002:328.

137. Patrick D, Erickson P. Health status and health policy: allocating resources to health care. New York: Oxford University Press; 1993.

138. Aaronson NK, Cull AM, Kaasa S, Spranger MA. The European Organization for Research and Treatment of Cancer (EORTC) modular approach to quality of life assessment in oncology: an update. In: Spilker B, ed. Quality of life and pharmacoeconomics in clinical trials. 2nd ed. Philadelphia (PA): Lippincott-Raven; 1996:179-89.

139. Cella DF, Bonomi AE. The functional assessment of cancer therapy (FACT) and functional assessment of HIV infection (FAHI) quality of life measurement system. In: Spilker B, ed. Quality of life and pharmacoeconomics in clinical trials. 2nd ed. Philadelphia (PA): Lippincott-Raven; 1996:203-10.

140. Clinch JJ. The functional living index-cancer: ten years later. In: Spilker B, ed. Quality of life and pharmacoeconomics in clinical trials. 2nd ed. Philadelphia (PA): Lippincott-Raven; 1996:215-25.

141. Guyatt GH, Jaeschke R, Feeny DH, Patrick DL. Measurements in clinical trials: choosing the right approach. In: Spilker B, ed. Quality of life and pharmacoeconomics in clinical trials. 2nd ed. Philadelphia (PA): Lippincott-Raven; 1996:44-5.

142. Juniper EF, Guyatt GH, Jaeschke R. How to develop and validate a new health-related quality of life instrument. In: Spilker B, ed. Quality of life and pharmacoeconomics in clinical trials. 2nd ed. Philadelphia (PA): Lippincott-Raven; 1996:49-56.

143. International Society for Pharmacoeconomics & Outcomes Research Consensus Group. ISPOR quality of life regulatory guidance issues. ISPOR Website. 1999 [cited 2013 Apr 2]: [26 screens]. Available from: http://www.ispor.org/workpaper/consensus/index.asp

144. Samsa G, Edelman D, Rothman ML, Williams GR, Lipscomb J, Matchar D. Determining clinically important difference in health status measures. A general approach with illustration to the Health Utilities Index Mark II. Pharmacoeconomics. 1999;15:141-55.

145. Bowling A. Measuring health: a review of quality of life measurement scales. 2nd ed. Philadelphia (PA): Open University Press; 1997:159.

146. Spilker B. Quality of life and pharmacoeconomics in clinical trials. New York: Lippincott-Raven; 1996:1259.

147. Gill TM, Feinstein AR. A critical appraisal of the quality of quality of life measurements. JAMA. 1994;272:619-26.

148. Guyatt GH, Naylor CD, Juniper E, Heyland DK, Jaeschke R, Cook DJ. User's guides to the medical literature. XII. How to use articles about health-related quality of life. JAMA. 1997;277:1232-7.

149. Sanders C, Egger M, Donovan J, Tallon D, Frankel S. Reporting on quality of life in randomized controlled trials: bibliographic study. BMJ. 1998;317:1191-4.

150. Stoney CM, Coates P, Briggs JP. Integrity of active components of botanical products used in complementary and alternative medicine. JAMA. 2008;300(17):1995.

151. Bailey RL, Gahche JJ, Lentino CV, Dwyer JT, Engel JS, Thomas PR, et al. Dietary supplement use in the United States 2003–2006. J Nutr. 2011;141(2):261-6.

152. Stones M. US supplement sales up 3% last year. NUTRA Ingredients USA website. May 23, 2011 [cited 2013 Mar 12]: [3 screens]. Available from: http//www.nutraingredients-usa.com/.

153. Croom M, Bryant PJ, Pace HA, Schnabel L. A comparative analysis of identified hierarchical categorizations of evidence. Paper presented at: Innovations in Drug Information Session. Proceeding of the 42nd American Society of Health-System Pharmacists Midyear Clinical Meeting; 2007 Dec 3; Las Vegas, Nevada.

154. Cook DJ, Guyatt GH, Laupacis A, Sackett DL. Rules of evidence and clinical recommendations on the use of antithrombotic agents. Chest. 1992;102(Suppl 4):305S-11S.

SUGGESTED READINGS

1. Bryant PJ, Pace HA, eds. The pharmacist's guide to evidence based medicine for clinical decision making. Bethesda (MD): American Society of Health-System Pharmacists; 2009.

2. Chiquette E, Posey LM, eds. Evidence-based pharmacotherapy. Washington, DC: American Pharmaceutical Association; 2007.

3. Walter RW. The application of statistical analysis in the biomedical sciences. In: Malone PM, Kier KL, Stanovich JE, Malone MJ, eds. Drug information: a guide for pharmacists. 5th ed. New York: McGraw-Hill Medical; 2014.

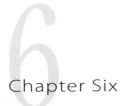

Chapter Six

Pharmacoeconomics

James P. Wilson ● Karen L. Rascati

Learning Objectives

After completing this chapter, the reader will be able to

- Describe the four types of pharmacoeconomic analysis: cost-minimization analysis (CMA), cost-benefit analysis (CBA), cost-effectiveness analysis (CEA), and cost-utility analysis (CUA).
- Describe the advantages and disadvantages of the different types of pharmacoeconomic analyses.
- List and explain the 10 steps that should be found in a well-conducted pharmacoeconomic study.
- List the six steps in a decision analysis.
- Give examples of the application of the pharmacoeconomic evaluation techniques to the formulary decision process, including decision analysis.
- Apply a systematic approach to the evaluation of the pharmacoeconomic literature.

Key Concepts

1 Pharmacoeconomics has been defined as the description and analysis of the costs of drug therapy to health care systems and society—it identifies, measures, and compares the costs and consequences of pharmaceutical products and services.

2 Pharmacoeconomic studies categorize costs into four types: direct medical, direct non-medical, indirect, and intangible.

3 Perspective is a pharmacoeconomic term that describes whose costs are relevant based on the purpose of the study.

4 There are four ways to measure outcomes: cost-minimization analysis (CMA), cost-benefit analysis (CBA), cost-effectiveness analysis (CEA), and cost-utility analysis (CUA). Each type of outcome management is associated with a different type of pharmacoeconomic analysis.

⑤ There are two common methods that economists use to estimate a value for health-related consequences, the human capital approach and the willingness-to-pay approach.

⑥ A CUA takes patient preferences, also referred to as utilities, into account when measuring health consequences.

⑦ All four types of analyses described (CMA, CBA, CEA, and CUA) should follow 10 general steps.

⑧ A sensitivity analysis allows one to determine how the results of an analysis would change when these best guesses or assumptions are varied over a relevant range of values.

⑨ Decision analysis is the application of an analytical method for systematically comparing different decision options. Decision analysis graphically displays choices and performs the calculations needed to compare these options.

Introduction

Many changes have recently taken place in health care. The continued introduction of new technologies, including many new drugs, has been among these changes. During 2012, over 150 new drugs formulations were approved by the Food and Drug Administration (FDA).[1] New biotechnology drugs can cost over $10,000 per course of therapy. The increase in the number of new drugs combined with the increase in costs of drugs provides a great challenge for all health care. The new organizations created by the Affordable Care Act to provide access to health care insurance for Americans, in addition to existing managed care organizations (MCOs), all desire to deliver quality care while minimizing costs.[2]

Pharmacy and therapeutics (P&T) committees are responsible for evaluating these new drugs and determining their potential value to organizations. Evaluating drugs for formulary inclusion can often be an overwhelming task. The application of pharmacoeconomic methods to the evaluation process may help streamline formulary decisions.

This chapter presents an overview of the practical application of pharmacoeconomic principles as they apply to the formulary decision process. Students and health professionals are often asked to gather and evaluate literature to support the decision process.

Pharmacoeconomics: What Is It and Why Do It?

❶ *Pharmacoeconomics has been defined as the description and analysis of the costs of drug therapy to health care systems and society—it identifies, measures, and compares the costs and consequences of pharmaceutical products and services.*[3] Decision makers can use these methods to evaluate and compare the total costs of treatment options and the outcomes associated

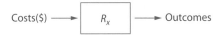

Figure 6–1. The pharmacoeconomic equation.

with these options. To show this graphically, think of two sides of an equation: (1) the inputs (costs) used to procure and use the drug and (2) the health-related outcomes (see Figure 6–1).

The center of the equation, the drug product, is symbolized by *Rx*. If only the left-hand side of the equation is measured without regard for outcomes, this is a cost analysis (or a partial economic analysis). If only the right-hand side of the equation is measured without regard to costs, this is a clinical or outcome study (not an economic analysis). In order to be a true pharmacoeconomic analysis, both sides of the equation must be considered and compared.

Relationships of Pharmacoeconomics to Outcomes Research

Outcomes research is defined as an attempt to identify, measure, and evaluate the end results of health care services. It may include not only clinical and economic consequences, but also outcomes such as patient health status and satisfaction with their health care. Pharmacoeconomics is a type of outcomes research, but not all outcomes research is pharmacoeconomic research.[4]

Models of Pharmacoeconomic Analysis

The four types of pharmacoeconomic analyses all follow the diagram shown in Figure 6–1; they measure costs or inputs in dollars and assess the outcomes associated with these costs. Pharmacoeconomic analyses are categorized by the method used to assess outcomes. If the outcomes are assumed to be equivalent, the study is called a **cost-minimization analysis** (CMA); if the outcomes are measured in dollars, the study is called a **cost-benefit analysis** (CBA); if the costs are measured in natural units (e.g., cures, years of life, blood pressure), the study is called a **cost-effectiveness analysis** (CEA); if the outcomes take into account patient preferences (or utilities), the study is

TABLE 6–1. FOUR TYPES OF PHARMACOECONOMIC ANALYSIS

Methodology	Cost Measurement Unit	Outcome Measurement Unit
Cost-minimization analysis (CMA)	Dollars	Assumed to be equivalent in comparable groups analysis
Cost-benefit analysis (CBA)	Dollars	Dollars
Cost-effectiveness analysis (CEA)	Dollars	Natural units (life years gained, mmHg blood analysis (CEA) pressure, mmol/L blood glucose)
Cost-utility analysis (CUA)	Dollars	Quality-adjusted life year (QALY) or other utilities

called a **cost-utility analysis** (CUA) (Table 6–1). Each type of analysis includes a measurement of costs in dollars. Assessment of these costs is discussed first, followed by further examples of how outcomes are measured for these four types of studies.

Assessment of Costs

First, the assessment of costs (the left-hand side of the equation) will be discussed. A discussion of the four types of costs and timing adjustments for costs follows.

TYPES OF COSTS

Costs are calculated to estimate the resources (or inputs) that are used in the production of an outcome. ❷ *Pharmacoeconomic studies categorize costs into four types.* **Direct medical costs** are the most obvious costs to measure. These are the medically related inputs used directly in providing the treatment. Examples of direct medical costs would include costs associated with pharmaceutical products, physician visits, emergency room visits, and hospitalizations. **Direct nonmedical costs** are costs directly associated with treatment, but are not medical in nature. Examples include the cost of traveling to and from the physician's office or hospital, babysitting for the children of a patient, and food and lodging required for patients and their families during out-of-town treatment. **Indirect costs** involve costs that result from the loss of productivity due to illness or death. Please note that the accounting term indirect costs, which is used to assign overhead, is different from the economic term, which refers to a loss of productivity of the patient or the patient's family due to illness. **Intangible costs** include the costs of pain, suffering, anxiety, or fatigue that occur because of an illness or the treatment of an illness. It is difficult to measure or assign values to intangible costs.

Treatment of an illness may include all four types of costs. For example, the cost of surgery would include the direct medical costs of the surgery (medication, room charges, laboratory tests, and physician services), direct nonmedical costs (travel and lodging for the preoperative day), indirect costs (cost due to the patient missing work during the surgery and recuperative period), and intangible costs (due to pain and anxiety). Most studies only report the direct medical costs. This may be appropriate depending on the objective or perspective of the study. For example, if the objective is to measure the costs to the hospital for two surgical procedures that differ in direct medical costs (e.g., using high-dose versus low-dose aprotinin in cardiac bypass surgery), but that are expected to have similar nonmedical, indirect, and intangible costs, measuring all four types of costs may not be warranted.

In order to determine what costs are important to measure, the perspective of the study must be determined. ❸ *Perspective is a pharmacoeconomic term that describes whose costs are relevant based on the purpose of the study.* Economic theory suggests that the most appropriate perspective is that of society. Societal costs would include costs to the insurance company, costs to the patient, and indirect costs due to the loss of productivity. Although this may be the most appropriate perspective according to economic theory, it is rarely seen in the pharmacoeconomic literature. The most common perspectives used in pharmacoeconomic studies are the perspective of the institution or the perspective of the payer. The payer perspective may include the costs to the third-party plan, the patient, or a combination of the patient copay and the third-party plan costs.

TIMING ADJUSTMENTS FOR COSTS

When costs are estimated from information collected for more than a year before the study or for more than a year into the future, adjustment of costs is needed. If retrospective data are used to assess resources used over a number of years, these costs should be adjusted to the present year. For example, if the objective of the study is to estimate the difference in the costs of antibiotic A versus B in the treatment of a specific type of infection, information on the past utilization of these two antibiotics might be collected from a review of medical records. If the retrospective review of these medical records dates back for more than 1 year, it may be necessary to adjust the cost of both medications by calculating the number of units (doses) used per case and multiplying this number by the current unit cost for each medication.

If costs are estimated based on dollars spent or saved in future years, another type of adjustment, called discounting, is needed. There is a time value associated with money. Most people (and businesses) prefer to receive money today, rather than at a later time. Therefore, a dollar received today is worth more than a dollar received next year—the time value of money. **Discount rate**, a term from finance, approximates the cost of capital by taking into account the projected inflation rate and the interest rates of borrowed money and then estimates the time value of money. From this parameter, the present value (PV) of future expenditures and savings can be calculated. The discount factor is equal to $1/(1 + r)^n$, where r is the discount rate and n is the year in which the cost or savings occur. For example, if the costs of a new pharmaceutical care program are $5000 per year for the next 3 years, and the discount rate is 5%, the present value (PV) of these costs is $14,297 ($5000 year one + $5000/1.05 year two + $5000/$[1.05]^2$ year three) (note that discounting does not start until year two). The most common discount rates currently seen in the literature are 3% to 5%, the approximate cost of borrowing money today.

Assessment of Outcomes

The methods associated with measuring outcomes (the right-hand side of the equation) will be discussed in this section. ❹ *As shown in Table 6–1, there are four ways to measure outcomes: CMA, CBA, CEA, and CUA. Each type of outcome measurement is associated with a different type of pharmacoeconomic analysis.* The advantages and disadvantages of each type of analysis will be discussed in this section.

COST-MINIMIZATION ANALYSIS

For a CMA, costs are measured in dollars, and outcomes are assumed to be equivalent. One example of a CMA is the measurement and comparison of costs for two therapeutically equivalent products, such as glipizide and glyburide.[5] Another example is the measurement and comparison of using prostaglandin E2 on an inpatient versus an outpatient basis.[6] In both cases, all the outcomes (e.g., efficacy, incidence of adverse drug interactions) are expected to be equal, but the costs are not. Some researchers contend that a CMA is not a true pharmacoeconomic study, because costs are measured, but outcomes are not. Others say that the strength of a CMA depends on the evidence that the outcomes are the same. This evidence can be based on previous studies, publications, FDA data, or expert opinion. The advantage of this type of study is that it is relatively simple compared to the other types of analyses because outcomes need not be measured. The disadvantage of this type of analysis is that it can only be used when outcomes are assumed to be identical.

Examples
A hospital needs to decide if it should add a new intravenous antibiotic to the formulary, which is therapeutically equivalent to the current antibiotic used in the institution and has the same adverse event profile. The advantage of the new antibiotic is that it only has to

be administered once per day versus three times a day for the comparison antibiotic. Because the outcomes are expected to be nearly identical, and the objective is to assess the costs to the hospital (e.g., the hospital perspective), only direct medical costs need to be estimated and compared. The direct medical costs include the daily costs of each medication, the pharmacy personnel time used in the preparation of each dose, and the nursing personnel time used in the administration of each dose. Even if the cost of the new medication is a little higher than the cost of the current antibiotic, the lower cost of preparing and administering the new drug (once a day versus three times per day) may offset this difference. Direct nonmedical, indirect, and intangible costs are not expected to differ between these two alternatives and they need not be included if the perspective is that of the hospital, so these costs are not included in the comparison.

Mithani and Brown[7] examined once-daily intravenous administration of an aminoglycoside versus the conventional every 8-hour administration (Table 6–2). The drug acquisition cost was in Canadian dollars ($Can) 43.70 for every 8 hours dosing, and $Can 55.39 for the single dose administration. Not including laboratory drug level measurements, the costs of the intravenous bag ($Can 29.32), preparation ($Can 13.81), and administration ($Can 67.63) were $Can 110.76 for the three-times daily administration versus $Can 42.23 (intravenous bag $Can 10.90, preparation $Can 6.20, and administration $Can 25.13) for the single daily dose. With essentially equivalent clinical outcomes, the once-daily administration of the aminoglycoside minimized hospital costs ($Can 97.62 versus $Can 154.46).

COST-BENEFIT ANALYSIS

A CBA measures both inputs and outcomes in monetary terms. One advantage to using a CBA is that alternatives with different outcomes can be compared, because each outcome is converted to the same unit (dollars). For example, the costs (inputs) of providing a pharmacokinetic service versus a diabetes clinic can be compared with the cost savings (outcomes) associated with each service, even though different types of outcomes are expected for each alternative. Many CBAs are performed to determine how institutions

TABLE 6–2. **EXAMPLE OF COST MINIMIZATION**

Type of Cost	Every 8 Hours	Once Daily
Drug acquisition cost	$43.70	$55.39
Minibag cost	$29.32	$10.90
Preparation cost	$13.81	$6.20
Administration costs	$67.63	$25.13
Total cost	$154.46	$97.62

NOTE: Costs are presented in Canadian dollars.

can best spend their resources to produce monetary benefits. For example, a study conducted at Walter Reed Army Medical Center looked at costs and savings associated with the addition of a pharmacist to its medical teams.[8] Discounting of both the costs of the treatment or services and the benefits or cost savings is needed if they extend for more than a year. Comparing costs and benefits (outcomes in monetary terms) is accomplished by using one of two methods. One method divides the estimated benefits by the estimated costs to produce a benefit-to-cost ratio. If this ratio is more than 1, the choice is cost beneficial. The other method is to subtract the costs from the benefits to produce a net benefit calculation. If this difference is positive, the choice is cost beneficial. The example at the end of this section will use both methods for illustrative purposes.

Another more complex use of CBA consists of measuring clinical outcomes (e.g., avoidance of death, reduction of blood pressure, and reduction of pain) and placing a dollar value on these clinical outcomes. This type of CBA is not often seen in the pharmacy literature, but will be discussed here briefly. This use of the method still offers the advantage that alternatives with different types of outcomes can be assessed, but a disadvantage is that it is difficult to put a monetary value on pain, suffering, and human life. ❺ *There are two common methods that economists use to estimate a value for these health-related consequences: the human capital (HC) approach and the willingness-to-pay (WTP) approach.* The HC approach assumes that the values of health benefits are equal to the economic productivity that they permit. The cost of disease is the cost of the lost productivity due to the disease. A person's expected income before taxes and/or an inputted value for nonmarket activities (e.g., housework and child care) is used as an estimate of the value of any health benefits for that person. The HC approach was used when calculating the costs and benefits of administering a meningococcal vaccine to college students. The value of the future productivity of a college student was estimated at $1 million in this study.[9] There are disadvantages to using this method. People's earnings may not reflect their true value to society, and this method lacks a solid literature of research to back this notion. The WTP method estimates the value of health benefits by estimating how much people would pay to reduce their chance of an adverse health outcome. For example, if a group of people is willing to pay, on average, $100 to reduce their chance of dying from 1:1000 to 1:2000, theoretically a life would be worth $200,000 [$100/ (0.001–0.0005)]. Problems with this method include the issue that what people say they are willing to pay may not correspond to what they actually would pay, and it is debatable if people can meaningfully answer questions about a 0.0005 reduction in outcomes.

Example

An independent pharmacy owner is considering the provision of a new clinical pharmacy service. The objective of the analysis is to estimate the costs and monetary benefits of two possible services over the next 3 years (Table 6–3). Clinical Service A would cost $50,000 in start-up and operating costs during the first year, and $20,000 in years two and three.

TABLE 6–3. CBA EXAMPLE CALCULATIONS

	Year 1 Dollars (No Discounting in Year 1)	Year 2 Dollars (Discounted Dollars)	Year 3 Dollars (Discounted Dollars)	Total Dollars (Discounted Dollars)	Benefit-to-Cost Ratio Dollars (Discounted Dollars)	Net Benefit Dollars (Discounted Dollars)
Costs of A	$50,000	$20,000	$20,000	$90,000	$120,000/$90,000 = 1.33:1	$120,000 − $90,000 = $30,000
	($50,000)	($19,048)	($18,140)	($87,188)	($114,376/87,188 = 1.31:1)	($114,376 − 87,188 = 27,188)
Benefits of A	$40,000	$40,000	$40,000	$120,000		
	($40,000)	($38,095)	($36,281)	($114,376)		
Costs of B	$40,000	$30,000	$30,000	$100,000	$135,000/100,000 = 1.35:1	$135,000 − 100,000 = 35,000
	($40,000)	($28,571)	($27,211)	($95,782)	($128,673/95,782 = 1.34:1)	($128,673 − 95,782 = 32,891)
Benefits of B	$45,000	$45,000	$45,000	$135,000		
	($45,000)	($42,857)	($40,816)	($128,673)		

Clinical Service A would provide an added revenue of $40,000 each of the 3 years, Clinical Service B would cost $40,000 in start-up and operating costs the first year and $30,000 for years two and three. Clinical Service B would provide added revenue of $45,000 for each of the 3 years. Table 6–3 illustrates the comparison of both options using the perspective of the independent pharmacy with no discounting and when a discount rate of 5% is used. Although both services are estimated to be cost beneficial, Clinical Service B has both a higher benefit-to-cost ratio and a higher net benefit when compared to Clinical Service A.

COST-EFFECTIVENESS ANALYSIS

This is the most common type of pharmacoeconomic analysis found in the pharmacy literature. A CEA measures costs in dollars and outcomes in natural health units such as cures, lives saved, or blood pressure. An advantage of using a CEA is that health units are common outcomes practitioners can readily understand and these outcomes do not need to be converted to monetary values. On the other hand, the alternatives used in the comparison must have outcomes that are measured in the same units, such as lives saved with each of two treatments. If more than one natural unit outcome is important when conducting the comparison, a cost-effectiveness ratio should be calculated for each type of outcome. Outcomes cannot be collapsed into one unit measure in CEAs as they can with CBAs (outcome = dollars) or CUAs (outcome = **quality-adjusted life years [QALYs]**). Because CEA is the most common type of pharmacoeconomic study in the pharmacy literature, many examples are available. Bloom and others[10] compared two medical treatments for gastroesophageal reflux disease (GERD), using both healed ulcers confirmed by endoscopy and symptom-free days as the outcomes measured. Law and others[11] assessed two antidiabetic medications by comparing the percentage of patients who achieved good glycemic control as the outcome measure.

A cost-effectiveness grid (Table 6–4) can be used to illustrate the definition of cost-effectiveness. In order to determine if a therapy or service is cost-effective, both the costs and effectiveness must be considered. Think of comparing a new drug with the current standard treatment. If the new treatment is (1) both more effective and less costly (cell G), (2) more effective at the same price (cell H), or (3) has the same effectiveness at a lower price (cell D), the new therapy is considered cost-effective. On the other hand, if the new drug is (1) less

TABLE 6–4. COST-EFFECTIVENESS GRID

Cost-Effectiveness	Lower Cost	Same Cost	Higher Cost
Lower effectiveness	A	B	C
Same effectiveness	D	E	F
Higher effectiveness	G	H	I

TABLE 6–5. LISTING OF COSTS AND OUTCOMES

Alternative	Costs for 12 Months of Medication	Lowering of LDL in 12 Months (mg/dL)
Current preferred medication	$1000	25
New medication	$1500	30

LDL = low-density lipoprotein.

effective and more costly (cell C), (2) has the same effectiveness but costs more (cell F), or (3) has lower effectiveness for the same costs (cell B), then the new product is *not* cost-effective. There are three other possibilities: the new drug is (1) more expensive and more effective (cell I)—a very common finding, (2) less expensive but less effective (cell A), or (3) has the same price and the same effectiveness as the standard product (cell E). For the middle cell E, other factors may be considered to determine which medication might be best. For the other two cells, an **incremental cost-effectiveness ratio** (ICER) is calculated to determine the extra cost for each extra unit of outcome. It is left up to the readers to determine if they think the new product is cost-effective, based on a value judgment. The underlying subjectivity as to whether the added benefit is worth the added cost is a disadvantage of CEA.

Example

An MCO is trying to decide whether to add a new cholesterol-lowering agent to its preferred formulary. The new product has a greater effect on lowering cholesterol than the current preferred agent, but a daily dose of the new medication is also more expensive. Using the perspective of the MCO (e.g., direct medical costs of the product to the MCO), the results will be presented in three ways in Tables 6–5 to 6–7 to illustrate the various ways that costs and effectiveness are presented in the literature. Table 6–5 presents the simple listing of the costs and benefits of the two alternatives. Sometimes for each alternative, the costs and various outcomes are listed but no ratios are conducted—this is termed a **cost-consequence analysis** (CCA).

The second method of presenting results includes calculating the average cost-effectiveness ratio (CER) for each alternative. Table 6–6 shows the cost-effectiveness

TABLE 6–6. COST-EFFECTIVENESS RATIOS

Alternative	Costs for 12 Months of Medication	Lowering of LDL in 12 Months	Average Cost per Reduction in LDL
Current preferred medication	$1000	25 mg/dL	$40 per mg/dL
New medic ation	$1500	30 mg/dL	$50 per mg/dL

LDL = low-density lipoprotein.

TABLE 6–7. INCREMENTAL COST-EFFECTIVENESS RATIO

Alternative	Costs for 12 Months of Medication	Lowering of LDL in 12 Months	Incremental Cost per Marginal Reduction in LDL
Current preferred medication	$1000	25 mg/dL	($1500 − $1000)/ (30 mg/dL − 25 mg/dL) = $100 per mg/dL
New medication	$1500	30 mg/dL	

LDL = low-density lipoprotein.

ratio for the two alternatives. The CER is the ratio of resources used per unit of clinical benefit and implies that this calculation has been made in relation to doing nothing or no treatment. In this case, the current medication costs $40 for every 1 mg/dL decrease in LDL while the new medication under consideration costs $50 for the same decrease. In clinical practice, the question is infrequently: "Should we treat the patient or not?" or "What are the costs and outcomes of this intervention versus no intervention?" More often the question is: "How does one treatment compare with another treatment in costs and outcomes?" To answer this more common question, an incremental cost-effectiveness ratio (ICER) is calculated. The ICER is the ratio of the difference in costs divided by the difference in outcomes. Most economists agree that an ICER (the extra cost for each added unit of benefit) is the more appropriate way to present CEA results. Table 6–7 shows the incremental cost-effectiveness (the extra cost of producing one extra unit) of the new medication compared to the current medication. For the new medication, it costs an additional $100 for every additional decrease in LDL of 1 mg/dL. The formulary committee would need to decide if this increase in cost is worth the increase in benefit (improved clinical outcome). In this example, the costs and benefits of the medications are estimated for only 1 year; discounting is not needed. If incremental calculations produce negative numbers, this indicates that one treatment is both more effective and less expensive, or dominant, compared to the other option. The magnitude of the negative ratio is difficult to interpret, so it is suggested that authors instead indicate which treatment is the dominant one. As mentioned earlier, when one of the alternatives is both more expensive and more effective than another, the ICER is used to determine the magnitude of added cost for each unit in health improvement (see CEA grid, cell I, Table 6–4).

Clinicians must then wrestle with this type of information—it becomes a clinical call. Many economists will argue that this uncertainty is why cost-effectiveness may not be the preferred method of pharmacoeconomic analysis.

COST-UTILITY ANALYSIS

❻ *A CUA takes patient preferences, also referred to as utilities, into account when measuring health consequences.*[12] The most common unit used in conducting CUAs is QALYs. A QALY is a health-utility measure combining quality and quantity of life, as determined by some valuations process. The advantage of using this method is that different types of health outcomes can be compared using one common unit (QALYs) without placing a monetary value on these health outcomes (like CBA). The disadvantage of this method is that it is difficult to determine an accurate QALY value. This is an outcome measure that is not well understood or embraced by many providers and decision makers. Therefore, this method is not commonly seen in the pharmacy literature. One reason researchers are working to establish methods for measuring QALYs is the belief that 1 year of life (a natural unit outcome that can be used in CEAs) in one health state should not be given the same weight as 1 year of life in another health state. For example, if two treatments both add 10 years of life, but one provides an added 10 years of being in a healthy state and the other adds 10 years of being in a disabled health state, the outcomes of the two treatments should not be considered equal. Adjusting for the quality of those extra years is warranted. When calculating QALYs, 1 year of life in perfect health has a score of 1 QALY. If health-related **quality of life** (HR-QOL) is diminished by disease or treatment, 1 year of life in this state is less than 1 QALY. This unit allows comparisons of morbidity and mortality. By convention, perfect health is assigned 1 per year and death is assigned 0 per year, but how are scores between these two determined? Different techniques for determining scales of measurement for QALY are discussed below.

There are three common methods for determining QALY scores: rating scales (RS), **standard gamble** (SG), and **time trade-off** (TTO). A rating scale consists of a line on a page, somewhat like a thermometer, with perfect health at the top (100) and death at bottom (0). Different disease states are described to subjects, and they are asked to place the different disease states somewhere on the scale indicating preferences relative to all diseases described. As an example, if they place a disease state at 70 on the scale, the disease state is given a score of 0.7 QALYs.

The second method for determining patient preference (or utility) scores is the standard gamble method. For this method, each subject is offered two alternatives. Alternative one is treatment with two possible outcomes: either the return to normal health or immediate death. Alternative two is the certain outcome of a chronic disease state for life. The probability (p) of dying is varied until the subject is indifferent between alternative one and alternative two. As an example, a person considers two options: a kidney transplant with a 20% probability of dying during the operation (alternative one) or dialysis for the rest of his life (alternative two). If this percent is his or her point of indifference

TABLE 6–8. SELECTED QALY ESTIMATES

Disease State	QALY Estimate
Complete health	1.00
Moderate angina	0.83
Breast cancer: removed breast, unconcerned	0.80
Severe angina	0.53
Cancer spread, constant pain, tired, not expected to live long	0.16
Death	0.00

(he or she would not have the operation if the chances of dying during the operation were any higher than 20%), the QALY is calculated as $1 - p$ or 0.8 QALY.

The third technique for measuring health preferences is the TTO method. Again, the subject is offered two alternatives. Alternative one is a certain disease state for a specific length of time t, the life expectancy for a person with the disease, then death. Alternative two is being healthy for time x, which is less than t. Time x is varied until the respondent is indifferent between the two alternatives. The proportion of the number of years of life a person is willing to give up $(t - x)$ to have his or her remaining years (x) of life in a healthy state is used to assess his or her QALY estimate. For example, a person with a life expectancy of 50 years is given two options: being blind for 50 years or being completely healthy (including being able to see) for 25 years. If the person is indifferent between these two options (he or she would rather be blind than give up any more years of life), the QALY for this disease state (blindness) would be 0.5. Table 6–8 contains examples of disease states and QALY estimates for each disease state listed.

As one might surmise, QALY measurement is not regarded as being as precise or scientific as natural health unit measurements (such as blood pressure and cholesterol levels) used in CEAs. Some issues in the measurement of QALYs are debated in the literature. One issue concerns whose viewpoint is the most valid. An advantage of having patients with the disease of interest determine health state scores is that these patients may understand the effects of the disease better than the general population, whereas, some believe these patients would provide a biased view of their disease compared with other diseases they have not experienced. Some contend that health care professionals could provide good estimates because they understand various diseases and others argue that these professionals may not rate discomfort and disability as seriously as patients or the general population.

Another issue that has been addressed regarding patient preference or utility-score measures is the debate over which is the best measure. Utility scores calculated using one method might differ from those using another. Finally, utility measures have been criticized for not being sensitive to small, but clinically meaningful, changes in health status.

Example

An article by Kennedy and associates[13] assessed the costs and utilities associated with two common chemotherapy regimens (vindesine and cisplatin [VP], and cyclophosphamide, doxorubicin, and cisplatin [CAP]) and compared the results with the costs and utilities of using best supportive care (BSC) in patients with nonsmall cell lung cancer. The perspective was that of the health care system or the payer. Using the TTO method, treatment utility scores were estimated by personnel of the oncology ward. Although the chemotherapy regimens provide a longer survival (VP = 214 days, CAP = 165 days) than BSC (112 days), the quality-of-life TTO score was higher for BSC (0.61) compared with the chemotherapy regimens (0.34). When survival time is multiplied by the TTO scores, the use of BSC results in an estimated 0.19 QALYs, which is similar to VP (0.19 QALYs), but higher than CAP (0.15 QALY). The costs to the health care system for the three options are about $5000 for BSC, $10,000 for VF, and $7000 for CAP (the authors reported median costs instead of average costs due to the abnormality of the cost data). Cost-utility ratios are calculated similarly to **cost-effectiveness ratios**, except that the outcome unit is QALYs. Therefore, the cost-utility ratio is about $26,000/QALY for BSC and about $44,000 to $52,000/QALY for the chemotherapy regimens. Because BSC is at least as effective, as measured by QALYs, and is less expensive than the other two options, a **marginal (or incremental) cost-utility ratio** does not need to be calculated. Marginal cost-utility ratios only need to be calculated to estimate the added cost for an added benefit, not when the added benefit comes at a lower cost.

Performing an Economic Analysis

Conducting a pharmacoeconomic analysis can be challenging. Resources (time, expertise, data, and money) are limited. Data used to construct a model may be impossible to obtain due to lack of computer automation. Comparative studies of drug treatments may not be available or poorly designed. Results of clinical trials may not apply at the institution performing the analysis due to lack of resources.

Methods for conducting a pharmacoeconomic analysis have been described. ❼ *All four types of analyses described (CMA, CBA, CEA, and CUA) should follow 10 general steps.* See Table 6–9. A modified practical approach to these steps based on the work developed by Jolicoeur and others[14] will be reviewed.

TABLE 6–9. **STEPS IN PERFORMING AN ECONOMIC ANALYSIS**

Step 1	Define the problem
Step 2	Determine the study's perspective
Step 3	Determine specific treatment alternatives and outcomes
Step 4	Select the appropriate pharmacoeconomic method or model
Step 5	Measure inputs and outcomes
Step 6	Identify the resources necessary to conduct the analysis
Step 7	Establish the probabilities for the outcomes of the treatment alternatives
Step 8	Construct a decision tree
Step 9	Conduct a sensitivity analysis
Step 10	Present the results

● STEP 1: DEFINE THE PROBLEM

This step is self-explanatory. What is the question or objective that is the focus of the analysis? An example might be, "The objective of the analysis is to determine what medications for the treatment of urinary tract infections (UTIs) should be included on formulary." Perhaps one of the drugs being evaluated is a new drug recently approved by the FDA. Should the new drug be added to the drug formulary? The important thing to remember with this step is to be specific.

● STEP 2: DETERMINE THE STUDY'S PERSPECTIVE

It is important to identify from whose perspective the analysis will be conducted. As mentioned in the Assessment of Costs section, this will determine the costs to be evaluated. Is the analysis being conducted from the perspective of the patient, health system, clinic, accountable care organization, or society? Depending on the perspective assigned to the analysis, different results and recommendations based on those results may be identified. If deciding on whether to add a new antibiotic to a formulary for treating UTIs, the perspective of the institution or payer would probably be used.

● STEP 3: DETERMINE SPECIFIC TREATMENT ALTERNATIVES AND OUTCOMES

In this step, all treatment alternatives to be compared in the analysis should be identified. This selection should include the best clinical options and/or the options that are used most often in that setting at the time of the study. If a new treatment option is being considered, comparing it with an outdated treatment or a treatment with low efficacy rates is a waste of time and money. This new treatment should be compared with the next best alternative or the alternative it may replace. Keep in mind that alternatives may include drug treatments and nonpharmacologic treatments. For the UTI example, a new antibiotic would probably be compared with fluoroquinolones or sulfa drugs, or even the use of cranberry juice—old or gold standard therapy—but still the usual and most commonly used therapy. Today's expensive new chemical entities are very unlikely to cost less than standard therapy, and because of this, newer drugs are sometimes compared to the most recent, more expensive drugs used as alternative therapy.

The outcomes of those alternatives should include all anticipated positive and negative consequences or events that can be measured. Remember, outcomes may be measured in a variety of ways: lives saved, emergency room visits, hospitalizations, adverse drug reactions, dollars saved, QALYs, and so forth. For the UTI example, cure rates would be the most important outcome.

STEP 4: SELECT THE APPROPRIATE PHARMACOECONOMIC METHOD OR MODEL

The pharmacoeconomic method selected will depend on how the outcomes are measured (see Table 6–1). Costs (inputs) for all four types of analyses are measured in dollars. When all outcomes for each alternative are expected to be the same, a CMA is used. If all outcomes for each alternative considered are measured in monetary units, a CBA is used. When outcomes of each treatment alternative are measured in the same nonmonetary units, a CEA is used. When patient preferences for alternative treatments are being considered, a CUA is used. For the UTI example, cure rates are a natural clinical unit measure, so a CEA would be conducted.

STEP 5: MEASURE INPUTS AND OUTCOMES

All resources consumed by each alternative should be identified and measured in monetary value. The cost for each alternative should be listed and estimated (see the Assessment of Costs section). The types of costs that will be measured depend on the perspective chosen in Step 2. When evaluating alternatives over a long period of time (e.g., greater than 1 year), the concept of discounting should be applied. For the UTI example, if the perspective is an acute care hospital, only inpatient costs of treatment are measured. If the perspective is that of the third-party payer, all direct medical costs for the treatment are included whether they are provided on an inpatient or outpatient basis.

Measuring outcomes can be relatively simple (e.g., cure rates) or relatively difficult (e.g., QALYs). Outcomes may be measured prospectively or retrospectively. Prospective measurements tend to be more accurate and complete, but may take considerably more time and resources than retrospective data retrieval. Prospectively it is possible to define exactly what data to capture, but because it is necessary to wait for the patients to complete therapy, these types of studies may take months to years to complete. A data set on the shelf (computer) can be available now, and may have all the data fields of interest. For the UTI example, cure rates attributed to the new product may be estimated from previous clinical trials, expert opinion, or measured prospectively in the population of interest.

STEP 6: IDENTIFY THE RESOURCES NECESSARY TO CONDUCT THE ANALYSIS

The availability of resources to conduct the study is an important consideration. Lack of access to important data can severely limit the validity of an analysis, as can the accuracy of the data itself. Data may be obtained from a variety of sources, including clinical trials, medical literature, medical records, prescription profiles, or computer databases. Before proceeding with the project, evaluate whether reliable sources of data are accessible or the data can be collected within the timeframe and budget allocated for the project.

STEP 7: ESTABLISH THE PROBABILITIES FOR THE OUTCOMES OF THE TREATMENT ALTERNATIVES

Probabilities for the outcomes identified in Step 3 should be determined. This may include the probability of treatment failures or success, or adverse reactions to a given treatment or alternative. Data for these can be obtained from the medical literature, clinical trials, medical records, expert opinion, prescription databases, as well as institutional databases. For the UTI example, probabilities of a cure rate for the new medication can be found in clinical trials or obtained from the FDA-approved labeling information. See Table 6–10. Probabilities of cure rates for the previous treatments (e.g., sulfas) can also be found in clinical trials or by accessing medical records. If prospective data collection is conducted, the probabilities of all alternatives will be directly measured instead of estimated.

STEP 8: CONSTRUCT A DECISION TREE

Decision analysis can be a very useful tool when conducting a pharmacoeconomic analysis (see the section on decision analysis for a step-by-step review). Constructing

TABLE 6–10. **STEPS IN DECISION ANALYSIS**

Step 1	Identify the specific decision (therapeutic or medical problem)
Step 2	Specify alternatives
Step 3	Specify possible outcomes and probabilities
Step 4	Draw the decision analysis structure
Step 5	Perform calculations
Step 6	Conduct a sensitivity analysis (vary cost estimates)

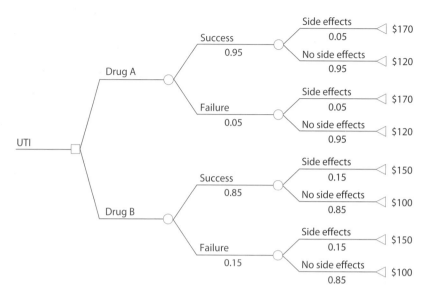

Figure 6–2. Decision tree for UTI example.

a decision tree creates a graphic display of the outcomes of each treatment alternative and the probability of their occurrence. Costs associated with each treatment alternative can be determined and the respective cost ratios derived. An example using a decision tree is provided in Figure 6–2.

STEP 9: CONDUCT A SENSITIVITY ANALYSIS

Whenever estimates are used, there is a possibility that these estimates are not precise. These estimates may be referred to as assumptions. For example, if the researcher assumes the discount rate is 5%, or assumes the efficacy rate found in clinical trials will be the same as the effectiveness rate in the general population, this is a best guess used to conduct the calculations. ❽ *A sensitivity analysis allows one to determine how the results of an analysis would change when these best guesses or assumptions are varied over a relevant range of values.* For example, if the researcher makes the assumption that the appropriate discount rate is 5%, this estimate should be varied from 0 to 10% to determine if the same alternative would still be chosen within this range. In order to vary many assumptions at one time, a **probabilistic sensitivity analysis** (changing each variable at random and recalculating) can be conducted that simulates many patients randomly being processed through the decision model using a range of estimates chosen for the analysis.[15]

STEP 10: PRESENT THE RESULTS

The results of the analysis should be presented to the appropriate audience, such as P&T committees, medical staff, or third-party payers. The steps outlined in this section should be employed when presenting the results. State the problem, identify the perspective, and so on. It is imperative to acknowledge or clarify any assumptions.

Although none of the models presented above are perfect, their utility may lead to better decision making when faced with the difficult task of evaluating new drugs or technology for health care systems.

What Is Decision Analysis?

Decision analysis is a tool that can help visualize a pharmacoeconomic analysis. ❾ *It is the application of an analytical method for systematically comparing different decision options. Decision analysis graphically displays choices and performs the calculations needed to compare these options.* It assists with selecting the best or most cost-effective alternative. Decision analysis is a tool that has been utilized for years in many fields, but has been applied to medical decision making more frequently in the last 10 years. This method of analysis assists in making decisions when the decision is complex and there is uncertainty about some of the information.

Discussions of the medical uses of decision analysis have been included in collections of pharmacoeconomic bibliographies,[16-20] and in such specific topic areas as CEAs,[21] CUAs,[22] CBAs,[23] CMAs,[24] policies,[25] formulary processes,[26] pharmacy practices,[27] and drug product development.[28]

STEPS IN DECISION ANALYSIS

The steps in the decision process are enumerated in greater detail in several articles,[29-33] and are relatively straightforward, especially with the availability of computer programs that greatly simplify the calculations.[33] Articles reporting a decision analysis should include a picture of the decision tree, including the costs and probabilities utilized. The steps in a decision analysis will be outlined using the UTI example. The six steps involved in performing a decision analysis are provided below and in Table 6–10.

Step 1: Identify the Specific Decision

Clearly define the specific decision to be evaluated (what is the objective of the study?). Over what period of time will the analysis be conducted (e.g., the episode of care, a year)?

Will the perspective be that of the ill patient, the medical care plan, an institution/ organization, or society? Specifying who will be responsible for the costs of the treatment will determine how costs are measured. For the UTI example, the decision was whether to add a new antibiotic to the formulary to treat UTIs. The perspective was that of the institution and the time period is 2 weeks.

● **Step 2: Specify Alternatives**

Ideally, the two most effective treatments or alternatives should be compared. In pharmacotherapy evaluations, makers of innovative new products may compare or measure themselves against a standard (older or well-established) therapy. This is most often the case with new chemical entities. For pharmaceutical products, dosage and duration of therapy should be included. When analyzing costs and outcomes of pharmaceutical services, these services should be described in detail. For the UTI example, the use of the new medication (drug A) will be compared with that of a sulfa drug (drug B).

● **Step 3: Specify Possible Outcomes and Probabilities**

Consequences, and outcomes calculated in dollars yield a cost per outcome in natural medical units, such as mg/dL, which is a CEA. For each potential outcome, an estimated probability must be determined (e.g., 95% probability of a cure or a 7% incidence of adverse events).

Table 6–11 shows the outcomes and probabilities for the UTI example. The probabilities represent the chances or likelihood of treatment success or adverse events, and the costs associated with them.

● **Step 4: Draw the Decision Analysis Structure**

Lines are drawn to joint decision points (branches or arms of a decision tree), represented as either choice nodes, chance nodes, or final outcomes. Nodes are places in the decision tree where decisions are allowed; a branching becomes possible at this point. There are three types of nodes: (1) a choice node is where a choice is allowed (as between two drugs or two treatments), (2) a chance node is a place where chance (natural occurrence) may influence the decision or outcome expressed as a probability, and (3) a terminal node is

TABLE 6–11. OUTCOMES AND PROBABILITIES, UTI EXAMPLE

	Drug A	Drug B
Effectiveness probability	0.95	0.85
Side effect probability	0.05	0.15
Cost of medication	$120	$100
Cost of side effects	$50	$50

TABLE 6–12. DECISION ANALYSIS CALCULATIONS FOR DRUG A

	Cost	Probability	Probability × Cost ($)
Outcome 1	$120 + $50 = $170	0.95 × 0.05 = 0.0475	8.08
Outcome 2	$120	0.95 × 0.95 = 0.9025	108.30
Outcome 3	$120 + $50 = $170	0.05 × 0.05 = 0.0025	0.42
Outcome 4	$120	0.05 × 0.95 = 0.0475	5.70
Total		1	122.5

the final outcome of interest for that decision. Probabilities are assigned for each possible outcome, and the sum of the probabilities must add up to one. Most computer-aided software programs utilize a square box to represent a choice node, a circle to represent a chance node, and a triangle for a terminal branch or final outcome. Figure 6–2 illustrates the decision tree for the UTI example.

Step 5: Perform Calculations

The first consideration should be the present value, or cost, of money. If the study is over a period of less than 1 year, actual costs are utilized in the calculations. If the study period is greater than 1 year, then costs should be discounted (converted to PV). For each branch of the tree, costs are totaled and multiplied by the probability of that arm of the tree. These numbers (costs × probabilities) calculated for each arm of the option are added for each alternative. Example calculations are given in Tables 6–12 to 6–14. The UTI example would be a cost-effectiveness type of study, so the difference in the cost for each arm would be divided by the difference in effectiveness for each arm to produce a marginal cost-effectiveness ratio (see Table 6–14).

Step 6: Conduct a Sensitivity Analysis (Vary Cost Estimates)

Because these decision trees or models are constructed with best guesses, a sensitivity analysis is conducted. The highest and lowest estimates of costs and probabilities are inserted into the equations, to determine the best case and worse case answers. These estimates should be sufficiently varied to reflect all possible true variations in values.

TABLE 6–13. DECISION ANALYSIS CALCULATIONS FOR DRUG B

	Cost	Probability	Probability × Cost ($)
Outcome 1	$100 + $50 = $150	0.85 × 0.15 = 0.1275	19.12
Outcome 2	$100	0.85 × 0.85 = 0.7225	72.25
Outcome 3	$100 + $50 = $150	0.15 × 0.15 = 0.0225	3.38
Outcome 4	$100	0.15 × 0.85 = 0.1275	12.75
Total		1	107.50

TABLE 6–14. INCREMENTAL COST-EFFECTIVENESS RATIO

	Alternative Costs of Drug and Treating Side Effects ($)	Effectiveness in Treating UTI (%)	Incremental Cost per Treatment Success
Drug A	$122.50	95	($122.50 − $107.50)/ (0.95 − 0.85) = $150
Drug B	$107.50	85	

For the UTI example, the new drug (drug A) would be added to the formulary if the committee thought the added cost ($150) was worth the added benefit (one more successful treatment) (see Table 6–12). Some might not agree with the probability of the adverse events of drug A; because the therapy is new, they may believe 5% may be an underestimate. If the estimate is increased to a 10% adverse event rate for the new drug and the marginal cost-effectiveness ratio is recalculated, the recalculated ratio would be $175 per added treatment success. Again, the committee would have to decide if the added cost is worth the added benefit.

Decision analysis is being used more commonly in pharmacoeconomic evaluations. The use and availability of computer programs[32] to assist with the multiple calculations makes it fairly easy for someone to automate their evaluations. Examples of software available for this purpose include TreeAge Pro (http://www.treeage.com), DPL (http://www.syncopation.com), and DecisionPro® (http://www.decisionpro.biz). The prices for these software packages range from less than $100 for student versions to over $1000 for professional versions. Decision analyses can also be conducted using Microsoft Excel (http://office.microsoft.com/en-us/excel).

Example

An article by Botteman and others[34] used a decision tree analysis to model the cost-effectiveness of enoxaparin compared to warfarin for the prevention of complications (deep vein thrombosis, venous thromboembolisms, and postthrombotic syndromes) due to hip replacement surgery. Data for this model were obtained through published literature and expert opinion. The model was created to assess both short-term (immediately after surgery) and long-term (followed until death or 100 years old) costs and consequences. The perspective was that of the payer, and a discount rate of 3% was used for the long-term analysis. Results: for the short-term model, therapy with enoxaparin was more expensive (+$133 per patient), but had a better outcome (+0.04 QALY per patient). For the long-term model, therapy with enoxaparin saved money (−$89 per patient) and had a better outcome (+0.16 QALY per patient), and was, therefore, the dominant (saves money and has a better outcome) choice. Both univariate (one item varied) and probabilistic (multiple items varied) sensitivity analyses were conducted and indicated that the results were robust.

Steps in Reviewing Published Literature

It is more likely that a practicing pharmacist will be asked to evaluate published literature on the topic of pharmacoeconomics, rather than actually conduct a study. When evaluating the pharmacoeconomics literature for making a formulary decision, or selecting a best product for an institution, a systematic approach to evaluating the pharmacoeconomics literature can make the task easier.

Several authors[14, 35-40] cite methodology to assist in systematically reviewing the pharmacoeconomic literature. If a study is carefully reviewed to ensure that the author(s) included all meaningful components of an economic evaluation, the likelihood of finding valid and useful results is high. The steps for evaluating studies are similar to the steps for conducting studies, because the readers are determining if the proper steps were followed when the researcher conducted the study. When evaluating a pharmacoeconomic study, at least the following 10 questions should be considered.

1. Was a well-defined question posed in an answerable form? The specific questions and hypotheses should be clearly stated at the beginning of the article.

2. Is the perspective of the study addressed? The perspective should be explicitly stated, not implied.

3. Were the appropriate alternatives considered? Head-to-head comparisons of the best alternatives provide more information than comparing a new product or service with an outdated or ineffective alternative.

4. Was a comprehensive description of the competing alternatives given? If products are compared, dosage and length of therapy should be included. If services are compared, explicit details of the services make the paper more useful. Could another researcher replicate the study based on the information given?

5. What type of analysis was conducted? The paper should address if a CMA, CEA, CBA, or CUA was conducted. Some studies may conduct more than one type of analysis (i.e., a combination of a CEA and a CUA). Some studies, especially older published studies, incorrectly placed the terms benefit or effectiveness analysis in the title of the article, when many were actually CMA studies.

6. Were all the important and relevant costs and outcomes included? Check to see that all pertinent costs and consequences were mentioned. The clinician needs to evaluate his or her situation and compare it to his or her practice situation.

7. Was there justification for any important costs or consequences that were not included? Sometimes, the authors will admit that although certain costs or consequences are important, they were impractical (or impossible) to measure in their study. It is better that the authors state these limitations, than to ignore them.

8. Was discounting appropriate? If so, was it conducted? If the treatment cost or outcomes are extrapolated for more than 1 year, the time value of money must be incorporated into the cost estimates.

9. Are all assumptions stated? Were sensitivity analyses conducted for these assumptions? Many of the values used in pharmacoeconomic studies are based on assumptions. For example, authors may assume the adverse event rate is 5%, or that adherence with a regimen will be 80%. These types of assumptions should be stated explicitly. For important assumptions, was the estimate varied within a reasonable range of values?

10. Was an unbiased summary of the results presented? Sometimes, the conclusions seem to overstate or exaggerate the data presented in the results section. Did the authors use unbiased reasonable estimates when determining the results? In general, are the study results believable?

Case Study 6–1

Title: Cost-Utility Analysis of Best Supportive Care versus Oncoplatin and Oncotaxel in the Treatment of Recurrent Metastatic Breast Cancer

Background: For patients diagnosed with recurrent metastatic breast cancer, the prognosis is grim. Two agents, Oncoplatin and Oncotaxel, have been used to help prolong the lives of these patients (authors would cite clinical literature here for real pharmaceutical products). As with other chemotherapy treatments, the toxic effects of the medications can be severe and vastly decrease the patient's quality of life. Some would argue that the small increase in life expectancy from these agents might not be worth the trade-off in suffering from the adverse effects of the agents during the treatment period. Instead of chemotherapy, palliative treatments, such as best supportive care (BSC), have been suggested as an option. BSC includes measures to keep the patient comfortable. These may include medications to alleviate pain, antibiotics, or radiotherapy to reduce tumor size. The objective of this study was to compare the costs and utility of two chemotherapy treatments, Oncoplatin and Oncotaxel, with those of BSC in patients with recurrent metastatic breast cancer.

Methods: The practice sites for data collection included three oncology clinics that are part of a multihospital, multiclinic health care system. Utility scores were collected via the time trade-off (TTO) method. A panel of experts helped create descriptions of the health states of patients undergoing the different treatment options. Based on these descriptions, utility scores were elicited from two sources: oncology nurses at the three clinics and a random sample of patients from general (nononcology) clinics associated with the health care system.

Data on treatment and survival time were collected for the past 3 years from a retrospective analysis of charts at three oncology clinics. Medical services and procedures associated with these treatment options were recorded. Treatment data included medications and their administration, as well as laboratory, radiology, and various types of medical visits (physician, clinic, emergency room, and hospital). Charges listed by the health care system in 2013 were used to estimate current costs for each service or procedure.

Results: Table 6–15A lists the costs and survival times found by the review of charts. Using the TTO method, treatment utility scores were estimated by nurses from the oncology clinics and a random sample of patients who did not have cancer. Although the chemotherapy regimens provided a longer survival (Oncoplatin, 200 days; Oncotaxel, 160 days) than BSC (130 days), the utility score was higher for BSC (0.60 to 0.61) compared with the chemotherapy regimens (0.32 to 0.35). Oncology nurses gave similar estimates compared with the group of nononcology patients.

If the difference in quality of life is not incorporated into the analysis, cost-effectiveness calculations based on survival time alone (life years saved [LYS]) indicate that chemotherapy is more effective but at a higher cost (Table 6–15B). When survival time is adjusted for the differences in utilities (preferences) for treatment, the use of BSC is dominant over both chemotherapy treatments because of its lower cost and higher QALY estimate.

Sensitivity analyses were conducted by reducing cost estimates using the clinic's cost-to-charge ratio of 0.83:1 and by varying the days of survival by their 95% confidence

TABLE 6–15A. COMPOSITE ARTICLE DATA

	BSC	Oncoplatin	Oncotaxel
	(N = 29)	(N = 36)	(N = 35)
Treatment Charges			
Mean	$5,000	$10,000	$7,000
(SD)	($1,000)	($2,000)	($2,000)
Survival (days)			
Mean	130 days	200 days	160 days
Range	110-140 days	180-215 days	110-190 days
Utility Scores			
Oncology Nurses	0.60	0.35	0.35
Utility Scores			
Nononcology Patients	0.61	0.32	0.32

TABLE 6–15B. COMPOSITE ARTICLE CALCULATIONS

	BSC	Oncoplatin	Oncotaxel
	(N = 29)	(N = 36)	(N = 35)
Cost Effectiveness			
Cost per LYS = (cost/ days) × 365 days/year	$14,038	$18,250	$15,969
Incremental cost per LYS = [Δcosts/Δdays] × 365 days/year		Oncoplatin vs. BSC = $26,071 per additional LYS	Oncotaxel vs. BSC = $24,333 per additional LYS
Cost Utility $QALY = \dfrac{days \times utility}{365\ days\ /year}$	O = 0.21 QALY P = 0.22 QALY	O = 0.19 QALY P = 0.17 QALY	O = 0.15 QALY P = 0.14 QALY
Average cost per QALY	O = $23,809	O = $52,631	O = $46,667
Cost/QALY	P = $22,727	P = $58,823	P = $50,000
Incremental cost per QALY = [Δcosts/ΔQALYs]	Both Oncoplatin and Oncotaxel dominated by BSC For both O and P estimates	Oncoplatin vs. Oncotaxel = $75,000 per additional QALY P = $100,000 per additional QALY	

BSC = best supportive care; LYS = life-years saved; O = based on utility scores from oncology nurses; P = based on utility scores from nononcology patients; QALY = quality-adjusted life-year

intervals. As with the comparison of oncology nurses versus patient utility estimates, the results were robust.

Conclusion: There are some limitations to this study. The data were collected from a small sample of patients. Although data were collected from three clinics, these clinics were all part of the same health care system. Oncology treatment in other clinics may vary in both costs and outcomes. Although utility scores were collected from health care professionals and general patients, they were not collected from patients with metastatic breast cancer. We believed that administering the instrument to these women might have placed an undue burden on patients with a poor prognosis. Actual cost data were not available, so charge data were used as a proxy, and a sensitivity analysis was conducted on this variable.

As with previous research, using BSC was found to be less expensive than using chemotherapy agents to treat advanced cancer. Although best supportive care may not be as effective as chemotherapy in traditional measures of effectiveness (e.g., survival time, progression-free survival time), when preferences for a less toxic treatment are factored into the decision, BSC may become the preferred treatment, and it should be considered as an option.

■ CRITIQUE OF CUA ARTICLE

1. Complete title: The title identified the type of study (CUA), the treatments that were being compared (BSC, Oncoplatin, and Oncotaxel), and the disease state (metastatic breast cancer).

2. Clear objective: The objective of this study was "to compare the costs and utility of two chemotherapy treatments, Oncoplatin and Oncotaxel, with those of best supportive care." This was clear.

3. Appropriate alternatives: The three alternatives were BSC, Oncoplatin, and Oncotaxel. A case was made that BSC is sometimes overlooked as a valid option. Based on the clinical literature cited, the readers would determine if the two chemotherapy options were appropriate.

4. Alternatives described: Chemotherapy dosing is very individualized, and data were collected from three clinics; average doses of agents were not included. BSC was defined as keeping the patient comfortable, including providing pain medications, antibiotics, and radiotherapy, if needed.

5. Perspective stated: The perspective of the study was not explicitly stated. Because the researchers only report measuring direct medical costs, the perspective could have been that of the payer or health care system, which included the three oncology clinics. Charges were measured, so the perspective is still unclear. If actual costs to the health system were estimated, the perspective could have been the health care system. If reimbursed costs were used, the perspective could have been that of the average third-party payer.

6. Type of study: The study was correctly identified as a CUA because outcomes were valued in QALYs. For comparison purposes, incremental cost-effectiveness ratios were also calculated based on length of survival for the three options, so the answer could be that both a CUA and a CEA were conducted.

7. Relevant costs: Because we are unsure of the perspective of the study, it is difficult to determine if relevant costs were measured. It seems as if all relevant direct medical costs were measured. Patient costs, such as time traveling to and from the clinic, might be different for BSC than for chemotherapy, but these costs were not measured.

8. Relevant outcomes: Outcomes of the treatment were measured by determining the length of life from chart reviews and utilities via two groups, oncology nurses and general patients. The TTO technique was used to elicit utility scores. A description of the health states used in eliciting these responses would have been a helpful addition to the article.

9. Adjustment or discounting: Data were collected from charts that spanned a 3-year period. To adjust for this, units of service were multiplied by current charges for each service. Discounting was not needed because neither costs nor outcomes were extrapolated into the future.

10. Reasonable assumptions: One assumption was that utility scores from the oncology staff would be accurate. To test this assumption, scores were also obtained from another group (a random sample of nononcology patients). Another assumption was that charges were a valid substitute for actual costs.

11. Sensitivity analyses: Sensitivity analyses were conducted. Utility scores from two groups were compared, and costs and survival time were varied. Although the authors indicated that results were insensitive to these analyses, a table with the numbers based on these new calculations would have been useful.

12. Limitations addressed: The authors did address some of their limitations at the beginning of the conclusion section. One limitation that was not addressed is that patients were not randomized to the three treatment options. It is possible that patients who received BSC were different from those who received chemotherapy. They may have been older or may have been in a more advanced stage of the disease.

13. Generalizations appropriate: Because data on both costs and outcomes were collected from only one health care system (albeit from three clinics within the system), caution should be used when extrapolating to other populations who are treated in other settings.

14. Unbiased conclusions: The authors state that when survival is adjusted for patient preferences, BSC is a valid option for treating patients with recurrent metastatic breast cancer. BSC costs less than chemotherapy treatments and provides a higher QALY score. Sensitivity analyses found the results to be robust (i.e., not sensitive to changes in estimates).

Many articles, several journals, and numerous texts have been devoted to pharmacoeconomics. Research and further development and refinement of the analysis tools are ongoing. It can be expected that the literature on pharmacoeconomics will continue to expand rapidly, not only for use in proving the value of new therapies, but for invalidating the worth of standard therapies. Grutters,[35] Husereau,[36] Doran,[37] Chiou,[38] Ofman,[39] Edwards,[40] among others,[41] cite references to assist readers in understanding and assessing economic analyses of health care as well as providing checklists (with examples and explanations) to evaluate published articles.

TABLE 6–16. SELECTED WEB SITE REFERENCES

Canadian Coordinating Office of Health Technology Assessment	http://www.cadth.ca/en
Cochrane Collaboration Home Page	http://www.cochrane.org
Department of Defense Pharmacoeconomic Center	http://www.pec.ha.osd.mil/
Institute of Health Economics	http://www.ihe.ca
International Society for Pharmacoeconomics and Outcomes Research	http://www.ispor.org/links_index.asp

Selected Pharmacoeconomic Web Sites

Articles that provide an overview of the field of pharmacoeconomics, its changing methodologies, and recent advances can often be found readily at Internet sites devoted to this area of specialization. These sites usually highlight articles that are not necessarily drug or therapy specific, but many present an overview or validation of methodologies. Several pharmacoeconomic Web sites are included as references. They were selected because they all have multiple links to other pharmacoeconomic-related sites (see Table 6–16).

Educational opportunities in pharmacoeconomics have grown tremendously over the past 15 years, especially in United States (U.S.) Colleges of Pharmacy.[42] A Web site that lists links to over 60 other Web sites that offer pharmacoeconomic education can be found at http://www.healtheconomics.com/resources/a-g/other-resources/.[43]

Conclusion

Many health care organizations continue to be challenged with managing costs of pharmacotherapy. With the proliferation of health care programs under the Affordable Care Act, each entity will be building pharmacoeconomic models that can be useful tools for evaluating the costs of pharmaceuticals in these plans. The ability to objectively measure and compare costs may also produce better decisions about the choice of pharmaceuticals for a formulary. Decision analysis is one of the many tools finding increased utilization in the field of medicine, and pharmacoeconomics specifically. As the science of pharmacoeconomics becomes more standardized, rigorous comparisons among several papers on the same topic will be possible (and necessary). For a more in-depth review of the principles and concepts of pharmacoeconomics, see textbooks devoted to the topic, such as *Essentials of Pharmacoeconomics*[44] or *Methods for the Economic Evaluation of Health Care Programmes*.[45]

Self-Assessment Questions

1. A patient is anxious about waiting 2 weeks for a test result—this can be categorized as what type of cost?
   a. Direct medical cost
   b. Direct nonmedical cost
   c. Indirect cost
   d. Intangible cost

2. A parent staying home from work to care for their sick child is categorized as what type of cost?
   a. Direct medical cost
   b. Direct nonmedical cost
   c. Indirect cost
   d. Intangible cost

3. For which of the following would Alternative A be considered cost-effective when compared to the standard Alternate B.
   a. Alternative A costs less than Alternative B.
   b. Alternative A is more effective than Alternative B.
   c. Alternative A is more effective than Alternative B, and Alternative A costs less than Alternative B.
   d. Alternative A is less effective than Alternative B, but Alternative A costs more than Alternative B.

4. When an article states that the results of an analysis are *insensitive* to a particular variable this means:
   a. The results vary depending on the range of that variable, thereby strengthening your confidence in the study results.
   b. The results vary depending on the range of that variable, thereby weakening your confidence in the study results.
   c. The results do not vary depending on the range of that variable, thereby strengthening your confidence in the study results.
   d. The results do not vary depending on the range of that variable, thereby weakening your confidence in the study results.

5. If Project A costs $30,000 this year, $40,000 in year two, and $50,000 in year three, what are the total 3 years costs in present value (PV) terms using a 5% discount rate. Do not begin discounting until year two. Round to the nearest $1000.
   a. $100,000
   b. $113,000

c. $120,000
d. $127,000

6. If a researcher evaluates cost per quality-adjusted life year saved, what type of study is being conducted?
   a. CEA
   b. CBA
   c. CMA
   d. CUA

7. Most economists agree that the most appropriate way to present cost-effectiveness data is using:
   a. An incremental cost-effectiveness ratio
   b. A simple cost-effectiveness ratio
   c. A net benefit ratio
   d. A benefit-to-cost ratio

8. In order to estimate utilities, researchers use:
   a. Rating scale methods
   b. Time trade-off methods
   c. Standard gamble methods
   d. Any of the above methods may be used

9. A disadvantage of using the human capital method to value health is:
   a. The value estimated depends on a person's earning potential.
   b. People may not pay what they indicate they are willing to pay.
   c. Both of the above.
   d. None of the above.

10. Drug A costs $3000 and saves $5000. What is the benefit-to-cost ratio for Drug A?
    a. 0.60:1
    b. 0.80:1
    c. 1.67:1
    d. 2.50:1

11. Drug B costs $5000 and saves $4000. What is the benefit-to-cost ratio for Drug B?
    a. 0.75:1
    b. 0.80:1
    c. 1.67:1
    d. 1.33:1

12. Based on these results from questions 10 and 11, which option would you choose?
    a. Drug A is the most cost-beneficial option.
    b. Drug B is the most cost-beneficial option.
    c. They are equally cost-beneficial.
    d. Not able to calculate based on information given.

For questions 13 to 15, use the following abstract:

Title: Cost utility of asthmazolimide (fictitious drug) in the treatment of severe persistent asthma.

Backgound: Some patients with severe persistent asthma are not controlled with standard treatment (defined in this study as a combination of long-acting beta-agonists [LABAs] and inhaled corticosteroids [ICS]). Clinical trials have shown improved outcomes for these patients if asthmazolimide is added to their regimen.

Objective: The objective of this study was to estimate the cost per quality-adjusted life year (QALY) of the addition of asthmazolimide to standard treatment for patients enrolled in a randomized controlled trial. The perspective of the study was the third-party payer.

Methods: Patients with severe persistent asthma in a health plan were enrolled in the study using a pre-post study design. The index date for each patient was his or her date of enrollment. Two years of preindex utilization and costs of medical services were recorded using retrospective data collection, and patients were followed prospectively for 1 year after their index date. For the first 12 months after enrollment, patients recorded their use of any asthma-related medical services and prescriptions and kept a daily symptom diary. Then patients had asthmazolimide added to their regimen for the next 12-month period and again kept track of their asthma-related medical services and prescriptions and a diary of daily symptoms. Costs of preindex services were adjusted to 2008 costs to the health plan. QALYs were calculated using utility weights for various asthma-related symptoms that were estimated from a previous study using the time trade-off (TTO) method.

Results: A total of 216 patients were enrolled in and completed the study. Asthma-related health plan costs increased after the addition of asthmazolimide (mostly from an increase in prescription costs) by an average of $800 per year. Fewer symptoms and less severe symptoms were reported after the addition of the new drug, resulting in an average increase of 0.1 QALY, for an incremental cost per QALY ratio of (for calculating the answer, see question 13, below).

Conclusion: For these 216 patients, the addition of asthmazolimide to their medication regimen resulted in a reduction of symptoms at a reasonable cost to the health plan.

13. What number should be included in the blank in the abstract?
    a. $800
    b. $8,000
    c. $80
    d. $80,000

14. In the abstract, was discounting needed? Was it conducted?
    a. Not needed, not conducted
    b. Needed, not conducted
    c. Needed, conducted
    d. Not needed, conducted

15. In the abstract, was adjustment needed? Was it conducted?
    a. Not needed, not conducted
    b. Needed, not conducted
    c. Needed, conducted
    d. Not needed, conducted

REFERENCES

1. CenterWatch: Clinical trials listing service [Internet]. [cited 2013 Oct 26] Available from: http://www.centerwatch.com/drug-information/fda-approvals/default.aspx?DrugYear=2012

2. Wang Z, Salmon JW, Walton SM. Cost effectiveness analysis and the formulary decision-making process. J Manag Care Pharm. 2004;10(10):48-59.

3. Bootman JL, Townsend RJ, McGhan WF. Introduction to pharmacoeconomics. In: Bootman JL, Townsend RJ, McGhan WF, eds. Principles of pharmacoeconomics. 2nd ed. Cincinnati (OH): Harvey Whitney Books; 1996: 5-11.

4. Rascati KL. Essentials of pharmacoeconomics. Philadelphia (PA): Wolters Kluwer/ Lippincott Williams & Wilkins; 2009: 3.

5. Nadel HL. Formulary conversion from glipizide to glyburide: a cost-minimization analysis. Hosp Pharm. 1995;30(6):467-9, 472-4.

6. Farmer KC, Schwartz WJ, Rayburn WF, Turnball G. A cost-minimization analysis of intra-cervical Prostaglandin E2 for cervical ripening in an outpatient versus inpatient setting. Clin Ther. 1996;18(4):747-56.

7. Mithani H, Brown G. The economic impact of once-daily versus conventional administration of gentamicin and tobramycin. Pharmacoeconomics. 1996;10(5):494-503.

8. Bjornson DC, Hiner WO, Potyk RP, Nelson BA, Lombardo FA, Morton TA, et al. Effects of pharmacists on health care outcomes in hospitalized patients. Am J Hosp Pharm. 1993;50:1875-84.

9. Jackson LA, Schuchat A, Gorsky RD, Wenger JD. Should college students be vaccinated against meningococcal disease? A cost-benefit analysis. Am J Public Health. 1995;85(6): 843-5.

10. Bloom BS, Hillman AL, LaMont B, Liss C, Schwartz JS, Stever GJ. Omeprazole or raniti-dine plus metoclopramide for patients with severe erosive oesophagitis. Pharmacoeco-nomics. 1995;8(4):343-9.

11. Law AV, Pathak DS, Segraves AM, Weinstein CR, Arneson WH. Cost-effectiveness analy-sis of the conversion of patients with non-insulin-dependent diabetes mellitus from glipi-zide to glyburide and of the accompanying pharmacy follow-up clinic. Clin Ther. 1995;17(5):977-87.

12. Kaplan RM. Utility assessment for estimating quality-adjusted life years. In: Sloan FA, ed. Valuing health care: costs, benefits, and effectiveness of pharmaceuticals and other medi-cal technologies. Cambridge (NY): Cambridge University Press; 1995.

13. Kennedy W, Reinharz D, Tessier G, Contandriopoulos AP, Trabut I, Champagne F, et al. Cost-utility analysis of chemotherapy and best supportive care in non-small cell lung can-cer. Pharmacoeconomics. 1995;8(4):316-23.

14. Jolicoeur LM, Jones-Grizzle AJ, Boyer JG. Guidelines for performing a pharmacoeco-nomic analysis. Am J Hosp Pharm. 1992;49:1741-7.

15. Shaw JW, Zachry WM. Application of probabilistic sensitivity analysis in decision analytic modeling. Formulary (USA). 2002;37:32-34, 37-40.

16. McGhan WF, Lewis NJW. Basic bibliographies: pharmacoeconomics. Hosp Pharm. 1992;27:547-8.

17. Wanke LA, Huber SL. Basic bibliographies: cancer therapy pharmacoeconomics. Hosp Pharm. 1994;29:402.

18. Skaer TL, Williams LM. Basic bibliographies: biotechnology pharmacoeconomics I. Hosp Pharm. 1994;29:1053-4.

19. Skaer TL, Williams LM. Basic bibliographies: biotechnology pharmacoeconomics II. Hosp Pharm. 1994;29:1136.

20. McGhan WF. Basic bibliographies: pharmacoeconomics. Hosp Pharm. 1998;33:1270, 1273.

21. Duggan AE, Tolley K, Hawkey CJ, Logan RF. Varying efficacy of Helicobacter pylori erad-ication regimens: cost effectiveness study using a decision analysis model. BMJ. 1998;316:1648-54.

22. Messori A, Trippoli S, Becagli P, Cincotta M, Labbate MG, Zaccara G. Adjunctive lamotrig-ine therapy in patients with refractory seizures: a lifetime cost-utility analysis. Eur J Clin Pharmacol. 1998;53(6):421-7.

23. Ginsberg G, Shani S, Lev B. Cost benefit analysis of risperidone and clozapine in the treat-ment of schizophrenia in Israel. Pharmacoeconomics. 1998 Feb 13;231-41.

24. Sesti AM, Armitstead JA, Hall KN, Jang R, Milne S. Cost-minimization analysis of hand held nebulizer LC vs UC metered dose inhaler protocol for management of acute asthma exacerbations in the emergency department. ASHP Midyear Clinical Meeting; 32: MCS-7: 1997 Dec 8–12; New Orleans, Louisiana.

25. Hinman AR, Koplan JP, Orenstein WA, Brink EW. Decision analysis and polio immuniza-tion policy. Am J Pub Health. 1988;78:301-3.

26. Kessler JM. Decision analysis in the formulary process. Am J Health Syst Pharm. 1997;54:S5-S8.

27. Einarson TR, McGhan WF, Bootman JL. Decision analysis applied to pharmacy practice. Am J Hosp Pharm. 1985;42:364-71.

28. Walking D, Appino JP. Decision analysis in drug product development. Drug Cosmet Ind. 1973;112:39-41.

29. Rascati KL. Decision analysis techniques practical aspects of using personal computers for decision analytic modeling. Drug Benefit Trends. 1998;July:33-36.

30. Richardson WS, Detsky AS. Users' guides to the medical literature. Part 7. How to use a clinical decision analysis. Par t A. Are the results of the study valid? JAMA. 1995;273:1292-5.

31. Richardson WS, Detsky AS. Users' guides to the medical literature. Part 7. How to use a clinical decision analysis. Part B. What are the results and will they help me in caring for my patients? JAMA. 1995;273:1610-3.

32. Baskin LE. Practical pharmacoeconomics. Cleveland (OH): Advanstar Communications; 1998.

33. Sacristán JA, Soto J, Galende I. Evaluation of pharmacoeconomic studies: utilization of a checklist. Ann Pharmacother. 1993;27:1126-32.

34. Botteman MF, Caprini J, Stephens JM, Nadipelli V, Bell CF, Pashos CL, et al. Results of an economic model to assess cost-effectiveness of enoxaparin, a low-molecular-weight heparin, versus warfarin for the prophylaxis of DVT and associated long-term complications in total hip replacement surgery in the United States. Clin Ther. 2002:24(11):1960-86.

35. Grutters J, Seferina S, Tjan-Heijnen V, van Kampen R,Goettsch W, Joore M. Bridging trial and decision: a checklist to frame health technology assessments for resource allocation decisions. Value Health [serial online]. July 2011;14(5):777-84.

36. Husereau D, Drummond M, Loder E, et al. Consolidated Health Economic Evaluation Reporting Standards (CHEERS) statement. Value Health [serial online]. March 2013; 16(2):e1-5.

37. Doran C. Critique of an economic evaluation using the Drummond checklist. Appl Health Econ Health Policy [serial online]. 2010;8(6):357-9.

38. Chiou C, Hay J, Ofman J, et al. Development and validation of a grading system for the quality of cost-effectiveness studies. Medical Care [serial online]. January 2003;41(1):32-44.

39. Ofman J, Sullivan S, Hay J, et al. Examining the value and quality of health economic analyses: implications of utilizing the QHES. J Manag Care Pharm [serial online]. January 2003;9(1):53-61.

40. Edwards R, Charles J, Lloyd-Williams H. Public health economics: a systematic review of guidance for the economic evaluation of public health interventions and discussion of key methodological issues. BMC Public Health [serial online]. October 24, 2013;13(1):1001.

41. Mullins CD, Flowers LR. Evaluating economic outcomes literature. In: Grauer DW et al. eds. Pharmacoeconomics and outcomes: applications for patient care. 2nd ed. Kansas City (MO): American College of Clinical Pharmacy; 2003.

42. Rascati KL, Drummond MF, Annemans L, Davey PG. Education in pharmacoeconomics: an international multidisciplinary view. Pharmacoeconomics. 2004;22(3):139-47.

43. HealthEconomics.com. [cited 2013 Oct 26] Available from: http://www.healtheconomics.com/resources/a-g/other-resources/
44. Rascati KL. Essentials of pharmacoeconomics. 2nd ed. Philadelphia (PA): Wolters Kluwer/Lippincott Williams & Wilkins; 2013.
45. Drummond MF, Sculpher MJ, Torrance GW, O'Brien BJ, Stoddart GL. Methods for the economic evaluation of health care programmes. 3rd ed. Oxford (NY): Oxford University Press; 2005.

SUGGESTED READINGS

1. Bingefors K, Pashos CL, Smith MD, Berger ML, Hedbloom EC, Torrance GW. Health care costs, quality, and outcomes ISPOR book of terms. Lawrenceville (NJ): International Society for Pharmacoeconomics and Outcomes Research; 2003.
2. Drummond MF, Sculpher MJ, Torrance GW, O'Brien BJ, Stoddart GL. Methods for the economic evaluation of health care programmes. New York: Oxford University Press; 2005.
3. Edwards R, Charles J, Lloyd-Williams H. Public health economics: a systematic review of guidance for the economic evaluation of public health interventions and discussion of key methodological issues. BMC Public Health [serial online]. October 24, 2013;13(1):1001.
4. Husereau D, Drummond M, Loder E, et al. Consolidated Health Economic Evaluation Reporting Standards (CHEERS) statement. Value Health [serial online]. March 2013;16(2):e1-5.
5. Rascati KL. Essentials of pharmacoeconomics. 2nd ed. Philadelphia (PA): Wolters Kluwer/Lippincott Williams & Wilkins; 2013.

7

Chapter Seven

Evidence-Based Clinical Practice Guidelines

Kevin G. Moores • Vicki R. Kee

Learning Objectives

After completing this chapter, the reader will be able to

- Define clinical practice guidelines.
- Define evidence-based medicine.
- Discuss the role of the pharmacist in development and use of these evidence-based clinical practice guidelines.
- Explain the methodology for development of evidence-based clinical practice guidelines.
- Describe the GRADE system for grading the quality of evidence and strength of recommendations.
- Describe the AGREE II instrument for evaluating clinical practice guidelines.
- Identify the key issues involved in the implementation of clinical practice guidelines.
- Identify sources of published clinical practice guidelines.

Key Concepts

1. Clinical practice guidelines are recommendations for optimizing patient care that are developed by systematically reviewing the evidence and assessing the benefits and harms of health care interventions.

2. Evidence-based medicine (EBM) is a philosophy of practice and an approach to decision making in the clinical care of patients that involves making individual patient care decisions based on the best currently available evidence.

❸ Evaluation of the quality of a guideline and the appropriateness of its use in a given setting depends primarily on an ability to distinguish methods that minimize potential biases in development.

❹ The definition of the clinical questions to be addressed by a guideline is a key step that provides direction for the activities to follow.

❺ The quality of the evidence that forms the basis for recommendations is a key aspect for interpretation and use of a practice guideline.

❻ The advantage of the Grading of Recommendations, Assessment, Development and Evaluation (GRADE) system is that all of the evidence that is most important for making the decision has been judged with explicit criteria, the judgments are made transparent, evidence profiles and summary of findings tables have been created, consequently facilitating the use of best evidence.

❼ Prior to selecting a clinical practice guideline for implementation in a health care system or for personal use by a health care professional, it is important that the quality of published guidelines be evaluated. Perhaps the most useful tool available for evaluating clinical practice guidelines is the one created by the Appraisal of Guidelines for Research and Evaluation (AGREE) collaboration.

❽ The most effective methods for implementing guidelines to achieve the desired effects of improved quality of care have not been determined.

❾ Complete clinical practice guidelines can be found on Web sites such as the National Guideline Clearinghouse and in the peer-reviewed medical literature located by use of secondary databases.

Introduction

❶ *Clinical practice guidelines are recommendations for optimizing patient care that are developed by systematically reviewing the evidence and assessing the benefits and harms of health care interventions.*[1] These interventions may include not only medications but other types of therapy, such as radiation, surgery, and physical therapy. Clinical practice guidelines are developed by a variety of groups and organizations including federal and state government, professional associations, managed care organizations, third-party payers, quality assurance organizations, and utilization review groups. The purpose of the guidelines, methods used to develop them, format of the documents, and the strategies for implementation vary widely. Considering the potential for clinical practice guidelines to influence thousands to millions of decisions on medical interventions, it is incumbent for all health care practitioners to be thoroughly familiar with criteria to judge the validity of guidelines and to be skilled in determining their appropriate application.

Development and implementation of clinical practice guidelines have many characteristics in common with traditional activities performed by drug information specialists, such as evaluation of new drugs for formulary consideration, medication use evaluation, and quality improvement. Many of the skills required for guideline development are required of pharmacists, including clear specific definition of clinical questions, literature search and evaluation, epidemiology, biostatistics, clinical expertise, writing, editing, and formatting. Drug information specialists benefit from the use of clinical practice guidelines as information resources for their work, and based on their skills they are logical professionals to participate in guideline development and implementation. Pharmacists and health care professionals should also be using clinical practice guidelines whenever possible in their practices.

The primary attraction for all health care professionals in properly developed, valid clinical practice guidelines is that they provide a concise summary of current best evidence on what works and what does not when considering specific health care interventions. New information and new technology in health care are developed at a rapid pace. It is very difficult for individual practitioners to systematically evaluate the benefits and risks of all new technology, including new medications. By presenting a summary of best evidence, guidelines assist the practitioner in decision making for specific patients and also facilitate discussion of care options most consistent with individual patient needs and preferences. Guidelines may also enhance provider communication and continuity of care, especially when decisions are made by multiple providers in different care settings.[2]

A significant time lag occurs in getting research information into practice, and one of the goals of development and implementation of evidence-based clinical practice guidelines is to help speed up the process of getting evidence into practice. There are several examples of treatments that have been well studied and proven effective but are substantially underutilized and interventions that have been proven ineffective or harmful but continue to be done.[3] One of the goals of development and implementation of evidence-based clinical practice guidelines is to help speed up the process of getting evidence into practice.

Clinical practice guidelines to assist with health care decision making and to identify indicators for monitoring quality of care are frequently mentioned in connection with efforts to improve quality and efficiency of services. The key issues in reforming the United States (U.S.) health care system are access to care, cost, and quality. Quality and safety are a major focus as evidenced by landmark reports published by the Institute of Medicine (IOM) regarding quality of care problems in the United States, recommendations to focus on improvements in patient safety, and recommendations to reduce preventable medical errors.[4-7] The central concepts in these reports and recommendations relate to using the best available evidence, providing decision support tools, use of informatics, and participation of patients in health care decisions and responsibilities. The most recent reports from the IOM deal specifically with standards for clinical practice guidelines, systematic reviews of comparative effectiveness research, and providing care at a lower cost.[1,8,9] All of these documents and standards highlight improvements in technology, information technology, quality of access to electronic records, and greater ability to use the data from processes of care to provide valuable new information to learn what works best. These concepts are central to improving the validity and usefulness of clinical practice guidelines.

Methods currently recommended as the most valid for development of clinical practice guidelines emphasize an evidence-based approach, formal quantitative techniques to calculate risks and benefits, and incorporation of the patient's preference. The concepts of an evidence-based approach and use of methods to grade the quality of evidence and strength of recommendations are critical elements that will be reviewed in more detail in this chapter. The evidence-based health care movement and the implementation of continuous quality improvement (CQI) programs stimulated growth in guideline development. Advancements continue to be made in methods of evaluation and summarizing the best available evidence. Development of information databases of systematic reviews and new informatics resources has facilitated the production of clinical practice guidelines and improved access to this information.

This chapter presents a review of the background of clinical practice guidelines and evidence-based medicine; review evidence-based methods for guideline development, evaluation, and implementation; and provide directions to locate sources of guidelines.

Evidence-Based Medicine and Clinical Practice Guidelines

❷ *Evidence-based medicine (EBM) is a philosophy of practice and an approach to decision making in the clinical care of patients that involves making individual patient care decisions based on the best currently available evidence.*[10] The practice of EBM refers to integrating individual clinical expertise with the best available published clinical evidence from systematic research. EBM is often mistaken for, or reduced to, just one of its several components, critical appraisal of the literature. However, EBM requires both clinical expertise and an intimate knowledge of the individual patient's situation, beliefs, priorities, and values to be useful. External evidence must be used to inform, but not replace, individual clinical expertise. It is clinical expertise that determines if the external evidence may be applied to the individual patient and, if so, how it should be used in decision making by the patient and the health care provider. The development and application of clinical practice guidelines are among the tools used in EBM. In fact, the first published use of the term *evidence-based* was in the context of clinical guidelines.[11] An understanding of EBM is necessary to understand recommended methods for production and implementation of guidelines.

The term evidence-based medicine was first used by physicians at McMaster University in Hamilton, Ontario. This group, the Evidence-Based Medicine Working Group, published a description of what they considered a new paradigm for medical practice and teaching.[12] Their article presented their views on changes that were occurring in medical practice relating to the use of medical literature to more effectively guide decision making. They stated that the foundation for the paradigm shift rested in significant advances in clinical research, such as the development of the randomized controlled trial and meta-analysis.

The practice of EBM has been described as focusing on five linked activities: (1) converting the information need into a clearly defined answerable clinical question, (2) conducting a search for the best available evidence for the problem, (3) critically appraising the validity, impact, and applicability of the evidence, (4) incorporating the critical appraisal with clinical expertise and the patient's unique characteristics, and (5) evaluating effectiveness and efficiency in executing the first four activities and identify ways to improve them.[13] Those who are familiar with the literature in drug information practice will recognize that these activities are remarkably similar to the systematic approach to drug information requests as outlined by Watanabe and colleagues in 1975.[14] This process is still very similar to the approach used to answer drug information questions today.

Following their original paper on EBM,[12] the lead individuals in the Evidence-Based Medicine Working Group published a description of how evidence-based care practitioners should be trained to locate, evaluate, and apply the best evidence.[15] This description recognizes that not all practitioners will have the time or an interest in using primary literature. The description notes that sources of appropriately preappraised evidence may be used. Examples of preappraised evidence would include clinical practice guidelines and systematic reviews that have been produced with evidence-based methods. These authors noted that skill in interpreting the medical literature is still necessary to judge the quality of the preappraised resources, to know when the recommendations in the preappraised resources are not applicable to selected patients, and to use the original literature when preappraised resources are unavailable.[15]

In a review of the philosophy of EBM, Eddy described an approach that is similar to the Evidence-Based Medicine Working Group.[11] The Evidence-Based Medicine Working Group's original description of the practice is referred to as evidence-based individual decision making. Eddy refers to a second approach to EBM as being evidence-based guidelines. This second approach has four important features: (1) small, specially trained groups should analyze the evidence and develop the guideline, (2) an explicit, rigorous process should be used, (3) the guideline should not be specific to an individual patient but rather should be applicable to a class or group of patients, and (4) the guideline should indirectly help, guide, or motivate health care providers to deliver certain types of care to people, not directly determine the care for a specific patient.[11] Eddy went on to explain that the most appropriate definition of EBM is a combination of these two approaches. The combination provides for medical practice that will achieve the most efficient and effective use of evidence.

Health care professionals face the complicated reality of constantly changing and increasing medical knowledge. To practice effective, high quality medicine, it is not necessary to memorize vast quantities of information; what is necessary are the skills to acquire and critically assess the specific information that is necessary to make clinical decisions.[16] The philosophy of EBM is consistent with the philosophy of clinical practice guidelines. The decision-making process of EBM is supported by access and use of clinical practice guidelines.

Guideline Development Methods

A thorough understanding of the methodology used for clinical practice guideline development is critical for health care practitioners. Although relatively few practitioners actually participate in guideline development, this understanding will prepare them for involvement in appropriate evaluation and implementation of these guidelines. ❸ *Evaluation of the quality of a guideline and the appropriateness of its use in a given setting depends primarily on an ability to distinguish methods that minimize potential biases in development.* A lack of understanding of the requirements for guideline development could lead to inappropriate interpretation, or acceptance of inappropriate levels of enforcement of biased guideline recommendations. Application of biased guidelines may result in provision of ineffective or harmful therapy. Because of the central importance of guideline development methods, a significant portion of this chapter is devoted to this topic.

Although many organizations produce clinical practice guidelines, there are no uniformly endorsed standards for their development. In 2008, the IOM was charged with developing and promoting standards for systematic reviews of comparative effectiveness research and evidence-based clinical practice guidelines.[1] Two committees were formed: the Committee on Standards for Systematic Reviews of Comparative Effectiveness Research and the Committee on Standards for Developing Trustworthy Clinical Practice Guidelines. In 2011, the committees published their proposed standards for systematic reviews of comparative effectiveness research[8] and for developing rigorous, trustworthy clinical practice guidelines.[1]

The IOM proposed eight standards (Table 7–1) for developing evidence-based clinical practice guidelines. The major steps in their proposed standards include the following (additional details for each of these steps are described below)[1]:

- Establish transparency.
- Manage conflict of interest.
- Establish a multidisciplinary guideline development group.
- Conduct a systematic review for qualifying evidence.

TABLE 7–1. STANDARDS FOR DEVELOPING TRUSTWORTHY CLINICAL PRACTICE GUIDELINES[1]

1. Establishing Transparency
    1.1 The processes by which clinical practice guidelines are developed and funded should be detailed explicitly and publicly accessible.

2. Management of Conflict of Interest (COI)
    2.1 Prior to selection of the guideline development group (GDG), individuals being considered for membership should declare all interests and activities, potentially resulting in COI with development group activity, by written disclosure to those convening the GDG:
       • Disclosure should reflect all current and planned commercial (including services from which a clinician derives a substantial proportion of income), noncommercial, intellectual, institutional, and patient–public activities pertinent to the potential scope of the clinical practice guideline.
    2.2 Disclosure of COIs within GDG:
       • All COIs of each GDG member should be reported and discussed by the prospective development group prior to the onset of his or her work.
       • Each panel member should explain how his or her COI could influence the clinical practice guideline development process or specific recommendations.
    2.3 Divestment
       • Members of the GDG should divest themselves of financial investments they or their family members have in, and not participate in marketing activities, advisory boards, or entities whose interests could be affected by clinical practice guideline recommendations.
    2.4 Exclusions
       • Whenever possible GDG members should not have COI.
       • In some circumstances, a GDG may not be able to perform its work without members who have COIs, such as relevant clinical specialists who receive a substantial portion of their incomes from services pertinent to the clinical practice guideline.
       • Members with COIs should represent not more than a minority of the GDG.
       • The chair or cochairs should not be a person(s) with COI.
       • Funders should have no role in clinical practice guideline development.

3. Guideline Development Group Composition
    3.1 The GDG should be multidisciplinary and balanced, comprising a variety of methodological experts and clinicians, and populations expected to be affected by the clinical practice guideline.
    3.2 Patient and public involvement should be facilitated by including (at least at the time of clinical question formulation and draft clinical practice guideline review) a current or former patient, and a patient advocate or patient/consumer organization representative in the GDG.
    3.3 Strategies to increase effective participation of patient and consumer representatives, including training in appraisal of evidence, should be adopted by GDGs.

4. Clinical Practice Guideline–Systematic Review Intersection
    4.1 Clinical practice guideline developers should use systematic reviews that meet standards set by the Institute of Medicine's Committee on Standards for Systematic Reviews of Comparative Effectiveness Research.
    4.2 When systematic reviews are conducted specifically to inform particular guidelines, the GDG and systematic review team should interact regarding the scope, approach, and output of both processes.

continued

TABLE 7–1. STANDARDS FOR DEVELOPING TRUSTWORTHY CLINICAL PRACTICE GUIDELINES[1] (*CONTINUED*)

5. Establishing Evidence Foundations for and Rating Strength of Recommendations
   5.1 For each recommendation, the following should be provided:
   - An explanation of the reasoning underlying the recommendation, including:
     ○ a clear description of potential benefits and harms
     ○ a summary of relevant available evidence (and evidentiary gaps), description of the quality (including applicability), quantity (including completeness), and consistency of the aggregate available evidence
     ○ an explanation of the part played by values, opinion, theory, and clinical experience in deriving the recommendation.
   - A rating of the level of confidence in (certainty regarding) the evidence underpinning the recommendation
   - A rating of the strength of the recommendation in light of the preceding bullets
   - A description and explanation of any differences of opinion regarding the recommendation

6. Articulation of Recommendations
   6.1 Recommendations should be articulated in a standardized form detailing precisely what the recommended action is, and under what circumstances it should be performed.
   6.2 Strong recommendations should be worded so that compliance with the recommendation(s) can be evaluated.

7. External Review
   7.1 External reviewers should comprise a full spectrum of relevant stakeholders, including scientific and clinical experts, organizations (e.g., health care, specialty societies), agencies (e.g., federal government), patients, and representatives of the public.
   7.2 The authorship of external reviews submitted by individuals and/or organizations should be kept confidential unless that protection has been waived by the reviewer(s).
   7.3 The GDG should consider all external reviewer comments and keep a written record of the rationale for modifying or not modifying a clinical practice guideline in response to reviewers' comments.
   7.4 A draft of the clinical practice guideline at the external review stage or immediately following it (i.e., prior to the final draft) should be made available to the general public for comments. Reasonable notice of impending publication should be provided to interested public stakeholders.

8. Updating
   8.1 The clinical practice guideline publication date, date of pertinent systematic evidence review, and proposed date for future clinical practice guideline review should be documented in the clinical practice guideline.
   8.2 Literature should be monitored regularly following clinical practice guideline publication to identify the emergence of new, potentially relevant evidence and to evaluate the continued validity of the clinical practice guideline.
   8.3 Clinical practice guidelines should be updated when new evidence suggests the need for modification of clinically important recommendations. For example, a clinical practice guideline should be updated if new evidence shows that a recommended intervention causes previously unknown substantial harm; a new intervention is significantly superior to a previously recommended intervention from an efficacy or harms perspective; or a recommendation can be applied to new populations.

- Establish evidence foundations for and rate strength of recommendations.
- Articulate recommendations.
- Conduct an external review.
- Establish a plan for updating the guideline.

ESTABLISH TRANSPARENCY

The standard for this step calls for the processes by which the guideline is developed and funded to be transparent, i.e., how the guideline is developed and funded should be explicitly detailed and the public should have access to this information. Transparency helps users understand how the recommendations were made and who developed them. The clinical experience of the guideline development group's members and potential conflicts of interest (COIs) should be stated as well.[1]

MANAGE CONFLICT OF INTEREST

The standard for this step provides details for managing of potential COIs by members of the guideline development group. COIs not only include financial COIs, but also intellectual conflicts that may occur as a result of previous research published by the individual, institutional COIs, and patient–public activities.[1]

Individuals being considered for membership on a guideline development panel should be asked to declare potential COIs. Individuals with a potential conflict of interest may still be considered for participation on a panel depending on the type and degree of conflict, along with appropriate levels of management and disclosure.[17] Rigid adherence to exclusion of any possible conflict could result in guideline panels excluding the majority of individuals with the critical expertise needed. Surveys have shown the need for attention to this issue as guideline authors frequently have some relationship with pharmaceutical manufacturers.[18] Controversies over the sponsorship of guideline development and publication[19] and potential COIs by panel members[20] have occurred.

The American College of Chest Physicians is one prominent guideline development group that placed an emphasis on dealing with conflict of interest in their most recent edition of their guideline on Antithrombotic Therapy and Prevention of Thrombosis.[21] The primary leadership and responsibility for authorship of each article was assigned to a methodologist with no COIs, who in most cases was also a practicing physician, but not an expert on the topic of thrombosis. Some experts nominated to participate in a panel were not accepted because of the magnitude of financial COIs. Panel members who had conflicts, either financial or intellectual, could be limited to some extent in their participation in discussions and could not participate in the final process of decisions regarding the direction or strength of a recommendation.[21,22]

ESTABLISH A MULTIDISCIPLINARY GUIDELINE DEVELOPMENT GROUP

The standard for this step relates to the composition of the group to develop the guideline and includes patient and public involvement in the process. Patient involvement is especially important in helping to formulate and prioritize the questions to be addressed by the guideline. This standard also provides direction for how to obtain input from panel members, reach consensus, and make decisions through the group process.[1]

The development of a clinical practice guideline should involve a multidisciplinary team. Ideally, all groups that have a stake in the development and implementation of a guideline are represented in the process. Participants should include physicians with special expertise in the condition being considered; primary care practitioners involved in the treatment of patients with the identified condition; representatives of other health care disciplines involved in providing care for the identified condition (e.g., pharmacy, physical therapy, respiratory therapy, nursing, occupational therapy, social work, dentistry); experts in research methods applicable to the topic; individuals, such as drug information specialists, with expertise in conducting a systematic search for evidence; individuals with administrative, health services, economics, and other health care systems expertise; and patient representatives or caregivers. Organizational skills, project management, and editorial ability are also key to successfully developing a guideline.

Case Study 7-1

You have been selected to lead the formation of a panel to be involved in the development of clinical practice guidelines in your institution. No additional information or guidance has been provided to you. You would like to follow the Institute of Medicine's proposed process for developing evidence-based clinical practice guidelines. As you sit in your office thinking about the many different activities that are going to be required of this panel, what are the first *three* steps that should be performed and what do they entail?

CONDUCT A SYSTEMATIC REVIEW FOR QUALIFYING EVIDENCE

The standard for this step acknowledges the overlap between clinical practice guidelines and systematic reviews (see Chapter 5 for more information on systematic reviews). It recognizes that systematic reviews are important for preparing a synthesis of evidence for the guideline development group to use in formulating recommendations that will be based on the best and most complete available evidence.[1] This standard recommends that clinical practice guideline developers conduct systematic reviews that meet the standards recommended in the IOM's previously mentioned companion publication for systematic reviews of comparative effectiveness research. A few key steps in the companion publication for systematic reviews of comparative research include the following (these are described in more detail below)[8]:

- Select an appropriate topic for creation of a guideline.
- Define the clinical questions to be addressed.
- Determine the study screening selection criteria.
- Conduct a systematic search for evidence.
- Critically appraise individual studies (see Chapters 4 and 5).
- Synthesize the body of evidence.

Select an Appropriate Topic for Creation of a Guideline

Selection of a topic for guideline development has aspects in common with selection of topics for a medication use evaluation program, or in a broader sense for any quality improvement program (see Chapter 14). Considering that guidelines are intended to improve the quality of care process and outcomes of care, it is important to consider the potential to achieve this improvement when a topic is chosen. As with a clinical management decision, the potential benefits of development and implementation of a guideline should be assessed. Disease states with the maximum potential for benefit from guideline development and implementation share common characteristics including the following:

- High prevalence
- High frequency and/or severity of associated morbidity or mortality
- Availability of high-quality evidence for the efficacy of treatments that reduce morbidity or mortality
- Feasibility of implementation of the treatment based on expertise and other resources required
- Potential cost-effectiveness
- Evidence that current practice is not optimal
- Evidence of practice variation; patients with similar characteristics are provided with different services or a substantially different frequency of services in different locations
- Availability of personnel, expertise, and resources to develop and implement the practice guideline

As an example, the AHA identified the following reasons for developing evidence-based guidelines for cardiovascular disease prevention in women[23]:

- Cardiovascular disease is the leading cause of death of women in the United States.
- It is essential that coronary heart disease (CHD) be prevented because CHD is often fatal, and the majority of women who die suddenly have not had any previous symptoms.
- There was an increased need to review and develop strategies for the prevention of CHD in women following the Women's Health Initiative and the Heart and Estrogen/Progestin Replacement Study.
- The number and percentage of women participating in clinical trials has been increasing, which provides more evidence of efficacy of different treatment strategies.
- Because the characteristics of patients seen in clinical practice may not be similar to those of clinical trial participants, it is necessary to evaluate the ability to apply these data in practice.

Define the Clinical Questions to Be Addressed

After the topic has been selected, the next step is to further define the specific issues for which recommendations will ultimately be provided. The guideline development group will consider what specific decision-making or action steps related to disease surveillance or screening methods for disease detection, confirmation of the diagnosis, or treatment can be improved with specific recommendations. The decision-making points can be expressed as clinical questions. ❹ *The definition of the clinical questions to be addressed by a guideline is a key step that provides direction for the activities to follow.* The questions are important to provide direction to the systematic review of the literature, and they also provide the outline for the recommendations that the guideline will provide. The importance of this phase cannot be overemphasized. Just as in the systematic approach to a drug information question, it is critical to first clearly define the question to be successful in searching for the necessary evidence, and subsequently be able to provide useful valid conclusions.

A clear description of the questions to be addressed by the guideline is also a good starting point for a practitioner to determine if a guideline could be useful in his or her practice. Depending on the overall goals of a guideline, questions may be about the best diagnostic test, methods of screening, what forms of treatment or prevention are most effective, quantification of the potential harms of treatment, what comorbidities change recommendations, or what costs are associated with different management strategies.

One of the important steps for guideline developers, and perhaps even more important for guideline users, is the careful framing of the clinical questions. Many guideline development groups use the Patients-Interventions-Comparison-Outcomes (PICO) model for framing the questions, which includes the following parts[13]:

- **P**atients: Which patients are being considered for the guideline, how can they be described, and are there any subgroups that require special consideration? (similar to inclusion and exclusion criteria in a clinical study, however, usually not as restrictive)
- **I**nterventions: Which intervention or treatment should be considered?
- **C**omparison: What other interventions or treatment should be compared with the intervention being considered?
- **O**utcome: What is most important to the patient (e.g., mortality, morbidity, treatment complications, rates of relapse, physical function, quality of life, and costs)?

The clinical questions should define the relevant patient population, the management strategies that will and will not be considered, and the outcomes of care that the guideline intends to achieve. All the questions that are necessary for consideration of patient management in a given clinical scenario are delineated to make sure that the recommendations provided by the guideline will be of sufficient scope to avoid important gaps in decision making. There is no specific standard for the number of questions required for each guideline; however, most guideline development groups state that if the number exceeds 30, or in some cases 40 questions, it may be necessary to break the guideline into subtopics. Subtopics may be determined to construct a guideline for making recommendations for screening or diagnosis in one guideline and recommendations for treatment in another. Or subtopics may be based on differentiation of populations that have different levels of severity of disease, for example, New York Heart Association classes of heart failure, or based on other demographic factors that might call for different recommendations for care of those patients. The American College of Chest Physicians guidelines on antithrombotic therapy created several subtopics such as antithrombotic therapy in pregnancy, persons with peripheral artery disease, ischemic stroke, valvular disease, and atrial fibrillation.

In some instances, a preliminary review of the literature may be necessary to assist with delineation of the focused clinical questions to be considered in the guideline. Clinical experts in the field as well as patients provide critical input in formulating the clinical questions.

Determine the Study Screening Selection Criteria

It is necessary to define the admissible evidence, i.e., the types of published or unpublished research to be considered so that an appropriate literature search may be performed. Key words from the focused clinical questions define the types of patients, interventions, comparators, and outcomes of studies that are considered to provide useful evidence. The guideline panel may decide that it will consider evidence from previous guidelines, meta-analyses or systematic reviews, and randomized controlled trials. The panel may also decide to consider evidence from observational studies, diagnostic studies, economic studies, and qualitative studies. This direction is necessary for the information specialists that will conduct the search for evidence. Detailed criteria are also important in this step so that evidence will be retrieved and selected for inclusion in the review with a minimum of bias, so that the search is reproducible, and so that the entire process is as transparent as possible. In most cases, more than one person is involved in searching for evidence and selecting evidence for consideration in the review. Clear criteria must be used so that there is consistency among all individuals involved in this process. Inconsistency in the retrieval of evidence between evaluators would add a potential for bias in the review.

The process to define admissible evidence may also be revisited at a later stage of guideline development depending on the results of the initial search. It is conceivable, and in fact common, that based on the initial review of evidence, the questions may be modified or new questions formed, and a decision may be made to expand the scope of admissible evidence. Documentation of these decisions, and the reasons for any changes, is another indicator of a guideline that has been developed with rigorous methods.

Conduct a Systematic Search for Evidence

Evidence-based guidelines require that all relevant evidence is located and appraised; therefore, a thorough literature search must be conducted. Many guideline development groups will first conduct a search to identify previously completed guidelines or systematic reviews of the same or closely related questions. The literature retrieval process should include a search of the available bibliographic resources such as MEDLINE®, Current Contents®, EMBASE, Science Citation Index, Cochrane Library, and Cumulative Index to Nursing and Allied Health Literature (CINAHL). A number of specialized databases exist and should be considered depending on the subject of the search. Also evidence may be obtained from citations listed in published bibliographies, textbooks, and any literature that may be identified by researchers and other individuals on the expert list that the panel may create. Specific keywords and other search constraints, for example, **M**edical **S**ubject **H**eadings (MeSH) terms from MEDLINE®, limits by publication year, language, randomized controlled trials or other study types, and so forth should be recorded to allow verification of the process. Each retrieved article should then be judged for its relevance and compliance to criteria for inclusion as predetermined by the panel. A log should be kept of excluded studies and the rationale for their rejection.

A review of all the details regarding search strategies, such as controlled vocabulary searching, text word searching, truncation of terms, use of the vocabulary tree structures to explode select terms, and adjacency of terms are beyond the scope of this chapter. Most guideline development groups use highly trained methodologists and librarians to perform this critical search for evidence. Drug information specialists are also well qualified to complete this task. A carefully planned and executed search is necessary to obtain a result that is very sensitive to avoid missing important evidence and at the same time as specific as possible to avoid the requirement to manually screen many irrelevant citations.

Critically Appraise Individual Studies

There are a variety of methods for evaluating individual studies. The purpose of this process is to identify issues with the trial design or any biases that would affect internal or external validity. Issues to consider include the basic trial design (i.e., randomized, controlled, clinical trial, cohort study, and case-control study), sample size, statistical power, selection bias, inclusion/exclusion criteria, choice of control group, randomization methods, comparability of groups, definition of exposure or intervention, definition of outcome measures, accuracy and appropriateness of outcome measures, attrition rates, data collection methods, methods of statistical analysis, confounding variables, unique characteristics of the study population, and adequacy of blinding. Other factors to be considered in the overall body of evidence are, for example, if the results of different trials are consistent with each other or if there is significant heterogeneity. The amount of evidence is also an important consideration—how many individuals have been evaluated over what length of time. The amount of available evidence is particularly important in consideration of the safety of treatments. Potentially serious adverse events that occur infrequently will not be identified in a database that does not contain a sufficient sample size or in a sample population that is too narrowly defined. See Chapters 4 and 5 for information on how to evaluate the literature. It may also be necessary to review Chapter 6 for information on how to evaluate cost information.

Synthesize the Body of Evidence

The evidence from the selected studies should be summarized in a format that facilitates the panel to begin developing conclusions. The best formats facilitate consideration of the characteristics and quality of individual studies, the consistency of the results between studies, the overall size of the evidence database, and the size of the treatment effects for benefits and harms. If the necessary evidence is available, it may be appropriate to perform a meta-analysis to present the summary estimate of the size of a treatment effect (see Chapter 5 for more information on meta-analyses).

Case Study 7–2

Building on Case Study 7–1, you have formed a practice guideline panel. As the panel moves forward, what is the next step that should be performed and what does it entail?

ESTABLISH EVIDENCE FOUNDATIONS FOR AND RATING STRENGTH OF RECOMMENDATIONS

The standard for this step focuses on the very important process of rating the quality of the evidence and the strength of the recommendations of the guideline produced. The Grading of Recommendations, Assessment, Development, and Evaluation (GRADE) Working Group has developed the most accepted system for determining strength of recommendations and rating quality of evidence.[24] The **GRADE system**, although not specifically endorsed by IOM, meets essential qualities of the IOM recommended standards. This is also the system used with minor modification by the American College of Chest Physicians[22] and by many other developers of high-quality guidelines. Because the approach to rating the quality of evidence (or the confidence in the estimates of the effects) and the approach for grading the strength of the recommendations are key characteristics for the clinical use of a guideline, greater detail on the GRADE system is provided below.

GRADE System of Grading Quality of Evidence and Strength of Recommendations

The GRADE working group began in 2000 as an informal international collaboration of people who recognized the shortcomings of the grading systems available at that time and wished to offer recommendations for improvement.

The GRADE working group first published standardized grading methods for the quality of the evidence and the strength of recommendations in practice guidelines in 2004.[25] The working group stated the belief that consistent judgments about the quality of evidence and strength of recommendations, combined with better communication about those judgments, would be achieved by use of the GRADE system. Ultimately, the working group felt that use of the GRADE system would support better informed choices in health care.[25] A five-part series of updated information on GRADE was published in 2008,[26] and a 22-part series was started in 2011.[24]

❺ *The quality of the evidence that forms the basis for recommendations is a key aspect for interpretation and use of a practice guideline.* However, before deciding to implement a guideline recommendation it is also necessary for the user to have information for consideration of the balance between benefits and harms and to have the ability to translate the evidence to specific circumstances (i.e., external validity). A system to communicate the strength of a recommendation should consider all of these factors. The designated strength of a recommendation should convey the amount of confidence one can have that adherence to that recommendation will do more good than harm.[25]

The system proposed by GRADE uses explicit definitions of what is meant by quality of evidence and strength of recommendation. The quality of evidence indicates the degree of confidence that an estimate of effect is correct. The strength of a recommendation indicates the degree of confidence that following the recommendation will do more good than harm.[25] Use of the GRADE system requires assessment of the validity of the results of individual studies for important outcomes and sequential judgments about the following[25]:

- The quality of evidence across studies for each important outcome
- Which outcomes are critical to a decision
- The overall quality of evidence across these critical outcomes
- The balance between benefits and harms
- The strength of the recommendations

The GRADE system starts with clearly defined clinical questions using the PICO model and considers all outcomes that are important to patients.[27] The GRADE system classifies each outcome as critical, important but not critical, or of limited importance. Guideline developers may also use a 9-point scale with 7-9 representing critical outcomes, 4-6 representing important outcomes, 1-3 representing outcomes of limited importance. Critical outcomes are given more weight in the final recommendation. Outcomes related to possible harms of therapy must also be considered.[27]

The quality of evidence for each outcome should be judged on the basis of a systematic review using explicit criteria. The GRADE system initially considers randomized trials to be high-quality evidence and observational studies to be low-quality evidence.[28] These ratings may then be increased or decreased based on additional factors (Table 7–2). There are five reasons for lowering the level of confidence rating (risk of bias, inconsistency, indirectness, imprecision, publication bias), and three reasons for rating the level of confidence higher (large effect, dose response, all plausible confounding).[28]

Basic study design does not tell the whole story of the quality of evidence. The risk for bias is assessed by the guideline panel based on several factors.[29] Randomization, when it is used correctly, has tremendous power to reduce the potential bias in the results. However, there are randomized controlled trials in which other aspects of the study design are seriously flawed, and there are observational studies (e.g., follow-up, case-control, interrupted time series, and controlled before and after) with very strong methods that may produce high-quality evidence. Consideration of the quality of study methods must include criteria such as adequacy of allocation concealment, blinding, completeness of follow-up, selective outcome reporting, stopping early for benefit, use of unvalidated outcome measures, and other design or execution errors in the study.[29]

The inconsistency of results between different studies can also reduce the confidence that the results are valid. If the point estimates of results vary widely across studies, confidence intervals show minimal overlap, or statistical tests for heterogeneity are significant and the differences are not explained, the quality of evidence will be rated lower.[30]

The directness of the results refers to the extent to which the subjects, interventions, and outcomes of a study are similar to the target population for a given treatment

TABLE 7–2. GRADE SYSTEM TO RATING CONFIDENCE IN EFFECT ESTIMATES[28]

1. Establish initial level of confidence		2. Consider lowering or raising level of confidence		3. Final level of confidence rating
Study design	Initial confidence in an estimate of effect	Reasons for considering lowering or raising confidence		Confidence in an estimate of effect across those considerations
		↓ Lower if	↓ Higher if	
Randomized trials →	High confidence	Risk of bias −1 Serious −2 Very serious Inconsistency −1 Serious −2 Very serious Indirectness −1 Serious −2 Very serious	Large effect +1 Large +2 Very large Dose response +1 gradient found	High ⊕⊕⊕⊕ Moderate ⊕⊕⊕○ Low ⊕⊕○○ Very low ⊕○○○
Observational studies →	Low confidence	Imprecision −1 Serious −2 Very serious Publication bias −1 Likely −2 Very likely		

GRADE = Grading of Recommendations Assessment, Development, and Evaluation.
Reproduced from Journal of Clinical Epidemiology, Vol 64, Howard Balshem, Mark Helfand, Holger J. Schunemann, Andrew D. Oxman, Regina Kunz, Jan Brozek, et al. GRADE guidelines: 3/ Rating the quality of evidence. Pp. 401–406, Copyright 2011, with permission from Elsevier.

recommendation.[31] If study subjects differ from the patients treated by a particular health care professional in ways that may predict a different level of response based on factors such as age, gender, race, other comorbidities or severity of illness, the quality of evidence for the clinician's decision making is not as great. In addition, studies using **surrogate endpoints**, or intermediate outcomes, are not as reliable for estimation of ultimate treatment benefits. Surrogate endpoints are laboratory values or physical assessments that are markers that predict the actual clinical events, but the time from the presence of the surrogate outcome and the ultimate clinical outcome may be long in some cases, and they may also be an imperfect predictor of the important clinical outcome. Surrogate endpoints include measurements such as changes in bone mineral density rather than incidence of fractures and effects of a medication on pulmonary function rather than on mortality. Another example in which indirect evidence must be used is when there are no studies comparing different interventions directly and the evaluation must be made across different studies. This is a common problem with new drugs that have been studied only in comparison to placebo and not to other effective treatments. With this type of evidence comparison, it is difficult to determine which treatment is more effective, and it is even more difficult to estimate the size of a potential treatment difference.[31]

The measure of imprecision in study results is primarily assessed by examination of the 95% confidence interval (see Chapter 8).[32] Certainly if the 95% confidence interval crosses the boundary of benefit versus harm the treatment is not considered to be proven effective. For example, with a relative risk of a clinical event measured as 0.8, but a 95% confidence interval of 0.5 to 1.1, the result is not considered to be statistically significant. Such a confidence interval does not exclude the possibility of either a reduction or an increase in risk of the event. Also, if the confidence interval extends into a point in which the size of the clinical benefit no longer would be judged to be greater than the potential adverse effects, burden of treatment and costs, the level of evidence should be graded down. It is also recommended that the absolute risk difference or number needed to treat (NNT) be the value for consideration of the size of the treatment benefit.[32] Absolute risk differences take into consideration the baseline risk, or the risk of the event with no treatment, and are, therefore, a more meaningful value to represent the size of the potential treatment benefits for a specific patient.

Publication bias may also be a reason to rate the quality of evidence lower. The risk of publication bias is generally greatest early in the development of a new therapy when there are relatively few studies published and particularly when the sample size is small.[33] Many factors may contribute to publication bias. Industry sponsors may be reluctant to publish negative results. Authors, journal editors, and peer reviewers all have been implicated in a bias against publication of negative results. Negative results are often slower to be published and are more likely to be published in non-English or limited-circulation journals. One method to assess the potential of publication bias is the funnel plot; however, it is not very sensitive or precise.[33] See Chapter 5 for more information about publication bias and funnel plots.

The level of confidence rating of the evidence may be increased in the GRADE system for one of three reasons. The most common reason to increase the confidence rating of evidence is for a large treatment effect.[34] Another reason for increasing the level of confidence in an observational study by one level is if it shows at least a twofold increase or decrease in risk (odds ratio or relative risk—see Chapters 4 and 5) and by two levels if the effect is a fivefold difference in risk. The third reason to increase the rating level is if a dose-response relationship has been demonstrated in the treatment effect.[34] A dose-response relationship has been considered a factor in causality assessment since the Bradford Hill criteria[35] were published in 1965. If all plausible confounding factors would predict that an observational study in fact underestimated the size of a beneficial treatment effect, that would also be reason to increase the level of confidence rating of the evidence.[34] In general, decisions to rate the quality of evidence at a higher level should only be considered in the absence of one or more of the five factors mentioned above which are causes for rating the evidence lower.

Based on consideration of the components described above, the GRADE system arrives at one of the following grades of evidence that express the degree of confidence that the true effect is close to the estimate of the effect[28]:

- High = very confident
- Moderate = moderately confident
- Low = limited confidence
- Very low = very little confidence

The evidence for harms should be graded using the same system as the evidence for benefits. This creates somewhat of a challenge when making judgments about the balance of benefits and harms because the quality of evidence for harms is rarely on the same level as the evidence for benefits. One only has to look at the evidence for harms for rosiglitazone (Avandia®) to note that obtaining high-quality evidence about harm is a more difficult process. The magnitude of the balance of the benefits compared to the harms, as well as value judgments of the desirability of the benefits and harms, must also be considered for treatment recommendations. In addition, information should be provided to demonstrate how the evidence translates into specific circumstances, and what adjustments may be necessary for individuals with different baseline risks, or who are receiving treatment in different settings. The GRADE working group recommends the following definitions to categorize the trade-offs between benefits and harms[25]:

- Net benefits: The intervention clearly does more good than harm.
- Trade-offs: There are important trade-offs between the benefits and harms.

- Uncertain trade-offs: It is not clear whether the intervention does more good than harm.
- No net benefits: The intervention clearly does not do more good than harm.[25]

Factors that should be considered in arriving at one of these designations include the estimated size and confidence intervals of the effect for the main outcomes, quality of the evidence, ability to extrapolate the evidence to different patients or care settings, and uncertainty of the baseline risk of disease events in the population of interest.[25]

Finally, the GRADE system assigns one of the following categories for a recommendation for an intervention: strong recommendation for using an intervention, weak recommendation for using an intervention, weak recommendation against an intervention, or a strong recommendation against using an intervention.[24] Factors involved in arriving at one of these four categories include the balance of benefits to risk, the quality rating of the evidence, the variability in the values and preferences that may occur between different patients in different circumstances, and resource use implications. The implications on resource use are often the most difficult to use in making a recommendation for political as well as scientific reasons because they can change substantially over time and in different settings.[24]

❻ *The advantage of the GRADE system is that all of the evidence that is most important for making the decision has been judged with explicit criteria, the judgments are made transparent, evidence profiles and summary of findings tables have been created, consequently facilitating the use of the best evidence.*

Although the system recommended by the GRADE working group may appear complex with the number of steps involved, it provides a balance of the need for simplicity with a need for full explicit consideration of important issues in clinical decision making, as well as transparency for the judgments made in arriving at recommendations. The evidence profile[36] and summary of findings tables[36-38] produced with the GRADE process are especially useful for documentation of the judgments made in making the recommendations and also for the clinical use of the guideline. See Appendix 7–1 for an example of an evidence profile.

ARTICULATE RECOMMENDATIONS

This step addresses the details of how the guideline recommendations should be phrased, specifying what actions should be taken and in what settings and circumstances. Standardized language should be used to detail exactly what the recommendation is and when it should be done. When justified by the evidence, these recommendations should be clear and concise with statements that are actionable and employ active voice, with avoidance of vague and nonspecific language.[1] This section also calls for strong recommendations to be worded so that the implications for quality of care monitoring systems can incorporate these recommendations into criteria for care.[1] The specifics of the expected clinical behavior of who should do what, for whom, under what circumstance is also necessary to permit the guideline recommendations to be incorporated into computerized clinical decision support tools. Of course, if the evidence does not support a specific action but only different options for consideration, it is important that the guideline recommendation reflect that. That is a feature of the GRADE system mentioned previously as well. Following the GRADE system a strong recommendation would be introduced by terms such as "We recommend" or "Clinicians should" and a weak recommendation would begin with the terms "We suggest," "Clinicians might," or "Clinicians may."

The basis of the draft document is provided by the graded recommendations. A formal narrative summary should also be provided with all relevant details of decisions made in the development of the guideline. It is highly desirable for the finished guideline to include details of the scope of the guideline including target patient population, restrictions on the population, interventions considered, specific outcomes or performance measures, who are the intended users of the guideline (e.g., specialty and care setting), and the overall objective of the guideline. A clear description of authorship, sponsorship, and any potential COIs should be provided. In addition, a detailed description should be provided of all production methods used, decision-making methods, recommendations for consideration in applying the guideline in practice (e.g., patient variables, setting, provider, and estimates of how the effects of these factors will alter outcomes are helpful for users to apply the guidelines locally), comments about ongoing studies which may affect recommendations, and any plans for updating the guideline.

It is also desirable for a guideline to be written in different formats and levels of detail for different audiences and purposes. Many guideline developers produce quick reference guides, which give the essentials of the recommendations without the detailed background. These documents are more convenient to use as quick reminders and decision aids in a patient care setting than a full guideline document. It is important, however, for users of the quick reference guides to review the full document before deciding that the guideline is valid for their use, and to recognize any specific limitations in how they may wish to use that particular guideline. Another format that is useful is a guideline summary that may be used for patient education purposes.

Reaching clear decisions on recommendations for clinical practices is often difficult because the data are not adequate to clearly label the practice as appropriate or inappropriate. Unfortunately, many practices fall into this gray zone category because of uncertainties about the benefits and harms, variability in patients and their responses to treatment, and differences in patient preferences about the desirability of outcomes and aversion to risk. The use of rigid language in an effort to produce clear-cut recommendations can be dangerous, particularly when presented as simplistic algorithms that fail to recognize the complexity of medical decision making and the need for individual clinical judgment. This danger can be avoided by describing uncertainty and providing broad boundaries for appropriate practice that allows for legitimate differences of opinion. Attempts to develop rigid guidelines, when the data are not conclusive, are clearly worse than having no written guidelines.

It is important to consider the information needs of the guideline's user. Practitioners will want specific, quantitative estimates of the relevant health outcomes if a recommendation is followed, a statement of the strength of the evidence and expert judgment supporting the guidelines, information on patient preferences, projections of cost, details of the reasoning behind the recommendations, and the ability to review the data independently if they so choose. Guidelines should be written such that they may be perceived as an explanation of the thinking process that is used in evaluating and applying the information. If guidelines are perceived as information only, they may be rejected out of fear that they will become cookbooks for managing specific conditions/disease states. Such guidelines would also not achieve the educational goals to focus further research efforts (outcomes research or other) on gaps in the current evidence.

Depending on the subject of the clinical practice guideline, more or less emphasis may be placed on the various sections of the guideline document. In addition, recommendations for future research may be included with the document. The process of developing practice guidelines often calls attention to the gaps in scientific information. The direction provided for future research is one of the important results of the practice guideline development process. Practice guidelines that fail to address research priorities may discourage innovation and negatively influence funding decisions for needed research in the involved area. For the few examples that exist in which clear answers are already provided by high-quality scientific evidence, waste of research resources may be avoided by stopping generation of data that would not increase understanding of a disease process or its treatment.

CONDUCT AN EXTERNAL REVIEW

The standard for this step details how the guideline should undergo external review, categories for types of stakeholders and participants to be involved in the review, and calls for a draft to be made available for general public comment.[1] All relevant stakeholders should be involved in the external review. Based on feedback from external review, revisions may be required for the guideline to meet its intended goals. As with many steps in the guideline development process, one of the key activities in this step is documentation. The decisions and actions taken in response to the recommendations from external review should be carefully documented. If there are critical recommendations that the guideline panel decides to reject, it is particularly important that the reason for that decision be documented.

ESTABLISH A PLAN FOR UPDATING THE GUIDELINE

The standard for this step addresses the need to keep guidelines up to date with new information as it becomes available. It calls for clarity of the publication date, dates of systematic reviews utilized in the guideline, regular review of the literature to identify new technology or new evidence that may impact the guideline recommendation, and a specific plan for updating or expiration of a guideline.[1]

A review interval to update the guideline should be established by the panel. The duration of the interval is dependent on the topic and knowledge of ongoing studies.

Case Study 7–3

Referring back to Case 7–1, the practice guideline panel has now performed a systematic review for evidence. What are the final *four* steps needed to develop the guideline and what does each step entail?

Guideline Evaluation Tools

❼ *Prior to selecting a clinical practice guideline for implementation in a health care system or for personal use by a health care professional, it is important that the quality of published guidelines be evaluated. Perhaps the most useful tool available for evaluating clinical practice guidelines is the one created by the Appraisal of Guidelines for Research and Evaluation (AGREE) collaboration.* The AGREE collaboration is an international group of researchers and policy makers. This collaboration has produced a structured instrument which can be used for critical appraisal of clinical practice guidelines. The collaboration refined the original instrument, which has resulted in the **AGREE II instrument**.[39,40] The purpose of the AGREE II instrument is to provide a framework to assess the quality of guidelines, provide a methodological strategy for the development of guidelines, and inform what and how information ought to be reported in guidelines.[40] For organizations or individuals who wish to perform an assessment of a guideline, the AGREE II instrument provides a tool that is structured, reliable, and reasonable to use. It should be noted that the AGREE II instrument does not assess clinical content or the quality of evidence; its purpose is to assess the quality of the process of guideline development methods and the reporting quality.

The AGREE II instrument addresses 23 quality items organized in six domains and two global rating items for overall assessment (Table 7–3). Individual items for consideration in developing the instrument are grouped into the following six quality domains: (1) scope and purpose, (2) stakeholder involvement, (3) rigor of development, (4) clarity and presentation, (5) applicability, and (6) editorial independence.[39,40] Each of the 23 items and the two global rating items are rated on a 7-point scale with 1 representing strongly

TABLE 7–3. AGREE II DOMAINS AND ITEMS FOR ASSESSMENT[40]

Domain 1. Scope and Purpose

1. The overall objective(s) of the guideline is (are) specifically described.

2. The health question(s) covered by the guideline is (are) specifically described.

3. The population (patients, public, etc.) to whom the guideline is meant to apply is specifically described.

Domain 2. Stakeholder Involvement

4. The guideline development group includes individuals from all the relevant professional groups.

5. The views and preferences of the target population (patients, public, etc.) have been sought.

6. The target users of the guideline are clearly defined.

Domain 3. Rigor of Development

7. Systematic methods were used to search for evidence.

8. The criteria for selecting the evidence are clearly described.

9. The strengths and limitations of the body of evidence are clearly described.

10. The methods for formulating the recommendations are clearly described.

11. The health benefits, side effects, and risks have been considered in formulating the recommendations.

12. There is an explicit link between the recommendations and the supporting evidence.

13. The guideline has been externally reviewed by experts prior to its publication.

14. A procedure for updating the guideline is provided.

Domain 4. Clarity of Presentation

15. The recommendations are specific and unambiguous.

16. The different options for management of the condition or health issue are clearly presented.

17. Key recommendations are easily identifiable.

Domain 5. Applicability

18. The guideline describes facilitators and barriers to its application.

19. The guideline provides advice and/or tools on how the recommendations can be put into practice.

20. The potential resource implications of applying the recommendations have been considered.

21. The guideline presents monitoring and/or auditing criteria.

Domain 6. Editorial Independence

22. The views of the funding body have not influenced the content of the guideline.

23. Competing interests of guideline development group members have been recorded and addressed.

Overall Guideline Assessment

Rate the overall quality of the guideline 1 lowest possible quality – 2,3,4,5,6 – 7 highest possible quality.

I would recommend this guideline for use Yes, Yes with modifications, No.

AGREE = Appraisal of Guidelines for Research and Evaluation.

disagree and 7 representing strongly agree.[39] The user's manual[40] provides more detail for each of the 23 items, guidance on how to rate each item, and directions on where to look in the guideline for information on the item.

Guideline users may benefit from using this instrument to evaluate the quality of guidelines before choosing to adopt them. Although the primary intent of the AGREE II instrument is to provide a tool for evaluation of a guideline by users, guideline developers may also use the AGREE II instrument to ensure that the methods used to develop a guideline and the documentation provided with the guideline will meet minimum standards.

Implementation of Clinical Practice Guidelines

❽ *The most effective methods for implementing guidelines to achieve the desired effects of improved quality of care have not been determined. Institutional, organizational, local practice, political characteristics, and even individual practitioner characteristics should be considered when planning an implementation strategy for a practice guideline.* It was previously believed that implementation strategies using multiple methods would be the most likely to succeed. In a systematic review of the adoption of clinical practice guidelines, variables that affected the success of implementation included qualities specific to the guidelines, characteristics of the health care professional, characteristics of the practice setting, incentives, regulation, and patient factors.[41] The implementation methods shown to be weak were traditional continuing medical education (CME) and mailings. Audit and feedback were moderately effective, especially if it was concurrent, targeted to specific providers, and delivered by peers or key opinion leaders. Strong methods were reminder systems, the use of multiple intervention systems, and academic detailing. Academic detailing is a process by which a health care educator visits a physician to provide a 15- to 20-minute educational intervention on a specific topic. Information provided is based on the physician's prescribing patterns and EBM.[41] See Chapter 23 for more information on academic detailing.

However, a subsequent extensive review of guideline dissemination and implementation strategies did not support the conclusion that multiple intervention methods are more effective. Grimshaw and colleagues conducted a systematic review of 235 studies that reported 309 comparisons of strategies for guideline dissemination and implementation.[42] Overall, multifaceted interventions were involved in 73% of the comparisons. Eighty-four of the 309 comparisons (27%) were performed on a single intervention compared to no intervention or usual care. One hundred thirty-six (44%) of the comparisons were of multifaceted interventions compared to no intervention or a usual care group. Multifaceted interventions were compared to a control intervention, which was either a single intervention or an alternative multifaceted intervention, for 85 (27%) of the comparisons in the identified studies. Of the single interventions compared to no intervention, the most common strategies used and the percentage of all comparisons in the systematic review were reminders (13%), educational materials (6%), audit and feedback (4%), and patient-directed interventions (3%). The most frequent strategies used in multifaceted interventions and corresponding percentage of all comparisons were educational materials (48%), educational meetings (41%), reminders (31%), audit and feedback (24%), and patient-directed interventions (18%).[42]

The effect size of the interventions were described in one of four categories on the basis of the absolute difference in the postintervention measures, which were generally process measures of care. The four categories of effect size were: small—an effect size ≤5%; modest—an effect size >5% and ≤10%; moderate—an effect size >10% and ≤20%; and large—an effect size >20%. Examples of the process measure of care included the frequency of prescribing a specific therapy, providing patient education, or test ordering that was in accordance with the guideline. Overall, 86% of interventions tested achieved positive improvements in process of care measures. There was considerable variation in the effect size of the interventions in different studies and in some studies between different interventions. The majority of interventions produced modest to moderate improvements in care. The lack of consistency of the differences between and within interventions did not permit any conclusion regarding the most effective strategy for guideline implementation. Multifaceted interventions were not found to be consistently more effective than single intervention strategies, and the number of components in the multifaceted interventions did not appear to be associated with effect size. The authors of this systematic review also noted that the overall quality of the methodology and reporting of the included studies were poor.[42]

This systematic review concluded that further research is required to develop and validate systems for estimation of the efficacy and efficiency of different strategies to implement patient, health professional, and organizational behavior change. Decision makers will have to evaluate the choice for implementation strategies carefully. Local factors, potential facilitators, and barriers to implementation are recommended for prominent consideration in this decision.[42]

As noted above, barriers to guideline implementation should be considered when making plans for this effort. Cabana and colleagues conducted a systematic review of the literature regarding barriers to physician adherence to clinical practice guidelines.[43] A barrier was defined as any factor that limits or restricts complete physician adherence to a guideline. The authors identified seven general categories of barriers and provided examples or a description of each (Table 7–4). The relative importance of different barriers will vary depending on the characteristics of the specific guideline and on many local health care system characteristics.[43] Paying appropriate attention to

TABLE 7–4. SEVEN CATEGORIES OF BARRIERS[43]

Barrier Category	Examples of Barriers Identified or Description of Barrier
Lack of awareness	Did not know the guideline existed
Lack of familiarity	Could not correctly answer questions about guideline content or self-reported lack of familiarity
Lack of agreement	Difference in interpretation of the evidence
	Benefits not worth patient risk, discomfort, or cost
	Not applicable to patient population in their practice
	Credibility of authors questioned
	Oversimplified cookbook
	Reduces autonomy
	Decreases flexibility
	Decreases physician self-respect
	Not practical
	Makes patient–physician relationship impersonal
Lack of self-efficacy	Did not believe that they could actually perform the behavior or activity recommended by the guideline, e.g., nutrition or exercise counseling
Lack of outcome expectancy	Did not believe intended outcome would occur even if the practice was followed, e.g., counseling to stop smoking
Inertia of previous practice	This barrier relates primarily to motivation to change practice, whether the motivation is professional, personal, or social. It was also noted that guidelines that recommend eliminating a behavior are more difficult to implement than guidelines that recommend adding a new behavior
External barriers	Patient resistance/nonadherence
	Patient does not perceive need
	Perceived to be offensive to patient
	Causes patient embarrassment
	Lack of reminder system
	Not easy to use, inconvenient, cumbersome, confusing
	Lack of educational materials
	Cost to patient
	Insufficient staff, consultant support or other resources
	Lack of time
	Lack of reimbursement
	Increased malpractice liability
	Not compatible with practice setting

these potential barriers in the planning and development of guidelines will facilitate successful implementation.

An observational study of general practice in the Netherlands identified the following characteristics that influenced the use of guidelines: (1) specific attributes of the guidelines determine whether they are used in practice, (2) evidence-based recommendations are better followed in practice than those not based on scientific evidence, (3) precise definitions of recommended performance improve use, (4) testing the feasibility and acceptance of clinical guidelines among target groups is important, and (5) the people setting the guidelines need to understand the attributes of effective evidence-based guidelines.[44]

A **computerized clinical decision support system (CDSS)** is an information system designed to improve clinical decision making[45] and is one method thought to facilitate guideline implementation. Garg and colleagues conducted a systematic review of controlled trials assessing the effects of CDSSs.[45] Of the 100 trials they reviewed, 88% were randomized; 49% of these were cluster randomized; and 40% used a cluster as the unit of analysis or adjusted for clustering. The methodological quality of the trials was noted to improve over time. Twenty-nine studies involved drug dosing or prescribing. Of the 24 studies involving systems for single-drug dosing, 15 (62%) demonstrated improved practitioner performance with guidelines, and two of the 18 studies assessing patient outcomes showed positive improvement. Of the five systems using computer order entry for multidrug prescribing, four improved practitioner performance, but none improved patient outcomes. There were 40 studies of systems for disease management of conditions such as diabetes, cardiovascular disease prevention, urinary incontinence, human immunodeficiency virus infection, and acute respiratory distress. Thirty-seven of these studies evaluated practitioner performance with 23 (62%) demonstrating improvement. Only five (18%) of the 27 disease management trials evaluating patient outcomes demonstrated improvement. Of 21 trials of reminder systems for preventive care, 16 (72%) found improvements in practitioner performance according to practice guidelines. Of the 10 trials that evaluated CDSSs for diagnostic systems, only 4 (40%) found improvements in practitioner performance. Of the five trials of diagnostic systems that evaluated patient outcomes, none found improvement.[45]

The authors also reported that improved practitioner performance was associated with CDSSs that automatically prompted the practitioner compared to systems that required the practitioner to initiate system use.[45] Improved performance was noted in 73% of trials of automated systems compared to 47% of user initiated systems ($p = 0.02$). It was also interesting to note that the best predictor of success of CDSSs was a study in which the authors were also the developers of the system. Studies conducted by the developer of the system were more likely to find success (74%), compared to 28% when the authors were not the developers ($p = 0.001$).[45]

It is clear that as with other methods for implementation of guidelines and achieving performance or behavior change, further research is needed on the use of CDSSs to provide clear guidance on predictable success rates. Many individual factors will need to be considered in the decision making for implementation of these systems.[46]

A randomized, controlled trial of CQI and academic detailing to implement clinical guidelines for the primary care of hypertension and depression produced mixed results.[47] The authors concluded that both academic detailing and CQI interventions involve complex social interactions that produce varied implementation success across the different organizations.

Grimshaw and Russell published one of the first systematic literature reviews and evaluations of the effect of practice guidelines.[48] They conducted an extensive literature search and identified 59 studies considered to have appropriate methods to evaluate the effect of guidelines on either physician behavior or patient outcomes. All but four of the studies showed some benefit from the guidelines; however, the magnitude of the benefit and the patient care significance was not impressive in all cases.

Clinical practice guidelines represent an early application of decision support systems to facilitate the provision of quality clinical care. When done well, clinical practice guidelines should contain all the necessary elements of routine care for most individuals with a specific condition. They should prompt consideration of what specific characteristics of an individual patient might warrant departures from the guideline. When effectively implemented, such systems save clinicians time. They should be assisted by computerized systems that, among other functions, can catalog past histories, check orders for medications against measures of hepatic and renal function, and schedule reminders for screening tests or preventive services. They should be part of the continuous improvement of systems of care. Guidelines will not be perfect at the outset; systems that use them must be constructed so that experience can be applied to improve the guidelines, just as the guidelines indicate where care delivery can be improved.[16]

Case Study 7–4

Referring back to Case 7–1, the practice guideline panel finally has a new practice guideline ready to be implemented. As you already know, the most effective methods for implementing guidelines have not been determined. You are also aware that barriers have been identified to guideline implementation that should be considered when developing the implementation plan. Since the most effective methods for implementing guidelines have not been determined, the successful implementation plan may very well include those methods that address these barriers. With this in mind, what are the seven categories of barriers to guideline implementation that have been identified to limit or restrict complete prescriber adherence to a practice guideline?

Sources of Clinical Practice Guidelines

❾ *Complete clinical practice guidelines can be found on Web sites such as the National Guideline Clearinghouse and in the peer-reviewed medical literature located by use of secondary databases.* Systematic reviews that can be helpful in developing or assessing specific practice guidelines are available from organizations such as the Cochrane Library, in addition to other Web sites that collect and provide health care–related information designed to support EBM such as the Agency for Healthcare Research and Quality (AHRQ).

There are several mechanisms to locate completed clinical practice guidelines or systematic reviews. The National Guideline Clearinghouse (NGC) (http://www .guideline.gov) is maintained by the AHRQ. The mission of the NGC is to provide an accessible mechanism for obtaining objectives and detailed information on clinical practice guidelines and to further their dissemination, implementation, and use. Components of the NGC include structured abstracts about the guideline and its development, a utility for comparing attributes of two or more guidelines in a side-by-side comparison, synthesis of guidelines covering similar topics, highlighting areas of similarity and difference, links to fulltext guidelines where available and/or ordering information for print copies, and annotated bibliographies on guideline development methodology implementation and use. The NGC has published criteria for guidelines to be considered for inclusion in the Clearinghouse (http://www.guideline.gov/about/ inclusion-criteria.aspx). There are also criteria published at that location that will be effective in June 2014. These criteria provide useful information for quality consideration for guidelines. There are links that also present very useful commentary for further understanding of what guidelines are, characteristics for guideline developers, how guidelines should be produced and formatted, and expectations for documentation of these details. The new criteria reflect the most recent recommendations from the IOM that have been described in this chapter.

Many guidelines have been published in the peer-reviewed medical literature and can, therefore, be located in MEDLINE®. A variety of search techniques may be used, but the most efficient may be to search for *practice guideline* in the publication type field of the record, or use the MeSH term *practice guideline* in conjunction with other terms for the specific disease or therapy of interest. Additional publication types in the record that may be searched include the terms: consensus development conference, guideline, and meta-analysis. Systematic review articles are also useful in preparation of clinical practice guidelines. The key differences with systematic reviews compared to the narrative review articles are that the systematic review begins with a focused clinical question, involves a comprehensive search for evidence, uses criterion-based selection that are uniformly applied to include evidence in the review, performs rigorous critical appraisal of the studies chosen, and provides a quantitative summary of the evidence.[49] Literature search strategies have been published for locating systematic reviews.[50,51]

The National Institutes of Health (NIH) consensus statements, the U.S. Preventative Services Task Force (USPSTF) guides to clinical preventive services and evidence syntheses, AHRQ evidence reports and summaries, comparative effectiveness reviews, technical reviews and summaries, publications and reports of the Surgeon General, and other resources are available from their respective Web sites and also collectively at the Health Services/Technology Assessment Texts (HSTAT) Web site (http://www .ncbi.nlm.nih.gov/books/NBK16710), which is published by the National Library of Medicine.

The Guidelines International Network (G-I-N) (http://www.g-i-n.net) is an international nonprofit association of international organizations and individuals involved in clinical practice guidelines. The G-I-N Library provides access to the International Guideline Library, development and training resources, relevant literature, health topic collection, relevant links, and other tools. Some of the resources from this Web site require membership for access.

Multiple professional organizations, academic centers, independent research centers, and government agencies are involved in development of clinical practice guideline activities. Updated information may be obtained by contacting these organizations directly and many have provided access to their guidelines on their Web sites. Finally, the Cochrane Collaboration has a list of databases offering online access to medical evidence (http://www.cochrane.org/about-us/evidence-based-health-care/webliography/ databases).

Conclusion

Clinical practice guidelines have become a significant tool in health care with the focus on evidence-based practice. Guidelines have the potential to assist medical decision making and ultimately improve the quality of care, improve patient outcomes, and make more efficient use of resources. Significant advances have been made in the methodology to produce valid guidelines. Information technology and greater understanding of optimal methods for implementation of guidelines will maximize their effect to improve quality of care. Pharmacists' active involvement in preparation and implementation of evidence-based clinical practice guidelines is vital. A thorough understanding of evidence-based methodology will prepare the pharmacist to participate in this process. A drug information trained pharmacist is an ideal person to help prepare and/or implement evidence-based clinical practice guidelines.

Self-Assessment Questions

1. Which of the following groups or types of organizations have been involved in development of clinical practice guidelines?
   a. Federal and state governments
   b. Professional societies and associations
   c. Managed care organizations
   d. Third-party payers
   e. All of the above

2. Which of the following is a common characteristic of practice guideline development and traditional drug information practice activities?
   a. Decision making and recommendations based on individual experience
   b. Assurance of cost savings
   c. Clear specific definition of clinical questions
   d. Lack of interdisciplinary participation
   e. All of the above

3. Clinical practice guidelines are important to getting research information into practice because:
   a. Well studied new treatments proven effective are substantially underutilized
   b. Interventions proven ineffective or harmful continue to be provided
   c. Research information is not readily available for implementation into practice
   d. a and b only
   e. b and c only

4. Recommendations for optimizing patient care that are developed by systematically reviewing the evidence and assessing the benefits and harms of health care interventions is the definition for:
   a. Strengths of recommendations
   b. Evidence-based medicine
   c. Conflicts of interest
   d. Clinical practice guidelines
   e. Systematic reviews

5. Which of the following are included in the five core competencies for health professionals as recommended in a landmark Institute of Medicine report?
   a. Deliver patient-centered care
   b. Participate in interdisciplinary teams
   c. Emphasize evidence-based practice
   d. Utilize informatics
   e. All of the above

6. The first step in the Institute of Medicine's proposed standards for developing evidence-based clinical practice guidelines is:
   a. Conduct a systematic review for qualifying evidence.
   b. Establish a multidisciplinary guideline development group.
   c. Establish transparency.
   d. Manage conflict of interest.
   e. Conduct an external review.

7. Development of a clinical practice guideline should:
   a. Include a hospital administrator
   b. Be a multidisciplinary process
   c. Be made up of panel members without any conflicts of interest
   d. Have a pharmacist leading the effort
   e. All of the above

8. Which of the following characteristics associated with a disease would suggest that it would be a good topic for development and implementation of a practice guideline?
   a. Low prevalence
   b. Evidence that current practice is optimal
   c. Evidence of little variation in current practice
   d. Availability of high-quality evidence for the efficacy of treatments that reduce morbidity or mortality
   e. Low frequency and/or severity of morbidity or mortality

9. In the PICO model for framing clinical questions, the C represents:
   a. Collaboration
   b. Comparison
   c. Clinical
   d. Control
   e. Cohort

10. When using the GRADE system, which of the following information should be incorporated with guideline recommendations?

a. Quality of evidence across studies for each important outcome
b. Strength of the recommendations
c. Balance between benefits and harms
d. a and b only
e. a, b, and c

11. When using the GRADE system, all of the following are reasons for lowering the level of confidence rating *except*:
a. Risk of bias
b. Publication bias
c. Imprecision
d. Indirectness
e. Consistency

12. When using the GRADE system, which of the following is/are reason(s) for rating the level of confidence higher?
a. Dose response
b. Large effect
c. All plausible confounding
d. b and c only
e. a, b, and c

13. All of the following are true regarding the AGREE II instrument for guideline evaluation *except*:
a. Created by an international group of researchers and policy makers
b. Provides a framework to assess the quality of guidelines
c. Assesses the quality of the clinical content
d. Intended for use by organizations and individuals
e. Provides a methodological strategy for the development of guidelines

14. External barriers to clinical practice guideline implementation include all of the following *except*:
a. Lack of familiarity with the guideline
b. Cost to patient
c. Increased malpractice liability
d. Insufficient staff, consultant support, or other resources
e. Lack of reimbursement

15. All of the following statements about clinical practice guidelines are true *except*:
a. They should contain all the necessary elements of routine care for most individuals with a specific condition.

b. They should not prompt consideration of what specific characteristics of an individual patient might warrant departures from the guideline.

c. They represent an early application of decision support systems to facilitate providing quality clinical care.

d. They will not be perfect at the outset.

e. They should be part of the continuous improvement of systems of care.

REFERENCES

1. Institute of Medicine, Committee on Standards for Developing Trustworthy Clinical Practice Guidelines. Clinical practice guidelines we can trust. Graham R, Mancher M, Wolman DM, Greenfield S, Steinberg E, eds. Washington, DC: National Academies Press; 2011. Available from: http://www.iom.edu/Reports/2011/Clinical-Practice-Guidelines-We-Can-Trust.aspx

2. Jones RH, Ritchie JL, Fleming BB, Hammermeister KE, Leape LL. 28th Bethesda Conference. Task Force 1: Clinical practice guideline development, dissemination and computerization. J Am Coll Cardiol. 1997;29:1133-41.

3. President's Advisory Commission on Consumer Protection and Quality in the Health Care Industry. Quality first: better health care for all Americans. [cited: 2012 Dec 14]. Available from: http://archive.ahrq.gov/hcqual/final/.

4. Institute of Medicine, Committee on Quality Health Care in America. Crossing the quality chasm: a new health system for the 21st century. Washington, DC: National Academy Press; 2001. Available from: http://www.iom.edu/Reports/2001/Crossing-the-Quality-Chasm-A-New-Health-System-for-the-21st-Century.aspx

5. Institute of Medicine, Committee on Data Standards for Patient Safety. Patient safety: achieving a new standard for care. Aspden P, Corrigan JM, Wolcott J, Erikson SM, eds. Washington, DC: National Academies Press; 2004. Available from: http://www.iom.edu/Reports/2003/Patient-Safety-Achieving-a-New-Standard-for-Care.aspx

6. Institute of Medicine, Committee on Quality of Health Care in America. To err is human: building a safer health system. Kohn LT, Corrigan JM, Donaldson MS, eds. Washington, DC: National Academy Press; 2000. Available from: http://iom.edu/Reports/1999/To-Err-is-Human-Building-A-Safer-Health-System.aspx

7. Institute of Medicine, Committee on Identifying and Preventing Medication Errors. Preventing medication errors. Aspden P, Wolcott J, Bootman JL, Cronenwett LR, eds. Washington, DC: National Academies Press; 2007. Available from: http://iom.edu/Reports/2006/Preventing-Medication-Errors-Quality-Chasm-Series.aspx

8. Institute of Medicine, Committee on Standards for Systematic Reviews of Comparative Effectiveness Research. Finding what works in health care: standards for systematic reviews. Eden J, Levit L, Berg A, Morton S, eds. Washington, DC: National Academies Press; 2011. Available from: http://www.iom.edu/Reports/2011/Finding-What-Works-in-Health-Care-Standards-for-Systematic-Reviews.aspx

9. Institute of Medicine, Committee on the Learning Health Care System in America. Best care at lower cost: the path to continuously learning health care in America. Smith M, Saunders R, Stuckhardt L, McGinnis JM, eds. Washington, DC: National Academies Press; 2012. Available from: http://www.iom.edu/Reports/2012/Best-Care-at-Lower-Cost-The-Path-to-Continuously-Learning-Health-Care-in-America.aspx

10. Sackett DL, Rosenberg WM, Gray JA, Haynes RB, Richardson WS. Evidence based medicine: what it is and what it isn't. BMJ. 1996;312:71-2.

11. Eddy DM. Evidence-based medicine: a unified approach. Health Aff (Millwood). 2005;24:9-17.

12. Evidence-Based Medicine Working Group. Evidence-based medicine. A new approach to teaching the practice of medicine. JAMA. 1992;268:2420-5.

13. Straus SE, Glasziou P, Richardson WS, Haynes RB. Evidence-based medicine: how to practice & teach it. 4th ed. New York: Churchill Livingstone; 2011.

14. Watanabe AS, McCart G, Shimomura S, Kayser S. Systematic approach to drug information requests. Am J Hosp Pharm. 1975;32:1282-5.

15. Guyatt GH, Meade MO, Jaeschke RZ, Cook DJ, Haynes RB. Practitioners of evidence based care. Not all clinicians need to appraise evidence from scratch but all need some skills. BMJ. 2000;320:954-5.

16. Chassin MR. Is health care ready for Six Sigma quality? Milbank Q. 1998;76:510,565-91.

17. Fye WB. The power of clinical trials and guidelines, and the challenge of conflicts of interest. J Am Coll Cardiol. 2003;41:1237-42.

18. Choudhry NK, Stelfox HT, Detsky AS. Relationships between authors of clinical practice guidelines and the pharmaceutical industry. JAMA. 2002;287:612-7.

19. Curtiss FR. Consensus panel, national guidelines, and other potentially misleading terms. J Manag Care Pharm. 2003;9:574-5.

20. Van der Weyden MB. Clinical practice guidelines: time to move the debate from the how to the who. Med J Aust. 2002;176:304-5.

21. Guyatt GH, Akl EA, Crowther M, Schunemann HJ, Gutterman DD, Zelman LS. Introduction to the ninth edition: antithrombotic therapy and prevention of thrombosis, 9th ed: American College of Chest Physicians evidence-based clinical practice guidelines. Chest. 2012;141:48S-52S.

22. Guyatt GH, Norris SL, Schulman S, Hirsh J, Eckman MH, Akl EA, et al. Methodology for the development of antithrombotic therapy and prevention of thrombosis guidelines: antithrombotic therapy and prevention of thrombosis, 9th ed: American College of Chest Physicians evidence-based clinical practice guidelines. Chest. 2012;141:53S-70S.

23. Mosca L, Appel LJ, Benjamin EJ, Berra K, Chandra-Strobos N, Fabunmi RP, et al. Evidence-based guidelines for cardiovascular disease prevention in women. J Am Coll Cardiol. 2004;43:900-21.

24. Guyatt GH, Oxman AD, Schunemann HJ, Tugwell P, Knottnerus A. GRADE guidelines: a new series of articles in the Journal of Clinical Epidemiology. J Clin Epidemiol. 2011;64:380-2.

25. Atkins D, Best D, Briss PA, Eccles M, Falck-Ytter Y, Flottorp S, et al. Grading quality of evidence and strength of recommendations. BMJ. 2004;328:1490.

26. Guyatt GH, Oxman AD, Vist GE, Kunz R, Falck-Ytter Y, Alfonso-Coello P, et al. GRADE: an emerging consensus on rating quality of evidence and strength of recommendations. BMJ. 2008;336:924-6.

27. Guyatt GH, Oxman AD, Kunz R, Atkins D, Brozck J, Vist G, et al. GRADE guidelines: 2. Framing the question and deciding on important outcomes. J Clin Epidemiol. 2011;64:395-400.

28. Balshem H, Helfand M, Schunemann HJ, Oxman AD, Kunz R, Brozek J, et al. GRADE guidelines: 3. Rating the quality of evidence. J Clin Epidemiol. 2011;64:401-6.

29. Guyatt GH, Oxman AD, Vist G, Kunz R, Brozek J, Alfonso-Coello P, et al. GRADE guidelines: 4. Rating the quality of evidence-study limitations (risk of bias). J Clin Epidemiol. 2011;64:407-15.

30. Guyatt GH, Oxman AD, Kunz R, Woodcock J, Brozek J, Helfand M, et al. GRADE guidelines: 7. Rating the quality of evidence—inconsistency. J Clin Epidemiol. 2011;64:1294-302.

31. Guyatt GH, Oxman AD, Kunz R, Woodcock J, Brozek J, Helfand M, et al. GRADE guidelines: 8. Rating the quality of evidence-indirectness. J Clin Epidemiol. 2011;64:1303-10.

32. Guyatt GH, Oxman AD, Kunz R, Brozek J, Alfonso-Coello P, Rind D, et al. GRADE guidelines 6. Rating the quality of evidence-imprecision. J Clin Epidemiol. 2011;64:1283-93.

33. Guyatt GH, Oxman AD, Montori V, Vist G, Kunz R, Brozek J, et al. GRADE guidelines: 5. Rating the quality of evidence-publication bias. J Clin Epidemiol. 2011;64:1277-82.

34. Guyatt GH, Oxman AD, Sultan S, Glasziou P, Akl EA, Alfonso-Coello P, et al. GRADE guidelines: 9. Rating up the quality of evidence. J Clin Epidemiol. 2011;64:1311-6.

35. Hill AB. The environment and disease: association or causation? Proc R Soc Med. 1965;58:295-300.

36. Guyatt G, Oxman AD, Akl EA, Kunz R, Vist G, Brozek J, et al. GRADE guidelines: 1. Introduction-GRADE evidence profiles and summary of findings tables. J Clin Epidemiol. 2011;64:383-94.

37. Guyatt GH, Oxman AD, Santesso N, Helfand M, Vist G, Kunz R, et al. GRADE guidelines: 12. Preparing summary of findings tables-binary outcomes. J Clin Epidemiol. 2013;66:158-72.

38. Guyatt GH, Thorlund K, Oxman AD, Walter SD, Patrick D, Furukawa TA, et al. GRADE guidelines: 13. Preparing summary of findings tables and evidence profiles-continuous outcomes. J Clin Epidemiol. 2013;66:173-83.

39. Brouwers MC, Kho ME, Browman GP, Burgers JS, Cluzeau F, Feder G, et al. AGREE II: advancing guideline development, reporting and evaluation in health care. CMAJ. 2010;182:E839-42.

40. AGREE Next Steps Consortium. Appraisal of Guidelines for Research & Evaluation (AGREE) II Instrument. [cited: 2012 Dec 14]. Available from: http://www.agreetrust

.org/wp-content/uploads/2013/10/AGREE-II-Users-Manual-and-23-item-Instrument_2009_
UPDATE_2013.pdf

41. Davis DA, Taylor-Vaisey A. Translating guidelines into practice. A systematic review of theoretic concepts, practical experience and research evidence in the adoption of clinical practice guidelines. CMAJ. 1997;157:408-16.

42. Grimshaw JM, Thomas RE, MacLennan G, Fraser C, Ramsay CR, Vale L, et al. Effectiveness and efficiency of guideline dissemination and implementation strategies. Health Technol Assess. 2004;8:iii-72.

43. Cabana MD, Rand CS, Powe NR, Wu AW, Wilson MH, Abboud PA, et al. Why don't physicians follow clinical practice guidelines? A framework for improvement. JAMA. 1999;282:1458-65.

44. Grol R, Dalhuijsen J, Thomas S, Veld C, Rutten G, Mokkink H. Attributes of clinical guidelines that influence use of guidelines in general practice: observational study. BMJ. 1998;317:858-61.

45. Garg AX, Adhikari NK, McDonald H, Rosas-Arellano MP, Devereaux PJ, Beyene J, et al. Effects of computerized clinical decision support systems on practitioner performance and patient outcomes: a systematic review. JAMA. 2005;293:1223-38.

46. Wears RL, Berg M. Computer technology and clinical work: still waiting for Godot. JAMA. 2005;293:1261-3.

47. Horowitz CR, Goldberg HI, Martin DP, Wagner EH, Fihn SD, Christensen DB, et al. Conducting a randomized controlled trial of CQI and academic detailing to implement clinical guidelines. Jt Comm J Qual Improv. 1996;22:734-50.

48. Grimshaw JM, Russell IT. Effect of clinical guidelines on medical practice: a systematic review of rigorous evaluations. Lancet. 1993;342:1317-22.

49. Cook DJ, Mulrow CD, Haynes RB. Systematic reviews: synthesis of best evidence for clinical decisions. Ann Intern Med. 1997;126:376-80.

50. Hunt DL, McKibbon KA. Locating and appraising systematic reviews. Ann Intern Med. 1997;126:532-8.

51. Montori VM, Wilczynski NL, Morgan D, Haynes RB. Optimal search strategies for retrieving systematic reviews from Medline: analytical survey. BMJ. 2005;330:68.

SUGGESTED READINGS

1. AGREE Next Steps Consortium. Appraisal of Guidelines for Research & Evaluation (AGREE) II Instrument. Available from: http://www.agreetrust.org/wp-content/uploads/2013/10/AGREE-II-Users-Manual-and-23-item-Instrument_2009_UPDATE_2013.pdf

2. Guyatt GH, Oxman AD, Schunemann HJ, Tugwell P, Knottnerus A. GRADE guidelines: a new series of articles in the Journal of Clinical Epidemiology. J Clin Epidemiol. 2011;64:380-2.

3. Institute of Medicine Committee on Standards for Developing Trustworthy Clinical Practice Guidelines. Clinical practice guidelines we can trust. In: Graham R, Mancher M, Wolman DM, Greenfield S, Steinberg E, eds. Washington, D.C.: National Academies Press; 2011. Available from: http://www.iom.edu/Reports/2011/Clinical-Practice-Guidelines-We-Can-Trust.aspx

4. Institute of Medicine Committee on Standards for Systematic Reviews of Comparative Effectiveness Research. Finding what works in health care: standards for systematic reviews. In: Eden J, Levit L, Berg A, Morton S, eds. Washington, D.C.: National Academies Press; 2011. Available from: http://www.iom.edu/Reports/2011/Finding-What-Works-in-Health-Care-Standards-for-Systematic-Reviews.aspx

Chapter Eight

The Application of Statistical Analysis in the Biomedical Sciences

Ryan W. Walters

Learning Objectives

● *After completing this chapter, the reader will be able to*

- Define the population being studied and describe the method most appropriate to sample a given population.
- Identify and describe the dependent and independent variables and indicate whether any covariates were included in analysis.
- Identify and define the four scales of variable measurement.
- Describe the difference between descriptive and inferential statistics.
- Describe the mean, median, variance, and standard deviation and why they are important to statistical analysis.
- Describe the properties of the normal distribution and when an alternative distribution should be, or should have been, used.
- Describe several common epidemiological statistics.
- Identify and describe the difference between parametric and nonparametric statistical tests and when their use is most appropriate.
- Determine whether the appropriate statistical test has been performed when evaluating a study.

Key Concepts

❶ There are four scales of variable measurement consisting of nominal, ordinal, interval, and ratio scales that are critically important to consider when determining the appropriateness of a statistical test.

❷ Measures of central tendency are useful to quantify the distribution of a variable's data numerically. The most common measures of central tendency are the mean, median, and mode, with the most appropriate measure of central tendency dictated by the variable's scale of measurement.

❸ Variance is a key element inherent in all statistical analyses, but standard deviation is presented more often. Variance and standard deviation are related mathematically.

❹ The key benefit to using the standard normal distribution is that converting the original data to z-scores allows researchers to compare different variables regardless of the original scale.

❺ The last observation carried forward (LOCF) technique used often with the data from clinical trials introduces significant bias into the results of statistical tests.

❻ The central limit theorem states when equally sized samples are drawn from a non-normal distribution, the plotted mean values from each sample will approximate a normal distribution as long as the non-normality was not due to outliers.

❼ There are numerous misconceptions about p values and it is important to know how to interpret them correctly.

❽ Clinical significance is far more important than statistical significance. Clinical significance can be quantified by using various measures of effect size.

❾ The selection of the appropriate statistical test is based on several factors including the specific research question, the measurement scale of the dependent variable (DV), distributional assumptions, the number of DV measurements as well as the number and measurement scale of independent variables (IVs) and covariates, among others.

Introduction

Knowledge of statistics and statistical analyses is essential to constructively evaluate literature in the biomedical sciences. This chapter provides a general overview of both descriptive and inferential statistics that will enhance the ability of the student or evidence-based practitioner to interpret results of empirical literature within the biomedical sciences by evaluating the appropriateness of statistical tests employed, the conclusions drawn by the authors, and the overall quality of the study.

Alongside Chapters 4 and 5, diligent study of the material presented in this chapter is an important first step to critically analyze the often avoided methods or results sections of published biomedical literature. Be aware, however, that this chapter cannot substitute for more formal didactic training in statistics, as the material presented here is not exhaustive with regards to either statistical concepts or available statistical tests. Thus, when reading a journal article, if doubt emerges about whether a method or statistical test was used and interpreted appropriately, do not hesitate to consult appropriate references or an individual who has more formal statistical training. This is especially true if the empirical evidence is being considered for implementation in practice. Asking questions is the key to obtaining knowledge!

For didactic purposes, this chapter can be divided into two sections. The first section presents a general overview of the processes underlying most statistical tests used in the biomedical sciences. It is recommended that all readers take the time required to thoroughly study these concepts. The second section, beginning with the Statistical Tests section, presents descriptions, assumptions, examples, and results of numerous statistical tests commonly used in the biomedical sciences. This section does not present the mathematical underpinnings, calculation, or programming of any specific statistical test. It is recommended that this section serve as a reference to be used concurrently alongside a given journal article to determine the appropriateness of a statistical test or to gain further insight into why a specific statistical test was employed.

Populations and Sampling

When investigating a particular research question or hypothesis, researchers must first define the population to be studied. A population refers to any set of objects in the universe, while a sample is a fraction of the population chosen to be representative of the specific population of interest. Thus, samples are chosen to make specific generalizations about the population of interest. Researchers typically do not attempt to study the entire population because data cannot be collected for everyone within a population. This is why a sample should ideally be chosen at random. That is, each member of the population must have an equal probability of being included in the sample.

For example, consider a study to evaluate the effect a calcium channel blocker (CCB) has on blood glucose levels in Type 1 diabetes mellitus (DM) patients. In this case, all Type 1 DM patients would constitute the study population; however, because data could never be collected from all Type 1 DM patients, a sample that is representative of the Type 1 DM population would be selected. There are numerous sampling strategies, many beyond the scope of this text. Although only a few are discussed here, interested readers are urged to consult the list of suggested readings at the end of this chapter for further information.

A random sample does not imply that the sample is drawn haphazardly or in an unplanned fashion, and there are several approaches to selecting a random sample. The most common method employs a random number table. A random number table theoretically contains all integers between one and infinity that have been selected without any trends or patterns. For example, consider the hypothetical process of selecting a random sample of Type 1 DM patients from the population. First, each patient in the population is assigned a number, say 1 to N, where N is the total number of Type 1 DM patients in the population. From this population, a sample of 200 patients is requested. The random number table would randomly select 200 patients from the population of size N. There are numerous free random number tables and generators available online; simply search for random number table or random number generator in any search engine.

Depending on the study design, a random sample may not be most appropriate when selecting a representative sample. On occasion, it may be necessary to separate the population into mutually exclusive groups called strata, where a specific factor (e.g., race, gender) will create separate strata to aid in analysis. In this case, the random sample is drawn within each stratum individually. This process is termed stratified random sampling. For example, consider a situation where the race of the patient was an important variable in the Type 1 DM study. To ensure the proportion of each race in the population is represented accurately, the researcher stratifies by race and randomly selects patients within each stratum to achieve a representative study sample.

Another method of randomly sampling a population is known as cluster sampling. Cluster sampling is appropriate when there are natural groupings within the population of interest. For example, consider a researcher interested in the patient counseling practices of pharmacists across the United States. It would be impossible to collect data from all pharmacists across the United States. However, the researcher has read literature suggesting regional differences within various pharmacy practices, not necessarily including counseling practices. Thus, he or she may decide to randomly sample within the four regions of the United States (U.S.) defined by the U.S. Census Bureau (i.e., West, Midwest, South, and Northeast) to assess for differences in patient counseling practices across regions.[1]

Another sampling method is known as systematic sampling. This method is used when information about the population is provided in list format, such as in the telephone book, election records, class lists, or licensure records, among others. Systematic sampling uses an equal-probability method where one individual is selected initially at random and every nth individual is then selected thereafter. For example, the researchers may decide to take every 10th individual listed after the first individual is chosen.

Finally, researchers often use convenience sampling to select participants based on the convenience of the researcher. That is, no attempt is made to ensure the sample is representative of the population. However, within the convenience sample, participants may be selected randomly. This type of sampling is often used in educational research. For example, consider a researcher evaluating a new classroom instructional method to increase exam scores. This type of study will use the convenience sample of the students in their own class or university. Obviously, significant weaknesses are apparent when using this type of sampling, most notably, limited generalization.

Variables and the Measurement of Data

A variable is the characteristic that is being observed or measured. Data are the measured values assigned to the variable for each individual member of the population. For example, a variable would be the participant's biological sex, while the data is whether the participant is male or female.

In statistics, there are three types of variables: dependent (DV), independent (IV), and confounding. The DV is the response or outcome variable for a study, while an IV is a variable that is manipulated. A confounding variable (often referred to as covariate) is any variable that has an effect on the DV over and above the effect of the IV, but is not of specific research interest. Putting these definitions together, consider a study to evaluate the effect a new oral hypoglycemic medication has on glycosylated hemoglobin (HbA1c) compared to placebo. Here, the DV consists of the HbA1c data for each participant, and the IV is treatment group with two levels (i.e., treatment versus placebo). Initially, results may suggest the medication is very effective across the entire sample; however, previous literature has suggested participant race may affect the effectiveness of this type of medication. Thus, participant race is a confounding variable and would need to be included in the statistical analysis. After statistically controlling for participant race, the results may indicate the medication was significantly more effective in the treatment group.

SCALES OF MEASUREMENT

❶ *There are four scales of variable measurement consisting of nominal, ordinal, interval, and ratio scales that are critically important to consider when determining the appropriateness of a statistical test.*[2] Think of these four scales as relatively fluid; that is, as the data progress from nominal to ratio, the information about each variable being measured is increased. The scale of measurement of DVs, IVs, and confounding variables is an important consideration when determining whether the appropriate statistical test was used to answer the research question and hypothesis.

A **nominal scale** consists of categories that have no implied rank or order. Examples of nominal variables include gender (e.g., male versus female), race (e.g., Caucasian versus African American versus Hispanic), or disease state (e.g., absence versus presence). It is important to note that with nominal data, the participant is categorized into one, and only one, category. That is, the categories are mutually exclusive.

An **ordinal scale** has all of the characteristics of a nominal variable with the addition of rank ordering. It is important to note the distance between rank ordered categories cannot be considered equal; that is, the data points can be ranked but the distance between them may differ greatly. For example, in medicine a commonly used pain scale is the Wong-Baker Faces Pain Rating Scale.[3] Here, the participant ranks pain on a 0 to 10 scale; however, while it is known that a rating of eight indicates the participant is in more pain than rating four, there is no indication a rating of eight hurts twice as much as a rating of four.

- An **interval scale** has all of the characteristics of an ordinal scale with the addition that the distance between two values is now constant and meaningful. However, it is important to note that interval scales do not have an absolute zero point. For example, temperature on a Celsius scale is measured on an interval scale (i.e., the difference between $10°C$ and $5°C$ is equivalent to the difference between $20°C$ and $15°C$). However, $20°C/10°C$ cannot be quantified as twice as hot because there is no absolute zero (i.e., the selection of $0°C$ was arbitrary).
- Finally, a **ratio scale** has all of the characteristics of an interval scale, but ratio scales have an absolute zero point. The classic example of a ratio scale is temperature measured on the Kelvin scale, where zero Kelvin represents the absence of molecular motion. Theoretically, researchers should not confuse absolute and arbitrary zero points. However, the difference between interval and ratio scales is generally trivial as these data are analyzed by identical statistical procedures.

CONTINUOUS VERSUS CATEGORICAL VARIABLES

- Continuous variables generally consist of data measured on interval or ratio scales. However, if the number of ordinal categories is large (e.g., seven or more) they may be considered continuous.[4] Be aware that continuous variables may also be referred to as quantitative in the literature. Examples of continuous variables include age, body mass index (BMI), or uncategorized systolic or diastolic blood pressure values.
- **Categorical variables** consist of data measured on nominal or ordinal scales because these scales of measurement have naturally distinct categories. Examples of categorical variables include gender, race, or blood pressure status (e.g., hypotensive, normotensive, prehypertensive, hypertensive). In the literature, categorical variables are often termed discrete or if a variable is measured on a nominal scale with only two distinct categories it may be termed binary or **dichotomous**.

Note that it is common in the biomedical literature for researchers to categorize continuous variables. While not wholly incorrect, categorizing a continuous variable will always result in loss of information about the variable. For example, consider the role participant age has on the probability of experiencing a cardiac event. Although age is a continuous variable, younger individuals typically have much a lower probability compared to older individuals. Thus, the research may divide age into four discrete categories: <30, 31–50, 51–70, and 70+. Note that assigning category cutoffs is generally an arbitrary process. In this example, information is lost by categorizing age because after categorization the exact age of the participant is unknown. That is, an individual's age is defined only by their age category. For example, a 50-year-old individual is considered identical to a 31-year-old individual because they are in the same age category.

Descriptive Statistics

There are two types of statistics—descriptive and inferential. Descriptive statistics present, organize, and summarize a variable's data by providing information regarding the appearance of the data and distributional characteristics. Examples of descriptive statistics include measures of central tendency, variability, shape, histograms, boxplots, and scatterplots. These descriptive measures are the focus of this section.

Inferential statistics indicate whether a difference exists between groups of participants or whether an association exists between variables. Inferential statistics are used to determine whether the difference or association is real or whether it is due to some random process. Examples of inferential statistics are the statistics produced by each statistical test described later in the chapter. For example, the t statistic produced by a t-test.

MEASURES OF CENTRAL TENDENCY

❷ *Measures of central tendency are useful to quantify the distribution of a variable's data numerically. The most common measures of central tendency are the mean, median, and mode, with the most appropriate measure of central tendency dictated by the variable's scale of measurement.*

The **mean** (indicated as M in the literature) is the most common and appropriate measure of central tendency for normally distributed data (see the Common Probability Distributions section later in chapter) measured on an interval or ratio scale. The mean is the arithmetic average of a variable's data. Thus, the mean is calculated by summing a variable's data and dividing by the total number of participants with data for the specific variable. It is important to note that data points that are severely disconnected from the other data points can significantly influence the mean. These extreme data points are termed outliers.

The **median** (indicated as Mdn in the literature) is most appropriate measure of central tendency for data measured on an ordinal scale. The median is the absolute middle value in the data; therefore, exactly half of the data is above the median and exactly half of the data is below the median. The median is also known as the 50th percentile. Note that the median can also be presented for continuous variables with skewed distributions (see the Measures of Distribution Shape section later in chapter) and for continuous variables with outliers. A direct comparison of a variable's mean and median can give insight into how much influence outliers had on the mean.

Finally, the **mode** is the most appropriate measure of central tendency for nominal data. The mode is a variable's most frequently occurring data point or category. Note that it is possible for a variable to have multiple modes; a variable with two or three modes is referred to as bimodal and trimodal, respectively.

MEASURES OF VARIABILITY

Measures of variability are useful in indicating the spread of a variable's data. The most common measures of variability are the range, interquartile range, variance, and standard deviation. These measures are also useful when considered with appropriate measures of central tendency to assess how the data are scattered around the mean or median. For example, consider the two histograms in Figure 8–1. Both histograms present data for 100 participants that have identical mean body weight of 185 pounds. However, notice the variability (or dispersion) of the data is much greater for Group 2. If the means for both groups were simply taken at face value, the participants in these two groups would be considered similar; however, assessing the variability or spread of data within each group illustrates an entirely different picture. This concept is critically important to the application of any inferential statistical test because the test results are heavily influenced by the amount of variability.

The simplest measure of variability is the range, which can be used to describe data measured on an ordinal, interval, or ratio scale. The range is a crude measure of variability calculated by subtracting a variable's minimum data point from its maximum data point. For example, in Figure 8–1 the range for Group 1 is 30 (i.e., 200–170), whereas the range from Group 2 is 95 (i.e., 235–140).

The interquartile range (indicated as IQR in the literature) is another measure of dispersion used to describe data measured on ordinal scale; as such, the IQR is usually presented alongside the median. The IQR is the difference between the 75th and 25th percentile. Therefore, because the median represents the 50th percentile, the IQR presents the middle 50% of the data and always includes the median.

The final two measures of variability described are the variance and standard deviation. These measures are appropriate for normally distributed continuous variables measured on interval or ratio scales. ❸ *Variance is a key element inherent in all statistical analyses, but standard deviation is presented more often. Variance and standard deviation are related mathematically.* Variance is the average squared deviation from the mean for all data points within a specific variable. For example, consider Figure 8–1, where the mean for both Group 1 and 2 was 185 pounds. Say a specific participant in Group 1 had a body weight of 190 pounds. The squared deviation from the mean for this participant would be equal to 25 pounds. That is, $190 - 185 = 5$ and $5^2 = 25$. To calculate variance, the squared deviations are calculated for all data points. These square deviations are then summed across participants and then divided by the total number of data points (i.e., N) to obtain the average squared deviation. Some readers may be asking why the deviations from the mean are squared. This is a great question! The reason is that summing unsquared deviations across participants would equal zero. That is, deviations resulting from values above and below the mean would cancel each other out.

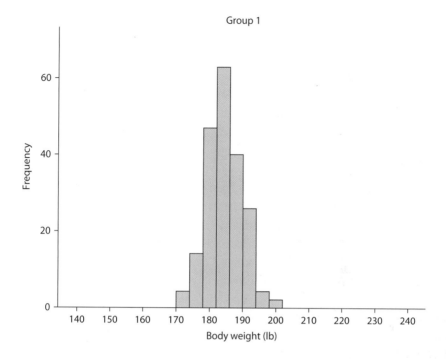

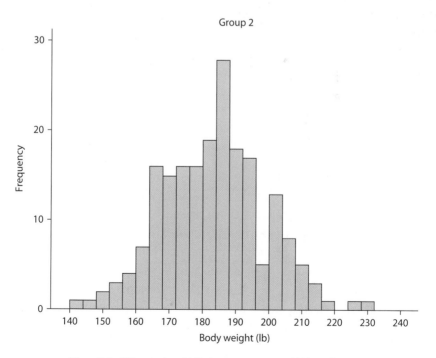

Figure 8–1. Differences in variability between two groups with identical means.

While the calculation of variance may seem esoteric, conceptually all that is required to understand variance is that larger variance values indicate greater variability. For example, the variances of Group 1 and 2 in Figure 8–1 were 25 and 225, respectively. While the histograms did not present these numbers explicitly, the greater variability in Group 2 can be observed clearly. The importance of variance cannot be overstated. It is the primary parameter used in all parametric statistical analyses, and this is why it was presented in such detail here. With that said, variance is rarely presented as a descriptive statistic in the literature. Instead, variance is converted into a standard deviation as described in the next paragraph.

As a descriptive statistic, the standard deviation (indicated as SD in the literature) is often preferred over variance because it indicates the average deviation from the mean presented on the same scale as the original variable. Variance presented the average deviation in squared units. It is important to note that the standard deviation and variance are directly related mathematically, with standard deviation equal to the square root of the variance (i.e., $SD = \sqrt{variance}$). Thus, if the standard deviation is known, the variance can be calculated directly, and vice versa. When comparing variability between groups of participants, the standard deviation can provide insight into the dispersion of scores around the mean, and, similar to variance, larger standard deviations indicate greater variability in the data. For example, from Figure 8–1, Group 1 had a standard deviation of 5 (i.e., $\sqrt{25}$) and Group 2 had a standard deviation of 15 (i.e., $\sqrt{225}$). Again, the greater variability within Group 2 is evident.

MEASURES OF DISTRIBUTION SHAPE

Skewness and kurtosis are appropriate measures of shape for variables measured on interval or ratio scales, and indicate asymmetry and peakedness of a distribution, respectively. They are typically used by researchers to evaluate the distributional assumptions of a parametric statistical analysis.

Skewness indicates the asymmetry of distribution of data points and can be either positive or negative. Positive (or right) skewness occurs when the mode and median are less than the mean, whereas negative (or left) skewness occurs when mode and median are greater than the mean. As stated previously, the mean is sensitive to extremely disconnected data points termed outliers; thus, it is important to know the difference between true skewness and skewness due to outliers. True skewness is indicated by a steady decrease in data points toward the tails (i.e., ends) of the distribution. Skewness due to outliers is indicated when the mean is heavily influenced by data points that are extremely disconnected from the rest of the distribution. For example, consider the histogram in Figure 8–2. The data for Group 1 provides an example of true positive skewness, whereas the data for Group 2 provides an example of negative skewness due to outliers.

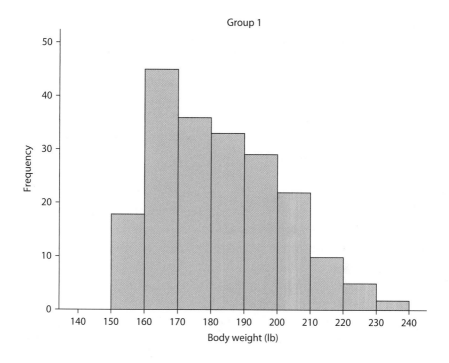

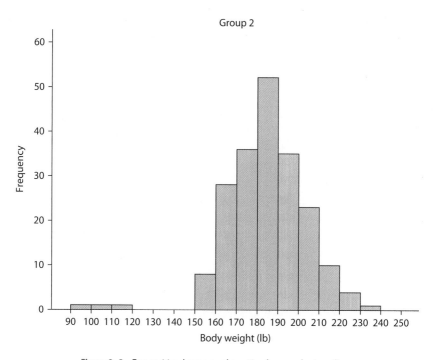

Figure 8–2. True positive skewness and negative skewness due to outliers.

Kurtosis indicates the peakedness of the distribution of data points and can be either positive or negative. Plotted data with a narrow, peaked distribution and a positive kurtosis value is termed leptokurtic. A leptokurtic distribution has small range, variance, and standard deviation with the majority of data points near the mean. In contrast, plotted data with a wide, flat distribution and a negative kurtosis value is referred to as platykurtic. A platykurtic distribution is an indicator of great variability, with large range, variance, and standard deviation. Examples of leptokurtic and platykurtic data distributions are presented for Group 1 and 2, respectively, in Figure 8–2.

GRAPHICAL REPRESENTATIONS OF DATA

Graphical representations of data are incredibly useful, especially when sample sizes are large, as they allow researchers to inspect the distribution of individual variables. There are typically three graphical representations presented in the literature—histograms, boxplots, and scatterplots. Note that graphical representations are typically used for continuous variables measured on ordinal, interval, or ratio scales. By contrast, nominal, dichotomous, or categorical variables are best presented as count data, which are typically reported in the literature as frequency and percentage.

A histogram presents data as frequency counts over some interval; that is, the x-axis presents the values of the data points, whether individual data points or intervals, while the y-axis presents the number of times the data point or interval occurs in the variable (i.e., frequency). Figures 8–1 and 8–2 provide examples of histograms. When data are plotted, it is easy to observe skewness, kurtosis, or outlier issues. For example, reconsider the distribution of body weight for Group 2 in Figure 8–2, where each vertical bar represents the number of participants having body weight within 10-unit intervals. The distribution of data has negative skewness due to outliers, with outliers being participants weighing between 90 and 120 pounds.

A boxplot, also known as a box-and-whisker plot, provides the reader with five descriptive statistics.[5] Consider the boxplot in Figure 8–3, which presents the same data as the Group 2 histogram in Figure 8–2. The thin-lined box in a boxplot indicates the IQR, which contains the 25th to 75th percentiles of the data. Within this thin-lined box is a thick, bold line depicting the median, or 50th percentile. From both ends of the thin-lined box extends a tail, or whisker, depicting the minimum and maximum data points up to 1.5 IQRs beyond the median. Beyond the whiskers, outliers and extreme outliers are identified with circles and asterisks, respectively. Note that other symbols may be used to identify outliers depending on the statistical software used. Outliers are defined as data points 1.5 to 3.0 IQRs beyond the median, whereas extreme outliers are defined as data points greater than 3.0 IQRs beyond the median. The boxplot corroborates the information provided by the histogram in Figure 8–2 as participants weighing between 90 and 120 pounds are defined as outliers.

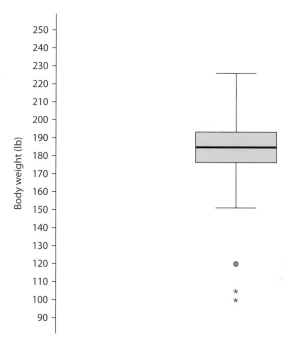

Figure 8–3. Boxplot of body weight with outliers. (Circle represent values 1.5 to 3.0 IQRs, asterisks represent values >3.0 IQRs.)

Finally, a scatterplot presents data for two variables both measured on a continuous scale. That is, the *x*-axis contains the range of data for one variable, whereas the *y*-axis contains the range of data for a second variable. In general, the axis choice for a given variable is arbitrary. Data are plotted in a similar fashion to plotting data on a coordinate plane during an introductory geometry class. Figure 8–4 presents a scatterplot of height in inches and body weight in pounds. The individual circles in the scatterplot are a participant's height in relation to their weight. Because the plot is bivariate (i.e., there are two variables), participants must have data for both variables in order to be plotted. Scatterplots are useful in visually assessing the association between two variables as well as assessing assumptions of various statistical tests such as linearity and absence of outliers.

Common Probability Distributions

Up to this point, data distributions have been discussed using very general terminology. There are numerous distributions available to researchers; far too many to provide a complete listing, but all that needs to be known about these available distributions is that each has different characteristics to fit the unique requirements of the data. Globally, these

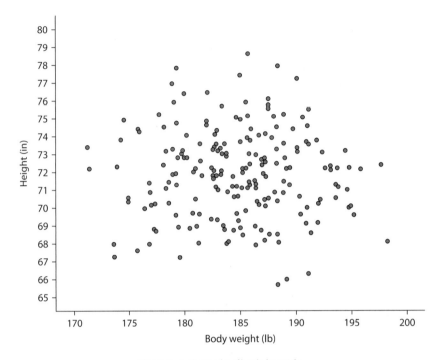

Figure 8–4. Scatterplot of height by weight.

distributions are termed probability distributions, and they are incredibly important to every statistical analysis conducted. Thus, the choice of distribution used in a given statistical analysis is nontrivial as the use of an improper distribution can lead to incorrect statistical inference. Of the distributions available, the normal and binomial distributions are used most frequently in the biomedical literature; therefore, these are discussed in detail. To provide the reader with a broader listing of available distributions, this section also presents brief information about other common distributions used in the biomedical literature and when they are appropriately used in statistical analyses.

THE NORMAL DISTRIBUTION

The normal distribution, also called Gaussian distribution, is the most commonly used distribution in statistics and one that occurs frequently in nature. It is used only for continuous variables measured on interval or ratio scales. The normal distribution has several easily identifiable properties based on the numerical measures of central tendency, variability, and shape. Specifically, this includes the following characteristics:

1. The primary shape is bell-shaped.
2. The mean, median, and mode are equal.

3. The distribution has one mode, is symmetric, and reflects itself perfectly when folded at the mean.
4. The skewness and kurtosis are zero.
5. The area under a normal distribution is, by definition, equal to one.

It should be noted that the five properties above are considered the gold standard. In practice, however, each of these properties will be approximated; namely, the curve will be roughly bell-shaped, the mean, median, and mode will be roughly equal, and skewness and kurtosis may be evident but not greatly exaggerated. For example, the distribution of data for Group 2 in Figure 8–1 is approximately normal.

Several additional properties of the normal distribution are important; consider Figure 8–5. First, the distribution is completely defined by the mean and standard deviation. Consequently, there are an infinite number of possible normal distributions because there are an infinite number of mean and standard deviation combinations. In the literature, this property is often stated as the mean and standard deviation being sufficient statistics for describing the normal distribution. Second, the mean can always be identified as the peak (or mode) of the distribution. Third, the standard deviation will always dictate the spread of the distribution. That is, as the standard deviation increases, the distribution becomes wider. Finally, roughly 68% of the data will occur within one standard deviation above and below the mean, roughly 95% within two standard deviations, and roughly 99% within three standard deviations.

THE STANDARD NORMAL DISTRIBUTION

Among the infinite number of potential normal distributions, only the standard normal distribution can be used to compare all normal distributions. Although this may seem

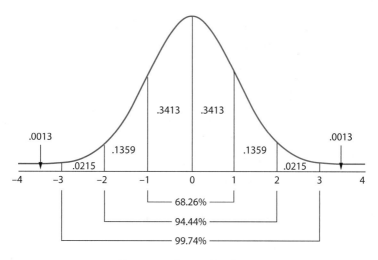

Figure 8–5. The normal distribution.

confusing on the surface, a clearer understanding of the standard normal distribution is made possible by considering the standard deviation. Initially, when converting a normal distribution to a standard normal distribution, the data must be converted into standardized scores referred to as **z-scores**. A z-score converts the units of the original data into standard deviation units. That is, a z-score indicates how many standard deviations a data point is from the mean. When converted to z-scores, the new standard normal distribution will always have a mean of zero and a standard deviation of one. The standard normal distribution is presented in Figure 8–5.

It is a common misconception that converting data into z-scores creates a standard normal distribution from data that was not normally distributed. This is never true. A standardized distribution will always have the same characteristics of distribution from which it originated. That is, if the original distribution was skewed, the standardized distribution will also be skewed.

❹ *The key benefit to using the standard normal distribution is that converting the original data to z-scores allows researchers to compare different variables regardless of the original scale.* Remember, a standardized variable will always be expressed in standard deviation units with a mean of zero and standard deviation of one. Therefore, differences between variables may be more easily detected and understood. For example, it is possible to compare standardized variables across studies. It should go without stating that the only requirement is that that both variables measure the same construct. After z-score standardization, the age of two groups of participants from two different studies can be compared directly.

THE BINOMIAL DISTRIBUTION

Many discrete variables can be dichotomized into one of two mutually exclusive groups, outcomes, or events (e.g., dead versus alive). Using the binomial distribution, a researcher can calculate the exact probability of experiencing either binary outcome. The binomial distribution can only be used when an experiment assumes the four characteristics listed below:

1. The trial occurs a specified number of times (analogous to sample size, n).
2. Each trial has only two mutually exclusive outcomes (success versus failure in a generic sense, x). Also, be aware that a single trial with only two outcomes is known as a Bernoulli trial, a term that may be encountered in the literature.
3. Each trial is independent, meaning that one outcome has no effect on the other.
4. The probability of success remains constant throughout the trial.

An example may assist with the understanding of these characteristics. The binomial distribution consists of the number of successes and failures during a given study period.

When all trials have been run, the probability of achieving exactly *x* successes (or failures) in *n* trials can be calculated. Consider flipping a fair coin. The coin is flipped for a set number of trials (i.e., *n*), there are only two possible outcomes (i.e., heads or tails), each trial is not affected by the outcome of the last, and the probability of flipping heads or tails remains constant throughout the trial (i.e., 0.50).

By definition, the mean for the binomial distribution is equal to the number of successes in a given trial. That is, if a fair coin is flipped 10 times and heads turns up on six flips, the mean is 0.60 (i.e., 6/10). Further, the variance of the binomial distribution is fixed by the mean. While the equation for the variance is not presented, know that the variance is largest at a mean of 0.50, decreases as the mean diverges from 0.50, and is symmetric (e.g., the variance for a mean of 0.10 is equal to the variance for a mean of 0.90). Therefore, because variance is fixed by the mean, the mean is the sufficient statistic for the binomial distribution.

In reality, the probability of experiencing an outcome is rarely 0.50. For example, biomedical studies often use all-cause mortality as an outcome variable, and the probability of dying during the study period is generally lower than staying alive. At the end of the trial, participants can experience only one of the outcomes—dead or alive. Say a study sample consists of 1000 participants, of which 150 die. The binomial distribution allows for the calculation of the exact probability of having 150 participants die in a sample of 1000 participants.

OTHER COMMON PROBABILITY DISTRIBUTIONS

As mentioned in the introduction to this section, there are numerous probability distributions available to researchers, with their use determined by the scale of measurement of the DV as well as the shape (e.g., skewness) of the distribution. When reading journal articles, it is important to know whether the appropriate distribution has been used for statistical analysis as inappropriate use of any distribution can lead to inaccurate statistical inference.

Table 8–1 provides a short list of the several commonly used distributions in the biomedical literature. Of note here is that alternative distributions are available when statistically analyzing non-normally distributed continuous data or data that cannot be normalized such as categorical data. The take away message here is that non-normal continuous data does not need to be forced to conform to a normal distribution.

The only DV scale presented in Table 8–1 that has not been discussed thus far is count data. An example of count data would be a count of the number of hospitalizations during a 5-year study period. It is clear from the example that count data cannot take on negative values. That is, a participant cannot have a negative number of hospitalizations. Both the Poisson and negative binomial distributions are used when analyzing count data.

TABLE 8–1. COMMON PROBABILITY DISTRIBUTIONS AND WHEN THEY ARE APPROPRIATE TO USE

Distribution Name	DV Scale	Distribution Characteristics	Comments
Normal	Continuous		
Gamma	Continuous	Positive skew	
Inverse Gaussian	Continuous	Positive skew	
Exponential	Continuous	Positive skew	Data has to be > 0
Log-normal[a]	Continuous	Positive skew	Data has to be > 0
Weibull	Continuous	Positive or negative skew	
Gompertz	Continuous	Positive or negative skew	
Poisson	Count	Mean = variance	Data ≥ 0
Negative binomial	Count	Mean ≠ variance	Data ≥ 0
Bernoulli	Binary		One trial; 2 categories
Binomial	Binary		Repeated Bernoulli trials; 2 categories
Categorical	Categorical		One trial; > 2 categories
Multinomial	Categorical		Repeated trials; > 2 categories

[a]Log = natural log or ln.

The Poisson distribution assumes the mean and the variance of the data are identical. However, in situations where the mean and variance are not equal, the negative binomial distribution allows the variance of the distribution to increase or decrease as needed. As a point of possible confusion, the negative binomial distribution does not allow negative values. The negative in negative binomial is a result of using a negative exponent in its mathematical formula.

TRANSFORMING NON-NORMAL DISTRIBUTIONS

Transformations are usually employed by researchers to transform a non-normal distribution into a distribution that is approximately normal. Although on the surface this may appear reasonable, data transformation is an archaic technique. As such, transformation is not recommended for the three reasons provided below.

First, although parametric statistical analyses assume normality, the distribution of the actual DV data is not required to be normally distributed. As stated in the previous section, and highlighted in Table 8–1, if non-normality is observed, alternative distributions exist allowing proper statistical analysis of non-normal data without transformation. For this reason alone, transformation is rarely necessary.

Second, transforming the DV data potentially prevents effects of an IV from being observed. As an overly simplistic example, consider the bimodal distribution of body weight data presented in Figure 8–6. Say the body weight data were collected from a

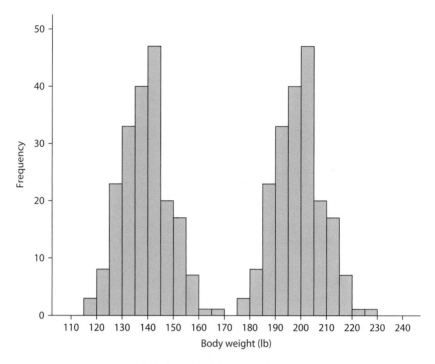

Figure 8–6. Body weight data for a group of men and women.

sample of men and women. Obviously, the data in Figure 8–6 is bimodal and not normally distributed. In this situation, a researcher may attempt to transform the data, but transformation would obscure the effects of an obvious IV—gender. That is, women tend to be lighter compared to men, and this is observed in these data, with women being grouped in the left distribution and men grouped in the right distribution. If transformation were performed successfully, inherent differences between men and women would be erased.

Third, while data transformation will not affect the rank order of the data, it will significantly cloud interpretation of statistical analyses. That is, after transformation all results must be interpreted in the transformed metric, which can become convoluted quickly making it difficult to apply results to the untransformed data used in the real world. Thus, when reading a journal article where the authors employed any transformation, be aware the results are in the transformed metric and ensure the authors' interpretations remain consistent with this metric.

Although transformation is not recommended, it can be correct, and it will inevitably be encountered when reading the literature, especially for skewed data or data with outliers. Therefore, it is useful to become familiar with several of the techniques used to transform data. Transformations for positive skewness differ from those suggested for negative skewness. Mild positive skewness is typically remedied by a square root transformation.

Here, the square root of all data is calculated and this square root data is used in analysis. When positive skewness is severe, a natural log transformation is used. When data are skewed negatively, researchers may choose to reflect their data to make it positively skewed and apply the transformations for positive skewness described above. To reflect data, a 1 is added to the absolute value of the highest data point and all data points are subtracted from this new value. For example, if the highest value in the data is 10, a 1 is added to create 11, and then all data points are subtracted from 11 (e.g., 11 − 10 = 1, 11 − 1 = 10, etc.). In this manner, the highest values become the lowest and the lowest become the highest. It should be clear that this process considerably convolutes data interpretation!

Epidemiological Statistics

The field of epidemiology investigates how diseases are distributed in the population and the various factors (or exposures) influencing this distribution.[6] Epidemiological statistics are not unique to the field of epidemiology, as much of the literature in the biomedical sciences incorporates some form of these statistics such as odds ratios. Thus, it is important to have at least a basic level of understanding of these statistics. In this section, the most commonly used epidemiological statistics are discussed briefly including ratios, proportions, and rates, incidence and prevalence, relative risk and odds ratios as well as sensitivity, specificity, and predictive values.

RATIO, PROPORTIONS, AND RATES

Ratios, proportions, and rates are terms used interchangeably in the medical literature without regard for the actual mathematical definitions. Further, there are a considerable number of proportions and rates available to researchers, each providing unique information. Thus, it is important to be aware of how each of these measures are defined and calculated.[7]

- A ratio expresses the relationship between two numbers. For example, consider the ratio of men to women diagnosed with multiple sclerosis (MS). If, in a sample consisting of only MS patients, 100 men and 50 women are diagnosed, the ratio of men to women is 100 to 50, or 100:50, or 2:1. Remember, that the order in which the ratio is presented is vitally important; that is, 100:50 is not the same as 50:100.

- A proportion is a specific type of ratio indicating the probability or percentage of the total sample that experienced an outcome or event without respect to time. Here, the numerator of the proportion, representing patients with the disease, is included in the denominator, representing all individuals at risk. For example, say 850 non-MS patients are added to the sample of 150 MS patients from the example above to create a total sample of 1000 patients. Thus, the proportion of patients with MS is 0.15 or 15% (i.e., 150/1000).

A rate is a special form of a proportion that includes a specific study period, typically used to assess the speed at which the event or outcome is developing.[8] A rate is equal to the number of events in a specified time period divided by the length of the time period. For example, say over a 1-year study period, 50 new cases of MS were diagnosed out of the 850 previously undiagnosed individuals. Thus, the rate of new cases of MS within this sample is 50 per year.

INCIDENCE AND PREVALENCE

Incidence quantifies the occurrence of an event or outcome over a specific study period within a specific population of individuals. The incidence rate is calculated by dividing the number of new events by the population at risk, with the population at risk defined as the total number of people who have not experienced the outcome. For example, consider the 50 new cases of MS that developed from the example above from the 850 originally undiagnosed individuals. The incidence rate is approximately 0.06 (i.e., 50/850). Note the denominator did not include the 150 patients already diagnosed with MS because these individuals could longer be in the population at risk.

Prevalence quantifies the number of people who have already experienced the event or outcome at a specific time point. Prevalence is calculated by dividing the total number of people experiencing the event by the total number of individuals in the population. Note that the denominator is everyone in the population, not just individuals in the population at risk. For example, the diagnosed MS cases (i.e., 50 + 150 = 200) would be divided by the population that includes them. That is, the prevalence of MS in this sample is 0.20 (i.e., 200/1000).

Finally, it is important to consider both incidence and prevalence when describing events or outcomes. This is because prevalence varies directly with incidence and the duration of the sickness or disease. For example, consider influenza where the duration of the sickness is relatively short. Thus, while incidence of new influenza cases may be high the overall prevalence may be low because most individuals recover quickly. By contrast, consider individuals diagnosed with asthma. Because asthma is incurable, the prevalence of the disease may be high, whereas the incidence may be low depending on the total number of new cases diagnosed throughout the year.

RELATIVE RISK AND ODDS RATIO

Relative risk is defined as the ratio (or probability) of the incidence of an event occurring in individuals exposed to a stimulus compared to the incidence of the event in those not exposed to the stimulus. Relative risk can be calculated directly from the cohort study design (see Chapter 5). Briefly, this design is typically a prospective observational design comparing the incidence of experiencing an event in cohorts of exposed and unexposed individuals over time.

Relative risk is used when comparing the probability of an event occurring to all possible events considered in a study. For example, consider the risk of developing lung cancer in those who are exposed and unexposed to second-hand smoke over a 10-year study period. Upon study conclusion, the 2×2 contingency table, shown in Figure 8–7, is created containing frequency counts of events for two groups exposed and unexposed to the second-hand smoke stimulus. This table provides all data necessary to calculate the incidence of the event for both exposed and unexposed individuals. Relative risk is calculated by dividing the proportion of individuals who suffered the event in the exposed group (i.e., A/A + B) by the proportion of individuals who suffered the event in the unexposed group (i.e., C/C + D). Relative risk provides a single number ranging from zero to infinity, and there are three resulting interpretations provided below.[6]

1. If relative risk equals 1, the risk of experiencing the event was equal within the exposed and unexposed groups. Thus, there is no association of being exposed to the stimulus.

2. If relative risk is greater than 1, the exposed group has a greater risk of experiencing the event compared to the unexposed group. Thus, there is a positive association or detrimental effect (risk factor) of being exposed to the stimulus.

3. If relative risk is less than 1, the exposed group has a lower risk of experiencing the event compared to the unexposed group. Thus, there is a negative association or protective effect of being exposed to the stimulus.

When relative risk cannot be calculated, researchers will often present an odds ratio. Odds are calculated by dividing the proportion of people experiencing an event by the proportion of people not experiencing an event. Thus, an odds ratio is a ratio of two odds; one for individuals exposed to the stimulus and the other for those not exposed to the stimulus. Odds ratios range from zero to infinity. They have three interpretations identical to those presented above for relative risk, simply substitute the odds ratio for relative risk.

	Event	No Event	
Exposed	A	B	A+B
Unexposed	C	D	C+D
	A+C	B+D	A+B+C+D

Figure 8–7. Example of a 2×2 contingency table.

Odds ratios can be calculated for both cohort and case-control designs. A case-control study compares cases that have experienced the event and controls who have not, and then assesses whether each individual was exposed to a stimulus or not. Thus, a case-control study is retrospective.

Odds ratios are used when comparing events to nonevents with its calculation depending on the study design. For example, consider comparing a group of individuals who developed measles to those who did not and then determining whether they received all recommended vaccinations. In a cohort study, the odds ratio is calculated by dividing the odds of experiencing the event in the exposed group (i.e., A/B) by the odds the unexposed group who experienced the event (i.e., C/D). In a case-control study, the odds ratio is calculated by dividing the odds that cases were exposed to the risk (i.e., A/C) by the odds that the controls were exposed (i.e., B/D).

Relative risk and odds ratios are comparable in magnitude only when the outcome under study is rare (e.g., some cancers). It is important to consider that odds ratios consistently overestimate risk when the outcome is more common (e.g., hyperlipidemia). As a result, relative risk should be used if possible and caution should be exhibited when interpreting odds ratios.

SENSITIVITY, SPECIFICITY, AND PREDICTIVE VALUES

Sensitivity, specificity, and positive and negative predictive values indicate the ability of a test to identify correctly those experiencing the event and those who did not. For example, consider the ability of a blood glucose screening test to correctly identify individuals with diabetes. Four outcomes result from this test, which are required for the calculation of sensitivity, specificity, and the predictive values:

1. True positives (TP) have the disease and have a positive test result.
2. False positives (FP) do not have the disease, but have a positive test result.
3. True negatives (TN) do not have the disease and have a negative test result.
4. False negatives (FN) have the disease, but have a negative test result.

Sensitivity is the probability a diseased individual will have a positive test result and is the true positive rate of the test. It is calculated by dividing true positives by all individuals who actually have the disease (i.e., TP/TP + FN). Specificity is the probability a disease-free individual will have a negative test result and is the true negative rate of the screening test. It is calculated by dividing true negatives by all disease-free individuals (i.e., TN/TN + FP).

Positive and negative predictive values are calculated to measure the accuracy of the screening test. Both predictive values are directly related to disease prevalence; that is, the higher the prevalence, the higher the predictive value.[6] Positive predictive value provides the proportion of individuals who test positive for the disease that actually have the disease. It is calculated by dividing true positives by all individuals with a positive test result (i.e., TP/TP + FP). Negative predictive value provides the proportion of individuals who test negative who are actually disease-free. It is calculated by dividing true negatives by all individuals with a negative test result (i.e., TN/TN + FN).

It is important to identify the implications all four values have to new and existing research. When designing a study involving a screening test, researchers must indicate a standard cutoff score for their screening. That is, qualify who is to be considered diseased and who will be considered disease-free. This decision clearly reflects the repercussions of classifying individuals as false negatives or false positives. For example, consider a screening tool for early stage breast cancer, where there are considerable consequences for both false positives and false negatives. On the one hand, a patient with a false positive may be referred for unnecessary testing that is painful and expensive, not to mention emotionally taxing. On the other hand, a false negative has more serious implications, since the patient may not receive any treatment until the disease has progressed.

Types of Study Design

The distinction between experimental, quasi-experimental, and nonexperimental research is important, both from a study design perspective and when evaluating literature. Although experimental designs are considered the gold standard by many, do not discount research conducted using quasi-experimental and nonexperimental designs, as long as the limitations are considered. Each of these types of designs will be discussed below.

EXPERIMENTAL DESIGNS

In the biomedical sciences, experimental designs are typically referred to as a randomized controlled trial (RCT). A full treatment of experimental design is presented in Chapters 4 and 5, so the discussion provided here will only touch the tip of the iceberg on experimental designs. Interested readers are encouraged to consult the suggested readings provided at the end of this chapter for more information.

First, experimental designs always allow the researcher to manipulate levels of an IV. For example, consider a drug trial assessing the effectiveness of a new cancer medication. For this trial, four groups of participants are randomly assigned to a different dose of a medication. Thus, there are four levels of the IV. The researcher, within ethical and theoretical constraints, can manipulate the size of the dose, if the participants will be measured multiple times, and the length of the study period.

Second, in experimental design participants are randomly assigned to levels of the IV; thus, any participant has a chance of being placed in any single group. There are many different methods and theories of randomization and the chance of being in one group versus another does not necessarily have to be equal. For example, consider a study that has two treatment groups and one placebo group where the researcher is interested in the difference between the treatment groups. Because the difference in the DV between the placebo and either treatment group will usually be larger than the difference in the DV between the treatment groups, the researcher may randomize more participants to the treatment groups to increase statistical power to detect the difference between treatments. Note that the concept of statistical power is discussed in the Statistical Inference section below as well as in Chapter 4. Often a 2:2:1 or 3:3:1 randomization schedule will be used with two or three times as many participants, respectively, being randomized to treatment as opposed to placebo.

Third, causality can be determined with proper experimental control of error. For example, the effectiveness of a cancer drug can be better explained by reducing sources of error due to the participant (e.g., age, health status), setting (e.g., prescriber's office), or diagnostic tests (e.g., measurement accuracy).

Finally, it should be noted RCTs have limitations. The primary limitation is cost, as RCTs are extremely costly requiring many considerations including space, personnel, and participants. RCTs also may have limited external validity and generalizability due to extreme control over experimental conditions (e.g., efficacy study) that do not necessarily translate to real world situations (e.g., effectiveness study). Third, it is difficult, if not impossible, to study rare events with an RCT due to ethical concerns and the considerable sample size required.

QUASI-EXPERIMENTAL DESIGNS

Quasi-experimental designs are used more often in the social sciences, but they can be observed in the biomedical literature. On the surface, these types of designs appear to be experimental; however, they lack one key aspect, random assignment.

For example, consider examining the effectiveness of a new dialysis treatment. Most dialysis patients are already in the care of a nephrologist at a specific clinic. Because nephrologists typically see numerous patients, randomizing patients to specific levels of treatment (i.e., the IV) within a group that is under the care of the same nephrologist may be unfeasible logistically or may lead to medication errors. Thus, the entire clinic must be randomized. That is, all patients within a specific clinic will receive one treatment.

Advantages of quasi-experimental designs include reduced cost and a quicker time-line compared to RCTs with the addition of possible increases in external validity due to conditions being more consistent with the real world. The disadvantages, however, are considerable. This is most notable with the lack of random assignment. Nonrandom assignment may create dissimilar groups based on any number of characteristics that are potentially related to the success of the treatment. For example, consistent differences in patient demographics (e.g., sickness) may result from a dialysis clinic in the suburbs being compared to a dialysis clinic in a more urban setting. Further, causation cannot be implied and statistical analysis can potentially be rendered uninformative.[9]

NONEXPERIMENTAL DESIGNS

Nonexperimental designs have several advantages over RCTs, primarily lower cost, a quicker timeline to publication, and a broader range of participants.[10] The advantages of nonexperimental studies over RCTs have prompted their widespread use in the biomedical sciences. Overall, these studies tend to be nonrandomized, retrospective, and correlational in nature and are distinct because the researcher cannot manipulate the IV(s).

For example, consider a 5-year retrospective study assessing the effectiveness of statin therapy on preventing cardiac events. The researcher has knowledge of which patients initiated statin therapy, but has no control over the drug, dose, adherence, etc. Although the researcher may assign patients to groups based on dose size, the researcher cannot randomly assign patients to a specific drug nor can they manipulate the dose. In addition, nonexperimental research often fails to indicate causality, which is due to lack of experimental control and randomization as well as inability to identify all confounding variables. Finally, it is important to note that while nonexperimental designs are ubiquitous in the biomedical sciences, treatment effects may be different when compared to RCTs.[11]

Case Study 8–1

The human body needs vitamin D to absorb calcium. Without sufficient calcium absorption the body will extract calcium from its bone stores thereby weakening bone and increasing the probability of bone fractures. An endocrinologist interested in bone metabolism is considering a 6-month prospective study to evaluate whether differing doses of vitamin D will affect rates of calcium absorption in postmenopausal women. The researcher plans to enroll her own patients from those seen at her clinic. Calcium absorption will be measured by the dual isotope tracer method and vitamin D will be measured as serum 25-hydroxyvitamin D (25OHD). Both will be treated as continuous variables in statistical analysis. After baseline calcium absorption and 25OHD measurements are collected, participants will be randomized into four groups—one placebo group and three groups ingesting a different orally administered vitamin D supplement daily for 6 months (i.e., 500 international units, 2500 international units, and 5000 international units). At the end of the 6-month study period, calcium absorption will be measured again.

1. Describe the population of interest.
2. What sampling strategy or strategies were used?
3. Would this study be considered a randomized controlled trial? Why or why not?
4. What is the DV for this study? What is the scale of measurement for the DV?
5. What is the IV for this study? What is the scale of measurement for the IV? How many levels does the IV have? What about the IV is manipulated by the researcher?
6. Based on the study description, were any confounding variables or covariates considered for this study?
7. The researcher is planning on using the binomial distribution to evaluate the probability the participant is calcium deficient. Is this correct given the scale of the DV? If not, what distribution would be a better option to consider?
8. The researcher is planning on presenting calcium absorption and 25OHD as median and IQR. Is this the most appropriate measure of central tendency for these variables?
9. A histogram of the calcium absorption variable indicated severe positive skewness, but no outliers. The researcher is considering using a square root transformation of the DV prior to analysis. Is a data transformation appropriate? Why or why not?

The Design and Analysis of Clinical Trials

The U.S. National Institutes of Health (NIH) defines five different types of clinical trials—treatment, prevention, diagnostic, screening, and quality of life.[12] In this chapter, two specific types of treatment clinical trials are discussed—the randomized controlled trial (RCT) and adaptive clinical trial (ACT). The experimental design of RCTs and ACTs are discussed at length in Chapters 4 and 5, so the descriptions provided in this chapter are minimal. Briefly, RCTs and ACTs are both protocol based, meaning that every step of the study from design to analysis is identified *a priori*. They are prospective studies where participants are followed over time using strict experimental control to indicate reliably the causality between the DV and manipulated IV.

THE DESIGN OF CLINICAL TRIALS

Parallel-Groups Design
The most common RCT is a parallel-groups design, where the IV typically involves participants randomized into fixed levels of treatment, also known as treatment arms, with

each arm indicating a different treatment or comparison.[13–16] That is, participants are randomly assigned to one, and only one, treatment arm. As stated in the previous section, the sample size within each group does not have to be equal and can vary depending on estimated statistical power to detect treatment effects.

There are two parallel-groups designs frequently used in the biomedical sciences—group comparison and matched pairs.[15] Briefly, a group comparison design simultaneously compares at least two groups of participants after each group is randomized to a different level of the IV. In a matched pairs design, participants are matched based on one or more characteristics (e.g., age, race) and then randomized to levels of the IV.

Crossover Design

The second most common RCT is a crossover design. A crossover design has the primary advantage of each participant serving as his or her own control.[13,15] The primary advantage of a crossover design is that it requires fewer participants in comparison to a parallel-groups design due to the fact that at the end of the study all participants will have received all treatment arms. A disadvantage is that a crossover design cannot be used in a study where the first drug may cure the participant (e.g., an antibiotic given for an infection), since there would be no reason for the participant to crossover to the other agent.

For example, consider a 1-month study that includes two treatment arms. For a parallel-groups design, say 20 participants are required; that is, 10 participants are randomized to each treatment arm. By contrast, in a crossover design, only 10 subjects are required because each participant receives both treatments—10 participants receive the first treatment and the same 10 participants receive the second treatment. While both designs have two total measurements, in the parallel-groups design, two individual groups of participants provide one measurement each, whereas in the crossover design the same group of participants provides both measurements.

At this point, a common question is whether the effect of the first treatment carries over to influence the effect of the second treatment. This is a considerable concern in crossover designs and is dealt with by including a washout period between treatments. While the maximum duration of the washout period is arbitrary so long as the effect of the first treatment to be absent prior to beginning the second treatment, but not be so long that participant attrition becomes a concern.

Adaptive Design

A more recent advancement to the RCT is the adaptive design or ACT. Although an ACT is possibly cheaper and more ethical than an RCT, this design is much more complex to both implement and analyze. Briefly, ACTs implement changes or adaptations in the design of the study based on the results of a predetermined set of interim statistical analyses. Interim analyses can be based on blinded or unblinded data, with the resulting adaptations aimed at establishing a more efficient, safer, and informative trial that is more likely to demonstrate treatment effects.[17]

For example, consider a 3-year study examining the effect of three different large doses of vitamin D on parathyroid hormone. Because implementing large doses of vitamin D is controversial, ethical considerations require this study to be adaptive. Here, the interim analyses would provide important information regarding the effectiveness and safety of the doses. Say, for example, that the ACT has interim analyses scheduled quarterly. Further, say that at the end of the second quarter of the first year the interim analyses indicated that the group receiving the highest dose of vitamin D had twice the risk of developing kidney stones compared to the other two groups. Thus, the group receiving the highest dose of vitamin D could have their dose reduced or the group could be dropped from the study completely. After these adaptations are implemented, the study continues as designed.

THE ANALYSIS OF CLINICAL TRIALS

The analysis of clinical trials typically involves evaluating repeated measures data where participants are followed prospectively over time or conducting an endpoint analysis using only the last observation or measurement. Regardless of the study design, the choice of the appropriate statistical test to analyze these data is based primarily on the scale of measurement of the DV, but other factors should also be considered (see the Selecting the Appropriate Statistical Test section later in the chapter).

Because an endpoint analysis is straightforward conceptually, a brief discussion of repeated measures design and analysis considerations is presented. Using a repeated measures design allows researchers to study the treatment effects over time in a smaller sample of participants due to the increased statistical power. Briefly, a repeated measures design increases statistical power by removing the error variance due to the participant. That is, each participant serves as their own control. Removing error variance is important because it results in larger test statistics and an increased probability of achieving statistical significance. However, a repeated measures design has limitations relevant to clinical trials, primarily participant attrition and nonadherence.

Attrition and nonadherence can assume many forms in a clinical trial. For example, participants may drop out of the study, fail to complete all required measurements, receive incorrect treatment or doses, or a myriad of other possible protocol violations. Thus, the first part of this section will discuss how the analysis of clinical trials typically handles missing data due to attrition and nonadherence. The final sections discuss the analysis of parallel-group, crossover, and adaptive designs.

Intent-to-Treat and Per-Protocol Approaches

Two analytical approaches exist for clinical trials—intent-to-treat (ITT) and per-protocol (PP). The ITT approach is often employed in the presence of violations to protocol or patients being lost to follow-up. ITT is the approach most often used in the biomedical literature. ITT requires the analysis to include all participants in the arm to which they were randomized originally. That is, treatment effects are best evaluated by the planned treatment protocol rather than the actual treatment given.[18]

For example, consider a participant randomized to receive treatment A but instead receives treatment B. For analysis, this participant would be considered as receiving treatment A. It should be noted that if a large number of protocol violations of this nature occur, the study would be discontinued; thus, these occurrences are relatively rare. It is important to note that for ITT has considerable weaknesses. Most notably, for ITT to be unbiased, attrition and nonadherence are considered to occur completely at random.[14] However, this is an untestable hypothesis. Further, the ITT approach can dilute treatment effects simply by including nonadherent participants by employing the last observation carried forward (LOCF) technique discussed later in this section.

By comparison, the PP approach evaluates only compliant participants with complete data. Although this analysis is straightforward analytically and allows researchers to evaluate a more accurate treatment effect, it has substantial limitations, primarily, reduced statistical power compared to an ITT approach, because participants with incomplete data are not considered in analysis.[18]

Because the ITT approach considers all participants with at least one measurement, an imputation or replacement method is often employed for missing measurements. The LOCF technique is one of the most commonly used imputation methods. This method uses the last recorded measurement for a participant for every missing measurement. For example, consider a study measuring HbA1c measured on six occasions over a 1-year study period. If a participant had only the first three measurements, the third (i.e., last) measurement would be imputed for measurements four through six. **❺** *From this example, it is clear the LOCF technique may not only dilute treatment effects, but also introduce significant bias into the results of statistical tests.* Therefore, be cautious when evaluating a study that has employed the LOCF technique. As a result of these limitations, better imputation approaches have been suggested including multiple imputation and the use of maximum likelihood estimation. These techniques are beyond the scope of this chapter, but are valid and produce unbiased estimates if data are considered missing at random.[19,20]

Analyzing Parallel-Groups Designs

When analyzing a parallel-groups design, the traditional approach is to conduct an endpoint analysis using only the final measurement. If the DV is continuous, analysis will typically require an independent samples t-test for two groups, one-way analysis of variance (ANOVA) for more than two groups, or analysis of covariance (ANCOVA) for two or more groups, statistically controlling for a baseline DV measurement. If the DV is categorical, an endpoint analysis will typically require a chi-square test or logistic regression analysis. Note that these analyses are discussed in detail in the Statistical Tests section later in the chapter.

For example, consider a study designed to assess the effect of lubiprostone compared to placebo in treating chronic constipation associated with Parkinson disease. Following randomization, this 1-month study will assess constipation symptoms twice—at the end of the second and fourth week. An endpoint analysis would only consider the treatment effect at the end of week 4, ignoring the measurement at the end of week 2. Thus, it is clear that this type of analysis does not consider the repeated measures, and, as a result, does not consider the changes occurring over time. Further, an endpoint analysis does not take full advantage of statistical power increases from a longitudinal design as discussed in the Design and Analysis of Clinical Trials section.

By contrast, to assess for change over time using repeated measures for a continuous DV, researchers often employ a mixed between-within ANOVA or mixed-effects linear regression. Briefly, these analyses assess differences between treatment groups as well as changes over time within treatment groups. The major benefit of these analyses is provided by the interaction effect, which evaluates whether the change over time was different between the two treatment arms (see Figure 8–8). To evaluate group differences in change over time for a categorical DV, researchers are required to employ a mixed-effects logistic regression. This analysis allows the researcher to evaluate group differences and interaction effects. In general, mixed-effects analyses are extremely complex and even a brief overview of this analysis is well beyond the scope of this chapter. With that said, when these analyses are most appropriate is provided in the Selecting the Appropriate Statistical Tests section. Interested readers are encouraged to consult the suggested readings at the end of the chapter for a treatment of this analysis.

As an example of analyzing a parallel-groups design, reconsider the lubiprostone example. Say the results are presented graphically in Figure 8–8. Notice that two groups experience drastically different change in constipation symptoms between the end of week 2 and the end of week 4. The between-group difference in constipation symptoms over time is the interaction effect. Because a lower number of symptoms are indicative of treatment success, Figure 8–8 shows that the effect of lubiprostone is more effective compared to placebo over the study period.

Following a statistically significant interaction effect, researchers can conduct follow-up or *post hoc* tests to determine where the significant difference occurred. In Figure 8–8, there is likely no statistically significant difference in constipation symptoms between groups at the end of week 2, but there is a likely statistically significant difference at the

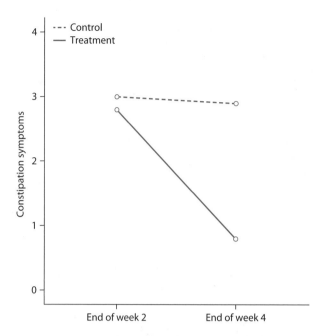

Figure 8–8. Statistically significant interaction effect.

end of week 4. Therefore, *post hoc* tests can assist researchers in identifying the shortest treatment time or minimum effective dose by indicating where treatment effects diminish (e.g., the slope plateaus) or indicating when differences between doses converge and are no longer statistically significant.

Analyzing Crossover Designs

The purpose of the crossover design is to study treatment effects using the participant as his or her own control. Remember, in a crossover design each participant receives all treatment arms, with an adequate washout period occurring between arms to prevent the carryover of treatment effects. For example, consider the lubiprostone example described in the Analyzing Parallel-Groups Designs section. Instead of having two treatment arms as in a parallel-groups design, the crossover design would randomize participants into a different treatment order. That is, Group A would receive lubiprostone and Group B would receive placebo for the first 2 weeks. At the end of the 2-week study period, constipation symptoms are assessed. Next, all participants are required to have a 3-week washout period purported to effectively eliminate any carryover effects of the lubiprostone. Note that during the washout period the placebo is not given either. After the washout period, Group A would receive placebo and Group B would receive lubiprostone for 2 weeks. At the end of this second 2-week study period, constipation symptoms are assessed again.

Statistically, a crossover design requires an initial test for order effects. If the DV is continuous, order effects are assessed by evaluating the interaction effect between order of treatment and the IV using a mixed between-within ANOVA or a mixed-effects linear regression. These analyses are described in detail in the Selecting the Appropriate Statistical Test section later in the chapter, but for now consider both analyses useful when evaluating interaction effects. When testing for order effects, a statistically significant interaction indicates that the order in which the treatments were received influenced the treatment effect. For example, say that receiving lubiprostone prior to placebo had a different treatment effect than receiving placebo prior to lubiprostone. A clear order effect is presented in Figure 8–9. Notice the effect of placebo differs depending on the order in which it was received. The presence of a statistically significant order effect can have multiple explanations. Considering the example and Figure 8–9, it is clear the washout period may not have been long enough, as the effectiveness of lubiprostone carried over to measurement of the placebo. In addition, the groups may have been initially different following randomization. Whenever a statistically significant order effect is identified, no further analysis is conducted as any subsequent analyses are biased by this order effect. However, if the interaction is nonsignificant and the DV is continuous, an endpoint analysis is typically evaluated via paired-samples t-test (also explained in detail in the Selecting the Appropriate Statistical Test section later in the chapter). That is, treatment differences between lubiprostone and placebo are assessed without respect to the order in which the treatments were received.

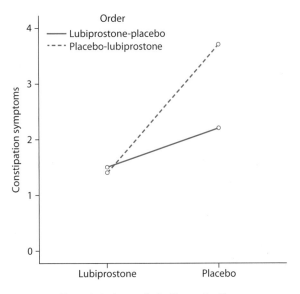

Figure 8–9. Statistically significant order effect.

Analyzing Adaptive Designs

The statistical analyses and considerations used when analyzing adaptive designs are similar to parallel-groups and crossover designs. If the DV is continuous, statistical tests used during the interim analyses or on the study endpoint typically include an independent-samples t-test for comparing two groups, one-way ANOVA for comparing more than two groups, or ANCOVA for statistically controlling baseline DV measurement. Note that the DV for the interim analyses is the most recent measurement. If the DV is categorical, an interim analysis will typically require a chi-square test or logistic regression analysis. All of the analyses mentioned are discussed in detail in the Statistical Tests section later in chapter.

Several important considerations are required when analyzing and interpreting the results from adaptive designs.[17] First, all interim and endpoint analyses suffer the potential risk of inflated Type I errors. Briefly, a Type I error can be thought of as a false positive. That is, the statistical test could indicate a statistically significant result when the result is actually not significant. Type I error has been discussed in Chapter 4 and in the Statistical Inference section later in this chapter. With this definition in mind, as the number of interim analyses increase the probability of finding a false positive might increase as well. To adjust for this possibility, researchers will often make the criteria for achieving statistical significance more conservative by adjusting alpha (see the Statistical Inference section later in chapter for a full description of alpha). Note that adjusting alpha is not a ubiquitous practice and there is no universal recommendation for doing so. Just be aware that inflated Type I errors may be an issue in an ACT.

Second, estimates of population parameters may be biased. That is, any adaptation can reduce the generalizability to the original population sampled, produce underestimated or overestimated parameter estimates, and produce misleading confidence intervals. Researchers must carefully document and provide rationale for adaptations resulting from interim analysis. Failure to do so will indicate results should be viewed with extreme caution.

Finally, when all adaptations are considered, the overall results of the endpoint analyses may actually be invalid, providing inaccurate support for treatment effects. Consumers of research are urged strongly to consider these factors when interpreting and evaluating research using adaptive designs.

Statistical Inference

Inferential statistics provide the probability a difference or association is actually observed in the population based on the analysis of sample data. Inferential statistics allow researchers to make rational decisions in the presence of random processes and variation. This section presents several requirements that need to be considered prior to conducting and evaluating the result of a statistical test. First, the sampling distribution and application of the **central limit theorem** are discussed, followed by hypothesis testing, as well as Type I and Type II errors and statistical power. Then, the difference between statistical and clinical significance is presented. Finally, the appropriate uses of parametric and nonparametric statistical tests are provided as well as a brief description of degrees of freedom.

SAMPLING DISTRIBUTIONS AND THE CENTRAL LIMIT THEOREM

Statistical inference uses sampled data to make conclusions about a specific population. Because quality samples are chosen randomly, the means produced from these samples are also random.[21] Given this information, it is important to remember that the mean may not be exactly representative of the population and will vary from sample to sample. However, the law of large numbers states as the size of the sample increases, the sample mean will move closer to the population mean. Further, as the number of samples increases, the mean of the sample means will begin to approximate the population mean. **❻** *The central limit theorem states when equally sized samples are drawn from a non-normal distribution, the plotted mean values from each sample will approximate a normal distribution as long as the non-normality was not due to outliers.*

A distribution of the sampled means calculated from repeated samples is termed the distribution of sampling means. For example, consider a study to analyze the mean value of blood urea nitrogen (BUN) in the general, healthy population, where the researcher selects 100 random samples of 10 healthy participants. Each sample of 10 will provide a mean BUN value. Although mean BUN will vary from sample to sample, when the 100 sample means are plotted in a histogram, this distribution of sampling means will begin to approximate the actual population distribution.

The central limit theorem states sufficiently large samples should approximate a normal distribution of sampling means as long as the data do not contain outliers. A sufficiently large sample is generally considered to consist of 30 or more participants or a situation where the degrees of freedom for the statistical test are greater than 20.[22] Note that degrees of freedom are discussed later in this section. In addition, researchers must be careful not to confuse the issue of having a large enough sample to achieve statistical significance and a large enough sample to be representative of the population.

As with any normal distribution, the standard deviation of the distribution of sampling means can be calculated. This is termed the standard error of the mean (SEM). The SEM is equal to the standard deviation divided by the square root of the sample size, and reflects variability within the sample means. Further, standard error is used in the majority of statistical tests. It is important when evaluating the literature to understand the relationship between the standard deviation and the SEM. Researchers often present the SEM to show variability or noise in their data. Note that the SEM will always be smaller than the standard deviation. Thus, the use of SEM will suggest the data is less variable and often more appealing.

HYPOTHESIS TESTING

A hypothesis indicates a theory about the population regarding an outcome the researcher is interested in studying. The statistical analyses discussed in this chapter evaluate two types of hypotheses, the **null hypothesis** and the alternative or research hypothesis. That is, the analyses discussed employ procedures generally known as null hypothesis significance testing (NHST). The null hypothesis (H_0) assumes no difference or association between the different study groups or variables, whereas the **alternative hypothesis** (H_A or H_1) states there is a difference or association between the different study groups or variables. A representative, ideally random, sample is then drawn from the population of interest to estimate the difference or relationship and test whether this difference or relationship rejects or fails to reject the null hypothesis. It is important to note that failing to reject the null hypothesis does not indicate the null hypothesis is true. This is a common misconception observed frequently in the literature. There are often many other reasons for failing to reject the null hypothesis including inadequate experimental design, inadequate control over extraneous variables, and inadequate sample size to detect the effect of interest, among others.

When testing a specific hypothesis, a researcher is required to determine whether their hypothesis is directional or not. A directional hypothesis requires a **one-tailed** hypothesis test, whereas a nondirectional hypothesis requires a **two-tailed** hypothesis test. For example, consider a hypothesis which states that initiating statin therapy will lower low-density lipoproteins (LDL). Note that use of the term lower implies directionality and requires a one-tailed test. If, however, the researchers were looking for any effect of statin therapy, whether lowering or raising LDL, the hypothesis is nondirectional and would require a two-tailed test. In the literature, it is generally more acceptable to use a two-tailed test, even if the hypothesis is directional because a two-tailed test is more conservative statistically, thereby reducing the probability of a spurious statistical significance.

ERROR AND STATISTICAL POWER

It is essential that researchers establish how much error they are willing to accept before initiating a study. NHST can only result in four possible outcomes, which can be observed in Table 8–2. Type I and Type II have been discussed at length in Chapter 4, but briefly, a **Type I error** occurs when a statistical test rejects the null hypothesis by indicating a statistically significant difference when, in fact, the null hypothesis is true (i.e., false positive). A **Type II error** occurs when the researcher fails to reject the null hypothesis by not indicating a statistically significant difference when, in fact, the null hypothesis is false (i.e., false negative). Type I and Type II errors are interconnected; that is, as the probability

TABLE 8–2. FOUR POSSIBLE OUTCOMES OF NULL HYPOTHESIS SIGNIFICANCE TESTING (NHST)

	Truth	
Decision	**False H_0**	**True H_0**
Reject H_0	Correctly reject H_0	Type I error
Fail to reject H_0	Type II error	Correctly fail to reject H_0

of one error increases the other decreases. Researchers must consider these two errors carefully when designing studies, weighing whether a false positive is more or less concerning than a false negative.

Statistical power was developed as a method allowing researchers to calculate the probability of finding a statistically significant result, when, in fact, one actually exists. This topic has been discussed in Chapter 4. Essentially, increasing statistical power reduces the probability of committing a Type II error; however, it can also increase the probability of committing a Type I error as described in the previous paragraph. Statistical power is influenced by four factors: alpha defined as the probability value at which the null hypothesis is rejected, effect size defined as the size of the treatment effect (discussed later), error variance defined as the precision of the measurement instrument, and the sample size. Statistical power can be increased by increasing alpha, effect size, or sample size as well as by decreasing error variance. Note that statistical power of 0.80 has been defined as adequate.[23] However, some researchers use 0.90 or higher in the biomedical sciences, indicating that a false negative is more detrimental than a false positive, such as when evaluating the effectiveness of a novel breast cancer treatment.

STATISTICAL VERSUS CLINICAL SIGNIFICANCE

Alpha and p Values

The next step in the research process is to employ a statistical test to assess whether a difference or relationship is due to random variation. The researcher is interested in determining whether the observed difference or relationship rejects or fails to reject the null hypothesis. **Alpha** (α) is the conventionally designated decision criterion for rejecting the null hypothesis and ranges from 0 to 1. Alpha is defined as the theoretical probability of rejecting the null hypothesis conditional on the null hypothesis being true. Alpha does not represent the exact Type I error rate; instead, alpha is the upper bound of the Type I error rate. Although most studies typically set alpha at 0.05, this value is arbitrary. A more conservative (i.e., $\alpha = 0.01$) or liberal ($\alpha = 0.10$) alpha may be used in an attempt to show greater support for rejecting or retaining the null hypothesis, respectively. As an example, conservative alpha levels are often used to protect against Type I errors, whereas liberal alpha values are often used in drug equivalency trials where researchers are using data to show nonsignificant differences between the drugs.

Conceptually related to alpha is the probability value (i.e., **p value**). Statistical tests produce p values that range from 0 to 1. The formal definition of a p value is the probability of obtaining a test statistic as large as or larger than the one obtained, conditional on the null hypothesis being true. Graphically, a p value is directly indicative of the area under the probability distribution used by the statistical test. Note that the area under any proper probability distribution is 1. A quick glance at the appendices of any introductory statistics textbook will provide area under the curve values for various distributions. In more general terms, $p = 0.05$ indicates 5% of the distribution's area is to the left or right of the associated test statistic depending on whether it is positive or negative. For example, consider a one-tailed statistical test with a positive test statistic and reconsider Figure 8–5. A z-score of 1.645 leaves approximately 5% of the distribution to the right of this value. This example highlights how a p value less than 0.05 indicates that less than 5% of the values (or area) lies beyond a specific test statistic value. As an alternative example, consider a two-tailed (i.e., nondirectional) statistical test. A z-score of 1.96 leaves approximately 2.5% of the distribution to the right this value, whereas a z-score of -1.96 leaves approximately 2.5% of the distribution to the left of this value. Thus, a two-tailed test also leaves 5% of the area under the distribution when the two parts are aggregated. Regardless of whether a one- or two-tailed test was used, in general, if a p value is less than the specified alpha, the researcher rejects the null hypothesis and the difference or relationship is considered statistically significant. Alternatively, if the p value is equal to or greater than alpha, the researcher has failed to reject the null hypothesis and the difference or relationship is not considered statistically significant.

❼ *Be aware that there is continuing difficulty when interpreting* p *values, even among statisticians.*[24] *Therefore, it is important to be cognizant of several misconceptions about* p *values that are stated commonly in the literature.* First, a p value is not the exact probability of committing a Type I error. Second, the p value is not the probability that the null hypothesis is true, nor is $1 - p$ the probability that the alternative hypothesis is true. Third, a small p value is not evidence that the results will replicate nor can p values be compared directly across studies. Fourth, a p value indicates nothing about the magnitude of a difference or relationship. For example, a small p value (e.g., $p = 0.00001$) does not indicate a larger treatment effect than a larger p value (e.g., $p = 0.049$). Finally, for better or worse, alpha in NHST is treated like a cliff. For example, if alpha is set at 0.05 and a p value of 0.051 is obtained, a researcher will often state that a p value of 0.051 was trending toward significance or that the p value indicated marginal or moderate significance. These statements are often wholly incorrect! Thinking back to the discussion of one-tailed versus two-tailed significance tests provided in the Hypothesis Testing section, trending can only occur if the hypothesis is directional using a one-tailed test and the result obtained was in the hypothesized direction. Results can never be trending toward significance if the hypothesis was nondirectional using a two-tailed test because the alternative claim that the result was trending away from significance cannot be challenged.

Confidence Intervals

Statistical significance can also be established by calculating a confidence interval around the estimated population parameters (e.g., sample means, slopes) or test statistics (e.g., t). A confidence interval provides a range of scores likely to contain the unknown population parameter, and generally, a confidence interval is reported using a 95% confidence level. The calculation of confidence intervals includes both sample size and variability where smaller confidence intervals indicate less variability in the data. A 95% confidence interval is calculated by multiplying 1.96 by the SEM and adding or subtracting this value from the estimated parameter to find the upper and lower confidence limits, respectively. A 95% confidence interval indicates that if repeated random sampling occurs within the population of interest under consistent conditions (e.g., sample size), the true population parameter would be included in the interval 95% of the time. Thus, every value within the interval is considered a possible value of the population parameter.

Confidence intervals can be used it indicate statistical significance without the use of statistical tests. This process varies according to whether the researcher is examining population parameters or test statistics. For example, consider Figures 8–10, 8–11, and 8–12. In each figure, HbA1c values are being compared for a treatment and placebo group. Further, mean HbA1c for each group is presented as the circle, while the 95% confidence intervals are the whiskers extending above and below the means. The overlap of the confidence intervals between groups is directly related to p values; that is, less overlap is indicative of larger differences resulting in smaller p values. In Figure 8–10, notice that the confidence intervals do not overlap; thus, this difference can be assumed statistically significant at least at $p < 0.05$. Statistical significance can also be indicated

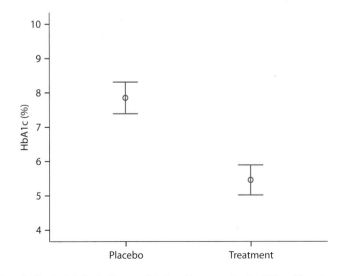

Figure 8–10. Statistically significant result indicated by non-overlapping 95% confidence intervals.

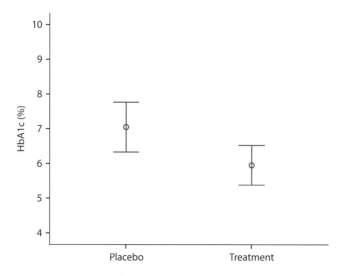

Figure 8–11. Statistically significant result indicated by overlapping 95% confidence intervals.

when the confidence intervals overlap as long as the overlap is less than approximately 50% of a whisker, as in Figure 8–11.[25] Finally, as shown in Figure 8–12, substantial overlap in confidence intervals indicates a nonstatistically significant difference (i.e., $p > 0.05$).

Determining statistical significance using confidence intervals around test statistics (e.g., t) uses procedures that vary based on the statistical test employed. For most parametric tests of group differences and correlation, a 95% confidence interval around the test statistic containing zero is not considered statistically significant at an alpha of 0.05.

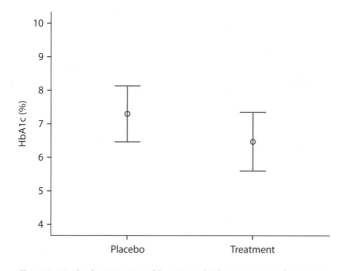

Figure 8–12. Overlapping 95% confidence interval indicating a nonsignificant result.

That is, statistical significance for these types of analyses are essentially testing that the differences or relationship are different from zero (i.e., $H_0 = 0$). Thus, a 95% confidence interval containing zero essentially indicates that it is plausible the true population differ-ence or relationship could be zero.[26] For example, consider the commonly used indepen-dent-samples t-test to evaluate for a difference between two group means (this statistical test is discussed in the Statistical Tests section below). Say that the test statistic pro-duced was 2.0, but the confidence interval ranged from –0.50 to 4.50. Based on this sample, the difference would not be considered statistically significant because it is plau-sible that in 95% of samples of the same size the true population parameter could in fact be zero.

Alternatively, the 95% confidence interval for test statistics based on ratios (e.g., odds ratios) that contain 1 are not considered statistically significant at an alpha of 0.05. Remember from the Epidemiological Statistics section, that an odds ratio or relative risk of 1 indicates no difference. Thus, a 95% confidence interval for a relative risk or an odds ratio that contains 1 indicates that it is plausible the true population parameter could in fact be an odds ratio or relative risk of 1. For example, say the result of a logistic regres-sion analysis produced an odds ratio of 2.5 (this statistical test is discussed in the Statisti-cal Tests section below). This value is greater than 1 indicating an increase in odds of experiencing the event. However, say the 95% confidence interval ranged from 0.50 to 15.0. Because the confidence interval contains 1, the odds ratio of 2.5 is not statistically significant using an alpha of 0.05.

Clinical Significance and Effect Size

❽ *When evaluating the significance of the finding, keep in mind that statistical significance (e.g., $p < 0.05$) does not indicate clinical significance. Statistical significance can be manip-ulated in several ways, most easily by increasing sample size drastically.* A sample size increase may artificially reduce error variance, which in turn reduces the standard error on which the test statistic is based. Reducing the standard error increases the value of the test statistic necessarily resulting in a smaller p value.

As an example, using a sample of 10,000 patients, researchers may find a CCB reduced blood glucose significantly in Type 1 DM patients. However, on examining the estimated parameters, the statistically significant difference in blood glucose was only 2 mg/dL, a decrease considered clinically insignificant.

This example highlights the importance of identifying and interpreting the clinical significance or effect size of all studies. While a complete discussion of effect size is beyond the scope of this chapter, larger effect size values are always preferred. Briefly, two different types of effect sizes exist. First, standardized difference effect sizes indicate a standardized difference between groups in standard deviation units. Examples commonly seen in the literature include Cohen's **d**, Glass' Δ, and Hedges' **g**.

As indicated by their name, standardized difference effect sizes are used when evaluating mean differences between groups. Further, because the effect sizes are standardized it may be easier to think of them as z-scores. Standardized difference effect sizes range from $-\infty$ to $+\infty$, with larger absolute values indicating larger effects. Second, effect size may also be reported as the proportion of variance explained. That is, how much of the reason a participant had a specific value of the DV is due to the IV. Examples commonly observed in the literature include R^2, ω^2, and η^2. Proportion of variance effect sizes is specific to tests of relationships or association as described in the Statistical Tests section below. Their values range from 0 to 1, with higher values indicating larger effects.

Given this information, it is important to remember that the definition of clinical significance varies by substantive area; thus, the definition of clinically significant to a bench researcher may be qualitatively different from an evidence-based practitioner. Finally, not all studies will provide an effect size estimate, especially in the biomedical sciences. Thus, research must be viewed with warranted skepticism until it can be determined whether the statistically significant difference or relationship is clinically meaningful.

PARAMETRIC VERSUS NONPARAMETRIC TESTING

The primary difference between parametric and nonparametric statistical tests is that parametric tests make assumptions regarding the descriptive characteristics of the normal distribution (i.e., mean, variance, skewness, and kurtosis). Nonparametric tests make a few or no distributional assumptions. In general, **parametric tests** are used only for interval and ratio scales, whereas **nonparametric tests** can be employed for any scale of measurement. Regardless, if the DV is measured on a continuous scale, the decision of which statistical test to employ typically begins with parametric tests. Because they assume a normal distribution, all parametric tests have several conservative and easily violated assumptions. These assumptions are testable, but vary depending on the statistical test employed. Therefore, in the Statistical Tests section below, all assumptions are described for each statistical test. It is important to know that employing a parametric test in the presence of a nondefined distribution will lead to inaccurate, biased, and unreliable parameter estimates. Therefore, when reading a journal article, if the authors neglect to provide information regarding assumption testing, caution should be exercised as it is unknown how much bias exists in their results.

Some assumption violations challenge the robustness of parametric tests greater than others. **Robustness** is defined as the ability of the statistical test to produce correct inferences in the presence of assumption violations. In most situations, any assumption violation requires the researcher to employ a nonparametric test, and most parametric tests have a widely used nonparametric alternative. Most, but not all, nonparametric statistical tests are distribution free, meaning they do not make inferences based on a defined probability distribution. Further, additional strengths of nonparametric tests include the ability to assess small sample sizes and the ability to assess data from several different populations.[27] However, it must be noted if the assumptions of a parametric test are tenable, parametric tests have greater statistical power to detect real effects compared to their nonparametric alternative(s).[28]

DEGREES OF FREEDOM

Degrees of freedom (df) are a vital component of all statistical tests, as most probability distributions, and statistical significance are based on them. Degrees of freedom are provided for all statistical tests and are a useful indicator of adequate sample size in the presence of assumption violations. For example, recall that the central limit theorem states the distribution of sampling means is approximately normal with degrees of freedom greater than 20. Thus, the central limit theorem operates independently of the distribution of the actual raw data. Therefore, if a researcher indicates that degrees of freedom for the statistical test are greater than 20, the results can typically be viewed as robust.

The definition of degrees of freedom is obscure and beyond the scope of this chapter; however, a brief description is provided. Degrees of freedom are conceptually defined as the number data points that are free to vary. Not all data is free to vary because values may have to be fixed by a specific sample parameter, such as the group mean. For example, consider a group of three participants who have a mean age of 50. Because the mean is 50, two of the participants can be of almost any age greater than zero. The third participant, however, must be the age that creates the mean of 50. Thus, if participant A is 40 and participant B is 45, participant C must be 65. That is, $[40 + 45 + 65]/3 = 50$. If instead, participant A is 75 and participant B is 40, then participant C must be 35. Therefore, because the age of two of the three participants could be just about any age greater than zero, there are two degrees of freedom (i.e., 2df)

Calculating degrees of freedom become increasingly complex in accordance with the complexity of the statistical test. That is, degrees of freedom for bivariate tests, such as those evaluating the difference between two group means, are easier to calculate and conceptualize than multivariate tests with multiple DVs. For the analyses described in the Statistical Tests section later in chapter, calculation of degrees of freedom is not explained explicitly, but it is important to note the distribution, probability, and statistical significance of all statistical tests are based on degrees of freedom. Further, degrees of freedom will usually be subscripted next to the test statistic for all parametric tests as well as for some nonparametric tests, such as the chi-square test. Subscripted degrees of freedom should be provided in the brief results section for all statistical tests described.

Selecting the Appropriate Statistical Test

While the information presented in this chapter has outlined the underlying processes of most statistical tests used in the biomedical sciences, the remainder of the chapter uses all previous information as a base to begin to integrate more directly useful information. This section presents decision trees that allow for determination of whether the appropriate statistical test was used in a journal article.

9 *The selection of the appropriate statistical test is based on several factors including the specific research question, the measurement scale of the DV, distributional assumptions, the number of DV measurements as well as the number and measurement scale of IVs and covariates, among others.* Tables 8–3 and 8–4 provide decision trees to identify the most appropriate statistical test based on the unique set of factors for statistical tests of group differences and statistical tests of association, respectively.

The first factor that needs to be addressed when selecting the most appropriate statistical test is whether the research question is phrased to evaluate differences or associations. In general, the last paragraph of the Introduction to any journal article should explicitly state the research questions, so give close attention to the phrasing of these questions. This may seem mundane, but it is important to note that all parametric tests of group differences are mathematically equivalent to parametric tests of association. Therefore, various parametric statistical tests can often be used interchangeably to answer the same research question. This can be seen in Tables 8–3 and 8–4 where one-way ANOVA can be used in the same situations as simple linear regression analysis. The overall statistical inference would be identical. This can be an overwhelmingly confusing concept for those with more novice statistical backgrounds. However, in general, when a research question is phrased to evaluate group differences (e.g., to determine whether three treatment groups differ on some outcome) follow the decision tree provided in Table 8–3, and when a research question is phrased to evaluate associations between variables (e.g., to determine whether a patient's age is associated with some outcome), follow Table 8–4.

The second factor to consider is the measurement scale of the DV. This is a much more concrete concept, but requires a thorough understanding of the four scales of variable measurement. Remember, nominal and ordinal scales are roughly classified as discrete or categorical, whereas interval and ratio scales are classified as continuous. Although it is often inappropriate, continuous variables may be also categorized into discrete variables. For example, categorization often occurs in the biomedical sciences with variables such as blood pressure, where exact systolic or diastolic blood pressure values are combined and categorized into low, normal, or high blood pressure.

The distributional assumptions of a statistical test involve complex explanations beyond the scope of this chapter. However, there are a few concepts to remember regarding

TABLE 8–3. CHOOSING THE MOST APPROPRIATE STATISTICAL TEST OF GROUP DIFFERENCES

	DV Scale	Distributional Assumptions Met	Repeated DV Measurements	Number of DV Measurements	Number of IVs	IV Levels	Covariates Allowed	Appropriate Statistical Test
Differences from known population	Continuous	Yes	No	1	0		No	One-sample z test
	Continuous	Yes	No	1	0		No	One-sample t-test
	Dichotomous		No	1	0		No	Binomial test
	Continuous		No	1	0		No	Kolmogorov-Smirnov test
Between-group differences	Continuous	Yes	No	1	1	2	No	Independent-samples t-test
	Ordinal or higher	No	No	1	1	2	No	Mann-Whitney test
	Ordinal or higher	No	No	1	1	2	No	Median test
	Continuous	Yes	No	1	1	≥ 2	No	One-way ANOVA
	Ordinal or higher	No	No	1	1	≥ 2	No	Kruskal-Wallis test
	Continuous	Yes	No	1	1	≥ 2	Yes	ANCOVA
	Continuous	Yes	No	1	≥ 2	≥ 2	No	Factorial ANOVA
Within-group differences	Continuous	Yes	Yes	2	0		No	Paired-samples t-test
	Ordinal or higher	No	Yes	2	0		No	Signed-rank test
	Ordinal or higher	No	Yes	2	0		No	Sign test
	Continuous	Yes	Yes	≥ 2	0		No	One-way RM-ANOVA
	Ordinal or higher	No	Yes	≥ 2	0		No	Friedman test
	Continuous	Yes	Yes	≥ 2	1	≥ 2	No	Mixed BW-ANOVA
	Dichotomous		Yes	2	0		No	McNemar test
	Dichotomous		Yes	≥ 2	0		No	Cochran Q test

TABLE 8–4. CHOOSING THE MOST APPROPRIATE STATISTICAL TEST OF ASSOCIATION

	DV Scale	Distributional Assumptions Met	Number of IVs	IV Scale	Covariates Allowed	Appropriate Statistical Test
One-sample association	Categorical		1	Categorical	No	Chi-square test
	Categorical		1	Categorical	No	Fisher's exact test
	Categorical		1	Categorical	Yes	Mantel-Haenszel test
Correlation and regression	Continuous	Yes	1	Continuous	No	Pearson's correlation
	Continuous	No	1	Continuous	No	Spearman's rank order correlation
	Continuous	Yes	1	Any	No	Simple linear regression
	Continuous	Yes	≥2	Any	Yes	Multivariable linear regression
	Dichotomous		1	Any	No	Simple logistic regression
	Dichotomous		≥2	Any	Yes	Multivariable logistic regression
Within-group regression	Continuous	Yes	≥0	Any	Yes	Mixed-effects linear regression[a]
	Dichotomous		≥0	Any	Yes	Mixed-effects logistic regression[a]
Time-to-event	Continuous	Yes	≥2		Yes	Cox proportional-hazards model
Reliability	Nominal		0		No	Kappa

[a]Mixed-effects linear and logistic regression models are complex analyses beyond the scope of this chapter. Therefore, they are not described in the Statistical Tests section. However, be aware that these analyses are available. Also, note that there is varying terminology used among researchers when describing these types of models; thus, in the literature mixed-effects models may be termed multilevel, hierarchical, nested, random effects, random coefficient, or random parameter models. The actual procedure for conducting the analyses remains identical regardless of the label attached to them.

distributions, most of which have been described in the Common Probability Distributions section above. First, distributional assumptions are required for all statistical tests using a continuous DV. Remember, the search for the most appropriate statistical test usually begins with parametric options, and all parametric statistical tests require a normal distribution (or application of the central limit theorem). Second, the distribution of the actual DV data is never considered when assessing distributional assumptions. Distributional assumptions are based on residual values, which represent the difference between the outcome predicted by the statistical model and the actual, observed outcome. Residuals are discussed in detail later in the simple linear regression analysis section. Third, if the distributional assumptions are violated, two options are generally available. First, the researcher could use a more appropriate distribution (see Table 8–1) or, second, they could employ a nonparametric statistical test. It is also common to see data transformation to attempt to force a normal distribution, but the considerable downside of this archaic technique was discussed previously in the Transforming Non-Normal Distributions section. It is more common in the biomedical literature to see a nonparametric test used, but be aware more statistically savvy researchers will use alternative distributions if the distributional assumption is violated.

The number of DV measurements is critically important to determine whether an appropriate statistical test was used. Note that studies using one DV measurement are known as **cross-sectional**, whereas studies using two or more DV measurements are known as **longitudinal**. If the DV was measured on multiple occasions, there is inherent association or correlation across DV measurements. That is, DV values from the same person inherently have a higher correlation compared to DV values from different people. Therefore, if a statistical test does not account for this correlation, the standard errors will be biased and improper statistical inference will occur.

It is also critically important to consider the number of IVs and covariates, their scale of measurement, the number of categorical IV levels, and whether the IVs and/or covariates interact. Note that the distribution of the IV or covariate is never considered in the statistical analysis. With that said, the scale of measurement for each IV and covariate is important when deciding which statistical test to employ. In general, ANOVA will usually be employed for categorical IVs, whereas regression analysis is required for continuous IVs. Note that the wording of the last sentence was chosen specifically. That is, although it was stated earlier that ANOVA and regression are mathematically equivalent, ANOVA cannot be used with continuous IVs. However, regression analysis can be used with any combination of IVs and covariates measured on any scale. This can be a confusing distinction. Another important concept is the number of levels for each categorical IV. Remember, a level can be thought of as the number of groups being studied and evaluated. When testing group differences, researchers will typically employ a t-test for two levels and ANOVA for three or more groups. Determining the number of levels is important because with three or more groups, the statistical test is an **omnibus test**. That is, an overall test result will be provided indicating a difference between at least two of the groups, but the test will not indicate specifically which groups differ. The concept of an omnibus test is discussed throughout the Statistical Tests section later in the chapter. Finally, whether an IV interacts with another IV or covariate is critically important. It is important to note that ANOVA can handle interactions between categorical IVs. Remember, an interaction indicates that the value of one IV is dependent on the value of another IV. For example, treatment group differences may be smaller in older patients (i.e., a treatment group-by-age interaction). However, if there is an interaction between a categorical IV and a continuous covariate, an ANOVA-type analysis, such as ANCOVA, cannot be used and a form of regression analysis must be used instead. Whether an interaction exists is an empirical question that is testable and described in the ANCOVA section later in the chapter.

Finally, other factors exist when determining whether the appropriate statistical test was used, but many are beyond the scope of this chapter. One key factor worth considering, however, is based on the concept of clustering (also known as nesting). Classic examples of clustering include children nested within the same classroom or patients nested within the same doctor. Clustering creates statistical issues that are similar to using a cross-sectional analysis on longitudinal data. That is, DV measurements from children nested within the same classroom have greater associations compared to DV measurements from children in different classrooms. Failing to account for clustering will result in biased standard errors and incorrect statistical inference. Although a description of the statistical analysis for clustered data is too complex for this chapter, recognizing when an analysis should account for (or should have accounted for) clustering is relatively easy, and the number of clustering levels can get as complex as the researcher desires. For example, patients could be nested within a doctor, the doctor could be nested within a clinic, the clinic could be nested within a hospital system, the hospital system could be nested within a city, and so on. When reading a journal article, take time to consider whether clustering should have been considered by the researchers. Do not be disheartened by the possibility of seeing an exorbitant number of clustering levels in any journal article. If clustering is considered, most studies in the biomedical sciences will only use two or three clustering units. The takeaway message is that careful thought must be undertaken when evaluating a study, especially when considering clustering. If clustering levels were not considered, but should have been, interpret all results with caution.

As an example of how to use Tables 8–3 and 8–4, say a researcher wanted to examine the effect a new statin medication had on the number of low-density lipoproteins (LDL) using a sample of 200 healthy patients. Although LDL has received a bad reputation, research has shown that the size of the LDL particles carrying the cholesterol is more predictive of future cardiovascular problems than the absolute LDL value measured in mg/dL.[29] More specifically, cholesterol carried by large, buoyant LDLs (i.e., Pattern A) has little association with cardiovascular problems, whereas cholesterol carried by small, dense LDLs (i.e., Pattern B) has been associated with a myriad of cardiovascular problems.[30] Therefore, a statin that only targets cholesterol carried by small, dense LDL is needed. Based on lipoprotein particle profile (LPP) testing, patients were placed into one of two groups based on LDL particle size (i.e., the IV: Pattern A versus Pattern B). The outcome for the study was LDL measured in mg/dL. Baseline measurements and demographic data were used as covariates and included categorized age (i.e., 40–49, 50–59, etc.), race, socioeconomic status indicated by whether the patient's mother graduated from high school, comorbid conditions, concurrent medications, and baseline LDL. The researchers hypothesized that the statin should reduce LDL significantly more in Pattern A patients compared to Pattern B patients. The analysis was completed at the end of a 6-month study period. In the method section, the researchers stated that baseline characteristics and demographic data were compared between the two groups of patients. Due to the presence of outliers, Mann-Whitney tests were used for all continuous variables and chi-square tests were used for categorical variables. For the primary analysis, multiple linear regression was used. No assumption violations were indicated.

The example above contains similar information to what is typically provided in the overwhelming majority of published literature. Thus, using the example information above, Tables 8–3 and 8–4 can be used to determine whether the statistical tests employed were appropriate. Note that all three of these tests are described in detail later in the chapter. For the baseline and demographic data, using Table 8–3, the Mann-Whitney test was used because the DV scale was continuous, distributional assumptions were not met due to outliers, the DV was only measured on one occasion, there was one IV with two levels, and no covariates were considered. Further, using Table 8–4, chi-square tests were used because both the DV and IV were categorical and no covariates were considered. For the primary analysis, using Table 8–4, multiple linear regression analysis was used because the scale of the DV was continuous, the distributional assumptions were met, there was one IV with two levels, covariates were considered measured on both categorical and continuous scales, and although the DV was measured twice, the baseline measurement was used only as an additional covariate. Based on this information, all three statistical tests were used appropriately.

Case Study 8–2

Tranexamic acid (TXA) and epsilon-aminocaproic acid (EACA) are two antifibrinolytics used to reduce blood loss following total joint arthroplasty. Because TXA is considerably more expensive than EACA, researchers at a local hospital currently dosing patients with TXA are interested in whether they can reduce costs by dosing EACA with no additional risk of blood loss. Therefore, a study was designed evaluate to differences in blood loss prevention between TXA and EACA following total joint arthroplasty. A sample of patients will be consented to participate in the study, with equal numbers randomized to receive either TXA or EACA. Blood loss will be measured using hemoglobin (Hbg). On the day of surgery, during the preoperative process, blood will be drawn to measure the patient's baseline Hbg to serve as a covariate in analysis. Hbg will be measured again from blood drawn 2 days post-operatively to serve as the primary outcome. Hbg will be treated as a continuous variable for analysis.

Because the local hospital only has three orthopedic surgeons who complete total hip and knee replacements, the decision was made to recruit orthopedic surgeons from other hospitals in the metropolitan area to participate in the study. Thirty additional orthopedic surgeons within five hospitals agreed to participate. Because surgeons often have privileges to perform surgery at multiple hospitals, they were asked to include surgeries at only one hospital of their choosing.

Questions:

1. Would you consider this study to be a randomized controlled trial?
2. Is the design parallel-groups, crossover, or adaptive? Why?
3. The researchers plan to use a one-tailed hypothesis for this study. Is this appropriate? Could the researchers have specified a two-tailed hypothesis?
4. Are the researchers interested in a statistical test of differences or association?
5. How many times was the DV measured?
6. The distributional assumptions have been met and authors have indicated they will use an independent-samples t-test to analyze their data. Is this correct given the study design? If so, why? If not, indicate which statistical test(s) of group differences would be more appropriate.
7. The distributional assumptions have been met and the authors have indicated they will use some form of regression analysis to analyze their data. Is this appropriate? What type of regression is most appropriate?
8. Should the researchers have been concerned with clustering or nesting? Why or why not? If so, describe the levels of nesting within their study design.

Statistical Tests

The remainder of this chapter describes the application and assumptions of numerous parametric and nonparametric statistical tests commonly used in the biomedical sciences. Note that this section only covers statistical tests applicable to study designs with one measured DV; no truly multivariate tests are discussed. A description and list of assumptions are provided for each statistical test as well as an example with an associated results section as it would likely appear in the literature. It is important to take careful note of the assumptions for each statistical test, as these assumptions are vital in determining whether correct statistical inference can be inferred from the statistical test results. The discussion of statistical tests begins with tests for nominal and categorical data, followed by statistical tests for evaluating group differences and associations.

TESTS FOR NOMINAL AND CATEGORICAL DATA

Nonparametric Tests

Pearson's chi-square test

Pearson's chi-square test (or simply the chi-square test) is one of the most common statistical tests used in the biomedical sciences. It is used to assess for significant differences between two or more mutually exclusive groups for two variables measured on a nominal scale. Note that the data may also be ordinal, if the number of rank ordered categories is small; however, the test does not consider rank order. The chi-square test assesses for differences between actual or observed frequency counts and the frequency count that would be expected if there actually was no differences in the data.

As an example, consider a study to determine whether a significant difference in gender exists between three treatment groups. In most journal articles, a 2×3 (i.e., gender by treatment group) contingency containing the observed frequency counts within each cell will typically be presented. This table would appear similar to Figure 8–7 but with another row or column. The expected frequencies are rarely presented in the literature. Next, a chi-square (χ^2) statistic should be presented with appropriate degrees of freedom subscripted next to the chi-square symbol (e.g., χ^2_2 for two degrees of freedom). As stated above, the number of degrees of freedom will vary based on the analysis. If the probability of the difference is below alpha; that is, if the observed frequencies are different from the expected frequencies, the test is considered statistically significant indicating a significant gender difference between the groups. The results of a statistically significant gender difference are presented as follows:

> *The results of the chi-square test indicated a statistically significant gender difference between treatment groups* ($\chi^2_2 = 11.59$, $p < 0.05$).

When the chi-square test is based on a contingency table larger than 2×2, the test is considered an omnibus test. That is, in the example above for the 2×3 table the chi-square test indicated a statistically significant gender difference existed between at least two treatment groups, but failed to indicate specifically which treatment groups differed. In these situations, *post hoc* chi-square tests (or Fisher's exact tests if expected frequencies are low, see the next section) are used to determine where statistically significant differences occurred. For example, in the 2×3 chi-square above, three 2×2

post hoc chi-square tests are required. Specifically, gender compared between groups A and B, gender compared between groups A and C, and gender compared between groups B and C. A sample results section including the *post hoc* chi-square test results is presented below:

> *Statistically significant gender differences were indicated across the three treatment groups ($\chi^2_2 = 11.59$, $p < 0.05$). Post hoc chi-square tests indicated statistically significant gender differences between groups A and B ($\chi^2_1 = 6.54$, $p < 0.05$) and between groups B and C ($\chi^2_1 = 10.26$, $p < 0.05$), with group B including significantly more males compared to both groups A and C. Further, no statistically significant gender difference was indicated between groups A and C.*

The assumptions of the chi-square test include:

1. Data for both variables being compared must be categorical.
   a. Note that continuous data can be categorized; however, information will be lost via categorization.
2. The categories must be mutually exclusive.
   a. That is, each individual can fall into one, and only one, category.
3. The total sample size must be large.
   a. The expected frequencies in each cell must not be too small. For chi-square tests with degrees of freedom greater than 1 (i.e., when the number of columns and/or rows are greater than 2), no more than 20% of the cells should have expected frequencies less than 5. Further, no cell should have an expected frequency less than 1.[31] This is a difficult assumption to verify from the literature, outside of calculating the expected frequencies by hand. However, if an article fails to indicate this assumption was tested, view results with caution.

Fisher's exact test

Fisher's exact test is ubiquitous in the biomedical literature. The test can only be applied to 2×2 contingency tables and is most useful when the sample size is small. It is often used when the third assumption of the chi-square test is violated. Conceptually, Fisher's exact test is identical to the chi-square test, in that, the two variables being compared must be nominal and have mutually exclusive categories.

For example, consider a study assessing for differences in cardiac events in dialysis patients who initiated beta blocker therapy compared to patients who did not initiate therapy. Note, both variables are dichotomous (i.e., event versus no event; beta blocker versus no beta blocker). Fisher's exact test provides the exact probability of observing this particular set of frequencies within each cell of the contingency table. Results of a statistically significant Fisher's exact test are presented below. Notice only a *p* value is provided:

The results of a Fisher's exact test indicated patients initiating beta blocker therapy had significantly fewer cardiac events compared to patients failing to initiate therapy ($p < 0.05$). The assumptions of Fisher's exact test include:

1. Data for both variables being compared must be dichotomous.
   a. Note that continuous data can be dichotomized; however, information will be lost via categorization.
2. The dichotomous categories must be mutually exclusive.
   a. That is, each individual can fall into one, and only one, category.

Mantel-Haenszel chi-square test

The Mantel-Haenszel chi-square test (also known as Cochran-Mantel-Haenszel test or Mantel-Haenszel test) measures the association of three discrete variables, which usually consists of two dichotomous IVs and one categorical confounding variable or covariate used as a stratification variable.

For example, consider a study assessing the presence or absence of lung cancer in smokers and nonsmokers (the IVs) after stratifying for frequent exposure to secondhand smoke (the dichotomous covariate; exposure versus no exposure). A 2×2 contingency table is created at each level of secondhand smoke. That is, a contingency table for exposure and another for no exposure. This test produces a chi-square statistic (χ^2_{MH}), with a statistically significant result indicating a significant difference in the presence of lung cancer for smokers and nonsmokers across the levels of the covariate (i.e., exposed versus unexposed). A statistically significant result is presented as follows:

The results of a Mantel-Haenszel chi-square test indicated the proportion of nonsmokers developing lung cancer was significantly greater for those exposed to second hand smoke ($\chi^2_{MH} = 29.67$, 1 df, $p < 0.05$).

The assumptions of the Mantel-Haenszel chi-square test include:

1. Data of the IVs must be dichotomous.
   a. Note that continuous data can be dichotomized; however, information will be lost via categorization.
2. The dichotomous categories must be mutually exclusive.
   a. That is, each individual can fall into one, and only one, category.
3. Data of the covariate must be categorical.
   a. Again, note that continuous data can be dichotomized; however, information will be lost via categorization.

The kappa statistic

The kappa statistic (also known as Cohen's kappa or κ) is a measure of inter-rater reliability or agreement for a categorical variable measured on a nominal scale. That is, kappa indicates how often individual raters using the same measurement scale indicate identical scores. Kappa provides the proportion of agreement corrected for chance and ranges from 0 indicating no agreement to 1 indicating perfect agreement. Be aware that there are no methodological studies defining a threshold for what could be considered good agreement. The definition of good agreement varies by substantive area. That is, what is considered good agreement in medical literature may not be considered good agreement in psychology, or vice versa. In general, however, a higher kappa is always better.

Because this statistic corrects for chance agreement, it is more appropriate than simply calculating overall percent agreement.[32] In fact, percent agreement should rarely be used and published results using percent agreement should be viewed with caution. Kappa can be applied to a variable with any number of categories, with the understanding that as the number of categories increase, overall agreement will undoubtedly decrease. That is, the more choices two raters have, the less likely they are to agree.

As an example, consider 100 professional school applicants, who each interview with two faculty members. After the interview is complete, each faculty member rates the applicant as accept, deny, or waitlist. Kappa is then used to calculate the agreement between faculty members. Results using the kappa statistic are presented as follows:

Cohen's kappa was employed to measure the agreement between faculty members in determining whether applicants should be accepted, denied, or waitlisted. Results indicated moderate agreement between faculty members ($\kappa = 0.75$).

The assumptions of the kappa statistic include:

1. Each object (e.g., the applicant in the example above) is rated only one time.
2. The outcome variable is nominal with mutually exclusive categories.
   a. That is, each individual can fall into one, and only one, category.
3. There are at least two independent raters.
   a. That is, each rater provides one, and only one, response for each applicant.

TESTING FOR DIFFERENCES FROM THE POPULATION

Parametric Tests

One-sample z test

The one-sample z test is used to assess for a difference between the mean of the study sample and a known population mean using a continuous DV.

For example, consider data collected from a random sample of 1000 patients with borderline high cholesterol, for which their mean serum total cholesterol was 210.01 mg/dL. The researcher is interested in determining whether the total cholesterol of this sample is significantly higher than the mean total cholesterol within the general population.

The 2007-2008 National Health and Nutrition Examination Survey (NHANES) determined the mean serum total cholesterol level for individuals in the United States aged 6 years and older is 186.67 mg/dL with a standard deviation of 42.15.[33] A one-sample z test provides a z-score indicating how many standard errors the sample mean is from the known population mean and if this difference is large enough to be considered statistically significant based on specific degrees of freedom. Note that degrees of freedom will be subscripted next to the z-score (e.g., z_{999}). Results of a statistically significant one-sample z test with no assumption violations are provided as follows:

Results of a one-sample z test indicated a statistically significant difference in total cholesterol between the study sample and population ($z_{999} = 2.10$, $p < 0.05$), with the study sample having significantly higher total cholesterol compared to the general population (210.01 mg/dL versus 186.67 mg/dL, respectively).

Assumptions of the one-sample z test include:

1. The DV is measured on an interval or ratio scale.
2. The sampling distribution of means for the DV is normal.
   a. This can be ensured by applying the central limit theorem.
3. The population mean and standard deviation is known.
4. The observations are independent.
   a. That is, each participant provides one, and only one, observation (i.e., data or response).

One-sample t-test

Only in rare cases is the population standard deviation known; thus, test statistics often must be based on sample data (i.e., standard deviation and sample size). The one-sample t-test is used in situations where only the population mean is known, or can at least be estimated by very large amounts of data. It is used only for a continuous DV.

For example, consider a study to compare the mean total cholesterol of a random sample of 1000 adults aged 20 years of age or older with borderline high cholesterol (e.g., 231.26 mg/dL) to the mean total cholesterol of the general population. In 2006, the National Center for Health Statistics determined the mean serum total cholesterol for adults in the United States aged 20 years and older was 199.00 mg/dL.[34] Notice, no population standard deviation is available; thus, a one-sample t-test is required. Note that this test produces a t statistic, which can be considered similar to a z-score when samples are large. In general, a t-test will approximate a z-test with a sample size of around 30. The result of a statistically significant one-sample t-test with no assumption violations is presented as follows:

Results of a one-sample t-test indicated a statistically significant difference in total cholesterol between the study sample and population ($t_{999} = 2.23$, $p < 0.05$), with the study *sample having significantly higher total cholesterol compared to individuals aged 20 or older in the general population (231.26 mg/dL versus 199.00 mg/dL, respectively).*

Assumptions of the one-sample t-test include:

1. The DV is measured on an interval or ratio scale.
2. The sampling distribution of means for the DV is normal.
    a. This can be ensured by applying the central limit theorem.
3. The population mean is known.
4. The observations are independent.
    a. That is, each participant provides one, and only one, observation (i.e., data or response).

Nonparametric Tests

Binomial test

The binomial test is used when the DV is dichotomous and all of the possible data or outcomes fall into one, and only one, of the two categories. The binomial test uses the binomial distribution to test the exact probability of whether the sample proportion differs from the population proportion. Further, the binomial test is often used in the literature when sample sizes are small and violate the assumptions of the chi-square test, specifically low expected frequencies.[27]

For example, say a fair coin is flipped 10 times, and lands on heads 6 of the 10 flips. The expected population proportion is 0.50; that is, if the coin is fair, as the number of flips increases the coin should land on heads 50% of the time. Because the coin landed on heads 6 of the 10 flips, the statistical test is whether this proportion (i.e., 6/10 or 0.60) is statistically different from the expected proportion (i.e., 0.50). In this case, the binomial test indicates the difference between these proportions is not significant and results are presented as follows:

Results of the binomial test indicated the probability of flipping 6 heads in 10 flips was not statistically different from the expected population proportion of 0.50 ($p > 0.05$).

The assumptions of the binomial test include:

1. Data for both variables being compared must be dichotomous.
    a. Note that continuous data can be dichotomized; however, information will be lost via categorization.
2. The dichotomous categories must be mutually exclusive.
    a. That is, each individual can fall into one, and only one, category.
3. The population proportion is known.
4. The observations are independent.
    a. That is, each participant provides one, and only one, observation (i.e., data or response).

Kolmogorov-Smirnov one-sample test

The Kolmogorov-Smirnov one-sample test is a goodness-of-fit test used to determine the degree of agreement between the distribution of a researcher's sample data and a theoretical population distribution.[27] That is, it allows researchers to compare the distribution of their sample data against a given probability distribution for a continuous DV (see Table 8–1).

For example, consider a study where HbA1c data was collected for a random sample of 100 patients with diabetes. The researcher is interested in determining whether the distribution of HbA1c data was sampled from a population of patients with an underlying normal distribution. That is, the researcher is interested in whether the sample data is normally distributed. A nonsignificant Kolmogorov-Smirnov test indicates the sample distribution and the hypothesized normal distribution are not statistically different; that is, the distribution of sample data can be considered normally distributed. Results of the Kolmogorov-Smirnov test are presented as follows:

Results of the Kolmogorov-Smirnov test indicated HbA1c variable had a nonsignificant departure from normality ($p > 0.05$); thus, the data are considered to result from a normal distribution.

The assumptions of the Kolmogorov-Smirnov one-sample test include:

1. The DV is measured on an interval or ratio scale.
2. The underlying population distribution is theorized or known.
   a. That is, the researcher must specify the correct probability distribution to test the sample data against. If the distribution is unknown, the test is inappropriate.
3. The observations are independent.
   a. That is, each participant provides one, and only one, observation (i.e., data or response).

TESTING FOR DIFFERENCES BETWEEN GROUPS

Parametric Tests

Independent-samples t-test

The independent-samples t-test (also known as Student's t-test) is used to assess for a statistically significant difference between the means of two independent, mutually exclusive groups using a continuous DV.

For example, consider testing for a mean difference in a methacholine challenge at the end of an 8-week study period in two groups of asthma patients receiving either rosiglitazone or placebo. Methacholine challenge was measured by a 20% decrease in forced expiratory volume in one second (FEV1; PC20). The independent-sample t-test provides the *t* statistic and probability of obtaining a difference of this size or larger based on specific degrees of freedom, which are usually subscripted (e.g., t_{31}). Results of a statistically significant independent-samples t-test with no assumption violations are presented as follows:

The results of an independent-samples t-test indicated a statistically significant difference between groups (t_{31} = 9.654, p < 0.05), with asthma patients receiving rosiglitazone displaying significantly better lung function compared to placebo (mean PC20 = 10.7 mg/mL versus 3.8 mg/mL, respectively).

The assumptions of the independent-samples t-test include:

1. The DV is measured on an interval or ratio scale.
2. The sampling distribution of means for the DV within each level of the IV (i.e., group) is normal.
   a. This can be ensured by applying the central limit theorem.
3. The IV is dichotomous.
   a. Note that continuous data can be dichotomized; however, information will be lost via categorization.
4. The IV categories are mutually exclusive.
   a. That is, each individual can fall into one, and only one, category.
5. Homogeneity of variance is ensured.
   a. That is, the variance within each group is similar. A crude indicator of a violation of this assumption (i.e., heterogeneity) is the ratio of the largest variance to smallest variance being greater than 10:1.[22] For example, most studies do not provide the variance for each variable; however, the standard deviation is reported consistently. Remember, variance is simply the standard deviation squared. Thus, consider two variables with standard deviations of 5 and 10. The homogeneity of variance assumption can be tested by squaring the standard deviations (i.e., $5^2 = 25$ and $10^2 = 100$, respectively) and finding their ratio (i.e., $100/25 = 4$). In this case, the ratio is less than 10:1; thus, the assumption is not violated.
6. The observations are independent.
   a. That is, each participant provides one, and only one, observation (i.e., data or response).

One-way between-groups analysis of variance

A one-way between-groups analysis of variance (ANOVA) is an extension of the independent-samples t-test to situations, where researchers want to assess for mean differences between three or more mutually exclusive groups using a continuous DV.

For example, consider the rosiglitazone example from the Independent-Samples t-Test section above, but in addition to the placebo group, include two groups receiving different doses of rosiglitazone (e.g., 4 and 8 mg). The use of three independent-samples t-tests to test for mean differences between groups (i.e., 4 mg versus placebo, 8 mg versus placebo, 4 mg versus 8 mg) is inappropriate due to a possible increase in Type I error. Instead, one-way ANOVA is used to partition the variance between and within groups to determine if a statistically significant group difference exists. This partitioning can be observed in the two numbers presented for degrees of freedom (i.e., $F_{2,27}$ indicates 2 between-group degrees of freedom and 27 within-group degrees of freedom). The result of a statistically significant one-way ANOVA with no assumption violations is presented as follows:

Results of a one-way ANOVA indicated a statistically significant difference between groups ($F_{2,27} = 6.89$, $p < 0.05$).

ANOVA provides an omnibus F test; that is, an overall test assessing the statistical significance between the three or more group means. A statistically significant omnibus F test indicates a statistically significant difference between at least two group means. To determine which groups differ specifically, a series of *post hoc* tests are conducted. *Post hoc* tests are simply tests comparing individual groups to one another; thus, *post hoc* tests can be viewed as a series of independent-samples t-tests. That is, two-group comparisons. Because *post hoc* tests increase the number of statistical tests used, they often use a more conservative alpha to control for potential Type I errors. With this in mind, the significant one-way ANOVA in the example above would require three adjusted *post hoc* tests. That is, 4 mg versus placebo, 8 mg versus placebo, and 4 mg versus 8 mg. The most commonly used *post hoc* tests in the literature include the Tukey and Scheffé tests. Be aware that the Scheffé test is the most conservative *post hoc* test available and some methodologists argue that the test may be too conservative increasing the probability of committing a Type II error. A suitable alternative is the Tukey test, which is conservative but to a lesser degree. In most cases, the two tests will indicate similar results and both are viewed as acceptable.

The results of a statistically significant one-way ANOVA including *post hoc* tests are presented as follows:

Results of a one-way ANOVA indicated a statistically significant difference between groups ($F_{2,27} = 6.89$, $p < 0.05$). Post hoc Tukey tests indicated statistically significant differences (at $p < 0.05$) between placebo (3.8 mg/mL) and 4 mg dose of rosiglitazone (10.7 mg/mL) as well as between placebo and the 8 mg dose of rosiglitazone (12.2 mg/mL). No statistically significant differences were indicated between the 4 mg and 8 mg doses of rosiglitazone.

The assumptions for one-way ANOVA include:

1. The DV is measured on an interval or ratio scale.
2. The sampling distribution of means for the DV within each level of the IV is normal.
   a. This can be ensured by applying the central limit theorem.

3. The levels of the IV are mutually exclusive.
   a. That is, each individual can fall into one, and only one, category.
4. Homogeneity of variance is ensured.
   a. That is, the variance within each group is similar. A crude indicator of a violation of this assumption (i.e., heterogeneity) is the ratio of the largest variance to smallest variance being greater than 10:1.[22] For example, most studies do not provide the variance for each variable; however, the standard deviation is reported consistently. Remember, variance is simply the standard deviation squared. Thus, consider two variables with standard deviations of 5 and 10. The homogeneity of variance assumption can be tested by squaring the standard deviations (i.e., $5^2 = 25$ and $10^2 = 100$, respectively) and finding their ratio (i.e., $100/25 = 4$). In this case, the ratio is less than 10:1; thus, the assumption is not violated.
5. The observations are independent.
   a. That is, each participant provides one, and only one, observation (i.e., data or response).

Factorial between-groups analysis of variance

A factorial between-groups analysis of variance (also known as factorial ANOVA) is an extension of the one-way between-groups ANOVA to a study with more than one IV using a continuous DV.

For example, consider a study to evaluate for differences in heart rate measured by beats per minute (bpm) between men and women following either a 25-mg dose of pseudoephedrine or placebo. In the literature, this may be described as a 2×2 factorial design indicating two IVs (i.e., gender and treatment) each with two levels (i.e., male versus female; pseudoephedrine versus placebo). This type of design produces two main effects—one for gender and one for treatment—and an interaction effect between gender and treatment. Thus, three separate F tests are provided, one for each effect, with statistical significance determined separately for each effect.

It is extremely important to note that if the interaction effect is statistically significant, the results of the main effects cannot be interpreted directly, as the IVs are dependent on each other. From the example, a statistically significant interaction effect indicates treatment effects differ depending on the gender of the participant. That is, pseudoephedrine had a different effect for males than it did for females. However, if the interaction effect is not significant, main effects can and should be interpreted. When interpreting the main effect of an IV, the levels of the other IV are averaged or marginalized. That is, interpreting the main effect of gender is done irrespective of whether the participants received pseudoephedrine or placebo. Likewise, interpreting the main effect of treatment is done irrespective of the participant's gender.

Similar to one-way between-groups ANOVA, following a statistically significant main effect or interaction, *post hoc* tests may be required to identify where statistically significant differences occurred. There are a number of *post hoc* tests available depending on whether the interaction or main effects are statistically significant including the Tukey and Scheffé tests.[35] Each *post hoc* test adjusts alpha more or less conservatively to reduce potential Type I errors. *Post hoc* tests for factorial ANOVA used in the literature are often termed simple comparisons, simple contrasts, simple main effects, or interaction contrasts. While each uses a slightly different procedure, they are used to accomplish the same goal—identify group differences.

In the biomedical sciences, the results of a nonsignificant interaction effect for a 2×2 factorial between-groups ANOVA with no assumption violations are presented as follows:

Results of a 2 (gender; male versus female) × 2 (treatment; pseudoephedrine versus placebo) factorial between-groups ANOVA indicated a nonsignificant interaction effect between gender and treatment ($p > 0.05$). However, the main effect for gender was statistically significant ($F_{1,26} = 21.36$, $p < 0.05$), with males having significantly higher heart rates than females (91.6 bpm versus 84.3 bpm, respectively). Further, the main effect of treatment was also statistically significant ($F_{1,26} = 15.24$, $p < 0.05$), with pseudoephedrine resulting in a significantly higher heart rate compared to placebo (70.3 bpm versus 65.2 bpm, respectively).

The results of a 2×2 factorial between-groups ANOVA with a statistically significant interaction and no assumption violations are presented as follows:

Results of a 2 (gender; male versus female) × 2 (treatment; pseudoephedrine versus placebo) factorial between-groups ANOVA indicated a statistically significant interaction effect between gender and treatment ($F_{1,26} = 15.42$, $p < 0.05$). Simple main effects were assessed to identify at which treatment level gender differed. Results indicated pseudoephedrine increased heart rate significantly higher for males compared to females (90.5 bpm versus 82.4 bpm, respectively). No statistically significant gender difference in heart rate was indicated for the placebo group.

The assumptions of factorial between-groups ANOVA include:

1. The DV is measured on an interval or ratio scale.
2. The sampling distribution of means for the DV within each level of the IV is normal.
   a. This can be ensured by applying the central limit theorem.
3. The levels of the IVs are mutually exclusive.
   a. That is, each individual can fall into one, and only one, category.
4. Homogeneity of variance is ensured.
   a. That is, the variance within each group is similar. A crude indicator of a violation of this assumption (i.e., heterogeneity) is the ratio of the largest variance to smallest variance being greater than 10:1.[22] For example, most studies do not provide

the variance for each variable; however, the standard deviation is reported consistently. Remember, variance is simply the standard deviation squared. Thus, consider two variables with standard deviations of 5 and 10. The homogeneity of variance assumption can be tested by squaring the standard deviations (i.e., $5^2 = 25$ and $10^2 = 100$, respectively) and finding their ratio (i.e., $100/25 = 4$). In this case, the ratio is less than 10:1; thus, the assumption is not violated.

5. The observations are independent.

   a. That is, each participant provides one, and only one, observation (i.e., data or response).

Analysis of covariance

Analysis of covariance (ANCOVA) is an extension of both one-way between-groups ANOVA and factorial between-groups ANOVA. ANCOVA evaluates main effects and interactions using a continuous DV after statistically adjusting for one or more continuous confounding variables. That is, ANCOVA adjusts all group means to create the situation as if all participants scored identically on the covariate.[22]

For example, consider a study comparing atenolol to placebo (IV) and assessing their effects on systolic blood pressure (DV). The researchers note, however, that previous research has shown systolic blood pressure and BMI to be highly correlated.[36] Thus, the analysis will include BMI as a covariate assessing the effect of atenolol on systolic blood pressure over and above the effect of BMI on systolic blood pressure. If the atenolol group has greater BMI values compared to the placebo group, ANCOVA will adjust the systolic blood pressure within both groups to account for this initial difference in BMI.

In ANCOVA, covariates are continuous, measured before the DV, and correlated with the DV. It should be noted that ANCOVA is closely related to linear regression. Thus, although not completely necessary, it may be useful to revisit this section after reading the sections on Simple and Multivariable Linear Regression presented later in the chapter. In ANCOVA, group means are statistically adjusted by the magnitude of the association (i.e., slope) between the DV and covariate.[37] That is, the greater the association, the more useful the covariate and better the adjustment. Thus, the goal of the covariate is to reduce error variance thereby increasing the statistical power of the test. From the example, mean systolic blood pressure for the atenolol and placebo groups are adjusted by the association between BMI and systolic blood pressure. Because previous research has shown the association between systolic blood pressure and BMI to be considerable, the statistical power of this test will undoubtedly be increased.

When presenting the results of ANCOVA, researchers should provide adjusted means; that is, the mean of the DV at each level of the IV after adjusting for the covariate. Published research that does not present adjusted means should be viewed with caution. Further, the effect of the covariate must also be presented which provides information regarding the effectiveness of the covariate in adjusting group means. Finally, it should be noted that ANCOVA is more suited for experimental design in which participants are randomized to groups, as opposed to nonexperimental designs without randomization. Remember, ANCOVA is used to adjust group means as if all participants had identical covariate values. However, in nonexperimental research, important covariates may have been missed and causality is difficult to infer—a characteristic intrinsic to all nonexperimental work. Thus, the limitations may be significant when applying ANCOVA to nonexperimental designs and results must be viewed cautiously.[9]

In the biomedical sciences, the results of a statistically significant ANCOVA with no assumption violations are presented as follows:

Results of a one-way ANCOVA indicated a statistically significant group differences in systolic blood pressure after adjusting for BMI ($F_{1,17} = 7.98$, $p < 0.05$), with patients receiving atenolol having significantly lower systolic blood pressure compared to placebo (adjusted means = 118 mm Hg versus 141 mm Hg, respectively). The relationship between systolic blood pressure and BMI was also statistically significant after adjusting for group ($F_{1,17} = 39.85$, $p < 0.05$) with a pooled within-group correlation of 0.61.

The assumptions of ANCOVA include:

1. The DV is measured on an interval or ratio scale.
2. The sampling distribution of means for the DV and covariate(s) within each level of the IV is normal.
   a. This can be ensured by applying the central limit theorem.
3. The levels of the IV are mutually exclusive.
   a. That is, each individual can fall into one, and only one, category.
4. Homogeneity of variance is ensured.
   a. That is, the variance within each group is similar. A crude indicator of a violation of this assumption (i.e., heterogeneity) is the ratio of the largest variance to smallest variance being greater than 10:1.[22] For example, most studies do not provide the variance for each variable; however, the standard deviation is reported consistently. Remember, variance is simply the standard deviation squared. Thus, consider two variables with standard deviations of 5 and 10. The homogeneity of variance assumption can be tested by squaring the standard deviations (i.e., $5^2 = 25$ and $10^2 = 100$, respectively) and finding their ratio (i.e., $100/25 = 4$). In this case, the ratio is less than 10:1; thus, the assumption is not violated.
5. Homogeneity of regression is ensured.
   a. This assumption requires the association between the DV and covariate to be the same within each level of the IV. A violation of this assumption renders ANCOVA inappropriate, and the authors should use linear regression instead. However, violation is difficult to detect from the literature, as most authors fail

to provide the appropriate information in the narrative. Thus, when reading a journal article employing ANCOVA, if the author fails to indicate whether this assumption was tested, results must be viewed with caution.

6. The covariate(s) is measured reliably and without error.
7. The observations are independent.
    a. That is, each participant provides one, and only one, observation (i.e., data or response).

Nonparametric Tests

Mann-Whitney test

The Mann-Whitney test is the nonparametric alternative to the independent-samples t-test and is one of the most powerful nonparametric tests.[27] It is used when the distributional assumptions for the parametric test are violated or when the DV is measured on an ordinal scale. The Mann-Whitney test is based on ranked data. That is, instead of using the actual values of the DV, as an independent-samples t-test does, each participant's DV value is ranked with the highest value receiving the highest rank and the lowest value receiving the lowest rank. The ranks within each group are then summed and the test assesses whether the difference in ranked sums between groups is statistically significant.

For example, consider a performance improvement study assessing gender differences in patient satisfaction of hospital stay following total hip replacement surgery. The measurement instrument uses a Likert-type scale with four possible responses anchored from Strongly Disagree to Strongly Agree. A statistically significant Mann-Whitney test indicates gender differences in patient satisfaction, with the group with the highest ranked sums indicating higher satisfaction. The results of the Mann-Whitney test are presented as follows:

The results of a Mann-Whitney test indicate a statistically significant gender difference in patient satisfaction following total hip replacement surgery ($z = 2.65$, $p < 0.05$), with males indicating higher satisfaction scores compared to females.

The assumptions of the Mann-Whitney test include:

1. The DV is measured on an ordinal, interval, or ratio scale.
2. The IV is dichotomous.
    a. Note that continuous data can be categorized into a dichotomous variable; however, information will be lost.
3. The levels of the IV are mutually exclusive.
    a. That is, each individual can fall into one, and only one category.
4. The observations are independent.
    a. That is, each participant provides one, and only one, observation (i.e., data or response).

Median test

The median test is used to assess whether two mutually exclusive groups have different medians. There is no parametric alternative to the median test; however, the nonparametric Mann-Whitney test can be used as an adequate alternative. The test calculates the medians within each group and then classifies the data within each group as either above or below the respective group median. Further, because the test is based on the median, it can be used appropriately for skewed distributions or data containing outliers.

For example, consider a study evaluating gender differences in childhood autism as measured by the Childhood Autism Spectrum Test (CAST).[37] The CAST measures difficulties and preferences in social and communication skills using the total score a 37-item questionnaire, with lower scores indicating fewer symptoms. Because autism is a relatively rare disorder, the distribution of CAST scores is expected to have severe positive skewness due to outliers. That is, most children will score low, while a few autistic children will have high scores. The median test was used to determine whether statistically significant gender differences existed in CAST scores. The results of a statistically significant median test are presented as follows:

The results of the median test indicated gender differences in CAST scores ($p < 0.05$), with boys having a significantly higher median score compared to girls (median = 5 versus median = 4, respectively).

Assumptions of the median test include:

1. The DV is measured on an ordinal, interval, or ratio scale.
2. Samples sizes are sufficiently large.
   a. If sample sizes are small, say less than 5 in each group, Fisher's exact test should be used instead. From the example, this means using a 2 (Group; male versus female) $\times$ 2 (Median; above versus below) contingency table.
3. The observations are independent.
   a. That is, each participant provides one, and only one, observation (i.e., data or response).

Kruskal-Wallis one-way ANOVA by ranks

The Kruskal-Wallis one-way ANOVA by ranks (or simply, the Kruskal-Wallis test) is the nonparametric alternative to the one-way between-groups ANOVA. The test is an extension of the Mann-Whitney test to assess group differences between three or more mutually exclusive groups. The Kruskal-Wallis test is typically used when distributional assumptions are violated or when the DV is measured on an ordinal scale. Further, the Kruskal-Wallis test is based on rank sums similar to the Mann-Whitney test. The DV scores are ranked from highest to lowest, summed, and statistically significant of group differences are evaluated based on these rank sums.

For example, consider a study evaluating regional differences in whether volunteer preceptors believe they have adequate time available to dedicate to their experiential pharmacy students.[38] In this study, the DV was measured on an ordinal 4-point Likert-type scale; thus, the Kruskal-Wallis test was used in lieu of one-way between-groups ANOVA. The results of the statistically significant Kruskal-Wallis test are presented as follows:

Results of the Kruskal-Wallis test indicated regional differences regarding whether volunteer preceptors believe they have adequate time to dedicate to experiential students ($\chi_6^2 = 33.07$, $p < 0.05$).

Similar to a one-way between-groups ANOVA, the Kruskal-Wallis test is an omnibus test. That is, the test will determine whether an overall statistically significant difference exists between groups, but will not indicate specifically which groups differed statistically. Thus, *post hoc* tests are required. In this situation, the Mann-Whitney test is used to compare all two-group combinations. From the example, *post hoc* tests would include West versus Midwest, West versus South, West versus Northeast, and so on for a total of six *post hoc* tests. The results of the Kruskal-Wallis test including Mann-Whitney *post hoc* tests are presented as follows:

Results of the Kruskal-Wallis test indicated regional differences regarding whether volunteer preceptors believe they have adequate time to dedicate to experiential students ($\chi_6^2 = 33.07$, $p < 0.05$). Post hoc Mann-Whitney tests indicated preceptors in the West disagreed more compared to preceptors located in the Midwest ($p < 0.05$) and agreed less with preceptors in the South ($p < 0.05$). No other statistically significant group differences were indicated.

The assumptions of the Kruskal-Wallis test include:

1. The DV is measured on an ordinal, interval, or ratio scale.
2. The IV is categorical.
   a. Note that continuous data can be categorized; however, information will be lost.
3. The levels of the IV are mutually exclusive.
   a. That is, each individual can fall into one, and only one category.
4. Each group has approximately the same distribution.
   a. Although the Kruskal-Wallis test does not assume data are distributed normally, if the distribution for one level of the IV is skewed negatively and the other levels are skewed positively, the results produced by the test may be inaccurate.
5. The data do not include a large number of ties.
   a. Tied values are given average ranks. Typically, if less than 25% of the data are ties, the test is unaffected.[27]
6. The observations are independent.
   a. That is, each participant provides one, and only one, observation (i.e., data or response).

TESTING FOR WITHIN-GROUP CHANGE

Parametric Tests

Paired-samples t-test

The paired-samples t-test (also known as matched t-test or nested t-test) is used when one group of participants in measured twice or two groups of participants are matched on specific characteristics. In both cases, the assumption of independence, or mutually exclusive groups, is violated. This statistical test is only appropriate using a continuous DV.

When one group of participants is measured twice, it is known as a repeated measures design. Repeatedly measuring participants is a valid method for reducing error and increasing statistical power, which requires fewer participants. The simplest repeated measures design is termed a pretest-posttest design. For example, consider measuring the therapeutic knowledge of 20 fourth-year pharmacy (P4) students prior to clinical rotations (i.e., pretest) and following rotations (i.e., posttest) to assess for increases in therapeutic knowledge. Therapeutic knowledge was measured using a discriminating 20-question test. The paired-samples t-test assesses for a statistically significant change in correct responses from pretest to posttest.

When two groups of participants are matched on specific characteristics, it is called a matched design. For example, when studying the effects of a new statin medication on hyperlipidemia, researchers would identify a group of patients to receive the statin and then identify a matched control group by matching individuals based on age, race, gender, BMI, and years with diagnosis. Note that the matched control group does not receive any medication. Matching participants serves the same purpose as repeated measures—reduce error variance—but is often more difficult because as the number of matching criteria increases the probability of finding a suitable match decreases.

Results of a statistically significant paired-samples t-test with no assumption violations using the pretest-posttest design example above is presented as follows:

The results of a paired-samples t-test indicated a statistically significant difference in therapeutic knowledge between pretest and posttest scores ($t_{19} = 3.25$, $p < 0.05$). Therapeutic knowledge increased significantly following clinical rotations (mean = 10.4 correct responses at pretest versus a mean of 16.5 at posttest).

The assumptions of the paired-samples t-test include:

1. The DV is measured on an interval or ratio scale.
2. The two DV measurements are associated.
3. The sampling distribution of means for both DV measurements is normal.
   a. This can be ensured by applying the central limit theorem.
4. Homogeneity of variance for both DV measurements is ensured.
   a. That is, the variance within each group is similar. A crude indicator of a violation of this assumption (i.e., heterogeneity) is the ratio of the largest variance to

smallest variance being greater than 10:1.[22] For example, most studies do not provide the variance for each variable; however, the standard deviation is reported consistently. Remember, variance is simply the standard deviation squared. Thus, consider two variables with standard deviations of 5 and 10. The homogeneity of variance assumption can be tested by squaring the standard deviations (i.e., $5^2 = 25$ and $10^2 = 100$, respectively) and finding their ratio (i.e., $100/25 = 4$). In this case, the ratio is less than 10:1; thus, the assumption is not violated.

One-way repeated measures analysis of variance

A one-way repeated measures ANOVA (aka, repeated measures ANOVA) is an extension of the paired-samples t-test to situations where the continuous DV is measured three or more times. Again, this can occur when the same participants are measured repeatedly or when three or more matched groups are measured once. A repeated measures ANOVA is used to indicate whether statistically significant change occurred between the repeated measurements.

For example, reconsider the pretest-posttest design described in the Paired-Samples t-Test section early in the chapter. Briefly, a researcher is interested in testing whether therapeutic knowledge of 20 pharmacy students in their last year of college changes before and after clinical rotations. To be applicable to repeated measures ANOVA, students would be tested on a third occasion 6 months after posttest to assess knowledge retention. That is, the design measures therapeutic knowledge at pretest, posttest, and 6-month follow-up. The repeated measures ANOVA is then used to test whether a statistically significance change occurred between the repeated measurements.

It should be noted that some researchers prefer to use repeated measures ANOVA over paired-samples t-tests when participants are only measured twice. This is an appropriate use of repeated measures ANOVA as repeated measures ANOVA can be used in any situation when a paired-samples t-test is appropriate. The results would be identical. However, the test statistic from the repeated measures ANOVA will be an F value instead of a t value produced by the paired-samples t-test. This is a nonissue, though, as the F value in this situation is simply t^2.

In most cases, repeated measures ANOVA has more statistical power than a paired-samples t-test. This has been alluded to in the Analysis of Clinical Trials and Paired-Samples t-test sections earlier in the chapter. In general, increasing the number of repeated measures further reduces error, which allows for more precise measurement and decreases the overall probability of committing a Type I error. With that said, increasing the number of repeated measurements has diminishing returns in statistical power. That is, for most studies, statistical power will increase drastically by adding a few additional repeated measurements, but the magnitude of this increase weakens rapidly between four and six measurements, with little to no increases in statistical power beyond the seventh measurement.[39] Finally, if a study has more than 10 repeated measurements, a time series analysis may be more appropriate than repeated measures ANOVA.

In addition, a brief discussion of the key assumption of repeated measures ANOVA is useful as a basic understanding this assumption will assist in determining whether the test statistics produced from the analysis are correct. This key assumption, known as sphericity, states that the variances of the differences between repeated measurements are equal. For example, consider a study with three repeated measurements. For the sphericity assumption to be satisfied, the variance of the difference between the first and second measurements must be similar to the variance of the difference between the first and third and second and third. This assumption tends to be restrictive, as most differences closer in time tend to have less variability compared to measurements further apart in time. Sphericity is a testable assumption using Mauchly's test, and a violation can severely bias the statistical inference. Therefore, when reading a journal article, if the authors fail to provide information regarding the assurance or violation of the sphericity assumption, results and interpretations must be viewed with caution.

Briefly reconsider the example provided above, where 20 pharmacy students in their final year have therapeutic knowledge measured before clinical rotations (i.e., pretest), once immediately after rotations (i.e., posttest), and at a 6-month follow-up. That is, therapeutic knowledge is measured on three separate occasions. A statistically significant repeated measures ANOVA with no assumption violations will be presented as follows:

The results of a one-way repeated measures ANOVA indicated a statistically significant difference in therapeutic knowledge between pretest, posttest, and 6-month follow-up ($F_{2,38} = 9.87$, $p < 0.05$).

With more than two repeated measurements, the one-way repeated measure ANOVA is an omnibus test. That is, the F test will identify whether a statistically significant difference exists between repeated measures, but will not indicate specifically which repeated measurements differ. Thus, *post hoc* tests, known as pairwise comparisons, are required. Similar to other analysis requiring *post hoc* tests, there are numerous adjusted pairwise comparisons available. Each type of pairwise comparison adjusts alpha differently, with some being more conservative. It may be simpler to think of these comparisons as a series of paired-samples t-tests with adjusted alpha values. That is, adjusted paired-samples t-tests comparing the first and second repeated measurements, the first and third, the second and third, and so on. The additional information required to present results of a statistically significant one-way repeated measures ANOVA with no assumption violations are presented as follows:

The results of a one-way repeated measures ANOVA indicated a statistically significant difference in therapeutic knowledge between pretest, posttest, and 6-month follow-up ($F_{2,38} = 9.87$, $p < 0.05$). Results of the pairwise comparisons indicated a statistically significant increase in therapeutic knowledge from pretest to posttest (mean = 5.50 versus 15.90, *respectively, p < 0.05). Further, no statistically significant difference was indicated from post-test to 6-month follow-up (mean = 15.90 versus 15.50, respectively) indicating therapeutic knowledge was retained for 6 months following clinical rotations.*

The assumptions of the one-way repeated measures ANOVA include:

1. The DV is measured on an interval or ratio scale.
2. All DV measurements are associated.
3. The sampling distribution of means for all DV measurements is normal.
    a. This can be ensured by applying the central limit theorem.
4. Homogeneity of variance for all DV measurements is ensured.
    a. That is, the variance within each group is similar. A crude indicator of a violation of this assumption (i.e., heterogeneity) is the ratio of the largest variance to smallest variance being greater than 10:1.[22] For example, most studies do not provide the variance for each variable; however, the standard deviation is reported consistently. Remember, variance is simply the standard deviation squared. Thus, consider two variables with standard deviations of 5 and 10. The homogeneity of variance assumption can be tested by squaring the standard deviations (i.e., $5^2 = 25$ and $10^2 = 100$, respectively) and finding their ratio (i.e., $100/25 = 4$). In this case, the ratio is less than 10:1; thus, the assumption is not violated.
5. Sphericity is ensured for designs with three or more repeated measurements.
    a. This is a complex assumption discussed above. In general, sphericity is violated when the variance of the differences between measurements are not similar.

Mixed between-within analysis of variance

A mixed between-within analysis of variance (also known as factorial ANOVA with repeated measures or split-plot ANOVA) is a combination of factorial between-groups ANOVA and repeated measures ANOVA. The mixed terminology highlights this combination, and indicates that the design considers two or more levels of the IV when a continuous DV is measured repeatedly. It is important to note that a mixed between-within ANOVA is qualitatively different from a mixed-effects analysis involving random effects (see Table 8–4). The simplest case is a 2×2 pretest-posttest design, using two mutually exclusive treatment groups measured on two separate occasions. The primary advantage of this analysis is that it allows researchers to assess the interaction effect evaluating whether two groups changed differently over time in addition to between-subjects main effect indicating the overall effect irrespective of measurement and within-subjects main effect indicating the overall effect irrespective of group.

As an example, consider a study examining the effectiveness of a relatively new FDA-approved tricyclic antidepressant (TCA) compared to amitriptyline over a 12-week study period. The researcher hypothesizes that the new TCA is more effective than amitriptyline in reducing symptoms of clinical depression. Prior to initiating treatment, 20 patients with diagnosed clinical depression are measured on the Beck Depression Inventory II (BDI-II).[40] Following this pretest or baseline measurement, each patient is randomized to receive one of two treatment options, the new TCA or amitriptyline, with 10 patients in each group. Patients then initiate the prescribed medication therapy and at the end of the 12-week study period BDI-II scores are measured again. A mixed between-within ANOVA provides researchers with a separate F tests for the interaction effect, between-groups main effect, and within-groups main effect each evaluated with specific degrees of freedom. Within this example, the primary effect of interest is the interaction effect, evaluating whether BDI-II scores changed differently within the new TCA group compared to the amitriptyline group from pretest to posttest.

Similar to factorial ANOVA discussed above, only if the interaction effect is nonsignificant can the researcher evaluate the statistical significance of overall group mean difference or between-group main effect and the overall change in BDI-II scores or within-group main effect. That is, a statistically significant interaction effect indicates that the change in BDI-II scores from pretest to posttest changed differently in the group receiving the new TCA group compared to the group receiving amitriptyline or vice versa. Stated another way, the reduction in symptoms from pretest to posttest was dependent on whether the patient received the new TCA or amitriptyline. In this example, the researcher's hypothesis would be supported by a statistically significant interaction effect; that is, the new TCA was more effective at reducing the symptoms associated with clinical depression compared to amitriptyline.

Although the example above was for a 2 (group: new TCA versus amitriptyline) × 2 (measurement: pretest versus posttest) design, a mixed between-within ANOVA can be used for a design with any number of IVs with any number of levels or repeated measures. This is often seen in the literature. For example, consider the pretest-posttest study evaluating the effectiveness of three treatment groups (e.g., new TCA, amitriptyline, and placebo) in reducing symptoms of clinical depression. This would be considered a 3×2 design. Or, consider the same study evaluating for additional gender differences within these three treatments. This would be considered a $3 \times 2 \times 2$ design. It must be noted that as the number and levels of the IVs increase so does the complexity of interpreting results. Thus, extreme care must be taken when interpreting results and implementing suggestions supported by these types of designs. Consultation with an individual well versed in research methodology and statistical analysis is advised prior to implementing findings into an evidence-based practice.

Because a mixed between-within ANOVA is an extension of factorial between-groups ANOVA and repeated measures ANOVA, *post hoc* tests or pairwise comparisons may be required for any IV with three or more levels. That is, when there are more than three levels of the between-groups IV (e.g., new TCA, amitriptyline, and placebo), the between-groups main effect is an omnibus test. A statistically significant between-groups main effect indicates that a statistically significant difference in BDI-II scores exists, but does not indicate specifically which groups differ significantly. Further, with three or more repeated measures, a statistically significant within-groups main effect indicates a difference between repeated measures, but fails to indicate specifically which measurements differ significantly. The *post hoc* tests and pairwise comparisons for factorial between-groups ANOVA and repeated measures ANOVA, respectively, are also appropriate for a mixed between-within ANOVA.

The results of a 2×2 mixed between-within ANOVA with no assumption violations for a nonsignificant interaction effect and statistically significant between- and within-groups main effects is presented as follows:

The results of a 2 (group: new TCA versus amitriptyline) $\times$ 2 (measurements: pretest versus posttest) mixed between-within ANOVA failed to indicate a statistically significant interaction ($F_{1,18} = 1.215$, $p > 0.05$). However, both main effects were statistically significant. Overall, patients receiving the new TCA had lower BDI-II scores compared to patients receiving amitriptyline ($F_{1,18} = 27.97$, $p < 0.05$; mean = 29.41 versus 47.50, respectively). Further, an overall decrease in depressive symptoms was indicated from pretest to posttest ($F_{1,18} = 24.74$, $p < 0.05$; mean = 49.86 versus 35.72, respectively).

With a statistically significant interaction effect, results of the mixed between-within ANOVA with no assumption violations are presented as follows:

The results of a 2 (group: new TCA versus amitriptyline) $\times$ 2 (measurements: pretest versus posttest) mixed between-within ANOVA indicated a statistically significant interaction effect ($F_{1,18} = 10.37$, $p < 0.05$). Simple main effects were assessed to identify statistically significant treatment differences at pretest and posttest individually. Results indicated no statistically significant difference between the new TCA and amitriptyline at pretest (mean = 48.53 versus 50.23, respectively). However, at posttest, a statistically significant difference was indicated, with the new TCA having significantly lower BDI-II scores compared to amitriptyline (mean = 24.63 versus 47.53, respectively).

The assumptions of a mixed between-within ANOVA include:

1. The DV is measured on an interval or ratio scale.
2. All DV measurements are associated.
3. The sampling distribution of means at each level of the IV(s), collapsed across the repeated DV measurements, is normal.
   a. This can be ensured by applying the central limit theorem.
4. Homogeneity of variance for all DV measurements within each level of the IV(s) is ensured.
   a. That is, the variance within each group is similar. A crude indicator of a violation of this assumption (i.e., heterogeneity) is the ratio of the largest variance to

smallest variance being greater than 10:1.[22] For example, most studies do not provide the variance for each variable; however, the standard deviation is reported consistently. Remember, variance is simply the standard deviation squared. Thus, consider two variables with standard deviations of 5 and 10. The homogeneity of variance assumption can be tested by squaring the standard deviations (i.e., $5^2 = 25$ and $10^2 = 100$, respectively) and finding their ratio (i.e., $100/25 = 4$). In this case, the ratio is less than 10:1; thus, the assumption is not violated.

5. Sphericity is ensured for designs with three or more repeated measurements.
   a. This is a complex assumption discussed briefly above for one-way repeated measures ANOVA. In general, sphericity is violated when the variance of the differences between measurements are not similar.

Nonparametric Tests

Wilcoxon signed-rank test

The Wilcoxon signed-rank test (also known as signed-rank test) is the nonparametric alternative to a paired-samples t-test. The test is used typically to assess for differences between two repeated measurements or two matched groups when distributional assumptions are violated or when the DV is measured on an ordinal scale. The signed-rank test is based on ranked difference scores (e.g., difference between pretest and posttest), with the highest difference score receiving the highest rank and the lowest difference score receiving the lowest rank.

For example, consider single group pretest-posttest study evaluating the secondary effect of weight loss in pounds while on exenatide therapy in a sample of 20 Type 1 DM patients. Prior to initiating exenatide therapy, all patients are weighed (i.e., pretest). At the end of a 1-year study period, patients are weighed again (i.e., posttest). For this study, the DV has numerous outliers; thus, the signed-rank test is used in lieu of paired-samples t-test to assess for a change in patient weight from pretest to posttest. The result of a statistically significant signed-rank test is presented as follows:

The results of the signed-rank tests indicated a statistically significant decrease in body weight from pretest to posttest ($z = 2.32$, $p < 0.05$).

The assumptions of the signed-rank test include:

1. The DV measured repeatedly on an ordinal, interval, or ratio scale.
2. The two DV measurements are associated.
3. The two measurements come from populations with the same median.
4. There should not be a large number difference scores equal to zero.
   a. That is, the number of participants having no change (i.e., difference score of zero) should be low.

Friedman two-way ANOVA by ranks

The Friedman two-way ANOVA by ranks test (also known as Friedman's test) is the non-parametric alternative to the one-way repeated measures ANOVA and is an extension of the signed-rank test to a situation with three or more repeated measurements. Similar to the other nonparametric tests, it is most often used when distributional assumptions are violated or the DV is measured on an ordinal scale. The Friedman test is based on ranked data, with higher scores receiving higher ranks, and is used to assess for statistically significant differences between repeated measurements.

For example, reconsider the exenatide example described in the Wilcoxon Signed-Ranks section above. Briefly, the example consisted of a one-time pretest-posttest study evaluating the secondary effect of weight loss in pounds while on exenatide therapy in a sample of 20 Type 1 DM patients. To extend this design to be applicable to Friedman's test, consider a study where patients are weighed prior to initiating exenatide therapy, 6 months after initiation, and 1-year after initiation. Thus, each patient is weighed on three occasions. Because the distribution of weight has numerous outliers, Friedman's test is employed. The results of a statistically significant Friedman's test are presented as follows:

The results of Friedman's test indicated statistically significant differences in body weight between the three repeated measurements ($\chi_2^2 = 15.21$, $p < 0.05$).

Similar to the one-way repeated measures ANOVA, Friedman's test is an omnibus test. That is, it assesses whether a statistically significant difference exists between the repeated measurements but does not indicate specifically which measurements differ significantly. Thus, a series of *post hoc* tests are required. For the example above, three signed ranks tests are required to test for differences between measurements: pretest versus 6 months, pretest versus 1 year, and 6 months versus 1 year. The results of a statistically significant Friedman's test including the additional *post hoc* tests are presented as follows:

The results of Friedman's test indicated statistically significant differences between the three repeated measurements ($\chi_2^2 = 15.21$, $p < 0.05$). Post hoc signed-rank tests indicated a statistically significant decrease in body weight from pretest to 6-month follow-up ($z = 2.65$, $p < 0.05$), with no statistically significant difference between the 6-month and 1-year follow-up ($z = 0.51$, $p > 0.05$). Thus, results suggest weight loss occurred rapidly, within 6 months of initiating exenatide therapy, and was sustained through 1 year of therapy.

The assumptions of the Friedman test include:

1. The DV is measured repeatedly on an ordinal, interval, or ratio scale.
2. All DV measurements are associated.
3. The DV measurements come from populations with the same median.

The sign test

The sign test is another nonparametric alternative to the paired-samples t-test. Similar to the signed-rank test, the sign test is used typically when distributional assumptions are violated or when the DV is measured on an ordinal scale. The sign test is used to assess for differences between two repeated measurements or two matched groups. It must be noted that the sign test is typically less powerful than the signed-rank test as the signed-rank test uses more information from the data to calculate the test statistic. Nevertheless, the sign test is presented here because it is seen in the literature; however, in most situations, the signed-rank test should have been used.

For example, consider a pretest-posttest study to evaluate change in BMI following a physical activity intervention in a sample of 20 third grade students. In this study, BMI was measured at the beginning of the school year (i.e., pretest) and again after school year was complete (i.e., posttest). The sign test assesses whether statistically significant change occurred between the two measurements. The results of a statistically significant sign test are presented below. Notice that no test statistic is presented, only a p value.

The results of the sign test indicated a statistically significant decrease in BMI from pretest to posttest ($p < 0.05$).

The assumptions of the sign test include:

1. The DV is measured repeatedly on an ordinal, interval, or ratio scale.
2. The two DV measurements are associated.

The McNemar test of change

The McNemar test of change (also known as McNemar's test) is an extension of the chi-square and Fisher's exact test when participants are measured on two separate occasions and assesses the statistical significance of observed changes between the two repeated measurements. McNemar's test is only applicable to a DV measured on a nominal scale; however, continuous variables can be artificially dichotomized, with the understanding that information will be lost.[27,41]

McNemar's test is often used for pretest-posttest studies to assess change following an intervention or treatment. For example, consider a study to determine the effectiveness of an influenza vaccination across two consecutive flu seasons. At the beginning of the first flu season, 20 participants are randomized to receive either vaccination or placebo with ten in each group. At the end of the first flu season, participants are asked whether they were diagnosed with the flu or not (i.e., yes versus no). Then, at the beginning of the second flu season, participants who received the vaccination originally will receive placebo and those who received placebo originally will receive the vaccination. At the end of the second flu season, participants are asked again whether they were diagnosed with flu. McNemar's test is used in this study to statistically test whether the flu vaccination was effective, where participants diagnosed with flu while taking placebo should not have developed flu with the vaccination. That is, the participant's outcome changed depending on the treatment received.

A critically important caveat is that McNemar's test only considers participants who changed between the two repeated measurements, with participants who did not change removed from analysis. Thus, if a researcher believes that change will be rare, the McNemar test may be inappropriate because the statistical power of this test may be extremely reduced due to the sample size decrease from removing participants who did not change.

Based on the example above, the results of a statistically significant McNemar test are presented below. Notice that no test statistic is provided, only the p value.

The results of a statistically significant McNemar's test indicated a statistically significant change between treatment and placebo ($p < 0.05$), with the vaccination significantly reducing influenza diagnoses compared to placebo.

The assumptions of the McNemar test include:

1. The DV is measured repeatedly on a dichotomous scale.
2. The two DV measurements are associated.

The Cochran Q test

The Cochran Q test (also known as Cochran's Q) is an extension of McNemar's test to situations where participants are measured repeatedly on three or more separate occasions.[27] Similar to McNemar's test, the DV must be measured repeatedly on a nominal scale.

In the biomedical literature, Cochran's Q is often used to assess stability of a treatment over time or to compare the effectiveness of several treatments. For example, consider a study evaluating the effectiveness of the combination treatment sildenafil and psychotherapy in reducing symptoms of erectile dysfunction (ED).[42] Eight patients with psychogenic ED attended weekly psychotherapy sessions and ingested 50 mg of sildenafil citrate orally as needed over a 6-month period. Symptoms of ED were assessed at baseline, 6 months (i.e., end of treatment), and at a 3-month posttreatment follow-up. For this study, Cochran's Q was used to evaluate a change in the stage of remission for patients dichotomized into ED versus no ED. A statistically significant finding indicated change from baseline and the possibility of sustaining effects at posttreatment follow-up. That is, all patients were diagnosed with ED at baseline, thus a statistically significant change indicates patients indicated remission of ED symptoms at some point.

In the literature, the results of the Cochran Q test may be presented with a χ^2 statistic and a p value; however, in other studies, the results may only present a p value. Although failing to include the test statistic provides less information, it does not necessarily damage the integrity of results. The result of a statistically significant Cochran's Q for the example above is presented as follows:

The results of Cochran's Q indicated a statistically significant change in psychogenic ED symptoms from baseline (p < 0.05) suggesting a combination of psychotherapy and 50 mg sildenafil are effective in reducing ED symptoms.

Because Cochran's Q is used to assess change over three or more repeated measures, it is an omnibus test. That is, the test will determine whether a statistically significant change occurred between the repeated measurements, but will not indicate where the change occurred. Thus, *post hoc* tests are required. For Cochran's Q, a series of McNemar tests comparing each repeated measurement serve as *post hoc* tests. In this example, three separate McNemar tests are required comparing baseline versus 6 months, baseline versus posttreatment follow-up, and 6 months versus posttreatment follow-up. The results of a statistically significant Cochran's Q including results of *post hoc* McNemar tests are presented as follows:

The results of the Cochran Q test indicated a statistically significant change in psychogenic ED symptoms from baseline (p < 0.05). Post hoc McNemar tests indicated statistically significant changes from baseline at 6 months as well as at posttreatment follow-up (all p < 0.05). These results suggest the combination of psychotherapy and sildenafil are effective in reducing ED symptoms and this effect continued to reduce ED symptoms up to 3 months following treatment completion.

The assumptions of the Cochran test include:

1. The DV measured repeatedly on a dichotomous scale.
2. All DV measurements are associated.

TESTING FOR RELATIONSHIPS OR ASSOCIATIONS

When exploring the association or relationship between two or more variables, two specific types of analyses are employed—correlation or regression. These analyses are applied to determine the magnitude and direction of an association or relationship. Correlation analysis indicates the co-relationship of two variables. That is, correlation described how one variable changes in relation to another. It is critically important to note that correlation cannot imply causation.

For example, consider the positive association between creatinine and BUN. In most cases, as creatinine increases so does BUN, but increasing creatinine does not cause BUN to increase or vice versa. Instead, the cause of the BUN and creatinine increase might be due to renal failure.

Regression analysis is a type of correlational analysis used to predict the value of one variable from the value of another variable. In this type of analysis, researchers attempt to determine the amount of variance in the DV that is explained by the IVs or covariates. Note that regression analysis can also permit multiple IVs and/or covariates measured on any scale. With the inclusion of multiple IVs or covariates this type of analysis is often referred to as multivariable regression analysis. While the definition of an IV and covariate is not always concrete, it is easier to think of an IV as the primary variable of interest and a covariate as a variable correlated with the DV, but not of specific interest.

For example, consider a multivariable analysis assessing the effect statin use (IV) had on all cause mortality due to heart failure (DV) during a 5-year study period after statistically controlling for age, gender, race, comorbid conditions, and concurrent medications (covariates). The covariates may explain the reason a patient died, but are not of specific research interest.

This section begins by discussing bivariate, or two variable, techniques followed by multivariable techniques. The discussion in this section will progress in a similar fashion to the statistical tests already presented where parametric tests will be discussed first, followed by the nonparametric alternatives.

Parametric Tests

Pearson's product-moment correlation

Pearson's product-moment correlation (also known as Pearson's correlation or Pearson's r) is one of the most commonly used correlation measures. It measures the direction and strength of a linear relationship between two continuous variables. Pearson's r ranges from -1 and $+1$, with r of 0 indicating no relationship. That is, as the correlation is stronger as it approaches -1 or 1. A positive correlation (e.g., 0.30 or 0.99) indicates that as the values of one variable increase so do the values of the other variable, while a negative correlation (e.g., -0.50 or -0.80) indicates that as the values of one variable increase, the values of the other variable decrease. Pearson's r tests whether the correlation of two variables is different from 0 (i.e., no relationship); thus, a statistically significant r indicates the slope of the linear relationship is not horizontal.

For example, research has shown a moderate, but statistically significant, positive correlation ($r = 0.25$) between weight in kilograms and platelet count in men aged 20 to 55.[43] Thus, in men, as weight increases, so does platelet count. However, the magnitude of this increase varies from person to person. That is, for any individual man, a 1-kg increase in body weight may indicate an increase in platelet count that is different from the platelet count increase for another man. It should be noted the value of r is dimensionless because it is based on standardized scores. That is, measuring weight in pounds or kilograms in the example above will not change the value of the correlation. Finally, be aware that r is substantially affected by outliers, so researchers must identify and remove them from analysis or use the nonparametric Spearman's rho discussed below.

The relationship between two variables can be assessed visually by plotting the data on a scatterplot. In fact, this practice is highly recommended.[5] The magnitude of the correlation is directly related to the strength of the linear relationship. Take a moment to consider Figures 8–13 and 8–14. In Figure 8–13, the value of Pearson's r is approximately 1 indicating

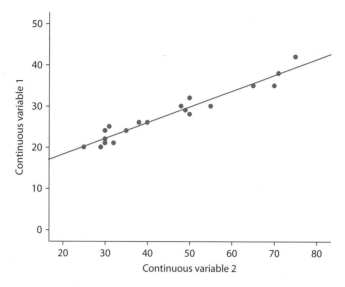

Figure 8–13. Scatterplot showing a positive correlation.

a near perfect relationship between the two variables. Notice the dots on the scatterplot lay near the best fit line and that the slope of this line is fairly steep. The positive correlation coefficient indicates that as the values of continuous variable 1 increase so do the values of continuous variable 2. In Figure 8–14, Pearson's r is approximately 0. Here, notice the dots are scattered all over the plot with no real direction, and the best fit line is almost perfectly horizontal, which indicates no relationship between the two continuous variables.

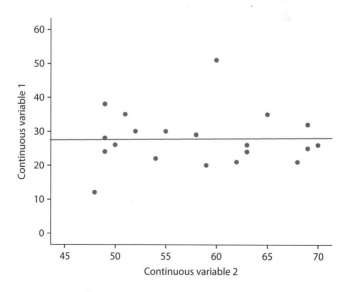

Figure 8–14. Scatterplot showing no correlation.

To highlight the substantial effect outliers have on Pearson's *r*, take a moment to draw an outlier on Figure 8–13, say, a value of 45 for continuous variable 1 and a value of 25 for continuous variable 2. Visualize what effect this outlier has on the previously strong positive correlation and how it would pull the best fit line toward horizontal significantly weakening the correlation.

The result of a statistically significant Pearson's product-moment correlation with no assumption violations using the example above is presented as follows:

The results of Pearson's product-moment correlation indicates a statistically significant moderate relationship between body weight in kilograms and platelet count ($r_{81} = 0.252$, $p < 0.05$) indicating body weight increased in concordance with platelet count.

Assumptions of Pearson's product-moment correlation include:

1. Both variables are measured on an interval or ratio scale.
2. There are no outliers.
3. The relationship between the variables is linear.
4. **Homoscedasticity** is ensured.
    a. The assumption states that the variability around the best fit line of the linear relationship is the same for all data. A violation of this assumption can be seen within a scatterplot. For example, consider a scatterplot where the lower values for a variable fall near the best fit line and higher values for this same variable fall far from the best fit line. In this situation, the variability around the line is not constant. The tenability of this assumption is difficult to ascertain in a journal article; thus, ensure the authors noted that it was tested.
5. The observations are independent.
    a. That is, each participant provides one, and only one, observation (i.e., data or response) for each variable.

Simple linear regression

As stated in the previous section, the magnitude or size of the correlation is directly related to the strength of the linear relationship. The pattern of this linear relationship is typically indicated by the regression line, which is another name for the best fit line presented in Figures 8–13 and 8–14. The regression line is a best fit line describing how the continuous DV changes as values of the IV change. Similar to Pearson's *r*, the statistical test in simple linear regression is whether the slope of the regression line is statistically different from zero, or, stated another way, whether the regression line has no slope or is horizontal. Simple linear regression, however, takes Pearson's *r* one step further, where the regression line is used to predict values of the DV for a given value of the IV.[21] This is incredibly useful to evidence-based practitioners looking to implement findings into their practice.

The algebraic linear regression equation is: $\hat{y} = a + bx$. Here, a is the intercept of the regression line with the y-axis, b is the slope of the regression line, x is the value of the IV, and $\hat{y}$ (pronounced y-hat) is the predicted value of the DV. The intercept is interpreted as the predicted value of the DV when the value of the IV is zero. The slope is interpreted as the overall change in the DV for a one-unit increase in the IV. Further, it is important to note that the value of Pearson's correlation between the DV and IV is incorporated into the mathematical equation for the slope.

As an example, consider the association between systolic blood pressure measured in millimeters of mercury (mm Hg) and height in centimeters for 100 children aged 5 to 7 years.[44] The results of this study indicated a positive Pearson correlation between height and systolic blood pressure of 0.33. Moving beyond basic correlation, the researchers used a simple linear regression analysis to predict a child's systolic blood pressure from their height. Results indicated an intercept value of 46.28 mm Hg and a slope of 0.48. Using these values, the linear regression equation would be: $\hat{y} = 46.28 + (0.48*\text{Height})$. Using the interpretation of the intercept and slope provided above, the intercept value of 46.28 is the predicted systolic blood pressure for a child 0 cm tall, whereas the slope indicates that a 1-cm increase in height increases systolic blood pressure 0.48 mm Hg. From this interpretation, it is obvious that a child with a height of 0 cm is impossible. This is a prime example of the awareness readers must have when interpreting the intercept. That is, unless it makes theoretical sense to have a meaningful zero point for the IV, the interpretation of the intercept is never useful. This situation, however, should not suggest the intercept is meaningless to prediction. Instead, the intercept is simply a starting point for predicting the outcome. For example, say we want to predict systolic blood pressure for a child that is 115 cm tall; the linear regression equation becomes: $\hat{y} = 46.28 + (0.48*115)$, which equals 101.48 mm Hg.

It is important to note that the predicted values of the DV are rarely identical to the actual observed values. That is, a child 115 cm tall in this sample may actually have a systolic blood pressure of 105 mm Hg, but have a predicted value of 101.48 mm Hg. The difference between the actual and predicted scores is referred to as a **residual value** or residual error. For the example child above, the residual value is 3.52 mm Hg (i.e., 105–101.48). Residual values are always calculated for all participants included in the regression analysis, and one of the assumptions of linear regression is that the residual values follow a normal distribution; this is where the assumption of normality originates for all parametric statistical tests. The tenability of this assumption is a key indicator of the reliability of the results. Therefore, if a researcher fails to describe the distribution of residuals alongside their results, the study should be read and interpreted with caution.

In addition, the interpretation of slope used in the above example is only appropriate for IVs measured on a continuous scale. If instead the IV is categorical, interpretation is slightly different. For example, consider replacing height in the example above with the dichotomous IV gender. In this situation, the researcher must specify which level of gender will serve as the reference or comparison category that is coded 0 for analysis. That is, specify which level of the IV the calculated slope represents. Note that every published study should indicate which group served as the reference category, and if the authors fail to provide a reference category, interpretation becomes impossible. Continuing, if females are specified as the reference category, the slope for gender provides the overall difference in predicted systolic blood pressure for males compared to females. Interpretation follows this logic. For example, using an example similar to the above, say a simple linear regression analysis indicated the intercept was 115.54 and the slope for gender was 15.20 with females considered the reference category. The new linear regression equation would be: $\hat{y} = 115.54 + 15.20*Male$. Thus, the intercept value of 115.54 now represents the average systolic blood pressure for a women (i.e., when Male = 0) and the slope indicates that the predicted value of systolic blood pressure will be 15.20 mm Hg higher for a man (i.e., when Male = 1) compared to a woman. Admittedly, these interpretations can be confusing, but understanding this concept is critically important to proper interpretation of study results.

The primary test used in simple linear regression is an omnibus between-groups ANOVA. It may seem esoteric, but linear regression and ANOVA are mathematically equivalent. The omnibus ANOVA provides an F test indicating whether the IV explains a statistically significant amount of variance in the DV. Stated another way, the omnibus test determines whether the IV reliably predicts the DV. Only if the ANOVA is statistically significant is the slope of the individual IV interpreted. Most research studies will provide the results of the ANOVA prior to presenting the slope of the IV. Further, the ANOVA results presented in simple linear regression will be presented identically to the one-way between-groups ANOVA examples discussed above. The statistical significance of the IV will most often be presented with the regression slope and potentially an associated t value. The slope is critical to proper interpretation of any regression analysis; thus, if the slope is not presented in the narrative portion or in a table complete interpretation of the regression analysis is impossible and the study is essentially useless.

Finally, the amount of variance in the DV explained by the IV must also be considered. That is, how much of the reason why a participant has a particular value on the DV is attributable to their IV value. As a side note, the word "explained" should not and does not imply causality, as causality in correlational studies is extremely difficult to determine. The amount of variance explained in simple linear regression is quantified by an effect size estimate termed the coefficient of determination. This coefficient is calculated by squaring Pearson's r between the IV and DV (i.e., r^2). In the literature it will often be referred to simply as r^2, or identically as R^2. Note that how this value is referred to in a study is dependent on the researcher, but regardless of whether r^2 or R^2 is reported, their values will be identical and, thus, interpreted identically. The coefficient will often be presented as a proportion, ranging from 0 to 1, with higher values indicating more reliable prediction. From the example above, remember the correlation between a child's height and systolic blood pressure was 0.33. Thus, approximately 0.11 (i.e., 0.33^2) of the child's measured systolic blood pressure can be explained by the child's height. Said another way, approximately 11% of the reason a child has a particular systolic blood pressure value is explained by his or her height.

In the literature, the result of a statistically significant simple linear regression analysis with no assumption violations will be presented as follows:

The results of a simple linear regression analysis indicated a child's height significantly predicts systolic blood pressure ($F_{1,98} = 12.03$, $p < 0.05$, $r^2 = 0.11$), with a 1-cm increase in height resulting in a 0.48 mm Hg increase in systolic blood pressure.

The assumptions of simple linear regression include:

1. The DV is measured on an interval or ratio scale.
2. There are no outliers.
3. The relationship between the DV and IV is linear.
4. Homoscedasticity is ensured.
   a. The assumption states that the variability around the regression line is the same for all data. A violation of this assumption can be seen within a scatterplot. For example, consider a scatterplot where the lower values for a variable fall near the regression line and higher values for this same variable fall far from the regression line. In this situation, the variability around the regression line is not constant. The tenability of this assumption is difficult to ascertain in a journal article; thus, ensure the authors noted that it was tested.
5. Residuals are distributed normally.
   a. Residuals are the difference between the actual and predicted values. Authors will need to state that they tested this assumption.
6. The observations are independent.
   a. That is, each participant provides one, and only one, observation (i.e., data or response) for each variable.

Multivariable linear regression

Multivariable linear regression (also known as multiple linear regression) is an extension of simple linear regression for designs with one continuous DV and multiple IVs or covariates measured on any scale. Remember, an IV is defined as an explanatory variable of specific research interest, while a covariate is a nuisance variable that is significantly associated with the DV but not of specific research interest. That is, covariates are typically included because they are related to the DV or because previous research has indicated they are important. In multiple linear regression, IVs can be any combination of continuous or discrete variables (e.g., height, gender). Further, this analysis is often a better option than simple linear regression because the inclusion of additional IVs often explains a higher percentage of variance in the DV. That is, multiple linear regression produces higher R^2 values.

For example, previous research has shown a statistically significant negative Pearson's correlation between serum 25-hydroxyvitamin D (25OHD; ng/mL) and serum parathyroid hormone (PTH; pg/mL) of −0.28.[45] Based on this correlation, the percentage of variance in serum PTH explained by serum 25OHD is 8% (i.e., $−0.28^2$). That is, 8% of the reason a participant has a predicted serum PTH value is due to their serum 25OHD level. In an effort to increase this percentage of variance explained, a new study is designed to determine the effect serum 25OHD has on serum PTH after statistically adjusting for age, BMI, total calcium intake, and serum creatinine. Thus, a multiple linear regression analysis will be used to determine whether there is an effect of serum 25OHD on serum PTH over and above the effect of the covariates. That is, multiple linear regression assesses the unique correlation between 25OHD and serum PTH after removing the effects already accounted for by age, BMI, total calcium intake, and serum creatinine.

The percentage of variance explained in multiple linear regression is always referred to as R^2, where the R indicates the multiple correlation. That is, R is the multivariate extension of Pearson's r and is defined as the combined or total correlation between all IVs and the DV. Similar to Pearson's r, R ranges from −1 to 1, with 0 indicating no relationship. Thus, as R approaches −1 or 1, the association between the IVs and DV becomes stronger. In addition, most studies will also present an adjusted R^2 value, sometimes labeled R^2_{adj} in the literature. Adjusted R^2 is interpreted exactly the same as R^2, but it is adjusted for the sample size used in the study. When reading a study, comparing R^2 and adjusted R^2 is incredibly useful to interpretation, as large differences between the two indicates significant issues with the analysis, such as inadequate sample size, which essentially render the regression model useless and not generalizable to the population. Finally, it should be noted a multiple linear regression model will never explain 100% of the variance in the DV. However, do not disregard studies reporting low values of R^2 because the definition of what constitutes a large R^2 value varies by research arena. That is, lower R^2 values are expected when using human participants because measurement error is usually high. For example, consider a study using participant self-reported daily calorie intake. Large R^2 values are expected for bench research studies because in well conducted bench research measurement error is typically not an issue. For example, think about a biomedical research study using analytic chemistry.

In general, the results of a multiple linear regression model are interpreted in an almost identical fashion to simple linear regression. As a result, please reconsider the section on simple linear regression if necessary. Similar to simple linear regression, multiple regression produces a regression equation allowing for prediction of DV values based on the y-intercept and the slope of the regression line for each IV or covariate. Briefly, the intercept is the predicted value of the DV when all values of the IVs and covariates are 0, while the slope quantifies the change in the predicted DV with a one-unit increase in the IV or covariates. Again, the regression equation is incredibly useful to evidence-based practitioners looking to implement findings into their practice. For example, consider the multiple regression example above, where serum PTH was predicted from 25OHD and a set of covariates. Based on the regression equation from this study, the practitioner can provide the patient with empirical evidence regarding which variables (i.e., age, BMI, total calcium intake, serum creatinine, and serum 25OHD) to increase or decrease, if possible, in an effort to optimize serum PTH levels and increase bone production.

The overall test of the multiple linear regression model is an omnibus between-groups ANOVA, which indicates at least one of the IVs or covariates significantly predicts the DV. However, this omnibus test fails to indicate which IVs or covariates significantly predict the DV. Thus, the statistical test for each IV or covariate is considered. Each of the statistical tests for the IVs and covariates can be considered similar to a *post hoc* test; however, unlike the *post hoc* tests discussed for ANOVA-type models above, alpha remains unadjusted. In most studies, the results of the individual IVs or covariates are presented as regression slope or *t* values. Note that regardless of which result an author presents, the *p* values will be identical. Further, interpretation of the slopes for the individual coefficients is also slightly different compared to simple linear regression. In multiple linear regression, interpretation of a particular IV or covariate is statistically adjusted for all other IVs and covariates in the regression model similar to ANCOVA.

An example may help clarify this information. Consider a situation where the result of a statistically significant multiple linear regression analysis based on the example above indicates 25OHD has a statistically significant slope of –1.5 pg/mL. Because the analysis is multivariable, this slope must be interpreted considering all covariates included in the model. Thus, the slope of –1.5 pg/mL indicates that after adjusting for age, BMI, total calcium intake, and serum creatinine, a 1-ng/mL increase in 25OHD decreases predicted serum PTH 1.5 pg/mL.

Based on the example, the results of a statistically significant multiple linear regression analysis with no assumption violations are presented below. Notice the effects of statistically significant covariates (i.e., BMI and serum creatinine) are also described; however, authors will vary on which covariates, if any, they choose to interpret.

The results of a multivariable linear regression analysis indicated age, BMI, total calcium intake, serum creatinine, and 25OHD significantly predicted serum PTH ($F_{5,472}$ = 21.82, p < 0.05, adjusted R^2 = 0.18). After adjusting for covariates, 25OHD significantly predicted serum PTH (slope = –1.5, p < 0.05). That is, with all else held constant, a 1-ng/mL increase in serum 25OHD resulted in a 1.5-pg/mL decrease in serum PTH. Regarding the individual covariates, after adjustment, increases in BMI and serum creatinine (slope = 0.75 and 2.12, respectively, both p < 0.05) resulted higher serum PTH levels. Finally, after adjustment, age and total calcium intake were not associated with serum PTH.

The assumptions of multiple linear regression include:

1. The DV is measured on an interval or ratio scale.
2. Absence of **multicollinearity** is ensured.
   a. That is, no Pearson's r between any IVs and covariates should be greater than 0.90, as correlations this high indicate the variables are redundant. That is, high correlations indicate the variables may be measuring the same construct. Including redundant variables will significantly bias results. Most published studies provide Pearson correlations between the DV, IVs, and covariates; thus, a violation of this assumption is easy to identify.
3. There are no outliers.
4. The relationship between the DV and IVs and between the DV and covariates is linear.
5. Homoscedasticity is ensured.
   a. The assumption states that the variability around the regression line is the same for all data. A violation of this assumption can be seen within a scatterplot. For example, consider a scatterplot where the lower values for a variable fall near the regression line and higher values for this same variable fall far from the regression line. In this situation, the variability around the regression line is not constant. The tenability of this assumption is difficult to ascertain in a journal article; thus, ensure the authors noted that it was tested.
6. Residuals are distributed normally.
   a. Residuals are the difference between the actual and predicted values.
7. The observations are independent.
   a. That is, each participant provides one, and only one, observation (i.e., data or response) for each variable.

Nonparametric Tests

Spearman rank-order correlation coefficient

The Spearman rank-order correlation coefficient (r_s), also known as Spearman's rho (ρ), is the nonparametric alternative to Pearson's r. This correlation is used when two continuous variables have outliers, when the variables are measured on an ordinal scale, or when the relationship is nonlinear. Similar to the other nonparametric statistical tests discussed previously, this correlation is based on rank ordered data as opposed to the actual values. The value of r_s ranges between -1 and 1, with 0 indicating no association. Thus, as r_s approaches -1 or 1, the association between the two variables becomes stronger. A statistically significant r_s indicates that the association is significantly different from 0.

As an example, consider a study assessing the association between triglyceride content and lag time in LDL oxidation in a sample of 18 renal transplant patients.[46]

Spearman's rank-order correlation was used in this study because outliers were identified in the sample, and because the sample was small, removing outliers was not a viable option. The study found a statistically significant negative r_s of –0.502, suggesting that as triglyceride content increased, LDL oxidation decreased.

Based on the example above, the result of a statistically significant Spearman rank-order correlation coefficient is presented as follows:

The Spearman rank-order correlation analysis was employed in lieu of Pearson's correlation due to the presence of outliers and small sample size. Results indicated a statistically significant negative association between triglyceride content and lag time in LDL oxidation ($r_s = -0.502$, $p < 0.05$), which suggest increases in triglyceride content translates into decreases in LDL oxidation.

The assumptions of the Spearman rank-order correlation coefficient include:

1. The two variables are measured on an ordinal, interval, or ratio scale.
2. The relationship between the two rank-ordered variables is linear.
   a. Although the relationship between the two variables based on their actual values may be nonlinear, the relationship based on rank-ordered data must be linear. This assumption typically cannot be tested by what the authors provide in the narrative. Thus, when authors fail to indicate whether the assumption was tested results should be viewed with caution.
3. The observations are independent.
   a. That is, each participant provides one, and only one, observation (i.e., data or response) for each variable.

Logistic regression

The interpretation of a logistic regression analysis is similar to linear regression; thus, a basic understanding of the interpretation of simple and multiple linear regression is extremely useful. Please reconsider reading the sections discussing simple and multivariable linear regression as much of the material discussed here is simply an extension of the material described in detail previously.

Logistic regression is used when the DV is measured on a dichotomous scale and the relationship between the DV and IV is nonlinear. This analysis is ubiquitous in the biomedical sciences. It is important to note that in any logistic regression analysis, the measurement scale of the DV is always considered unordered. That is, the dichotomous DV is always considered to be measured on a nominal scale. While the logistic regression analyses discussed here are only for a dichotomous DV, an extension of logistic regression is available for a categorical DV with three or more categories. This analysis is termed multinomial logistic regression, with the definition of multinomial being multiple nominal categories. Interpretation of results from this analysis is similar to the analyses discussed in this section and interested readers are encouraged to consider the suggested readings at the end of the chapter.

As an example of a design requiring a simple logistic regression analysis, consider a 5-year study designed to assess the effect that the duration of statin use measured as percentage of time on any statin during the study period has on all-cause mortality in a sample of Veterans Administration patients previously experiencing congestive heart failure. Note that the DV is dichotomous (i.e., dead versus alive). Further, a simple logistic regression analysis can always be extended to a multivariable analysis by including additional IVs and covariates in an effort to explain more of the reason why patients experienced the outcome of interest. For example, consider a multivariable extension to the study above where the effect duration of statin use has on all-cause mortality is assessed after controlling for age, race, gender, concurrent medications, and comorbid conditions.

For all logistic regression models, researchers must choose a reference category for the DV. When identified, the reference category is used as a comparison group for the primary outcome of interest. In most situations, the reference category is typically the category determined by the researcher to be of less specific interest. For example, consider all-cause mortality, a dichotomous DV (i.e., dead versus alive). Most studies are interested in the individuals who died; essentially the researcher wants to identify the primary reasons for death. Thus, with patients alive at the end of the study period considered the reference category, all regression slopes are calculated for patients who died compared to patients who lived. Thus, the first step in properly interpreting the results of logistic regression analysis is to identify the primary outcome of interest and the reference category within the DV. It should be noted that most authors will not explicitly identify the primary outcome of interest or the reference category; however, this information can be obtained easily as all results and interpretations are typically written in relation to the primary outcome of interest.

Similar to linear regression, a logistic regression analysis provides a regression equation that can be used to predict the probability of experiencing primary outcome of interest. Briefly, the regression equation contains a y-intercept and slope values for all IVs included in the analysis. This equation is interpreted slightly different from linear regression because the association between the DV and IV is nonlinear. That is, because probability is bounded between 0 and 1, the slope has to essentially shut off at these bounds. However, the usefulness of the equation is the same. That is, the equation can be used to assist evidence-based practitioners in instructing patients regarding what changes need to be made to optimize or prevent a specific outcome.

The primary statistical test in logistic regression determines whether the logistic model including all IVs or covariates better predicts the probability of experiencing the outcome of interest compared to the model with no IVs or covariates. That is, a logistic regression analysis determines whether the IVs significantly predict the primary outcome of interest. Similar to linear regression, this overall test is an omnibus chi-square test. If this omnibus chi-square test is statistically significant, the statistical significance of each IV or covariate is assessed and interpreted. These tests of individual predictors can be thought of as *post hoc* tests, and typically no adjustment is made to alpha. When interpreting the results for individual predictors, authors typically provide two values, the slope and odds ratio.

The slope is interpreted similar to linear regression; however, slopes in logistic regression indicate changes in the **log-odds** (also known as **logits**) of experiencing the outcome of interest. That is, a one-unit increase in the IV indicates a change in the predicted log-odds of experiencing the primary outcome of interest. While a full description of log-odds or logits is beyond the scope of this chapter, they can be thought of simple as a linear transformation of probability. That is, after transformation, log-odds or logits are linear; thus, their values can be interpreted similarly to slopes in linear regression. For example, reconsider the 5-year study assessing the effect duration of statin use, measured as percentage of time on any statin during the study period, has on all-cause mortality. Say, the slope for statin use is –0.25. With death considered the primary outcome of interest and alive serving as the reference category, this slope suggests that a 1% increase in statin use during the study period resulted in a 0.25 unit decrease in the log-odds of dying. Note this was a decrease because the slope was negative. Based on this interpretation, a common question is, what does a 0.25 unit decrease in log-odds mean? While the slope is integral in producing the regression equation, the interpretation in log-odds can be fairly convoluted. Thus, logistic regression provides an alternative value that some individuals find easier to interpret—the odds ratio.

The odds ratio produced by a logistic regression analysis is calculated and interpreted similarly to the odds ratios discussed in the Epidemiological Statistics section earlier in the chapter. Briefly, odds ratios range from 0 to infinity, with 1 indicating no association. Therefore, an odds ratio above 1 indicates an increase in the odds of experiencing the primary outcome of interest, whereas an odds ratio below 1 indicates a decrease in the odds of experiencing the primary outcome of interest. For example, reconsider the example above with a slope of –0.25. The associated odds ratio for this slope is 0.78. Because the odds ratio is below 1, a 1% increase in statin use is associated with a 22% (i.e., 1–0.78) decrease in the odds of dying during the study period.

It is important to be aware that authors will vary the information they present in journal articles, as one article may only provide slopes as log-odds and another article may provide odds ratios. This is not an issue, however, because there is a direct mathematical relationship between slopes and odds ratios. That is, the slope is the natural log of the odds ratio (i.e., $\ln 0.78 = -0.25$) and the odds ratio is simply the exponentiated slope (i.e., $e^{-0.25} = 0.78$). It should become clear that this mathematical relationship is where the definition of log-odds originates; they are literally the log of the odds. Given this relationship, if an author provides log-odds, the odds ratio can be easily calculated to ease interpretation. Also, note that regardless of which value the authors present, the associated p value will be identical. That is, a statistically significant slope will have a statistically significant odds ratio, and vice versa.

Finally, similar to linear regression, the primary reason a researcher includes additional IVs and covariates in a multivariable logistic regression model are to increase the amount of variance explained in the primary outcome of interest. That is, multivariable logistic regression models aim to better identify the reason why participants experienced the outcome of interest. However, unlike R^2 in linear regression, there is no accepted measure for quantifying explained variance in logistic regression. While a detailed description regarding why is beyond the scope of this chapter, it has to do with the fixed variance of the logistic distribution used to model the residual values. However, be aware that several pseudo-R^2 values may be presented in the literature, with the most common including the Nagelkerke R^2 and the Cox and Snell R^2. These pseudo-R^2 values are used to approximate R^2 from linear regression and are interpreted in similar fashion. For example, reconsider the 5-year study assessing the effect of statin use on all-cause mortality. Say the Nagelkerke R^2 value from the logistic regression analysis was 18%. This value indicates that 18% of the reason why patients died was due to their statin use. Again, it is important to note that these pseudo-R^2 values will never be near 100%, and the definition of a large or small pseudo-R^2 value is determined by the specific research arena, as discussed in the section on multivariable linear regression.

Based on the example described above, the result of a simple logistic regression analysis is presented as follows:

The results of a simple logistic regression analysis indicated a statistically significant association between duration of statin use and all-cause mortality. ($\chi_1^2 = 13.65$, $p < 0.05$) where a 1% increase in duration of statin use resulted in a 22% decrease in the odds of dying during the study period.

An example of a multivariable logistic regression analysis, with the addition of age, race, gender, concurrent medications, and comorbid conditions as covariates is presented below. Notice in this example, the researcher is not interested in the individual effects of the covariates, as they are not interpreted.

The results of a multivariable logistic regression analysis indicated a statistically significant overall association between the variables as a set and all-cause mortality ($\chi_1^2 = 156.02$, $p < 0.05$). After controlling for age, race, gender, concurrent medications, and comorbid conditions, duration of statin use significantly predicted all-cause mortality (OR = 0.62, $p < 0.05$). Thus, holding all variables constant, a 1% increase in statin use resulted in a 38% decrease in all-cause mortality.

The assumptions of logistic regression include:

1. The DV is discrete with mutually exclusive categories.
2. The sample size is large.
    a. A very rudimentary rule is to have at least 50 participants per variable included in the model. A large sample is required so that the parameters (e.g., slopes, standard errors) are estimated accurately.[47] Using this rule, a model with 10 IVs or covariates requires a minimum of 500 participants (i.e., $10 \times 50 = 500$).
3. Adequacy of expected frequencies is ensured.
    a. This assumption applies only to categorical IVs and is the same assumption as the chi-square test. That is, no more than 20% of cells can have expected frequencies less than 5. This is a difficult assumption to verify, outside of calculating the expected frequencies by hand. Thus, if an article fails to indicate this assumption was tested, view results with caution. However, most studies using logistic regression will have large sample sizes and this assumption is rarely violated.
4. Linearity in the logit is ensured.
    a. Remember, logit and log-odds are synonyms. This is a convoluted assumption, and difficult to explain without getting into mathematical detail. However, the logit is defined as the linear transformation of probability. This assumption is tested by determining whether the relationship between continuous IVs or covariates and the DV is linear. This is a key assumption, and a violation severely biases results. Thus, if authors do not mention the assumption was ensured in the methods or results sections, view results with caution.
5. Absence of multicollinearity is ensured.
    a. That is, no Pearson's r between any continuous IVs and covariates should be greater than 0.90, as correlations this high indicate the variables are redundant. That is, high correlations indicate the variables may be measuring the same facet. Including redundant variables will significantly bias results.
6. There are no outliers.
7. The observations are independent.
    a. That is, each participant provides one, and only one, observation (i.e., data or response) for each variable.

SURVIVAL ANALYSIS

Survival analysis (or failure analysis) consists of three of the most commonly used statistical techniques in the biomedical sciences—life tables, the Kaplan-Meier method, and Cox proportional-hazards model or Cox regression. Survival analysis is concerned with time-to-event data; that is, the time to experience an outcome of interest. For example, consider a study designed to examine whether a new hormone therapy, in comparison to chemotherapy, prolongs remission in women previously diagnosed with breast cancer over a 20-week study period.

In survival analysis, participants who do not experience the outcome of interest are considered to survive, while those who experience the event are considered to fail. Although this is fairly grim terminology, survival and failure do not necessarily imply living or dying. For example, in the example above failure was defined as breast cancer recurrence, not death. In survival analysis, the outcome will typically be dichotomous, patients do not need to enter the study at the same time because enrollment can be continuous, and patients are followed until the study ends which is known as end of follow-up.

Patients who do not experience the event by the end of follow-up, who are lost to follow-up, or who drop out of the study are termed censored. The key advantage survival analysis has over the analyses presented above, particularly logistic regression, is it can handle censored data, which is essentially incomplete data. That is, censored data are considered incomplete because the researcher does not know when or if participants experienced the event. Survival analysis can handle censored data because the DV is time, which is a continuous variable allowed to vary for each participant. Thus, as long as a participant has a survival time indicated, they are included in analysis. The key point here is that survival time for a censored participant is the time until they were censored, whether that is end of follow-up or whether they left the study for reasons other than suffering the event. Thus, all participants who entered the study are included in analysis regardless of whether they experienced the event or are censored because the analysis only considers the time they were in the study.

Life Tables

Life tables present time-to-event data in table format. That is, a life table tabulates the time that has elapsed until an event is experienced. Life tables are used to indicate the proportion of individuals surviving or not experiencing the event based on fixed or varying time intervals.

For example, reconsider the example above evaluating the effectiveness of the new hormone therapy in preventing recurrence of breast cancer. A life table allows the researcher to tabulate the cumulative proportion of women who do not have a recurrence of breast cancer at any interval, whether it is 6 months, 1 year, or 3 years.

As stated in the introduction to this section, life tables can be based on fixed or varying time intervals. Life tables based on fixed time intervals have a significant weakness, as they do not consider the exact time within the specified interval when the patient experienced the event. Thus, depending on the length of the time interval, a great amount of information could be lost regarding the exact time the event was experienced. That is, the longer the time interval, the less precise a researcher can be regarding the exact moment the event occurred. Thankfully, better methods have emerged, particularity the Kaplan-Meier method.

The Kaplan-Meier Method

The Kaplan-Meier method is the most widely used estimator of survival time in the biomedical sciences.[48] The Kaplan-Meier method is an extension of the life table using varying time intervals. Using this method, the cumulative proportion surviving is recalculated every time an event occurs.[49]

As an example, instead of assessing the total number of women who have a breast cancer recurrence at fixed intervals of 6 months, the Kaplan-Meier method recalculates the proportion of women surviving every time a woman in the study has a recurrence. In most studies, Kaplan-Meier data is presented as a graph of the cumulative survival over the study period known as a Kaplan-Meier curve. The Kaplan-Meier curve presents either a survival or hazard functions, where the survival function is the cumulative frequency of participants not experiencing the event, whereas the hazard function is the cumulative frequency of participants experiencing the event. A Kaplan-Meier curve is provided in the vast majority of published literature using survival analysis and will appear similar to the survival curve presented in Figure 8–15. Note that for ease of interpretation the curve in Figure 8–15 only presents data for the sample of women initiating the new hormone therapy and does not include data for women initiating chemotherapy. Notice the y-axis indicates the cumulative proportion of women surviving, while the x-axis indicates the total number of weeks of the study. The solid line represents the survival function. That is, the

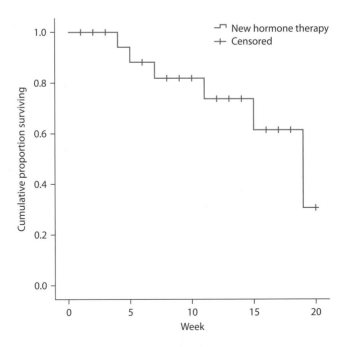

Figure 8–15. Kaplan-Meier curve.

cumulative proportion of women not experiencing the event at any given time. The survival function indicates when a woman experienced the event when the function steps down. For example, by week 5, two women have experienced the event, indicated by the two steps in the survival function. Further, notice the vertical dashes throughout the survival function. These dashes indicate individual women who were censored. That is, women who dropped out of the study for reasons other than experiencing the event such as side effects or they simply were lost to follow-up by moving out of the area. Few studies provide explicit information regarding censored participants on the Kaplan-Meier curve because most survival analyses involve large samples. Thus, the dashes in Figure 8–15 are usually omitted from the curve; however, frequency counts of censored participants are always provided within the narrative or in table format.

The Kaplan-Meier curve can also be presented for multiple groups. For example, consider the overall survival of women initiating the new hormone therapy compared to women initiating chemotherapy. Figure 8–16 presents a Kaplan-Meier curve where the survival functions for both treatment groups are presented simultaneously. Interpretation of these survival functions is identical to the methods described above for Figure 8–15. However, with two or more treatment groups, a statistical test must be conducted to assess for a statistically significant group difference in survival rate. The most common

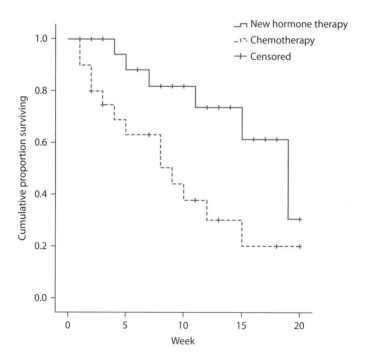

Figure 8–16. Kaplan-Meier curve—comparing groups.

test in the biomedical literature is the log-rank test (aka, the Mantel-Cox test).[49] A statistically significant log-rank test indicates there is a significant difference in survival rate between the groups. However, it is important to note that a Kaplan-Meier curve and associated log-rank test have no way of indicating why the breast cancer recurred beyond the possibility of the therapy being ineffective.

Based on the survival functions presented in Figure 8–16, the results of a statistically significant log-rank test are presented as follows:

Based on Kaplan-Meier curves, the results of the log-rank test indicated a statistically significant difference in duration of breast cancer remission between the new hormone therapy and chemotherapy groups ($\chi_1^2 = 5.68$, $p < 0.05$), with women initiating the new hormone therapy experiencing significantly longer breast cancer remission.

It should be noted that when more than two treatment groups are being compared the log-rank test is an omnibus test. That is, with three or more groups, a statistically significant log-rank test will indicate that a statistically significant difference exists between groups, but will not indicate specifically which groups differ. Thus, *post hoc* log-rank tests are required to determine where a significant difference in survival occurred.

For example, consider the addition of another treatment group to the breast cancer example, say, women who do not want to initiate any therapy. Following a statistically significant omnibus log-rank test, three *post hoc* log-rank tests would be required to determine whether statistically significant differences in survival rate occurred between hormone therapy versus chemotherapy, hormone therapy versus no therapy, and chemotherapy versus no therapy.

The results of statistically significant *post hoc* tests are presented as follows:

Based on Kaplan-Meier curves, the results of the log-rank test indicated a statistically significant difference in breast cancer recurrence between the three treatment groups ($\chi_2^2 = 9.76$, $p < 0.05$). Post hoc log-rank tests indicated women initiating the new hormone therapy experienced significantly longer breast cancer remission compared to women receiving chemotherapy or women choosing not to receive therapy (both $p < 0.05$). No statistically significant difference was indicated between women initiating chemotherapy and women receiving no therapy.

Cox Proportional-Hazards Model

Although the Kaplan-Meier method is effective in assessing for overall differences in survival, the analysis is unable to identify the association between covariates and survival. That is, the Kaplan-Meier method cannot identify whether the IV significantly predicts survival, and for many studies prediction is a far more important consideration. Thus, a form of regression analysis is required. The Cox proportional hazards model (also known as Cox regression) is a semiparametric method used to predict the time to experience an event of interest. Note that the DV is time-to-event, the event is usually a dichotomous variable, and the analysis is considered semiparametric because it includes both parametric and nonparametric components. In addition, all predictor variables in a Cox regression are termed covariates. That is, in the literature, authors will not identify a distinction between IVs and covariates. Finally, it should also be noted that most published studies progress from Kaplan-Meier curves and log-rank tests to Cox regression analysis. That is, the Kaplan-Meier curve will first present the survival functions for the covariate of interest as well as associated log-rank tests and then authors will present the results of a Cox regression assessing for the relationship between covariates and the event of interest.

The interpretation of Cox regression can be considered a combination of linear and logistic regression; however, the primary difference is that in Cox regression results are considered time dependent. That is, Cox regression is concerned with the time-dependent risk of experiencing the event instead of the overall occurrence of events as in logistic regression. Remember, the DV is time. For example, consider a study designed to assess the effect duration of statin use, measured as percentage of time in any statin during the study period, has on all-cause mortality in a sample of Veterans Administration patients previously experiencing congestive heart failure. If the researchers were interested in the effect duration of statin use had on prolonging the time until death during the study period a Cox regression analysis is the analysis of choice. Again, the primary consideration in Cox regression is time-to-event, not in the overall probability of the event as in logistic regression.

Similar to linear and logistic regression, Cox regression can be simple or multivariable. For example, in the example above a simple Cox regression analysis was required because only duration of statin use was used to predict the risk of death. However, if the study was extended to statistically control for age, gender, race, comorbid conditions, and concurrent medications, a multivariable Cox regression is appropriate. That is, assess the effects duration of statin use had on the risk of death over and above the effects of the other covariates.

Similar to logistic regression analysis, within the DV the researcher must choose the primary event of interest and the associated reference category. When identified, the reference category is used as a comparison group for the event of interest. In most situations, the reference category is typically the category determined by the researcher to be of less specific interest. For example, consider all-cause mortality, a dichotomous outcome variable, in which most studies are interested in the individuals who died. Thus, patients who lived are usually considered the reference category and all regression slopes are calculated for patients who died compared to patients who lived. Therefore, the first step in properly interpreting the results of a Cox regression analysis is to identify the event and the reference category. If an author does not explicitly state the reference category, this information can be obtained easily as all results and interpretations are typically written in relation to the primary event of interest.

It is critically important to note that in the literature authors will report using one of two different Cox regression analyses—with or without time varying covariates. The decision of which model to use is based on whether the proportionality of hazards assumption was violated. This assumption typically applies to all categorical covariates and states that, although events can begin to occur at any time during the study period, when events do begin, the rate at which events occur between levels of a categorical covariate must remain constant over time. That is, when events begin to occur, the survival functions for the groups must be the same or roughly parallel.

For example, reconsider Figure 8–16. Here, the proportionality of hazards assumption is not violated because events occur at approximately the same rate in each group. Notice women initiating the new hormone therapy did not begin experiencing breast cancer recurrence until week 4, as indicated by no steps in the curve until week 4, whereas women in the chemotherapy group began experiencing the recurrence at week 1, steps occurred immediately. However, when events began to occur in either group, they occurred at approximately the same rate. That is, the slopes of the survival functions are roughly parallel. Thus, the proportionality of hazards assumption is not violated and the treatment group covariate is assumed to have constant survival rates over time. More specifically, in this situation a Cox regression without time varying covariates is appropriate.

By contrast, a violation of the proportionality assumption is provided in Figure 8–17. Notice that in this figure, events began occurring at roughly around weeks 3 and 4 within both treatment groups. However, the survival functions are drastically different, and in fact intersect twice. In general, any time survival functions intersect, the proportionality of hazards assumption can be considered violated, because the rate of survival within each group varies across time. In this situation, Cox regression with time varying covariates would be required.

In conclusion, when reading a journal article, take careful notice of the Kaplan-Meier curves presented prior to the Cox regression analysis. Clear violation of this assumption is apparent any time survival functions intersect. If a violation is observed, identify whether the appropriate Cox regression analysis was employed. That is, if a violation is indicated, Cox regression with time-varying covariates must be used. If Cox regression without time varying covariates was used in the presence of a violation, results and interpretations are extremely misleading.

Similar to the other forms of regression discussed, Cox regression allows researchers to produce a regression equation useful in determining the overall risk score for a patient based on specific characteristics. The primary difference in Cox regression, however, is that there is no y-intercept representing the baseline hazard function. Thus, overall risk is calculated simply by using the slopes for the covariates. Even without the intercept, however, this regression equation remains useful for evidence-based practitioners when consulting their patients on changes required decreasing the risk of experiencing an unfavorable event.

Identical to logistic regression, the overall statistical test in Cox regression is whether the model including the covariates predicts the time elapsed prior to experiencing the event significantly better than the model with no covariates. That is, a Cox regression analysis determines whether the covariates significantly predict the time elapsed prior to experiencing the primary event of interest. This overall test is an omnibus chi-square test. Only if this omnibus chi-square test is statistically significant does the researcher evaluate the statistical significance of each covariate. The tests of individual predictors are usually more important and these will be presented in all studies using a Cox regression model. Tests of individual predictors will be presented by regression slopes and/or hazard ratios.

In Cox regression, slopes are interpreted similar to logistic regression. However, for this analysis, a one-unit increase in a covariate results in an increase or decrease in the log-hazard or log-risk of experiencing the event. While a full description of log-risk is beyond the scope of this chapter, they can be thought of simply as a linear transformation of probability of experiencing the event. That is, after transformation, log-risks are linear and their values can be interpreted similarly to slopes in linear regression. For example, say the slope for women initiating the new hormone therapy was –0.65. That is, women initiating chemotherapy served as the reference or comparison group. Thus, the slope represents a 0.65 unit decrease in the log-risk of breast cancer recurrence for the new

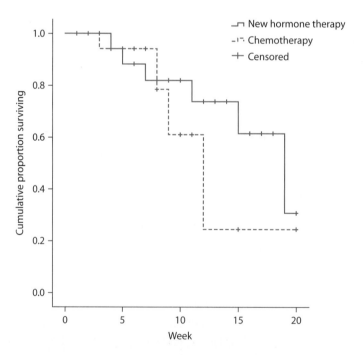

Figure 8–17. Kaplan-Meier curve showing violation of proportionality of hazards assumption.

hormone therapy compared to chemotherapy. A 0.65 unit decrease in log-hazard is diffi-cult to explain and beyond the scope of this chapter; thus, the presentation and interpreta-tion of hazard ratios are often a useful alternative.

The hazard ratio produced by a Cox regression analysis is calculated and interpreted similarly to the relative risk discussed in the Epidemiological Statistics section above. However, it is important to note that a hazard ratio is not identical to relative risk. Briefly, hazard ratios range from 0 to infinity, with 1 indicating no association. Therefore, a hazard ratio above 1 indicates an increase in the risk of experiencing the event, whereas a hazard ratio below 1 indicates a decrease in the risk of experiencing the event. For example, reconsider the example above where the slope for the new hormone therapy was –0.65. The associated hazard ratio for this slope is 0.52. Because the hazard ratio is below 1, initiating the new hormone therapy resulted in a 48% (i.e., 1 to 0.52) decrease in the risk of breast cancer recurrence compared to chemotherapy.

It is important to consider that authors may vary the information they present in jour-nal articles, as one study may only provide slopes and another study may only provide haz-ard ratios. This is not an issue because there is a direct mathematical relationship between slopes and hazard ratios. That is, the slope is simply the natural log of the hazard ratio (i.e., ln 0.52 = –0.65), whereas the hazard ratio is simply the exponentiated slope (i.e., $e^{-0.65}$ = 0.52). It should become clear that this mathematical relationship is where the definition of log-risk originates; they are literally the log of the risk. Thus, if an author only provides slopes, the hazard ratio can be easily calculated to ease interpretation. Also, note that regard-less of which value the authors present, the associated p value will be identical. That is, a statistically significant slope will have a statistically significant hazard ratio, and vice versa.

Finally, no pseudo-R^2 exists for Cox regression to indicate proportion of variance explained. Although several have been suggested they are not interpreted as the percent-age of variance explained and these values do not indicate how much of the overall reason why a participant experienced the event.[46] Thus, when reading a journal article, do not be discouraged by authors failing to provide this information.

Based on the breast cancer example above, a statistically significant multivariable Cox regression analysis is presented below. Note that this Results section will typically be presented in addition to the results of the Kaplan-Meier analysis above.

No violation of the proportionality of hazards assumption was indicated; thus, a Cox regression without time dependent covariates was conducted to assess the effectiveness of a new hormone therapy compared to chemotherapy in preventing breast cancer recurrence after adjusting for age, concurrent medications, and comorbid conditions. Results indicated the covariates, as a set, significantly predicted time to breast cancer recurrence ($\chi^2_8 = 63.12$, p < 0.05). Holding age, concurrent medications, and comorbid conditions constant, women initiating the new hormone therapy experienced a 48% decrease in the risk of breast cancer recurrence compared to women initiating chemotherapy.

The assumptions of Cox regression include:

1. Time is measured on an interval or ratio scale.
2. Sample size must be large.
   a. A very rudimentary rule is to have at least 50 participants per variable included in the model. A large sample is required so that the parameters (e.g., slopes, standard errors) are estimated accurately.[45] Using this rule, a model with 10 IVs and covariates requires a minimum of 500 participants (i.e., $10 \times 50 = 500$).
3. Proportionality of hazards is ensured.
   a. The survival functions for all categorical covariates must be similar.
4. No differences between withdrawn and remaining cases exist.
   a. Because Cox regression can handle censored data, participants who are lost to follow-up must not differ from those whose outcome is known. That is, participants who dropped out of the study must not be different from those who completed it. For example, women who dropped out of the new hormone group because they are experiencing unbearable side effects that do not occur in the chemotherapy group.
5. Absence of multicollinearity is ensured.
   a. That is, no Pearson's r between any continuous covariates should be greater than 0.90, as correlations this high indicate the variables are redundant. High correlations indicate the variables may be measuring the same facet. Including redundant variables will significantly bias results.
6. There are no outliers.
7. Observations are independent.
   a. That is, each participant provides one, and only one, observation (i.e., data or response) for each variable.

Conclusion

A thorough understanding of statistical methods is integral to effectively evaluating medical literature. Being cognizant of the effect study design has on results, interpretation, and generalization is incredibly important to implementing evidence-based practice. Statistical analyses are simply a piece of the puzzle when evaluating literature, since the study design and research question determine the appropriate analyses. It must be noted that simply because a study is published does not define it as a quality study. Further, all research has flaws, some trivial, others significant. A reader's task is to determine whether these flaws prevent the research from being credible.[50] Thus, when reviewing an empirical study, the following steps must be considered carefully:

1. Thoughtfully consider the study design (see Chapters 4 and 5). This includes, but is not limited to, the theory, specific research question(s), randomization, sample characteristics, data collection methods, variables, and outcomes. A poor design will lead to inaccurate or biased estimates, leading to an inferior study.
2. Evaluate the statistical test. Is it appropriate for the research question? Did the author test for assumption violations? If no assumption tests are stated, can violations be determined from the descriptive statistics provided? Was the test interpreted properly? Were effect size (i.e., clinical significance) measures provided?
3. Evaluate the discussion section. Are the results interpreted within the context of the sample and population? Are generalizations accurate? What were the limitations? How does the study lend itself to future research?

Finally, to reiterate, this chapter is by no means exhaustive of all statistical tests, nor does it provide a complete overview of statistical tests. Interested readers are encouraged to consult any of the suggested readings below for a more thorough treatment of the topics discussed.

Self-Assessment Questions

1. A pharmacy professor wants to know whether a new instructional method improves test scores during her class. She uses all students in her classroom as participants. This is an example of which type of sampling?
   a. Convenience sample
   b. Cluster sample
   c. Stratified random sample
   d. Multistage sample

2. Say the DV in the study described in question 1 is whether the student passed or failed the test using a cutoff of 70%? This is an example of which scale of measurement?
   a. Binary
   b. Categorical
   c. Dichotomous
   d. Discrete
   e. All of the above

3. Say a continuous variable such as board scores from the North American Pharmacist Licensure Examination (NAPLEX) are categorized into pass versus not pass, where ≥75 is determined to be the cutoff for passing. If this new categorical variable were included in a statistical analysis, pharmacists who passed the NAPLEX with a score of 80 would be considered identical to pharmacists who passed with a score of 130.
   a. True
   b. False

4. The most appropriate measure of central tendency for binary data is:
   a. Mean
   b. Median
   c. Mode
   d. Range

5. Variance is an incredibly important descriptive statistic that is used in all statistical analyses. Although, most journal articles will only report the standard deviation, it is easy to translate between variance and standard deviation. For example, say the standard deviation of a continuous variable is reported to be 25. What is the variance?
   a. 100
   b. 250
   c. 50
   d. 625

6. A histogram is appropriate to present data for variables measured on which scale of measurement?
   a. Nominal
   b. Interval
   c. Categorical
   d. Ratio
   e. Both b and d

7. A z-score of 1.5 indicates that a specific data point is what?
   a. The data point is 1.5 interquartile ranges the variable's median.
   b. The variable has a range of 1.5.
   c. The data point is 1.5 standard deviations above variable's mean.
   d. The data point is 1.5 standard deviations below the variable's mean.

8. An odds ratio of 1 indicates that:
   a. There is a 100% increase in the odds of experiencing some outcome.
   b. There is no increase or decrease in the odds of experiencing some outcome.

    c. There is a 1% increase in the odds of experiencing some outcome.

    d. There is a 1% decrease in the odds of experiencing some outcome.

9. An example of nonexperimental research would be:

    a. A randomized controlled trial

    b. An observational study

    c. A situation where some clinics receive an intervention and others do not

    d. A doctor doses some patients with a treatment and gives others a placebo

10. A study where participants eventually receive all treatments is an example of what type of study design?

    a. A crossover design

    b. A randomized controlled trial

    c. A parallel-groups design

    d. An adaptive design

11. A statistical test is used to evaluate for differences between two treatment groups. Alpha is set at 0.05. The statistical test indicates $p = 0.0001$, which is statistically significant. This statistically significant result unanimously indicates a large treatment effect.

    a. True

    b. False

12. A nonparametric test is most appropriate when:

    a. The distributional assumptions of a parametric statistical test is violated.

    b. There are larger numbers of outliers.

    c. The sample size is small.

    d. All of the above.

13. Parametric statistical tests always assume normality.

    a. True

    b. False

14. A study is published evaluating the differences across several treatment arms. The DV is continuous, the IV has three levels, and one continuous covariate is considered. No interaction is observed between the IV and covariate. Which statistical analysis is most appropriate?

    a. Independent-samples t-test

    b. ANCOVA

    c. Multivariable linear regression

    d. Simple linear regression

    e. Both b and c

15. A study is designed to evaluate time-to-death in a group of patients suffering from congestive heart failure over a 2-year study period. Two of the three researchers think they should use the Cox proportional-hazards model for analysis, the third researcher wants to use logistic regression. Which analysis is correct given the research question?

   a. The Cox proportional-hazards model is appropriate because the researchers are interested in time-to-death.

   b. The logistic regression analysis is appropriate because the researchers are interested in time-to-death.

   c. The Cox proportional-hazards model cannot be used to model a dichotomous outcome, so logistic regression should be used.

   d. Logistic regression is not appropriate to use with a binary DV.

REFERENCES

1. United States Census Bureau. Census regions and divisions of the United States [Internet]. Available from: http://www.census.gov/geo/www/us_regdiv.pdf. Accessed June 24, 2010.

2. Stevens SS. On the theory of scales of measurement. Science. 1946;103(2684):677-80.

3. Hockenberry MJ, Wilson D. Wong's essentials for pediatric nursing. 8th ed. St. Louis (MO): Mosby; 2009.

4. Tabachnick BG, Fidell LS. Using multivariate statistics. 5th ed. Boston (MA): Pearson Education Inc.; 2007.

5. Tukey JW. Exploratory data analysis. Reading (MA): Addison-Wesley; 1977.

6. Gordis L. Epidemiology. Philadelphia (PA): Saunders Elsevier; 2009.

7. Hennekens CH, Buring JE, Mayrent SL, eds. Epidemiology in medicine. Philadelphia (PA): Lippincott, Williams, and Wilkins; 1987.

8. Friis RH. Epidemiology 101. Sudbury (MA): Jones and Bartlett Publishers; 2010.

9. Campbell DT, Stanley JC. Experimental and quasi-experimental designs for research. Boston (MA): Houghton Mifflin Company; 1966.

10. Feinstein AR. Epidemiologic analyses of causation: the unlearned scientific lessons of randomized trials. J Clin Epidemiol. 1989;42(6):481-89.

11. Ioannidis JP, Haidich AB, Pappa M, Pantazis N, Kokori SI, Tektonidou MG, et al. Comparison of evidence of treatment effects in randomized and nonrandomized studies. JAMA. 2001;286(7):821-30.

12. United States National Institutes of Health. Understanding clinical trials [Internet]. Available from: http://clinicaltrials.gov/ct2/info/understand#Q18. Accessed June 25, 2010.

13. Hopewell S, Dutton S, Yu L-M, Chan A-W, Altman DG. The quality of reports of randomized trials in 2000 and 2006: comparative study of articles indexed in PubMed. BMJ. 2010;340(c723):1-8.

14. Everitt BS, Pickles A. Statistical aspects of the design and analysis of clinical trials. 2nd ed. River Edge (NJ): Imperial College Press; 2004.

15. Chow S, Liu J. Design and analysis of clinical trials: concepts and methodologies. 2nd ed. Hoboken (NJ): John Wiley & Sons; 2004.

16. International Conference on Harmonisation of Technical Requirements for Registration of Pharmaceuticals for Human Use (ICH). Statistical principles for clinical trials E9 [Internet]. Available from: http://www.ich.org/fileadmin/Public_Web_Site/ICH_Products/Guidelines/Efficacy/E9/Step4/E9_Guideline.pdf. Accessed June 26, 2010.

17. United States Department of Health and Human Services. Guidance for industry: adaptive design clinical trials for drugs and biologics [Internet]. Available from: http://www.fda.gov/downloads/Drugs/GuidanceComplianceRegulatoryInformation/Guidances/UCM201790.pdf. Accessed June 18, 2010.

18. Lachin JM. Statistical considerations in the intent-to-treat principle. Control Clin Trials. 2000;21(3):167-89.

19. Enders CK. A primer on the use of modern missing-data methods in psychosomatic medicine research. Psychosom Med. 2006;68(3):427-36.

20. Rubin DB. Inference and missing data. Biometrika. 1976;63(3):581-92.

21. Moore DS. The basic practice of statistics. 2nd ed. New York (NY): W. H. Freeman and Company; 2000.

22. Tabachnick BG, Fidell LS. Experimental design using ANOVA. Belmont (CA): Duxbury Press; 2007.

23. Cohen J. Statistical power analysis for the behavioral sciences. 2nd ed. Hillsdale (NJ): Lawrence Erlbaum Associates Inc.; 1988.

24. Nickerson RS. Null hypothesis significance testing: a review of an old and continuing controversy. Psychol Methods. 2000;5(2):241-301.

25. Cumming G, Finch S. Inference by eye: confidence intervals and how to read pictures of data. Am Psychol. 2005;60(2):170-80.

26. Cumming G, Finch, S. A primer on the understanding, use, and calculation of confidence intervals that are based on central and noncentral distributions. Educ Psychol Meas. 2001;61(4):532-74.

27. Siegel S, Castellan NJ. Nonparametric statistics for the behavioral sciences. 2nd ed. New York (NY): McGraw-Hill Inc.; 1988.

28. Sheskin DJ. Handbook of parametric and nonparametric statistical procedures. 3rd ed. Boca Raton (FL): CRC Press; 2000.

29. Krauss RM, Burke DJ. Identification of multiple subclasses of plasma low density lipoproteins in normal humans. J Lipid Res. 1982;23(1):97-104.

30. Austin MA, King MC, Vranizan KM, Krauss RM. Atherogenic lipoprotein phenotype. A proposed genetic marker for coronary heart disease risk. Circ. 1990;82:495-506.

31. Cochran WG. Some methods for strengthening the common χ^2 tests. Biometrics. 1954;10(4):417-51.

32. Cohen J. A coefficient of agreement for nominal scales. Educ Psychol Meas. 1960;20(1): 37-46.

33. United States Centers for Disease Control and Prevention. National health and nutrition examination survey [Internet]. Available from: http://www.cdc.gov/nchs/nhanes/nhanes2007-2008/lab07_08.htm. Accessed June 24, 2010.

34. Schober SE, Carroll MD, Lacher DA, Hirsch R. High serum total cholesterol—an indicator for monitoring cholesterol lowering efforts; U.S. adults, 2005–2006. NCHS data brief no. 2. Hyattsville(MD): National Center for Health Statistics; 2007.

35. Keppel G. Design and analysis: a researcher's handbook. 3rd ed. Englewood Cliffs (NJ): Prentice Hall; 1991.

36. Hardy R, Kuh D, Langenberg C, Wadsworth ME. Birthweight, childhood social class, and change in adult blood pressure in the 1946 British birth cohort. Lancet. 2003;362(9391): 1178-83.

37. Williams JG, Allison C, Scott FJ, Bolton PF, Baron-Cohen S, Matthews FE, et al. The Childhood Autism Spectrum Test (CAST): sex differences. J Autism Dev Disord. 2008; 38:1731-9.

38. Skrabal MZ, Jones RM, Walters, RW, Nemire RE, Soltis DA, Kahaleh AA, et al. National volunteer preceptor survey of experiential student loads, quality of time issues, and compensation: differences in responses based on region, type of practice setting, and population density. J Pharm Prac. 2010;23(3):265-72.

39. Vickers AJ. How many repeated measures in repeated measure designs? Statistical issues for comparative trials. Br Med Res Methodology. 2003;3(22):1-9.

40. Beck AT, Steer RA, Brown GK. Manual for Beck depression inventory-II. San Antonio (TX): Psychological Corporation; 1996.

41. Jekel JF. Epidemiology, biostatistics, and preventative medicine. 3rd ed. Philadelphia (PA): Asunders Elseiver; 2007.

42. Melnik T, Abdo CHN. Psychogenic erectile dysfunction: comparative study of three therapeutic approaches. J Sex Marital Ther. 2005;31(3):246-55.

43. Siebers RWL, Carter JM, Wakem PJ, Maling TJB. Interrelationship between platelet count, red cell count, white cell count and weight in men. Clin Lab Hematol. 1990;12(3): 257-62.

44. Petrie A, Sabin C. Medical statistics at a glance. 2nd ed. Malden (MA): Blackwell Publishing Ltd.; 2005.

45. Need AG, Horowitz M, Morris HA, Nordin BEC. Vitamin D status: effects of parathyroid hormone and 1,25-dihydroxyvitamin D in post menopausal women. Am J Clin Nutr. 2000; 71(6):1577-81.

46. Sutherland WH, Walker RJ, Ball MJ, Stapley SA, Robertson MC. Oxidation of low density lipoproteins from patients with renal failure or renal transplants. Kidney Int. 1995; 48(1):227-36.

47. Aldrich JH, Nelson FD. Linear probability, logit, and probit models. Sage University paper series on quantitative applications in the social sciences, series no. 07-045. Newbury Park (CA): Sage Publications, Inc.; 1984.

48. Allison PD. Survival analysis using the SAS system: a practical guide. Cary (NC): SAS Institute Inc.; 1995.

49. Kleinbaum DG, Klein M. Survival analysis: a self learning text. 2nd ed. New York (NY): Springer; 2005.

50. Simon SD. Is the randomized clinical trial the gold standard of research? J Androl. 2001; 22(6):938-43.

SUGGESTED READINGS

The suggested readings below are for interested readers to gain further insight into some of the topics covered in this chapter. Note that most of the information provided in the first half of this chapter can be obtained in any introductory statistics textbook.

Epidemiological Statistics

1. Gordis L. Epidemiology. Philadelphia (PA): Saunders Elsevier; 2009.

    Clinical Significance and Effect Size

1. Cohen J. Statistical power analysis for the behavioral sciences. 2nd ed. Hillsdale (NJ): Lawrence Erlbaum Associates Inc.; 1988.

    Study Design and Randomized Controlled Trials

1. Campbell DT, Stanley JC. Experimental and quasi-experimental designs for research. Boston (MA): Houghton Mifflin Company; 1966.

2. Chow S, Liu J. Design and analysis of clinical trials: concepts and methodologies. 2nd ed. Hoboken (NJ): John Wiley & Sons; 2004.

    Nonparametric Statistical Tests

1. Siegel S, Castellan NJ. Nonparametric statistics for the behavioral sciences. 2nd ed. New York (NY): McGraw-Hill, Inc.; 1988.

    ANOVA Designs

1. Keppel G. Design and analysis: a researcher's handbook. 3rd ed. Englewood Cliffs (NJ): Prentice Hall; 1991.

    Linear and Logistic Regression, Survival Analysis

1. Tabachnick BG, Fidell LS. Using multivariate statistics. 5th ed. Boston (MA): Pearson Education Inc.; 2007.

2. Stevens J. Applied multivariate statistics for the social sciences. 4th ed. Mahwah (NJ): Lawrence Erlbaum Associates, Inc.; 2002.

3. Cohen P, Cohen J, West SG, Aiken LS. Applied multiple regression/correlation analysis for the behavioral sciences. 3rd ed. Mahwah (NJ): Lawrence Erlbaum Associates Inc.; 2003.

4. Hosmer DW, Lemeshow S. Applied logistic regression. 2nd ed. New York (NY): John Wiley and Sons; 2000.

5. Kleinbaum DG, Klein M. Survival analysis: a self-learning text. 2nd ed. New York (NY): Springer; 2005.

Clustering and Nesting

1. Snijders TAB, Bosker RJ. Multilevel analysis: an introduction to basic & advanced multi-level modeling. 2nd ed. Thousand Oaks (CA): Sage Publications; 2011.

2. Hox J. Multilevel analysis: techniques and applications. 2nd ed. New York (NY): Routledge; 2010.

3. Raudenbush SW, Bryk AS. Hierarchical linear models: applications and data analysis methods. 2nd ed. Newbury Park (CA): Sage Publications; 2002.

Chapter Nine

Professional Writing

Patrick M. Malone • Meghan J. Malone

Learning Objectives

After completing this chapter, the reader will be able to

- State reasons both for and against writing professionally.
- Describe the various steps of professional writing.
- Identify the order for authors in a professional paper.
- Describe the importance of knowing the audience.
- Describe various writing styles and their differences.
- Explain where to find a publication's requirements for submission.
- Describe what an article proposal consists of and why it is used.
- Explain the need for continued practice to develop good writing skills.
- List the components of both a research and review paper.
- Explain the general guidelines for writing.
- Describe the peer-review process.
- Explain the absolute importance of revision.
- Explain the steps in creating a newsletter or Web site.
- Describe how to prepare audiovisual materials for a poster or platform presentation and place those items on a Web site.
- Describe techniques for creating an abstract for an article.
- Describe how to correctly cite reference materials.

Key Concepts

1 Essentially any time a professional takes pen, pencil, word processor, or any other writing implement in hand to fulfill professional duties, it is considered professional writing.

2 When writing, it is best to keep things as simple and direct as possible.

3 With the probable exception of policy and procedure documents, the two most important paragraphs in any document are the first and last.

4 If the information is taken from a particular source, even if it is reworded, the original author should be given credit via footnotes or endnotes.

5 In many cases, revision of a document will be necessary.

6 Instead of concentrating on the technology, it is best to concentrate on the message.

7 Professional writing is a skill necessary for every health professional.

Introduction

A common thought when considering the topic of **professional writing** is, "That doesn't apply to me, I'm not writing for a journal." But professional writing is certainly not limited to journal articles or books. It includes writing evaluations of medications for consideration on a hospital formulary, preparing written policies and procedures for the preparation of an intravenous admixture, reporting the results of the latest sales to the home office, preparing a written evaluation of a technician or clerk, writing in a chart, writing a term paper for a class, preparing slides or posters for a presentation, writing a letter of recommendation,[1] and many other things. **1** *Essentially any time a professional takes pen, pencil, word processor, or any other writing implement in hand to fulfill professional duties, it is considered professional writing.* When writing, although the format changes, the general principles remain the same. So whether the objective is to write the ultimate book on the practice of pharmacy or to type a label, a pharmacist must know how to write professionally.

Although some may say the purpose of writing is to keep a job or to pass a course, there are, generally, four larger purposes for the existence of written material. That material serves to inform, instruct, persuade, or entertain. The first three items are those usually considered in professional writing, although including the fourth, whenever possible, will help convince people to read what has been written.

There are also some advantages to professional writing, besides those mentioned above. For example, writing is often used to evaluate an employee for promotion in many jobs. In academia, there is always the concept of publish or perish. Even pharmacy technicians are encouraged to write as a means of advancement.[2] Also, writing gives the authors the opportunity to share their knowledge or ideas,[3] obtain gratification or satisfaction,[4] and improve their knowledge. It may even lead to some fame or notoriety in a field.

Unfortunately, there are disadvantages to professional writing. The major problem is that any significant amount of writing often involves a lot of potentially frustrating work, because few people are natural writers. The author must practice to become proficient at writing, which will involve false starts, numerous drafts, roadblocks, and other problems.[5] If that is not enough, writing exposes a person to criticism and possible rejection. Although at one time authors were paid to publish articles, today it is not unheard of that authors may actually have to pay to have their article published.[6,7] At best, the direct financial rewards are likely to be few, unless a best-selling novel is produced. Indirectly, writing may lead to pay increases and promotions. However, because writing is a professional necessity, it can be made easier by following the correct procedures, which will be covered in this chapter.

Steps in Writing

As each of the steps in professional writing are covered in this section, the emphasis will be on writing items likely to be encountered in a practice setting, although additional steps that are necessary when writing for publication will be mentioned.

PREPARING TO WRITE

The first step in writing is to know the purpose—why something needs to be written in the first place. It is necessary at this time to have a good idea of the expected endpoint, which is important, no matter what is being done. For example, someone learning to plow a field with a tractor may be concentrating on the ground near the tractor and end up wandering all over the field, thinking he or she is going straight. However, by concentrating on going to a specific point on the far end of the field, rather than looking just in front of the tractor, the row will probably be plowed fairly straight. Throughout this whole process it is necessary to keep in mind that endpoint, to keep from wandering all over the place. If the item being written is for publication, rather than something required for work, it will also be necessary to pick the topic and, perhaps, submit an **article proposal** (see Figure 9–1). Although the writing is considered to be more important than the idea, it is still essential to have a good idea or topic that is of interest to prospective readers before starting.[8] It can even cover an old topic, as long as the topic is covered in greater depth, in a new way, or is addressed to a different group. It should also be pointed out that in the case of clinical trial results, it can be important to publish articles showing that something did not work, although in the past such topics have often been avoided.[9]

Although relatively few professionals write articles for journals or books, those who do need to follow an occasional step in addition to those outlined in the main text of this chapter. One difference is the potential need to write an article proposal to the publisher. This simply is a letter asking the publisher whether there would be any interest in possibly publishing something on a particular topic written by the person who is inquiring. As might be expected, this step is generally not necessary if writing a description of original research, but would be important when writing a review article or even a descriptive article. The letter should contain certain information, which will be described below, and be addressed to an appropriate editor. If at all possible, it is also a good idea to talk to an editor before submitting a proposal. For example, the proposal for the first edition of this book originated after a discussion with the editor at the Appleton & Lange booth in the ASHP Midyear Clinical Meeting Exhibitor's Area.

In the written proposal, the prospective author should first briefly explain the basic idea that is to be covered in the article or book, including a working title. Similarly, a description of the approach the author wishes to take in covering the subject should be described. Although this description should be kept brief, it must provide enough information for the publisher to determine whether the topic and approach are even appropriate for their journal, etc. In the case of a book, it is important to include a table of contents that is descriptive enough to be useful to reviewers who will be advising the publisher on the need for such a book. Related to that need, it is also necessary to describe why the proposed article or book will be important to the publisher's customers. This is the sales pitch. It is necessary to briefly show that there is nothing similar, or as good, currently available in the literature for the audience being addressed.

Although the above is the meat of the proposal, there are several other items that should be included. These include the time necessary to complete the article/book (be realistic), the approximate length of the work, and a statement of the authors' qualifications, including any previous publications.

There are several good reasons for submitting a proposal. The first is simply to avoid work if the editor decides that there is no need for such a publication (although an author should not hesitate to send the proposal to another publisher, if it still seems that the topic is important). Second, and perhaps most important, it allows the editor(s) to make suggestions. By following those suggestions, an author is more likely to be successful in getting work published. Finally, if the idea is accepted, the acceptance letter will provide motivation.

Figure 9–1. Article proposal to publishers.

It is also necessary to decide whether there needs to be a **coauthor**. This may be easy to resolve, depending on who is working on the project. However, even if no one else has been involved, it may be a good idea to look for a coauthor. An inexperienced writer (e.g., a student or someone early in his or her career) would benefit from working with an experienced author.[10] Additionally, working with someone will give a different perspective (especially if working with practitioners from many disciplines) and, hopefully, lessen the work for each person. Finally, it is sometimes a necessity to include coauthors for political reasons (as in "Would you prefer to share the credit or work nights and holidays for the rest of your life?"). Although this last reason should not exist, it does. These may be considered honorary authors and are relatively common,[11] although this is considered to be inappropriate.[12] A variety of other problems with authorship credit are also seen.[13-15] The best outcome is that everyone must do part of the writing[16] and that authors be listed in the order of their contributions to the project. This does not always happen.[17,18] In some cases, pharmaceutical manufacturers may want ghost writers to write an article for the researchers, but even they agree that original authors must prepare the first draft of editorials or opinion pieces, although non-English speaking authors may be assisted by others after that.[19] The ghost writers should also be appropriately acknowledged.[9] Although arguments may be made,[20-26] there is no valid reason for people to be listed as an author in excess of their contribution to the writing and submission of the work for publication.[27-31] The only exception would be if the publisher has other specific rules. For example, some journals may want to list contributors with an explanation of what they contributed (e.g., writing, origination of study idea, data collection). Generally, all of the following must be met for an individual to be given credit as an author[30]:

- Conception and design of the study, or analysis and interpretation of the data in the study
- Writing or revising the article
- Final approval of the version that is published

Things that do not qualify a person to be listed as an author include[29,30]:

- Acquisition of funding
- General supervision of the research group

Individuals that do not meet the first qualifications should be listed in the acknowledgments section. Also, the **primary author** should be able to explain the order the authors are listed in and journals may require one or more authors to be guarantors, who will be taking responsibility for the work as a whole, including legally.[31]

It should also be mentioned that there can be too many authors and acknowledgments.[32] Some scientific papers list many, many authors for a particular paper, and the number of authors has grown over the years.[33] It is obvious that 20 authors could not have written a three-page paper. Some of this may be a result of job requirements that include publishing a certain number of articles, leading to demands by individuals to get their names listed on any article they can. Again, authors should contribute to the written work in some significant way, as defined above. In some cases, it may be necessary to just name the group performing the research, with a few of the most responsible individuals specifically named, and list others as acknowledgments, sometimes by group, institution, or type of contribution.[23,32,34] Others may be listed as clinical investigators, participating investigators, scientific advisors, data collectors, or other appropriate titles.[31] In relationship to authorship, remember the people taking credit are also taking responsibility—they need to make sure that the work is clear and not subject to misinterpretation (i.e., do not write something that is designed to mislead the reader into believing something that has not been proven).[35]

Before the first word is written, it is necessary to know the audience, which involves knowing the type of person who will be reading the final document and where it will be published. Keep in mind that the word published was picked for a specific reason. Whether the final product appears in *The New England Journal of Medicine*, the *IV Room Policy and Procedure Book*, or even the label on a prescription vial, it is published. It is necessary to aim the work at the audience. At a broad level, written work should not be submitted for possible publication in a journal that does not cover the topic; it is no more appropriate to submit an article on preparation of cardioplegic solutions to the *Journal of Urology* than it is to type a monthly fiscal report on prescription labels. So, be sure to review a journal and its Instructions for Authors before attempting to write an article for submission to that journal.[36]

More specifically, it is necessary to aim both the writing style and depth of information toward the audience. If something is written for physicians, it is not likely to be understood by lay people. Conversely, items written for lay people may not satisfy the needs of physicians. It is certainly appropriate to have a secondary audience in mind. For example, a report written for physicians may be of interest to pharmacists and nurses. However, make sure the secondary audience is not served at the expense of the primary audience.

In regard to writing style, there are three types commonly used by pharmacists and other health care professionals: **pure technical style**, **middle technical style**, and **popular technical style** (Table 9–1).[37]

Pure technical style is used by business or technical professionals when they are writing for other professionals in the same or similar fields. For example, an article published in the *American Journal of Health-Systems Pharmacy, American Journal of Nursing,* or *Journal of the American Medical Association* would normally be written in this style. There are several characteristics of this style. First, the authors can use technical jargon, because they can expect the readers will understand it. Second, it is written in formal English. Third, it is written in the third person; words such as I, we, us, and you are

TABLE 9–1. TYPES OF TECHNICAL WRITING

- Pure technical style—used by professionals addressing other professionals in the same field
- Middle technical style—used by professionals addressing professionals in other fields
- Popular technical style—used by professionals addressing lay people

eliminated. Finally, there is a general lack of slang or contractions. The great majority of writing done by health professionals will be in this style, because it is usually other health professionals who will be reading their work.

Middle technical style is very closely related to pure technical style. This style is used by authors when they are writing for readers with a variety of technical backgrounds, with everyone having some unifying factor. For example, a report regarding a pharmacy department's quality assurance activities might be presented to the hospital's pharmacy and therapeutics committee. That committee is made up of physicians, nurses, hospital administrators, and other professionals. Although each has a background that makes their membership on the committee appropriate, not all of them would understand what a HEPA filter is, as would most hospital pharmacists. Therefore, it is necessary to better explain, or sometimes avoid, some technical areas. Otherwise, this writing style is very similar in most respects to pure technical style.

Finally, popular technical style is used in anything meant for the general public. Common language is used throughout. For example, a patient information sheet would need to be written in this style. A widely available example would be the articles on medical subjects that have appeared in *Reader's Digest* over the years. Information that is written in this style will use less complicated words and be less formal in its presentation.

It should be pointed out that usual technical writing differs greatly from what most people learn in high school English class or college composition courses. Although there is often a tendency to protest the formality of professional writing styles at first, the reality of the situation is that those styles must be followed for a piece of written material to be accepted.

The next step is to know the requirements of the publisher. Whether the work is for the department's policy and procedure manual or a journal, chances are that there is a format that needs to be followed. In the case of a journal, directions on the format to follow will be published at least once a year, usually in the first journal publication of the year or on the journal's Web site. Also, specific guidelines are followed by a number of professional journals, both for general format and statistical reporting. Many journals have approved those guidelines and expect that all work submitted for publication will follow them. They are referred to as the "Uniform Requirements for Manuscripts Submitted to Biomedical Journals."[31] This standardization makes it easier on the prospective author; one style can be learned and followed, regardless of the journal. Other publications that can be helpful are *Scientific Style and Format: The CSE Manual for Authors, Editors, and Publishers* prepared by the Council of Science Editors, the *American Medical Association Manual of Style,* the *MLA Style Manual,* and the *Publication Manual of the American Psychiatric Association.*

In the case of reports, policy and procedure manuals, and similar documents, it is best to see what has been done in the past. If this is the first time a particular item is being prepared, it is advisable to try to see what has been done in other places, and prepare something similar that meets the perceived needs. If writing something for work, do not be afraid to try to improve the format to make it more usable. However, be aware that it may be necessary to get any changes in format approved by the appropriate individual(s) or committee(s). Whenever possible, follow the Uniform Requirements[31] format used by the medical journals, because it is the standard for biomedical writing.

GENERAL RULES OF WRITING

Once the preparation is completed, it is time to start writing. Unfortunately, there is no easy way to learn how to write professionally; it just requires a lot of practice. However, a number of rules can be followed (Table 9–2). This section covers some of the general rules, with information on how to prepare specific items (e.g., introduction, body, conclusion, references, **abstracts**) being covered later. The first step is to organize the information before starting to write. At risk of sounding like a high school English teacher, it is still true that this step should include preparing an outline.[5] In the past, that was an onerous task that few performed. However, with modern word processing software, the outline actually becomes part of the finished product, so it does not amount to any significant extra work. Minimally, the different sections should be listed to create some order to the layout of the work (remember, keep in mind the endpoint). Overall, the goal is to prepare a document that is clear, concise, complete, and correct. The two latter items depend, to a large part, on preparation. The former items, however, can be helped by following some simple rules.

TABLE 9–2. CHECKLIST FOR PREPARATION OF WRITTEN MATERIALS

- Do research first
- Put oneself in the reader's position
- Use proper grammar and spelling
- Make the document look professional
- Keep things simple and direct
- Keep the document as short as possible
- Avoid abbreviations and acronyms
- Avoid the first person (e.g., I, we, us)
- Use active sentences
- Avoid slash construction (e.g., he/she, him/her)
- Avoid contractions (e.g., don't, can't)
- Cite other references wherever appropriate (and get permission to do so where appropriate)
- Cover things in whatever order is easiest
- Get everything down on paper before revising
- Edit, Edit, Edit!

The first two rules actually apply to the organization step. First, do sufficient research before getting started. Research in this regard, means obtaining whatever information—whether records, articles, performance evaluations, or anything else—necessary to prepare the item. Although, it is likely that additional research will be necessary to fill in the fine points at some point in the process, most information should be gathered ahead of time. It is impossible to be organized if there is nothing collected, and a document that is not organized will generally not be worth much. The second rule is to put oneself in the reader's position. What does that reader want and how does he or she want it presented?

Although it should not need to be stated, it is very important to use proper spelling and grammar. This is easier than in the past, because word processing programs check both; however, it is still necessary to double check, because the computer is likely to overlook things. For example, a properly spelled, but incorrect, word will be missed (e.g., two instead of to, trail instead of trial, ration instead of ratio). Unfortunately for some writers, appearances count greatly. The writer may know more about a particular subject than anyone else, but if poor grammar and spelling permeate the document, it is unlikely that anyone will read or believe the information presented.[38] It will be dismissed as probably wrong, based on grammar and spelling alone. In a case where the finished product will be published in a language other than the writer's native language, the writer should have the work read and edited by someone for whom the language is their first language. It should also be mentioned that the writing should try to be entertaining. Although professional writing tends to be a bit dry, an attempt should be made to make it as enjoyable and easy to read as possible, although it is necessary to be cautious with humor and stay within limits of professionalism and good taste. It should also be unpretentious, direct, and accurate.[39]

Related to this, the document should look presentable. Some students are well known for turning in papers that are crumpled, creased, torn, dirty, or coffee stained. That is not professional and must be avoided. The sad truth is that people will assume that if an author was sloppy with the appearance of the document, he or she was probably sloppy with the information. That may not be so, but that assumption will kill a good, but sloppy, document.

❷ *When writing it is best to keep things as simple and direct as possible.*[40-43] This has been referred to as the KISS (Keep It Simple, Stupid) principle. There is a temptation to use big words that sound impressive, but doing so is more likely to confuse than impress.

Related to that, keep the paper as short as possible.[44] If a document is long, subheadings should be used. This can be part of the outline step mentioned earlier. Also, consider whether tables, figures, or graphs would make the document simpler and easier to understand. This can be particularly useful with documents containing a great deal of data that may be organized through the use of tables.

● When writing, avoid using abbreviations or acronyms. If it is necessary to do so, state the full form of the word or term the first time it is mentioned in the document, followed by the abbreviation in parenthesis (e.g., acquired immunodeficiency syndrome [AIDS]). The only exceptions to this rule are units of measurement (e.g., mL, mg). Units of measurement should be expressed in the metric system. Clinical chemistry and hematologic measurements should be in terms of the International System of Units (SI).

● Several rules apply to the wording that is used in professional writing.[37] First, completely avoid writing in the first person, and avoid the second person wherever possible. It is not a bad idea, at least at first, to ask the word processor to find all occurrences of *I, me, we, us,* and *you.* If those words are found, try to rewrite the sentence to avoid them.

● Also, it is preferable to avoid using the passive voice throughout[45]; again, a grammar

● checker can help. Avoid both contractions and slash construction (i.e., *and/or, he/she*

● [use *he or she*], *this/that*). Finally, in this politically correct era, avoid sexism. That includes words like *he* or *she,* although it is not always appropriate or desirable to delete those terms. For example, using *he* in a case report of a patient with testicular cancer is quite appropriate. It is also inappropriate to use *their* instead of *his or her* to get around the problem.

● When writing, be sure to give credit where it is due. This does not mean just making sure the listed authors wrote part of the document. It includes using endnotes, or possibly footnotes, for all information obtained from one or a limited number of sources. If there is extensive quoting, permission to do so should be obtained by writing to the person or organization holding the copyright on the material. Endnotes are something everyone dreaded in the past. They waited until the end, because the articles should be cited in the order they appear in the document. By that time it was difficult to go back and do it. Now, however, it is much easier with word processors; it is possible to insert the citations as the document is prepared and let the software worry about making sure they are in the correct order.

● Related to the endnotes, everything that is stated should be supported by objective evidence. When writing a paper based on scientific literature, that evidence must be shown in the endnotes. To reemphasize, any unreferenced statement of fact is for all practical purposes worthless. However, it is necessary to make sure information is extracted from the original article and expressed properly. Some writers will improperly twist facts, whether inadvertently or not, to support their assertions.[46]

● Finally, work through the document in whatever order seems easiest.[5] In preparing a drug evaluation for a pharmacy and therapeutics committee, a stack of 50 articles might be used. At first, the stack may look like an impossible task, but after sorting the articles into groups that correspond to the sections, start with the shortest stack or the easiest information. By the time the document is finished, the writer may be surprised to find out that they were all fairly short, easy stacks.

At first, a writer should simply try to make sure that all of the information is down on paper.[5] Once that occurs, go back and revise, and perhaps reorganize the document. Waiting a few days before revising the document can be very beneficial. After some time away from the project, errors practically jump off the page. It is also a good idea to have someone else who has not been involved with the writing, read the document. Something that seems quite clear to the author may not actually be clear at all. Also, the author may be mentally inserting words or even sentences that were inadvertently omitted. Having someone edit the document can be humbling, but helpful. Be sure to provide the product in a format that will make things easier for the person reviewing the document. A typed, double-spaced manuscript will make it easy to read and provide room for comments. Even better, electronic versions of a document can be reviewed directly on a computer using "comment" or "track changes" features. The reviewer can put in comments or suggested wording changes electronically and then return the document. The writer can then go through the document making changes or simply accepting proposed changes with the click of a mouse. Often, the use of the electronic reviewing mechanism will be quicker, easier, and provide much clearer suggestions.

The three most important things in real estate may be location, location, location, but the three most important things in writing are edit, edit, edit. This can be particularly important when multiple authors have contributed different sections, since it will be necessary to make sure that the various contributions fit well together, including the style of writing.[47] It may be best for either the first author or the most senior author to edit for consistency. Also, remember editing includes paring out unnecessary words, sentences, and larger sections. It is not sufficient to settle for good enough—do the best. Look at it this way: the boss or editor is only going to do so much editing before giving up. The trick is to make sure that the document is well prepared and does not need that much editing.

SPECIFIC DOCUMENT SECTIONS

A typical document consists of three main parts—the introduction, body, and conclusion. In the case of a clinical study, it is recommended to follow the IMRAD structure that divides a paper into Introduction, Methods, Results, and Discussion,[31] which is the standard for such papers.[48] Other parts, such as references, tables, figures, and abstracts may also be necessary. These will be discussed in later sections and in the appendices of this chapter. It should also be noted that a number of the points in Chapters 4, 5, and 8 are applicable to writing of journal articles, as are the contents of the Web sites for the International Committee of Medical Journal Editors (http://www.icmje.org), Consolidated Standards of Reporting Trials (CONSORT) statement (contains a checklist for contents of clinical trial to report when publishing and flow diagram illustrating recruitment, randomization, and analysis of subjects enrolled in a trial) (http://www.consort-statement.org),[49-59] Preferred

Reporting Items for Systemic Reviews and Meta-Analysis (PRISMA)[60,61] (http://www
.prisma-statement.org/), Conference on Guideline Standardization (COGS) standards
(http://gem.med.yale.edu/cogs/), and Good Publication Practice for Pharmaceutical
Companies (http://www.ismpp.org/gpp2),[62] and should be considered, along with this
material. An example question layout that includes an introduction, body, and conclusion
section is shown in Appendix 9–1.

Introduction

❸ *With the probable exception of policy and procedure documents, the two most important
paragraphs in any document are the first and last.* It is vital to start out strong, to encourage
the reader to continue reading. Otherwise, the work will end up in that stack of articles
everyone has that they intend to read someday. That first paragraph should also inform
the readers of what they can expect in the rest of the document; it should be similar to a
road map that shows what is to be accomplished in the document. The introduction
should have a clear objective for the existence of the document. Many people neglect the
need to state a clear objective, which leaves the reader to flounder and wonder whether
there really is a purpose to the document. In a research article, the introduction will also
contain the hypothesis being investigated. In a policy and procedure document, it may
simply be a description of what the remainder of the document will cover. The introduction should also contain background information about the topic that provides a good
information base for the reader. The amount of background information has to be a balance—enough to show the reader that the writer has done an appropriate amount of
research, but yet not so exhaustive as to bore or overwhelm the reader with unnecessary
details.[63] Overall, the introduction should be short but contain properly referenced background material and show the reader where the document is headed.

The introduction should generally not be a conclusion; some people are so anxious
to jump to the end that they put the conclusion first. Admittedly, the BLOT concept (bottom line on top) has its purpose in some documents (e.g., policy and procedures, formulary monographs), but that should be a conscious decision. If the introduction amounts to
a conclusion, many people will read no further, making the remainder of the document a
waste of time and paper.

Body

The body of the document contains all of the details. In a research article, the body may
be divided into the methods, results, and, possibly, discussion sections, although the latter section may be incorporated into the conclusion. Details of what should be included
are covered in Chapter 4. In other documents, the body will probably be divided into
whatever sections are appropriate or logical. A number of rules can be followed in preparing the body of a document.

The first rule is that, while it is important to be concise, all necessary information must be presented. Again, keep an eye on the desired endpoint, and do not stray from the subject unless it is absolutely necessary. Including unnecessary information, even if it is interesting, will tend to confuse or obscure the important points. Also, be sure to provide a balanced coverage of the material and avoid unsupported bias.[9]

It is important to cover the information in a logical order, so that it flows easily from one point to another. A common mistake, when learning to write professionally, is to skip back and forth between subjects. For example, someone might insert a point about dosing in the middle of indications, when dosing is discussed at another point in the document.

Material that can identify patients should be left out of any work, unless it is absolutely necessary to include. If that is not possible, informed consent must be obtained[31] and pertinent legal procedures must be followed (see Chapter 10). The authors should also disclose any approval of a study by institutional review boards and their following of other rules related to protection of study subjects (both humans and animals).[31]

Writers should also put the information in their own words. Perhaps out of lack of confidence, a number of professionals are tempted to simply quote other authors word for word. However, by presenting the information in their own words, writers demonstrate that they actually understand the topic. ❹ *Remember, though, that if the information is taken from a particular source, even if it is reworded, the original author should be given credit via footnotes or endnotes.*

It is necessary to expand on the topic discussed in the previous paragraph, because there seems to be much confusion about it and there are many cases where the rules against copyright infringement and plagiarism are broken. Plagiarism can be considered the copying of another's words or ideas, without properly giving credit. Copyright violations consist of copying another's work, even with appropriate quotations and citation, without permission. They are similar; however, it is possible to commit either plagiarism or copyright violations without committing the other. Self-plagiarism, where an author copies material that he or she previously had published in one journal for something in another journal, is a concern and can lead to copyright violations.[64] It appears that plagiarism is becoming more frequent and many people do not understand that it is wrong to copy work without proper attribution, even something from a source written by many anonymous people (e.g., Wikipedia, Yahoo! Answers, and Answers.com).[65,66]

Sometimes those infractions are rather blatant, such as the cases documented in the newspapers about students downloading papers from the Internet and presenting them as their own or simply retyping a previously published article (an attempt to prevent this can be seen on the Internet at http://www.plagiarism.com, http://www.plagiarism.org, or http://www.turnitin.com[67]).[68] Interestingly, although there might be suspicions that this is more prevalent with online classes, a study found that it was more likely to occur with traditional campus students.[69] Another Web site, http://www.ithenticate.com/ is a resource to check if published material is plagiarized. Other times, the infringement is quite accidental. For example, it was once brought to the attention of the famous science fiction writer, Isaac Asimov, that a short story he wrote was similar to an article that had been published 10 years previously.[70] Dr. Asimov went back and found the article and read it, realizing as he did so that he had read it when it first came out and had forgotten about it. When he wrote his story 10 years later, he did not realize that portions of it could be considered plagiarism. Although he had no intention of infringing upon the other author's work, Dr. Asimov made sure that the story was never reprinted and even wrote an article discussing the problem. This shows how easy it is to inadvertently cross the line into copyright infringement or plagiarism, and there are many examples that would fall in between the extremes given above.[71] Therefore, it is necessary for the author to be on guard and to try to prevent the problem in the first place. A few general rules can act as a guide.

- When copying wording directly from another's work, it should be in quotations (or otherwise shown to be a quote) and a citation should appear to give credit to the original author(s). Also, if a significant amount of a work published in the last 100 years is quoted, it is probably necessary to get permission from the copyright holder, which may require paying a fee.[72] Exactly what is a significant amount is debatable; however, it would be best to err on the side of asking for permission if a quotation is more than a few sentences. Reproducing an entire chart, table, figure, and so on should normally require asking for permission. A letter to the copyright holder will solve problems; publishers often have forms to request permission. Some special cases need to be mentioned. First, U.S. government documents are not copyrighted, so only quotation marks and citations are necessary. Second, if it is impossible to locate a copyright holder (e.g., the publisher went out of business without transferring copyrights), the writer should at least be able to document a thorough effort to obtain permission. Finally, there are special legal requirements for use of copyrighted materials in online education, covered in the Technology, Education, and Copyright Harmonization (TEACH) Act. Further information on this can be found in Chapter 10.
- Extensive quotations should be avoided. After all, if a writer cannot put something in his or her own words, does that person truly understand the material? In any writing, there really is very little reason to provide quotations. The author should try to put things in his or her own words whenever possible.
- Paraphrased information should have the original publication(s) cited, if it comes from one or a limited number of sources.
- Extensive paraphrasing, particularly without citations, may be considered plagiarism (i.e., copying the ideas of others).

- When citing an article, cite the one that the material comes from. If the material came from a review article, cite that article, not the original study that was not consulted. It is worth mentioning that in the case of unusual information, reading and citing the original study is preferable to just using a review article, because the review may be inaccurate.
- Be sure to follow publishers' rules or licenses, which may be stricter and may not allow any reproduction of material. Obtain permission from publisher, even if it is author's original work, for use in a different publication to avoid copyright violations.[64]
- Remember that it is necessary to always cite others' work, even on slides.[73] Always cite everything, even if it is the author's own previously published work to avoid self-plagiarism.[64]

In preparing certain documents (written answers to questions, for example), there may be very little information available. Perhaps only one or two research articles will have been written on the topic. If so, it will often be desirable to summarize the articles in detail, including most of the information presented in an abstract (see Appendix 9–2). In general, the information presented will summarize how many and what type of patients (i.e., inclusion and exclusion criteria), the drug or procedure being investigated, results (e.g., efficacy, adverse effects), and conclusions of authors of referenced articles. It is also important to point out any noticeable flaws in the paper. An example would be:

Smith and Jones performed a double-blind, randomized comparison of the effects of drug X and drug Y in patients with tsutsugamushi fever. Patients were required to be between 18 and 70 years old, and could not have any concurrent infection or disorder that would affect the immune response to the disease (e.g., neutropenia, AIDS). Twenty patients received 10 mg of drug X, three times a day for 15 days. Eighteen patients received 250 mg of drug Y, twice a day for 10 days. The two groups were comparable, except that the patients receiving drug X were an average of 5 years younger ($p < 0.05$). Drug X was shown to produce a cure, both in terms of symptoms and cultures in 85% of patients, whereas drug Y only produced a cure in 55.5% of patients. The difference was statistically significant ($p < 0.01$). No significant adverse effects were seen in either group. Although it appears that drug X was the better agent, it should be noted that drug Y was given in its minimally effective dose, and may have performed better in a somewhat higher or longer regimen.

A list of material to be covered in a review of an article similar to that above is found in Table 9–3.

Conclusion

- A conclusion should be placed at the end of the body of the document, except for certain documents (e.g., policy and procedures). This conclusion should follow logically from the

TABLE 9–3. ITEMS TO INCLUDE IN WRITTEN REVIEW OF A JOURNAL ARTICLE

Items to Include	Examples
Main author of article and a reference number	Johnson et al.[2] Smith and associates[24]
Type of article	Clinical study, case report, case series, review, meeting abstract
Research design (if appropriate)	Blinding, randomization, experience report, descriptive report
Objective or purpose of the report	
Description of group studied	Size of groups, age, sex, disease state(s), other pertinent demographic characteristics, inclusion and exclusion criteria
Any important confounding factors	Smoking, age, general health
Description of treatment being studied	Drug, dose, administration route, dosing interval, treatment duration
What was measured as an indicator of effect/ outcome variables	
Results	Efficacy, adverse effects
Author conclusions	
Strengths and weaknesses of the study	See Chapters 4 and 5

information presented and should serve to summarize that information. Remember, the conclusion should also correspond with the objective stated in the introduction.[74] It is also worth noting that in clinical consultations, a common mistake is to write the conclusion in a general manner, rather than addressing the specific patient in question, which is what the reader wants to hear about. The author must remember to address the specific patient's situation.

Many writers are tempted to avoid formulating a conclusion. Various reasons include not feeling qualified to make a conclusion for the reader, not wanting to restate what has already been stated, laziness, and so on. This is improper. The readers need something to bring their thoughts together at the end, and the author is in the perfect position to provide this closure. However, the author should also be careful to avoid extrapolating beyond the information available.

Other Items

If items include endnotes, the references should be found following the conclusion (see Appendix 9–3 for more information on how to prepare a **bibliography**). Use of bibliographic software, such as Reference Manager (Thomson Reuters; http://www.refman .com), ProCite (Thomson Reuters; http://www.procite.com), EndNote (Thomson Reuters; http://www.endnote.com), or Zotero (Center for History and New Media at

George Mason University; http://www.zotero.org/) can be helpful in this process.[19] Other items may also be necessary, depending on the document, such as tables, graphs, figures, and so forth. They will not be dealt with here, other than to say that those items should supplement or clarify (not distort or misrepresent), and not simply duplicate material in the text portion of a piece of written work, although there may be overlap as an author explains data or expands on the material presented.

SUBMISSION OF THE DOCUMENT

● Once the document is completed, proofread, and edited, it is ready to be submitted, whether this is to a supervisor or a journal. In the latter case, the author will need to include a cover letter that serves as an introduction to the document. In the former case, it will be possible to be less formal. Also, it should be noted that when submitting an item to a journal it may be necessary to include transfer of copyright forms, conflict of interest disclosures (including financial),[16,75–77] or other items, which will be found in the directions for authors for that journal (usually found in the first issue of each year and on the publication's Web site). The conflict of interest may be reported by the publisher in the final publication, but this is variable.[78] In addition, be sure to precisely follow the journal's Instructions for Authors to improve chances for acceptance.[79] It is also worth a word of warning that articles should very rarely, if ever, be submitted to more than one journal at the same time (Note: prior publication of an abstract does not mean that submission of a full article is duplication and publication in a second language is often considered acceptable).[9,16,80] If duplicate submission is felt to be appropriate and/or necessary, the rules outlined in the Uniform Requirements must be followed.[31] Also, the article should not be broken down into many small articles and submitted over time, unless submission as a whole would result in a publication that would be too long or complex.[81]

REVISION

● ❺ *In many cases, revision of the document will be necessary.* This may be due to a difference in opinion or different perception of need. Although an author should never change a document to say something he or she believes is wrong, minor revisions are often necessary to improve clarity or make the document more appropriate in some other manner. The comments given with the request for revision are likely to be helpful,[82] and they should be taken seriously. Even if it is felt that the person who read and commented on the paper is wrong, all concerns should be addressed. If a comment is truly wrong, it may still indicate that the work was not clear in a particular area and needs some other appropriate revision to clarify the material. Changes should be made, based on the comments and completed within the time limits given.

Sometimes, however, a document may be rejected entirely. This can be for any of the following reasons[37]:

1. The document is not up to standards (too much work to correct or edit).
2. The idea or research the document is based on is too weak.
3. The idea is inappropriate for that forum of publication.
4. A similar article has been recently prepared (and possibly published) by someone else in that forum.

In the case of the first item, major revisions would be necessary before resubmitting to the boss or a journal. The second reason may also prompt major revisions, or even cause an author to stop working on the document. An article submitted to a journal but rejected for the last two reasons is not necessarily bad. It may be possible to submit it to another appropriate journal after only minor changes.

GALLEY PROOFS

A term well known to authors who have published articles or books is **galley** (or page) **proofs**. This is a final copy of the article, as it is to appear when published. It is the responsibility of the author(s) to carefully check to make sure there have been no mistakes made in typesetting. Although it may seem like a lot of work, everything must be checked, including the references, which frequently contain errors.[83-88] This step is necessary to prevent problems later. Although documents ready for distribution at work are generally not referred to as galley proofs, it is still necessary to carefully check those items.

REFEREES

Although this term is more familiar to sports fans, **referees** (also referred to as reviewers) are used in writing. These are the individuals to whom journals send submitted articles for review and comments. This is also referred to as the peer-review process. On a local level, reviewers are the people who a writer may ask to look at a report before the boss gets it. Whatever arena, whether local or international, a person should also be willing to be a reviewer at that level. To be a reviewer for a journal (which produces **refereed publications**), a person usually can simply write a letter stating interests, qualifications, and experience to the editor of the journal, and ask to be considered for the journal's reviewer list. If the person has adequate credentials, the journal will usually be happy to have that person as a reviewer.

Anyone who is a reviewer should be up front about such things as lack of expertise, conflict of interest,[76] or inability to complete a review within a reasonable time, and should be willing to step aside as a reviewer of a particular paper if those are problems.[89] Also, a reviewer should treat anything submitted to him or her as a confidential document.

It should be pointed out that people who act as reviewers for papers should follow the procedures discussed in Chapters 4 and 5 to evaluate an article. Specific directions will also be received from the editor and may involve preparing comments for both the editor (to discuss matters, such as ethics, with the editor alone) and the author(s) (this latter document is also used by the editor). It may be required that the latter be signed or unsigned. Also, as with any quality assurance procedure, the reviewer should treat it as an opportunity to provide constructive, as opposed to destructive, criticism.[90] Finally, for those who are reviewers for journals, it is recommended to get new people involved in the process, such as residents or new practitioners, so that they can learn how to be a reviewer.[91]

It is beyond the scope of this chapter, but if further information is needed on being an editor of a biomedical journal, the reader should consult the Web site of the World Association of Medical Editors (http://www.wame.org).

Case Study 9–1

Your boss comes to you and lets you know that you are assigned to write a new policy and procedure for a product that is to be added to the formulary, but which requires specific safety precautions when administered to patients (e.g., premedication of the patient, availability of resuscitation equipment, unusual preparation for administration). This is to be available for approval at the next pharmacy and therapeutics committee meeting.

- *What are your first steps?*
- *You have progressed to the point where you have the material gathered to prepare your policy and procedure. What should be done at this stage?*
- *Once the document is written, what needs to be done next?*

Specific Documents

NEWSLETTERS AND WEB SITES

Newsletters have been considered to be a part of any pharmacy practice, but have probably been encountered most frequently in hospitals as a method for communicating pharmacy and therapeutics committee actions and other drug-related topics to the medical, pharmacy, nursing, and other health care provider staffs. Newsletters have also been seen from community pharmacies[92,93] (addressed to patients and/or physicians), nursing homes, drug companies, pharmacy organizations, and government or regulatory bodies. Wherever newsletters are found, their reason for existence is likely to be one or more of the following reasons: to communicate information to a target group, advertisement, and/or compliance with legal/accreditation standards.

In many cases, newsletters are now replaced by a Web site. Such sites can serve the same purposes, but can also have some specific advantages and disadvantages. For example, Web sites take very little effort for distribution, because all they take is a computer on the Internet. Also, the material can take a greater variety of forms, including audio and video. The Web site can actually be used to sell products, including prescriptions. Within institutions, the material can be kept available for health care providers to review for an indefinite time period, thereby preventing problems when somebody wants another copy of an old article or when nurses are trying to make sure they have all of the publications for an accreditation visit. In regard to disadvantages, it should be noted that consulting a Web site does take more effort, because it does not just fall into people's hands when they open their mailboxes. Also, there are still some people who do not use the Internet and would, therefore, not be able to consult the site.

Whatever the reason for the existence of a newsletter or Web site, the same set of steps generally applies to their preparation.[94-98] These steps will be covered individually in the remainder of this section.

Define the Audience

Who will, or at least should, be reading the newsletter or accessing the Web site? It may be physicians, pharmacists, nurses, other health care professionals, the lay public, other groups, or some combination of these. The target group(s) will have an effect on decisions made in the other steps.

Define the Goals of the Newsletter/Web Site

The goal can be any of the reasons mentioned previously, but generally includes informing and educating the reader, and also to report news (including changes in policies and procedures, laws, etc.). With Web sites, it can also be to directly sell products or gather information.

Identify Constraints

No matter what kind of newsletter or Web site is produced, there are always going to be constraints that limit what it can contain and how good it will be. One of the first constraints is time. It seems like every year people are busier and have less time to do things than they want or need to do. This includes preparing a newsletter or keeping up a Web site (must be done continuously), which can take a significant amount of time if it is done right. It will be necessary to have time to write, type, edit, typeset, and perform other functions in publishing the newsletter—and all of those things have to be done in time to get the finished result to the printer, so that it can be ready for distribution on time. With a Web site, it is necessary to write the material, figure out the layout or organization, and prepare it on the computer. It is generally best, when beginning publication of a newsletter, to have it come out at longer intervals. If the newsletter is well received and it is found that there is enough time and sufficient material, publication frequency can be increased. Overall, it is better to find it necessary to speed up publication frequency, rather than spread it out (people might get the idea the newsletter ceased publication).

Another constraint is the people who can, or will, be involved with publishing the newsletter or Web site, particularly the editor-in-chief and/or Web master. This is a case where the phrase, "many hands make light work" may be applicable. If a group of dependable people are willing to work together to make sure the articles get written, the job may be easier. Generally, there are two extremely hard parts to publishing a newsletter or Web site, neither of which is the actual writing. One of them is coming up with topic ideas; the other is to make it look good. If others are at least willing to help here, it can be a great aid to the editor of the newsletter. If at all possible, people from all groups served by the newsletter should be asked for topics, if not entire articles. If a health professional is in charge of the newsletter or Web site, some other possible places for help include an institution's public relations department, if available, and clerical help (to do the typing, formatting, copying, distribution, etc.). Keep an eye on the time necessary for health professional (e.g. pharmacy, nursing) staff to produce the newsletter or Web site, because this is likely to be the most costly item.

The third constraint is financial. As has been said, "There is no such thing as a free lunch." This also applies to newsletters and Web sites. There is always some cost involved. Although personnel costs are likely to be the largest expense, the computer equipment and printing or duplication charges (for newsletters) can be significant. If the printing is to be done by an outside agency, it is best to check on such items as the effect of order size (number of copies) and type of paper (e.g., plain versus glossy, $8\frac{1}{2} \times 11$ versus 11×17 versus A4, colors), stapling or binding on the cost. It is preferable to get bids from at least three printers. Another item to consider is method of delivery (e.g., personal versus first-class mail versus second-class mail). All of these items do add up and, depending on the budget, it may be necessary to sell advertising space to cover the costs.

Finally, it is necessary to look at what equipment is available. If at all possible, the use of a high-end word processing program or desktop publishing program with a laser or inkjet printer will allow production of a high-quality, professional newsletter quicker and at a lower cost. This equipment may be all that is necessary for a Web site, assuming that the computer has some type of Internet connection. Although a number of Web programs are now available for little cost, and are the preferable solution, many times it is possible to just use a word processor or Web browser to create and maintain the Web site.

Newsletter/Web Site Design

While it might be easy to believe substance is more important than appearance, it eventually becomes noticeable that many people do not bother looking at the substance if the appearance is poor or unprofessional. Therefore, one of the most important things is to make the publication look appealing.[99,100] People tend to throw away newsletters that look sloppy or unprofessional, and do not bother with Web sites that are not exciting, easy to use, and neat. Even if the publication looks good it may[101-103] or may not[104,105] have any impact on health professionals, but without looking professional it is highly unlikely to even have a chance.

A few general rules can help make a newsletter or Web site more appealing. These will be covered in the remainder of this section. However, for a more in-depth look at this subject, the reader is directed to references specializing in the subject.[106,107] A particularly detailed book is available on the Internet at http://www.usability.gov/guidelines/.

One of the first rules is to keep the publication consistent. This means not only from month to month, but also from page to page. This does not mean that improvements cannot be made from time to time. Nor does it mean that each page has to look exactly like the previous one. Instead, it means that it should have its own style that is recognizable by the reader, and that the various pages must fit with one another. The easiest way to do this, with either a newsletter or Web site, is to create a template, style sheet, or theme (these terms overlap somewhat). Many pieces of software make this possible for either type of publication. A *template* is a file that contains material that appears the same from issue to issue—the term is often associated with a newsletter. Examples of this can be the newsletter's masthead (first page heading), listing of editors, footers at the bottom of each page, number of columns, and so on. A *theme* should be similar to a template, but may be used more frequently when discussing a Web site. *Style sheets* define how specific paragraphs or other parts of the newsletter or Web sites will look (they would often be incorporated into the template or theme). For example, a style might be called "Heading 1," and by using this style for each article's title, the look remains the same from page to page, and issue to issue. This style can include such items as what the font looks like (e.g., typeface, font size, bold, italic, underlined, superscript, subscript, etc.), and what the paragraph looks like (e.g., left justified, right justified, centered, line spacing, space before or after, etc.), in addition to other items (e.g., whether the section is to be located in a particular part of the page, borders, etc.). A style manual should be established or at least a commercially available style manual, such as the *American Medical Association Manual of Style,* should be used. Whatever the editor(s) establish should be reasonably simple and elegant (i.e., do not get carried away—a couple of different fonts on a page are fine, but 10 fonts look terrible). In the case of Web sites, it might be useful to consult the publication *Elements of E-text Style,* which is available at http://w2.eff.org/Net_culture/Linguistics/e-style.guide.

- A second rule is to use appropriate software and equipment. A high-end word processor or desktop publishing program and a laser printer can be used to produce the master copy of the newsletter for reproduction.[108,109] This can allow a pharmacy to turn out a product that looks typeset at a fraction of the cost. As mentioned, there are a variety of low (or no) cost Web site software tools. Some are specific, whereas others are incorporated into word processors, Web browsers, or other software. Also, just using a text editor is possible, although that tends to be much more difficult.

- A third rule is to make the newsletter or Web site look good. For example, use white space properly. Do not just crowd in as much material as possible on the page. The reader will have a hard time following if it is too crowded, and may just give up. Layout really is a difficult problem, and requires at least a little artistic ability to do well. If lack of artistic ability is a problem, it is probably a good idea to look over other newsletters or Web sites from various sources to try to come up with ideas concerning what looks good. Minimally, most newsletters should at least be set up in two columns to allow easier reading. Other, more artistic, items to consider are asymmetrical layout (not having the two sides of each page look the same from a distance, perhaps using a narrow column for graphics or titles along one edge), different column widths, teasers (statements taken from the text that may pique the curiosity of the reader enough to read the article), surrounding boxes and columns with rules, and artwork/graphics.[110] The programs used to prepare either newsletters or Web sites can also have samples that can be used to prepare a professional looking end product.

- Next on the list for newsletters is to design a masthead. As mentioned, the masthead is essentially the part of the first page of the newsletter which gives the name of the publication, volume, issue, date, and so on. This may be at the top of the page or down one side of the first page. It is a good idea to consider having this done professionally, because it is a one-time expense and can be a major factor in the appearance of the newsletter. Sometimes it is good to have a multicolored masthead that is preprinted on blank stock paper. The newsletter text can then just be photocopied onto the paper and look much more professional. Material to be put into the masthead, or at least be included somewhere in the newsletter, includes the newsletter name (be descriptive, but do not get cute—remember this is a professional newsletter), name and address of the pharmacy or organization, names of editor and editorial staff (give credit or blame where it is due), and frequency of publication. The name of the publication, along with some way of identifying the issue and page, should be placed on every page of the newsletter, so that the source of information can be identified if the page is photocopied or torn out.

- Much of the material in a masthead should also be contained on the home page, if not every page, of a Web site. Again, getting professional design help, at least at first, may be of value. Also, following the guidelines of the Health on the Net Foundation Code of Conduct (http://www.hon.ch/HONcode/Conduct.html) in designing the Web page is appropriate.

In general, software themes available will help create a professional looking site, if professional help is not available. However, some specific items that need to be considered for a Web site include[111,112]:

- Provide information that is good, credible, timely, and original. Share everything possible.
- Custom tailor information to take into account user preferences.
- Break up tables for readability.
- Related to the previous item, optimize the other aspects of the page to improve download times.
- Make the page easy to read—good contrast between the text and the background including the colors (remember that some people are color blind and may not be able to distinguish some colors, rendering some things unreadable), not too busy.
- Use self-generating content—make the site interactive.
- Web pages should be well organized—both the pages by themselves and how the pages are interconnected on the site.
- Consider selling things, if appropriate.
- Make sure everything works, from all likely browsers.

In designing the newsletter or Web site, effort should also be placed in deciding on a name. A local or institutional newsletter will often have a name related to the organization and the purpose of the newsletter. A Web site may be similarly named, but there is an opportunity to go farther. In this case, the uniform resource locator (URL) should be considered. This is the address of the Web site on the intranet and/or the Internet. An institution may already have a registered URL, and the department Web page may simply be under that name (e.g., http://www.yourorganizationname.org/pharmacy). However, independent community pharmacies, ambulatory clinics, physician offices, etc. can also register an unused name on the Internet and have that address (e.g., http://www.johnspharmacy.com).

It has been alluded to, but it is necessary to make a very specific decision on how the newsletter is to be printed. While typesetting still produces the best looking newsletter, it is quite easy to get a good-looking final product using a good photocopy machine. Also, even if the department produces the original copy on its computer, the file can be taken to a service bureau that can essentially produce a typeset copy. It is necessary to determine the paper to be used (glossy paper is not going to be used if photocopying). Most newsletters are 8½ × 11 inches in size, but that does not mean the paper is that size. It is better to use 11 × 17 paper for multipage newsletters and just fold the sheets. That looks much better than simply stapling the corner. Also, it is possible to take an electronic storage medium (e.g., USB drive) with the newsletter file on it to some professional printers for them to print good looking final copies.

Newsletter/Web Page Content

Before getting into items that a newsletter or Web site should or can contain, it is necessary to discuss some general rules that deal with any article.[113]

First, it is a good idea to have a number of short articles, rather than one long article.[99,114] People will take a look at a short article and mentally decide they have the time to read it, whereas a long article may be dismissed immediately ("If I'm going to read something that long, it will be out of *The New England Journal of Medicine!*") or put aside to read when they have time (does house dust actually come from publications on the bottom of that read someday pile disintegrating from old age?). As a matter of fact, some recommend that newsletters should not exceed two pages (one sheet, front and back)[113] and one hospital cut their newsletter to one page (for P&T News) and replaced the remaining articles with a page to fit into a Drug Therapy Pocket Guide that consisted of useful tables (e.g., sodium content and neutralizing capacity of different antacids).[115] Related to the above, use catchy titles to draw the reader into reading the article right then.

Use proper writing techniques, as described earlier in this chapter. Be clear, concise, and complete—do not waste the reader's valuable time. Also, be unbiased—support the article with facts. Be positive—talk about 90% adherence, rather than 10% nonadherence.

Finally, be sure the newsletter or Web site is properly edited. Have multiple people read and edit the newsletter or Web pages before publication. Having more people read it makes it more likely that simple mistakes will be noticed and corrected. In particular, the editors should check for spelling, grammar, and readability. Also, it is a good idea to have people from each target group as editors, particularly physicians.[116]

The actual content of a newsletter or Web site is one of the two most difficult areas for the editor (the other being that the newsletter should look good). Coming up with new ideas on a regular basis can be rather difficult. A list of possible areas to cover is included in Table 9–4. If at all possible, material that was prepared for a different audience can be recycled for the newsletter or Web site readers. For example, material from the pharmacy and therapeutics committee meeting might be turned into a short review of a drug. Whenever possible, the material presented should be topics not available to the audience from another source, or material that is prepared in a format that will be of greater value to the readers than that same topic area as presented by other publications. Whatever the topics used, it is a good idea to survey the readers on a regular basis to make sure their needs are being met.

Newsletter Distribution

All of the above work will be for nothing if the readers do not get the newsletter. A good distribution system must be developed. Sometimes it can be as simple as sticking the

TABLE 9–4. NEWSLETTER OR WEB SITE TOPICS[93,94,99,112]

- Adherence
- Advances in therapeutics
- Adverse drug reactions
- Calendar of events
- Clinical guidelines
- Clinical pearls
- Compliance
- Drug shortages
- Drugs withdrawn from market
- Effects of external events on jobs
- FDA warnings
- Job-related information
- New information sources
- New legal or regulatory requirements
- New services
- News from other departments
- Organization's stand on issues
- Patient safety
- Personnel policies
- Pharmacoeconomics
- Pharmacogenomics
- Pharmacy and therapeutics committee actions and news
- Productivity improvement
- Professional announcements
- Review of drugs/drug classes
- Quality assurance

Data from references 93, 94, 99, and 112.

newsletters in individual mailboxes, setting out piles of newsletters, or using intraorganizational mail systems. If it is necessary to use the post office, it would be a good idea to check on the possibility of second-class or bulk mail, which can save money. Newer distribution methods are by electronic mail[117] or other computerized methods.[118] It may also be useful to distribute information with **QR (Quick Response) Codes** that will make it easier to download information via a smartphone or tablet. Whatever method used, it is important to make sure the readers actually get the newsletter. Also, make sure they get the newsletters on a regular cycle, so that they know when to anticipate the arrival of the publication.

Case Study 9–2

Your boss comes and lets you know that you are in charge of a new Web site for your department.

• *What are the first steps to do?*

PRESENTATIONS

A health professional may have the opportunity to give a formal presentation at some point in a career. This could be simply where the health professional works or at a national meeting. Although it is well known that fear of public speaking is an extremely common occurrence, a speaker who prepares should do well. The problem may simply be fear of the unknown and having some simple directions may be of immense help. Overall, the main concern should be to know the topic. If someone knows enough to be asked to talk, chances are that person will know quite a bit about a topic, or will be able to learn enough about the topic. Alternately, the potential presenter may volunteer to give a presentation on an interesting topic or one in which the person has done a lot of work (e.g., a new method of practice or a new practice area). After that, most of the concern will deal with looking good. This includes a variety of items, many of which involve professional writing, and will be dealt with in the remainder of this section.

In cases where a person is asking to speak, a proposal will need to be submitted. This describes the proposed topic, which should be of interest to the target audience. The directions given by the organization preparing the meeting will need to be followed. Beyond that, the skills described earlier in this chapter and appendices will need to be used.

Next, it may be necessary to write an abstract that the organization providing the presentation forum will use to inform potential attendees about the presentation. Each organization may have a format to be followed in creating the abstract. As to what should appear in the abstract, the writer might use the information presented in Appendix 9–2. Admittedly, an abstract should usually be prepared after the presentation is done to best reflect what will be said. However, abstracts may be requested more than 6 months before the presentation, so in this case it will serve more as a planning document. Actually, it is probably best to create a brief outline of the presentation (at least the topics to be covered) and then write the abstract.

Along with the abstract, it may be necessary to prepare learning objectives to describe what the attendee will be able to do as a result of participating in the program. The objectives should state that behavior in objective, measurable terms. For example, an objective may state that the attendee can explain, list, or identify something. It will not say that the attendee knows, understands, or learns, because those are not measurable. The objectives should relate directly to the program and should be adequately broken down to cover the different areas of the presentation. Refer to the beginning of any of the chapters of this book for examples of objectives. Also, refer to *Bloom's Taxonomy of Educational Objectives and Appropriate Verbs* for more details.[119] Also, this information could be used for objectives written for other documents.[120]

The presenter may be requested to provide self-assessment questions. Often these will be multiple choice or true/false, to simplify assessment. Those questions should be clearly stated and measure that the attendee has met the objectives. Efforts should be made to make the questions clear. Also, they should avoid the use of NOT or EXCEPT, because these terms can lead to confusion. Writing good questions can be extremely difficult, so testing the questions out on others before the presentation may help improve the quality.

The speaker may also have to prepare a brief biography to be used in the introduction. This includes a few items about the speaker's background, such as title and current position. Also, some information that gives the audience an idea of why the speaker is qualified to make a presentation is useful.

Presentations can usually be broken down into platform or poster presentations. The former is a more formal, oral presentation that typically requires some sort of audiovisual component and is often presented in a room set up for an audience. The latter requires the presenter to place a summary of the material to be presented on a poster (or series of small posters) that will be displayed on a bulletin board–type display (usually provided by the organization) that will be 3 to 4 feet high and 6 to 8 feet wide. In that situation, the attendees can walk through a group of such presentations, stopping to look at any that appeal to them and ask the presenter questions. Also, a QR code on the poster may allow the attendee to download further information or the poster itself using a smartphone or tablet.

Many of the rules described in the main part of this chapter relate to preparing the information to be presented, including slides, posters, and other audiovisual materials. However, a few other rules need to be mentioned.

- The presenter should learn the circumstances under which the presentation is to be given. That includes whether it is a platform or poster presentation.
- The presenter should learn what equipment is to be provided (e.g., computer projector, microphone, size of board for poster presentation).
- If the presenter needs other items, they should be made clear to the organization. For example, it is common for presenters to want to use computer slide projection equipment, which may present certain technical requirements for both the equipment and the support people. Also, the presenter may need such things as power

outlet strips, extension cords, wireless microphones (many good speakers prefer to move about on the stage or in the audience and are frustrated by a podium microphone that requires them to stand in one place behind a podium), Internet connection, connections from a computer to the room sound system, Bluetooth®, USB connection, DVD player, cables, device to advance slides, audience response systems, and other items. The presenter's own needs and desires should be taken into account, in addition to those of the audience. It is necessary to be very specific, since the people organizing the meeting may not understand the requirements. For example, a speaker requesting an Internet connection may arrive to find a connection that is too slow or one that has security restrictions, preventing access to necessary Internet sites. Also, even the resolution of a computer projector or type of connector for a network may need to be specified.

- If the speaker is doing a poster presentation, it is necessary to remember to bring pushpins to mount the poster on the provided display board.
- The audience should be taken into account. One common complaint when a speaker flies in for a presentation is that they may not know anything about local circumstances, including simple social skills that are expected (e.g., foreign countries). It is best if the speaker tries to find out more about the audience and the situation, adjusting the presentation to take those items into account.[121]
- If necessary, the setup of the room should be specified (e.g., theater style, discussion tables, screen placement).

All of the above should be double checked at the location of the presentation after arrival, but in plenty of time to correct any problems. Speakers may also want to take advantage of a speaker ready room that many organizations offer to check out slides, etc. As a side note, checking in with those arranging the presentation is necessary, so that they will not be worried about the speaker's arrival and will be able to clear up any last minute items.

The speaker then needs to prepare the presentation, doing appropriate research and preparation, using skills described earlier in this chapter and in the following sections. The presentation should also be rehearsed adequately. The next steps will discuss preparation of audiovisual materials, which can enhance the audience's ability to understand and retain the material.[122,123]

Platform Presentations

When giving platform presentations it is usually necessary to prepare audiovisual materials and, possibly, handouts. Most office software suites (e.g., Microsoft Office, Google Docs) have very powerful tools to create slides and other materials. These also have professionally designed templates that provide good layouts for materials, including color and background choices. The programs may also guide the user to follow general rules, such as avoiding a busy slide that will be unreadable from the back of a large room.[124] Also, the programs can be used to do everything from creating simple slides to multimedia extravaganzas—the former being learned in a few minutes, with the more advanced features available for those who need or desire them. Be aware, however, that it is necessary to use only those features that truly add to the presentation and to avoid having fancy effects in slides just for the sake of the effects.[124] ❻ *Instead of concentrating on the technology, it is best to concentrate on the message.*[125] This will also have the advantage of having fewer things that might go wrong in a presentation.

When starting to prepare audiovisuals, it is necessary to determine what type of equipment and situation will be found at the presentation. The most desirable type of audiovisual is the use of a computer with a projector and appropriate software to give the presentation. It is also possible to project slides from a smart phone or tablet (e.g., Android or iPad) that is properly equipped,[126] although the presentation may not be able to use any advanced features, such as the embedding of multimedia items.[127] When information or software is available on the Internet, it can be demonstrated. Also, in cases where a discussion ensues, it is possible for the presenter to use a word processor, presentation program, or other software to record items on the screen for users to read during or after the session. It is even possible to not only record the information on the screen during the presentation, but also to make it immediately available on the Internet at the end of the program, including audio and video. Some disadvantages include the cost of the equipment for the organizing group, the need for greater technical skills by both the presenter and the organizing group, and the potential for technological problems (e.g., a computer that refuses to boot, a corrupted data disk, an Internet connection that does not work), and it may be necessary for the presenter to bring a notebook computer with appropriate software and data. Fortunately, the technical support people for professional meetings are familiar with the equipment and the equipment itself is often more dependable.

When preparing the slides themselves, the presenter will have to prepare an outline to guide what is to be presented and determine the information to be presented in each slide. Some general rules can be mentioned.

- Limit each slide to a particular topic. Sometimes this will be an **overview**, but specifics should be limited to a discrete topic. One or two minutes of presentation material per slide is appropriate. If it is necessary to refer back to a previous slide, just make a duplicate that is inserted at the appropriate location.
- Keep things simple. The program may be able to do many things (e.g., 20 fonts in 16 million colors), but they may not be desirable. Typically use one font (perhaps with bold or underline in a few specific places for emphasis) and limited graphics.
- Limit the amount of information presented on each slide.[124] A rule of thumb is no more than about five bulleted points per slide and no more than about five words

per bulleted point. Any more than that quickly becomes confusing or unreadable. Generally, if someone in the back of the room has to squint or it takes more than 10 seconds to read a slide, there is too much information on it.[128] It has been theorized that a portion of the blame for the loss of the space shuttle, Columbia, was due to the information necessary for National Aeronautic and Space Administration (NASA) engineers being hidden in small print on an extremely busy slide.[129] While the consequences for most presentations are not nearly as large, it is still important that slides enhance the provision of the appropriate information, rather than obscure it.

- Consider using a theme in the program that will provide colors that go together well and contrast enough to be legible. Colors and color combinations have to be carefully considered, because they may have emotional overtones or, in cases of color-blind attendees, may not even be distinguishable.[130]

- Consider graphics. They can make the slide more pleasing to the eye, but they also need to be as simple as possible. If cartoons are included to entertain the audience, make sure they are related to the talk and, preferably, help to make a point. Also, pictures of landscapes or the presenter's institution may be desired by the presenter, but serve only to distract from the presentation and should be avoided. Also, remember that if copyrighted material is to be used, it is necessary to get permission to reproduce the material.

- Consider embedding sound or video in the presentation, if it adds to the presentation. That sounds difficult, but may be done with a few clicks of the mouse. It will be necessary in this case to make sure the computer for the presentation is hooked to the room's sound system so that attendees can hear the audio.

- Embed links to appropriate Web sites in the presentation. This can be particularly useful if an electronic version of the handout is provided to attendees.

- Save the presentation several ways. Even if it is on the computer hard drive, it may become corrupted or the computer can break. Perhaps also bring it on a USB drive, so that someone else's computer can be borrowed, if necessary. It is often useful to consider burning the presentation to a recordable (or read/write) CD-ROM or DVD, which will not be sensitive to magnetic fields that might have affected the original disk. Also, in case the computer to be used in the presentation does not have presentation software, it might be necessary to use the feature in many presentation software packages which creates a run-time presentation that does not require the actual software. In some cases, putting the slides on a Web server in presentation format may work, although accessing the slides and Web pages over the Internet can be a risky proposition. Also, as mentioned previously, the presentation might be given using a smart phone or tablet device.

Other items to consider include the following:

- Make sure to carry the presentation materials personally and do not check them as luggage, since they may be lost. Also, be careful not to damage the materials being carried.
- Make the presentation interactive—ask the audience questions and take input, or have the audience work on some project during the presentation. This is now a requirement of continuing education programs.
- In all but a very small room, be sure to use the microphone. Speakers may not want to be bothered or may feel it as a sign of weakness to use a microphone, but they need to remember that the microphone is to help the audience, not the speaker, and should be used so that everyone in the back of the room can hear over the ventilation system, etc.
- Keep to the slides, if at all possible, but do not read the slides—use the slides as speaking points for the oral presentation information and to organize thoughts.[123]
- Do not read a prepared script, unless it is considered to be the norm in a particular environment. Actors and politicians can read such scripts and sound natural, but most speakers cannot do so. Instead use the slides (preferable) or a simple outline. The presentation program will allow easy preparation of handouts and speakers notes that can be used.
- Consider the delivery of the material, including pitch, power, pace, poise, and confidence.[131]
- Be prepared for technological disaster.[124] Even when using something as simple as a projector, the bulb can burn out. When using more equipment and more complex equipment, the potential for equipment failure rapidly increases. Whenever possible, have backup equipment, but also have a backup plan so that the presentation can proceed without any equipment. Just making sure to have a printed copy of the slides can save a presentation.

It may be desirable to prepare a handout for the audience, in which case, the presenter can consider the following styles[132]:

- *Outline*—a reference document that gives the audience a guide to where the speaker is going in text form. This can often be prepared by importing the slide content from the presentation software to a word processor. Some presentation programs will also prepare the document itself.
- *Full-text handout*—this is essentially a transcription of the speech. While helpful as a reference document, it is probably of more use to politicians when they wish to avoid being misquoted. This is seldom seen in the health care field, because

the presenter will not be able to make last minute changes and the audience will likely read ahead and become bored. Interestingly, a comment heard when such documents are presented is that the speaker did not know the material, because all the person did was read the handout, even though the speaker was the one who wrote it!

- *Slide reproduction*—this is becoming more popular and easy; presentation programs allow easy slide handout preparation. This does give the attendee all of the information, including graphics, but will likely require more paper.
- *Partial text handout*—this can be something of a combination of the above, where only a portion of the presentation is on the handout.

In any of the above, it is good to consider the following[132]:

- Consider whether it is necessary to provide references or supplemental readings.
- Make sure the handout follows the order of the presentation. If it does not, the attendee may become confused and annoyed.
- Make it look good, using skills mentioned elsewhere in this chapter. By all means, allow plenty of room for the attendee to take notes.

The speaker may also use the handout as a set of speaker notes, but care should generally be taken to avoid just reading the handout to the audience, except in the case of full-text handouts, for the reasons previously mentioned.

The skills necessary to give the presentation itself are beyond the scope of this chapter that deals with the preparation and distribution of written material. New presenters may wish to read a book or pamphlet on how to give effective talks. Also, Toastmasters International (http://www.toastmasters.org) is a group that help individuals develop their speaking skills. Many organizations have a chapter of this organization. These aids provide guidance on such skills as what level of sophistication to use in speaking, how to stand (e.g., do not hide behind the podium, making eye contact), what language to use, how to use humor and other techniques to entertain the audience, how to address questions (including so-called sniper questions that tend to disrupt speakers due to level of difficulty and how they are thrown into the middle of the presentation),[133] how to avoid distractions by having everyone turn off phones and pagers,[134] and so forth. Also, some of the references used in preparation of this chapter provide many additional suggestions.[122,132]

Poster Presentations

Preparing a poster requires the presenter to first determine what is to be included. Typically, the information will be similar to that found in an abstract, but with an expansion of the various sections. There are likely to be tables, bulleted points, and figures. Overall, the information to be presented must be brief, so that it can be read within a couple of minutes by an individual passing by the display. Therefore, large amounts of text are undesirable. A poster presentation will not likely contain nearly as much information as a formal journal article, but will contain many of the same sections. It will serve as a place for discussion to begin between the presenter and interested individuals.

Preparing posters was at one time a very difficult prospect. This has changed with the availability of presentation and high-end word processing/publishing software on computers. A large, one-piece poster that is typically about 3 by 6 feet may be made using this software. Although the final poster must be printed by a graphics firm (e.g., printer, architectural drawing firm), the cost can be reasonable to produce a very good-looking poster. This may also be done over the Internet. The initial preparatory work can also be done by various firms, but it is less expensive for the presenters to do this themselves. The software necessary would be either desktop publishing software (e.g., Adobe® PageMaker, Microsoft Publisher, and Microsoft PowerPoint) or a high-end word processor (e.g., Microsoft Word). Essentially, what needs to be done is to lay out the page in these programs so that it is in landscape format (i.e., sideways from the normal typed page). The top of the page will have a centered title in large print, with the author names, institution, city, and so on centered in a smaller font below the title. Often, it is desirable to place graphics to one or both sides of that information, such as the symbol for the authors' institution(s). Under that, the page may be divided up into three or so columns and the information laid out in a logical order, including tables and figures. It may be desirable, once finished, to print out the final copy. One can produce a copy that fits on typical 8½ × 11 inch paper that can be reproduced and distributed to interested individuals at the meeting. It may also be on larger paper (e.g., 11 × 17 inches), if there is a suitable high-quality printer available.

Whatever method is used, the final product will need to be transported to the meeting (poster tubes are available for little or no cost from many graphics firms). It is preferable to carry such posters on airplanes, because they may be crushed in the baggage areas or lost. The presenter should also remember to bring pushpins to mount the presentation at the meeting. The presenter should show up early enough for the presentation to have the material mounted to the bulletin board before meeting attendees are allowed in the area and will be expected to remain with the presentation to answer questions for the assigned time. Although many people may be the authors of a presentation, it is not uncommon that only one or two actually attend the meeting and give the presentation.

Web Posting

After a presentation, consider making the material available on the Internet. Some organizations make at least some presentation materials available that way. Of course, copyright restrictions may prevent individuals from posting the material, but technology makes it easy when it is allowable. Text documents or graphic images, such as posters, are easily placed on a Web site. However, even full-slide presentations can be placed on a Web site, using streaming audiovisual. A variety of software can be used to prepare such streaming presentations that can include slides and an audiovisual recording of the presenter. This can even be done concurrently with the presentation (live streaming), with a recording being made for later viewing. The equipment needs are relatively minor (e.g., computer, presentation software, microphone, inexpensive computer video capture device). For the actual Internet streaming, the appropriate streaming software, running on a file server, is necessary. For those who do not have the appropriate streaming software, just placing the slides themselves, as a downloadable file or in presentation format, can be an easy process using the original software used to prepare the slides. Even the simplest Web site can then be used to give access to the material.

Case Study 9–3

You are preparing a platform presentation for a national professional meeting for the first time.

• *What are some things that should be considered in slide preparation?*

Conclusion

⦿ ❼ *Professional writing is a skill necessary for every health professional.* It simply consists of following the accepted rules for writing that have been established by the profession to prepare a written item that is clear, concise, complete, correct, and in the appropriate format.

Self-Assessment Questions

1. Which of the following items are considered to be a type of professional writing?
   a. An article published in a professional journal
   b. A budget report
   c. A label for a prescription vial
   d. A performance evaluation of a new technician
   e. All of the above

2. Which of the following is considered to be adequate for credit as an author?
   a. Acquisition of funding for the study
   b. Conception and design of the study
   c. Provision of equipment used in the study
   d. Supervision of the research group
   e. All of the above

3. When writing a document that is intended for an audience of physicians, pharmacists, nurses, and other health care practitioners, which style of writing should be employed?
   a. Pure technical style
   b. Middle technical style
   c. Popular technical style

4. Which guideline tends to be used the most in writing for medical and pharmacy journals?
   a. *American Medical Association Manual of Style*
   b. *MLA Handbook for Writers of Research Papers*
   c. *Publication Manual of the American Psychiatric Association (APA)*
   d. *Scientific Style and Format: The CBE Manual for Authors, Editors, and Publishers*
   e. *Uniform Requirements for Manuscripts Submitted to Biomedical Journals*

5. It is necessary to only define unusual abbreviations in a document, since nearly every reader will understand common abbreviations, such as the use of AIDS for Acquired Immunodeficiency Syndrome.
   a. True
   b. False

6. When writing a document, it is not necessary to provide a citation to a source such Wikipedia, since that only contains information that is considered to be common knowledge.
   a. True
   b. False

7. In most cases, when writing up an answer to a question for another health care practitioner, the first paragraph of the paper should contain the summary of the information contained in the body to make things simpler and faster to read.
   a. True
   b. False

8. Copyright violations and plagiarism are not the same. It is possible to commit one while avoiding the other.
   a. True
   b. False

9. Health on the Net Foundation provides what?
   a. A code of conduct for Web sites
   b. A Web-hosting site for medically related Web sites
   c. General drug information references
   d. b and c
   e. All of the above

10. Which of the following is an appropriate objective for a presentation? The attendee will:
    a. Explain the steps for preparation of the intravenous form of drug X.
    b. Know the steps for preparation of the intravenous form of drug X.
    c. Learn the steps for preparation of the intravenous form of drug X.
    d. Understand the steps for preparation of the intravenous form of drug X.
    e. None of the above are appropriate.

11. When preparing slides for presentations, it is best to provide as many details on each slide as possible, even if the font has to be smaller than normal.
    a. True
    b. False

12. You are going to provide a 1-hour CE presentation. How many slides should you likely be preparing?
    a. 10
    b. 50
    c. 100
    d. 150

13. Which of the following is true when giving a presentation?
    a. It is best to avoid the use of microphones, if possible, since most people do not know how to use them for the best effect and they are just another technology that may fail. Most of the time the speaker can just raise his or her voice so that everyone can hear.
    b. Microphones are placed in a room for the convenience of the audience, not the presenter. If there is a microphone present, the speaker should always use it.

14. Presentation handouts should:
    a. Follow the order of the presentation
    b. Provide the full text of the speech
    c. Supplement, but not replace the presentation
    d. a and c
    e. All of the above

15. It is necessary to always send an article proposal to a publisher, prior to sending in an article.
    a. True
    b. False

REFERENCES

 1. Kelley KW, Liles AM. Writing letters of recommendation: where should you start? Am J Health Syst Pharm. 2012;69:563-5.
 2. Thordsen DJ. Preparing an article for publication. J Pharm Technol. 1986 Nov/Dec:268-75.
 3. Generali JA. Why publish? Hosp Pharm. 2008;43(11):868.
 4. Moghadam RG. Scientific writing: a career for pharmacists. Am J Health Syst Pharm. 2003 Sept 15;60:1899-1900.
 5. Armbruster DL. Starting the writing process. J Pediatr Pharmacol Ther. 2003;8(3):210-1.
 6. Fye WB. Medical authorship: traditions, trends, and tribulations. Ann Intern Med. 1990;113:317-25.
 7. Gannon F. Ethical profits from publishing. EMBO Rep. 2004;5(1):1.
 8. Nahata MC. Publishing by pharmacists. DICP Ann Pharmacother. 1989;23:809-10.
 9. Wager E, Field EA, Grossman L. Good publication practice for pharmaceutical companies. Curr Med Res Opin. 2003;19(3):149-54.
10. Morris CT, Hatton RC, Kimberlin CL. Factors associated with the publication of scholarly articles by pharmacists. Am J Health Syst Pharm. 2011;68:1640-5.
11. Dotson B, Slaughter RL. Prevalence of articles with honorary and ghost authors in three pharmacy journals. Am J Health Syst Pharm. 2011;68:1730-4.
12. Sadler TR. Publishing in academia: woes of authorship, figures, and peer review. Drug Inf J. 2011;45:145-50.
13. Wilcox LJ. Authorship. The coin of the realm, the source of complaints. JAMA. 1998;280:216-7.
14. Hoen WP, Walvoort HC, Overbeke AJPM. What are the factors determining authorship and the order of the authors' names? A study among authors of the Nederlands. Tijdschrift voor Geneeskunde (Dutch Journal of Medicine). 1998;280:217-8.
15. Zoog HB, Chang T. Interpretation and implementation of good publication practice. Drug Inf J. 2011;45:137-44.

16. Committee on Publication Ethics (COPE). Guidelines on good publication practice. Cope Report. 2002:48-52.

17. Shapiro DW, Wenger NS, Shapiro MF. The contributions of authors to multiauthored biomedical research papers. JAMA. 1994;271:438-42.

18. Flanagin A, Carey LA, Fontanarosa PB, Phillips SG, Pace BP, Lundberg GD, et al. Prevalence of articles with honorary authors and ghost authors in peer-reviewed medical journals. JAMA. 1998;280:222-4.

19. Wager E. Raising the quality of publications: now we have GPP! Qual Assur J. 2003;7: 166-70.

20. Peterson AM, Lowenthal W, Veatch RM. Authorship on a manuscript intended for publication. Am J Hosp Pharm. 1993;50:2082-5.

21. Carbone PP. On authorship and acknowledgments. NEJM. 1992;326:1084.

22. Hart RG. On authorship and acknowledgments. NEJM. 1992;326:1084.

23. Pinching AJ. On authorship and acknowledgments. NEJM. 1992;326:1084-5.

24. Canter D. On authorship and acknowledgments. NEJM. 1992;326:1085.

25. Rennie D, Yank V, Emanuel L. When authorship fails. A proposal to make contributors accountable. JAMA. 1997;278:579-85.

26. Fathalla MF, VanLook PFA. On authorship and acknowledgments. NEJM. 1992;326:1085.

27. The International Committee of Medical Journal Editors. Statement from the International Committee of Medical Journal Editors. JAMA. 1991;265:2697-8.

28. Hasegawa GR. Spurious authorship. Am J Hosp Pharm. 1993;50:2063.

29. Rennie D, Flanagin A. Authorship! Authorship! Guests, ghosts, grafters, and the two-sided coin. JAMA. 1994;271:469-71.

30. International Committee of Medical Journal Editors. Uniform requirements for manuscripts submitted to biomedical journals. Med Educ. 1999;33:66-78.

31. International Committee of Medical Journal Editors. Uniform requirements for manuscripts submitted to biomedical journals: writing and editing for biomedical publication [Internet]. Philadelphia (PA): International Committee of Medical Journal Editors. 2009 Nov. [cited 2010 Nov 16]. Available from: http://www.icmje.org/index.html

32. Kassirer JP, Angell M. On authorship and acknowledgments. NEJM. 1991;325:1510-2.

33. Drenth JPH. Multiple authorship. The contribution of senior authors. JAMA. 1998;280: 219-21.

34. Kassirer JP, Angell M. On authorship and acknowledgments. NEJM. 1992;326:1085.

35. Foote MA. Medical writing: looking back, moving forward. Drug Inf J. 2011;45:121-3.

36. Foote MA. How to write a better manuscript. Drug Inf J. 2009;43:111-4.

37. McConnell CR. From idea to print: writing and publishing a journal article. Health Care Supervisor. 1984;2:78-94.

38. Burnakis TG. Advice on submitting papers. Am J Hosp Pharm. 1993;50:2523.

39. Higa GM. Scientific publications and scientific style. W V Med J. 1995;91:198-9.

40. Crichton M. Medical obfuscation: structure and function. NEJM. 1975;293:1257-9.

41. Jones DEH. Last word. Omni. 1980;2(12):130.

42. Hamilton CW. How to write effective business letters: scribing information for pharmacists. Hosp Pharm. 1993;28:1095-100.

43. Albert T. The fear of writing—it's not as hard as pharmacists seem to think. Pharmaceut J. 2003 Jan 11;270:55-6.

44. Baker SJ. Getting published. Aust J Hosp Pharm. 1994;24(5):410-5.

45. Hamilton CW. How to write and publish scientific papers: scribing information for pharmacists. Am J Hosp Pharm. 1992;49:2477-84.

46. Ingelfinger FJ. Seduction by citation. NEJM. 1976;295:1075-6.

47. Roederer M, Marciniak MW, O'Connor SK, Eckel SF. An integrated approach to research and manuscript development. Am J Health Syst Pharm. 2013 Jul 15;70:1211-8.

48. Sollaci LB, Pereira MG. The introduction, methods, results and discussion (IMRAD) structure: a fifty-year survey. J Med Libr Assoc. 2004;92(3):364-7.

49. Schulz F, Altman DG, Moher D. CONSORT 2010 statement: updated guidelines for reporting parallelgroup randomized trials. Ann Intern Med. 2010;152(11):1-7.

50. Moher D, Hopewell S, Schulz KF, Montori V, Gøtzsche PC, Devereaux PJ, et al. CONSORT 2010 explanation and elaboration: updated guidelines for reporting parallel group randomized trials. BMJ. 2010;340:c869. doi:10.1136/bmj.c869.

51. Campbell MK, Elbourne DR, Altman DG for the CONSORT Group. CONSORT statement: extension to cluster randomized trials. BMJ. 2004;328:702-8.

52. Piaggio G, Elbourne DR, Altman DG, Pocock SJ, Evans SJW for the CONSORT Group. Reporting of noninferiority and equivalence randomized trials. An extension of the CONSORT Statement. JAMA. 2006;295:1152-60.

53. Gagnier JJ, Boon H, Rochon P, Moher D, Barnes J, Bombardier C for the CONSORT Group. Reporting randomized, controlled trials of herbal interventions: an elaborated CONSORT Statement. Ann Intern Med. 2006;144:364-7.

54. Boutron I, Moher D, Altman DG, Schulz KF, Ravaud P for the CONSORT Group. Methods and processes of the CONSORT Group: example of an extension for trials assessing non-pharmacologic treatments. Ann Intern Med. 2008;148:W-60-6.

55. Ioannidis JPA, Evans SJW, Gøtzsche PC, O'Neill RT, Altman DG, Schulz K, et al. Better reporting of harms in randomized trials: an extension of the CONSORT Statement. Ann Intern Med. 2004;141:781-8.

56. Hopewell S, Clarke M, Moher D, Wager E, Middleton P, Altman DG, et al. CONSORT for reporting randomized controlled trials and conference abstracts: explanation and elaboration. PLoS Med. 2008;5(1): e20. doi:10.1371/journal.pmed.0050020.

57. von Elm E, Altman DG, Egger M, Pocock SJ, Gøtzsche PC, Vandenbroucke JP for the STROBE Initiative. The Strengthening the Reporting of Observational Studies in Epidemiology (STROBE) Statement: guidelines for reporting observational studies. Ann Intern Med. 2007;147:573-7.

58. Vandenbroucke JP, von Elm E, Altman DG, Gøtzsche PC, Mulrow CD, Pocock SJ, et al. Strengthening the Reporting of Observational Studies in Epidemiology (STROBE): explanation and elaboration. Ann Intern Med. 2007;147:W-163-94.

59. Zwarenstein M, Treweek S, Gagnier JJ, Altman DG, Tunis S, Haynes B, et al. Improving the reporting of pragmatic trials: an extension of the CONSORT Statement. BMJ. 2008;227:a2390. doi:10.1136/bmj.a2390.

60. Moher D, Cook DJ, Eastwood S, Olkin I, Rennie D, Stroup DF. Improving the quality of reports of meta-analyses of randomised controlled trials: the QUOROM statement. Lancet. 1999;354:1896-900.

61. Moher D, Liberati A, Tetzlaff J, Altman DG. The PRISMA Group (2009) preferred reporting items for systematic reviews and meta-analyses. The PRISMA Statement. PLoS Med. 2009;6(7):e1000097. doi:10.1371/journal.pmed.1000097.

62. Graf C, Battisti WP, Bridges D, Bruce-Winkler V, Conaty JM, Ellison JM, et al. Good publication practice for communicating company sponsored medical research: the GPP2 guidelines. BMJ. 2009;339:b4330. doiI 10: 10.1136/bmj.b4330.

63. Talley CR. Perspective in journal publishing. Am J Hosp Pharm. 1993;50:451.

64. LaRochelle JM, King AR. Avoiding plagiarism. Hosp Pharm. 2011;46(12):917-9.

65. Gabriel T. Plagiarism lines blur for students in digital age. New York Times. 2010 Aug 1 [cited 2010 Aug 2];[4 p.]. Available from: http://www.nytimes.com/2010/08/02/education/02cheat.html?_r=1&scp=1&sq=plagiarism%20lines%20blur&st=cse

66. Turnitin.com [Internet]. Oakland (CA): iParadigms, LLC; c1998-2012. Plagiarism and the web: a comparison of internet sources for secondary and higher education students; 2011 [cited 2012 Jun 13]; [about 10 p.]. Available from: http://pages.turnitin.com/rs/iparadigms/images/Turnitin_WhitePaper_SourcesSECvsHE.pdf

67. Mapes D. Net's plagiarism 'cops' are on patrol. MSNBC [Internet]. 2009 Sept 10 [cited 2009 Sep 11]: [3 p.]. Available from:http://www.msnbc.msn.com/id/32657885/ns/technology_and_science-tech_and_gadgets/.

68. Ware J. Cheat wave. Yahoo! Internet Life. 1999;5(5):102-3.

69. Stuber-McEwen D, Wiseley P, Hoggatt S. Point, click, and cheat: frequency and type of academic dishonesty in the virtual classroom. Online J Dist Learning Admin. 2009 Fall [cited 2009 Sep 17];XII(III):[10 p.]. Available from: http://www.westga.edu/~distance/ojdla/fall123/stuber123.html

70. Asimov I. Gold. The final science fiction collection. New York: HarperPrism; 1995.

71. Willful infringement. [cited 2004 Aug 9]. Available from: http://www.willfulinfringement.com/.

72. Ardito SC, Eiblum P, Daulong R. Conflicted copy rights. Online. 1999 May/Jun:23(3):91-5.

73. Crawford M. Are you committing plagiarism? Top five overlooked citations to add to your course materials [Internet]. Message to: Patrick M. Malone. 2010 Sep. 29. [4 p.].

74. Gousse G. Advice on submitting papers: I. Am J Hosp Pharm. 1993;50:2523.

75. World Association of Medical Editors. WAME policy statements [Internet]. Chicago (IL): World Association of Medical Editors; 2004 April 7 [cited 2004 Apr 14]. Available from: http://www.wame.org/wamestmt.htm

76. International Committee of Medical Journal Editors. Conflict of interest. Am J Hosp Pharm. 1993;50:2398.

77. Davidoff F, DeAngelis CD, Drazen JM, Hoey J, Højgaard L, Horton R, et al. Sponsorship, authorship, and accountability. Lancet. 2001 Sep. 15;358:854-6.

78. Krimsky S, Rothenberg LS. Financial interest and its disclosure in scientific publications. JAMA. 1998;280:225-6.

79. Laniado M. How to present research data consistently in a scientific paper. Eur Radiol. 1996;6:S16-8.

80. DeAngelis CD. Duplicate publication, multiple problems. JAMA. 2004;292:1745-6.

81. Stead WW. The responsibilities of authorship. J Am Med Inform Assoc. 1997;4:394-5.

82. Garfunkel JM, Lawson EE, Hamrick HJ, Ulshen MH. JAMA. 1990;263:1376-8.

83. Evans JT, Nadjari HI, Burchell SA. Quotation and reference accuracy in surgical journals. JAMA. 1990;263:1353-4.

84. Roland CG. Thoughts about medical writing. XXXVII. Verify your references. Anesth Analg. 1976;55:717-8.

85. Biebuyck JF. Concerning the ethics and accuracy of scientific citations. J Anesthesiol. 1992;77:1-2.

86. McLellan MF, Case LD, Barnett MC. Trust, but verify. The accuracy of references in four anesthesia journals. Anesthesiology. 1992;77:185-8.

87. de Lacy G, Record C, Wade J. How accurate are quotations and references in medical journals. BMJ. 1985;291:884-6.

88. Doms CA. A survey of reference accuracy in five national dental journals. J Dent Res. 1989;68:442-4.

89. Hasegawa GR. How to review a manuscript intended for publication. Am J Hosp Pharm. 1994;51:839-40.

90. Hoppe S, Chandler MJJ. Constructive versus destructive criticism. Am J Health Syst Pharm. 1995;52:103.

91. Baker DE. Peer review: personal continuous quality improvement. Hosp Pharm. 2004;39:8.

92. Seltzer SM. Desktop publishing in a drug store? Am Druggist. 1987;196:64, 66.

93. Srnka QM, Scoggin JA. 10 ways to distribute newsletters to build sales volume. Pharm Times. 1984;50:71-2, 74.

94. Making the media. The pharmacy newsletter. Hosp Pharm Connection. 1986;2(3):11-2.

95. Kaldy J. Effectively creating a pharmacy newsletter. Consult Pharm. 1992;7(6): 697-8, 700.

96. Goldwater SH, Haydon-Greatting S. How to publish a pharmacy newsletter. Am J Hosp Pharm. 1991;48:2121, 2125.

97. Almquist AF, Wolfgang AP, Perri M. Pharmacy newsletters—the journalistic approach. Hosp Pharm. 1988;23:974-5.

98. Schultz WL, Dendiak ST. Pharmacy newsletters: a needed service. Hosp Pharm. 1975;10(4):146-7.

99. Plumridge RJ, Berbatis CG. Drug bulletins: effectiveness in modifying prescribing and methods of improving impact. DICP Ann Pharmacother. 1989;23:330-4.

100. Appearance and content attract newsletter audience. Drug Utilization Review. 1988; 4(4):45-8.

101. Lyon RA, Norvell MJ. Effect of a P&T Committee newsletter on anti-infective prescribing habits. Hosp Formul. 1985;20:742-4.

102. Fendler KJ, Gumbhir AK, Sall K. The impact of drug bulletins on physician prescribing habits in a health maintenance organization. Drug Intell Clin Pharm. 1984;18:627-31.

103. May JR, Andrusko KT, DiPiro JT. Impact and cost justification of a surgery drug newsletter. Am J Hosp Pharm. 1984;41:1837-9.

104. Ross MB, Volger BW, Bradley JK. Use of "dispense-as-written" on prescriptions for targeted drugs: influence of a newsletter. Am J Hosp Pharm. 1990;47:2519-20.

105. Denig P, Haaijer-Ruskamp FM, Zijsling DH. Impact of a drug bulletin on the knowledge, perception of drug utility, and prescribing behavior of physicians. DICP Ann Pharmacother. 1990;24:87-93.

106. Parker RC. Looking good in print. 4th ed. Scotsdale (AZ): The Coriolis Group, LLC; 1998.

107. Baird RN, McDonald D, Pittman RK, Turnbull AT. The graphics of communication. Methods, media and technology. 6th ed. New York: Hartcourt Brace Jovanovich College Publishers; 1993.

108. Don't let cost prohibit publication of pharmacy-related newsletter. Drug Utilization Review. 1988;4(4):48-9.

109. Utt JK, Lewis KT. Using desktop publishing to enhance pharmacy publications. Am J Hosp Pharm. 1988;45:1863-4.

110. Pfeiffer KS. Award-winning newsletter design. Windows Mag. 1994;5(8):208-18.

111. What makes a great web site? [cited 1999 May 13];[1 screen]. Available from: http://www.webreference.com/greatsite.html

112. Tweney D. Don't be a slow poke: keep your site up to speed or lose visitors. InfoWorld. 1999;22:21(12):64.

113. Tullio CJ. Selecting material for your newsletter. Hosp Pharm Times. 1992;Oct:12HPT-16HPT.

114. Journalism pro offers editing tips for effective pharmacy newsletters. Drug Utilization Review. 1988;4(4):49-50.

115. Mitchell JF, Cook RL. Pharmacy newsletters: time for a new approach. Hosp Formul. 1985;20:360-5.

116. Ritchie DJ, Manchester RF, Rich MW, Rockwell MM, Stein PM. Acceptance of a pharmacy-based, physician-edited hospital Pharmacy and Therapeutics Committee newsletter. Ann Pharmacother. 1992;26:886-9.

117. Craghead RM. Electronic mail pharmacy newsletters. Hosp Pharm. 1989;24:490.

118. Mok MP, Castile JA, Kowaloff HB, Janousek JR. Drugman—a computerized supplement to a hospital's drug information newsletter. Am J Hosp Pharm. 1985;42:1565-7.

119. Bloom BS, ed. Taxonomy of educational objectives, handbook 1: cognitive domain. New York: David McKay; 1956.

120. Medina MS. Using the three e's (emphasis, expectations, and evaluation) to structure writing objectives for pharmacy practice experiences. Am J Health Syst Pharm. 2010 Apr 1;67:516-21.

121. Speaking abroad. How to prepare when you're presenting over there. Presentations. 1999;13(6):A1-15.

122. Spinler SA. How to prepare and deliver pharmacy presentations. Am J Hosp Pharm. 1991;48:1730-8.

123. Simons T. Multimedia or bust? Presentations. 2000;14(2):40-50.

124. Buchholz S, Ullman J. 12 commandments for PowerPoint. Teaching Prof. 2004;18(6):4.

125. Zielinski D. Technostressed? Don't let your gadgets and gizmos get you down. Presentations. 2004 Feb:28-35.

126. Malone PM. Slides, files and keeping up. Adv Pharm. 2004;2(2):175-80.

127. Goldstein M. PDA presenting has come a long way, but still has drawbacks. Presentations. 2003 Nov:22.

128. Endicott J. For the prepared presenter, fonts of inspiration abound. Presentations. 1999;13(4):22-3.

129. Bullet points may be dangerous, but don't blame PowerPoint. Presentations. 2003 Nov:6.

130. The psychology of presentation visuals. Presentations. 1998;12(5):45-51.

131. DeCoske MA, White SJ. Public speaking revisited: delivery, structure and style. Am J Health Syst Pharm. 2010 Aug 1;67:1225-7.

132. Engle JP, Firman SC. Perfecting pharmacist presentation skills. Am Pharm. 1994; NS34(7):60-4.

133. Simons T. For podium emergencies. Presentations. 2003 Nov:24-29.

134. Hill J. The attention deficit. Presentations. 2003 Oct:27-32.

10

Chapter Ten

Legal Aspects of Drug Information Practice

Martha M. Rumore

Learning Objectives

- *After completing this chapter, the reader will be able to*

- Describe the legal issues related to the provision of drug information (DI).
- Apply various legal theories that impose liability on pharmacists providing DI.
- Describe how pharmacists can help protect themselves from malpractice claims resulting from the provision of DI.
- Explain the Doctrine of Drug Overpromotion as it pertains to the 1997 Food and Drug Administration (FDA) Modernization Act (FDAMA).
- Identify the liability concerns inherent with off-label drug use and informed consent.
- Describe United States (U.S.) copyright law as it pertains to the provision of DI.
- Identify copyright, liability, and privacy issues arising from the Internet and social media.
- Describe the legal and ethical challenges emerging in telemedicine and cybermedicine.
- Describe the DI plan that addresses the Health Insurance Portability and Accountability Act (HIPAA) of 1996.
- Explain the legal issues involved with industry support for pharmaceutical educational activities.

Key Concepts

① Currently, most litigation concerning pharmacists involves negligence.

② There are a number of ways in which tort liability can relate to the provision of DI: incomplete information, inappropriate quality information, outdated information, inappropriate analysis or dissemination of information.

③ There are at least three key areas of labeling and advertising liability: the learned intermediary rule, which is a defense to failure to warn actions; the doctrine of overpromotion, under which adequate warning is alleged to have been diluted by communications failing to adequately convey the full impact of the warning; and promotion of off-label use or FDA-unapproved indications.

④ Drug information is currently being obtained from a number of Wikis, blogs, and search engines and there is the possibility of drug information liability for information obtained from other Internet sources.

⑤ Pharmacists providing drug information must have a working knowledge of copyright law both to avoid liability and to protect their own literary works.

⑥ The Health Insurance Portability and Accountability Act of 1996 (HIPAA) Privacy Rule is not intended to disrupt or discourage adverse event reporting or drug information in any way.

⑦ The FDA, the American Council for Continuing Medical Education (ACCME), and the Pharmaceutical Research and Manufacturers of America (PhRMA) have established educational policies, guidelines, or guidances which allow communication between industry and the continuing medical education (CME) providers.

Introduction

An understanding of the legal aspects of drug information (DI) can help practitioners in day-to-day practice, as well as provide some possible ways to protect himself or herself in the legal system. This chapter is intended to examine legal issues and should not be considered legal advice.

There are a myriad of legal issues confronting the various facets of DI. These legal issues cross over a number of traditional legal specialties, including computer law, advertising law, privacy law, intellectual property law, telecommunications law, and tort law. This chapter provides an overview and discussion of the key legal issues involving intellectual property rights, torts, privacy, and advertising and promotion that may arise in the provision of DI.

Decades after the genesis of DI services, the legal duties of pharmacists providing DI are still evolving. Today, most pharmacy curriculums, board certifications, and postgraduate year one (PGY-1) residencies include DI, realizing that whether a student specializes in DI or not, it is an integral part of pharmacist-supervised patient care. Pharmacists can and will be held liable for their conduct relating to DI. This chapter begins with an examination of the expanded liability of the DI specialist, which is defined as those pharmacists who either work in DI centers or who spend the majority of their working day providing DI (e.g., clinical managers, DI specialists, and PGY-1 and postgraduate year two [PGY-2] residents). The liability inherent in the provisions of DI to patients as an integral component of pharmacist-supervised patient care will be covered in this chapter. The chapter will examine and provide recommendations for prevention and mitigation of liability for the non-DI specialist. The chapter then explores copyright, privacy, unique legal issues pertaining to the Internet, direct-to-consumer-advertising, off-label use, as well as industry support for educational activities.

Tort Law

DI is a specialized discipline of pharmacy practice. Specialists are held to the highest degree of care by the law. Because of the DI pharmacists' greater expertise in the area of DI, it is likely that the courts would expand their legal and professional liability beyond that of other pharmacists. The liability of the DI specialist versus generalist differs for a number of reasons, the most obvious of which are the nature of the information provided and the recipients of the information. The DI specialist is most often providing DI to other health professionals and often has the title Drug Information Specialist or Clinical Manager.[1]

Functions such as online searching, monitoring or recommending drug therapy, preparing drug alerts and pharmacy bulletins, participating in pharmacy and therapeutics (P&T) committees, conducting medication use evaluations (MUE), writing and revising medication policies, training residents, pharmacy students, and pharmacy staff, and identifying adverse drug events entail legal obligations of proper performance.

Minimal practice standards for specialists have been put forth to delineate functions and activities that may be considered essential to the provision of DI services and the expected competencies of DI specialists. Position papers and standards of the American Society of Health-System Pharmacists (ASHP) and The Joint Commission (TJC), as well as DI curriculum and residency standards, and literature regarding appropriate management of DI requests remove any doubt about the level of expertise needed for DI specialists and standards for DI centers.[2-4] Minimal standards of performance and a consistent level of competence must be ensured by pharmacists promoting or offering this service regardless of the practice site. Although there are no standards to accredit DI centers, professional standards of performance may be used by courts as an objective measuring tool for the standard of care.

In the latter part of the nineteenth century, the locality rule or community rule was followed. This doctrine stated that the local defendant practitioner would have his or her standard of performance evaluated in light of the performance of other peers in the same or similar communities.[5] This is no longer the case and a DI center in a rural area will be held to the same standard as one in New York City. Creation of standards of practice and the disappearance of the locality rule make it easier for plaintiffs to prevail.

In addition to the DI specialist, the pharmacy profession is assuming an increased legal responsibility to provide DI in the daily practice of pharmacist-supervised patient care. The physician has been considered the learned intermediary, responsible for communicating the manufacturer's warnings to the patient. However, failure to counsel or warn cases are showing a trend in pharmacist liability.[6] Although most cases still maintain the pharmacist has no duty to warn, a minority of cases in various jurisdictions demonstrate the pharmacist's duty to warn of foreseeable complications of drug therapy is becoming a recognized part of the expanded legal responsibility of pharmacists. Courts have been more willing to apply a duty to warn where the pharmacist voluntarily assumes the duty, or has special knowledge about a patient, or the prescription is dangerous as written.[7]

Where the patient is at higher risk than the general population, the courts have uniformly found liability. There are many such cases against physicians for failure to disclose material risks of medical procedures or treatments to their patients.[8-10] Today pharmacists providing DI, be they generalists or DI specialists, are more likely to be held to the same standards as physicians when determining standard of care.

❶ *Currently, most litigation concerning pharmacists involves negligence.* Traditionally, physicians remain responsible for their patients and must exert **due care**; that is, a physician who knows or should have known that the information provided was improper may be held liable for negligence. Therefore, it is safe to assume that a legal cause of action pertaining to the provision of DI will be founded on the theory of negligence as the direct or **proximate cause** of personal injury or death. Malpractice liability based on negligence refers to failure to exercise the degree of care that a prudent (reasonable) person would exercise under the same circumstances. Elements of negligence include the four Ds: (1) duty breached, (2) damages, (3) direct causation, and (4) defenses absent. To establish a negligent failure, actual conduct must be compared to what is considered standard professional conduct. Typically, this is accomplished by introducing evidence of the relevant professional standards or testimony from expert witnesses such as college of pharmacy faculty or other DI practitioners. Once the duty of care is established, the plaintiff would need a preponderance of evidence to prove that (1) the information provided was materially deficient, (2) the deficient information was a proximate cause of injury suffered (or at least a substantial contributing factor), (3) the recipient reasonably relied on the information provided, (4) the information deficiency was due to failure to exercise reasonable care, and (5) the pharmacist knew or should have known that the safety or health of another may have depended on the accuracy of the information provided.

Expanding on the first element of negligence, duty breached, it is important to be aware of the fact that the duty must be a legal duty, not a moral or ethical duty. Although there are many ethical dilemmas pertaining to the provision of DI by pharmacists and they can sometimes give rise to a cause of action, an ethical breach is not necessarily a legal breach. Similarly, conduct that is considered unprofessional in the broad sense (e.g., rudeness) is distinct from legal duty. An example of an ethical breach that could result in liability for the pharmacist would be a breach of patient confidentiality, if that disclosure caused damages (e.g., loss of employment or the misuse of information gained in the course of employment).

In a study of DI requests, calls from consumers raised more ethical issues than calls from health professionals.[11] For example, should a pharmacist respond to a drug identification request for someone else's medication? Is the situation different if the medication is a drug of abuse and the inquiry is from a parent, relative, teacher, or police officer? Current law provides little guidance for disclosure of DI for questionable purposes and pharmacists must exercise independent professional judgment and assume legal responsibility for that judgment when exercised.

Case Study 10–1

The anticoagulation clinical pharmacist receives an order for enoxaparin in a patient who is receiving warfarin. The patient's current INR is 5.2. The anticoagulation pharmacist is a board-certified pharmacotherapy specialist (BCPS). The pharmacist dispenses the enoxaparin and the patient is harmed.

- *What factors favor finding the pharmacist liable for negligence?*
- *Is the prescription dangerous as written?*
- *Is the specialist more liable than the generalist?*
- *Who may be liable in this situation—the pharmacist, the physician, or the clinic?*

It is necessary to expand on the reasonable care aspect to provide a case of negligence. Reasonable care is that which would be considered acceptable and responsible. Suppose a patient develops a reaction that is believed to be caused by a drug, and the pharmacist is consulted to find any case reports of this drug causing the reaction. If the case is available online, but not in print, and the pharmacist had access to online databases, but did not consult them, was the pharmacist required to do so? Did the pharmacist exert reasonable care? What if the pharmacist searched MEDLINE® but not Embase® databases, or vice versa, and thereby failed to retrieve the case? Should the pharmacist have searched both? There are no clear answers here. Who can say what a reasonable search might have been on a given day? However, using outdated references or old editions of textbooks would more likely constitute an inadequate search. In a German case, a court held a Business and Patent Information Service to be responsible for not having used updated materials.[12]

In a highly publicized case involving a clinical trial being conducted at the Johns Hopkins University, a researcher conduced an incomplete search for lung damage from hexamethonium on PubMed®, which was searchable only back to 1966 and an open Web search.[13] Although articles published in the 1950s and other sources such as TOXLINE® and Micromedex® warned of such dangers, the researcher had not consulted these references resulting in a patient's death.

Recent cases against pharmacists have held that pharmacists who gain information about the unique susceptibility of a patient are liable for failure to warn of the risks. In *Dooley v. Everett,* the court held the pharmacist liable for failing to warn a patient of the interaction of theophylline with erythromycin that produced seizures and consequent brain damage.[14] Similarly, in *Hand v. Krakowski,* the pharmacist failed to alert either the patient or the physician of the drug interaction between the patient's psychotropic drug and alcohol.[15] The fact that the medication profile indicated that the patient was an alcoholic created a foreseeable risk of injury and, therefore, a duty to warn on the part of the pharmacist.

Case Study 10–2

The health system pharmacist receives a prescription order for metformin 500 mg twice daily for a 55-year-old male patient who has severe renal impairment. The pharmacist dispenses the drug without checking the patient's renal function in the computer. The pharmacy department medication use manual policy for metformin requires the pharmacist to check and document the patient's creatinine clearance prior to dispensing metformin.

• *If the patient is harmed, did the pharmacist fall below the standard of care? Could the*
pharmacist be judged negligent?

In *Baker v. Arbor Drugs, Inc.*, the court ruled that by advertising its drug interaction software, the defendant pharmacy voluntarily assumed a duty to use its computer technology with due care. The pharmacy technician had overridden the drug interaction between tranylcypromine (Parnate®) and clemastine fumarate/phenylpropanolamine hydrochloride (Tavist-D®) that the system detected from the patient's medication profile. The patient committed suicide after suffering a stroke from the combination.[16] In another case, the pharmacist chose to override the computer alert regarding an interaction between tramadol and methadone, resulting in the patient's death. A $6 million verdict was returned against the pharmacy for failure to warn.[17]

❷ *There are a number of ways in which* tort liability *can relate to the provision of DI: incomplete information, inappropriate quality information, outdated information, inappropriate analysis, or dissemination of information.*

INCOMPLETE INFORMATION

Is the pharmacist liable when the DI provided is incomplete? Should the pharmacist provide all the medication information via a DI sheet or patient package insert (PPI)? There have been several cases against pharmacists for failure to dispense mandatory PPIs for certain drugs that later caused harm. In *Parkas v. Saary,* the court addressed the issue of whether the pharmacist's failure to dispense the FDA mandated PPI for progesterone was the proximate cause of a congenital eye defect that occurred.[18] Because congenital defects, but not eye deformities, were specified in the PPI, failure to provide the PPI could not be proven to be the proximate cause. Therefore, judgment was in favor of the pharmacy. In *Frye v. Medicare-Glaser Corporation,* the pharmacist counseled the patient regarding drowsiness with Fiorinal® (aspirin, butalbital, caffeine), but failed to provide a warning not to consume alcohol. The patient died presumably as a result of combining the drug with beer. Here, the DI provided was incomplete. The trial court did not find the pharmacist had a duty to warn in this instance.[19] Although this case was decided before Omnibus Budget Reconciliation Act of 1990 (OBRA'90), with its mandatory patient counseling provisions in effect, its outcome would not seem to have changed as a result.

In a number of cases where the plaintiffs asserted that the pharmacist breached a duty to warn as required under OBRA'90, the courts have held that OBRA does not create an independent or private cause of action.[20-22]

Other cases are finding pharmacists have a responsibility for patient counseling and drug therapy monitoring.[23] In *Sanderson v. Eckerd Corporation*, the pharmacy promised in its advertising that its computer system would detect drug interactions or warn patients about adverse drug reactions; the pharmacists were held liable when they failed to detect and warn the patient of a potential adverse reaction.[24] In *Horner v. Spalitto*, the court imposed a duty on a pharmacist to alert the prescriber when the dose prescribed is outside the therapeutic range.[25] In *Happel v. Wal-Mart Stores,* the pharmacy's computer system was overridden, and the pharmacist failed to warn a patient allergic to aspirin and ibuprofen of the potential for cross-allergenicity with ketorolac.[26] The court found the pharmacist has a duty to warn when a contraindicated drug is prescribed. In *Morgan v. Wal-Mart Stores*, where the plaintiffs alleged that the pharmacist's failure to properly warn of the known dangers of desipramine was the proximate cause of the patient's death, the court held that pharmacists have a duty beyond accurately filling a prescription "based on known contraindications, which would alert a reasonably prudent pharmacist to a potential problem."[27] However, the court did not find for the plaintiff opining that pharmacists do not have knowledge that desipramine may cause hypereosinophilic syndrome.

Liability could also attach where there is a risk evaluation and mitigation strategy (REMS) requirement where either a pharmacist is required to provide a MedGuide or patient consent is required for failure to adhere to some other component of the REMS program, such as patient or provider enrollment.

Clearly, these cases demonstrate an expansion of pharmacist's duties from the nondiscretionary standard of technical accuracy to a discretionary standard which requires pharmacists to perform professional functions—that is, from a technical model to a pharmacist-supervised patient care model. Knowledge of, or access to, DI is becoming an important factor that courts consider in determination of the pharmacist's duty to warn.

In a case of first impression, a court decided whether a hospital pharmacist contacting a physician regarding the dosage of colchicine had a duty of care to the physician to provide complete DI.[28] While the pharmacist advised what a correct oral dosage would consist of, he did not advise of the correct dose in a renally impaired patient. The plaintiff alleged that the hospital pharmacy's voluntary undertaking to provide DI, and the pharmacist's voluntary intervening between the patient and the physician created a duty on the part of the pharmacist to the physician. This is different from other duty to warn cases where plaintiff alleges the pharmacist has a duty to warn to the patient. In the present case, the plaintiff alleged the hospital's pharmacy voluntarily undertook to be a DI resource and the hospital pharmacist voluntarily intervened between the patient and the physician, thereby creating a duty on the part of the pharmacist to the physician. The court, however, rejected the argument that a voluntary undertaking of a duty to a physician was created based on a pharmacist's interaction with the patient's physician. The court further held that the learned intermediary doctrine forecloses any duty of care on the part of the pharmacist to the patient, based on the pharmacist's statements to the physician. Significantly, the court commented that even if such a duty were placed on the pharmacist, the duty was not breached inasmuch as the pharmacist correctly followed the hospital's intervention policy.

While pharmacists are in a position to provide DI, providing the patient with all information may have a detrimental effect. In fact, it is the FDA's position that the information contained in professional labeling can be safely used only under the supervision of the licensed prescriber. It has, therefore, been the practice not to provide the patient with the professional labeling unless the patient specifically requests it. With regard to the duty to disclose to the patient low percentage risks, the court rulings have been inconsistent. One court has allowed **strict liability** against a pharmacy. In *Heredia v. Johnson,* the pharmacist dispensed an otic solution without warning of the risk of tympanic membrane rupture and the need to discontinue the drug if certain symptoms appeared. The plaintiff claimed that because of the lack of warning he suffered from severe and permanent injury including brain damage.[29] However, in *Marchione v. State,* a prison inmate alleged lack of informed consent based on the failure of the prison physician to inform him about the adverse effects of prazosin (Minipress®), which caused permanent impotence. The physician argued that his duty was only to warn of severe or frequent adverse effects. The *Marchione* court concluded that the physician need not disclose a laundry list of 31 remote drug adverse effects. The adverse effect had a reported incidence of only two or three cases out of several million prescriptions and was, therefore, rare. The plaintiff also did not have any unique risk factors that would increase the likelihood of the reaction occurring.[30] The courts seem to look at risk factors unique to the patient in deciding whether the health professional is required to indicate the likelihood of occurrence of the risks.

RISK ASSESSMENT AND RISK MANAGEMENT

Brushwood and Simonsmeier[31] delineate two responsibilities with regard to patient counseling: risk assessment and risk management. Risk assessment is judgmental and occurs before prescribing when a decision is made to accept or forego drug therapy. Although this has traditionally been the responsibility of the physician, the current scope of pharmacy practice is expanding, as many states permit independent, dependent, and collaborative prescribing, the latter is also known as collaborative drug therapy management (CDTM).[32] Each level of prescriptive authority is characterized by a specific level of liability. For example, independent prescribers are professionally accountable for their own prescribing decisions. Dependent prescribing, which involves the delegation of authority from an independent prescriber, as is typical of therapeutic interchange and CDTM protocols in health care facilities, involves a shared accountability. Similarly, in CDTM, where there is a collaborative practice agreement that allows pharmacists to initiate and/or modify patients' medication regimens pursuant to an approved protocol, both the physician and pharmacists share accountability.[33] In addition, employers remain vicariously liable for the actions and decisions of their staff.

The authority granted via CDTM depends on the pharmacy practice acts of the individual states that recognize CDTM, as such specific risk issues are difficult to identify. Liability risks for CDTM include exceeding the scope of the agreement or beyond the scope of practice, malpractice, practicing medicine without a license, unlawfully prescribing controlled substances, committing Medicare or Medicaid fraud, HIPAA and patient consent issues. Pharmacists undertaking CDTM should be well trained, not exceed the scope of the agreement, document all activities completely, be certain patients signed an affirmative written consent, and are aware you are not a physician. Pharmacists involved with CDTM should ensure coverage under their malpractice insurance for such activity. Unfortunately, several lawsuits have already occurred regarding CDTM. In *Reeves v. Pharmaject, Inc.*, a needleless injector was used to administer influenza vaccines and the patient developed swelling and hematomas at the injection site. FDA had, in fact, issued a warning advising against use of needleless injectors to administer vaccines. While the pharmacy had advertised needleless flu shots, it was not named in the lawsuit.[34]

Risk management after prescribing is nonjudgmental and assists the patient in proper drug use to maximize benefits and minimize potential problems.[35,36] Drug risk management, but not drug risk assessment information, should be provided to patients. The drug management information provided to patients should be accurate and in a form that the patient understands.

Hall and Honey[37] divided the risks associated with a particular drug into two groups: inherent or noninherent. Inherent risks are unavoidable, unique to the drug, and usually identified in the package insert (PI), but do not include probable or common adverse effects. However, well a drug is researched, manufactured, and prescribed, it still may have the ability to produce certain adverse effects. Examples of inherent drug risks are stroke from oral contraceptives or teeth discoloration from tetracyclines. Noninherent risks are created by the particular drug in combination with some extrinsic factor about which the pharmacist should reasonably know, and include maximum safe dosages, interactions, patient characteristics influencing pharmacokinetics, and probable or common adverse effects. Examples of noninherent risks would be nephrotoxicity from aminoglycosides in patients with renal impairment. The responsibility of the pharmacist to provide DI about noninherent risks is expanding.

What liability does the pharmacist incur for information outside of the PI? Physicians may prescribe drugs as they see fit, without adhering to the specific therapeutic indications or dosing guidelines within the labeling. The FDA regulates the manufacture and promotion of drugs, not the practice of medicine. However, it has been held that a physician's deviation from the PI was **prima facie** (i.e., not requiring further support to establish validity, on its face value) evidence of negligence if the patient's injury resulted from the failure to adhere to the recommendations.[38] However, the states appear to be split on whether recommendations in a PI are *prima facie* evidence of the standard of care. It would be prudent for the pharmacist to consult the PI when responding to an inquiry and include such information in the response, especially if the response is contrary to what is contained in the PI.

A disciplinary action by a state pharmacy board highlights the importance of checking the PI or literature concerning the proposed use of a product. In *re Michael A. Gabert*,[39] a pharmacist received a prescription for 5% silver nitrate for bladder instillation. The pharmacist contacted a DI center and was told there was no literature supporting the proposed use of the product. The pharmacist then asked the physician what evidence he had for such use and the physician referred to a published Mayo Clinic newsletter. The pharmacist did not ask to see a copy of the letter, or have a copy of it for the pharmacy records. Significant patient harm resulted when the solution was instilled into the patient's bladder. The Mayo Clinic newsletter pertained to silver argyrol, not silver nitrate.

INAPPROPRIATE QUALITY INFORMATION

It has long been recognized by law that false information provided to another could result in harm to the recipient if the recipient acted relying on the false information. Although **negligent misrepresentation** has not been applied to DI, there is no guarantee that it will not be in the future.[40] The relevant law is the *Restatement (Second) of Torts, §311, Negligent Misrepresentation Involving Risk of Physical Harm*, which states:

> "One who negligently gives false information to another is subject to liability for physical harm caused by action taken by the other in reasonable reliance upon such information[...] Such negligence may consist of failure to exercise reasonable care in ascertaining accuracy of the information, or in the manner in which it is communicated."[41]

Thus, the DI itself may be faulty for one or more reasons: it may be dated; it may simply be wrong; it may be incomplete and, therefore, misleading; or none may have been provided because of an incomplete search or incompetent searcher. Information negligence may occur because of (1) **parameter negligence** (failure to consult the correct source) or (2) **omission negligence** (consulting the correct source, but failure to locate the correct answer[s]). A study evaluated the accuracy of a drug identification response by 56 DI centers. Approximately, 30% correctly identified the investigational drug product; 67% could not make the identification; most importantly, 3.6%

(two DI centers) made an incorrect identification. The study found inconsistencies in responses of DI centers.[42] Another study evaluated the quality of DI responses provided by 116 DI centers to multiple queries. The correct response rates varied from 5% for a question pertaining to erythromycin for diabetic gastroparesis to 90% for a drug interaction question pertaining to didanosine-dapsone. For each of three patient-specific questions, the percentages of centers eliciting vital patient data were 5%, 27%, and 86%. The findings suggest that many DI centers continue to fail to elicit patient-specific information necessary for informed responses and focus instead on procedural and technical matters.[43] As an example, despite the peer-review process, the structure of bilirubin was found to be incorrect in an article and the three leading biochemistry textbooks in the United States.[44]

Inappropriate quality information may be the result of ghostwriting or publication marketing. Ghostwriting occurs when a pharmaceutical company develops the concept for an article to counteract criticism of a drug or embellish its benefits, hires a professional writing company to draft the article, retains a health professional to sign off as the author, and finds a publisher to unwittingly publish the work. In a recent product liability case, the court ordered the pharmaceutical company to disclose its documents pertaining to its ghostwriting practices.[45] In some instances, posters and meeting abstracts may actually be pharmaceutical industry generated or incomplete and lacking in peer review. For example, the reader has no way of knowing whether the abstract results are reflective of the entire study population or merely a small subset.

Can pharmacists providing DI be held responsible for retrieving information that is itself inaccurate? What responsibility does the information producer incur for errors in information sources? An unskilled searcher or one with insufficient searching knowledge may not find correct or complete information, which can lead to the wrong answer. The fault can lie anywhere in the information dissemination chain, publication, collection, storage, retrieval, dissemination, or utilization. Errors are often encountered in DI databases.[46] DI pharmacists are constantly finding errors and reporting the errors to the vendor or publisher. For example, when completing a class review of potential probiotic agents for the drug formulary it was noted that only capsules were listed for one of the products, although the product was available as a liquid and granules. Although very few cases have been brought before courts concerning the liability of print or online information sources, there is some case law to guide (see below). The issue concerns strict liability.

Strict liability applies where a defective product proximately causes physical harm. Where the service rendered is deemed to be a professional service, the courts exhibit a reluctance to impose strict liability. With exceptions, persons physically injured because of their reliance on defective and unreasonably dangerous information have only negligence as a cause of action, and only against the author, not the publisher[47]; only if the publisher is negligent or offers intentionally misleading information could it be held liable. This was tested in *Jones v. J.B. Lippincott Co.*, where a nursing student was injured after consulting and relying on a nursing textbook that recommended hydrogen peroxide enemas for the treatment of constipation. The courts rejected the plaintiff's claim that strict liability should be applied to the publisher.[48] Similarly, in a German case, a misprint in a medical textbook resulted in the injection of 25% rather than 2.5% sodium chloride solution, injuring a patient. Again, the court rejected strict liability for the publisher on the basis that any medically educated person should have noticed the misprint.[49] In *Roman v. City of New York*, the plaintiff sued for an alleged misstatement in a booklet distributed by a Planned Parenthood organization that resulted in a "wrongful conception." The court found that "a publisher cannot assume liability for all misstatements, said or unsaid, to a potentially unlimited public for a potentially unlimited period."[50] In *Winter v. G.R Putnam's Sons*, two people required liver transplants after collecting and eating poisonous wild mushrooms. They had relied on an *Encyclopedia of Wild Mushrooms* in choosing to eat the mushrooms that caused this severe harm.[51] The court refused to hold the publisher liable and found that a publisher has no duty to investigate the accuracy of the information it publishes.

In *Delmuth Development Corp. v. Merck & Co.*, the plaintiff claimed lost sales because of the publication of erroneous information in the *Merck Index*. The court considered the duty of a publisher to a reader to publish accurate information in a compendium.[52] The court noted a publisher's right to publish without fear of liability is guaranteed by the First Amendment and societal interest. It further held that even if it had a duty to publish with care, the plaintiff could not claim it suffered damages because of reliance on this information.

What liability is incurred by an author or publisher for publication of product comparisons? Recently, a pharmacy journal publisher and article author were sued for defamation by a device manufacturer where the publication compared and opined on the performance of devices for compounding sterile products.[53] The court granted the defendants motion to dismiss stating lack of actual malice (a necessary element of defamation). In this ruling, the court protected the First Amendment rights of scientists to report product comparisons and the rights of publishers regarding the peer-review process and publication of such comparisons.[54]

In *Libertelli v. Hoffman La Roche, Inc. & Medical Economics Co.*, the plaintiff became addicted to diazepam (Valium®) and sued the publisher of the *Physician's Desk Reference* (PDR).[55] The claim was based on the absence of warnings in the PDR regarding the addictive nature of the drug. The court dismissed the case against the publisher. Under a long line of cases, a publisher is not liable for matters of public interest if it has no knowledge of its falsity. Although some effort should be made to verify search results, the pharmacist cannot be held responsible for knowing and verifying the contents of all sources, whether in print or online. However, checking a second reference to verify information is prudent.

Strict liability would appear applicable to software that is licensed without significant modification as a standard packaged system, as has been found with defective medical computer programs.[56] Pharmacists providing DI should be aware of computer-related lawsuits that have arisen involving defects (or bugs) in software that caused erroneous results. These cases result in greater damage awards based on **consequential damages** (i.e., special as opposed to actual) suffered. An example of consequential damages would be damage to a firm's reputation. Perhaps the most widely cited software-related accidents involve malfunctioning computerized radiation machines where overdosages have caused patient deaths.[57] Radiation overdosages from faulty software continue to occur today; grim reminders of the problems faced by reliance on software.[58] In one particularly relevant case, the court held that the National Weather Service was liable for the deaths of four fishermen off Cape Cod, Massachusetts. The Weather Service had forecasted calm weather because of faulty software. Although the verdict was overturned on technical grounds, the U.S. District Court let stand the precedent holding an entity liable for information it provides.[59]

In another case, Jeppesen, an information provider, was held liable for an airplane crash caused by faulty data from the Federal Aviation Administration on flight patterns. A pilot used one of the faulty charts and crashed into a mountain, killing the crew and destroying the plane. The company paid $12 million in damages.[60] The court held the information provider strictly liable because the charts were considered a product. In *Jeppesen,* the mass production and mass marketing of the charts rendered them a product. Similarly, in *Greenmoss Builders v. Dun & Bradstreet,* the issue involved the erroneous listing of Greenmoss Builders as a company in bankruptcy in Dun & Bradstreet Business Information Report database. A jury awarded $350,000, including $300,000 in punitive damages. The case was appealed all the way to the Supreme Court, where Dun & Bradstreet lost the case.[61]

In *Daniel v. Dow Jones & Co., Inc.,* where a subscriber brought action against a provider of a computerized database alleging that he relied on a false news report in making investments, the court found that the subscriber did not have a special relationship with the database provider necessary to impose liability for negligent misstatements. First Amendment guarantees of freedom of the press also protected the provider from liability.[62]

As mentioned previously, DI provided may be inaccurate because it is dated, incomplete or wrong. For example, inappropriate quality information may occur because references are updated differently. Even electronic references are updated differently—some monthly, others weekly. Most DI services require documentation of an answer in at least two difference sources. The double-check procedure is common practice when preparing chemotherapy and avoiding drug administration errors. In many of the cases described above, liability could have been prevented by checking the information in more than one reference or source. Thus, checking a DI response in several references is the standard of practice.

INAPPROPRIATE ANALYSIS/DISSEMINATION OF INFORMATION

Is liability for providing DI a rhetorical supposition or a real possibility? The responsibility of pharmacists providing DI goes beyond that of mere information intermediary, the person between the information producer and the user. Published studies for DI centers have reported that 41% to 83% of requested information is patient specific or judgmental in nature.[63] In addition to liability for the negligent information retrieval and dissemination, the pharmacist's role involves information interpretation, evaluation, and giving advice. This role falls into a consultative model and differs greatly from that of librarians. Librarians are not equipped to give advice. The pharmacist's role as an evaluator and interpreter of the information creates a duty sufficient to sustain liability.

The paucity of case law in the area does not negate liability. The issue deserves consideration because of the potential for harm caused by the DI provided by the pharmacist. There have only been two cases involving poison information centers, one of which also was a DI center. In *Reben v. Ely,* the plaintiffs filed suit against the DI center for injuries sustained by inadvertent administration of cocaine solution instead of acetaminophen to a 10-year-old patient. The local pharmacy had colored the 10% cocaine solution red and labeled it red solution to thwart abuse. When the nurse realized the mistake she contacted the Arizona Poison and DI Center. The DI pharmacist described the symptomatology of cocaine overdose, but did not go far enough in recommending that the patient seek emergency care. The patient developed seizures and cardiopulmonary arrest with brain damage that required lifetime nursing care. At the trial, the expert witness testified that the DI center operated below the standard of care. The issue was not erroneous information, but whether the center went far enough in its responsibility in handling the call. The plaintiff was awarded $6.5 million; the DI center was held liable for $3.6 million.[64]

In another case, a lawsuit named a poison information center that was called for assistance when a student died after swallowing a toxic substance during a laboratory experiment. The poison center was named in the $2.5 million suit because it refused to release proof of its claim that the person who called had given the wrong name for the solution that the student drank.[65]

From a liability standpoint, there are disadvantages to the formal combination of poison control and DI centers. For example, poison inquiries usually require immediate answers in critical situations without written documentation and sometimes without supporting references.[66,67] The outcomes of poisonings (e.g., overdoses and suicide attempts) are more likely to result in patient morbidity and mortality and require medical backup for acute treatment decisions. Some states (e.g., Arkansas, Oregon, Washington, Arizona, New Jersey) have statutory provisions for joint poison control and DI centers. In several of these states, such as Arkansas, immunity from personal liability in judgment (in contrast to carelessness or inadvertence) would not be actionable as malpractice unless a lack of due care can be shown. However, not all DI centers are protected from liability. Additionally, there have been other lawsuits involving poison control centers but these have mostly involved medical toxicologists serving as poison control center consultants, not DI pharmacists.[68]

Defenses to Negligence and Malpractice Protection

Even if the plaintiff can establish all the necessary elements of negligence, legal defenses can avoid or reduce liability. Some defenses might include a statute of limitations, comparative or contributory negligence, informed consent, or governmental immunity. It is important to keep in mind that there may be differences in both types of defenses to negligence and insurance coverage for individuals and employers. Further information on defenses will be described in the following sections.

DEFENSES FOR INDIVIDUALS

Assumption of the risk via informed consent and comparative or contributory negligence are defenses to negligence for individuals. Under informed consent, the defendant could assert that the patient knowingly assumed the risk for a new or experimental therapy or regimen. However, the risks the patient assumes does not include negligence on the part of the physician or pharmacist. There is no assumption of the risk for negligent behavior.

Comparative negligence is the allocation of responsibility for damages incurred between the plaintiff and the defendant, based on the relative negligence of the two. **Concurrent negligence** is the wrongful acts or omissions of two or more persons acting independently, but causing the same injury. Under comparative or concurrent negligence, the pharmacist may also be held liable, either alone or together with the information requestor (e.g., physician and nurse), for inaccurate information or information that does not ensure maximal protection for the patient.

In the landmark case *Harbeson v. Parke Davis,* a federal court ruled that the doctrine of informed consent required a physician to furnish a patient contemplating pregnancy with information concerning the teratogenicity of the phenytoin she was taking. The physician had a duty to provide information reasonably available in the medical literature, but failed to do so. Even though the physician was not aware of the potential effects of phenytoin, studies were reported in the medical literature.[69] This case represents the only case in which a lack of a literature search resulted in liability.

• Cases of **vicarious liability** are not new to medical malpractice. Vicarious liability is the attribution of liability on one person for the actions of another. Through the doctrine of vicarious liability, a pharmacist could become associated with professional liability actions as part of a case against a hospital or physician. Physicians have been found negligent for the negligence of nurses, therapists, and others working under their supervision. Significantly, no cases were found where physicians were found negligent from the negligence of pharmacists working under them. If a physician requests DI, he or she would also be held liable if a patient suffers because the search was deficient or the information incorrect. For example, in the *Harbeson* case, if the physician had requested the pharmacist to search for information about the teratogenicity of phenytoin and no references were found because of a faulty search, the pharmacist would share in the negligence together with the physician. The institution would probably also be named as a party in such legal action.

• Delegation of authority does not mean abdication of responsibility. Under vicarious liability, a pharmacist who has not been personally negligent could be held responsible for the negligence of others. Supervision and adequate training of subordinates (e.g., interns, pharmacy technicians, other employees) are essential. Incompetence and substandard training of these individuals can lead to liability. An example might include a breach of confidentiality (e.g., revealing someone has a loathsome disease) by one of these employees.

From a legal standpoint, does charging a fee increase liability for the DI provider?
• Fee-based providers would appear to be at greater malpractice risk, especially if the relationship is a contractual one. If any of the contractual expectations are not met, the client has a contractual cause of action against the DI center. The courts will look to the terms of the agreement and the reasonable expectations of the parties. However, where bodily injury results, tort law may impose liability even where the defective information is given gratuitously and the DI provider derives no benefit from giving it.

Does providing DI services to consumers increase liability exposure? Many DI centers provide services to consumers; some via a hotline or health information lines, some via the Internet. Several studies have reported that more ethical questions to DI centers arise from consumers than any other group.[70-72] Such ethical questions may involve drug abuse and toxicologic effects, the safety of drugs in pregnancy or nursing, experimental
• therapy, or the appropriateness of prescribing decisions. A decision to comment on a physician's therapeutic recommendations, even if factually correct and in the patient's best interest, may result in a legal liability. The answers to this and other questions that the pharmacist providing DI encounter are not found in the legal precedent.

DEFENSES FOR EMPLOYERS

Is the provider the hospital, university, or pharmacy where the DI center is located, or the pharmacist providing the DI? The vast majority of DI centers are located in hospitals and universities. In addition, many pharmaceutical companies have DI departments staffed by pharmacists who handle inquiries on the company's products. There also exist independent information brokers who have liability under contract law, as well as tort law. The employer–employee relationship is a significant factor under either common law **respondeat superior** doctrine or, alternatively, a theory of negligent hire or supervision. Respondeat superior refers to the proposition that the employer is responsible for the negligent acts of its agents or employees. The injured party may also sue the employer for its negligence in hiring or supervising the employee. Under a negligent hire theory, it must be shown that the employee was unfit for the position and that a reasonable, preemployment interview or postemployment supervision would have discovered this fact.[73]

Although the person who provides the information is liable for the harm caused by it, the employer may also be held liable in the absence of sovereign or charitable immunity. For pharmacists providing DI employed by the government (e.g., Veteran's Administration [VA] or Public Health Service [PHS]), there are statutes providing governmental immunity, also called sovereign immunity, from **civil liability**. Such immunity, however, will not protect an intentionally or grossly negligent person.

Even if the lawsuit is nonmeritorious, DI centers affiliated with hospitals or universities provide another deep pocket for contribution to the settlement. With exceptions, suing the pharmacist alone would fail to provide a windfall settlement for plaintiffs. The board of directors/trustees of the hospital or university or director of the DI center or pharmacy department where the DI center is located would be jointly liable. Joint and several liability refers to the sharing of liabilities among a group of people collectively and also individually. If the defendants are jointly and severally liable, it means that the injured party may sue some or all of the defendants together, or each one separately, and may collect equal amounts or unequal amounts from each. In states where joint and several liability applies, the pharmacist provides additional assurance that there will be sufficient assets to recover. The DI provider will be held responsible for the standard of care in the response to DI inquiries and may be found negligent.

PROTECTING AGAINST MALPRACTICE

Methods to protect against lawsuits include contracts covering financial arrangements, adequate documentation, disclaimers, and insurance.[74] For example, a disclaimer can be placed on results of online searches stating that the data being provided are from a source believed to be reliable and factually correct.[74] The best way to avoid omission negligence is to learn from experience, anticipate mistakes that may appear in databases, and keep abreast of changes in DI sources. Even if the delivery of false information is the result of inaccurate information itself, the pharmacist would likely be named as a defendant if the database producer were sued.

Adequate documentation may spell the difference between refuting or not refuting an unfounded claim of malpractice. Such documentation includes responses to inquiries, as well as a record of steps taken in a search. Designing and following procedures to document the research process can help avoid negligence. In *Fidelity Leasing Corp. v. Dun & Bradstreet, Inc.,* the court looked at the operation procedures and adherence to them in the particular instance to determine liability for providing false information.[75]

The key to provision of quality DI in an information service is the availability of current, objective information. Procedures should be in place to ensure that data are continually reviewed and updated. Quality assurance (QA) standards for the timeliness, thoroughness, and accuracy of information could also insulate against liability. QA programs, although they exist, are inconsistent among DI centers.

Problem areas common to DI centers regardless of practice site include files not updated and incomplete documentation of responses to requests. With regard to inquiries about adverse reactions, details of the adverse event should be taken and reported to the FDA reporting program. Cases may be clinically urgent and the physician or nurse may have a patient waiting. Response via e-mail, even with alerts attached, is not prudent in such situations as there is no guarantee that the caller is at their desk to receive such e-mails. All statements made should be traceable to the literature. Additionally, information should be confirmed with other references to ensure consistency between various resources. DI centers should address at least some of the items in Table 10–1.

Insistence on a good educational background for entry-level positions including PGY-1 and, ideally PGY-2 residencies in DI, followed by the continuing education of DI professionals, certification in online training courses, and good interpersonal communication skills may also protect against malpractice. Several studies have shown that physicians who were sued frequently had poor interpersonal skills, i.e., patients did not like them.[76] It is also important to keep abreast of changes in sources of DI via regular advanced training, conferences, and reading. All courses in DI should teach situations in ethical conflict that will assist in the decision making and value judgments encountered in the provision of DI.

Under the tort law doctrine of *respondeat superior*, both the pharmacist providing DI and the employer are jointly and severally liable for the damages. This enables the plaintiff to have access to the pharmacist's personal assets where the employer's assets are not sufficient to cover an adverse judgment. Professional liability insurance provides protection to cover exactly this kind of liability. Consideration should be given to obtaining professional indemnity insurance for the DI pharmacist.

TABLE 10–1. QUALITY ASSURANCE AS A LIABILITY REDUCING FACTOR

- Identify scope of activities and personnel requirements.
- Develop and follow policies and procedures or formal call triaging protocols.
- Keep standard operating procedure manual available for consultation.
- Avoid violations of statutes and regulations.
- Unapproved uses or doses should be well documented and if a use or dose differs from the labeling, the requestor must be so notified.
- Do not recommend a use or dose of a drug based solely on foreign literature or animal studies or questionable resources or references that are not peer reviewed.
- Never extrapolate pediatric or geriatric dosages from usual adult dosages.
- Maintain knowledge of the current literature, new drug applications and supplemental approvals, labeling changes, and new warnings.
- Do not present inadequate data or ignore contrary data.
- Avoid overly enthusiastic or exaggerated efficacy and safety claims.
- Do not attempt to diagnose or treat acute poisoning—direct such inquiries to a poison control center or an emergency room.
- Know the circumstances of the case and appropriate background information (e.g., knowledge of causality assessment scales [e.g., Naranjo—see Chapter 15]), laboratory findings, concurrent drugs that are necessary for adverse drug reaction inquiries.
- Exert special care for drug identification questions in view of the growth of counterfeit drugs.
- Responses of new employees, students, residents should be checked—document, document, document.
- Maintain reasonable response time; if necessary prioritize requests.
- Obtain peer concurrence or outside professional consultation, if necessary.
- Develop a quality assurance (QA) mechanism to ensure that service is maintained at a high level of quality (e.g., periodic audits or surveys).
- Maintain up-to-date files and reference texts (e.g., paper files should be randomly checked to be sure they contain articles at least as recent as 2 years old).
- For Internet-specific data, check currency, authorship, publisher, length of time site has existed, site reviews, links to/from other sites, biases/objectiveness, intended audience, quality of the writing, references provided (information without references should receive little weight in clinical decision making), who maintains the site (owner/sponsor or whether the site has an expert advisory board), affiliations (commercial, organization "org", governmental "gov"), and seal of approval from organizations that review health care sites. (See Chapter 3 for further information regarding evaluating Internet Web sites.)

Most policies now provide coverage on either an occurrence or claims-made basis. Occurrence means any incident that occurs during the policy period, no matter when the claim is filed, within the applicable statute of limitations. Claims-made policies cover only claims that are filed while the policy is active. To cover claims that are filed after a claims-made policy is terminated, the DI pharmacist can purchase tail coverage from the insurer. Tail coverage insures for an incident that occurred while the insurance was in effect but was not filed by the time the insurer–policyholder relationship terminated. It is important to be aware of the limitations and exclusions in these policies, such as some policies no longer covering intravenous compounding. Many do not require the carrier to obtain the consent of the insured before settling a claim. In these policies, the right to protect one's reputation may conflict with the economic interest of the insurer to dispose of the claim as inexpensively as possible. Therefore, it is imperative that individuals obtain insurance coverage policies separate from those of their employers. Most common exclusions are coverage for dishonest, fraudulent, criminal, or malicious acts; property damage; and personal injury coverage. In these cases, the pharmacist faces such liability alone, and in certain situations can be ruined financially.

Finally, limiting language in subscriber contracts (i.e., **exculpatory clauses**) may serve to restrict monetary awards in certain circumstances. Such clauses could be included in either contracts for subscribers or signed on acceptance of responses to inquiries. A provision could be included that specifically disclaims any responsibility to a third party who might rely on the information. Written information (e.g., a bulletin) should carry a disclaimer specifying that the information provided is issued on the understanding that it is the best available from the resources available to the service at a particular time.

An attorney could draft a standard agreement providing that the application of the research by the recipient would not be subject to any implied warranty of fitness for that purpose. However, certain jurisdictions have held that contracts that purport to exculpate a party from negligence will be subjected to strict judicial scrutiny. Courts in certain jurisdictions have declared contracts that attempt to exempt a party's willful or grossly negligent conduct to be void. Further, no exculpatory clause will protect a pharmacist who is grossly or intentionally negligent.

Labeling and Advertising

The FDA defines labeling as written or oral information used to supplement or explain a product regardless of whether the information accompanies the product. As such, even literature, textbooks, reprints of articles, and scientific seminars may constitute labeling. Labeling requires full disclosure. Advertisements, on the other hand, require a fair balance, meaning there must be a discussion of both benefits and risks, so as not to be misleading, and substantial evidence from clinical trials must be included for comparative claims.[77]

❸ *There are at least three key areas of labeling and advertising liability: the* **learned intermediary rule**, *which is a defense to failure to warn actions; the doctrine of overpromotion, under which adequate warning is alleged to have been diluted by communications* *failing to adequately convey the full impact of the warning; and promotion of off-label use or FDA-unapproved indications.*

DIRECT-TO-CONSUMER DRUG INFORMATION AND EROSION OF THE LEARNED INTERMEDIARY RULE

In 1997, the FDA relaxed the standards for direct-to-consumer advertising (DTCA).[78] DTCA involves magazine, television, Web site, cell phone, and text advertisements, suggesting the use of various prescription drugs for medical conditions the viewer might experience and also suggesting the viewer ask their physician if the medication would be appropriate for them.

Today, prescription drug advertising is a multibillion dollar industry. Prescription drug advertising is governed by the Food, Drug & Cosmetic Act (FDCA) and 21 U.S.C. §331, which prohibits the misbranding of a prescription drug.[79] The primary regulation aimed at pharmaceutical product advertising is found at 21 C.F.R. § 202.1 that pertains to all "advertisements in published journals, magazines, other periodicals, newspapers, and other advertisements broadcast through media such as radio, television, and telephone communication systems." These implementing regulations specify that prescription drug advertisements cannot omit material facts, and must present a fair balance between effectiveness and risk information. Further, for print advertisements, the regulations specify that every risk addressed in the product's approved labeling must also be disclosed in the advertisements. The regulations further require that the advertisement contain a summary of "all necessary information related to adverse effects and contraindications" or provide convenient access to the product's FDA-approved labeling and the risk information it contains." DTCA of off-label uses of prescription drugs is prohibited.[80]

There is evidence that DTCA is becoming more aggressive.[81] The FDA has cited unsubstantiated safety claims and minimization of risk, including "websites that omit or bury important safety information," as areas of particular concern.[82] In some cases, the advertising does not focus on a product but rather on patient education. One company has developed a campaign to bring mental health educational forums to college campuses featuring free screenings for depression. In another case, a 24-hour television network directed to a captive audience (i.e., hospitalized patients) was launched. As federal regulations require patient education, this programming may be used by hospitals for patient education. Other manufacturers offer monetary rewards or gifts (e.g., free exercise video) to patients who visit their physician regarding the product or offer a rebate or sweepstakes opportunity if the patient completes a questionnaire. Manufacturers are also sending out video press releases about drugs that are often aired as news stories. Many advertisements provide an 800 number to encourage consumers to seek additional information about the products; others offer free videotapes, brochures, and information packets discussing the product.[83] There also exist DI search tools for use directly by consumers (e.g., PDR.net; http://www.pdr.net).[84]

Another popular DTC vehicle is blog posts. For example, YouTube™ videos about products from patients are being posted on pharmaceutical company Web sites without review. Often these patient testimonials go well beyond what a company is permitted to advertise about the product. In general, patient testimonials minimize product risks and adverse events and are unbalanced. However, the FDA has yet to establish formal regulations or guidance on such activity, even where the pharmaceutical company is hosting the blog.[85] In March 2012, the FDA issued a draft guidance on DTC television advertisements, but has not issued a final guidance. Nor has the FDA issued formal guidelines regarding online DTCA.

The advent of DTCA bypasses the advice of the physician. In 1999, the first lawsuit was brought against a pharmaceutical company in connection with DTCA. Other DTCA cases have followed where the attorney for plaintiffs have made some footholds in convincing courts to abandon the learned intermediary doctrine, greatly impacting pharmaceutical product liability law.[86]

In *Perez v. Wyeth Laboratories Inc.*,[87] the New Jersey Supreme Court created an exception to the learned intermediary doctrine on the ground that foundational tenets of the doctrine are no longer applicable in the context of DTCA. The court wrote, "...we believe that when mass marketing of prescription drugs seeks to influence a patient's choice of a drug, a pharmaceutical manufacturer that makes direct claims to consumers for the efficacy of its product should not be unqualifiedly relieved of a duty to provide proper warnings of the dangers or the adverse effects of the product." *Perez* involved Norplant®, an implantable contraceptive that provided contraception for up to 5 years, but was removable. The plaintiffs alleged personal injury and failure to warn of the contraceptive's adverse effects, including removal complications, which resulted in pain, and scarring. The plaintiffs asserted that based on the mass advertising campaign to women that the pharmaceutical manufacturer had a duty to warn patients directly. According to the majority in *Perez*, the learned intermediary doctrine has four theoretical premises: (1) a reluctance to undermine the physician–patient relationship, (2) an absence for the need for the patient's informed consent, (3) the inability of drug manufacturers to communicate with patients, and (4) the complexity of the subject matter. The court asserted that each of these bases, except the fourth, is obviated in DTCA of prescription drugs. According to *Perez*, when direct advertising influences a patient to request a particular drug, and the physician does not adequately consult with the patient, "neither the physician nor the manufacturer should be entirely relieved of their respective duties to warn."[88]

It is important for pharmacists providing DI to be aware of the emerging legal issues relating to DTCA, such as the erosion of the learned intermediary doctrine and the shifting of liability to pharmaceutical manufacturers.[89] Additionally, the erosion of the learned intermediary rule, as demonstrated in *Perez*, and the shifting of liability away from physicians has broad implications for pharmacists. Increasingly, the courts are holding that the pharmacist has a duty to warn patients and intervene on their behalf. In 1991, Pharmacists Mutual reported no claims involving drug utilization review. In 1999, drug review claims accounted for 9% of all pharmacist liability claims. A 2002 study by the same firm found that drug review claims were continuing in a straight-line increase.[90] In 2010, drug review claims at 7.9% represented the largest category of intellectual errors (as opposed to mechanical or dispensing errors). Counseling claims account for 1.6% of all claims.[91]

Multiple constitutionality issues have been raised regarding any government interference with DTCA of prescription drugs. In *Thompson v. Western States Medical Center*, the U.S. Supreme Court upheld the rights of pharmacists to advertise compounded prescription drugs.[92] In doing so, the court held that the Food and Drug Administration Modernization Act (FDAMA) prohibition of the promotion or advertisement of compounded drugs by pharmacists violated the First Amendment and that proposed restrictions would limit the First Amendment rights of pharmaceutical manufacturers as well as the implied constitutional right of patients to receive the information.

In any event, pharmacists must remain vigilant to ensure that DTCA does not promote false expectations. Clearly, DTCA achieves its goals of encouraging consumerism, whereby patients go to seek prescription information from health professionals. DTCA increasingly lead patients to seek information that will confirm or refute the manufacturer's claims that differentiate a product from its competitors. When confronted with the influences of such advertising, pharmacists are on the front lines educating patients regarding these products, including the cost-effectiveness of prescription drug options. Pharmacists have a responsibility to provide objective information, to educate the patient, and to serve as a DI resource.[93] Refer to Chapter 23 for additional information.

DOCTRINE OF DRUG OVERPROMOTION

The doctrine of overpromotion is based on liability where an adequate warning is alleged to have been diluted by communications that do not adequately convey the full impact of the warning and are so overpromoting of a drug that members of the medical profession prescribe it when it was not warranted. In other instances, overpromotion involves promoting a drug to a group for an off-label use. Recent examples include promoting an opioid indicated for cancer pain to nononcologists; promoting a birth control pill to treat premenstrual syndrome and/or acne; and promoting an antipsychotic approved for bipolar disorder and schizophrenia for anxiety, obsessive compulsive disorder, dementia, and autism.

On August 9, 2003, Prescription Access Litigation Project filed the first class action lawsuit against a pharmaceutical company in connection with DTCA. The class action was brought for allegedly deceptive advertising and overpricing of Claritin®.[94] Plaintiffs alleged that the company's DTCA overstated the limited efficacy of its product and that the company deliberately left out any information about the drug's efficacy.

In yet other cases, the overpromotion failed to warn of the potential for serious adverse effects. While product liability laws vary by jurisdiction, counts of fraud/intentional misrepresentation, negligent misrepresentation, and breach of warranty are often found in the lawsuit pleadings. Another DTCA lawsuit involves Paxil®, one of the top-selling drugs in the world.[95] Plaintiffs allege that the drug causes withdrawal symptoms, such as severe nausea and other psychological problems, and that the company failed to tell plaintiffs, their physicians, or the public of this adverse effect.[94] If the adverse reaction is not listed in the labeling, the health care prescriber (e.g., the physician) is exonerated, leaving the pharmaceutical company liable. Recent cases have involved tendon rupture from fluoroquinolone antibiotics, amputation from inadvertent promethazine intravenous extravasation,[96] and neuropathy and polyneuropathy from 3-hydroxy-3-methylglutaryl-coenzyme A (HMG CoA) reductase inhibitors.[97]

As evidenced by these DTCA cases, there is no doubt that there has been a narrowing of the learned intermediary doctrine in pharmaceutical liability litigation and the use of the doctrine in failure to warn claims.

OFF-LABEL USE AND INFORMED CONSENT

Off-label use involves use for indications not specifically approved by the FDA. It is an accepted principle that once FDA approves a drug for marketing, a physician's discretionary use of that product is not restricted to the uses indicated on FDA-regulated labeling. This is particularly important in the areas of oncology and acquired immunodeficiency syndrome (AIDS), where a significant portion of drug use is off-label. While patients and medical innovation, in general, benefit from having their physicians informed about off-label uses, off-label use information from manufacturers has been restricted. In fact, manufacturer promotion of off-label use constitutes misbranding under the FDCA.[98]

Under the 1997 FDAMA, specifically Section 401, the FDA attempted to strengthen regulation of information pertaining to off-label uses.[99] One requirement under FDAMA was FDA review of material to be disseminated to ensure that it does not pose a significant risk to public health and is not false and misleading.[100] However, the authority of the FDA under the FDAMA to regulate the promotion of off-label uses was successfully challenged and Section 401 ceased to be effective on September 30, 2006.[101] In favoring the commercial free speech doctrine, the court ruled that the FDA had to permit drug company–sponsored advertisements for off-label use, as long as they were directed at physicians and not consumers.[102] In 2009, FDA released a guideline allowing for distribution of reprints about off-label uses from peer-reviewed publications.[103] Major provisions of that guideline, which refer to what is considered "Good Reprint Practices" are found in Table 10–2. The FDA agrees that off-label uses by unbiased researchers in bona fide published literature should be discussed.

Moreover, medical science liaisons are permitted to provide off-label information in response to unsolicited medical inquiries. The types of nonpromotional information that can be provided include general education, report of a clinical trial, follow-up to a question originally posed to a sales representative, and advice for formularies. Problematic are responses to inquiries that are not really unsolicited or formulary advice that borders on preapproval promotion (known as new product seeding).[104] Additionally, pharmaceutical

TABLE 10–2. MAJOR PROVISIONS OF THE FDA GUIDANCE FOR INDUSTRY—GOOD REPRINT PRACTICES FOR THE DISTRIBUTION OF MEDICAL JOURNAL ARTICLES AND MEDICAL OR SCIENTIFIC REFERENCE PUBLICATIONS ON UNAPPROVED NEW USES OF APPROVED DRUGS

- Articles should:
  - Be published by an organization with an editorial board
  - Be peer-reviewed
  - Be an unabridged reprint, copy of an article, or reference publication
  - Be accompanied by the approved labeling and, when such information exists, a comprehensive bibliography of well-controlled clinical studies
  - Be disseminated with a representative publication which reaches contrary or different conclusions
- Article should not:
  - Be a special supplement or funded by a manufacturer of the product that is the subject of the article
  - Be primarily distributed by a manufacturer, but should be generally available via other distribution channels
  - Be written, edited, excerpted, or published specifically at the request of a manufacturer or edited or influenced by someone having a significant financial relationship with the manufacturer
  - Be false or misleading or discuss a clinical trial that the FDA has indicated is not adequate and well controlled
  - Post a significant risk to public health, if relied upon.
  - Be marked, highlighted, summarized or characterized by the manufacturer
- Not consistent with Good Reprint Practices are:
  - Letters to the editor
  - Abstracts of a publication
  - Reports of Phase I trials in healthy subjects
  - Reference publications with little/no substantive discussion of relevant investigation or data
- Articles should be distributed separately from information that is promotional:
  - They may not distribute in exhibit halls or during promotional speakers' programs
- Articles should be accompanied by a prominently displayed and affixed statement disclosing:
  - That the uses are off-label
  - The manufacturer's interest in the subject drug of the article
  - Any person known to the manufacturer who has funded the study
  - All significant risks/safety concerns known to the manufacturer
  - Any author who has received financial compensation from the manufacturer and the nature and amount of the same

companies may freely distribute to health professionals copies of articles from peer-reviewed professional journals or reference textbooks containing discussions of off-label product usage. However, sales representatives are not permitted to use this information to promote the company's products. In December 2011, the FDA issued a draft guidance for industry entitled "Responding to Unsolicited Requests for Off-Label Information about Prescription Drugs and Medical Devices."[105] An entire section of this document is devoted to unsolicited requests for off-label information through emerging electronic media. The FDA is recommending that the public DI response to off-label information be limited to providing the firm's contact information and should not include any off-label information. This will ensure that the communication occurs solely between the firm and the individual who made the request and circumvents both broad distribution and issues regarding the enduring nature of online responses.

Researchers continually conduct studies to determine new uses for already marketed drugs and effective combinations of drugs for new indications with the results being published in the literature. Additionally, with up to 40% of all prescriptions being for off-label use, off-label use comprises a large component of providing DI, especially for queries that involve pediatrics.[106] These queries are often from physicians seeking evidence to support a particular off-label use. Problems arise when the off-label use is not really off-label, but rather, crosses the line and is experimental (in which case an Investigational New Drug Application and/or Institutional Review Board [IRB] approval for study is required).[104] Refer to Chapter 17 for more detailed information.

Unfortunately, once an off-label use becomes rampant, the market drives it and there remains little incentive for the pharmaceutical company to provide more data or conduct further research regarding that off-label use. This disincentive arises not only because of the expense involved in conducting clinical trials but also because trial results could actually have an adverse effect on sales by showing lack of efficacy or safety. For example, it was a study of rofecoxib (Vioxx®) for an off-label use that first uncovered the cardiovascular risks that eventually led to market withdrawal.[107]

Medicare Parts B and D are required to cover off-label uses of drugs in cancer treatment when the use is supported by a citation in at least one of the following references: *AHFS Drug Information (AHFS-DI), The National Comprehensive Cancer Network's Drugs and Biologics Compendium (NCCN), Truven Health Analytics, Inc. DRUGDEX®, or Clinical Pharmacology*, or the use is supported by clinical research in peer-reviewed articles published in respected medical journals.[108] Medicaid utilizes only *AHFS Drug Information®* and *DRUGDEX®*.[109] When providing DI, it should be realized that not all compendia include revision dates for the monographs. Moreover, a recent study revealed that update policies were not followed, certain off-label indications were excluded without rationale, and for common off-label cancer treatments, old literature and scanty and inconsistent evidence was found in the compendia.[110] Under the Medicare Improvements for

Patients and Providers Act of 2008 (MIPPA), the criteria for medically accepted off-label uses are now the same for both Medicare Part B and Part D.[111] For noncancer Part B and D drugs, the off-label coverage is limited to uses in *DRUGDEX®, Clinical Pharmacology,* or *AHFS Drug Information,* but only if the FDA has approved the drug for some other use. Peer-review literature still may not be used to support off-label use for noncancer drugs.

Following these guidelines for DI queries pertaining to an off-label use would appear to be a prudent practice. Similarly, in providing responses to DI requests pertaining to off-label uses (including usages of off-label dosages), it is prudent to provide complete information, so that a decision may be made whether the information is enough to warrant a particular off-label use. For example, letters to the editor or abstracts would not be complete information. When there is another drug on the market with an approved-label use for the same indication that the off-label product is being considered, the response to the DI request should mention that labeled alternative.[112] Moreover, it is also important to be cognizant of the implications of disseminating off-label information in the context of patient safety and liability. Responding to consumer requests for information about off-label uses is not advised, simply because, unlike health professionals, most often they are not in a position to evaluate the literature and extrapolate to a particular situation.

Off-label use of pharmaceuticals has resulted in liability. For example, physicians have been the target of lawsuits involving coadministration of insulin with rosiglitazone (Avandia®) before the combination was approved by the FDA, and included in the labeling.

While there is no question that patients should be advised if a proposed treatment is truly investigational or experimental, off-label use is not necessarily experimental or investigational and informed consent is not necessary whenever an off-label use is proposed.[113] Federal informed consent regulations governing investigational drugs do not apply to off-label use.[114] State informed consent laws vary but usually require discussion of the nature, risks, benefits, and alternative modes of treatment. For example, the New York statute states:

> "Lack of informed consent means the failure of the person providing the professional treatment or diagnosis to disclose to the patient such alternatives thereto and the reasonably foreseeable risks and benefits involved as a reasonable medical ... practitioner under similar circumstances would have disclosed, in a manner permitting the patient to make a knowledgeable evaluation."[115]

Actions for informed consent are, therefore, limited to the nondisclosure of medical information. However, failure to disclose FDA status does not raise a **material issue of fact** as to informed consent.

Liability Concerns for Web 2.0 Information

❹ *DI is currently being obtained from a number of* Wikis, *blogs, and search engines and there is a possibility of DI liability for information obtained from other Internet sources.* Google Scholar, Wikipedia, RxWiki, PubDrug, and Web citations, in general, are increasingly being accessed for handling DI queries. Recently, these sources have appeared as references in publications.[116] More than 25% of the Internet's content involves health care and medical information.[117] The browser of Internet information resources can now expect to find full prescribing information for most heavily marketed drugs. The situation is complicated by links to investigational products or investigational uses and vice versa. The question is whether this is promotion of off-label uses.[118] Refer to Chapter 23 for further information on this topic.

Liability concerns arise in the area of whether a manufacturer's Web site content is considered labeling or advertising. It appears to be necessary to distinguish between Internet promotion directed to health professionals and consumers. DTCA on the Internet is considered labeling, rather than advertising and, as such, the FDA has principal authority to regulate it.[119]

On February 2004, the FDA issued new industry guidelines, entitled "Help-Seeking and Other Disease Awareness Communications by or on Behalf of Drug and Device Firms and Brief Summary: Disclosing Risk Information in Consumer-Directed Print Advertisements." While these guidelines are intended to improve the brief summaries of adverse effects that must be included in DTCA, they do not address Internet advertisements. The FDA has not issued guidelines on DTCA via the Internet. In fact, the FDA has stopped work on a planned guidance on Internet drug promotional activities because the Internet is changing so rapidly. The FDA now believes existing regulations can be followed.[79] For example, a drug's black box warning should be configured prominently on the Internet. A person should not have to click multiple times to get this important information. Additionally, there are liability risks inherent in DTCA via the Internet, mainly because the risks are ill-defined by sparse FDA guidance and judicial precedence commingled with jurisdictional and extraterritoriality issues.

QUALITY OF INFORMATION

Not all Web sites are reputable and currently there is no way to distinguish which sites providing DI are authoritative and which are not. Problems have arisen such as **hyperlink** obsolescence, defunct Web sites, broken links, altered content, and an inability to determine currency.[113] Moreover, it is common for Web sites to change or move.

Entries in Wikipedia, an encyclopedia project, recently ranked as one of the top 10 sites visited, can be the subject of erroneous entries, fraud, conflict of interest, or even criminal mischief.[120] For example, pharmaceutical companies may edit or delete their product information as the site is user edited. Thus, sites such as Wikipedia are not authoritative and can only be supplementary to, rather than the sole source of, DI.[121] Google Scholar includes both published and unpublished (hence not peer-reviewed) information and, unlike PubMed®, it may not contain the latest literature. However, as the number of Internet-only journals not indexed in PubMed® increases, there will be increased reliance on Google Scholar as an easy to use source for locating primary literature. In fact, in a recent comparison with PubMed®, no significant differences were found regarding the number of primary literature articles, although PubMed® did retrieve more specific articles.[122]

What about DI liability for information obtained from the Internet and electronic journals or apps (such as Epocrates®)? Is there a possibility of pharmacist liability occurring via cyberspace? As mentioned above, the Internet contains a growing hodgepodge of sources with little organization and uneven credibility. In fact, material on the Internet may contain innocent mistakes and/or deliberate fraud, as well as outdated material. Several situations may result in search results that are not comprehensive. Examples include faulty search strategies and failing to search for historical information. Many databases including PubMed® do not contain material prior to the 1940s. Searchers may not even be aware that pre-Internet or old nonelectronic material exists. Old MEDLINE® articles from 1949 through 1965 may not be updated with MeSH terms and may not contain searchable abstracts.[123] For e-books (e.g., online textbooks) with their own built-in search engine (e.g., Merck Manual), there is a possibility of patient harm occurring when the computer malfunctions. Currently, there are no laws pertaining to, and no means for, ensuring the accuracy of information posed on the Internet. It is possible for information on the Internet to be false, misleading, corrupted by an outside source, or otherwise harmful to the reader to apply it to their specific situation. There is a potential for misinformation to be disseminated, while the reader unknowingly assumes the information to be accurate and true via the Internet and related technologies.

The Health Summit Working Group, which consists of professional societies including ASHP, and the Health on the Net Foundation (HON) are currently working to improve the quality of DI on the Internet. HON has developed a code (HONcode) for quality and reliability which, if displayed, increases the likelihood that the information is reliable. A seal of approval may also be given from other organizations that approve health care sites such as Internet Healthcare Coalition, Verified Internet Pharmacy Practice Sites (VIPPS®), and Medical Matrix. Unfortunately, these instruments may be difficult to use and their actual validity is unclear. Additionally, a seal of approval should in no way replace critical clinical judgment of the content. Also, the application of the National Information Infrastructure to consumer health information is one of the priorities of the federal government. Examples of Web site QA criteria are included in Table 10–1 and are found in Chapter 3.

Another venue where the quality of DI may be suspect is e-mail communication. Both the American Medical Association and the American Medical Informatics Association have issued guidelines for physicians using e-mail to communicate with patients.[124] These guidelines encourage physicians to be cautious when using e-mail because of the possibility of liability due to misunderstanding and privacy concerns.[125] Perhaps in the near future, health insurers will cover calls made to online pharmacists providing DI, much the same way as Medicare now covers teleconferencing.

The Internet is at the forefront of practice, where pharmacists will consult with each other, thereby learning from one another and benefiting their DI clients and patients.[126] Web 2.0 is the term commonly associated since 2004 with Web applications that facilitate interactive information sharing, such as Wikis, blogs, hosted-services, and networking sites. Specific examples include the University Health System Consortium and Google Scholar. In the fast-paced practice of DI, Web 2.0 information may provide a quick starting point for an answer to a query. However, other non-Web-based references should also be consulted. DI professionals should never rely solely on a Google Scholar retrieved search to respond to a DI query. Additionally, when using Web citations, it is recommended to include the date accessed to provide readers with some indication of how current the information is (refer to Appendix 9–3).

TELEMEDICINE AND CYBERMEDICINE

Legal issues are emerging from e-health technologies, such as telemedicine and cybermedicine programs. **Telemedicine** is defined as the use of telecommunications and interactive video technology to provide health care services to patients who are at a distance. **Cybermedicine** is a broader concept that includes marketing, relationship creation, advice, prescribing, and selling pharmaceuticals and devices in cyberspace. Therefore, telepharmacy is a subset of telemedicine and the terms are used interchangeably here. As telemedicine and cybermedicine expand, questions regarding liability for pharmacists providing DI on the Internet will need to be addressed. For example, health professionals, such as pharmacists, are licensed by states. Which state law applies when the pharmacist is located in New York, the patient is in Florida, and the Web site is maintained by a company in California? Who is liable for technical problems that make it impossible for the information to be received in a timely manner or for breaches of confidentiality caused by those who would invade private files? Already some sites offer fee-based live physician offices and nurse triage services (e.g. OptumHealth Care NurseLine) for self-diagnosis and health screening. Additionally, some DI centers provide information over the Internet.

Although the courts have yet to test liability for medical malpractice involving the practice of pharmacy or medicine on the Internet, such a case is bound to surface soon. The most important determination of whether there is such malpractice is whether or not a health care provider–patient relationship has been created by the consultation in the absence of physical contact. Hard copy printouts of Internet discussions would be discoverable before trial and could be uncovered in the defendant's computer files by a plaintiff's attorney. It is likely that where a physician consults with a pharmacist for DI via telemedicine, the pharmacist will not be deemed to have established a pharmacist–patient relationship. Telephone consultations between physicians are most analogous and have not been held to create a physician–patient relationship.[127] Similarly, as previously mentioned no pharmacist–physician relationship has been found based on a provision of DI to the physician.[28] This is largely because of the public policy interest of promoting consultations, professional association, and education, as well as the assumed limited information conveyed to the consulting physician. However, in view of advancing technology where the patient's entire medical history and test results are available on the computer, this situation may change, especially where a consultation fee is involved. Also, where a pharmacist posts a Web site and is paid to provide DI, the courts will surely find such cybermedical consultation to create a pharmacist–patient relationship.

Although there have been several lawsuits for false information on online bulletin boards (e.g., Usenet News, CompuServe®), the basis of these lawsuits has been defamation, not malpractice.[128,129] The offering of general medical advice and judgments online (e.g., chat rooms) does not appear to be creating a formal physician–patient relationship. Nor does it appear that the giving of generic advice will generate liability for either the provider or the publisher. If, however, the information is fraudulent or quackery, then courts do have authority under both state and federal computer statutes to stop the activity. Similarly, Internet (or telephone) medical call centers, or triage services used by some healthcare plans can expect to be held liable when misdiagnosis occurs. On the other hand, liability is lessened where Internet discussions resemble an academic conference between health care providers, rather than a formal consultancy. Similarly, the issuance of a disclaimer in writing with the original subscription and with each message written may help insulate from any liability.

Some Web sites now carry disclaimers to protect the authors from liability. The limitation of the remedies available should be displayed prominently. A cap equal to the price of the service sold may be included. The following is an example: "Please read this agreement entirely and carefully before assessing this Web site. By accessing the site, you agree to be bound by the terms and conditions below. If you do not wish to be bound by these terms and conditions, you may not access or use this site. Our maximum liability to you under all circumstances will be equal to the purchase price you paid for any goods, services, or information."

This statement is then followed by disclaimers pertaining to accuracy, currency, copyright, no medical advice, no warranties, a disclaimer of endorsement, disclaimer regarding liability for third party content, and a general disclaimer of liability including negligence with a statement that the user assumes all responsibility and risk for use.[130] It may also be desirable to include a provision that any dispute will be brought in the city of the site owner's principal place of business.

SOCIAL MEDIA

There is a growing use of social media that allows large groups of individuals to share information, expand contact, and serve as a means for professional news and a tool for discussion of pharmacy-related issues. Examples include Facebook®, LinkedIn®, Amazon .com®, Twitter®, YouTube, Pinterest®, blogs, and forums. In fact, most state pharmacy organizations have a Twitter® presence. A number of legal issues for DI pharmacists who use social media warrant consideration—ranging from patient privacy under HIPAA and state privacy torts, creation of a pharmacist–patient relationship to antikickback issues. Privacy controls vary by site and change frequently, but patient information must never be disclosed on such sites. Breaches can occur easily such as inquiring about how a patient's diabetes is on Facebook® or discussing celebrities getting medications in pharmacies. Posting of comments and breaches of patient confidentiality, especially by students, are common.[131] There has been a recent increase in lawsuits brought under invasion of privacy. While there are no legal rules on this, friending patients is not a good idea. ASHP has developed a statement on use of social media by pharmacy professionals.[132] However, there is still no clear picture of issues such as the duty to warn in social media.[133]

Questions have also been raised whether providing DI over social media is tantamount to unlicensed practice in a state where the pharmacist is not licensed. Moreover, harmful patient-specific advice may lead to malpractice. Some pharmacists have placed a disclaimer on their blog to indicate "Reading this blog should not be construed to mean that you and I have a pharmacist–patient relationship." Besides privacy and negligence issues other liability may follow for defamation, copyright infringement, discrimination, or harassment.

Some pharmaceutical manufacturers have developed patient blogs and other social media Web sites, especially for patients with chronic illnesses such as diabetes. In some cases, testimonials by what appear to be patients are actually being made by people paid or allied with the pharmaceutical company. While the effect of social media on patient care is currently unclear, the FDA is currently drafting guidelines to cover drug companies' social media presence.

FRAUD AND ABUSE

Another consideration pertains to fraud and abuse laws, such as the antikickback laws.[134] The antikickback statute prohibits physicians participating in the Medicaid and Medicare programs from submitting any false remuneration, including any kickback, bribe, or rebate to induce referrals of patients.[135] Certain aspects of e-health promotional and marketing tools, such as per click payment arrangements, are particularly susceptible to violation of the antikickback statute. The violation occurs because the health care provider is receiving remuneration based on the referral rate provided by the fee charged per click. Likewise, promotional banners on a health care organization or pharmacist's Web site that link to a pharmacy or other type of patient care items are most likely in violation because the referring provider is receiving a benefit (i.e., per click arrangements involve the payment of a fee based on the clicking on a particular link on a Web site) in exchange for referrals.[136] Similarly, the provision of free e-mail services, online publications, computer equipment, or other types of computer ventures are in violation of the antikickback statute when these companies sell items or services reimbursable under Medicaid or Medicare programs.

Another area of uncertainty pertains to the handling of links between Web pages. A link is any component of a Web page that connects to another Web page. The issue of whether pharmaceutical manufacturers will be liable for material posted on sites they have not sponsored, but have merely linked to their own, is yet to be decided in the courts.

At least according to cases over the past few years, mere hyperlinking does not constitute copyright or trademark infringement.[137] Copyright law does not require that permission be obtained for linking, but if there is copyrighted graphic material, people will be reproducing and displaying copyrighted material they do not own. The copyright owner's permission needs to be obtained to use the graphic image, unless fair use is utilized (fair use is discussed further under the section for copyright). Where the information being linked to is violating the copyright law, it is also possible that a Web site owner who links to a site containing infringing material may be liable for contributory copyright infringement. Contributory copyright infringement is established when a defendant, with knowledge of another's infringing activity, causes or materially contributes to the infringing conduct.

Moreover, whether deep linking (i.e., bypassing the homepage and linking to an internal page of the linked site) is copyright infringement is currently unclear.[138] However, if a Web page specifically states, ask permission before linking, it is possible that linking to the site without the owner's permission may be trespass or breach of contract where there are terms of use to which were agreed.[139]

Additionally, certain businesses, which do not want their valuable content associated with or connected to certain sites, have brought legal action under theories of trademark, defamation, disparagement, unfair competition, false advertising, invasion of privacy, and other laws. In *Playboy Enterprises, Inc. v. Universal Tel-A-Talk, Inc.*, an X-rated Web site is linked to the Playboy Web site.[140] Playboy sued and proved that users of the site may be confused as to whether Playboy sponsored or endorsed the adult site. Playboy also proved that its trademark bunny logo would be blurred or tarnished by the association with the adult site. Also, in *Coca-Cola Co v. Purdy*, the Court entered judgment for several well-known trademark owners on their infringement claims where an antiabortionist used a host of domain names incorporating their famous marks.[141] The antiabortionist linked the domain names (e.g., mycoca-cola.com) with a Web site associated with abortionismurder.com. According to the decision, the "quick and effortless nature of 'surfing' the Internet makes it unlikely that consumers can avoid confusion through the exercise of due care."[142]

The practice of using framing to incorporate third-party content into a Web site is also an area of unsettled law. The framing site can surround the framed pages with its own advertising, logos or promotions. Framing may trigger a dispute under copyright and trademark law theories because a framed site arguably alters the appearance of the content and creates the impression that its owner endorses or voluntarily chooses to associate with the framer.[143] However, liability for framing has not been fully or clearly resolved by the courts.[144]

Advances in technology may render this dilemma moot. Technology now exists to keep undesired links or frames off a Web site. In any event, it is advisable not to link to or frame another Web site without the express permission of that site. However, if a Web site owner is concerned about liability for links or frames, a prominently placed disclaimer may be added. Additionally, if a Webmaster wants to obtain permission before someone links to their site, a request permission notice needs to be posted and require users to agree to the terms by clicking "I agree" on the homepage.

The Internet raises a variety of legal issues, most of which are unresolved but evolving. Future goals should be for pharmaceutical manufacturers to promote their products to consumers more responsibly, for the FDA to regulate DTCA more effectively, and for the medical and pharmacy communities to educate the public about prescription drugs more constructively.

Intellectual Property Rights

COPYRIGHT

The current copyright law is codified at 17 U.S.C.A. § 101 *et seq.* A copyright is a property right in an original work of authorship that is fixed in tangible form.[145] It is a statutory requirement that literary, dramatic, and musical works, for example, must have been recorded or produced in some physical object (or fixed) before copyright can subsist. A copyright holder in a work is granted certain exclusive rights to control use of the work created. A work of authorship must be original in order to qualify for copyright protection. This requirement has two facets. First, the author must have engaged in some intellectual endeavor of his or her own, and not just have copied from a preexisting source. Second, the work must exhibit a minimal amount of creativity. Copyright protection covers both published and unpublished works. Also, the fact that the previously published work is out of print does not affect its copyright. Works of authorship under copyright and items not entitled to copyright are found in Table 10–3.

⑤ *Pharmacists providing DI must have a working knowledge of copyright law both to avoid liability and to protect their own literary works.* Under the 1976 Copyright Act, an author is protected as soon as a work is recorded in some concrete way. The process of registering for a copyright involves depositing material with the Copyright Office to be reviewed by an examiner, followed by publication with a copyright notice, usually the symbol ©. Under the Copyright Term Extension Act (CTEA) of 1998, such work is protected until 70 years after the death of the author or for 95 years for corporate copyright holders. In effect, the CTEA retroactively extended copyright terms by 20 years.[146] The constitutionality of CTFA has been challenged and upheld by the Supreme Court. The author or copyright owner has the exclusive right to make copies of the work, control derivative works or adaptations, and sue for damages and injunctive relief (an **injunction** is a judicial remedy issues in order to prohibit a party from doing or continuing to do a certain activity) against infringers. Public domain works may be copied and distributed without copyright permission. Works of the U.S. government (e.g., General Accounting Office [GAO] reports, Congressional Record, FDA releases) are considered part of the public domain.

Ownership of copyright usually rests with the author at the time the work is created. The exception is a work made for hire (i.e., "a work prepared by an employee within the scope of the employment relationship, or is a work specially ordered or commissioned for use as a contribution to a collective work, as part of a motion picture or other audiovisual work, as a translation, as a supplementary work, as a compilation, as an instructional text,

TABLE 10–3. COPYRIGHT PROTECTION

Works of authorship entitled to copyright protection include the following:
- Literary works
- Musical works, including any accompanying works
- Dramatic works, including any accompanying music
- Pantomimes and choreographic works
- Pictorial, graphic, and sculptural works
- Motion pictures and other audiovisual works
- Sound recordings
- Architectural works

Not entitled to copyright protection:
- Ideas, concepts, principles, or discovery
- Procedures, processes, systems, methods of operation
- Mere compilations of facts

as a test, as an answer material for a test, or as an atlas, if the parties expressly agree in a written instrument signed by them that the work shall be a work made for hire"). (Copyright Law of the U.S., 17 U.S.C. Sec 106.)[147] Another exception is the first-sale doctrine, which in effect, permits intralibrary loan of materials. Under the first-sale doctrine, a person who legitimately owns a copy of a work is one who purchased the work or otherwise acquired ownership of the work with the permission of the copyright owner, and has full authority to "sell or otherwise dispose of the possession of that copy."[148]

Since the Berne Convention in 1989, the copyright formalities of registration and notice have lost almost all their legal significance. Registration, although not mandatory, affords the copyright claimant certain advantages. For example, it prevents an infringer from pleading innocent infringement. Similarly, the only substantive legal effect of copyright registration is that attorney fees and statutory damages are only recoverable for postregistration infringements. That is, U.S. authors must register before bringing suit. But for works prior to 1989 and the Berne Convention, copyright can be lost if notice was omitted and that omission was not cured within 5 years of publication by registration and affixation of notice to the remaining copies.

Under the fair use provision of the 1976 Copyright Act, if a use is fair, permission of the copyright owner need not be received, nor royalties paid. Fair use is determined by a four-pronged test: (1) nature and character of use, (2) nature of the work, (3) proportional amount copied, and, most importantly, (4) effect on the market for the copied work.[149]

The first factor in the fair use analysis is the nature and character of the use. Uses for research, teaching, scholarship, and news reporting are more likely to be considered fair than strictly commercial uses. In addition, there is a narrow special exemption for educators. The mere fact that the use is educational and not for profit does not insulate the use from a finding of infringement.

The second factor in the fair use analysis is the nature of the work. This factor centers on whether a copyrighted work is creative or informational, and whether it is published or unpublished. The scope of fair use is greater when the copyrighted work is informational because it is generally recognized that there is a greater need to disseminate factual material than works of fiction or fantasy.[150] An unpublished work is given greater copyright protection than a published work and is, therefore, less likely to be subjected to a valid assertion of fair use.[151] In *Harper & Row Publishers, Inc. v. Nation Enterprises, Nation* obtained an unauthorized manuscript of former President Ford's memoirs before they were published in a book form under a contract with Harper & Row. The fact that President Ford's memoirs had not yet been published by the time, *Nation* published them was a deciding factor.[152] That is, in looking at the nature of the work, an unpublished work seems to be entitled to greater protection than a published work.

The third factor is the amount copied. There does not appear to be a minimal amount or threshold quantity (e.g., five sentences) standard where fair use will be presumed.

Many copyrighted works are accessed through a campus license that overrides copyright. Libraries vigorously negotiate licenses for such materials. Although the statute itself does not set the maximum standards for educational fair use, Classroom Guidelines have been agreed upon by educational, author, and publisher organizations.[153] Multiple copies for classroom use, but not to exceed in any event more than one copy per pupil in a course, are permissible, provided each copy bears a copyright notice and meets the test of (1) brevity, (2) spontaneity, and (3) cumulative effect. For example, to meet the test of brevity the Classroom Guidelines prohibit multiple copying of complete articles longer than 2500 words. They prohibit copying excerpts longer than 1000 words or 10% of the work, whichever is shorter. For motion media, up to 10% or 3 minutes, whichever is less, in the aggregate of a copyrighted motion media work may be reproduced or otherwise incorporated as part of an educational multimedia project. To meet the test of spontaneity, the copying must be at the instance and inspiration of the individual teacher, where the teacher's decision to use the work in class does not allow for a timely reply to request for permission. To meet the cumulative effect requirement, the copying must be for only one course in the school, and except for current news periodicals, newspapers, and current news sections of periodicals, only one article or two excerpts therefrom may be copied from the same author, or three excerpts from the same collective work or periodical volume. Additionally, the copying must be for only one class term; and no more than nine instances of such multiple copying for one course during one class term. In other words, the copied material may only be used for one semester and permission for longer use must be obtained. Further, students may not be charged for the copy beyond the actual cost of photocopying.

Case Study 10–3

You are publishing a guide regarding "do not crush" drugs for which you will receive compensation. You are merely listing all drugs which should not be crushed. However, the material for this publication is derived from a number of published references, all of which are copyright protected. You adopt an entire table from one of the articles without permission. You also take several direct sentences without providing any source reference. One of the references you are using is out of print.

- *Which of these acts would constitute a violation of the copyright law? What steps should have been taken to avoid copyright violation?*

In *Association of American Publishers v. New York University,* the issue was the production and distribution of custom-made anthologies sold to students. Although the classroom guidelines allow students to make single copies for personal use, the court found infringement when anthologies were sold for profit.[154] The action was settled with the adoption of certain procedures by New York University.

The fourth factor in a fair use analysis is the impact the infringing work will have on the market or potential market of the copyrighted work.[155] The Supreme Court has decided that all four factors of the fair use test should be given equal weight.[156] Under the Copyright Act of 1976, these four fair use factors provide a broad and flexible defense against copyright infringement.

Fair use is an equitable defense to copyright infringement, determined by the courts on a case-by-case basis. Unfortunately, in court decisions on educational photocopying to date, the ruling in almost every case has been against fair use. Copying by nonprofit medical libraries has been held to be a fair use where the photocopying of medical journals by federal nonprofit institutions was made solely for the purpose of medical research. In *Williams & Wilkins Co. v. United States,* the library was copying a single copy for each request and the court found that "medical science would be seriously hurt if such library photocopying were stopped."[157] In *Williams & Wilkins,* the copying of medical journals was by two governmental libraries, i.e., the National Institutes of Health and the National Medical library, a repository of much of the world's medical literature.[157] The public benefits of fair use apparently held considerably more weight than any commercial considerations presented before the courts. However, where the photocopying of medical journals by scientists occurred in a large for-profit company, the court decided the making of unauthorized copies of copyrighted articles published in scientific journals for use by research scientists was not fair use. The court determined that the publishers had created through the Copyright Clearance Center, Inc., a viable market for institutional users to obtain licenses to allow photocopying of individual articles. However, in *Princeton University Press v. Michigan Document Services, Inc.,* the court held that a copy shop selling coursepacks, which are compilations of various copyrighted and uncopyrighted materials such as journal articles, sample test questions, course notes, and book excerpts, infringed the copyrights of several publishers.[158] In deciding this was not a fair use, the court noted that the copying was substantial and commercial. Similarly, in *Basic Books v. Kinko's Graphic Corp.,* the court held that a copy shop's reproduction and sale of coursepacks to students was not a fair use of the copyrighted material.[159]

Course management systems and digital coursepacks which post copyrighted articles, book excerpts, and research data are used today by 90% of U.S. colleges and universities. Simply because the material is online does not mean it is free from copyright protection. Unless fair use or some other exemption applies, permission is required before posting.[160] When fair use does not apply, the institution must obtain permission from the rightsholder, who may charge a fee for such permission based on the amount of content and the number of people, usually students, who will view the content. Additionally, reporting of the same material for use in a subsequent semester requires a new permission. Moreover, it violates the intent and spirit of copyright law to use course management systems as a substitute for the purchase of books, subscriptions, or other materials when substantial portions of the material are required for educational purposes. When scanning in paper materials (such as textbooks) to create electronic copies, be sure legally obtained copies of the work are used, either purchased or owned by the institution. All posted materials in a course management system should contain both the copyright notice from, and complete citation to, the original material, and a caution against further electronic distribution.[154] Instant permission may be obtained at http://www.copyright.com though the Copyright Clearance Center for use in course management systems, coursepacks, e-reserves, classroom handouts, and other formats.

The court has also ruled that there is only a limited copyright protection available to a compilation of works written by another author. In *Silverstein v. Penguin Putnam*, the plaintiff had compiled a collection of 122 unpublished Dorothy Parker poems.[161] He presented the compilation to Penguin which rejected it and subsequently inserted the poems into a new edition of Parker's work published by Penguin. The court held that Silverstein would not be entitled to injunctive relief as he did not hold the copyrights on the poems. Thus, his efforts to gather the poems were not protectable in copyright. Additionally, the court looked at Silverstein's arrangement of the poems and found that Penguin did not copy his arrangement.

In 2008, in *Warner Bros. Entm't Inc. v. RDR Books*, a lexicon of terms from the *Harry Potter* series of books, initially posted on a free Internet Web site and then scheduled for publication, was held as copyright infringement.[162] The legal issues involved were whether there is a distinction in the law between digital and printed copyright and what is a third party's right to create a new reference book designed to help others better understand the original work (i.e., a study guide). The court held the print version of the lexicon was not a derivative work, especially in view of the number of places where copying was deemed excessive. However, the court explicitly stated that authors do not have the right to stop the publication of reference guides and companion works.

Copyright infringement requires a showing of copying, which can be proven circumstantially by demonstrating that the defendant had access to the copyrighted work and that the defendant's work is substantially similar to that work. Copyright infringement for purposes of commercial advantage or private financial gain is punishable under 18 U.S.C. §2319. Although the act allows for damages of as much as $100,000 per infringement, innocent infringers (e.g., educators and universities) may be entitled to a remission of statutory damages. They are only liable for actual damages, such as profits earned by the infringer or profits denied to the copyright holder. This provision lowers the incentive for the publishing industry to sue. Recently, publishers have resorted to unsavory tactics in their attempts to control educational copying, such as sending letters threatening to sue copy shops for infringement unless they agree to pay royalties.

Newsletter copying is strictly prohibited and violators risk not only the statutory damages ($100,000) but can be subject to criminal penalties. These newsletters require a fee to be paid to the Copyright Clearance Center even for internal or personal copying and offer rewards to those who report violations. Washington Business Information, Inc. has won major payments in infringement actions against pharmaceutical manufacturers for photocopying its *Food & Drug Letter.*

Section 201(c) of the Copyright Act has produced electronic copyright issues for freelance articles and photography in electronic databases. Specifically, a series of cases involves whether or not permission is required from authors to place their articles on commercial databases or in the electronic public domain (e.g., MEDLINE®). In *New York Times v. Tasini*, the U.S. Supreme Court ruled that publishers cannot republish printed works electronically without obtaining permission from authors.[163] *Tasini* should not have much impact on new work as most publisher agreements now address electronic publication rights. Problematic, however, are older works published without a written agreement. The publishers argued unsuccessfully that the use of the articles in a database was no different from issuing a microfilm or microfiche copy of a newspaper. However, permissibility of electronic republication of an entire issue of a newspaper, magazine, newsletter without further payment to authors remains unresolved.[164] Rather than attempt to contact freelancers and offer compensation for articles, some database producers have already begun to purge their databases of freelance contributions.

Photocopies fall within the territory of the Copyright Act. When sending copies of original articles, a statement to the effect that the copies are only for personal or private use must be made. The most effective way for any DI facility to protect itself against copy infringement lawsuits is to copy the page with the copyright notice and stamp the first page of the copies with a statement that the enclosed document is protected by copyright, thus putting the burden of responsibility on the recipient of the one copy. Such a notice might state, "This material is subject to the United States Copyright Law (17 U.S. Code): unauthorized copying may be prohibited by law."

The Computer Software Act of 1980 amended the Copyright Act to extend protection to computer software. However, copyright laws do not provide sufficient protection for information transmitted over the Internet and other information networks. Although copyright protection applies when copyrighted material is converted into a digital form, the havoc that cyberspace can wreak on copyright owner's rights cannot be overestimated.

A debate is currently raging over whether existing copyright law can successfully adapt to the Internet.

Google recently settled two class action lawsuits regarding application of copyright protection to the indexing of scanned documents.[165,166] The lawsuits involve the Google Library Project where in 2004, the company announced it has entered into agreement with several libraries to digitalize books and other documents from those libraries collections. The books and documents were also to be indexed for search purposes. Thus, the legal question of whether indexing for search purposes is fair use. Google was sued by publishers and authors when attempting to create an unprecedented extensive digitalized library of books. The authors and publishers claimed the scanning and indexing was not fair use but commercial in nature.[167] The case was settled and not decided by a court. However, in March 22, 2011, the court denied the final settlement approval. The parties are currently considering their next steps. Until then, the question of the legal fair defense of unauthorized copying of the works remains unresolved. Meanwhile Google continues to scan books although some of the digitalization efforts have shifted to European collections perhaps because of the litigation.[168] By April 2013, the Google database encompassed 30 million scanned books.[169]

On October 3, 2002, Congress enacted the Technology, Education, and Copyright Harmonization (TEACH) Act, fully revising §110(2) of the U.S. Copyright Act governing the lawful uses of existing copyright materials in distance education. The TEACH Act defines the conditions and circumstances on which educators may clip pieces of text, images, sound, and other works and include them in distance education. Table 10–4 outlines the key provisions of the TEACH Act. If a particular use does not fit these conditions, one may still consider whether the use is a fair use.[170]

Access to works on the Internet or those publically available does not automatically mean that these can be reproduced and reused without permission or royalty

TABLE 10–4. MAJOR PROVISIONS OF THE TEACH ACT

- Expanded range of allowed works (e.g., nondramatic literary works; nondramatic musical works; audiovisual works).
- Expanded receiving locations. Educational institutions may now reach students through distance education at any location.
- Storage of transmitted content. Allows retention of the content and student access for a brief period of time, especially with regard to digital transmission systems.
- Allows for digitalizing of analog works but only if the work is not already available in digital form.
- Educational institutions must now institute policies regarding copyright although the details of content of those policies is not provided.
- Transmission of content must be made solely to students officially enrolled in a course for which the transmission is made. Technological restrictions on access are required.

payment and, furthermore, some copyrighted works may have been posted on the Internet without authorization of the copyright holder. Publically available is not to be confused with the legal concept of public domain which comprises all works that are either no longer protected by copyright or never were. With the ease of retrieval of material electronically, copyright holders are likely to uncover those who are violating their copyright. Publishers who did not previously press for royalty payments of small segments of works can now trace the borrowing of snippets of text and create systems of payment and collection. Research downloading, with deletion of material after use, appears to be a fair use of the material. However, downloading to create a personal database and avoid payment of connect fees and higher user fees is illegal unless covered under special agreements between the database owner and the subscriber. Also, linking to a work is always an option. Copyright law does not preclude anyone from linking to a copyright work on a Web site. But remember if the link contains copyrighted graphic material, you cannot use that without permission of the copyright holder. Further, although the Berne Convention is the principal copyright treaty, there is no such thing as an International copyright. The treaty obligates signatory countries to extend the protection of their copyright law to foreigners whose works are infringed within their borders.[171]

Current copyright law denies protection to compilations of facts unless such facts are arranged or organized with some minimal element of originality. Even then, it is the creative aspect of such arrangements or organizations that may be protected and not the underlying facts themselves. Legislation has been repeatedly introduced, advocated primarily by large database companies, aimed at codifying into law a new unique form of intellectual property protection for databases. The situation is different in Europe where the European Union (EU) 1996 Database Directive grants copyright protection for the selection and arrangement of information in a European database, and calls downloading and hyperlinking unfair extraction of information.

Related to copyright infringement is plagiarism and fictitious reporting. Plagiarism is a legal offense or crime. The owner of a copyright (i.e., author) could sue the plagiarist in federal court for violation of the copyright. Fictitious reporting may simply constitute poor journalism or it may rise to the level of fraud or libel. Plagiarism involves not citing material while factitious reporting involves citing things that do not exist.

The definition of plagiarism is subjective and vague. History, facts, and ideas are not copyrighted, although they may be plagiarized. The addition of original material by the plagiarist in no way excuses the act of plagiarism. In fact, trivial changes in copied text, in an attempt to avoid copyright infringement, is specifically prohibited by the copyright law. Additionally, there is no fixed number or percentage of words that can be used without exposure to charges of plagiarism.[172] Verbatim quotes are permitted, provided it falls within the fair use protection. Software and Web-based technologies (e.g., Turnitin®) now exist that can scan millions of documents almost instantly to compare what has been written before to what is being written today. Further information on plagiarism is contained in Chapter 9.

Privacy

HEALTH INSURANCE PORTABILITY AND ACCOUNTABILITY ACT OF 1996

Information security concerns are at the forefront of legal issues involved in electronic communications, specifically, questions of authenticity of medical or pharmacy records and confidentiality or privacy of the contents of medical and personal information of patients. Today an individual's health information is often used for payment, QA, research, peer review, accreditation, and a multitude of other purposes. In realizing that this creates significant privacy and security concerns, Congress enacted the Health Insurance Portability Act of 1996 (HIPAA).[173] While security and privacy under HIPAA are inextricably linked, there are distinctions. HIPAA *Privacy* Rule protects the privacy of individually identified health information. HIPAA *Security* Rule sets standards for the security of *electronic* protected health information.

The security rule standards define the administrative, physical, and technical safeguards (e.g., encryption) to protect the confidentiality, integrity, and availability of electronic PHI. HIPAA's security standards are intended to protect the security of the environment in which health care information is maintained and transmitted. The privacy rule, by contrast, sets standards for how PHI should be controlled by setting forth what uses and disclosures are authorized or required and what rights patients have with respect to their health information. The privacy rule applies to information in any form, whereas the security rule only applies to PHI in electronic form.

For pharmacies, the security standards are applicable only to electronic **protected health information**, not paper, facsimile, nor telephone transmissions. HIPAA's privacy standards govern the use and disclosure of protected health information. Many aspects of HIPAA fall outside the scope of this chapter. In any event, reasonable steps should always be taken to ensure that fax transmissions are sent to and received by the intended recipient. Examples of such steps include confirming with the intended recipient that the receiving fax machine is located in a secure area or the intended recipient is waiting by the fax machine; preprogramming and testing fax numbers for frequent recipients of DI faxes to avoid errors associated with misdialing; double checking the recipient's fax number prior to transmission; using a fax cover sheet with an erroneous transmission statement and advising to notify the sender immediately and arrange for return or destruction of the fax; promptly checking all fax confirmation sheets to determine that faxed material was received at the intended fax number.

Individually identifiable health information is information, including demographic data, that relates to the individual's past, present, or future physical or mental health or condition; the provision of health care to the individual, or the past, present, or future payment for the provision of health care to the individual, and that identifies the individual or for which there is a reasonable basis to believe it can be used to identify the individual.[174] Individually identifiable health information includes many common identifiers such as name, address, birth date, and social security number.

However, there are no restrictions on the use or disclosure of de-identified health information.[175] Deidentified health information neither identifies nor provides a reasonable basis to identify an individual. There are two methods for deidentifying protected health information: the statistical method and the safe-harbor method via removal of certain identifiers.[176] Deidentified data sets, which separate individuals' identities from their protected health information, are becoming increasingly available through the Centers for Medicare and Medicaid Services and the National Institutes of Health.[177] These data are proving useful for outcomes and medical error research not associated with the original data collection protocol.

Under HIPAA, a covered entity may engage in research activities in four ways: (1) by using or disclosing only deidentified information, (2) by obtaining a waiver or an authorization from the individual to use and disclose the information for research purposes, (3) by obtaining a waiver of an authorization from an IRB, or (4) by representing that the use or disclosure is solely of the protected health information of a deceased individual. Clinical investigators are most likely to choose option 3.[178]

HIPAA specifically permits covered entities such as health care professionals or hospitals to report adverse events and other information relate to the quality, effectiveness, and safety of FDA-regulated products to both the manufacturers and directly to FDA. Under this exception, a pharmacist need not obtain an authorization from a patient before notifying a pharmaceutical company and the FDA that the patient had an adverse reaction to a drug manufactured by the drug company.[179] **6** *It is important to keep in mind that the HIPAA Privacy Rule is not intended to disrupt or discourage adverse event reporting or DI in any way.*

In responding to DI questions, it is of utmost importance to obtain specific patient identification information including, but not limited to, patient name, age, height, weight, or medical record number. Nothing in HIPAA would diminish or affect that responsibility. In the DI arena, HIPAA allows disclosure of patient information for treatment, payment, and health care operations. Examples of health care operations include quality management, QA, outcomes evaluation, development of clinical guidelines, peer review, and credentialing. While not specifically mentioned, DI would appear to fall under both treatment and health care operations. In most instances, HIPAA should not affect DI requests from health care providers as patient identity is usually not required or is provided via medical record number only. However, when patient identifying information is communicated, protection of information within the DI center (or pharmacy) is an important HIPAA requirement. Policies and procedures governing use and disclosure of confidential information should be in place. These policies should include guidance on training and strategies for mitigating risks during all stages of the DI request processing (receipt, triage, and response). For example, procedures should be in place to verify the identity of the requestor of information. Patient information security safeguards should be in place, for example, requiring personal identifiers to be removed as soon as feasible, physical controls, software controls, and formal oversight.[180]

Case Study 10–4

A drug information question involves a patient who has a socially stigmatic disease. In responding to the question, the pharmacist needs to share the patient's personally identifiable health information with the laboratory and pharmacokinetic services. However, in sharing this information the pharmacist discusses it as well as the diagnosis in an area where it was easily overheard by others not entitled to know. Additionally, the patient's personal information is faxed by the pharmacist to a fax machine in an unsecured area where many people have access to the fax machine.

- *Does HIPAA prohibit any of the pharmacist's actions?*
- *What safeguards should be taken when discussing the patient and his or her information?*
- *What reasonable steps are necessary to ensure that fax transmissions are sent and recorded by the intended recipient?*

There are several other situations in pharmacy practice where HIPAA compliance issues may be triggered. For example, in clinical case reports, whether for publication or teaching purposes, the patient should only be referred to via his or her initials, age, or sex (e.g., RM, a 35-year-old female). When writing a case report or article for publication, always remove any patient identifiers. In some cases, the patient consent may be required to publish the report.

HIPAA permits a pharmacist to counsel individuals other than the patient (e.g., a friend, family member, or neighbor picking up the patient's prescription) even though some of the patient's protected health information may be revealed in such a situation. However, the regulation is clear that such disclosures must be limited and should only be

• made when the provider believes it is in the patient's best interest. For example, there can be no doubt that disclosing the medication picked up is for treatment of HIV infection would not be necessary. Under HIPAA, personal representatives, defined as individuals legally authorized, under state or other applicable law, to make health care decisions on behalf of a patient, are to be treated in the same way as a patient. However, in some cases the personal representative's authority is limited to a specific matter, such as treatment for a life-threatening illness. In these cases, the personal representative may only access protected health information directly related to that illness. Additionally, many states have enacted laws that protect persons with illnesses that are seen as particularly stigmatizing, such as HIV, mental illness, and drug addiction. The Public Health Service Act and implementing regulations govern the confidentiality of substance abuse records maintained by federally assisted drug and alcohol abuse programs.[181]

• Similarly, parents are considered the personal representative of a minor child and can access the minor's health records. Exceptions exist when the minor consents to health care and consent of the parent is not required under state or other law, or when the minor obtains health care at the direction of a court, or when the minor is emancipated. Other exceptions exist if a provider believes that a patient or minor is subject to abuse, neglect, or domestic violence by their personal representative.[182] Many states specifically authorize minors to consent to conceptive services, testing and treatment for HIV and other sexually transmitted diseases, prenatal care and delivery services, treatment for alcohol and drug abuse, and outpatient mental health care.

• HIPAA also requires that pharmacies make a good faith effort to obtain a patient's acknowledgment that they have received a copy of the Notice of Privacy Practices. The notice describes how the pharmacy uses and discloses protected health information to carry out treatment, payment, or health care operations and to protect the patient's rights. The notice is to be distributed to patients on or before the first treatment encounter. Where the prescription is being picked up by someone other than the patient, the pharmacy must attempt to deliver the notice to the patient. Examples of a good faith effort include providing the notice in the prescription bag or mailing the notice to the patient together with some type of return receipt means. However, the pharmacy is not in violation if the return receipt is not returned. The pharmacy need only document its efforts.[183]

Under HIPAA, pharmacists will be held accountable for handling confidential information properly. Civil and criminal penalties for violating patient confidentiality exist.

COMMUNICATION PRIVACY

The Telephone Consumer Protection Act (TCPA) sets rules prohibiting unsolicited commercial faxes. A Federal Communication Commission (FCC) regulation implementing the act requires businesses and nonprofit groups to get signed written permission from clients or members before faxing unsolicited materials containing advertisements. Litigation under the TCPA is increasing, particularly in the area of junk fax class actions and insurance coverage for TCPA damages. Claims may be brought in local state court, including small claims court. The statute provides statutory damages, generally from $500 to $1500 for each violation, which are paid to the consumer.

• Privacy is also an issue on the Internet (e.g., e-health sites) where the dominant privacy issue arises from the growing practice of data collection. Some Web sites are interactive; that is, they may require the patient to complete a survey or will send visitors a prescription refill reminder. These sites then link to privacy policies that address any concerns prospective patients may have about filling out an online survey. Disclosure of an online privacy policy together with an opt-out feature can provide assurances about the protection of consumer privacy and personal information. The policy should also address passive disclosure of information, e.g., from cookies (a feature which allows Web servers to recognize a specific user or computer to access the Web site) or Web server logs. Unfortunately, e-health sites were not included under HIPAA. Some of these e-health Internet sites violate their own privacy policies and transfer patient-identifiable information to third parties.[184]

• E-mail use in health care has developed without encryption and HIPAA does not directly address e-mail in any of its standards. However, because e-mail may involve protected health information in electronic form, both HIPAA's privacy and security rules apply. The security of unencrypted e-mail is low. Passwords, firewalls, and other conventional network security should exist to secure electronic DI communications.[185]

A number of broad consumer privacy bills have been introduced in Congress aimed at consumer surveys, mandated opt-in consents, and other privacy enhancing technological features.[186] Many of these bills implicate DTCA such as interactive Web sites which inherently have invasion of privacy liability issues. In 2012, the Obama administration announced its support for a consumer "privacy bill of rights" in its report, "Consumer Data Privacy in a Networked World: A Framework for Protecting Privacy and Promoting Innovation in the Global Digital Economy."[187]

There has also been litigation in this area. In *re Pharmatrak Inc. v. Privacy Litigation*, the plaintiffs alleged that numerous pharmaceutical companies secretly intercepted and accessed their personal information through the use of computer cookies and other devices,[188] in violation of state and federal laws such as the Electronic Communications Privacy Act.[189]

Industry Support for Educational Activities

Many pharmacists attend conferences, sometimes funded by pharmaceutical companies to further their professional education. Dialogue between health professionals and the pharmaceutical industry is an opportunity to pass along scientific and educational information, and product risks and benefits. Such dialogue encourages and supports medical research, while providing the health professional with an opportunity to address questions, discuss issues, and offer expertise.

GUIDELINES AND GUIDANCE

❼ *The FDA, the American Council for Continuing Medical Education (ACCME), and the Pharmaceutical Research and Manufacturers of America (PhRMA)*[190] *have established educational policies, guidelines, or guidances which allow communication between industry and the continuing medical education (CME) providers* with the proviso that the final decisions and control rest with the accredited provider. The Office of Inspector General (OIG) issued a guidance that prohibits the pharmaceutical industry from direct communication with CME providers and calls for an intermediary organization to develop CME programs.[191] The following factors are provided in the OIG Guidance: Does the arrangement skew clinical decision making? Is the information complete, accurate, and nonmisleading? Does the arrangement have the potential to be a disguised discount or result in inappropriate over- or underutilization? Does the arrangement raise patient safety, quality, or care concerns? Importantly, for pharmacists providing DI as industry clinical education consultants or medical liaisons, the Accreditation Council for Pharmacy Education (ACPE) no longer accredits pharmaceutical and biomedical manufacturers.[192] However, not all states actually require all of a pharmacist's continuing education activities to be accredited by the ACPE.[193]

The PhRMA Code, which became effective in July 2002, and updated in January 2009, is the most specific and stringent and deals with various interactions between industry and health care professionals, such as informational presentations, professional meetings, consultant activities, scholarships and educational funds, and educational and practice-related items.[194] Scholarships for pharmacists, students, and residents to attend selected educational conferences may be provided. Salient features of the latest PhRMA Code are found in Table 10–5 and at http://www.phrma.org/sites/default/files/pdf/phrma_marketing_code_2008.pdf.

The FDA guidance seeks to draw a distinction between educational activities that the FDA considers nonpromotional and those it considers promotional. The distinction is important, especially with regard to off-label uses, which can be an important component of educational activities. The FDA's factors to determine independence of the educational activity are found in Table 10–6.[195]

Some health care institutions have established their own best practices approach to developing ethical guidelines for pharmaceutical industry support. The practice involves a process similar to weighing the risks and benefits of a particular medication or therapeutic intervention, whereby each proposal for support can be viewed as having potential value, which may or may not outweigh any potential drawbacks inherent in the involvement of

TABLE 10–5. PhRMA CODE ON INTERACTIONS WITH HEALTH CARE PROFESSIONALS

- Gifts
  - Generally prohibited
  - Exceptions—$100 or less; must benefit patients or educate health care professionals, e.g., medical textbooks or anatomical models permitted, but not stethoscopes that are primarily used for treating patients
  - Pens, pads, etc. no longer permitted
  - Product samples allowed
- Meals
  - Modest meals accompanying informational presentations
  - Can only be offered occasionally
  - Can only *directly* provide in office or at hospital (no restaurants or resorts)
- Entertainment
  - Prohibited
  - May sponsor meals or reception at conferences
- Spouses
  - Never appropriate
- Consultants
  - Must be *bona fide* via written contract, appropriate venue, selection criteria related to purpose of service, must exclude spouses
  - Special disclosure requirements for health care professionals that set up formularies or develop clinical practice guidelines; disclosure requirements extend 2 years beyond the terms of any speaker or consultant arrangements
  - A legitimate need must be identified in advance of entering into agreement
  - Number of consultants cannot be greater than number reasonably needed to achieve purpose
- Financial Sponsorship of Educational Conferences
  - Support should be provided to continuing professional education sponsor, not individual speaker/author
  - Sponsor should control selection of content, faculty, educational materials, venue
  - Faculty, but not attendees or spouses, may be paid/reimbursed for time, travel, and lodging
  - Exception—companies may pay for travel/lodging for students to attend educational conferences; educational institution must select individual students
- Informational Presentations
  - Should be modest by local standards
  - Should occur in a venue and manner conducive to informational communication
  - Should provide scientific or educational value
  - Can recommend to continuing education providers topics of interest that manufacturer would sponsor

funding from a for-profit company. Often a committee assesses proposals based on the apparent balance between these factors and a set of guidelines developed by the institution.[196]

In general, most policies and procedures prohibit acceptance of commercial support of educational activities if such acceptance would appear to (1) create an atmosphere limiting academic freedom and the free exchange of ideas and information, (2) introduce bias or otherwise threaten objectivity, (3) create a conflict of interest, or (4) be in conflict with the mission and profit status of the health care organization.[197]

TABLE 10–6. FACTORS USED BY THE FDA TO DETERMINE INDEPENDENCE OF AN EDUCATIONAL ACTIVITY

- Control of content and selection of faculty: Is there scripting or other actions designed to influence the content by the supporting company?
- Disclosures: Does it include company funding the program, relationship between provider(s) and presenters to the supporting company, off-label discussion?
- Focus of the program: Does the title accurately represent the presentation; is there fair-balanced educational discussion?
- Relationship between provider and supporting company: Is there a legal, business, or other relationship between the parties?
- Provider involved in sales or marketing: Are provider employees also doing marketing or promotional programs?
- Provider's demonstrated failure to meet standards: Does the provider have a history of biased programs?
- Multiple presentations: Do they serve public health interests?
- Audience selection: Is the audience generated by sales or marketing departments to influence marketing goals?
- Opportunities for discussion: Is there an opportunity for meaningful discussion?
- Dissemination: Is the supporting company distributing additional information after the activity; unless requested by participant and then through an independent provider?
- Ancillary promotional activities: Are promotional activities taking place in the educational meeting room?
- Complaints: Are provider(s), faculty, or others complaining about the supporting company?

RELATIONSHIP TO THE ANTIKICKBACK STATUTE

Particular arrangements between pharmacists and the pharmaceutical industry pose potential risks under the antikickback statute. The antikickback statute makes it a criminal offense to knowingly and willfully offer, pay, solicit, or receive any remuneration (in cash or in kind) to induce (or in exchange for) the purchasing, ordering, or recommending of any good or service reimbursable by any federal health care program.[198] Funding that is conditioned, in whole or in part, on the purchase of product implicates the statute, even if the educational or research purpose is legitimate. Several cases hold that intent is improper if one purpose, not the sole or even primary purpose, is to induce the purchase or recommendation of a company's goods or services.[199,200] When a grant is provided to a customer or potential customer, it may violate the antikickback statute if one purpose is to induce the customer to buy the company's product. Educational grants, for example, were at the heart of the $161 million Caremark, LLC settlement[201] and research grants were at the heart of the $450,000 Hoffman-La Roche, Inc. settlement.[202] Furthermore, to the extent the manufacturer has any influence over the substance of an educational program or the presenter, there is a risk that the educational program may be used for inappropriate marketing purposes.

In the area of DI, specific practices that may be problematic under the antikickback statute include gifts, use of pharmacists who are customers as consultants or members of speaker's bureaus, and questionable research grants. Problems under the antikickback statute could arise where the DI pharmacist participates in any of these activities and also advises on formulary choices or is a member of a formulary committee or subcommittee or is involved with purchasing decisions. If a product or service is recommended and the recommender stands to make financial gain from it, and that service is paid for in part or in whole by the federal government, that person may be violating the antikickback statute. Similarly, no gifts should be accepted if there are strings attached.

Educational activities or speakers can be funded by the pharmaceutical industry, whereas promotional marketing activities that purport to be of an educational purpose but serve no direct patient benefit are prohibited. Hiring DI pharmacists under the guise of a consultant or advisor, or focus group participant or advisory board member, or even as a speaker at a meeting, could be considered payments for referrals. Similarly, compensating DI pharmacists as consultants, when all they do is attend conferences primarily in a passive capacity, is suspect. Other suspect activities include compensation for speaking, researching, listening to marketing pitches, or providing preceptor, shadowing or ghostwriting services. However, where the pharmacist is compensated for actual, reasonable, and necessary services, the activities may be considered legitimate.

The antikickback statute prohibits involvement with research contracts that come through a pharmaceutical company's marketing department, research not reviewed by the manufacturer's scientific or medical department, research that is unnecessarily duplicative or not needed for any purpose other than the generation of business, and postmarketing research used as a pretense for product promotion.[203] Manufacturers should use Chinese walls (i.e., ethical barriers prohibiting exchange of confidential information between different departments of an organization) for marketing and grant-funding activities to demonstrate that grants are bona fide and not improperly influenced by marketing considerations. The antikickback statute requires that grants be given in exchange for fair market value research consideration. This is often difficult to accomplish, since the precise costs and schedules of research activities are not knowable in advance and sometimes not conducive to being reduced to written agreements.

Conclusion

By now the reader has undoubtedly discovered that the liability aspects of DI include more than just negligence. Liability for off-label uses, consumer advertising, copyright infringement, liability issues unique to the Internet, privacy concerns, and industry support for educational activities are all connected to DI practice. The DI practitioner and pharmacists in general must at least have a working awareness of these areas. DI services provide a foundation for the provision of pharmacist supervised patient care. To date, pharmacists providing DI have only speculated about and not actually faced malpractice lawsuits. Hopefully, this chapter has shed some light on how courts would react to malpractice suits against pharmacists for negligent provision of DI. However, legal precedents cannot be relied on to predict the future. There is no way to predict how a court will rule in a particular case. What can be done to avoid malpractice and other causes of action? First, always strive for excellence. Second, have good relations with requestors and make sure they are aware of alterations or modifications in information systems and sources. Third, make no outrageous claims about the accuracy and thoroughness of the information provided. Finally, pharmacists should carry their own malpractice insurance policy.

The future of pharmacists as DI providers clearly lies in their ability to provide consultative DI services. While in the past, most of the reported appellate decisions against pharmacists have involved routine dispensing errors, not mistakes in DI or other expanded practice areas, in the future this situation may change. Pharmacists should not be preoccupied with the risk of incurring liability, but should take the necessary steps to limit exposure and develop an appreciation of modern legal philosophy. Definitive guidelines need not emerge only through court decisions. It remains most important that DI be recognized as a liability-reducing factor for the institution and personnel who provide health care to patients.

Self-Assessment Questions

1. All of the following would result in holding the pharmacist providing drug information to a higher standard *except*:
   a. The pharmacist wears a pin stating, "Ask me: I am the medication expert."
   b. The drug information query pertains to oncology and the pharmacist is a Board Certified Oncology Pharmacist (BCOP).
   c. The pharmacist knows the patient has previously had anaphylaxis from penicillin and ceftriaxone is prescribed.
   d. The pharmacist is the Drug Information Coordinator.
   e. The pharmacist is aware that the patient has severely impaired renal function and gentamicin is prescribed.

2. In which of the following scenarios would tort liability attach to the provision of drug information if harm occurs:
   a. A 1-year-old patient has been prescribed ketorolac for 7 days. The pharmacist contacts the prescriber to notify them that the duration of therapy should not

exceed 5 days. However, for children less than 2 years of age, treatment should not exceed 3 days.

b. The patient received the erythropoiesis-stimulating agent (ESA), epoetin alfa for an oncologic indication and developed a serious adverse drug reaction. Since the prescriber is not enrolled in the REMS program, the patient consequently never received the Medication Guide warning of the risk of the event and did not provide informed consent.

c. A patient with preexisting QT prolongation receives a 32-mg single dose of ondansetron intravenously. The maximum single dose has been lowered by the FDA to 16 mg. When a drug information query is received about whether to order the drug in dextrose 5% in water or normal saline, the pharmacist reviews the patient's profile and the medication order and fails to mention that the dose should be divided into 16 mg every 12 hours.

d. a and b only

e. a, b, and c

3. Which of the following drug information scenarios may result in vicarious liability?

a. The pharmacist undertakes to warn the patient about the adverse effects from simvastatin but fails to warn of myopathy.

b. The pharmacist is too busy to counsel the patient on the warning against sunbathing while on doxycycline. He or she instructs the pharmacy technician to counsel the patient instead. The technician tells the patient not to take a bath while taking the drug. The patient goes to the beach and harm results.

c. The pharmacist receives a drug information query from a prescriber asking what the common adverse effects of dabigatran (Pradaxa®) are. The pharmacist provides the correct response; the prescriber counsels the patient and gets it all wrong!

d. b and c

e. a and c

4. Which of the following is considered a noninherent risk?

a. The package insert for enoxaprin contains a typographical error.

b. The FDA recently placed a black box warning on zolpidem to lower the maximum dose in women and the patient is female and receiving a dose exceeding this maximum.

c. The patient is receiving dexamethasone for posttonsillectomy bleeding, an off-label use.

d. All of the above are inherent risks.

e. a and b are noninherent risks.

5. Which of the following statements is/are false?
   a. Checking the response to a drug information query in two or more references is the standard of practice.
   b. Since the drug information center does not charge a fee for providing the information, no liability can occur as the drug information provider derives no benefit.
   c. The pharmacist is working off the books in an effort to avoid payroll taxes. In case of liability, he or she is not covered by his or her employer but could be protected via his or her own professional liability insurance policy.
   d. b and c are false.
   e. a, b, and c are false.

6. A violation of the antikickback statute would occur when:
   a. A pharmacist attends a pharmacy conference and visits a pharmaceutical manufacturer's exhibitor booth. That manufacturer employs the pharmacist's brother.
   b. A hospital pharmacist receives a research grant in exchange for the hospital adding the agent to its formulary.
   c. Compensation is provided to a drug information pharmacist by a pharmaceutical editor to write a review article where there is complete independence of content.
   d. b and c.
   e. a, b, and c.

7. Which of the following is required for off-label use of a medication?
   a. Two pivotal clinical trials
   b. An investigational new drug application
   c. Isolated case reports
   d. Patient informed consent
   e. None of the above

8. Problems using the Internet for responding to drug information queries include:
   a. Information may contain innocent or deliberate mistakes.
   b. There are no laws for assuring the accuracy of information on the Internet.
   c. May include unpublished (not peer-reviewed) information.
   d. a and c only.
   e. a, b, and c.

9. Which of the following statements regarding telepharmacy are true?
   a. A drug information service Web site that charges patients for drug information consultation most likely creates a pharmacist–patient relationship.

b. Cybermedicine is a subset of telepharmacy.

c. Chat rooms create a formal pharmacist–patient relationship.

d. a and c are true.

e. a, b, and c are true.

10. Which of the following would constitute fair use under copyright law?

    a. Obtaining a copyright to prohibit use of a list of medications that cause QT prolongation.

    b. Scanning and distributing to all drug information colleagues an entire chapter from *Drug Information: A Guide for Pharmacists.*

    c. You, Professor X, photocopy an excerpt from an article which is about 6% of the work. You will only be using the excerpt for one lecture of a course, one semester only.

    d. You, Professor X, photocopy without permission multiple copies of a 6000-word article every semester for classroom use in both your ethics and law classes.

    e. Your colleague has written an article which is currently unpublished. He or she requests that you critique it and you borrow several paragraphs verbatim in your new book.

11. Which statement is accurate with regard to course packs or course management systems and copyright law?

    a. If the course pack material is online, it is free from copyright protection.

    b. If substantial amounts are from a textbook and the intent is to save students from purchasing the textbook, this constitutes fair classroom use.

    c. If permission to use any copyrighted material in the course pack was granted and a fee was paid to the copyright holder, fair use would apply.

    d. Where the course pack is sold every semester to students and contains uncopyrightable materials for which no permission to use was obtained, copyright law is violated.

    e. None of the above are accurate.

12. Which of the following statements is *inaccurate* under HIPAA?

    a. Permits pharmacists to report adverse events to manufacturers and directly to the FDA without patient authorization.

    b. HIPAA allows disclosure of patient information in the handling of drug information queries but requires protection of information within the drug information center.

    c. There are no restrictions on the use or disclosure of deidentified health information.

d. HIPAA privacy standards do not apply to facsimile or telephone communication, only electronic-protected health information.

e. All of the above statements are correct.

13. Which of the following actions would constitute a HIPAA violation?

a. You publish a case report and identify the patient by his or her initials.

b. You fax a response to a drug information query containing protected health information to an incorrect fax number.

c. You are conducting research using deidentified health information. You lose the flash drive containing this information.

d. A patient you are following develops a serious, unexpected adverse drug reaction. You report the reaction to the Food and Drug Administration.

e. a and b are HIPAA violations.

14. Which of the following is in compliance with the "PhRMA Code on Interactions With Health Care Professionals?"

a. Gifts from pharmaceutical manufacturers of $250 or less that benefit patients or educate health care professionals are permitted.

b. Pharmaceutical manufacturers may sponsor entertainment in university or nonprofit venues.

c. Pharmaceutical manufacturers may sponsor meals or receptions at conferences.

d. Consultant agreements must be in writing.

e. c and d are true.

15. In which of the following scenarios would education be considered promotional activities?

a. A portion of the presentation content is directed or scripted by the pharmaceutical company.

b. Promotional activities are taking place in the educational meeting room.

c. Disclosures do not mention that the pharmaceutical company has funded the program.

d. Educational session evaluations report that the session was biased toward a particular product.

e. All of the above.

REFERENCES

1. Brand KA, Kraus ML. Drug information specialists. Am J Health Syst Pharm. 2006;63:712-4.

2. American Society of Health-System Pharmacists. ASHP supplemental standard and learning objectives for residency training in drug information practice. Practice standards of ASHP. 1995-1996. Bethesda (MD): American Society of Health-System Pharmacists; 1995.

3. Southwick AF. The law of hospital and health care administration. 2nd ed. Ann Arbor: Health Administration Press; 1988.

4. Nathan JP, Gim S. Responding to drug information requests. Am J Health Syst Pharm. 2009;66:706, 710-1.

5. Dobbs DB, Hayden PT. Torts and compensation. 3rd ed. St. Paul: West Publishing Co.; 1997. p. 336.

6. Baker K. OBRA '90 mandate and its impact on pharmacist's standard of care. Drake Law R. 1996;44:503, 508.

7. Burns K, Spies A. A pharmacist's duty to warn: trying to make sense of all the legal inconsistencies. Rx Ipsa Loquitur. 2008;35:1-2.

8. Rosenberg v. Equitable Life Insurance Society of the United States, 595 N.E.2d 840 (N.Y. 1992).

9. Keller v. Manhattan Eye, Ear & Throat Hospital, 563 N.Y.S.2d 88, 89 (2nd Dept. 1990).

10. Kashkin v. Mt. Sinai Medical Center, 538 N.Y.S.2d 686 (Sup. Ct. 1989).

11. Kelly WN, Krause EC, Krowinski WJ, Small TR, Drane JF. National survey of ethical issues presented to drug information centers. Am J Hosp Pharm. 1990;47:2245-50.

12. Doppelparker Case, OLG Karllsrule GRUR 1979 P267.

13. Perkins E. Johns Hopkins' tragedy: could librarians have prevented a death? [Internet]. Medford (NJ): Information Today. 2001 Aug 7 [cited 2013 Mar 13]. Available at: http://newsbreaks.infotoday.com/NewsBreaks/Johns-Hopkins-Tragedy-Could-Librarians-Have-Prevented-a-Death-17534.asp

14. 805 S.W.2d, 380 (Tenn. Ct. App. 1991).

15. 453 N.Y.S.2d 121 (1987).

16. 544 N.W.2d 727, 731 (Mich. Ct. App. 1991).

17. Fink JL. Ignore computer alerts at your peril? Pharm Times. Jan 2013:56.

18. 191 A.D.2d 178, 594 N.Y.S.2d 195 (1993).

19. 579 N.E.2d 1255 (Ill. App. 1991) reversed by 605 N.E.2d 557 (Ill. 1992).

20. Moore v. Memorial Hospital & Winn Dixie, 825 So.2d 658 (Miss. 2002).

21. Deed v. Walgreens, 2004 WL 2943271 (Conn. Super. Ct.).

22. K-Mart v. Chamblin, 612 S.E.2d 25 (Ga. Ct. App. 2005).

23. Brushwood DB, Belgado BS. Judicial policy and expanded duties for pharmacists. Am J Health-Syst Pharm. 2002;59:455-7.

24. 780 So.2d 930 (Fla. App. 2001).

25. 1 S.W.3d 519 (Mo. App. 1999).

26. 737 N.E.2d 650 (Ill. App. 2000).

27. 30 S.W.3d 455 (Tex. App. 2000).

28. Larrimore v. Springhill Memorial Hospital. LEXIS 38:008 WL 54 2000 (Ala. 2008). CV-02-3205, 1051748.

29. 827 F. Supp. 1522 (D.Nev. 1993).

30. 598 N.Y.S.2d 592 (App. Div. 1993).

31. Brushwood DB, Simonsmeier LM. Drug information for patients. J Leg Med. 1986;7:279.

32. Howe A. Are independent prescribing rights for pharmacists set to increase in 2004? Prescr Pract. 2004;1(2 Suppl 1):5-6.

33. Canadian Society of Hospital Pharmacists [Internet]. Canada; 2009 [cited 2013 Mar 13]. Available from: http://www.cshp.ca/productsServices/officialPublications/type_e.asp

34. Reeves v. Pharmaject, Inc., 2012 WL 380186 (N.D. Ohio Feb 3, 2012).

35. Abood RR, Brushwood DB. Pharmacy practice and the law. New York: Aspen Pub.; 2001.

36. Berry M. The Canadian pharmacist's duty to counsel. Pharm Law Annual. 1992;19-75.

37. Hall M, Honey W. The evolving legal responsibility of the pharmacist. J Pharm Market Manage. 1994;8:27-41.

38. Brushwood DB. The pharmacist's drug information responsibility after McKee v. American Home Products. Food Drug Cosm Law J. 1993;48:377-410.

39. In re Michael A. Gabert, No. 92 PHM 21 (Wis. Pharmacy Examining Bd., Dec. 14, 1993).

40. Rees W, Rohde NF, Bolan R. Legal issues for an integrated information center. J Am Soc Info Sci. 1991;42:132-6.

41. Restatement (Second) of Torts, Section 311, 1982.

42. Beaird S, Coley R, Blunt JR. Assessing the accuracy of drug information responses from drug information centers. Ann Pharmacother. 1994;28:707-11.

43. Calis KA, Anderson DW, Auth DA, Mays DA, Turcasso NM, Meyer CC, et al. Quality of pharmacotherapy consultations provided by drug information centers in the United States. Pharmacotherapy. 2000;20:830-6.

44. McDonagh AF, Lightner DA. Attention to stereochemistry. Chem & Engin News. 2003 Feb 3:2.

45. In re Prempro Products, 03-CV-015070-WRW, U.S. Dist Ct., E.D. Arkansas, Jul 17, 2009.

46. Clauson KA. Pharmacists: are your drug information databases accurate? U.S. Pharmacist. 2008 Sept:54-63.

47. Gray JA. Strict liability for the dissemination of dangerous information? Law Lib J. 1990;82:497-517.

48. 694 F. Supp. 1216 (D. Md. 1988).

49. Bundesqe Richtsaf. Neue Juristische Wochenschrift (1970), 1973.

50. 110 Misc.2d 799, 442 N.Y.S.2d 945 (N.Y. Sup. 1981).

51. 938 F.2d 1033 (9th Cir. 1991).

52. 432 F. Supp. 990 (E.D.N.Y. 1977).

53. Containment Technologies v. ASHP, 2009 US Dist LEXIS 25421 (March 26, 2009), 2009 US Dist LEXIS 76270 (Aug 26, 2009).

54. Talley CR. Affirming science and peer-review publishing. Am J Health Syst Pharm. 2009;66:896.

55. Prod. Liab. Rep (CCH), Section 8968 (S.D.N.Y.Feb. 20, 1981).

56. Brannigan VM, Dayhoff RE. Liability for personal injuries caused by defective medical computer programs. Am J L Med. 1981;122:132-3.

57. Joyce EJ. Software bugs: a matter of life and liability. Datamation. 1987 May 15:88-92.

58. Gage D, McCormick J. Case 108-we did nothing wrong. Panama's Cancer Institute. Baseline. 2004;28:32-47.

59. Cuzamanes PT. Automation of medical records: the electronic superhighway and its ramifications for health care providers. J Pharm Law. 1997;6:19.

60. Brocklesby v. Jeppesen, 767 F.2d 1288 (9th Cir. 1985), cert. denied, 474 U.S. 1101 (1986).

61. 472 U.S. 749 (1985).

62. 137 Misc.2d 94, 520 N.Y.S.2d 334 (N.Y. Civ. Ct. 1987).

63. Amerson AB. Drug information centers: an overview. Drug Info J. 1986;20:173-8.

64. 705 P.2d 1360 (Ariz. Ct. App. 1985).

65. Rumore MM, Rosenberg JM, Costa JG. The pharmacist and the law: legal aspects of providing drug information. Wellcome Trends in Hosp Pharm. 1989 Dec;6-8.

66. Gough AR, Healey KM, Rupp SR. Poison control centers, from aspirin to PCBs and the scarlet runner beam: a study of legal anomaly and social necessity. Santa Clara L R. 1983;23:791-809.

67. Brushwood DB, Simonsmeier LM. Drug information for patients—duties of the manufacturer, pharmacist, physician, and hospital. J Leg Med. 1986;7:279-341.

68. Curtis JA, Greenberg MI. Legal liability of medical toxicologists serving as poison control center consultants: a review of relevant legal statutes and survey of the experience of medical toxicologists. J Med Toxicol. 2009;5(3):144-8.

69. 656 P.2d 483 (Wash. 1983).

70. Sigell LT, Bonofiglio JF, Siegel EG, et al. The role of drug information centers with consumers. Drug Info J. 1987;21:201-8.

71. Arnold RM, Nissen JC, Campbell NA. Ethical issues in a drug information center. Drug Intell Clin Pharm. 1987;21:1008-11.

72. Okasas RM. Hospital drug information centers: a new role in patient counseling. Pharma-Guide to Hospital Med. 1988;2:1-4.

73. Gray JA. The health sciences librarian's exposure to malpractice liability because of negligent provision of information. Bull Med Libr Assoc. 1989;77:33-7.

74. Mintz AP. Information practice and malpractice. Libr J. 1985:38-43.

75. Fidelity Leasing Corp. v. Dun & Bradstreet, Inc., 494 F. Supp. 786 (E.D. Pa. 1980).

76. Baker KR. Do people sue people who counsel? Drug Topics. 2007 Dec 3:4.

77. Food & Drug Administration [Internet]. Center for Drug Evaluation and Research, Office of Medical Policy, Division of Drug Marketing, Advertising and Communications, Comparative Advertising, Fair Balance, and the Patient-Consumer; c2003 [cited 2013 Mar 12]. Available from: http://www.fda.gov/downloads/AboutFDA/CentersOffices/OfficeofMedicalProductsand Tobacco/CDER/UCM213627.pdf

78. Food & Drug Administration, Guidance for Industry: Consumer-Directed Broadcast Advertisements, Aug 8, 1997.

79. 21 U.S.C. § 352(n).

80. 21 C.F.R. § 202.1(e).

81. Wilkes MS, Bell RA, Kravitz RL. Direct-to-consumer prescription drug advertising: trends, impact, and implications. Health Aff. 2000;19:110-28.

82. FDA officials describe agency actions on problematic drug promotion activity. BNA Pharm Law & Industry Report. 2003 Sept 19;1(35):1006.

83. Schwartz TM. Consumer-directed prescription drug advertising and the learned intermediary rule. Food Drug Cosm Law J. 1991;46:829-37.

84. PDRnet [Internet]. PDR Network. [cited 2013 Jun 27]. Available at http://www.pdrhealth.com.

85. FDLI Panel cautions firms on new media use. FDC Reports. The Pink Sheet. 2008 Sep 15:24.

86. Lyles A. Direct marketing of pharmaceuticals to consumers. Ann Rev Public Health. 2002;23:73-91.

87. 161 N.J. 1, 734 A.2d 1245 (N.J. 1999).

88. Ferrelli JJ. Perez creates exception to learned intermediary doctrine. New Jersey L J. Sep 20, 1999.

89. Heather JL. Liability for direct-to-consumer advertising and drug information on the internet: while the learned intermediary doctrine still lives, drug manufacturers can take some precautionary measures if it is ruled inapplicable. Defense Counsel J. 2001 Oct 24;68(4):1.

90. Gebhart F. Here comes the judge. Drug Topics. 2005 Jan 24;26-32.

91. Pharmacist's mutual [Internet]. [cited 2013 Mar 13]. Available at http://apps.phmic.com/RMNLFlipbook/06_2011/index.html

92. 122 S.Ct. 1497 (2002). No. 01-344.

93. Rumore MM. Direct-to-consumer advertising of prescription drugs: emerging legal and regulatory issues. Hosp Pharm. 2004;39:1058-68.

94. New Jersey Citizen Action v. Schering-Plough Corporation [Internet]. 367 N.J. Super. 8, 842 A.2d 174 (App. Div. 2004). Available from: http://www.prescriptionaccess.org/lawsuitssettlements/past_lawsuits?id=0011

95. Anderson v. SmithKline Beecham Corp., W.D. Wash. No. CV 03-2886-L, Sep 22, 2003.

96. Wyeth v. Levine 129 S. Ct. 1187, 1200 (2009).

97. Patsy BM, Furburg CD, Ray WA, Weiss NS. Potential for conflict of interest in the evaluation of suspected adverse drug reactions: cerivastin and risk for rhabdomyolosis. JAMA. 2004;292:2585-90.

98. FDC Act § 312.7.

99. 21 U.S.C. §§ 360.999, 403 (1998).

100. 21 C.F.R. § 99.101(a)(3)-(4).

101. Ward SM. WLF and the two-click rule: The First Amendment inequity of the Food and Drug Administration's regulation of off-label drug use information on the Internet. Food Drug L J. 2001;56:41-56.

102. Kennedy D. The old file-drawer problem. Science. 2004;305:451.

103. Good Reprint Practices for the Distribution of Medical Journal Articles and Medical-Scientific Reference Publications on Unapproved New Uses of Approved Drugs and Approved or Cleared Medical Devices. Dept. HHS, Food and Drug Administration, Office of the Commissioner, Jan. 2009.

104. The Medical Science Liaison: Examining the Role. CME Briefing, Jul-Sep 2002;3-5.

105. Guidance for Industry. Responding to Unsolicited Requests for Off-Label Information about Prescription Drugs and Medical Devices. Dept. HHS, Food and Drug Administration, Center For Drug Evaluation and Research, Center for Biologics Evaluation and

Research, Center for Veterinary Medicine, Center for Devices and Radiological Health. Dec 2011.

106. American Academy of Pediatrics. Policy Statement 2002;110-1, 2002 Jul 18:1-3.

107. Fugh-Berman A, Melnick D. Off-label promotion, on-target sales [Internet]. PLoS Medicine. 2008;5(10). Available from: http://www.medscape.com/viewarticle/704698. Accessed March 12, 2013.

108. Understanding the approval process for new cancer treatments [Internet]. Bethesda (MD): National Cancer Institute; c.2004 [cited 2013 Mar 12]. Available from: http://www.cancer.gov/clinicaltrials/learningabout/approval-process-for-cancer-drugs/page1

109. Brown L. Gain a solid understanding of compendia and its impact on patient access. Formulary. 2012;47:252-6.

110. Abernethy A, Raman G, Balk EM, Hammond JM, et al. Systematic review: reliability of compendia methods for off-label oncology indications. Ann Intern Med. 2009;150:336-43.

111. P.L. No. 110-275. Medicare Improvements for Patients and Providers Act of 2008. Jul 15, 2008.

112. Vivian JC. Off-label use of prescription drugs. US Pharm. 2003;28:508.

113. Beck JM, Azari ED. FDA, off-label use, and informed consent: debunking myths and misconceptions. Food Drug L J. 1998;53:71-103.

114. 21 C.F.R. pt. 50.

115. N.Y. Pub. Health L. § 2805-d(1) (McKinney 1993).

116. Edmunds MW, Scudder L. Using web citations in professional writing. J Prof Nursing. 2008;24:347-351.

117. Wood JM, Dorfman HL. Dot.com medicine—labeling in an Internet age. Food Drug L J. 2001;56;143-178.

118. Moberg MA, Wood JW, Dorfman HI. Surfing the Net in shallow waters: product liability concerns and advertising on the Internet. Food Drug Cosm Law J. 1998;53:213-24.

119. 21 U.S.C. §§ 351-354 (1994).

120. Deugan L, Powe N, Blakey B, Makary M. Wiki-surgery? Internal validity of Wikipedia as a medical and surgical reference. J Am Coll Surg. 2007;205(Suppl):576-7.

121. Clauson KA, Poten HH, Boulos MK, Dzeno Wagis JH. Scope, completeness, and accuracy of drug information in Wikipedia. Ann Pharmacother. 2008;42:1814-21.

122. Freeman MK, Lauderdale SA, Kendrach MG, Woolley TW. Google Scholar versus PUBMED in locating primary literature to answer drug-related questions. Ann Pharmacother. 2009;43:478-84.

123. Adams SR. Information quality-liability and corrections. Online. Sep/Oct 2003:16-22.

124. Kane B. Guidelines for the clinical use of electronic mail with patients. White paper. JAMA. 1998;5:104-11.

125. Gulick PG. E-health and the future of medicine: the economic, legal, regulatory, cultural, and organizational obstacles. Alb L J Sci & Tech. 2002;12:351-60.

126. Engstrom P. Can you afford not to travel the Internet? Med Econ. 1996;73:173-80.

127. Lopez, et al. v. Aziz, 852 S.W.2d 303, 304 (Tex. App. 1993).

128. Cubby v. Compuserve, 776 F. Supp. 135,140 (1990).

129. Stratton Oakmont Inc. and Daniel Porush v. Prodigy Services Co. & Others (NY Sup. Ct. 1995).

130. Terms of Use Agreement [Internet]. HealthActCHQ™ Inc. [cited 2013 Aug 8]. Available from: http://www.healthact.com/terms.php

131. Muhler MV, Ohno-Machado L. Reviewing social media use by clinicians. J Amer Med Inform Assoc. 2012;19:777-81.

132. American Society of Health System Pharmacists. ASHP statement on use of social media by pharmacy professionals. Am J Health Syst Pharm. 2010;74:145-8.

133. Clauson KA, Seamon MJ, Fox BI. Pharmacist's duty to warn in the age of social media. Am J Health Syst Pharm. 2010;67:1290-3.

134. Kalb PE, Bass IS. Government investigations in the pharmaceutical industry: off-label promotion, fraud and abuse, and false claims. Food Drug Cosm L J. 1998;53:63-70.

135. 42 U.S.C. § 1320a-7b(b)(1) (1994).

136. Huntington S. Presentation to the American Bar Association Health Law Section, Emerging professional liability exposures for physicians on the Web, Jun 8, 2001.

137. Warnecke M. Tested IP litigation storm of '04: fair use principles prove their pluck. Patent, Trademark, Copyright J. 2005;69:369.

138. Ticketmaster Corp. v. Tickets.Com, Inc., 2003 U.S. Dist. LEXIS 6483 (C.D. Cal. 2003).

139. eBay, Inc. v. Biddder's Edge, Inc., 100 F. Supp. 2d 1058 (N.D. Cal. 2000).

140. 1998 U.S. Dist. LEXIS 17282 (E.D. Pa. 1998).

141. D Minn., No. 02-1782 ADM/JGL, 2005 Jan 28.

142. Warnecke M. Effortless nature of Web surfing makes it unlikely consumers can avoid confusion. Patent, Trademark, Copyright J. 2005;69:363-4.

143. Millstein JS, Neuberger JD, Weingart JP. Doing business on the Internet. New York: Law Journal Press, 2004, §3.02[17][a][iii].

144. Futuredontics, Inc. v. Applied Anagramics, Inc., 1998 U.S. App. LEXIS 17012 (9th Cir. 1998).

145. 17 U.S.C. § 102.

146. Eldred v. Ashcroft, 239 F. 3d 373 (D.C. Cir. 2001).

147. 17 U.S.C. § 106.

148. 17 U.S.C. § 109(a).

149. 35 U.S.C. § 107.

150. College Entrance Examination Boear v. Pataki, 889 F. Supp. 554, 568 (N.D.N.Y. 1995).

151. Epstein E, Zulieve AJ. The fair use doctrine: commercial misappropriation and market diversion. Isaacson Raymond [Internet]. [cited 2013 Mar 12]. Available from http://www.isaacsonraymond.com/Articles/tabid/123/articleType/ArticleView/articleId/9/The-Fair-Use-Doctrine-Commercial-Misappropriation-And-Market-Diversion.aspx

152. 471 U.S. 539 (1985).

153. Guidelines for Classroom Copying in Not-for-Profit Educational Institutions. H.R. Rep. No. 1476, 94th Cong., 1st Sess. § 68-70 (1976).

154. Latman A, Gorman R, Ginsberg JC. Copyright for the nineties. 3rd ed. Charlottesville (VA): Michie;1989:655-6.

155. Campbell v. Acuff-Rose Music, 510 U.S. 569, 578 (1994).

156. 420 U.S. 376 (1975).

157. Perlman R. Williams & Wilkins Co. v. United States; photocopying, copyright, and the judicial process, 1975 Sup. Ct. Rev. 1976;355.

158. 74 F. 3d 1512 (6th Cir. 1996).

159. 758 F. Supp. 1552 (SDNY 1991).

160. Copyright Clearance Center. Using course management systems. Guidelines and best practices for copyright compliance. [cited 2013 Mar 13]. Available from: http://www .copyright.com/content/cc3/en/toolbar/education/resources/reprints_and_reports .html

161. 2004 WL 1008314 (2d Cir., May 7, 2004).

162. No. 07 Civ. 09667 (S.D.N.Y. Sept. 8, 2008).

163. FindLaw® for legal professionals [Internet]. Thomson Reuters; c2013. New York Times Co, Inc., et al. vs. Tasini et al. [cited 2013 Aug 27]. Available from: http://caselaw .lp.findlaw.com/scripts/getcase.pl?court=US&vol=000&invol=00-201

164. Greenberg v. National Geographic, 201 U.S. App. LEXIS 4270 (11th Cir. 2001).

165. The Authors Guild, Inc. et al. v. Google Inc, Case No.05 CV 8136 (S.D.N.Y.).

166. Google book search copyright class action settlement [Internet]. Available from: www .googlebooksettlement.com

167. Persky AS. Paper or plastic? Google's plan to digitalize materials pits book lovers v. book innovators. Wash Lawyer. 2009 Jun:35-40.

168. Google begins to scale back its scanning of books from university libraries [Internet]. The Higher Ed Chronicle. Mar 9, 2012. Available from: http://chronicle.Com/article/ Google-Begins-to-Scale-Back/131109/.

169. The National Digital Public Library is launched. The New York review of books [Internet]. April 25, 2013. Available from: http://www.nyBooks.com/articles/archives/2013/apr/ 25/national-digital-public-library-launched/.

170. American Libraries Association; c2004 [cited 2005 Feb 10]. Crews KD. New copyright law for distance education: the meaning and importance of the TEACH Act [Internet]. Am Libr Assoc. Available from: http://www.ala.org/Template.cfm?Section=distanceed

171. Smedinghoff TJ, ed. Online law. New York: Addison Wesley Press; 1996:139.

172. Pack R. Honest writers. Washington lawyer. 2004 Sep:21-6.

173. Health Insurance Portability and Accountability Act of 1996, Pub. L. No. 104-191, 110 Stat. 1936 (1996) (codified as amended in scattered sections of 18, 26, 29 and 42 U.S.C.A.); 42 U.S.C.A. § 1320d to 42 U.S.C.A. § 1320d-8.

174. 45 C.F.R. § 160.103.

175. 45 C.F.R. §§ 164.502(d)(2), 164.514(a) and (b).

176. Daniels JG. Health care privacy and HIPAA. In: Cronin KP, Weikers RN, eds. Data security and privacy law. Eagan (MN): West Group; 2002.

177. Clause SL, Triller DM, Bornhorst CP, et al. Conforming to HIPAA regulations and compilation of research data. Am J Health Syst Pharm. 2004;61:1025-31.

178. 45 C.F.R. § 164.512(i)(1)(i).

179. 45 C.F.R. § 164.512(b)(1)(iii).
180. Car J, Sheikh A. Email consultation in health care: 2. Acceptability and safe application. BMJ. 2004;329:439-42.
181. 42 U.S.C.A. § 290dd-2.
182. Bishop S. Interactions with individuals other than the patient, Part 2: Caregivers, personnel representatives, and minors. Pharm Today. 2003 Jul;4.
183. Bishop S. Interactions with individuals other than the patient, Part 1: Notice of Privacy Practices and medication counseling. Pharm Today. 2003 Jul;4.
184. California Healthcare Foundation. Achieving the right balance: privacy and security policies to support electronic health information exchange [Internet]. 2012 Jun. Available from: http://www.chcf.org/publications/2012/06/achieving-right-balance. E-health privacy policies. Oakland (CA): California Health Care Foundation; 2000.
185. Baker DB. Provider-patient e-mail: with benefits come risks. J Am Health Info Mgmt Assoc. 2003;74:22-9.
186. 2012 Association of National Advertisers Compendium of Legislative, Regulatory, and Legal Issues. Available from: www.ana.net/advocacy.com
187. Consumer data privacy in a networked world: a framework for protecting privacy and promoting innovation in the global digital economy [Internet]. c2012 [cited 2013 Mar 12]. Available from: http://www.whitehouse.gov/sites/default/files/privacy-final.pdf.
188. D. Mass, No. 00-11672-JLT, Nov 6, 2003.
189. 18 U.S.C. § 2510 *et seq.*
190. Pharmaceutical Research and Manufacturers of America Code on Interactions with Healthcare Professionals. Jul 2002 [Updated Jan 2009].
191. Health and Human Services, OIG Compliance Program for Pharmaceutical Industry, Apr 2003.
192. Accreditation Council for Pharmacy Education. Accreditation standards and criteria [Internet]; c2005 Jan [cited 2010 Jan 17]. Available from: http://www.acpeaccredit.org/ceproviders/standards.asp
193. 2011 National Association of Boards of Pharmacy (NABP) Survey of Pharmacy Law. Mount Prospect (IL): NABP; 2012.
194. Cutting the strings on gifts and other questionable marketing practices: PhRMA takes a stand. CME Briefing. 2002 Jul-Sep:1-6.
195. FDA Guidance for Industry-Supported Scientific and Educational Activities, 1997.
196. Steiner JL, Norko M, Devine S, Grottole E, Vinoski J, Griffith EE. Best practices: developing ethical guidelines for pharmaceutical company support in an academic health center. Psychiatr Serv. 2003;54:1079-89.
197. Rosner F. Pharmaceutical industry support for continuing medical education programs: a review of current ethical guidelines. Mt. Sinai J Med. 1995;62:427-30.
198. 42 U.S.C. § 1320a-7b(b).
199. U.S. v. Greber, 760 F.2d 68 (3d Cir. 1985).
200. U.S. v. LaHue, 261 F.3d 993 (10th Cir. 2001).
201. *In re* Caremark Int'l, Inc. Derivative Litig., 698 A. 2d 959 (1996).

202. Drug firm settles kickback charges. The Palm Beach Post, Sep 6, 1994, p. 4B.

203. Astrue MJ, Szabo DS. Pharmaceutical marketing and the anti-kickback statutes. Food Drug Cosmet Med Device Law Dig. 1993;10(2):57-60.

SUGGESTED READINGS

1. Brand KA, Kraus ML. Drug information specialists. Am J Health Syst Pharm. 2006;63:712-4.

2. Department of HHS, Food and Drug Administration, Center For Drug Evaluation and Research, Center for Biologics Evaluation and Research, Center for Veterinary Medicine, Center for Devices and Radiological Health. Guidance for industry, responding to unsolicited requests for off-label information about prescription drugs and medical devices [Internet]. Dec 2011. Available from: http://www.fda.gov/downloads/Drugs/Guidance-ComplianceRegulatoryInformation/Guidances/UCM285145.pdf

3. American Libraries Association [homepage on the Internet]; c2004. Crews KD. New Copyright law for distance education: the meaning and importance of the TEACH Act. Am Libr Assoc. Available from: http://www.knowyourcopyrights.org/resourcesfac/faq/online.shtml

4. American Society of Health System Pharmacists. ASHP statement on use of social media by pharmacy professionals. Am J Health Syst Pharm. 2010;74:145-8.

11

Chapter Eleven

Ethical Aspects of Drug Information Practice

Linda K. Ohri

Learning Objectives

After completing this chapter, the reader will be able to

- Explain characteristics that differentiate an ethical deliberation from other types of decision making.
- Interpret and make use of ethics rules, principles, and theories to analyze identified ethical dilemmas.
- Identify and analyze examples of ethical dilemmas that may arise for health professionals when providing drug information, in various practice settings and for various types of clients and circumstances.
- Identify micro, meso, and macro levels of ethical decision making that may occur during the provision of drug information.
- Use the described process of ethical analysis in order to propose and justify a specific decision or course of action in an ethical dilemma case.
- Describe resources and structures that can prepare, guide, and support clinicians faced with ethical dilemmas during the course of providing drug information.

Key Concepts

❶ Ethical deliberations may be differentiated by three characteristics: they are ultimate (fundamental), the issue is universal, and the welfare of all affected parties is considered.

❷ Ethical judgments may occur at micro, meso, or macro levels of health care decision making.

❸ Professional ethics is different than the law.

❹ The primary focus will be on the health professional's identification, interpretation, specification, and balancing of pertinent ethical rules and principles.

❺ The application of a proposed process of ethical analysis is demonstrated for identifying, analyzing, and resolving ethical dilemmas that may arise during health professionals' provision of drug information.

❻ The first process step requires identification and evaluation of pertinent background information to ensure that the facts of the specific case are understood, and to assess whether a true ethical dilemma exists.

❼ Sometimes, the professional will find it necessary and valuable to more consciously deliberate on how various ethical theories suggest that the relevant rules and principles should be prioritized or balanced.

❽ Health care professionals need training, resources, and support to prepare them to effectively address those ethical dilemmas they confront.

What Is Ethics and What Is Not

The Ethics Course Content Committee of the American Association of Colleges of Pharmacy (AACP) described **ethics** as "the philosophical inquiry of the moral dimensions of human conduct."[1] They mentioned that Aristotle taught ethics as "an eminently practical discipline". . . dealing . . . "with concrete judgments in situations in which action must be taken despite uncertainty."[1] These authors indicated that the term ethical is often used synonymously with the term moral to describe an action or decision as good or right. They further stated that ethics is not the study of moral development, and it is not the law.

Veatch stated that "an ethical, or moral, issue involves judgments between right and wrong human conduct or praiseworthy and blameworthy human character."[2] This author indicated that an ❶ *ethical deliberation may be differentiated from other endeavors by three characteristics: (1) it is ultimate or fundamental, there is no higher standard against which to measure the rightness of the decision or action; (2) the issue is universal, the parties involved in the dilemma do not consider it simply a difference of opinion or taste—each party believes there is a right or wrong answer—even if they disagree about what the answer is; and (3) the deliberation takes into account the welfare of all involved or affected by the judgment at hand.* Those who provide drug information (DI) typically rely on an intuitive sense of these characteristics: we have the feeling that the situation we are confronting is a big deal, and somehow anticipate that we should not address only personal preference in the matter at hand.

Over the past two decades evolving literature has described that ❷ *ethical judgments may occur at micro, meso, or macro levels of health care decision making*[3-15]: (1) a traditionally recognized **micro** level of health care–related decision making involves decisions made at the individual professional–patient level of health care; (2) a less commonly discussed **meso** level of decision making (with some literature using the term organizational for similar purpose) is variably described as occurring at the institutional/ organizational level or at community/regional levels; and (3) **macro** level decision making often sets policy for the health system, as a standard established for an entire profession, or through government as law/regulation for the society as a whole.

Health care providers may be involved in ethical decision making at each of these levels related to the provision of or access to drug information. Primarily, micro level ethical decision-making scenarios will be presented in this chapter. However, certain scenarios involving meso and macro level ethical decision making will also be addressed. For example, a physician, nurse, and pharmacist may all be participating on a pharmacy and therapeutics committee that is developing an organizational policy regarding use of pharmaceutical samples within hospital clinics, or in a large independent clinic practice. The policy also addresses use of in-house professionals versus industry detailers to provide information about new drug products. Each of these professionals may have competing priorities and concerns that add ethical dimensions to their decision making on this proposed policy.[11] This constitutes a meso level of ethical decision making for these professionals. A clinician participating on a national task force charged with developing policy related to **medication therapy management** services (with inherent drug information access) as part of a health care reform model will have macro level ethical decisions to make relative to balancing patient needs, professional identity, and societal economic constraints.[10]

❸ *Professional ethics is different than the law.* Law might be defined as rules of conduct imposed by society on its members. By contrast, professional ethics has been defined as "rules of conduct or standards by which a particular group in society regulates its actions and sets standards for its members."[16] Both constitute macro level policy making, across society or across an entire profession. Law involves written rules set by the whole society (or its representatives) that address responsibilities of that society's members. Professional ethics focuses on explicit or implicit rules and standards set by a professional subgroup of society, and addresses the responsibilities of only those who are members of that subgroup. Certain ethical standards of a given profession may be institutionalized as law by society as a whole. However, professional ethical standards (for example, do no harm or preserve life) are often impossible to fully regulate by law. Meeting an ethical standard also goes beyond legal requirements; indeed, our ethical beliefs may on occasion command our civil disobedience (e.g., a prison pharmacist who refuses to dispense drugs to be used in legal executions). On the other hand, as will be discussed further below, law also represents one aspect of the culture within which ethical decisions are made. In considering the cultural perspectives of a given dilemma, relevant legal requirements must be identified and considered when one seeks to make an ethical decision.

Ethical Dilemmas When Providing Drug Information

This chapter presents case scenarios representing ethical dilemmas. These scenarios will be utilized to demonstrate a specific method for analyzing ethical dilemmas confronted by health professionals providing drug information. The discussion will address ethical dilemmas encountered by generalist and specialist patient care providers providing drug information, as well as examples drawn from the experiences of drug information specialists. All health professionals provide drug information and must address the ethical dilemmas that arise in the course of providing this service. Many of these scenarios represent examples of micro level ethical dilemmas that primarily involve an interaction between a drug information provider and the direct recipient of the information. Other scenarios where health professionals may be providing or determining access to drug information occur at meso (organizational) or macro (societal) levels of ethical decision making. While perhaps less immediately obvious as an ethical dilemma to some individuals involved, these may constitute dilemmas that have even further reaching impacts for both individual professionals and impacted groups. These larger dilemmas may often seem beyond the scope of individual decision making, but indeed ultimately are primarily addressed through the contributed actions/ decisions of individuals, typically as they interact in some group process. Of course, it should also be recognized that all ethical dilemmas, by definition, have some implications beyond the welfare of the most immediate individuals involved. The list of example dilemmas provided in Table 11–1 includes scenarios from each of these levels. These dilemmas might arise in a wide variety of settings and circumstances where health care is practiced or health care policy is set. Please identify the level of ethical decision making that each example seems to represent, and consider what ethical issues might exist for each scenario.

In the fifth edition of their foundational text *Principles of Biomedical Ethics,*[17] Beauchamp and Childress address the following aspects of the moral life: principles and rules; rights, character and virtues; and moral emotions. The responsibilities (based on principles and rules) and rights of the health care provider and other involved parties will be addressed briefly in this chapter as considerations that must be dealt with in the course of responding to a specific dilemma. While acknowledging their importance, this chapter will not address the roles of character, moral virtue, or emotions in ethical decision

TABLE 11–1. EXAMPLE ETHICAL DILEMMAS

- The hospital practitioner is asked to provide information that might be used to speed the ending of a terminal patient's life.
- The community pharmacist or physician is requested by a patient to critique another health care provider's drug therapy recommendations.
- The emergency room nurse is asked to tell the patient's significant other that the administered medication is for other than the sexually transmitted disease being treated.
- The drug information specialist is confronted by an administrator, pressuring for a certain formulary recommendation that is more cost containment than evidence based.
- The home health care practitioner is asked to positively present questionably substantiated information on the efficacy of a given therapy, in order to support insurance reimbursement for a truly needy patient.
- The practitioners working in industry, who are asked to prepare a consumer product education and promotion piece according to directions that do not adhere to FDA or WHO guidelines for balanced presentation of both the benefits and the risks associated with the drug product being advertised.
- The health professional practicing in any patient care setting, who experiences another episode (in a repetitious pattern) where his or her patients would benefit from additional drug information, but who finds workload demands to be an impossible barrier to providing more than the minimum, legally required information.
- The health professional is enrolled by her professional organization to testify against a proposed health reform policy that mandates her profession to provide verbal drug information associated with a prescription refill, but does not set any requirements for third-party payer reimbursement of this service.

making by health professionals. One might say that they constitute the provider's inherent moral perspective that will direct and support his or her decision making. The interested reader is referred to the text referenced above for a fascinating discussion of these factors[17]; this discussion is continued in the 2008 edition of the same text for those wishing to review updated coverage of this material.[18] The remainder of this chapter is intended to prepare and assist the pharmacist and other health professionals providing drug information to analyze and address dilemmas, such as those listed above. ❹ *The primary focus will be on the health professional's identification, interpretation, specification, and balancing of pertinent ethical rules and principles* as he or she seeks to determine and justify what he or she considers the right decision or the best course of action.

Basics of Ethics Analysis

This section briefly presents relevant terminology and definitions used in the field of ethics, as well as an overview of a specific process of analysis that may be used in assessing ethical dilemmas. In the section following this one, specific case scenario demonstrations of this process for analysis will be presented.

DEFINITIONS USED IN THE FIELD OF ETHICS

Beauchamp and Childress[19] defined ethics as "a generic term for several ways of examining the moral life." These authors described a process of deliberation and justification that is necessary when confronting a moral dilemma. They stated, "When we deliberate . . . we are considering which judgment is morally justified...." They indicated that, "Particular judgments are justified by moral rules, which in turn are justified by principles, which ultimately are defended by an ethical theory." These authors presented a hierarchical diagram that depicts this approach to analysis (Figure 11–1). A later article by Beauchamp further addresses the need to consider these principles and rules within the specific context of the case at hand, in order to fully realize their action-guiding potential.[20]

The authors referred to these hierarchical levels of analysis (particularly rules and principles) as action-guides, which are utilized to justify a particular judgment. They describe a rule of ethics as specific to context and relatively restricted in scope; for instance, the moral rule about confidentiality that specifically addresses a patient's right to consent prior to release of privileged information.[19] Principles are more broad and fundamental in scope; for example, the principle of respect for **autonomy**, which is the patient's right to decide on personal issues. They describe ethical theories as "integrated bodies of principles and rules . . . that may include mediating rules that govern cases of conflicts." The prominent rules and principles guiding ethical decision making by health care professionals can generally be placed within one of two broad ethical theories: **consequentialist** theory or **deontological** (derived from the Greek word *deon*, meaning duty) theory.[19] Multiple versions exist of each of these broad categories. Consequentialist theories describe actions or decisions as morally right or wrong based on their consequences, rather than on any intrinsic features they may have. The two cardinal principles of consequentialist theory are **beneficence** (do that which promotes a good outcome) and **nonmaleficence** (do that which minimizes bad outcomes). Consequentialist theories focus on this one feature of an act, its consequences. For example, an informed consent ethical rule can be of value within consequentialist theory because consent generally results in improved compliance and outcome—good consequences.

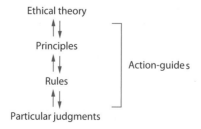

Figure 11–1.

However, if informed consent was likely to result in a bad outcome, it would not be justifiable within consequentialist theory. A mediating rule utilized by many advocates of consequentialist theory is to hold nonmaleficence as more important, or more foundational, than beneficence.

Duty-driven (deontological) theories look more to intrinsic qualities of an act or decision to assert its moral rightness or wrongness. Deontological theory considers other inherent features of an act, besides consequences, as also relevant and often of greater importance. For example, in various forms of deontological theory, the act is considered inherently wrong if it is dishonest or breaks confidentiality, or if it does not respect individual autonomy. Conflicts between different rules are mediated by appealing to more foundational, underlying principles such as adherence to justice or to respect for persons.

Conscious recognition of the pertinent action-guides, and understanding mediating rules that operate within the health professional's preferred ethical theory or theories, can help providers honestly and equitably analyze the ethical dilemma, and better comply with the imperative characteristics of ethical deliberation (see the beginning of this chapter).

OVERVIEW OF A SUGGESTED PROCESS OF ANALYSIS TO BE USED WHEN AN ETHICAL DILEMMA ARISES

In the article *Hospital Pharmacy: What Is Ethical?*, Veatch[2] indicated that often people reach a particular ethical decision without a great deal of conscious deliberation, through moral intuition, and without subsequent challenge from any external party. However, on occasion, when pondering a certain ethical judgment, they are called on (internally or externally) to analyze and justify the basis for their conviction. He suggested that when this occurs, it is first important to understand the facts of the specific case. He then described progression through three additional process stages of reflection (on ethical rules, principles, and theories) by which we may identify, analyze, and present reasons for our judgment. In the same report, the author also emphasized the importance in one's reflection of taking into account the points of view of all parties impacted. As stated earlier in this chapter, this is one of the key characteristics distinguishing an ethical deliberation. A survey of the text *Cross-Cultural Perspectives in Medical Ethics*, 2nd ed.[21] demonstrates that there are many commonalities, but also important differences across the ethical perspectives of different cultures. These cultural perspectives must be considered if all parties' points of view are to be taken into account.

In this section ❺ *the application of a proposed process of ethical analysis is demonstrated for identifying, analyzing, and resolving ethical dilemmas that may arise during health professionals' provision of drug information.* These steps of analysis are derived

from the writings of Veatch, Beauchamp, and Childress, as well as other authors.[2,19,21-23]
The process may be summarized as follows:

I. Identification of relevant background information
   A. Factual details of the issue at hand
   B. Consideration of who is affected by the ethical issue
   C. Learn and respectfully address the cultural perspectives (including applicable legal requirements) for those affected by the dilemma
II. Identification and justification of the relevant moral rules and principles (action-guides) pertinent to the case
III. Deliberation, through the use of moral intuition and application of ethical theory, on how to rank/balance the rules and principles pertinent to the case in order to resolve the ethical dilemma

Step I. Identification of Relevant Background Information

❻ *The first process step requires identification and evaluation of pertinent background information to ensure that the facts of the specific case are understood and to assess whether a true ethical dilemma exists.* This first step deserves careful consideration and research. Once the facts of a case are known, the moral concerns may be resolved. This step has been divided into three parts: (a) data gathering, (b) consideration of the welfare of all affected parties, and (c) respect for the cultural perspectives of these parties.

Health professionals already use data gathering when they apply a systematic approach to answering any drug information question (see Chapter 2). When addressing a potential ethical dilemma, the providers must learn about the factual details of the issue, who is directly involved, and whether there is conflict in factual understanding among the involved parties in the issue. For example, does the parent who calls to ask about the medication recently prescribed for her teenager already know that the teenager is taking a birth control pill prescribed by a gynecologist (rather than a dermatologist for acne) and simply wants to know the name of the product?

If the matter still seems to involve an ethical dimension once data gathering clarifies the facts, the next step is to consider the rights and responsibilities of all affected parties. As previously mentioned, this has been described as an essential component of any ethical deliberation.[2] The health care provider, the direct client (patient or parent in the case just described), other indirect but individual clients (e.g., any existing or unborn children, parent paying for service provided to the child patient, or the patient's spouse), other health professionals (e.g., the patient's physician), other societal groups (e.g., other patients who might be harmed by an incompetent practitioner), and any higher power recognized by the health professional have rights and/or responsibilities that should be considered.

Finally, during first consideration of any potential ethical issue, the provider should take into account the cultures of the affected parties.[22] In his reviews of the foundations of modern medical ethics theories, Veatch[21,23] described how the unique perspectives of Western, Chinese, Hindu, Jewish, Catholic, Protestant, and other cultural groups have affected the formulation of their dominant medical ethics traditions. Other cultural classifications might include socioeconomic status, political affiliation, age category, and racial or ethnic group. A report by Najjar et al.[24] demonstrates some important similarities (e.g., requests to assess physician recommendations) and differences (e.g., requests to serve as a primary health care provider) in the types of ethical dilemmas that are identified by drug information specialists functioning within the cultural environment of Saudi Arabia compared to those reported at the United States (U.S.) centers.

In a very interesting case study, Carrese et al.[25] discussed the ethical obligations of medical professionals in caring for those of a different ethnic culture. In this case, a young Laotian mother had utilized a traditional Mien folk cure to treat her infant. The treatment involved placing several small burns on the child's abdomen to treat gusia mun toe, an apparently transient, but very distressing, colic-like ailment. The cure resulted in several small scars, but no other obvious ill effects. The mother indicated that the cure worked. The physician recognized the value in supporting the positive impacts of the woman's attachment to her cultural support group. However, the physician was confronted with the dilemma of how to respond to this mother's revelation of a culturally promoted treatment measure that was not scientifically supported and could be dangerous. Sometimes, culturally based actions may conflict with the professional's goal to avoid harm and promote benefit. However, failing to consider a cultural perspective may also have harmful effects. An extended discussion of how differing cultural perspectives affect ethical decision making is beyond the scope of this chapter. However, the health professional should strive to be aware of and respect the cultural perspectives of the affected parties when contemplating an ethical dilemma. The interested reader is encouraged to refer to the resources cited here and above for further discussion of cultural factors in ethical analysis.[21,23]

One final issue should be addressed relative to cultural considerations. The legal requirements of the society within which an ethical dilemma occurs are part of the culture and must be identified. A specific ethical decision will not always exactly conform to the existing legal requirements of society. The ultimate nature of ethical deliberations may result in decisions that are more demanding than the legal requirements and, unfortunately, may even occasionally involve perceived or true conflict with specific legal requirements. This may involve, for instance, a decision not to divulge confidential communications between a professional and client, which may or may not be acceptable within the law. In another case, the health professional may decide not to provide information related to abortion or capital punishment, even though these activities are acceptable within the law. Obviously, legal requirements cannot be ignored or dismissed lightly when making a specific ethical decision.

Step II: Use of Rules and Principles (Action-Guides) to Assist in Analysis of an Ethical Dilemma

If the dilemma persists, once the available background information has been identified and considered, the process of full ethical deliberation should proceed. Veatch[2] suggests that the involved party/parties can proceed as far as necessary through successive stages of general moral reflection assessing at the level of moral rules and then at the level of ethical principles, within their accepted ethical theory. These might be described as the action-guides referred to by Beauchamp and Childress.[19] This second process step of analysis will look at moral rules that may apply to the specific case and more general pertinent ethical principles. Definitions are provided at the end of this section for a number of ethical rules and principles that are considered particularly relevant to decision making by practitioners.

It should be noted that specific action-guides may be considered a rule within one ethical theory and a principle within another. For example, **veracity** (truth telling) as mentioned above, may be considered by some ethicists to be a specific moral rule and by others to be a general principle, depending on which ethical theory is followed. For the practitioner immediately involved in analyzing a specific ethical dilemma, defining the relevant action-guides as rules or principles is important only to the extent that this helps in assessing which are more fundamental to the issue at hand. Therefore, in this chapter, both rules and principles will be included within the same process step of ethical analysis.

Examples of moral rules within biomedical ethics include a confidentiality rule dictating that patient-entrusted information should not be disclosed or an informed consent rule that addresses the individual's right to information before agreeing to a specific medical procedure. Unfortunately, there is no definitive list universally defining all moral rules and, sometimes, multiple pertinent rules can be in conflict. Furthermore, there are acceptable exceptions to most moral rules. For instance, disregarding the informed consent rule might be justifiable in an acute situation to protect the life of the client, suffering may be necessary in order to achieve cure of serious disease, and many consider killing justified under certain circumstances. Therefore, there may not be a specific rule that resolves a particular ethical dilemma.

When such a circumstance arises, the practitioner may begin a more general level of analysis by looking at the ethical principles that apply to the case. Sometimes, the involved parties can reach an acceptable resolution to an ethical dilemma once they recognize the more broad relevant ethical principles. In a given dilemma, the professional may decide that the primary principle is to respect the autonomy of the client and that requires providing complete information that enables the client to make an informed decision. In another dilemma, if do no harm is considered the most fundamental ethical principle, decisions or acts that deny this principle would be considered unethical. It becomes immediately obvious, however, that relevant ethical principles such as these may also come into conflict. This problem can be demonstrated by the following example:

The professional may believe that full disclosure will result in nonadherence by the patient, with significant risk of resultant harm. The practitioner, therefore, confronts two conflicting principles: respecting client autonomy versus the duty to do no harm.

Step III: Ethical Theory as a Means to Clarify or Resolve Ethical Dilemmas

This third step of ethical analysis reveals how relevant moral rules and principles interact within the preferred ethical theory to address the given dilemma. When confronted with conflicting ethical rules or principles, the practitioner may simply resolve the dilemma through his or her moral intuition of the right thing to do; even if unconsciously, this reflects the individual's at least temporary affiliation to some theory of what constitutes good versus bad or right versus wrong. ❼ *Sometimes, the professional will find it necessary and valuable to more consciously deliberate on how various ethical theories suggest that the relevant rules and principles should be prioritized or balanced.* According to Veatch,[2] this process step can lead to more rational and honest decision making or action taking. He suggests that these ultimate deliberations at the level of ethical theory will be affected by our most basic religious and/or philosophical commitments. It is important that the practitioner recognizes and acknowledges the impact on decision making of his or her own personal ethical perspective. Those dilemmas that cannot be fully resolved can at least be viewed with greater clarity.

Veatch[23] states that, "The components of a complete theory will answer such questions as what rules apply to specific ethical cases, what ethical principles stand behind the rules, how seriously the rules should be taken, and what constitutes the fundamental meaning and justification of the ethical principles." In this reference and another text, the author reviews the foundations of consequentialist, deontological, and other ethics theories particularly relevant to health professionals, including the Hippocratic tradition; Judeo-Christian and other religious-based traditions; the philosophies of the modern secular West; and medical ethics theories outside the Anglo-American West, including Socialist, Islamic, Hindu, African, Chinese, and Japanese traditions.[21,23] Frequently, versions of the broad consequentialist and deontological theories are expressed in various ways across these traditions. Particular note should be given to the core of the various **Hippocratic Oaths**, since this has been the central ethical tradition of Western medicine: "Those who have stood in that (Hippocratic) tradition are committed to producing good for their patient and to protecting that patient from harm."[23] In Hippocratic tradition, there is also a special emphasis placed on the responsibility of the medical professional to the specific patient versus obligations to other less directly affected parties or to society in general. A contract theory of medical ethics has also been proposed, which describes an implicit (unwritten) contract between health professionals and patients.[23] This modern theory is of special relevance to the pharmacist providing drug information as a service within an implicit pharmaceutical care contract.[23,26] First of all, this theory represents a shift in thinking for those pharmacists who might have considered their primary obligation to be to the prescriber rather than to the patient. Furthermore, this contract between patients and professionals suggests an obligation for more substantive communication with patients and a higher level of caregiving than some pharmacists have previously felt obligated to offer. The reader is referred to foundational writings by Veatch, as well as those of Beauchamp and Childress, for a more in-depth discussion of various medical ethics theories.[18,19,21,23]

AN ANNOTATED LISTING OF RULES AND PRINCIPLES (ACTION-GUIDES) APPLIED IN MEDICAL ETHICS INQUIRY

The following rules and principles of ethical conduct will be described and subsequently used in the analysis of case scenarios provided in the next section. Their description will necessarily be brief. The reader is referred to other sources to read more about these rules and principles.[19,23]

1. **Nonmaleficence**—A basic principle of consequentialist theory; encompasses the duty to do no harm. This tenet has a long history as part of the Hippocratic tradition, where it has often been described in terms of the health care provider's duty to the individual patient. The principle is also cited as justification for actions benefiting all. Sometimes, application of the principle requires addressing conflicts between the needs of one and all.[18]

2. **Beneficence**—Another basic principle of consequentialist theory that expresses the duty to promote good. Again, conflict can arise between what constitutes good for one individual versus the larger societal group. Good or bad consequences are also of importance within deontological theories, but are evaluated along with other principles that may be considered of equal or greater importance.[18]

3. *Respecting the patient–professional relationship*—A moral rule, often referring to respect for the physician–patient relationship, but also applicable to other professional–patient relationships. This rule has been mentioned in published reports of ethical dilemmas arising during the provision of drug information.[24,27-29] As expressed in Hippocratic traditions, this rule indicates that the physician's primary duty is to the patient and tends to give the physician, rather than the patient, control in the relationship, which may be judged paternalistic by some. This rule is particularly noted in duty-driven (deontological) ethical theories that consider the professional's duty to the patient, but also supports consequentialist theory to the extent that good outcomes are enhanced.

4. *Respect for autonomy*—A principle described particularly within deontological theory. This principle is founded on a belief in the right of the individual to self-rule. It speaks to the individual's right to decide on issues that primarily affect self.

5. **Consent**—A moral rule related to the principle of autonomy which states that the client has a right to be informed and to freely choose a course of action; for example, informed consent to receive a therapy or procedure.

6. **Confidentiality**—A moral rule, also related to the principle of autonomy, which specifically addresses the individual client's right to give or refuse consent relative to release of privileged information.

7. **Privacy**—Another rule within the principle of autonomy, more generally relating to the right of the individual to control his or her own affairs without interference from or knowledge of outside parties. This rule has been addressed in deliberations on the rights of individuals with AIDS versus those of their potential sexual contacts.

8. *Respect for persons*—A principle expressing duty to the welfare of the individual, particularly described within religion-based deontological theories. This principle may also be expressed within dignity of life or sanctity of human life principles. It has common elements with the respect for autonomy principle, but addresses more directly a belief in the inherent value of human life, independent of characteristics or abilities of the specific human being.

9. **Veracity**—This term addresses the obligation to truth telling or honesty. Veracity is considered an ethical principle within deontological theory. However, it is considered a useful rule within consequentialist theory, to the extent that it promotes good.

10. **Fidelity**—Another principle of moral duty in deontological theory that addresses the responsibility to be trustworthy and keep promises. This principle also relates to a duty of reciprocity—consideration of the other's point of view. Descriptions of pharmaceutical care have spoken of the need to develop an ethical **covenant** between the pharmacist and the client.[26] Nurses, physicians, and other health professionals undoubtedly also have various standards that call them to such ethical relationships with their patients. This covenant details the characteristics of a relationship requiring fidelity and reciprocity, in which each party takes on certain responsibilities and gives up certain rights in order to achieve specific good outcomes (consequentialist theory). Success of this contract depends in good measure on consideration by each party of the other's point of view.

11. **Justice**—This concept has been presented within various principles that relate to fairness and tendering what is due, resource allocation and providing that to which the individual is entitled. A number of more fundamental justice theories have also been developed to connect and justify these various principles.[18,19] Moral decision making at the meso and macro level will frequently cite justice as a main justification for particular decisions. A more thorough discussion on justice-related

principles and theories is beyond the scope of this chapter. However, recent texts that address this topic can provide much assistance to those health professionals preparing for roles at these levels of ethical decision making, or to those who teach such professionals.[18,30,31]

These are certainly not the only relevant rules or principles, nor are they necessarily universally accepted definitions. However, these action-guides seem particularly pertinent to medical ethics inquiry. Furthermore, several of these rules and principles have been specifically discussed in published reports that describe ethical dilemmas encountered by drug information specialists.[27,28] Such dilemmas have also been described in situations where practitioners are providing drug information directly to patients, either from a formal drug information center or during the process of providing patient care.

Demonstration of the Process for Analyzing Ethical Dilemmas

The following examples demonstrate ethical dilemmas that might arise for professionals providing drug information. These cases will be utilized to demonstrate the aforementioned process of analysis for the practitioner(s) addressing an ethical dilemma.

DEMONSTRATION OF CASE ANALYSIS

Example Case 11-1

(MICRO LEVEL CASE)

Mrs. Billings, a new patient at the medical center, calls the Drug Information Center (DIC), which the medical center advertises as a resource for both patients and professionals, and asks Dr. Ford, the drug information specialist, a question. She is concerned about whether she should take the metronidazole just prescribed for her by Dr. Meyers, her family practitioner (who practices at the center where the DI center is located).

■ ANALYSIS

Step #1 Identification of relevant background information

A. Factual details of the issue at hand. The drug information practitioner learns the following information through discussion with the patient:
    1. Mrs. Billings is approximately 8 weeks pregnant; she wonders if this medication is safe for the baby.
    2. She says she is being treated for a recently acquired vaginal infection.
    3. She states that this is the first vaginal infection that she has had in several years.

4. She mentions that she has only recently begun seeing Dr. Meyers as her family just moved into town about 3 months ago.

5. Mrs. Billings indicates that Dr. Meyers knows she is pregnant. He is managing her pregnancy.

6. She states that she asked him about the drug's safety, but he rather impatiently brushed off her questions by asking "don't you trust me?"

7. Dr. Ford may decide that it is necessary to consult professional resources to evaluate whether the therapy appears to be appropriate. She should not hesitate to ask the patient for some reasonable time period in which to investigate the pertinent information before providing an answer.

8. Dr. Ford will need to consider whether any identified risks are likely to be known to the physician.

9. Dr. Ford may decide that further facts must be obtained through direct discussion with Dr. Meyers.

B. Identification of who is affected by any ethical issue considered to be present. As the drug information provider reflects on this patient's inquiry, it is helpful to consider who might be impacted by her response.

1. Herself, relative to her own desire to do right; any relationship between her and her patient, any relationship between her and the physician.

2. Mrs. Billings, relative to the consequences of any harm to her infant or of inadequate treatment of the infection, and relative to her future relationships with both the physician and the drug information provider.

3. Mrs. Billings' infant, relative to the consequences of any harmful or beneficial effects of the drug, or of inadequate treatment of the mother's infection.

4. Dr. Meyers, relative to the consequences of prescribing a potentially inappropriate therapy during the woman's pregnancy, and relative to the effects of any drug information provided on the patient–physician relationship.

5. Mrs. Billings' family, significant others, and society in general relative to the impacts of either delivery or abortion of a child with harm from the therapy, or from inadequate treatment of the woman's infection.

C. Consideration for the cultural perspectives of those affected by the dilemma.

Dr. Ford will consciously or unconsciously act within her own cultural and religious framework, and her understanding of her legal obligations. Awareness of her own perspective, as well as consideration of the cultural perspectives of others who may be affected, is important if she is to pursue a truly ethical course of action. To repeat Veatch's words differentiating ethical deliberations, "The deliberation takes into account the welfare of all involved or affected."[1] Each involved party's welfare is affected by his or her cultural perspective. Cultural, religious, and legal perspectives that the clinician must be aware of in this case might include:

1. Perspectives regarding parental responsibility to the unborn infant versus self
2. Perspectives and legal requirements relative to both the DI provider's and physician's obligations to the patient and her infant
3. Perspectives about the role and authority of the physician and DI provider

D. Consideration of the level of decision making involved in responding to any ethical dilemma recognized by the DI practitioners.

Within the context of this DI professional's job description, or the charge of the particular case, it should be fairly obvious whether micro, meso, or macro level decision-making activities are involved. However, a clinician may be involved in micro level decision-making activities related to individual patients, but also have obligations to the pharmacy and therapeutics committee within the health organization (meso level), or perhaps even beyond as a policy committee member for his or her national professional organization (macro level). By definition, all ethical dilemmas tend to have implications beyond the context of just two individuals (note from the first page of this chapter that ethical deliberations take into account the welfare of all involved or affected by the judgment at hand), but meso and macro level decision making will always affect various population groups, as well as the individuals within those groups.

Step #2 Identification and justification of the relevant moral rules and principles (action-guides) pertinent to the case at hand

If the background facts of Mrs. Billings' inquiry do not dismiss the DI provider's ethical concerns, Dr. Ford will find it helpful to consider the various rules and principles discussed above in order to clarify the dimensions of her concern. It is most useful to first identify all potentially pertinent action-guides, and seek an understanding of how fundamentally each applies to the situation.

Ethical action-guides that seem pertinent to this inquiry include the following:

1. *Informed consent*—A moral rule supporting Mrs. Billings' right to be informed and freely choose whether to take the metronidazole in relation to other available options.
2. *Respect for the patient–professional relationship*—This rule addresses Dr. Ford's obligation to support the professional relationship between Mrs. Billings and Dr. Meyers. It also requires Dr. Ford to respect her own professional relationship with the patient. Increasingly, professionals within all health care professional groups are interpreting this ethical rule to define their obligation to the patient as primary. Such an interpretation represents a departure for many health care providers from a historical orientation of their primary obligation being to the physician.

3. *Veracity*—Addresses Dr. Ford's responsibility to tell the truth to Mrs. Billings. This may be considered a basic principle of obligation within deontological theory, or a useful rule within consequentialist theory (to the extent that it promotes good).

4. *Nonmaleficence*—A basic principle of consequentialist theory that would base a decision to divulge information on minimizing the potential for harm.

5. *Beneficence*—This consequentialist principle would base the decision regarding what information to divulge on the potential to promote good. Beneficence and nonmaleficence can be considered together in judging the ethical response to Dr. Ford's dilemma.

Dr. Ford must consider the potential benefits of the prescribed therapy for Mrs. Billings, and address the potential harm resulting from exposure of her infant to the metronidazole. Consideration of other available alternatives for therapy is also pertinent. Frequently such consideration takes place, at least initially, in the face of inadequate and conflicting information. Dr. Ford will also need to decide what constitutes harm and good for Mrs. Billings versus all others who may be affected.

6. *Fidelity/reciprocity*—A principle of obligation to an ethical covenant between Dr. Ford and Mrs. Billings (within deontological theory), which may suggest a requirement for full disclosure of information. However, to the extent that this covenant asks that each party take on certain responsibilities and give up certain rights in order to achieve specific good outcomes, full disclosure of potentially harmful information may not be required. For instance, if Dr. Ford were concerned that Mrs. Billings may decide to forgo any treatment, this could have strong potential of negative consequences for both Mrs. Billings and her infant.

7. *Justice*—This principle is considered of intrinsic value within certain deontological theories, and addresses Mrs. Billings' (and other affected parties') right to be given what is due—entitlement to information may be considered justice in this case. Certainly, Dr. Ford's time and expertise might be legitimately considered due to her patient.

8. *Autonomy*—This principle is directly applicable to Dr. Ford's dilemma, as was the related rule of informed consent, based on a belief in Mrs. Billings' right to decide on issues that primarily affect her. The principle of autonomy has support within both deontological (as an intrinsic good) and consequentialist (if it is likely to promote good consequences) theories. However, competing interests (for example, Mrs. Billings' and her child's), and the individual's capability to be truly autonomous (for example, the infant in this case), are factors that often complicate the application of this principle in medical ethics.

The reader may believe that other ethical rules or principles are pertinent to this case. If so, they should also be considered the analysis proceeds.

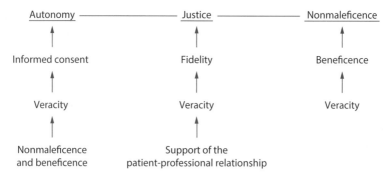

Figure 11–2.

Step #3 How should these rules and principles be ranked or balanced against each other in order to resolve the ethical dilemma?

- This step may sometimes be accomplished rather easily through the use of moral intuition. At other times, careful consideration of ethical theory can suggest the more fundamental action-guides to be applied. In some cases, it may be necessary to balance similarly weighted principles against each other, identifying when the weight of one versus another might be considered greater.

    The rules and principles that Dr. Ford considers pertinent to her dilemma over how to respond to Mrs. Billings' inquiry could be ranked as shown in Figure 11–2.

SUMMARY

- In the case of Dr. Ford and Mrs. Billings, autonomy, justice, and nonmaleficence could be considered the primary principles that must be balanced against each other. Autonomy and justice are both valued principles within various deontological theories. Nonmaleficence and beneficence are the cornerstone principles of consequentialist theory. The principle of justice also seems to be inherent in the contract theory of medical ethics described by Veatch.[2] The other relevant rules and principles above support these primary principles and inform how they apply to specific ethical dilemmas. The Code of Ethics for Pharmacists (see Appendix 11–1) approved in 1994 provides further support for these fundamental principles and clearly indicates that Dr. Ford's primary obligation is to Mrs. Billings rather than to Dr. Meyers.[16,17] It may be surmised that all of the fundamental principles seem to support honestly discussing the benefits and risks of the therapy with the patient. However, if there were no good alternative therapies for Mrs. Billings' infection, and Dr. Ford was concerned that probable nonadherence constituted a greater risk to her and/or her baby, the decision would become more difficult. Once Dr. Ford has considered the facts of the case, who will be affected by her action, the cultural perspectives and legal requirements for the affected parties, and the relevant action-guides, she should have more clarity on what constitutes the ethical action. Finally, Dr. Ford's personal beliefs and values relative to these principles of patient autonomy, promotion of justice, and the importance of potential consequences will all affect her ultimate ethical decision. It must be emphasized that she will make some response, even if only by avoiding the patient's question.

It is not likely that all will agree on the provided ranking or balancing of the pertinent rules and principles in this case, nor will there be universal agreement about what constitutes the right resolution to the ethical dilemma presented. It is necessary to remember that an ethical issue has been defined as one where most agree that there is a right answer, but cannot always agree on what that answer is.

Example Case 11–2

(MESO LEVEL CASE)

Drs. Chalmers, Bristow, and Harold are a physician, a nurse practitioner and a pharmacist, respectively. The practitioners are working for a multinational pharmaceutical company, as members of a project team, along with advertising, communications, legal, and technical production staff. The team has just been brought together and charged to prepare two versions of an education and promotion piece for a new cardiac combination product. The information piece is targeted toward prescribers. One version will meet the U.S. Food and Drug Administration (FDA) guidance on drug promotion rules by including a description of safety issues. The other version, for use in India which has more loosely monitored guideline adherence, will omit all safety information.

■ ANALYSIS

Step #1 Identification of relevant background information

A. Factual details of the issue at hand

During project group discussion, and based on their research, the health care professional members of the work group clarify their understanding of the current U.S. FDA guidance on drug promotion,[32,33] and World Health Organization (WHO) criteria for ethical medicinal drug promotion that are available to the world community.[34] They confirm that the FDA educates health care professionals about what constitutes misleading prescription drug promotion, and takes action in response to complaints about instances of nonadherence with promotion guidelines in the United States.[35] The health professionals of the project group also review two recent published reports analyzing compliance with

WHO guidelines in India.[36,37] It appears from this research and an earlier Indian study[38] that there has been an ongoing history of wide noncompliance with the WHO guidelines among companies marketing drugs in India.

B. Identification of who is affected by any ethical issue considered to be present. As these drug information developers work on creating this information/promotion piece, it is again helpful to consider who might be impacted by the information they do/do not provide.

Certainly the medical professionals prescribing the promoted drugs will be impacted in their ability to make evidence-based decisions on appropriate use of the drug, as well as in their credibility over time, if their prescribing practices are found to be deficient. Furthermore, the prescriber's patients may be impacted to the extent that lack of full knowledge of the drug's benefits and potential harms negatively affects the outcomes of their therapy. A 2007 report from Australia[39] also notes that the cost of drugs prescribed by physicians increased for those who gave more attention to drug promotion information from pharmaceutical sales representatives. This suggests the potential for society in general to be negatively impacted by drug promotion materials that encourage prescribing of higher cost drugs, as well as the potential for lost productivity from workers who do not gain optimal disease state management.

C. Consideration of the cultural perspectives of all those affected by the dilemma

The professional and cultural perspectives of both the project team professionals and the targeted prescribers must be considered, as well as the overall cultural norms of populations in the two countries.

The health professionals confronting this potential ethical dilemma will need to address the cultural and professional standards and codes that they have subscribed to as licensed members of their professions. Indeed, it might be argued that these standards, in addition to their clinical experience, are reasons for their presence on this work group. These norms may be different in India versus the United States with respect to prescriber use and dependence on promotional materials as a main source of information about new drugs available for prescribing. A 2009 report[40] evaluating drug promotional materials in Nepal commented that "unbiased and current drug references were not available in most clinical facilities for healthcare professionals," suggesting impacts of this lack resulting in use of irrational combinations of drugs, overuse of antibiotics, and other inappropriate prescribing. The typically wide gap in social and educational status between the medical practitioner in India and his or her patients may also result in a greater tendency to follow the physician's directions without question. By comparison, in the United States, attitudes are often quite different, and there is also greater access for the patient to secondary sources of information. These factors may all lead to somewhat greater risk of negative impacts felt by prescribers and patients in a country where provided promotional materials are incomplete and even misleading, but may be the only written drug information available.

D. Consideration of the level of decision making involved in responding to any ethical dilemma recognized by the DI practitioners.

This author designated the case above as one involving a meso level of ethical decision making by the concerned practitioners, because the activities involve workers within one specific drug manufacturing company. When considering the wide reach of actions taken by this group across the greater organizational system of the multinational company, and the multiple countries where the system operates, some might also appropriately judge this to involve a macro level of decision making.

Step #2 Identification and justification of the relevant moral rules and principles (action-guides) pertinent to the case at hand

Some might claim that the charge of this work group is wholly about advertising and marketing of a product, and as such claims no particular ethical demand on the producers of the advertising piece. Such an interpretation would require an assessment of the company's and the professional's obligations to the WHO Guidelines, as well as other governmental and professional guidelines on drug information. There appears to be fairly clear ethical issues for these health care professionals, as they consider their roles in determining content of the planned promotional material. A brief listing of a few ethical rules and principles is provided below that should probably be considered by them as they consider their ethical responsibilities in preparation of this material.

1. *Veracity*—Does this basic principle of obligation within deontological theory constitute a duty for these professionals, impelling them to advocate for complete and truthful information to be provided, in keeping with WHO guidelines? Within consequentialist theory, veracity also holds value as an ethical rule to the extent that it promotes better prescribing by the medical professionals using the promotional materials.

2. *Nonmaleficence*—A basic principle of consequentialist theory that would base a decision to divulge more complete and accurate information on minimizing the potential for harm. This principle appears to have relevance for the project group professionals to consider.

3. *Justice*—This principle within certain deontological theories addresses whether it is just to provide a higher level of educational content only subject to enforced regulation and guidelines, without regard to possible innate rights of access to such information by healthcare providers and patients in a country with less stringent safety protections. Basic fairness would seem to be relevant when the more informative and complete materials are being prepared and could perhaps be made available without a great deal of additional cost or effort.

The reader is encouraged to consider other ethical rules and principles that may apply to this case, as well as thinking about what seems to be a general tendency by some to dismiss the professional and ethical obligations of licensed health care professionals producing such materials for advertising purposes.

Step #3 How should these rules and principles be ranked or balanced against each other in order to resolve the ethical dilemma?

The reader should consider these rules and principles, as well as any others considered pertinent, in order to reach his or her own conclusions about the professionals' ethical responsibilities to the ultimate beneficiaries (or victims) of these information services. How does one think he or she would view his or her role and responsibilities if he or she were a health professional providing drug information in circumstances such as these? How might one's views be affected if the work group was producing direct-to-consumer advertising materials for this product?

SUMMARY

The reader is encouraged to apply this process of analysis to two additional case scenarios, found in Case Studies 11–1 and 11–2 of this chapter. Imagine a set of circumstances that might provide the background context behind each case, and carry out an ethical analysis in light of this context. The reader might perhaps then vary some important aspect of the background context to determine whether this affects the analysis of the ethical dimensions of the case. As each case is considered, also assess at what level of health care (micro, meso, or macro) does the ethical decision making seem to apply?

Case Study 11–1

A nurse on one of the medical-surgical units of your hospital calls you, the on-call nurse specialist who is a member of the hospital's pain management team, with a question. She has a patient who she believes is being undertreated for pain. He is a young man who was admitted from the emergency room (ER) the previous evening after a motorcycle accident. He is a frequent patient in the ER, known to have a drug problem, with use of a variety of street products. She does not believe that he is in withdrawal, but does think he is getting inadequate pain medications for the severe bruises, scrapes, and a broken leg. However, the admitting physician (coincidentally, the rather testy Chair of the Medical

Staff) is quite adamant that he will not enable the patient's drug habit, and maintains that perhaps living with some pain will encourage the patient to mend his ways. The nurse asks you to intervene with the physician to convince him that additional pain therapy is indicated, medically and ethically, for this patient.

- *Assess whether this drug information request constitutes a potential ethical dilemma, based on the three characteristics that differentiate such a situation.*
- *What background information might you want to obtain to clarify this information request? (Imagine a background with details that might establish this as an ethical dilemma for you.)*
- *If you can imagine this scenario to constitute an ethical dilemma for the pain management nurse, identify whether you consider it a situation requiring decision making at a micro, meso, or macro level.*
- *If, as a practitioner, this question constitutes an ethical dilemma, consider what moral rules and principles are likely to apply to this issue.*
- *Assuming that some of these relevant action-guides conflict with others describe further deliberations by which the clinician might prioritize or balance these conflicts in order to reach a decision on how to respond to the information request.*
- *What organizational strategies might best prepare this nurse specialist to most effectively respond to ethical dilemmas such as this one?*

Refer to the article *Ethical dilemmas: Controversies in pain management* by Janet Brown to read the analysis of a similar case.[60]

Case Study 11–2

Dr. Rich, who develops drug information materials for a managed care organization, is asked to review and strongly encouraged to recommend a policy to routinely deny coverage for an expensive drug therapy that has been used on an unlabeled basis to treat a difficult medical condition.

■ ANALYSIS

- *Assess whether this drug information request constitutes a potential ethical dilemma, based on the three characteristics that differentiate such a situation.*

- *What background information might you want to obtain to clarify this information request? (Imagine a background context with details that might establish this as an ethical dilemma for you.)*
- *If you can envision this scenario to constitute an ethical dilemma for this health care professional, identify whether you consider it a situation requiring decision making at a micro, meso, or macro level.*
- *If, as a practitioner, this question constitutes an ethical dilemma, consider what moral rules and principles are likely to apply to this issue.*
- *Assuming that some of these relevant action-guides conflict with others describe further deliberations by which the clinician might prioritize or balance these conflicts in order to reach a decision on how to respond to the information request.*
- *What organizational strategies might best prepare this pharmacist to most effectively respond to ethical dilemmas such as this one?*

Resources for Use by Professionals Seeking to Learn More about Medical Ethics, as Applied to Issues Involving Provision of Drug Information

8 *Health care professionals need training, resources, and support to prepare them to effectively address the ethical dilemmas they confront.* The first goal in learning more about medical ethics should be to learn to recognize opportunities for ethical deliberation when they are confronted. Situations will arise where ethical judgments will be made that have moral consequences—with or without the conscious understanding of the parties involved. It is just as important that professionals are prepared to deal with these situations, as it is for them to learn how to address efficacy and safety concerns relative to drug therapies. This section of the chapter offers a survey of medical ethics resources that can assist practitioners who personally desire to learn how to better recognize ethical situations and how to respond to them, or who will be teaching others in formal settings or informally in the workplace.

Formal coursework, in-services, or continuing education opportunities can teach skills that will aid professionals in handling ethical dilemmas related to work responsibilities that involve provision of drug information. Thornton et al.[22] discussed what should be taught in basic ethics education that takes place within and outside the academic environment. Their review of important elements to be included in ethics education is worthwhile reading for anyone who may desire to participate in these teaching activities. They also refer the reader to other useful resources on the topic. In Davis's manual on patient–practitioner interactions, the author presents an easy-to-understand description of the stages of moral development, comparing two commonly identified models proposed by Piaget and Kohlberg.[41] This information is valuable to assist in gaining insight into one's personal moral development, as well as that of others. This workbook, published by a physical therapist for the purpose of assisting in the professional socialization process, also offers a description of moral values associated with development as a professional. The author goes on to present a framework for resolving ethical dilemmas that has similar elements to those presented in this chapter; she also provides exercises that could be readily adapted for use in various health care professionals' education or even for professional in-services. Haddad et al.[1] have provided a comprehensive guideline on pharmacy ethics course content; this is also valuable reading for those wishing to address ethics topics in continuing education of health professionals. This guideline describes examples of educational methods including case presentation and debate; scenario building, with identification and discussion of potential ethical issues; and role-playing activities. The authors indicate that such educational methods should involve group participation to conduct the analysis of sample cases for the ethical issue being discussed. Writing techniques, such as a 5-minute write exercise prior to discussion can serve to focus the participant's ideas and facilitate the resultant discussion.[42] The guideline also provides an extensive bibliography of resource materials. Two other texts, one edited by Haddad[43] and the updated second edition of *Case Studies in Pharmacy Ethics* by Veatch and Haddad,[44] provide further discussion of teaching methods and many case examples of ethical dilemmas confronted by pharmacists. Pirl[16] described the use of role-playing assignments for pharmacy students. This article also listed case scenarios that could be used in continuing education programs for any practitioners who are exploring ways to resolve ethical dilemmas arising in their provision of drug information. Smith et al.[45] have written a book on pharmacy ethics that also provides background discussion and case examples that relate to many target areas of healthcare practice, including providing responses to drug information inquiries. This resource can be very useful for various practitioners who need to address ethical issues in their particular area of practice. Case discussion activities should always respect the privacy of individual practitioners and patients who have been involved in any specific case with ethical dimensions.

Students and practitioners also require education about their ethical obligations when receiving and passing on manufacturer's drug information, whether at micro, meso, or macro levels of practice. Monaghan et al. addressed this issue in their report, Student Understanding of the Relationship between the Health Professions and the Pharmaceutical

Industry.[46] This cross-sectional survey of pharmacy, nursing, and medical students identified deficiencies in student knowledge and attitudes about ethical aspects of professional interactions with drug companies. Overreliance on potentially biased or incomplete promotional materials provided by industry representatives can lead professionals to make less than optimal therapeutic decisions or recommendations for their patients. It can also lead professional consultants or institutional leaders to recommend institution-wide (meso level) therapeutic policies such as formulary approvals that do not reflect the best available evidence. A 1994 report by Chren and Landefeld investigated associations between physician-reported interactions with drug companies and their history of requests for additions to a hospital drug formulary.[47] Physicians were 13 times more likely to request that drugs manufactured by specific companies be added to the formulary if they had met with industry representatives from that company. The FDA provides information and tools for health care professional education on what to expect in compliant product promotion literature, and guidance on reporting "Bad Ad" materials.[33,35]

As they prepare drug information, health care professionals must also be vigilant about the potential for ethical lapses such as scientific misconduct to impact the evidence available to them from the drug therapy literature. Samp et al. identified 73 drug study articles published in the general biomedical literature between 2000 and 2011 that were classified as representing scientific misconduct.[48] While learning of such publication-related ethical lapses would not inherently constitute an ethical dilemma for the drug information provider, deciding whether and how to correct faulty drug information developed from such materials might indeed constitute such a dilemma.

Information technology is an integral part of the provision of drug information by health professionals. Sometimes technology is utilized as a tool to access literature and other information sources utilized by the professional responding to an inquiry. In other cases, the professional may utilize the Internet to offer drug information to various target audiences, both professional and the lay public. Anderson and Goodman have authored a text *Ethics and Information Technology: A Case-Based Approach to a Health Care System in Transition*.[49] This text addresses many ethical issues of pertinence to health care professionals, related to both Web-based services and drug information. Case studies on topics such as provision or use of inaccurate information, conflicts of interest, issues of confidentiality and data sharing, and ethical standards that have been set for health Web sites are presented.

Poirier and Laux[50] have discussed redesign of a drug information resources course to meet the needs of nontraditional Pharm. D. students; this report describes addition of a course section where ethical issues associated with drug information questions received at the author's practice site were utilized to demonstrate how to deal with such situations. The authors utilized self-study, computer-assisted instruction, and recitations to teach the course. Published descriptions of ethical dilemmas arising during the provision of drug information may be utilized to build case discussions; these scenarios are helpful for educators of both traditional and nontraditional students, as well as for in-services aimed at practicing health professionals.[24,27-29]

Structures That Support Ethical Decision Making

Berger describes the need for an ethical covenant between the pharmacist and the patient who is being provided pharmaceutical care.[26] This term suggests an implicit contract between the client and the health care provider that broadly describes the relationship involved whenever a pharmacist provides drug information. Within this contract, the service recipient has a right to receive competently provided information as well as respectful treatment. He or she also has the obligation to provide background information needed by the pharmacist. Likewise, the provider pharmacist has the right to adequate background information (and respectful treatment as well), and the obligation to give competent, trustworthy, and caring service. Recognition of this implicit contract can occasionally suggest corrective action to resolve or avoid perceived ethical dilemmas. Such recognition is especially helpful when there has been a failure to adequately communicate, or there has been a lack of mutual respect in the interaction. Pharmacists also have a revised Code of Ethics for Pharmacists available to them since 1994, which may serve as a general guide to those obligations implicit to the patient–pharmacist relationship.[51,52] The text of this code is provided in Appendix 11–1. While specific documents will not be reviewed here, certainly other health professionals practice under Codes and Ethical Standards that apply to rules of relationship with clients who are requesting drug information among other services.

It is also important to establish organizational structures that guide and support the practitioner providing drug information (in any setting), when he or she is faced with an ethical dilemma. Some formal structures, such as ethics committees[53,54] and other policy setting bodies, are generally available in larger hospitals. Formal attention to education and anticipatory planning activities on how to address ethical conflict situations is also needed within smaller institutions, the chain pharmacy setting, or in smaller organizations such as the independent community pharmacy. A report on a survey of medicine information pharmacists, conducted in the United Kingdom, assessed perceptions of possible ethical scenarios involving lay callers, and asked about respondents' training to address such situations.[55] The authors described considerable variation in how specific scenarios were addressed, and a minority of the respondents had received training in this area. It is also imperative that pharmacists and other health professionals participate in policy setting that may affect how they are expected to practice. Both the organization and the individual practitioner have an obligation to plan in advance how they will handle situations where ethical conflict might arise, particularly relative to compliance with any policy affecting the employee's patient care obligations. A February 2004 Associated Press news story demonstrates this message very clearly (and was one source for an example case analysis presented in this chapter for the third edition of this text).[56] The story describes an incident where a pharmacist on duty at a branch of the Eckerd pharmacy chain declined to fill a prescription written for an emergency contraception product for a rape victim. (Apparently all three pharmacists on duty refused to fill the prescription or to refer the patient to someone who would fill the prescription.) One pharmacist was fired for the action by Eckerd Drugs. His stated reason for declining the prescription was that he believed the product could cause an abortion if fertilization had already occurred, expressing his unwillingness to participate in such an action. A spokesman for the Eckerd chain indicated that their employment manual was clear that their pharmacists could not decline to fill a prescription for moral or religious reasons. The pharmacist claimed that he was not aware of the policy until he was fired; his attorney protested that such a policy violated part of the Civil Rights Act. The attorney said that this act "prohibits private companies from forcing employees to do something that violates their religious beliefs." Yet, another article, *Promising, Professional Obligations, and the Refusal to Provide Service*, by Alexander maintained that the professional "may not override the obligations derived from a prior act of promising to abide by the values, norms, and procedures that define their professional roles as instantiated within a specific practice;" suggesting that the professional should leave the organization if they can not conform to the expectations of their role within that practice.[57] In practice, pharmacists and other practitioners may have to deal with a specific ethical dilemma very rapidly and alone in order to decide or act in a timely manner. Policies and procedures to inform and support the clinician in overall client interactions, and in ethical analysis and decision making, can better prepare the practitioner to address the real-life dilemmas he or she will encounter. The emergency contraception case makes it clear that practitioners must also be involved early (whatever their side in the issue) to make their voices heard during initial policy development (a meso level activity within the organization, or perhaps a macro level one if contributing to policy development for the whole profession or in law). They must also keep themselves informed about existing organizational policies in order to protect themselves and their patients. In the opinion of this author, after the fact controversy over unfamiliar policies does not serve the needs of practitioners, patients, or organizations.

Organizations can assist professionals by sponsoring the creation of explicit policies addressing certain issues that have demonstrated a history of ethical controversy. For example, in the ASHP *Guidelines on the Provision of Medication Information by Pharmacists* it is explicitly stated, "Consideration should be given to the ethical and legal aspects of responding to medication information requests."[58] In relation to the emergency contraception case mentioned above, a written policy might state that clinicians may refer questions (to another practice colleague or perhaps at a minimum back to the prescriber), where provision of an answer would violate their personal ethics. This could at least partially resolve a potential dilemma for the practitioner who has been asked to provide information that involves ethical conflict. A policy that states practitioners are not required to answer questions from a client who refuses to provide required background information could guide response in the dilemma of dealing with an unidentified client who wants to know how long amphetamine can be detected in the urine. Another policy might address adequate staffing requirements to ensure the community pharmacist has adequate time to perform counseling services. Of course, the legal and ethical rights of clients have to be recognized during development of such policies. This author believes that all health professionals, including pharmacists, should demand the right to a major role in organizational policy development that affects their practice, preferably with input from client/patient representatives. To be useful, organizational policies must be developed with attention to avoiding or at least addressing what constitutes infringement on the domain of personal ethics (such as a personal prohibition against euthanasia).

Finally, institutions engaged in the professional education of health care practitioners must provide foundational education in the area of ethics, and organizations employing these practitioners should continue this education through the use of various continuing education programs that foster increasing skills in application of ethical principles to practical decision making.[59]

Conclusion

Many health care professionals will be called on to provide drug information. On occasion, they will encounter ethical dilemmas regarding what information, if any, should be provided. It is important that the practitioner approach such moments prepared to (often quickly) identify the pertinent facts, analyze relevant points of the situation, and rank or balance the pertinent ethical rules and principles that are involved. The individual professional must recognize his or her rights and responsibilities relative to the client, to other involved individuals and populations, to society as a whole, and to any higher power to whom the practitioner feels accountable. Organizations can assist employee professionals by formal orientation on certain implicit and explicit policies. Furthermore, opportunities for deliberate study and rehearsal of important analytic steps are important to help practitioners be prepared to address ethical dilemmas that arise when providing drug information.

Self-Assessment Questions

1. Characteristics that differentiate an ethical deliberation from other decision-making endeavors include which of the following? (Choose all that apply.)
   a. The issue is universal, with any parties involved agreeing that there is a right or wrong answer.
   b. The issue has been addressed in law, with penalties identified for failure to comply with the legal directive.
   c. The welfare of all parties affected by the judgment at hand is taken into account.
   d. The issue is fundamental, with no higher standard against which to measure the rightness of the decision.

2. A physician receives a call from one of his son's friends indicating that another friend fed him several brownies earlier that evening that contained marijuana. The caller asks if this could be dangerous, but states that he is feeling all right. He then notes that he has an appointment the next day for a drug test related to a new job, and asks for the name of a chemical that he understands will interfere with tests for marijuana in the blood or urine. The physician is nearly convinced that this is a legitimate call, but feels ethical qualms about how to deal with the information request. What level of ethical decision making would this constitute?
   a. Micro level
   b. Meso level
   c. Macro level
   d. None of the above

3. Assuming you decide that the case in question #2 involving the young patient who the physician knows personally does constitute an ethical dilemma for the medical practitioner, which of the following ethical rules or principles do you think would potentially apply to the situation (check all that apply, and consider your reasons for selection; you may also want to consider whether there are any others in the chapter list that you think could apply)?
   a. Respecting the patient–professional relationship
   b. Nonmaleficence
   c. Confidentiality
   d. Justice

4. A nurse member of the local hospital's pharmacy and therapeutics committee is directed by her nursing supervisor to vote in opposition to a proposed policy

(which she currently supports) that will designate pharmacists to screen patient immunization status and provide vaccine information to patients regarding indicated immunizations. If the nurse considered this an ethical dilemma, what level of ethical decision making would this constitute?

a. Micro level
b. Meso level
c. Macro level
d. None of the above

5. A practitioner is asked by administration to present an in-service for department colleagues on a recently approved drug product that may have applicability for use in the department's target population. The clinician is expected to present a set of materials provided by the administrator. What would be a first step in determining whether this is an ethical dilemma for the presenter?

a. Considering who might be affected by the dilemma
b. Considering the cultural perspectives of those attending the presentation
c. Determining what ethical rules seem to be at play in this situation
d. Seeking the factual details relative to the content provided by the administrator

6. Based on question #5, assume the practitioner does ultimately feel that he is confronting an ethical dilemma in being asked to present drug information with which he disagrees. Which of the following organization policies might be useful to support this professional in addressing his dilemma? (Choose all choices that apply.)

a. A policy that requires supervisor approval of all educational content presented by staff professionals
b. A policy that supports staff professional's freedom to independently develop educational content of drug information provided in group settings, subject to review by designated expert reviewers
c. A policy establishing a mediation process for resolving conflict between staff professionals and administrative supervisors
d. A policy mandating education for administrative and professional staff on shared governance and professional rights and responsibilities

7. Which of the following statements are true when describing *ethics*?

a. Philosophical inquiry on the moral dimensions of human conduct.
b. The terms ethical and moral have substantially different meaning.
c. Ethics involves the study of moral development.
d. Ethics involves concrete judgments on the legal aspects of situations.

8. Ethical issues might arise around which of the following kinds of issues in relationship to the provision of drug information?
   a. Decisions by the health professional on whether to provide drug information
   b. Decisions on policies related to access to drug information
   c. Both answers in a and b may involve ethical issues
   d. Neither answer in a or b is likely to involve ethical issues

9. Identification of relevant background information when analyzing an ethical dilemma includes which of the following statements? (Choose all that apply.)
   a. Determine the applicable moral rules in the case.
   b. Determine the factual details of the issue at hand.
   c. Consider who is affected by the ethical issue.
   d. Identify the cultural perspectives of the dilemma.

10. The purposes for identifying relevant background in analyzing a potential ethical dilemma include which of the following? (Choose all that apply.)
    a. Knowledge of available background information sometimes alleviates any moral concerns about the issue.
    b. Background information typically clarifies what parties might be affected by decisions made or actions taken.
    c. Background information generally leads to resolution of a recognized ethical dilemma without further analysis.
    d. Background information normally facilitates the drug information provider in addressing the dilemma in a culturally sensitive manner.

11. A hospital hotline nurse is contacted by a patient inquiring about a medication his physician has recently prescribed for him called Obecalp (placebo spelled backwards). Which of the following moral rules or principles will likely be of most immediate concern if the nurse has any ethical qualms about this situation? (Consider whether any other rules/principles from the chapter listing might also have relevance in this case.)
    a. Beneficence
    b. Veracity
    c. Nonmaleficence
    d. Confidentiality

12. A primary care physician is told by the mother of his 5-year-old patient that she regularly gives the child ground rhino horn in order to help him grow to be a strong man. After learning more background about the situation, if this

practitioner did feel he was facing an ethical dilemma, which of the following ethical principles or rules do you think would be most pertinent to this case? (Choose all that apply, and consider your reasons.)

a. Privacy

b. Justice

c. Veracity

d. Respect for persons

13. A physician in the endocrinology department of the hospital assists with development of a report for presentation to the pharmacy and therapeutics committee that addresses the use of growth hormone in children to treat short stature. This expensive agent is frequently also in short supply. If concern over resource allocation is an ethical concern for this practitioner, which of the following action guides (rule or principle) is likely to be prioritized?

a. Nonmaleficence

b. Respecting the patient–professional relationship

c. Justice

d. Veracity

14. Educational methods intended to prepare professionals to effectively and efficiently address ethical dilemmas that might confront them in their work should include a discussion of dilemmas that occur at which of the following levels of ethical decision making?

a. Micro level

b. Meso level

c. Macro level

d. All of the levels above

15. Preparation of health care professionals in an organization to address ethical dilemmas that may occur during the course of their providing drug information should generally include (choose all that apply):

a. Learning about existing standards, guidelines, and codes intended to assist professionals in understanding their ethical responsibilities

b. Involvement of the professionals in developing policies under which they will be practicing

c. Opportunities to practice decision making to resolve ethical dilemmas through case study discussions

d. Practice in discussions about cultural perspectives that may impact judgments when addressing ethical dilemmas

REFERENCES

1. Haddad AM, Kaatz B, McCart G, McCarthy RL, Pink LA, Richardson J. Report of the ethics course content committee: curricular guidelines for pharmacy education. Am J Pharm Educ. 1993;57(Winter Suppl):34S-43S.

2. Veatch RM. Hospital pharmacy: what is ethical? (Primer). Am J Hosp Pharm. 1989;46: 109-15.

3. Wilson R, Rowan MS, Henderson J. Core and comprehensive health care services: 1. Introduction to the Canadian Medical Association's decision-making framework. Can Med Assoc. 1995;152(7):1063-6.

4. Smith L, Morrissy J. Ethical dilemmas for general practitioners under the UK new contract. J Med Ethics. 1994;20:175-80.

5. Dierchx de Casterle B, Meulenbergs T, van de Vijver L, Tanghe A, Castmans C. Ethics meetings in support of good nursing care: some practice-based thoughts. Nurs Ethics. 2002;9(6):612-22.

6. Kirby J, Simpson C. An innovative, inclusive process for meso-level health policy development. HEC Forum. 2007;19(2):161-76.

7. Martin D, Singer P. A strategy to improve priority setting in health care institutions. Health Care Analysis. 2003;11(1):59-68.

8. Pentz RD. Expanding into organizational ethics: the experience of one clinical ethics committee. HEC Forum. 1998;10(2):213-21.

9. Goold SD. Trust and the ethics of health care institutions. Hastings Cent Rep. 2001;6: 26-33.

10. Nunes R. Evidence-based medicine: a new tool for resource allocation? Med, Health Care Phil. 2003;6:297-301.

11. Coyle SL, for the Ethics and Human Rights Committee, American College of Physicians-American Society of Internal Medicine. Physician-industry relations. Part 1: Individual physicians. Ann Intern Med. 2002;136:396-402.

12. Kenny N, Joffres C. An ethical analysis of international health priority-setting. Health Care Analysis. 2007;16:145-60.

13. Ruger JP. Ethics in American Health 1: Ethical approaches to health policy. Am J Pub Health. 2008;98(10):1751-6.

14. Ruger JP. Ethics in American Health 2: An ethical framework for health system reform. Am J Pub Health. 2008;98(10):1756-63.

15. Khushf G. The case for managed care: reappraising medical and socio-political ideals. J Med Phil. 1999;24(5):415-33.

16. Pirl MA. An ethics laboratory as an educational tool in a pharmacy law and ethics course. J Pharm Teach. 1990;1(3):51-68.

17. Beauchamp TLC, Childress JF. Principles of biomedical ethics. 5th ed. New York: Oxford University Press; 2001.

18. Beauchamp TLC, Childress JF. Principles of biomedical ethics. 6th ed. New York: Oxford University Press; 2008.

19. Beauchamp TLC, Childress JF. Principles of biomedical ethics. 4th ed. New York: Oxford University Press; 1994.

20. Beauchamp TL. Principles or rules? In: Kopelman L, ed. Building bioethics. Great Britain: Kluwer Academic Publishers; 1999. p. 15-24.

21. Veatch RM. Cross-cultural perspectives in medical ethics. 2nd ed. Sudbury(MA): Jones and Bartlett Publishers; 2000.

22. Thornton BC, Callahan D, Nelson JL. Bioethics education: expanding the circle of participants. Hastings Cent Rep. 1993;23(1):25-9.

23. Veatch RM. A theory of medical ethics. New York: Basic Books Publishers; 1981.

24. Najjar TA, Al-Arifi MN, Gubara OA, Dana MH. Ethical requests received by drug and poison information center in Saudi Arabia. J Soc Adm Pharm. 2000;17(4):234-7.

25. Carrese J, Brown K, Jameton A. Culture, healing, and professional obligations. Hastings Cent Rep. 1993;15:7.

26. Berger BA. Building an effective therapeutic alliance: competence, trustworthiness, and caring. Am J Hosp Pharm. 1993;50:2399-403.

27. Arnold RM, Nissen JC, Campbell NA. Ethical issues in a drug information center. Drug Intell Clin Pharm. 1987;21:1008-11.

28. Kelly WN, Krause EC, Krowsinski WJ, Small TR, Drane JF. National survey of ethical issues presented to drug information centers. Am J Hosp Pharm. 1990;47:2245-50.

29. Schools RM, Brushwood DB. The pharmacist's role in patient care. Hastings Cent Rep. 1991;12:7.

30. Powers M, Faden R. Social justice. The moral foundations of public health and health policy. New York: Oxford University Press; 2006.

31. Bayer R, Gostin LO, Jennings B, Steinbock B, eds. Public health ethics. Theory, policy and practice. New York: Oxford University press; 2007.

32. Food and Drug Administration. Guidance for industry presenting risk information in prescription drug and medical device promotion: draft guidance [Internet]. Food and Drug Administration; 2009 [cited 2013 Oct 18]. Available from: http://www .complianceonline.com/articlefiles/FDA_Guidance_Presenting_Risk_Information_ Labels_Drugs_Devices.pdf

33. Risk information in prescription drug & medical device ads, promotional labeling—what the FDA expects [Internet]. ComplianceOnline; Nov 2011 [cited 2013 Oct 17]. Available from: http://www.complianceonline.com/ecommerce/control/articleDetail?contentId= 12737&catId=10002

34. Ethical criteria for medicinal drug promotion [Internet]. Geneva: World Health Organization; 1988 [cited 2013 Oct 18]. Available from: http://apps.who.int/medicinedocs/documents/ whozip08e/whozip08e.pdf

35. Food and Drug Administration. Bad ad program: 2011–2012 year end report [Internet]. Food and Drug Administration; Jul 2012 [cited 2013 Oct 18]. Available from: http:// www.fda.gov/Drugs/GuidanceComplianceRegulatoryInformation/Surveillance/ DrugMarketingAdvertisingandCommunications/ucm258719.htm

36. Khakhkhar T, Mehta M, Shah R, Sharma D. Evaluation of drug promotional literatures using WHO guidelines. J Pharm Negative Results [Internet]. 2013;4:33-8. Available from: http://www.pnrjournal.com/text.asp?2013/4/1/33/116770

37. Dhanaraj E, Nigam A, Bagani S, Singh H, Tiwari P. Supported and unsupported claims in medicinal drug advertisements in Indian medical journals. Indian J Med Ethics. 2011;8(3):170-4.

38. Lal A. Information contents of drug advertisements: An Indian experience. Ann Pharmacother. 1998;32:1234.

39. Spurling G, Mansfield P. General practitioners and pharmaceutical sales representatives: quality improvement research. Qual Saf Health Care. 2007;16:266-70.

40. Alam K, Shah AK, Ojha P, Palaian S, Shankar PR. Evaluation of drug promotional materials in a hospital setting in Nepal. South Med Review. 2009;2(1):2-6.

41. Davis CM. Patient practitioner interaction: an experiential manual for developing the art of health care. Thorofare (NJ): Slack; 1989.

42. Coach R. 5-minutes to monitor progress. Teaching Prof. 1991;5(9):1-2.

43. Haddad AM, ed. Teaching and learning strategies in pharmacy ethics. 2nd ed. Binghamton(NY): Pharmaceutical Products Press; 1997.

44. Veatch RM, Haddad AM. Case studies in pharmacy ethics. 2nd ed. New York: Oxford University Press; 2008.

45. Smith M, Strauss S, Baldwin HJ, Alberts KT. Pharmacy ethics. New York: Pharmaceutical Products Press; 1991.

46. Monaghan M, Galt KA, Turner P, Houghton B, Rich E, Markert R, et al. Student understanding of the relationship between the health professions and the pharmaceutical industry. Teaching and Learning in Medicine: An International Journal [Internet]. 2009;15(1):14-20. Available from: http://dx.doi.org/10.1207/S15328015TLM1501_04

47. Chren M, Landefeld C. Physicians' behavior and their interactions with drug companies: a controlled study of physicians who requested additions to a hospital drug formulary. JAMA. 1994;271:684-9.

48. Samp JC, Schumock GT, Pickard AS. Retracted publications in the drug literature. Pharmacotherapy. 2012;32(7):586-95.

49. Anderson JG, Goodman KW. Ethics and information technology: a case-based approach to a health care system in transition. New York: Springer-Verlag; 2002.

50. Poirier TL, Laux R. Redesign of a drug information resources course: responding to the needs of nontraditional PharmD students. Am J Pharm Educ. 1997;61:306-9.

51. Vottero LD. Code of ethics for pharmacists. Am J Health Syst Pharm. 1995;52:2096-131.

52. American Pharmacists Association. Code of ethics 1994 [Internet]. [updated Oct 27, 1994 Mar 26, 2010]. Available from: http://www.pharmacist.com/code-ethics

53. Mappes TA, Zembaty JS, eds. Biomedical ethics. 3rd ed. New York: McGraw-Hill; 1991.

54. Mappes TA, Degrazia D, eds. Biomedical ethics. 5th ed. Boston: McGraw-Hill; 2001.

55. Wills S, Brown D, Astubry S. A survey of ethical issues surrounding supply of information to members of the public by hospital pharmacy medicines information centres. Pharm World Sci. 2002;24(2):55-60.

56. Austin L. Emergency contraception denial raises moral, legal issues. Associate Press State and Local Wire. 2004.
57. Alexander JK. Promising, professional obligations, and the refusal to provide service. HEC Forum. 2005;17(3):178-95.
58. American Society of Health-System Pharmacists. ASHP guidelines on the provision of medication information by pharmacists. Am J Health Syst Pharm. 1996;53:1843-5.
59. Gettman DA, Benson B, Nguyen V, Luu SN, eds. Use of motivational techniques by drug information center personnel to respond to calls involving perceived ethical dilemmas [Abstract]. ASHP Midyear Clinical Meeting; 2000.
60. Brown J. Ethical dilemmas: controversies in pain management. Adv Nurse Pract. 1997: 69-72.

SUGGESTED READINGS

1. Wills S, Brown D, Astbury S. A survey of ethical issues surrounding supply of information to members of the public by hospital pharmacy medicines information centres. Pharmacy World and Science (Netherlands). 2002;24(Feb):55-60.
2. Kelly WN, Krause EC, Krowsinski WJ, Small TR, Drane JF. National survey of ethical issues presented to drug information centers. Am J Hosp Pharm. 1990;47:2245-50.
3. Beauchamp TLC, Childress JF. Principles of biomedical ethics. 6th ed. New York: Oxford University Press; 2008.
4. Veatch RM, Haddad A. Case studies in pharmacy ethics. 2nd ed. New York: Oxford University Press; 2008.
5. Ethical criteria for medicinal drug promotion [Internet]. Geneva: World Health Organization; 1988 [cited 2013 Oct 18]. Available from: http://apps.who.int/medicinedocs/documents/whozip08e/whozip08e.pdf

12

Chapter Twelve

Pharmacy and Therapeutics Committee

Patrick M. Malone • Nancy L. Fagan • Mark A. Malesker
• Paul J. Nelson

Learning Objectives

After completing this chapter, the reader will be able to

- Describe the pharmacy and therapeutics (P&T) committee.
- Define the functions of the P&T committee.
- Describe attributes and structure of a P&T committee likely to promote its ability to function successfully.
- Describe where and how the P&T committee fits into the organizational structure of a health care institution or other groups.
- Describe how the pharmacy department participates in P&T committee activities.
- Describe and explain the concepts of drug formularies and drug formulary systems, and how pharmacy participates in their establishment and maintenance.
- Describe how P&T committee activities contribute to the quality improvement of medication use.
- Describe how to develop policies and procedures for the process of medication use.

Key Concept

❶ A **pharmacy and therapeutics (P&T) committee**, or its equivalent, oversees all aspects of medication use within an institution.
❷ Although it is common for pharmacists to downplay or misunderstand the importance of P&T committee support in comparison to other clinical activities, such support is vital for pharmacy to impact patient care.

❸ A P&T committee may find it necessary to create ad hoc committees to address various issues, depending on their complexity and size.

❹ Typically, P&T committee functions include determining what drugs are available, who can prescribe specific drugs, policies and procedures regarding drug use (including pharmacy policies and procedures, clinical protocols, standard order sets, and clinical guidelines), performance improvement as well as quality assurance activities (e.g., drug utilization review/drug usage evaluation/medication usage evaluation, as well as compliance surveillance), adverse drug reactions/medication errors, dealing with product shortages, and education in drug use.

❺ A variety of topics regarding the quality of medication use, inclusive of applicable medication metrics, are normally part of the activities of a P&T committee.

Introduction

When considering how a pharmacist can have an impact on a patient's drug therapy, it is common to consider the individual practitioner dealing with a specific patient or, perhaps, a small group of patients. Certainly the clinician can have a deep impact this way, but it does have the disadvantage of dealing with a very limited number of patients. In order for pharmacists to efficiently impact a population of patients, a different approach is necessary. Fortunately, pharmacists have the opportunity to participate in the activities of ❶ *a P&T committee or its equivalent, which generally oversees all aspects of medication use in an institution.* Physicians and pharmacists have collaborated to implement cost-effective prescribing practices and assess clinical outcomes through educational initiatives, administrative programs to restrict ordering practices, use of formularies and prescribing guidelines, and financial incentives.[1] There are data to show that P&T committee actions are useful.[2,3]

Before proceeding, it must be stated that while this chapter deals with the P&T committee, which is usually the group responsible for overseeing all aspects of drug therapy in an institution, there is sometimes a similar body referred to as the formulary committee. This latter group deals strictly with determining which drugs are carried within an institution or organization, whereas the P&T committee has numerous other tasks, covering all aspects of drug therapy (e.g., adverse drug reaction [ADR]/medication error monitoring, quality assurance, policy and procedure approval), although the exact group of functions may vary from place to place.[4] Some institutions use a formulary committee, since other bodies may perform the additional P&T committee tasks described later in this chapter. Also, some health care groups may use both committees, with one body addressing the issues for the group as a whole, while the other is located separately at various institutions to address issues specific to that location (e.g., only one institution in the group has an oncology unit, therefore, the committee for that individual institution will consider specific antineoplastic agents that are not of much use for the rest of the group). In this chapter, anything discussed regarding which drugs are available within an institution or group applies to both bodies, whereas all other items are for the P&T committee only.

It should be noted that while P&T committees have normally been associated with institutional pharmacy, other organizations have increasingly used P&T-type committees in an attempt to improve drug therapy while lowering costs. Some places where such committees are seen include **managed care organizations (MCOs)**,[5] insurance companies, pharmacy benefit management (PBM) companies, unions, employers,[6] state Medicaid boards, state departments of public institutions,[7] Medicare,[8] long-term care facilities,[9] ambulatory clinics,[10] and even community pharmacies.[11] Much of this chapter will use examples from institutional pharmacy and managed care, simply because much of the published literature deals with those areas of practice and it is the most likely setting in which a pharmacist will be directly involved in P&T committee activities. However, the concepts covered are applicable to any P&T-type committee and comply with recommendations of the American Medical Association (AMA),[12,13] the American Society of Health-System Pharmacists (ASHP),[14] The Joint Commission (formerly the Joint Commission for the Accreditation of Health Care Organizations) (TJC),[15] and the Academy of Managed Care Pharmacy (AMCP).[16]

The role of the P&T committee has been continuously expanded over the years and now encompasses a great number of functions and activities that cover all aspects of overseeing drug therapy. As some of these are of sufficient size and importance, they are covered separately in other chapters (e.g., drug monographs and quality assurance). In addition, there are a number of areas (e.g., investigational drugs) in which P&T committees play a secondary role, and these too are covered in other chapters. This chapter will serve to provide a base to tie together discussion of all of these areas and a number of smaller functions or activities that will be covered as a portion of this chapter. The information is appropriate both for those just learning about the concepts and also for those individuals who are involved with P&T committee activities.

Organizational Background

The concept of a P&T committee represents a unique niche within the structure of a hospital or hospital system. The current role of a hospital in Western countries[17] began about 200 years ago, at a time when very few efficacious medications were available, although drug formularies had been developed during the Revolutionary War to list the drugs available.[18] It has also been noted that a **drug formulary** was developed for all municipal hospitals in New York City at Bellevue Hospital in 1868.[19] Drug formularies were required for participation in the Medicare program in 1965.[20] The original hospital was a place to receive basic health care when a person had no extended family to provide the basic needs of good health. After infection control became a recognized concept and anesthesia for surgery evolved around 1900, the value of the modern hospital progressively became a recognized need for all segments of society. The origins for standards of how a hospital functioned subsequently developed during the first half of the twentieth century. This began with the early efforts of the American College of Surgeons in the United States (U.S.) to develop the first accreditation standards for hospitals. Later, the Joint Commission on Accreditation of Hospitals (JCAH), now known as TJC, evolved to centralize the basic requirements for the functional character of a U.S. hospital. The concept of the P&T committee originated and evolved to help hospitals meet various standards regarding drug therapy. The first P&T committee was formed at Bellevue Hospital in New York City in the mid-1930s.[18,21] While it dealt with true compounding formulas, it was originally founded to ensure quality and efficacy of those products, which is still a portion of the functions of P&T committees.

In keeping with the social origins of the hospital, the legally sanctioned or licensed privilege of being a professional health care provider evolved.[17] Both the physician and pharmacist were considered unique for the needs of society. Minimum standards evolved, including the accreditation of their training as a basis for being licensed. Originally, physicians and pharmacists functioned primarily as independent professionals. The nature of a physician's independence was legally defined to further support their obligations to a patient. Many states in the United States legally prohibited a physician from being employed by a corporation. Eventually, these laws were all repealed, but they had the effect of creating the basis for a medical staff as being a separate legal entity within a hospital. The medical staff reflected the legally evolving traditions of a physician, and indirectly the pharmacist, as being independent professionals committed only to the care of a patient without unnecessary outside influences. This evolution has had a major impact on the organizational structure of hospitals.

A typical hospital organization is shown in Figure 12–1. The board of directors divides the functions of its organization into two entities. First, the administration of the hospital operates as a typical business with a chief executive officer, chief operating officer, and so forth. Second, the board of directors authorizes that a medical staff be formed that reports separately to the board of directors. While the medical staff as a whole is ultimately in charge of all clinical aspects of care in the hospital, in most institutions this is unworkable without an administrative structure of some kind. Therefore, the medical staff may elect officers and either elect or appoint somebody to oversee all aspects of patient care. In this example, the term **medical executive committee** is used for that body, although the name and exact function may vary. The medical staff functions to certify the

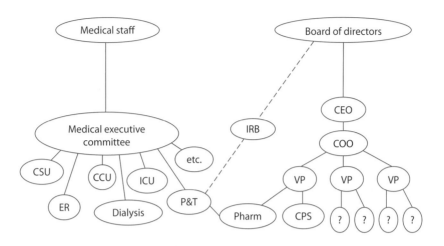

CCU	Coronary Care Unit Committee
CEO	Chief Executive Officer
COO	Chief Operating Officer
CPS	Central Processing & Supply
CSU	Cardiac Surgery Unit Committee
ER	Emergency Room Committee
ICU	Intensive Care Unit Committee
IRB	Institutional Review Board
Pharm	Pharmacy Department
P&T	Pharmacy & Therapeutics Committee
VP	Vice President
?	Other Hospital Departments

Figure 12–1. Hospital organization.

credentials of its members, establish their scope of practice where appropriate, monitor the quality of health care provided by its members, and maintain the means to collaborate with the administration of the hospital.

In modern medicine, there are so many clinical areas to consider that it is unrealistic for one committee to adequately oversee all aspects of patient care, except in very small institutions. For this reason, various subcommittees of the medical executive committee are usually necessary, as can be seen in Figure 12–1. As a means to coordinate the needs of the medical staff and the operation of the hospital pharmacy, the modern P&T committee developed. From the traditions established by TJC and ASHP, the P&T committee developed as a function of the medical staff's responsibilities. This committee or related committees may have other names, such as the drug and therapeutics committee in other countries,[22,23] but the functions are the same. While the P&T committee has been referred to in TJC accreditation standards in the past, it is no longer specifically required and may be replaced by some other committee or body,[15,24,25] although the P&T committee concept is supported by many national and professional organizations.[26] Given the continuing growth in the number, complexity, and expense of medications, both the importance and number of functions of the P&T committee have continued to increase. Policy and procedures to set up a P&T committee are described in Appendix 12–1, but the following will serve as a general description of P&T committees and their actions.

In some cases, the P&T committee may be part of a corporation of hospitals and medical centers, rather than just being for a specific institution. While the philosophy of operating one P&T committee within this corporate structure seems reasonable, this is not often accomplished without problems and decentralization of these efforts may be better.[27] Different patient populations, medication needs, cross hospital physician participation, meeting time, length and location of meetings, and differing clinical cultures within a specific institution are examples of barriers that may be present. The P&T model may need to be revised to work with these challenges.[28-33]

Although it is easy to assume from its name that the P&T committee is organizationally a part of the pharmacy department, such is not the case, as was mentioned above. Instead, it is usually a medical staff entity and, perhaps, only one or two pharmacists may actually be members of the committee (possibly *ex officio* members without voting privileges). Commonly, the pharmacy director or clinical coordinator, serving as the committee's secretary (e.g., taking minutes, collating, and arranging the agenda), may be the sole official pharmacy representative. Other pharmacists may also attend to act as consultants to the committee, often having great impact on the committee's decisions, even if they cannot officially vote. Fortunately, in larger hospitals, it appears that more pharmacists are now becoming full members of the P&T committee.[34]

Typically, the voting members of an institutional P&T committee are limited to members of the medical staff, although there may be a few voting or nonvoting members from other groups, including pharmacy. Membership is mostly physicians (preferably a wide variety of physicians from various areas of practice), but usually includes at least one pharmacist and often members from other areas of the hospital (e.g., nursing, administration, radiology, respiratory therapy, dietary, quality assurance, medical records, laboratory, and risk management).[35] A pharmacoeconomist also can be extremely helpful. There have also been recommendations to include other individuals, such as a medical ethicist or community pharmacist.[36] It may be best to try to keep down the number of physician members to encourage a smaller group to participate more fully, while taking care of addressing the wide variety of issues by calling in physicians to consult with the committee on an as needed basis.[37] In some cases, the pharmacy department is asked to recommend physicians for the committee. If possible, pharmacy should suggest physicians who are noted for their commitment to rational drug therapy.[38] As an example, the U.S. Department of Defense has procedures for appointment of members, including nonphysician members, of the P&T committee. The procedures are available on the Internet.[39] Also, efforts should be made to ensure that the physician chosen to be chairman of the committee is an advocate of the pharmacy department. It is possible for the medical executive committee of the medical staff to pass a resolution to approve a policy broadening the voting members of the P&T committee (e.g., director of pharmacy or hospital vice president) or delegating the functions of the P&T committee to the hospital. In this latter arrangement, the medical staff would reserve the right to terminate the policy if the P&T committee fails to support the needs of the medical staff. If the P&T committee is a hospital committee, rather than medical staff committee, a pharmacist or nurse might more easily obtain voting privileges, given appropriate physician quorum requirements in the authorizing policy.

The P&T committee of MCOs and government bodies often have similar membership to that in institutional committees; however, there may need to be a requirement for at least some of the members to be independent practitioners and retail pharmacists (i.e., having no financial ties to the organization or group that sponsors the P&T committee).[35,40,41] In accordance with the 2003 Medication Modernization Act, the use of formularies is an essential component to the PBM.[35]

Once the general organizational setting of the P&T committee has been determined, the operating policy of the P&T committee requires careful attention to two key issues. The first key issue is obvious—to whom does the P&T committee report and to what degree can the decisions of the P&T committee be overturned by another segment of the organization? It is important to point out that the P&T committee may act only as an advisory body to the medical executive committee. Decisions of the P&T committee may not be considered final (and, therefore, not be implemented) until they are reviewed and approved by the medical executive committee. In this situation, a report is forwarded from the P&T committee after each meeting to the medical executive committee. In addition, an annual report of the P&T committee may be prepared for both internal review and review by the medical executive committee. This annual report is time consuming in preparation, but is a very important means of tracking P&T activities and action over time.

The second issue is that the P&T committee will likely be successful based on the leadership qualities of its members and the chairperson. The role of the chairperson includes developing the respect and involvement of all members of the committee.

PHARMACY BENEFIT MANAGEMENT (PBM) P&T COMMITTEE ORIGIN

The origin of the PBM organizations dates back to the late 1960s. Their primary focus was on claims administration for insurance companies. Later, it became a challenge for the insurance companies to efficiently manage the increase in drug coverage in the private sector when the prescription volume was high and the cost per claim was low.[42] The plastic drug benefit card began in the 1970s and changed the way many prescriptions were bought and paid for by the insurance company and employee. From then on, any employee with an ID card, using a pharmacy network, only had a small copayment.[42] In addition, administrative costs for the **third-party payer**, whether it is the insurance company, health plan, or employer, were reduced, with the PBM creating pharmacy networks and mail service benefits. Pharmacy networks are a group of pharmacies that are under contract with the insurance company, health plan, and/or their contracted PBM partner to promote prescription services at a negotiated discounted fee.[43] Mail service is a program offered by the PBM, whereby pharmaceutical agents, both prescription and nonprescription, are offered through the mail.[43]

In the late 1980s, the introduction of real-time electronic claims processing began. Not only was there two-way communication between the pharmacy and the PBM for claim processing, but also for clinical information. In the 1990s, the PBMs moved toward a greater emphasis on patient health by offering a variety of new services in addition to the claims processing. Since 2000, there has been an emphasis on consumer behavior modification, enhanced patient interventions, physician connectivity, clinical consulting, disease management, and retrospective drug utilization review (DUR; see Chapter 14 for further information) to name a few.[42]

One of the key functions of a PBM is to design, implement, and administer outpatient drug benefit programs for employers, MCOs, and other third-party payers. PBMs manage prescription drug benefits separate from other health care services (i.e., physician and hospital services).[43] Determining which medications are most cost-effective, without compromising patient care, is one of the key elements for controlling the cost of a prescription drug benefit.[6,44] PBMs accomplish this by developing drug formularies.[6] Formularies define what medications are covered (i.e., paid for) and provide the main component of the pharmacy benefit. Specific PBM drug payment and management activities occur within this formulary structure, such as therapeutic interchange and disease management programs. Eighty to one hundred percent of PBM-covered lives receive some type of formulary management service.[6,43] The use of drug formularies is in flux due to the advantages and disadvantages identified over the last decade or so; however, they are likely to be continued for at least the foreseeable future, particularly due to the Medicare drug formulary requirements.[45]

Development and maintenance of drug formularies for third-party payers is an ongoing process. The formulary must be continuously updated to keep pace with new drugs, therapies, prices, recent clinical research, changes in medical practice, evidence-based treatment guidelines, and updated Food and Drug Administration (FDA) information.[46] PBMs use a panel of experts called the P&T committee to develop and manage their drug formularies. Many times individuals with special clinical expertise are consulted when considering medications within a specific therapeutic class.[46] Meetings are usually held on a quarterly basis, and not only are drug formulary recommendations made, but this group also provides input into other clinical areas, such as development of disease management programs.[6,42,43,45,46]

Many PBMs establish their own P&T committee to evaluate the efficacy, safety, uniqueness, cost of therapeutic equivalent drugs, and other appropriate criteria. In addition, PBMs work with the health plan, employer, or insurance company P&T committee to develop drug formularies using the same evaluation process. In either case, if the P&T committee determines that one drug provides a clear medical benefit over the other, therapeutically equivalent drugs in that same therapeutic category, the drug is usually added to the formulary.[6] However, if there are drugs in the same therapeutic category that have very similar efficacy and safety profiles and no unique properties that would make it a better drug, then the net cost becomes a deciding factor as to which drug should be added to the formulary.[6] There has been some discussion as to whether drug costs are weighted too heavily, while drug efficacy and other clinical information is weighted too lightly when it comes to drug formulary decisions.[42,43] The committee leadership needs to recognize the potential for conflicts of interest between efficacy and economic interests of the PBM and to establish collaboration as the basis for resolving conflicts that arise.

Me-too drugs are drugs that are structurally very similar to an already known drug that has only minor differences. Many drugs come in two versions: an L-isomer (left) and an R-isomer (right). An example of a me-too drug is esomeprazole (Nexium®), the L-isomer of omeprazole (Prilosec®, the R- and L-isomers). Both drugs are used to treat gastroesophageal reflux disease (GERD). When a comparative analysis was conducted looking at drugs approved for marketing between January 2007 and July 2008, those that had a different chemical entity and a separate mechanism of action accounted for 69%; however, they offered no clinical improvement over those already on the market. Forty-four percent offered some type of new convenience, but only 13% offered greater efficacy.[47]

In the case of a health plan, employer, or insurance company's own P&T committee, the drug formulary recommendations made by the PBM P&T committee are presented and reviewed by the organization's P&T committee. The PBM recommendations regarding drug formulary recommendations can be either accepted or denied by the organization's P&T committee and the organization's own decision made regarding formulary inclusion.

Pharmacy Support of the P&T Committee

❷ *Although it is not uncommon for pharmacists to downplay or misunderstand the importance of P&T committee support in comparison to other clinical activities, such support is vital for pharmacy to impact patient care.* P&T committee support and participation can have far-reaching effects on the overall quality of drug therapy in an institution and must be given a great deal of attention, since the benefits of its function serves to build collaboration, transparency, and trust among the institutional divisions of authority for drug therapy within health care. While such attention is time consuming,[48] it can be of value to the pharmacy since this is an opportunity to present recommendations to a decision-making body and P&T committees often accept pharmacy recommendations[49,50]; therefore, pharmacy departments can have a great and far-reaching impact on drug therapy through this mechanism.

Some pharmacists who participate in P&T committee activities feel they are serving their function by just providing information requested by physicians and considering drugs for formulary approval only following physician requests. This can rapidly deteriorate into crisis management, where the pharmacy department reacts to problems, fighting each fire as it occurs. It is much better for a pharmacy to be proactive,[51,52] seeking to address issues (e.g., changes in drugs carried on the formulary, new policies and procedures, quality assurance activities, and so forth) before they become problems. TJC accreditation requirements include annual evaluation of all drugs and/or drug classes.[15] Through prospective actions with the P&T committee it is possible for the pharmacy to get physician support for their clinical activities.

In the specific instance of P&T committee support, one or more pharmacists must be identified to conduct the necessary planning. This may consist of a pharmacy-based steering committee and might include administrators, purchasing agents, or clinicians, and, particularly, drug information specialists. These people must develop and regularly evaluate data sources to anticipate physicians' needs[53] (see Table 12–1). For example, it is necessary to assess what drugs have been recently FDA approved in order to identify drugs for possible formulary inclusion. FDA approval often occurs about 3 months before commercial availability and is published on the FDA Web site (http://www.accessdata.fda.gov/scripts/cder/drugsatfda/index.cfm). Therefore, there is time for the drug to be considered for formulary addition before the first orders arrive from the

TABLE 12–1. AREAS WHERE PHARMACISTS SHOULD BE SUPPORTING A PHARMACY AND THERAPEUTICS COMMITTEE

- Planning future agendas (including medications, policies and procedures, quality assurance, and other subjects to be addressed)
- Gathering data to create drug monographs and other necessary documents
- Evaluating medications for formulary adoption or deletion
- Preparing and conducting quality assurance programs (including drug usage evaluation and monitoring of adverse effects and medication errors)
- Preparing policies and procedures
- Communicating information from the P&T committee to other areas of the institution
- Creating hardcopy and electronic versions of the formulary

TABLE 12–2. FDA CLASSIFICATION BY CHEMICAL TYPE*

Type	Definition
1	New molecular entity not marketed in the United States
2	New salt, ester, or other noncovalent derivative of another drug marketed in the United States
3	New formulation or dosage form of an active ingredient marketed in the United States
4	New combination of drugs already marketed in the United States
5	New manufacturer of a drug product already marketed by another company in the United States
6	New indication for a product already marketed in the United States (Beginning in 1994, Type 6 new drug applications [NDAs] were tracked as efficacy supplements)
7	Drug that is already legally marketed without an approved NDA • First application since 1962 for a drug marketed prior to 1938 • First application for DESI (Drug Efficacy Study Implementation)-related products that were first marketed between 1938 and 1962 without an NDA • First application for DESI-related products first marketed after 1962 without NDAs. In this case, the indications may be the same or different from the legally marketed product.
8	Over-the-counter switch

*Drugs@FDA Frequently Asked Questions [Internet]. Washington, DC: Food and Drug Administration; [updated 2010 Jun 25; cited 2010 Oct 19]. Available from: http://www.fda.gov/Drugs/InformationOnDrugs/ucm075234.htm#chemtype_reviewclass

nursing units, which necessitates a review of some sort under TJC standards.[15] In a case where it is not possible to consider a drug before it is commercially available, it has been suggested by some that drugs rated P (priority) by the FDA be made available to physicians until the drug can be fully considered (the FDA classification codes are found in Tables 12–2 and 12–3, with the priority versus standard explanation found in Table 12–3).[54] This latter procedure may be effective, but considering the drug before commercial availability is preferable, because if the ultimate P&T committee decision is to leave the

TABLE 12–3. FDA CLASSIFICATIONS BY THERAPEUTIC POTENTIAL*

Type	Definition
P	Priority handling by FDA—before 1992 this was two categories: A—Major therapeutic gain B—Moderate therapeutic gain
S	Standard handling by FDA—before 1992 this was referred to as class C, which indicated the product offered only a minor or no therapeutic gain
O	Orphan drug

*Drugs@FDA Frequently Asked Questions [Internet]. Washington, DC: Food and Drug Administration; [updated 2010 Jun 25; cited 2010 Oct 19]. Available from: http://www.fda.gov/Drugs/InformationOnDrugs/ucm075234.htm#chemtype_reviewclass

drug off the drug formulary, there may be difficulties in helping physicians stop the use of the product. It is also a good idea to track older drugs. For example, the use of nonformulary drugs may be tracked within the hospital (Note: a nonformulary drug may be a product that has not been approved for use within an institution, but may also be a drug that has been approved for use, but has been prescribed in a particular situation for a use other than what was approved by the P&T committee when it was added to the drug formulary).[55-57] If patterns of increased use are noted, it is best to identify a reason for that use. If the use is inappropriate, the physician(s) should be contacted and given information about alternative formulary agents. In some cases, new information may be available showing a new advantage or use for an old agent, which can lead to its reconsideration for formulary adoption. Related to this is the necessity to regularly consider the material being promoted by the drug company representatives. It is worth mentioning that some hospitals will restrict drug representative access to the institution or restrict the drugs that may be promoted by those representatives to only items approved for use in the hospital in order to prevent this problem (see Chapter 24 for further information). There may also be new indications or other information that will increase demand for nonformulary items. If there are sufficient changes noted in the use(s) of a particular class of drugs, it is useful to review the class as a whole to decide which drug(s) are to be retained on the formulary. TJC now requires annual review of all medications,[10-15] which is useful because there may be new information (e.g., labeling changes or safety in terms of postmarketing surveillance) not otherwise noted that necessitates changes in formulary items in a particular class, both additions and deletions. However, these situations that have been noted above may necessitate moving up the review. Other items, such as trends in reported ADRs in the institution or published data for new products with little information in the literature on first approval may also be useful in determining products for P&T committee consideration or reconsideration.[58] Although there must be a mechanism by which physicians can request that drugs be added to the formulary, all of the above methods and others can help the pharmacy anticipate physician needs, allowing time for information gathering, evaluation of products, and P&T committee consideration before the need becomes too urgent to permit proper consideration.

   To guide the clinician into considering the logic of requesting the addition of items to the drug formulary, a specific request form may be useful. Items that a physician may be required to fill out or attach to the form can be seen listed in Table 12–4.[59] An example form is seen in Appendix 12–2.

   The P&T committee should be kept advised by the above-mentioned pharmacy-based steering committee of future plans, so that it can be aware that a rational planning process is governing its agenda. Also, it is a good idea for one or more representative(s) of this steering committee to meet with the pharmacy director, chairman of the P&T

TABLE 12–4. ITEMS THAT MAY BE ON A REQUEST FOR FORMULARY CONSIDERATION FORM

- Date and time of request
- Name of product (e.g., generic, brand, chemical)
- Source of product (e.g., manufacturer, distributor)
- Specific information about drug product (e.g., class of drug, mechanism, adverse effects, clinical studies)
- Anticipated use of drug (e.g., what type of patient, how often)
- Comparable drugs already on the formulary
- Why the product is needed
- What drugs could be removed from the formulary
- What restrictions, policies, cautions, etc., are necessary
- How the drug fits into any clinical guidelines
- Action requested (e.g., addition, deletion, restriction)

committee, and a representative of the hospital administration on a regular basis to assist with planning and ensure their concerns are addressed. This meeting could be held shortly before the P&T committee actually meets to present preliminary formulary evaluations, DUE material, and policy and procedure documents for an initial review, allowing modifications addressing physician and administration concerns to be made before formal committee review and action. During this meeting, plans for future months can be made or adjusted as the circumstances dictate. Other appropriate physicians or groups should also be consulted in order to ensure that their concerns are addressed. For example, if changes to the cephalosporins carried on the drug formulary or their permitted uses (e.g., restrictions to particular uses or prescribing groups) are considered, the infectious disease specialists should be contacted to provide input. (Note: This does not necessarily mean that recommendations are changed to account for physician preferences, but that their preferences and concerns are specifically addressed in the evaluation.)

Regarding quality assurance activities, the pharmacy department should obtain data to guide the selection of upcoming quality assurance programs. This will be covered in greater detail in Chapter 14.

The pharmacy should also investigate which medications need specific policies and procedures developed to guide their use and monitoring. This may be done when the drug is first being evaluated for formulary addition or later if problems (e.g., increased ADR reports, medication errors, and overuse) are noted. For example, concerns about a new thrombolytic agent leading to increased morbidity and mortality through improper use might prompt the P&T committee to approve specific protocols for the use of the agent. Policy and procedure documents are covered later in the chapter. Information on preparing policies and procedures can be found in Chapter 18.

Finally, it is extremely important for the P&T committee to make sure that physicians are informed about the actions taken. Often the pharmacy is heavily involved in providing this information to physicians. While a great deal of effort is placed on communication within the committee itself, it is also necessary to keep the entire medical staff informed. This may be accomplished through medical department meeting presentations, newsletters and Web sites (refer to Chapter 9), or other mechanisms.

AD HOC COMMITTEES

❸ *A P&T committee may find it necessary to create ad hoc committees to address various issues, depending on their complexity and size.* Some of the common committees are discussed below. Institutions may or may not use these committees (sometimes referred to as subcommittees) and their exact use varies from place to place, depending on their needs or desires.[4]

Adverse Reactions

A comprehensive ADR monitoring and reporting program is an essential component of the P&T committee (see Chapter 15 for further information about ADRs and how they are handled). A subcommittee may be helpful to review the entire ADR data for trends and any necessary actions that need to be taken. The P&T committee will usually report the ADR data on a monthly or quarterly basis. Following approval of this report, the P&T committee is responsible for the dissemination of information to the medical staff and other health professionals in the institution. This includes recommending processes to cut the rate of preventable ADRs. This subcommittee may be combined with the medication errors subcommittee.[15,60]

Anticoagulation

The anticoagulation subcommittee is responsible for policies and procedures to maintain compliance with TJC Goal 3E, now called the TJC National Patient Safety Goal 03.05.01.[15] This goal is to reduce the likelihood of patient harm associated with anticoagulation therapy. The subcommittee can also participate in improvement processes to maintain standards with quality organizations such as the National Quality Forum (NQF), and the Surgical Care Improvement Project (SCIP). Standard orders and policies to follow evidence-based guidelines of the American College of Chest Physicians (ACCP) are also developed by this subcommittee. Pharmacists have an important role on this committee. Most hospitals have pharmacists dedicated to anticoagulation monitoring and education.

Antimicrobials/Infectious Disease

Antibiotics can represent the largest category of formulary medications.[61] Frequent category review and revision is necessary and complex.[62] Cunha has defined five factors to consider when reviewing antimicrobial agents for formulary inclusion: microbiologic activity,[63] pharmacokinetics and pharmacodynamics profiles,[64] resistance patterns,[65,66] adverse effects,[67] and cost to the institution.[68] The P&T committee or a subcommittee of the P&T may be responsible for developing appropriate antibiotic selection and use in both inpatient and outpatient settings.[69,70] Some institutions may rely on input from the infection control committee regarding antibiotic formulary management and appropriate utilization. Multidisciplinary antibiotic use committees have limited inappropriate pre-scribing of antimicrobials and increased the medical staff's knowledge on appropriate antibiotic use.[68,71,72]

The main purpose of the antimicrobial/infectious disease subcommittee is to pro-mote antimicrobial stewardship to ensure cost-effective therapy and improve patient out-comes. Antimicrobial stewardship promotes and optimizes antimicrobial therapy consistent with the hospital's/health system's antibiograms. Guideline development and education is provided to the medical staff as well as to other health care professionals. The subcommittee is also involved in the enforcement of formulary agent use, substitution policies, and restrictions for antibiotics. In addition, review and feedback on prescribing patterns is provided to the medical staff regarding antibiotic therapy.[73-75] Use of P&T for-mulary and policy decisions has been shown to be successful in controlling antimicrobial use in hospitals.[76,77]

Medication Safety

A medication safety committee (sometimes called safety committee or medication mis-adventure subcommittee) should be multidisciplinary in nature. This subcommittee will review medication misadventures and medication errors that occur within the institution or health care system. They may also review adverse drug reactions (instead of an adverse reaction committee), drug–drug interactions, drug dispensing processes, medication errors (see Chapter 16 for more information), look-alike/sound-alike medications, and communication errors. It may also be appropriate for them to review protocols to improve medication safety, such as the settings for intravenous fluid pumps. A report will commonly be presented to the P&T committee on a quarterly or semiannual basis. Following approval of this report, the P&T committee is responsible for the dissemination of information to the medical staff and other health professionals in the institution. This includes recommending processes to cut the rate of preventable medication safety issues. In some places, a medication error reduction plan (MERP) is prepared to identify process improvements that have been made and those that are planned. When evaluating drug cost strategies, patient safety should always be a priority.[78] The 2013 Joint Commission Accreditation Process Guide for Hospitals addresses the potential for adverse drug events.[15] Also, as will be explained in the next chapter, patient safety will be evaluated whenever a product is considered for formu-lary addition.

Medical Devices

The P&T committee or a subcommittee may be responsible for the approval of some medical devices within an institution. This subcommittee is often multidisciplinary and is given the opportunity to review medical devices before purchases are made or contracts are signed. The committee is also responsible for reviewing the safety information associated with these devices because adverse medical device events are an important patient safety issue. Devices that contain medications, such as topical hemostats that contain thrombin, may also be reviewed by the committee or by the transfusion service committee described below.

Nutrition

As nutrition of the hospitalized patient evolved and became more complex, the role of the pharmacist on a nutrition support team became more justified. Their role started out improving the ordering process for parenteral nutrition, and communicating these changes to the pharmacy staff for proper preparation. Today, pharmacists on the nutritional team assist in the clinical management of parenteral nutrition patients, parenteral nutrition research, and continual involvement with improving the safety of parenteral nutrition use.[79] TJC, in their National Patient Safety Goals (NPSG), once addressed the safe use of parenteral nutrition feeding solutions,[80] but even though that has been removed, one of the responsibilities of the P&T committee is to oversee and approve the components of the parenteral nutrition solutions.

Quality Assurance of Medication Use

A subcommittee of the P&T committee may be placed in charge of planning and overseeing the plan for quality assurance regarding drug therapy. Details about this activity are found in Chapter 14. This committee may develop criteria for a drug use evaluation, collect the data, interpret the data, and recommend acting when necessary regarding the appropriate use of medication.

Tranfusion Service Committee

Hospitals often have a transfusion service committee charged with reviewing the use of blood and blood derivative products. Many of these products overlap with medications and may also be classified as medications. Therefore, it is necessary for this type of committee to work with or, possibly, be combined with the P&T committee in order to oversee the proper use of such products.[81]

Many times departments or service lines (e.g., oncology, cardiology, psychiatry/ mental health, radiology, anesthesiology, women's health) are asked for input regarding the formulary management within their specialty area of practice.

P&T COMMITTEE MEETING

Before beginning the description of a typical P&T committee meeting, it is important to note that a smoothly functioning P&T committee has certain needs. The committee will need the support of its parent organization. A room for the meetings should be carefully selected (see Appendix 12–3). The agenda for the meeting should be prepared in advance by the committee's secretary and sent to the members. Most often, as mentioned previously, an informal meeting of the supporting pharmacists and others is required between P&T committee meetings to plan the activities necessary to support the agenda. The chair of the committee may also attend such planning meetings to ensure that priority issues are addressed before the meeting. Formulary reviews represent a special concern when sending out an agenda, since they may trigger the outside influences of dedicated pharmaceutical marketing efforts if companies learn from committee members that their products or their competitor's products are being evaluated. Efforts must be made to make sure the committee is not distracted by outside influences, such as the pharmaceutical industry and advertisements. This consideration should be reflected in the selection of members and it may be necessary to avoid sending out some materials ahead of time, to lessen the chance of them being obtained by pharmaceutical company representatives. Also, if it is possible to prevent pharmaceutical representatives from knowing the membership of the committee, many of these problems may be avoided. If materials are sent out, it may be found that sending minutes from the previous P&T committee meeting is not always appropriate, since it may be difficult to adequately describe the full basis of a decision in a set of minutes. As a result, the minutes might be open to inappropriate projection regarding the basis for the P&T committee decision process. Some institutions simply make the minutes a pure recording of the decisions, eliminating any information about the discussion to avoid this problem. A sample set of minutes is seen in Appendix 12–4. Along with sending an agenda to members, a reminder phone call, fax, and/or e-mail may be useful to facilitate attendance. Each P&T committee meeting will require extensive preparation by the pharmacists involved in its affairs. Specifically, management of the formulary requires extensive background research and the preparation of written reports for any addition or deletion. Similarly, quality-related functions require time-consuming review of patient records. Finally, the P&T committee functions will be peripherally related to other affairs of the parent organization, for example, the standard order set preparation by other segments of a hospital. This requires special attention in order to prevent the use of nonformulary products. These items will be discussed in greater detail in the next section. Finally, the chairperson should be skilled at guiding an efficient meeting (see Appendix 12–5). In respect of the time commitment for members, meetings should always start and end at the scheduled times.

P&T COMMITTEE FUNCTIONS

● ❹ *Typically, P&T committee functions include determining what drugs are available, who can prescribe specific drugs, policies, and procedures regarding drug use (including pharmacy policies and procedures, clinical protocols, standard order sets, and clinical guidelines—see Chapter 7 for the latter), performance improvement as well as quality assurance activities (e.g., drug utilization review/drug usage evaluation/medication usage evaluation, as well as compliance surveillance—see Chapter 14), adverse drug reactions/medication errors (see Chapters 15 and 16), dealing with product shortages, and education in drug use.*[15,82,83] Many of those functions are related to quality assurance activities, because they are designed to improve the quality of drug therapy. Because the functions may improve drug therapy quality, they may actually provide some legal protection for an institution, as long as the reason for decisions is not strictly based on financial considerations.[84] P&T committee functions can also include investigational drug studies; however, that is often delegated to the **Institutional Review Board (IRB)** that oversees all investigational activities in the hospital (see Chapter 17). In addition, some P&T committee functions may be delegated to subcommittees (e.g., quality assurance, antibiotic, and medication errors subcommittees)[85]; however, this can be cumbersome and is often avoided, except in larger institutions. P&T committees should recognize principles of epidemiology and pharmacoeconomics in the decision making whenever possible.[86-88] A standardized safety assessment tool has been developed to evaluate potential formulary agents.[89]

According to TJC, the medical staff, pharmacy, nursing, administration, and others are to cooperate with each other in carrying out the previously mentioned functions.[15] Although the medical staff normally takes overseeing drug therapy very seriously and expects to approve all activities of the P&T committee, it is common for the pharmacy department to do much of the preparation work for the committee. Although it is tempting to say the reason pharmacies are charged with all of the work is that they are the drug experts, which is usually true, it is probably more realistic that the reason is that pharmacists are paid to do this as part of their salary. Physicians usually do not obtain any direct monetary compensation for this committee's work, although such compensation may be considered by an institution to encourage more physician participation.

Case Study 12–1

You are the clinical pharmacist assigned to be the Secretary of the pharmacy and therapeutics committee (P&T). You are asked to develop an agenda for each monthly meeting, prepare each agenda topic, present each agenda item in a presentation, take notes, and provide follow-up to the meeting.

- *What steps do you need to take to prepare an agenda?*
- *What steps are needed to prepare a medication monograph, including the summary page?*
- *What methods are used to disseminate the information once approved by the committee?*

FORMULARY MANAGEMENT

Drug Formulary

Wherever a **drug formulary system** is in place, there is usually a drug formulary published, as a hardcopy book and/or more commonly in electronic format (e.g., Web site, intranet, or other software). In its simplest form, the drug formulary contains a list of drugs that are available under that formulary system, which reflects the clinical judgment of the medical staff.[90,91] This list will be arranged alphabetically and/or by therapeutic class (American Hospital Formulary Service [AHFS] classification usually), and usually contains information on the dosage forms, strengths, names (e.g., generic, trade, and chemical), and ingredients of combination products. Many drug formulary publications contain a great deal more material related to the drugs, including a summary of indications, side effects, dosing, use restrictions, and other clinical information.[92] Formularies may also be referred to as preferred medication lists or preferred drug lists.[18]

A related term, the formulary system, can be thought of as a method for developing the list, and sometimes even as a philosophy.[93] In theory, a well-designed drug formulary can guide clinicians to prescribe the safest and most effective agents for treating a particular medical problem, at the most reasonable cost.[94-99] Some people argue that the formulary system itself does not work because it is not properly implemented and recommend replacing it with counterdetailing by pharmacists or computers at the time a prescription order is written (see Chapter 23 for further information).[100] However, whether or not that is true has yet to be determined. The most well-known article indicating that formularies may ultimately result in higher patient costs was written by Horn and associates.[101] While this may be one of the best articles on the topic and the author has defended criticism of the article,[102] there are nevertheless various deficiencies in the study that make it uncertain whether it was truly the drug formulary or other factors that lead to increased costs.[103-106] Horn and associates[107] also published a similar study conducted in the ambulatory environment, which appears to have similar results and deficiencies. In the case of national drug formularies, there has been a positive[108] effect on prescribing habits shown in Canada. A study of formulary use in the western Pacific region found that they are commonly used in hospital, but questioned their effectiveness, since in that area the products on the formulary are often not connected to treatment guidelines or the best evidence for treating disease.[109] Further research is needed before a definite conclusion may be reached on the effectiveness of formulary management.[110] For now, a well-constructed formulary is still believed to improve patient care while decreasing costs. It serves as a focus for building comprehensive drug therapy options.

The goal of the formulary system is to provide a decision-making process leading to the selection of medications necessary for the treatment of any disease states likely to be seen in that institution.[95] In some cases, decisions for formulary addition can be made for entire groups of institutions, for example, the U.S. Veteran's Administration has combined the formularies of all of its component parts.[111] These formulary medications should be the most efficacious and cost-effective agents with the fewest side effects or drug interactions.[15] Other factors should also be taken into consideration, such as the variety of dosage forms available for the medication, estimated use, convenience, dosing schedule, compliance, abuse potential, physician demand, ease of preparation, storage requirements, and risks.[112] Economic factors should not be the sole basis for this evidence-based process.[95] Typically, only two or, perhaps, three drugs from any drug class are added to the formulary. Some people would argue that only one agent is necessary from any class; however, some individuals will not respond and/or tolerate certain agents, so at least one secondary agent is usually desirable. Therapeutic redundancy must be minimized, however, by excluding superfluous or inferior preparations. This should improve the quality of prescribing and also lead to improved cost-effectiveness, both by eliminating less cost-effective agents that do not improve patient care and by assisting patients to become well faster. To analyze potentially conflicting literature and strength of recommendation, a grading system has been developed for review of potential formulary additions.[113]

Whether an institution has a very strict formulary with a minimum number of items or a less-restricted formulary that excludes items that are significantly inferior is sometimes a matter of philosophy. The former will cut down the pharmacy department's inventory and often save money through avoidance of highly priced products, but may only be practical in closed **health maintenance organizations (HMOs)** where the same formulary is used in both the inpatient and ambulatory environments. In cases where physicians are free to prescribe whatever products they prefer in the ambulatory environment, they have been shown to have difficulty in remembering what products are contained on the formularies of third-party payers.[114] Therefore, the increased time necessary for pharmacists to contact physicians for order changes may lead to the disruption of patient care. As a result, a less-restricted formulary may be more practical. As an example, a patient is admitted to the hospital on a nonformulary medication. While there would be other satisfactory medications in the same therapeutic category on the formulary, it may be best to simply allow use of the nonformulary product, rather than adding another complicating factor to the patient's hospital treatment by attempting to change therapy. Pharmacist and physician time would also be saved.

Even in cases where an institution has a strict and enforced drug formulary, it should be noted that there are occasions when it is necessary to prescribe a drug that is not on the drug formulary. This might be due to a patient with a rare illness, a patient who does not respond or has intolerable side effects to the formulary drugs, a patient stabilized on a nonformulary medication where it would be difficult or dangerous to change, a conflict between the institutional formulary and the patient's insurance company formulary,[115] or some other valid reason. A mechanism must be in place to promptly obtain the particular drug when it is shown to be necessary (the National Committee for Quality Assurance [NCQA] requires such a mechanism for HMOs,[116] as does TJC for other hospitals,[15] but it must try to prevent physicians from ordering nonformulary drugs "because I said so!"). Some institutions require specific request forms to be filled out (see example in Appendix 12–2), sometimes with a cosignature from the physician's department head, or at least require a consultation between a pharmacist and the physician before the drug is obtained. Also, patients may be charged more for the nonformulary medications. In some HMOs and insurance company plans, the physicians or pharmacies may be financially penalized for use or overuse of nonformulary medications.[117] Whatever mechanism is used, it is important to make it easy to obtain necessary nonformulary medications, but difficult to obtain unnecessary medications, otherwise the benefits of the formulary system may be negated.[56] Also, it is necessary to track which nonformulary drugs are being used regularly and why that is happening because it may be worthwhile to add an agent to the drug formulary.[118]

Some physicians feel that a drug formulary serves only to keep costs down, at the expense of good patient care.[119] These physicians must be reassured that there is evidence to support that a good formulary does keep expenses down[120] without negatively affecting care,[121] although in some cases the costs are merely transferred to other hospital expenses.[122,123] One study demonstrated that a well-controlled formulary or therapeutic substitution (substituting a different medication that is effective for the disease being treated for the one ordered by the physician) results in 10.7% lower drug costs per patient day, and both a well-controlled formulary and therapeutic substitution together could cause 13.4% lower drug costs per day.[124] Some physicians do not like formularies because they consider them to be a limitation to their authority.[119] It is necessary to keep in mind that when physicians become a part of a medical staff or sign up to participate in some managed care group they are given privileges not rights. The privileges generally do include limitations on what medications they can prescribe, and when and how they can prescribe them. If a drug formulary system is run well, there is little reason to feel there are inadequate drugs available; however, it does take some effort for the physician to learn to use the drugs available rather than the drugs they normally prescribe. An effort must be made to collaborate with physicians in this regard and to reassure them that every effort is being made to ensure the best drugs are available for the patients. Additionally, all changes to the drug formulary must be quickly and effectively communicated to the physicians to avoid confusion. A lack of such communication can negate some of the benefits of the formulary and lead to poor physician/pharmacist relations.[122] Also, it is important for physicians to be aware that it is the medical staff that makes these decisions, in order to avoid pharmacy being perceived as the policeman who is waiting to jump on the unsuspecting physician.[125] Increasingly, physicians will enter prescription orders into the computer, which can quickly inform the physician of formulary drug choices and guide therapeutic decisions. Currently, however, pharmacists often have to tactfully contact the physician about nonformulary drugs in order to make a formulary system work.

Similarly, pharmacies filling prescriptions for an HMO must be kept informed of the formulary status of drugs. One suggestion is to have a help desk to answer pharmacist questions and to provide information.[126]

Oftentimes, the drug formularies will have a number of other sections that may include information about the P&T committee and pharmacy department, policy and procedure information (e.g., how to obtain nonformulary drugs, how to request a drug be placed on the formulary), laboratory test information, dietary supplement charts, pharmacokinetics information, approved abbreviations, sodium content, nomograms, dosage equivalency charts, apothecary/metric equivalents, drug–food interactions, skin test directions, cost data, antimicrobial therapy charts, and any other brief clinical information tables felt to be necessary. Use of linking in Web sites can make such information much more readily available and usable, since users can navigate back and forth between these tables and the drug list. MCOs may need to include the procedure they use to limit choice of drugs by physicians, pharmacists, and patients.[16,127]

In institutional pharmacies, a hardcopy book was normally published once a year in the past. Often it was published in a pocket-size format that could be carried in lab coats by physicians, pharmacists, and nurses. There may also have been a larger loose-leaf binder published that could be updated regularly throughout the year. Such a book is no longer justified.[128] It is now common for this reference to be available electronically. The electronic form can be made more widely available and can be kept continually up to date by making changes, as necessary, at one central location. Also, the electronic formulary coupled with physician order entry may lead to the most efficient and effective way to encourage or enforce the use of formulary items,[129-131] although there is some evidence that electronic messages may be ignored by physicians.[132] Also, other information can be included to improve drug therapy. For example, this may include a requirement for a consultation by a specialist or pharmacokinetic monitoring. For outpatient drug formularies this may include quantity level limits and requirements for **prior authorizations**.

Preferably, the pharmacy can use the information on their computer system to create a formulary that is constantly up-to-date. The information can be accessed as part of the prescription order software and/or it may be interfaced with Web software.[133] The latter makes it possible to embed other information easily, but may take further work by the pharmacist. In any case, this information should be available to the physician and other health care professionals wherever necessary—even by wireless connection. As a side note, many institutions do not want information about their formularies readily available to individuals not directly associated with the institution (e.g., pharmaceutical manufacturers, pharmaceutical representatives), but this should not be a problem using Virtual Private Network (VPN) software and firewalls to secure the data—allowing access to only qualified individuals. Increasingly, physicians access this information using iPads or Google Android devices.

PBMs, in conjunction with an organization, may publish a **patient pocket formulary** or informational Web site in addition to the formulary published for physicians and provided online for pharmacies. These patient pocket formularies or Web sites may contain the top therapeutic categories and other information as well. Within these categories are the key drugs in that specific therapeutic class as well as the designated preferred products and the associated patient cost index. Patients are encouraged to take the pocket formularies on their physician visits as a means of ensuring formulary compliance when discussing therapeutic options. Physicians may also have the capability of prescribing online, whereby the physician enters the prescription in an electronic device and instant messaging occurs alerting the physician to potential drug interactions or formulary status of the prescription, allowing the physician to change the prescription immediately and eliminating the need for a pharmacist to call.[43,134]

In addition to pocket formularies, one method whereby the pharmacist educates the physician about formulary drugs is academic detailing. Through mailings, phone conversations, and personal visits the pharmacist discusses with the physician his or her prescribing patterns and, using evidence-based medical literature, supports the rational for preferred formulary product selection and clinically appropriate, cost-effective prescribing without compromising quality.[43]

It is recommended to use a combination of methods to make sure prescribers are informed about formulary information, including electronic resources, academic detailing, educational programs, and any other available methods.[135]

Evaluating Drugs for Formulary Inclusion

The establishment and maintenance of a drug formulary requires that drugs or drug classes be objectively assessed based on scientific information (e.g., efficacy, adverse effects, cost, contribution to some critical treatment pathway,[136] ease of preparation/use, and other appropriate items), not anecdotal physician experience.[93,137] Also, it must be noted that the safety of medications is an important consideration and that decisions must not be made purely based on cost.[138] Also, when costs are considered, it needs to be an evaluation of all costs to the institution, not just the cost of the medication itself, and may include such diverse things as laboratory monitoring costs, length of therapy, nursing care demands, and rehospitalization rates.[139] Medication selection and procurement were specifically added to the TJC accreditation process under medication management in the 2009 standards.[140] There is an emphasis in the literature that P&T committee activities should be a result of evidence-based decisions.[95,141] Regarding the formulary process, 2013 TJC standard MM.02.01.01 calls for written criteria for addition or deletion of medications.[15] Any health care practitioner who is involved with ordering, dispensing, administering, and monitoring medications needs to be involved with the development of the criteria.[15,140] A process must also be in place to monitor patient responses to a new medication. All formulary medications are to be reviewed at least annually based on safety and efficacy information. This means that in addition to new formulary additions, all categories of the AHFS therapeutic classification should be reviewed at least yearly.

According to the 2013 TJC, the criteria used for approving addition of a drug to a formulary need to minimally include the following[15]:

- Indications for use
- Effectiveness
- Risks (e.g., adverse effects, drug interactions, and potential for medication errors)[142]
- Cost

A procedure for preparing the written evaluation of drug products is found in the next chapter; however, this section will go further into how the P&T committee should use that information and other items to do the actual evaluation.

When a P&T committee considers a drug for formulary adoption, it is quite common for the discussion to include statements such as "In my clinical experience...," which leads the discussion into rather subjective areas. Commonly, physicians are most likely to request drugs after they have met with the pharmaceutical company representative or received compensation from the drug company (e.g., speaking fees and travel funds to a meeting).[132,143] In addition, medications may be requested and added to a formulary simply because they are new, even when they clearly are not superior and cost more.[144] Valid formulary decisions should be based on objective evidence, particularly clinical studies,[145] rather than a few cases of clinical experience by a physician attending a meeting.[95] Efforts must be made to guide discussions to scientific information when it wanders into vague subjective areas.[94] In some cases this is rather difficult because many new drugs have limited published information when they are first commercially available. The information that is available is generally placebo-controlled studies that are funded by the manufacturer. In situations such as this, the decision on formulary addition may need to be postponed until adequate information is available. It may be recommended that consideration of any new product be delayed until it has been on the market at least 1 year, unless it is a treatment that is significantly different from those already available.[146] In at least one case it has been bluntly stated that a P&T committee should show leadership by restricting the availability of a drug product if there is no convincing evidence that the product offers meaningful benefits over other available products.[147] Sometimes the decision cannot wait, as is the case with many managed care companies, which need to review a drug before a patient picks up the drug from the pharmacy so that appropriate coverage determination can be made, or in hospitals in response to the new TJC accreditation standards.[15,140]

Then the P&T committee's decision-making process needs to be structured in a manner that is very objective and data driven, and takes into account the lack of data.[95] In these cases, a committee may make a decision and then place the product on a 6-month follow-up for an additional review, after which time additional prescribing and patient use data or clinical trial data may be available.

While there is a temptation to think that anything new is better, which is an attitude that is certainly pushed by drug company representatives with new products to sell, it cannot be assumed and must be proven. In some cases, experts have determined that the new products pose no significant advantages to the patients to justify the costs.[148-150] Often, manufacturers are trying to get products approved and on the market that may be in a different strength or dosage form, single isomer of a product, a new indication for a product, or even an extended release version of a product (sometimes several different extended-release versions).[151] All of the products potentially need to be given consideration by a P&T committee. However, with a lack of published trials and, in many cases, objective and reliable data, the P&T committee faces the challenge of creating a sound drug formulary that represents the needs of an organization or patient population in an objective manner that encompasses current clinical practice, established guidelines of patient care, and a thorough risk-benefit analysis of the drug product.[26] Some places have even tried computerized methods to make more objective decisions[152,153]; however, there does not seem to be any data demonstrating the superiority of such a method. Similarly, there are processes called System of Objectified Judgment Analysis (SOJA), which uses a computer program to score different aspects of drugs in the same class to determine the best product,[154,155] and multiattribute utility technology.[156] A Web-based tool for designing pediatric vaccine formularies has been developed (http://www.vaccineselection.com).[157]

The 2013 Joint Commission Accreditation Process Guide for Hospitals also addresses the elements of performance for selecting and procuring medications.[15]

Elements of this performance that provide additional information to that already covered are the following:

1. Members of the medical staff, licensed independent practitioners, pharmacists, and staff involved in the ordering, dispensing, administering, and/or monitoring the effects of medications develop written criteria for determining which medications are available for dispensing or administering to patients.
2. Before using a new medication, the hospital establishes processes to monitor patient response (see MM.07.01.01, EP 2).

Conflict of Interest

Also, it is necessary to determine whether people involved in the discussion and decision about a drug's formulary status have some conflict of interest (i.e., would receive some direct or indirect compensation from having a drug available, e.g., stock in a company, honoraria for speaking, consulting fees, and gifts or grants from a company[83,146,158-160]) and avoid that biasing factor. Nationally, this is considered to be a significant problem.[161] The P&T committee has the responsibility to identify and address conflict of interest issues in the decision-making process.[95] Perhaps a conflict of interest policy, requiring regular disclosure of any possible conflicts, needs to be established.[26,162,163] An example form to gather information about conflicts of interest is found in Appendix 12–6. Also, the ProPublica Web site (http://projects.propublica.org/docdollars/) discloses payments to prescribers from some pharmaceutical companies. In certain cases, regular voting P&T committee members may have to abstain from the vote if they disclose a possible conflict of interest or the committee may vote to determine whether the conflict is considered to be significant enough to prevent voting by the individual in question. There is concern at a federal, state, and institutional level regarding potential conflict of interest. In 2009, some drug manufacturers made public their financial relationship with health care providers.[164] There is also concern that the PBMs P&T committees may be financially influenced by drug manufacturers.[165] Unlike the traditional health insurers, the U.S. Department of Defense solicits input from various providers and beneficiaries. In addition, they provide beneficiaries and their representatives with an opportunity to comment on the committee recommendations prior to final approval. However, this has not deterred their placement in a category where they will provide the lowest reimbursement for the product.[166]

Other Aspects of Formulary Evaluation

Several other areas need to be considered, which will be explained below.

Patent expiration is a common question that should be considered for all products or drug classes undergoing formulary review, since the introduction of generic products after that date may lead to decreasing prices. Patent expiration information can be found at http://www.fda.gov/cder/ob/default.htm.

TJC Medication Management Standards for 2013 are focused on medication safety. The definition of a medication goes beyond prescription products and the FDA classification as drugs. Also considered medications are herbal/alternative therapies, vitamins, nutraceuticals, nonprescription products, vaccines, diagnostic and contrast agents, radioactive agents, respiratory treatments, parenteral nutrition, blood derivatives, intravenous (IV) solutions, anesthetic gases, sample medications, and anything else deemed by the FDA to be a drug.[140] The pharmacist is required to review the appropriateness of all medication orders before a medication is dispensed.[15,140,167]

While it is desirable to evaluate herbal or other alternative medicine products,[168-170] some institutions may instead handle them as nonformulary requests or investigational drugs.[171] Although alternative and herbal medications seem somewhat unusual to the P&T committee, they can still be treated much the same way as any drug product, perhaps with additional evaluation of the purity and composition of the products (see the Dietary Supplement Medical Literature section of Chapter 5 for additional details regarding how to evaluate for these products).[172] Some pharmacies also have other policies and procedures,[173] perhaps some that are highly restrictive,[174] including requiring pharmacists to verify labeled product ingredients.[175]

The possibility of a new drug product leading to medication errors should also be considered in the evaluation of products. Such things as difficulty in dosing or administration (including programming intravenous infusion pumps), black box warnings, look-alike and sound-alike names, the need for extra monitoring, unusual storage requirements, and other issues may be considered.[176]

In addition to considering the cost of drug products in the institution, it is necessary to consider the cost to the patient, once he or she returns home. If a product is so expensive that an uninsured or underinsured patient cannot afford it in the ambulatory environment, it may not be good to place the patient on that drug in the hospital. However, in some cases pharmaceutical companies may offer assistance to this type of patient.

Open versus Closed Formularies

When setting up a drug formulary there are several things to consider. First, whether it will be an open or **closed formulary**.[177] The open (or voluntary) formulary essentially means any drug on the market is available, and some would argue that the term **open formulary** is really an oxymoron.[94] One exception to this definition is that the NCQA states that an open formulary for an MCO can be a list of recommended drugs, as long as there are no requirements concerning its use.[178] A closed (or restricted) formulary means that only a limited number of agents are available.[90] This is certainly preferable, because such agents should be chosen by objective evidence in the scientific literature. The evidence should support the superiority of the agents over other similar drugs and because closed formularies can result in cost savings.[179] Closed formularies are becoming much more common in HMOs.[180,181] In some instances of closed formularies, patients may have access to these nonformulary or **nonpreferred drug products** by paying a substantially higher copayment, the difference between the formulary and nonformulary products in addition to the copayment, or the nonformulary drug in its entirety unless there is a prior authorization to allow this drug.[42]

Issues may arise with a closed or restricted formulary in that it may be too restrictive for those patients who cannot afford the drug, even though the drug is still available on a closed formulary. A growing health policy concern is the ability to successfully appeal for coverage of a nonformulary product. Newer breakthrough medications and biotechnology products are making their way onto the market. Although clinically valuable, they are very expensive. In addition, PBMs have managed or preferred formularies. In a managed or preferred formulary, interventions may be used to encourage physicians to use the preferred products. Some of these interventions for physicians include academic detailing, prior authorizations, and coverage rules. For pharmacies this may mean a higher dispensing fee for formulary compliance. For the patient this may mean higher copayments if the formulary or preferred product is not used.

Unlike hospitals, PBMs along with their clients (i.e., health plans) place their formulary and nonformulary medications into tiers with an associated copayment with each tier. This tier copayment structure came about in response to the rising cost of prescription drugs. The first tier is generally reserved for generic drug products. This tier usually has the lowest copayment (e.g., $10.00). The second tier is usually reserved for those name brand drugs that are formulary (e.g., $15.00). This tier has a higher copayment than the first tier due to the added cost of the brand name drug. The third tier is reserved for those drug products that are nonformulary brand names. This copayment is significantly higher than the other two tiers (e.g., $30). However, some third tier copayments may be calculated as a proportion of the drug cost, even as much as one-third as a form of coinsurance, or require paying for the drug in its entirety. The reason for the copayment structure is to encourage the patient to use the most clinically appropriate, cost-effective drug without compromising quality care.[42] Decisions as to the tier placement of a drug product may be dependent on comparative effectiveness research.[182]

The closed formulary can also be broken down into what is referred to as **positive or negative formularies**. This is the method by which the formulary is developed. A positive formulary effectively starts with a blank sheet of paper and specifically adds agents. While this is probably the best method to limit the number of drugs available, it is often not very popular when first implementing the formulary because every agent must be considered. That means the physicians must even make specific decisions on whether they should add such things as acetaminophen and amoxicillin to the formulary. Therefore, in hospitals just establishing a formulary, it is often more popular and easier to use a negative formulary system. This essentially starts with the current hospital drug stock, with each drug class being evaluated to eliminate agents that are not necessary.[183] The first steps in this process may be as simple as eliminating multiple salts/esters of the same drug. Then classes of drugs with multiple similar products could be addressed (e.g., analgesics, antacids, laxatives, vitamins, and topical steroids). While in some ways this process is easier, it is also likely to result in a much bigger formulary, since the decision will be made as to what drugs are definitely not needed, rather than which drugs the institution definitely needs. However, the specific institution's situation will need to be assessed before the method of determining the formulary items can be decided on. Overall, the goal is to provide an optimal array of agents. It is easy to end up with too many duplicative agents; however, having a greater number of agents to choose from can lead to better patient care in some areas.[184,185]

Therapeutic Interchange

The AMA[12,177] defines therapeutic interchange as "authorized exchange of therapeutic alternatives in accordance with previously established and approved written guidelines or protocols within a formulary system." An example would be the use of cefazolin in specific doses whenever any other first-generation injectable cephalosporin is ordered. Please note that this concept is different than biosimilar substitution in which the FDA has determined that specific biologic products (i.e., not drugs in general) are similar except for minor differences in clinically inactive components, with no meaningful differences between the biologics in safety, purity, and potency.[186] Biosimilar substitution may allow something very similar to therapeutic interchange, even in community pharmacies, depending on state laws that are being updated to allow for it; however, it does not require action of a P&T committee. Therapeutic interchange is used in nearly 90% of U.S. hospitals[187] for reasons that include cost savings,[188,189] improved patient outcomes, decreased adverse effects, decreased inventory, fewer medication errors,[190] or other benefits. Therapeutic interchange has been shown to decrease costs without adversely affecting patient outcomes.[52,191] There is even reason to believe that when therapeutic interchange is properly performed, and not entirely based on financial considerations, it may produce lower legal liability on an institution,[84] although there are no published legal cases regarding therapeutic interchange to demonstrate either increased or decreased legal liability.[192] The concept of therapeutic interchange through collaborative interactions with interdisciplinary teams to develop protocols and comprehensive therapeutic assessments has been described. Several medication classes may be the target of therapeutic interchange and an aggressive intravenous to oral conversion may be part of this process.[193] The most common classes of drugs for therapeutic interchange are, in order: H_2 antagonists, proton pump inhibitors, antacids, quinolones, potassium supplements, cephalosporins, and hydroxymethylglutaryl-coenzyme A reductase inhibitors.[194] Some drugs classes, such as low-molecular weight heparins, that at first glance may appear to be possible places for therapeutic interchange, may be found to be unacceptable after a closer inspection.[194]

Therapeutic interchange is considered acceptable to the AMA, unlike therapeutic substitution, which they define as the "act of dispensing a therapeutic alternative for the drug product prescribed without prior authorization of the prescriber" (Note: prior authorization may be a blanket authorization, not a specific authorization for each case).[195,196] Therapeutic interchange has also been found to be acceptable by other organizations, including the American College of Clinical Pharmacy (ACCP), American College of Physicians (ACP) (they require immediate prior consent by the physician),[197] ASHP, American Pharmacists Association (APhA), American Association of Colleges of Pharmacy (AACP), AMCP,[198] and the American Society of Consultant Pharmacists (ASCP).[199,200] The ACCP spells out the concept of therapeutic interchange in great detail and suggests that it not only be conducted under the auspices of a P&T-type committee, but also that it specifically include DUE, a set method for informing the physicians and other staff that interchange is taking place (should be well planned and thorough[201]), and a mechanism under which the therapeutic interchange policies may be overridden in specific cases. Evaluations for therapeutic interchange should also consider medical, legal, and financial evaluations.[194] Other practical aspects, such as communication forms, policies and procedures, medical staff bylaw changes, and other items may need to be addressed by the institution.[202] Electronic means to provide authorization for a therapeutic interchange may be a future option.[203] Outside of an institution (e.g., ambulatory environment), therapeutic interchange may not be as easy to implement due to practical procedure methods and because patients are not as closely monitored; however, it may still be possible.[204,205] In the ambulatory situation, the AMA states that therapeutic interchange recommendations must be approved by the majority of physicians affected and must otherwise follow similar standards to that described for inpatient settings.[177]

The consideration of certain therapeutic agents for interchange may result in strong differences of opinion among medical staff members regarding their appropriate use. The process for evaluating any product, especially those having deeply held physician opinions, should be followed, along with efforts being made by committee members to actively approach appropriate influential individuals before a crisis occurs. Through anticipatory, structured negotiation, it is more likely that rational and balanced decisions will be made. Also, it is necessary to take into consideration whether a short-term interchange of products, while the patient is in a hospital, may cause confusion or other difficulties when the patient returns to the outpatient environment and may be restarted on the original agent.[206] Working with the physicians to resolve this issue is a necessity for the long-term care of patients.

Generic substitution can also be considered by the P&T committee, but many pharmacies consider generic substitution to be one of their responsibilities and do not take such decisions to a P&T committee for approval. The one exception may be drugs with narrow therapeutic indexes (e.g., anticonvulsants), where a P&T committee may determine a list of products where generic substitution is not allowed,[207] although the FDA insists that such precautions are unnecessary.[208] In relation to generic substitution, it must be mentioned that pharmacies must determine quality suppliers. The ASHP has guidelines for this function.[209] Also, states may have a variety of laws governing generic substitution. They may also publish so-called positive and negative formularies, which differ in definition from those terms used elsewhere in this chapter in that they are lists of drugs that may or may not be substituted for one another, respectively.[192]

In some instances, physicians may prefer that no generic substitution or therapeutic substitution occur on a written order or prescription by indicating "Dispense as Written" (DAW) on that document. This can occur in the inpatient setting as well as the outpatient setting. Depending on the state, dispense as written is synonymous with the following: no substitution, do not substitute, medically necessary, brand necessary/medically necessary, no drug product selection, brand medically necessary, substitution prohibited without permission of physician or patient, or no substitution/brand necessary.

In most states, the law provides that pharmacists can use a generic version of any medication on a prescription or medication order if the physician has not precluded that action by indicating DAW. In the outpatient setting, in general, if a patient wants a generic medication, they should be sure that their pharmacist knows of their desire.

In some benefit plans, if the physician requests a brand name medication when a generic equivalent is available, the patient member may be responsible to pay the difference in cost in addition to the generic copayment. In some instances, members may not be required to pay this cost difference, if their physician documents that the brand name medication is necessary.

Nonformulary Usage

Many institutions track the drug use patterns of prescribers, as was mentioned previously in describing the tracking of nonformulary drug products.[210] Annually, a listing of nonformulary products and expenses should be made available to the P&T committee. It is helpful if the pharmacy director can report the total cost of nonformulary items as a percent of the total budget, particularly since the cost can exceed the cost of carrying the nonformulary product on the formulary.[211] Also, as part of this, it is good to check on whether nonformulary drug usage has led to medication errors, since there was at least one report that such nonformulary use resulted in a 28% error rate.[210] Ideally, a report of the number involved and costs of nonformulary orders will be made available to each prescriber. This process is helpful in improving the appropriate use of medications and has also been linked to the prescriber credentialing process.[212] The process can also be used to reevaluate whether nonformulary items should be made available on the drug formulary.

Unlabeled Uses

While some third-party payers may attempt to limit the use of drugs to only FDA-approved indications, this may unnecessarily restrict use of products for indications that may have significant literature support. This should not be supported.[213] However, as will be discussed in more detail in the next chapter, it is sometimes necessary for institutions to specifically restrict drugs to specific uses when they may be used inappropriately. While at first glance, this seems to be the same, in reality, such restrictions may be totally unrelated to approved labeling. In this situation, it may be found that products are permitted to be used for unlabeled indications where there is adequate literature support and, conversely, may not be permitted to be used, at least without special approval within the institution, for FDA indications when there may be more appropriate drugs available.

New Product Introductions

When new drug products are added to the formulary, it is best to prepare physicians, nurses, and others.[132] Initially, it is necessary to inform affected individuals that the drug will be available as of a specific date. That could be immediately or at some time in the near future. There are various reasons for a delay. For example, a drug may have been approved by both the FDA and the P&T committee, but the company may not have yet made it commercially available because they have not yet produced a sufficient supply or they are not yet ready to start their marketing efforts. In some cases, it is necessary for specific equipment to be obtained and installed. Such was the case a number of years ago when Fluosol®-DA was made available for a limited period of time. This parenteral product required very specialized preparation method involving a warm water bath and percolating a mixture of gases through an IV bag under sterile conditions. Few, if any, pharmacies had the necessary equipment at the time of introduction and it would have taken some time to get the equipment, set it up, and train pharmacists and technicians in its use, requiring a delay in making the product available in an institution. Most commonly, the reason for the delay is likely to be the time it takes to inform all individuals likely to be involved in the prescribing, preparing, and administering of the drug that the drug will be available and to educate them in the proper use, including applicable policies and procedures. These education efforts may be provided through newsletters, Web sites, portals, e-mail, memos, educational programs, RSS (Really Simple Syndication) **aggregators** (programs that pull together information from a variety of sources, such as news resources—an example is Google

Reader), or other methods. The method chosen should generally be a standard method used within the institution and should be appropriate for the specific medication product introduction. In cases where a product is particularly complicated, dangerous, or prone to misuse, several methods of instruction, perhaps along with prescribing restrictions, should probably be employed. Further information about newsletters and Web sites is found in Chapter 9.

Case Study 12–2

You are the only pharmacist assigned to work the evening shift in the main pharmacy doing electronic order entry. The physician writes an order for dexlansoprazole. From the order you cannot tell if the dexlansoprazole is a patient home medication or a new order. The clinical pharmacist on that particular floor has gone home for the day. The hospital where you practice has a closed formulary. Your formulary agent is pantoprazole. Your hospital has a policy and procedure for nonformulary drug orders as well as a therapeutic interchange program that includes this class of drugs. You call the physician and explain to him that pantoprazole is the formulary agent. He states that dexlansoprazole is what he prefers for this patient.

- *In order for dexlansoprazole to be dispensed, what form does the physician have to fill out?*
- *On receiving the nonformulary request, you notice the reason for the dexlansoprazole order is efficacy. Is this consistent with what you know about the products?*
- *You call the physician and explain what you found and the approved therapeutic interchange. You inform the physician that per the nonformulary medication policy it may take 24 hours or longer to obtain the nonformulary medication. The physician approves the interchange this time, but wants a formal review of the drug at P&T. How would you document the therapeutic interchange?*
- *Knowing that the physician wants a formal review of dexlansoprazole, how do you proceed with the request in the pharmacy records or medical records?*

POLICIES AND PROCEDURES

Occasionally, policies and procedures must be developed to support the rational use of medications. While the pharmacy department may decide they need to have their own policies and procedures for internal functions that is not the focus of this discussion.[214]

Instead, policies and procedures for the use of medications in an institution, clinic, and so forth will be discussed, since that is often provided through a P&T committee.

TJC has specifically stated that they expect policies and procedures for the following types of orders[15]:

- As needed (prn) medications
- Standard order sets
- Automatic stop
- Titrating
- Taper
- Range
- Compounded or admixed drugs
- Medication-related devices
- Investigational medications
- Herbal/natural products
- Discharge medications
- Anticoagulation dosing[55]

Some examples of policies and procedures can be found on the Internet at http://www.hosp.uky.edu/pharmacy/departpolicy/departmentalpolicies.html

To begin this discussion, the definitions for policies and procedures should be considered.[215] A policy is a broad general statement that describes the goals and purposes of the document. The procedures are specific actions to be taken. In some ways, policies and procedures may resemble a cookbook-type approach, in that a set of steps to be accomplished are described in order. Taken together, these policies and procedures may be a logical, step-by-step explanation of why and where a product may be used, how to use it, and who is to follow the policy (i.e., there may be different portions of the document addressed to pharmacists, technicians, nurses, and prescribers),[216] along with a brief introductory statement describing why the process is necessary.

Before developing a specific policy and procedure, the first step should be deciding whether it is necessary at all. In other words, is there a good reason for the existence of that particular policy and procedure and is it likely to be used? This can be looked at as a risk-benefit decision. For example, is there sufficient risk that a particular medication will be used incorrectly (e.g., prepared wrong, administered wrong, and used for an inappropriate indication) to make it worthwhile to develop a policy and procedure? Generally, the answer will be no, but in a certain number of cases, policies and procedures may be necessary. Examples of where a policy and procedure may be necessary include thrombolytic agents (where the drug can cause serious or fatal effects if used improperly), antibiotics (where it is found that expensive, broad-spectrum antibiotics are being used where amoxicillin should suffice), injectable drugs (where specific individuals who will administer the medication and the process, including programming infusion devices, will be defined),[217] and even for drugs where reimbursement may be a problem.

Once a decision is reached to develop the policy and procedure, a logical and orderly course should be followed. It is undesirable to wait until after problems occur before deciding that policies and procedures are necessary. This process should follow the drug formulary process, where a mechanism is set up to help determine that a policy and procedure is necessary. In many cases, a policy and procedure for use of drugs likely to be misused may be developed in conjunction with its consideration for addition to the drug formulary.

As in any process, it is first necessary to decide who will be coordinating the effort and the likely endpoint. That person, or designee, will then need to investigate various sources for background material necessary to develop the policy and procedure. This might include doing a literature search, talking to experts in the field, talking to other institutions that have already developed policies on the same topic, reviewing published professional (e.g., http://www.ashp.org/Import/PRACTICEANDPOLICY/ PolicyPositionsGuidelinesBestPractices.aspx) or clinical guidelines (e.g., http://www .guideline.gov), and checking the institution's requirements for developing policies and procedures. If the policy and procedure is for a hospital group, other institutions in the group must also be involved. In particular, it is necessary for the person developing the policy and procedure to have good communications with those who will be affected. After all, if the final product is looked at as being more trouble than it is worth, it is not likely to be followed. Where the policy and procedure fits in relation to other institutional policies and procedures will also have to be evaluated. Finally, a document should be written, reviewed, and revised, using many of the skills outlined in Chapter 9.

As part of the process of preparing the policy, it is important to be clear as to when it is applicable and where there may be exceptions. For example, institutions have policies for the automatic stop of specific medications (e.g., stopping an antibiotic after 7 days). There needs to be careful consideration of only applying that policy in cases where it will be likely to improve drug therapy. There also needs to be a mechanism to make sure that such an automatic stop, which may be programmed into the computer system, may not cause harm to particular patients[218] (e.g., patients with osteomyelitis receiving antibiotics for an extended period of time).

Once the policy and procedure is finished, it will need to be approved by the same mechanism that drug formulary changes go through (i.e., P&T committee, medical executive committee, and so forth). The approval and/or effective date for the policy and procedure should be recorded on the document itself to ensure it is not confused with earlier or later documents. A plan for implementing the policy and procedure will need to be developed. Forms may need to be prepared and distributed. Copies of the policy and procedure will have to be distributed to those affected (preferably on the computer network), and educational programs will need to be planned and given. At that point, the policy and procedure can be implemented, perhaps in conjunction with the first appearance of a particular agent on the drug formulary. That is not the end of the process, however. At some point, the policy and procedure should be evaluated to determine if it is being properly followed and having the desired effect as a part of a quality assurance plan. A method to enforce compliance with the policies and procedures is required and it is necessary for legal reasons to demonstrate that this enforcement method is used.[216] Also, the policy and procedure will need to be reviewed, revised (if necessary), and reapproved on a regular basis (preferably once a year). As part of that process, the actual need for the policy and procedure should be reconsidered. The policy and procedure should be eliminated if no longer needed. One way to determine whether the policy and procedures are consulted is if they are on a Web server, where the number of times the specific page is opened is recorded. Superseded copies (i.e., previous versions) of the policies and procedures should be kept on file for background and legal purposes.

It is also necessary to have policies and procedures for the operation of the P&T committee itself (see Appendix 12–1 for policies and procedures for setting up a P&T committee). Some examples of other policies and procedures that may need to be developed include how new drugs are requested for addition to the formulary, how nonformulary drugs can be used, what procedure is used to evaluate new drugs,[140] the composition of the committee, and other committee functions (e.g., conflict of interest). These have been discussed elsewhere in the chapter and will not be dealt with further at this point. For more information on writing policies and procedures, refer to Chapter 18.

Clinical Guidelines

P&T committees may be involved with the development, alteration (to fit local circumstances), and/or approval of evidence-based clinical guidelines. The reader is directed to Chapter 7 to obtain further information.

Standard Order Set Development

Many prescribers, both in their offices and in institutions (e.g., hospital and nursing home), make use of something called standard orders. This usually consists of some sort of form, preprinted hardcopy, or electronic checklist, which lists various orders that are often written for specific patients under certain circumstances. This can include medications, laboratory tests, x-rays, other diagnostic tests, diet restrictions, preoperative preparation, restrictions, and many other things. For example, there may be a specific set of orders for all patients a prescriber admits to the hospital in general or for a specific diagnosis, or a set of orders for a patient who is scheduled to undergo a specific procedure, such as an operation. Standard order sets are commonly used for some medications, such as total parenteral nutrition solutions and oncology agents, where the order can be complex and confusing, perhaps resulting in potential medication errors. The prescribers using the standard order sets can simply indicate which of the items they wish their patients to receive and provide various necessary details, such as dose or duration. The use of standard order sets can be a very good practice, since they act like checklists used by pilots or astronauts—saving time and ensuring that important items are not inadvertently missed or misused. This can be particularly important in the use of drugs that can be dangerous or ineffective if not properly used, such as chemotherapeutic regimens in oncology patients. However, the disadvantage is that the standard order sets do take time to establish and maintain, and may not keep up with actual practice standards, therefore, contributing to the perpetuation of outdated or inappropriate practices. While many P&T committees do not address standard order sets directly, leaving them to the individuals or groups that use them, it is something that still needs to be considered for several reasons.

First, P&T committees are responsible for overseeing all things related to medication use in an institution. Second, the standard order sets may contain medications that may be removed from the formulary for various reasons. This requires the P&T committee to make a special effort to communicate with those individuals or groups with standard order sets that contain drugs that may be eliminated from the formulary. This communication should begin prior to recommendation for removal of a product from the formulary, in order to find out the reason for the use of the product and the acceptability of available substitutes. By maintaining copies of standard order sets, the pharmacy department can help facilitate this process. Also, once it has been decided that a particular product on standard order sets is to be removed from the formulary, that decision must be quickly communicated to the affected individuals and groups, with enough time allocated before the removal becoming effective for the standard order sets to be updated and the new ones be put into use. This process may be delayed by the frequency of meetings of the groups affected, the time it takes to have new standard order set sheets either printed or put on the computer system, and the necessity to adequately train personnel in the use of the replacement products. In all likelihood, it may take several months after a decision by the P&T committee before the changes can be put into effect. Finally, P&T committees may find that products on standard order sets may be used in ways that are not supported by the medical literature and/or hospital policy, which means that they need to make sure the prescribers or groups that use those orders make necessary changes.

Optimally, individuals or groups using standard orders should be required to review and reapprove their use on a regular basis (probably at least once a year). It may also be necessary to have standard order sets go through an institutional standard order sets committee. In any case, TJC requires a specific policy and procedure for how institutions handle standard order sets.[140] Any changes should be reported to both the affected groups (e.g., nursing units, pharmacy, and information technology) and the P&T committee in cases where the standard order sets include drugs. All printed sets of the standard order sets must include their revision date, to make sure that that old copies are not inadvertently used. Old copies of the orders must be maintained for medicolegal purposes, with the length of time for keeping such records to be determined by the institution's legal counsel.

Credentialing and Privileges

Health care institutions are required by various groups to verify that physicians and other health care professionals have the credentials to practice.[219] This can include degrees, licenses, training, and experience. Based on the credentials, professionals may be given privileges to practice within that institution and perform certain activities.[220] Please note that this term is privilege, not right. For example, while all physicians may have the same license, only those trained in surgery may be allowed to do more than very minor surgical procedures (e.g., suturing lacerations and removing minor skin growths). There may be even more specific rules, such as those preventing a chest surgeon from performing neurosurgery. These privileges can also extend to drugs. For example, it may be decided within the P&T committee that only oncologists have privileges to prescribe most antineoplastic agents. This type of policy and procedure is the basis for some restrictions that may be placed when a drug is considered for formulary addition. In addition to restrictions placed within an institution, restrictions may be enforced from outside the institution. For example, the use of dofetilide (Tikosyn®) requires the credentialing of both the prescriber and the hospital by the company; see http://www.tikosyn.com/ for details.

It also must be mentioned that policies and procedures may be in place within an institution to require pharmacists to perform certain operations, whether that is the preparation of particular agents or performing specific clinical functions (e.g., pharmacokinetics and warfarin dosing).[219] Institutions may have a method by which pharmacists are credentialed to perform such services. Further credentialing of pharmacists may be necessary in the future if pharmacist interdependent prescribing becomes more common.[221]

Quality Improvement Within the P&T Committee— Internal Audit

❺ *A variety of topics regarding the quality of medication use, inclusive of applicable medica-tion metrics, are normally part of the activities of a P&T committee*, especially timely com-munication issues. Many of these activities are covered in Chapter 14; however, the items described in the following sections may be considered to be specific to the P&T committee.

MEDICATION QUALITY ASSURANCE

In addition to determining which medications are available and providing direction in their use, it is required that the quality of use is regularly measured in whatever areas are felt to be necessary, including medication use evaluation (MUE), drug use evaluation (DUE), and other similar activities. The P&T committee will likely be involved in this, although coordina-tion of such efforts, including preparing an annual plan of quality assurance activities, may be through other groups, such as a quality assurance committee. The initial plan may be devel-oped by pharmacists, but multidisciplinary feedback is essential before the focused areas of evaluation are finalized. Ideally, all practice areas of the medical staff are given opportunity for input into these focused evaluations. The project list should be continually reviewed and allow for special urgent projects when necessary. If a project is not completed during the year, it may be reconsidered for the next year. DUE criteria should be selected that can be used for continuous improvements that meet TJC accreditation requirements. DUE activities may be used to identify ADRs, contain cost, and expand clinical pharmacy activities.[222] Even if the P&T committee does not direct quality assurance efforts, they must be kept informed of the information gathered and the medication-related quality improvement efforts that are being instituted. This way the P&T committee can be supportive of such efforts directly (e.g., making changes to the drug formulary or policies and procedures to improve medication use) or less directly (e.g., providing statements supporting such activities). Quality assur-ance is a large topic and further information is available in Chapter 14.

ADVERSE DRUG REACTIONS

The P&T committee has a responsibility to review adverse reaction data in an institution to identify trends. One tool they can employ is to monitor the use of medications, sometimes referred to as tracer drugs, to treat the symptoms and side effects of other medications,[223] for example, the monitoring of epinephrine, flumazenil, phytonadione, or protamine to try to detect allergic responses, benzodiazepine overdoses, warfarin overdoses, or heparin overdoses, respectively. The topic of ADRs is covered more in Chapter 15.

MEDICATION ERROR INCIDENTS

Data collected regarding medication errors may be reported to the P&T committee and, probably, for investigational drugs, to the IRB. A systematic method to collect data about medication errors must be set up within an institution, perhaps using internal incident report forms employed by the institution to track all unusual occurrences regarding patients. All incidents are reviewed by severity (none, minimal, moderate, major, death) and process (prescribing, transcription, dispensing, administration, other). A multidisciplinary review of all incidents should take place and trends in the specific quality indicators should be shared with the entire professional staff. High-alert medications (e.g., narcotics, patient-controlled analgesia, insulin, anticoagulants, electrolytes, neuromuscular blockers, thrombolytics, and chemotherapy) should be benchmarked and followed to identify trends to improve the medication management system and ultimately enhance patient safety.

Another monitoring consideration is related to errors with medical devices and may also be monitored by these committees. A study completed in a 520-bed tertiary teaching institution demonstrated that more intensive surveillance methods yielded higher rates of medical device problems as compared to voluntary reporting.[224]

The topic of medication errors is covered in more detail in Chapter 16.

ILLEGIBLE HANDWRITING, TRANSCRIPTION, AND ABBREVIATIONS

It is important to work with the medical staff and all other health professionals regarding illegible handwriting and transcription errors. Typically, a task force assigned by the P&T committee is given the charge of evaluating and trending illegible handwriting, followed by developing process improvement measures. A report can be made to the P&T on an ongoing or quarterly basis. An education process must be in place for those individuals who consistently demonstrate poor handwriting. Hands-on reminders have been helpful or, in some extreme cases, handwriting school is recommended. In addition, institutions have adapted TJC unapproved abbreviation list.[15] Unacceptable abbreviations may have an intended meaning but often are potentially misinterpreted and can lead to serious complications. In many institutions, the nurse or pharmacist must clarify the order with the prescriber when an unapproved abbreviation is written. In some cases, the only effective prevention of this problem has been when the medical staff has determined through the P&T committee that orders containing unapproved abbreviations are invalid and must be rewritten by the physician.[225] The addition to the formulary of look-alike, sound-alike medications is discouraged.[226-229] Increasingly, institutions are implementing computerized physician order entry (CPOE), which eliminates the problem of illegible handwriting and decimal point errors, thus reducing medication errors,[230] although implementation costs are considerable and some institutions may currently feel that it is not yet worth the effort and expense.[231]

TIMELINESS

The time for medication orders to be filled and sent to the floor may be tracked by the P&T committee. One area of importance is the response time sequence for a stat (immediate) order. The time should be evaluated from the time the order was written, to when the order was filled, to when the patient receives the medication. There are many obstacles in the order process and getting the medication to the patient. Each institution should have a standard expectation of the turnaround time for stat orders and a policy that will ensure that the medication is dispensed and administered promptly. Benchmarking should be done to make sure the policy is followed.

Although not quite as imperative, the timeliness of ordinary order fulfillment must also be evaluated for appropriateness.

COUNTERFEIT DRUG PRODUCTS

Counterfeit drugs can be considered to be those that do not contain the ingredients claimed on the labeling, perhaps having no active ingredients, incorrect dose, or even other drugs.[232] Counterfeit drugs appear to be an increasing problem, although the actual incidence is unknown.[233] The ASHP announced in February 2004 that it would partner with the FDA in a program to keep pharmacists informed about entrance of counterfeit drug products into the nation's drug supply. The ASHP planned to provide rapid alerts to hospital pharmacy departments about counterfeit drug incidents.[234] Also, there are methods being developed or implemented that will help ensure the pedigree of products, particularly those imported from foreign countries, to help avoid counterfeit products. This may include the use of radio frequency identification (RFID) tags to help track products.[235]

The FDA Web site may be consulted at http://www.fda.gov/Safety/MedWatch/SafetyInformation/SafetyAlertsforHumanMedicalProducts/default.htm for an updated list of counterfeit products. Because of the potential problems associated with counterfeit drug products, the P&T committee must be kept informed of any situations that affect the institution, as should the medical staff as a whole.[233] This topic also may be handled with medication errors, since it leads to such errors.

SAFETY ALERT

A variety of other safety-related items are also important to P&T committees, including recalls, black box warnings, risk evaluation and mitigation strategies (REMS) (see Chapter 22),[138] and product shortages, which will be covered in the following subsections. The items covered in this section can also be considered related to ADRs and medication errors, since some portions fit under those categories.

Recalls

The 2013 Joint Commission Accreditation Process Guide for Hospitals requires that a policy and procedure be in place, and be implemented when necessary, to retrieve recalled or discontinued medications. This policy must involve notification of prescribers and patients.[15] The pharmacy department constantly reviews medication products recalled by the manufacturer or the FDA due to a safety issue.[236] This information is provided to the pharmacy by the wholesaler and manufacturer. If a product lot number involved in the recall is found in the pharmacy inventory, that product should be removed from the inventory immediately and recalled from other areas of the institution that may stock it.[140] In the outpatient environment, a recall from consumers may be necessary. A report of medications that have been pulled from the pharmacy inventory should be made available to the P&T committee and the committee may need to decide whether or not to identify patients who may have been affected by the safety issue. Further actions would be based on these findings. The P&T committee chair should be contacted when a patient has significant consequences in relation to a product recall. When a product recall requires the removal of a product treating a disease with limited alternative treatments from the pharmacy inventory, therapeutic alternatives must be made known to the prescribers.[10]

The safety of medications is under constant evaluation and the safety of new agents cannot be known until the product has been on the market for a period of time.[237] Some newly reported serious adverse effects result in black box warnings being inserted in the product labeling or REMS, due to requirements of the FDA, which may necessitate action up to the withdrawal of the medication from the market, as was done with propoxyphene.[238] The reason for this name is that the warning is set off from the rest of the information in the package insert by a thick black box that is drawn around it. It is the responsibility of the P&T committee to review safety data for every medication on the formulary. Many P&T committees have a standing agenda item to review all new black box warnings or newly released FDA safety alerts for medications (obtainable from http://www.fda.gov/Safety/MedWatch/default .htm). The P&T committee needs to review the safety data and make any formulary, policy and procedure, and/or other changes as required. The black box safety data of formulary products need to be disseminated to the medical staff, including any special restrictions or actions taken on a specific product. 2013 TJC Standard MM.02.01.01 addresses the hospital's role in selecting and procuring medications and their annual review for safety and efficacy.[15]

Product Shortages

Product shortages should be continuously monitored by the pharmacy department in an organized fashion; this is a TJC requirement.[83,140,236] Information on this can be found at http://www.fda.gov/Drugs/DrugSafety/DrugShortages/default.htm or http://www.ashp.org/shortages. It is possible to get a free e-mail of these shortages or subscribe to an RSS feed. In recent years, there has been a trend toward more frequent medication shortages.[239] In some cases, evaluation of information may show that acceptable alternative products or treatments may be interchanged for products affected by a shortage. The appropriate health care professionals (e.g., physicians, drug information service, pharmacy director, and buyer) need to be immediately notified of product shortages that may have an effect on therapeutic outcomes, along with plans or recommendations on how to address the situation.[240] In some instances, the chief of the medical staff and even the ethics committee may be consulted when policies need to be put into place to ration drug supplies. The shortage of intravenous immunoglobulin (IVIG) in the 1990s necessitated a complete medical staff and pharmacy department agreement for appropriate patient selection for treatment.[241] This shortage required product rationing with the available supply. Unfortunately no therapeutic alternatives were available for the IVIG shortage. Methods of alerting medical staff of shortages include personal communication, the use of posters or message boards in key areas of the hospital (e.g., medical staff lounge, dictation area, parking garage, and high traffic areas), e-mail, smartphone notification, computer/tablet notification during physician order entry, and the use of newsletters or faxes. A guideline is available from the ASHP to aid in determining how to handle a variety of types of shortages.[236]

In today's health care environment, it is essential to keep medication shortages as a standard agenda item for each P&T meeting. Products with limited availability and products that are not available need to be evaluated constantly. Formulary alternatives for these product shortages then need to be communicated to the medical staff.

Case Study 12–3

You are the pharmacist medication buyer for the health system. Your wholesaler has notified you that there is a product shortage of intravenous furosemide and there is no timeframe when it will be available. You check the Food and Drug Administration (FDA) Web site as well as the American Society of Health-System Pharmacists (ASHP) Web site for further information. Information is available for estimated resupply dates, implications for patient care, safety and alternative agents, and management of this shortage. You are asked to develop a plan to manage this shortage.

- *What health care personnel should be notified of this shortage?*
- *What methods should be used to alert the medical staff?*

- *What information should you provide to the P&T committee regarding this drug shortage?*
- *What steps do you need to develop a plan to manage this shortage and ensure that patient care is not compromised?*

Communication Within an Organization

INVESTIGATIONAL REVIEW BOARD ACTIONS

While P&T committees are generally responsible for overseeing all aspects of medication use in a hospital, they often turn the major responsibility for overseeing investigational drug use over to an IRB. The IRB should provide a regular overview of its actions to the P&T committee for review, but oftentimes this is all that is done. Further information about IRBs can be found in Chapter 17.

COST, BUDGET, AND FORECASTING

How does the P&T committee actively balance its quality promoting activities as well as the economic requirements of its parent organization? For an individual hospital, this is probably an easier task as long as the economic pressures on the hospital's margin are manageable. As previously mentioned, a closed formulary can result in lowered costs within an institution.[179] However, the P&T committee decisions will be more difficult for the PBM function of a health insurance company or HMO. In the latter situation, the pressures of cost containment, the contents of an insurance plan's Certificate of Benefits, and the applicable payer regulations represent formidable obstacles for building broad support for the decisions of a PBM's P&T committee. In comparison to institutional formularies, PBMs have instituted tier-based formularies that encourage the use of more cost-effective agents to control prescription costs and improve therapy.[242,243] In spite of the economic influences on the P&T committee functions of a PBM, there is no end to opportunities for quality improvement by a PBM since there is no other organization that has the ability to access outpatient medication use to the same extent. Regardless of the organizational setting, the requirements for quality as a basis for decisions should be the chief focus of a P&T committee. Obviously, this is a potentially moving target because of the need to achieve a balance between the ethical standards involved in health care. The vested interests of the parent organization, patient's needs and expectations, the professional activities of physicians, pharmacists and nurses, the pharmaceutical companies, and the requirements of society may be very difficult to reconcile.

National drug expenditure projection data, and the factors likely to influence drug costs for a particular year, can be reviewed by the P&T committee on a yearly basis. Also, it is necessary to keep hospital administrators informed of drug costs.[244] An understanding of current trends is essential for formulary management.[245-247]

LIAISON WITH OTHER ELEMENTS OF THE ORGANIZATION

Within any organization, it is often found that the root of problems is communications or, perhaps more often, a lack thereof. Unfortunately, the solution is not simply an increase in communication efforts in general. Instead, the need is for increasing appropriate communication, along with decreasing inappropriate communication. Some specific things have to be kept in mind.

First, make sure that everyone involved in any way in drug therapy receives some communication about medication-related matters.[160,248] Often, this may simply be a list of new drugs available being given to practitioners, along with any policies and procedures. Newsletters and educational presentations may also be valuable, depending on the circumstances. Electronic methods of communication are increasingly important, but the use of in-person counterdetailing may be necessary (see Chapter 23).[135]

Second, be sure the amount of material is not overwhelming, otherwise it will be ignored. A news program on television a number of years ago described a situation that the military found regarding its pilots in Vietnam. They had a tape from the cockpit of an aircraft that had been shot down. Those listening to the tape could clearly hear the warning alarm letting the pilot know that a radar missile was locked on his aircraft and posing an imminent danger; however, it was also clear that the pilot did not even realize that warning was happening because of everything else going on. He mentally tuned out the warning and was shot down as a result. It became clear to those training pilots that it was necessary to limit the amount of information to whatever is most important, so that those items were noticed. This is also important in communicating P&T committee materials.

In addition, it is important to keep certain materials confidential for various reasons. In the case of quality assurance materials, keeping materials suitably confidential may protect that data from legal discovery in court (see Chapter 10 and consult attorneys for specifics). Also, some P&T committees keep the agenda and handouts confidential by not sending them to committee members in advance and by collecting the materials at the end of the meeting in order to destroy them. By doing so, they can often avoid pressure put on the committee by pharmaceutical company representatives, who may be trying to have their products included on the formulary, while having their competitor's products excluded. The disadvantage, of course, is that committee members are not able to prepare for a meeting in advance. In relationship to this, it is often a good idea to make sure the pharmaceutical company representatives do not know the members of the committee and who is preparing the evaluation of a particular product, since that can lead to the evaluator being pressured to sway his or her opinion about a particular product. Many hospitals even fully ban pharmaceutical representatives from the hospital to avoid issues.

Finally, an annual report of the P&T committee may be prepared for both internal review and review by the medical executive committee. This annual report is time consuming in preparation but is a very important means of tracking P&T activities and actions over time.

Overall, it is necessary for the chair person and secretary of the P&T committee to work in cooperation with other appropriate individuals and groups to make sure that essential information is provided wherever needed, while minimizing the amount of extraneous material.

SYNCHRONIZATION OF DATABASES

Although it is more common to think of communication in regard to people, another important area of communications to be addressed is that between electronic databases. The pharmacy computer system may have to communicate with a whole hospital system or other computer systems. It is important to make sure all of these electronic systems are also synchronize, preferably automatically, although that may prove to be a problem.[249]

Conclusion

The pharmacy department can have a major impact on the quality of drug therapy in an institution through participation in P&T committee functions and activities described in this chapter; many of which are related to the management of information or are commonly performed by drug information practitioners. While there are many appropriate ways that may be used in addition to those outlined above, those described can be successfully used to improve drug therapy.

Discussion Questions

1. What is the P&T committee, what are its functions, and how does the committee relate to a pharmacy department?
2. How should a pharmacy/pharmacist be involved in supporting a P&T committee?

3. Define drug formulary and formulary system. How do those items relate to one another?
4. Define open versus closed formularies, including the specific types of closed formularies.
5. How does a P&T committee improve the quality of medication use in a hospital?
6. Define policy. Define procedure.
7. What are the steps in preparing a policy and procedure?
8. Name and briefly explain four policies and procedures that may be implemented by a P&T committee.
9. How does an institutional P&T committee differ from one in a PBM?
10. Who must a P&T committee communicate with? What should they communicate and how should they communicate?
11. What is considered a conflict of interest?

Self-Assessment Questions

1. The pharmacy and therapeutics (P&T) committee can be defined as:
   a. A committee that oversees all aspects of medication therapy in an institution
   b. A committee that oversees all procedures of the institution
   c. A committee that oversees only the medications that are carried in a hospital
   d. A committee that oversees only the quality of medication utilization

2. The P&T committee may act only as:
   a. An advisory body to the medical executive committee
   b. An advisory body to the administration
   c. An advisory body to the board of trustees
   d. An advisory body to the pharmacy

3. The functions of a P&T committee include:
   a. Determining what medications are available
   b. Quality assurance activities
   c. Policies and procedures regarding drug use
   d. All of the above

4. Pharmacy/pharmacists support the P&T committee by:
   a. Having the P&T committee part of the pharmacy department
   b. Serve as chairperson
   c. Involvement in the rational planning process for each meeting agenda
   d. Only addressing medications to be carried on the formulary

5. A drug formulary and a formulary system relate to each other in that:
   a. A drug formulary is a list of available medications under the formulary system which is the method for developing the drug list that reflects the clinical judgment of the medical staff.
   b. A drug formulary comes before a formulary system.
   c. The formulary system provides for a drug formulary that serves only to keep costs down at the expense of patient care.
   d. Where there is a drug formulary system in place there is never a drug formulary published.

6. A closed formulary differs from an open formulary in that:
   a. A closed formulary includes all medications on the market.
   b. Closed formularies may not result in cost savings.
   c. Only certain medication classes are available in a closed formulary.
   d. It is restrictive.

7. Which of the following does not describe the benefits of a therapeutic interchange?
   a. Decrease cost
   b. Improve patient outcomes
   c. Decrease inventory
   d. Increased medication errors

8. The P&T committee improves the quality of medications used in the hospital by:
   a. Objectively assessing medications based on the scientific evidence
   b. Anecdotal physician experience
   c. Manufacturer sponsored information
   d. Occasional review of formulary medications

9. A policy differs from a procedure in that a policy:
   a. Is a broad general statement that describes the goals and purpose of a document
   b. Provides specific action to be taken
   c. Is usually developed after a problem occurs
   d. Is not required by The Joint Commission

10. Taken together policies and procedures may be a logical, step-by-step explanation of why and where a product may be used, how to use it, and who is to follow the policy.
    a. True
    b. False

11. Policies and procedures that may be implemented by the P&T committee include:
    a. As needed (prn) medications
    b. Hold medications
    c. Resume medications
    d. All of the above

12. A conflict of interest is considered when people involved in the drug decision process:
    a. Receive direct or indirect compensation from having the drug available
    b. Have stock in the company
    c. Receive honoraria for speaking, consulting fees, and gifts or grants from the company
    d. All the above

13. A pharmacy benefit management (PBM) P&T committee differs from an institutional P&T by the following:
    a. Members consist of physicians, pharmacists, and nurses
    b. Work with health plans, insurers, and employers to develop drug formularies
    c. Meet on a monthly basis

14. Pharmacy networks are a group of pharmacies that are under contract with insurance companies, health plans, and/or contracted PBM parties to promote pharmacy services at negotiated discount fees.
    a. True
    b. False

15. PBMs place their formulary and nonformulary medications into tiers with an associated copayment with each tier.
    a. True
    b. False

Acknowledgment

Debra Lee, PharmD, from Alegent Creighton Health Creighton University Medical Center is acknowledged for her assistance in preparing this chapter.

REFERENCES

1. Shulkin DJ. Enhancing the role of physicians in the cost-effective use of pharmaceuticals. Hosp Formul. 1994;29:262-73.

2. Nair KV, Ascione FJ. Evaluation of P&T committee performance: an exploratory study. Hosp Formul. 2001;3:136-46.

3. Zellmer WA. Dr. Avorn's wake-up call to pharmacy. Am J Health Syst Pharm. 2004;61:2010.

4. Nair KV, Coombs JH, Ascione FJ. Assessing the structure, activities, and functioning of P&T committees: a multisite case study. P&T. 2000;25(10):516-28.

5. Redman RL, Mays DA. Data analysis. Drug information services in the managed care setting. Drug Benefit Trends. 1997;9:28-40.

6. Sroka CJ. CRS report for Congress: pharmacy benefit managers. Washington, DC: Library of Congress; 2000 Nov 29.

7. Gourley DR, Halbert MR, Hartmann KM, Malone PM. Development and implementation of a P&T committee for state institutions. Hosp Formul. 1981;16(2):143-4, 149-51, 154-5.

8. McCutcheon T. Medicare prescription drug benefit model guidelines. Washington, DC: United States Pharmacopeial Convention; 2004.

9. Stefanacci RG. The expanding role of P&T committees in long-term care. P&T. 2003;28:720-3.

10. Feldman L. Pharmacists' role in the pharmacy and therapeutics committee. Pharm Times. 2004 Feb:26.

11. Jenkins A. Formulary development by community pharmacists. Pharmaceutical J. 1996;256:861-3.

12. AMA Board of Trustees. Drug formularies and therapeutic interchange. Recommendations adopted at the American Medical Association (AMA) House of Delegates Interim Meeting 1993. Chicago (IL): American Medical Association; 1993.

13. H-125.991 drug formularies and therapeutic interchange. Chicago (IL): American Medical Association; 2000 [cited 2004 Mar 9]:[2 p.]. Available from: http://www.ama-assn.org/apps/pf_new/pf_online?f_n=browse&doc=policyfiles/HnE/H-125.991.HTM

14. Formulary management (medication-use policy development). Bethesda: American Society of Health-System Pharmacists; 2004 [cited 2004 Mar 9]:[1 p]. Available from: http://www.ashp.org/bestpractices/formulary.cfm?cfid=497523&CFToken=39106216

15. TJC—The Joint Commission comprehensive accreditation and certification manual. Accreditation requirements for hospitals [Internet]. Oakbrook Terrace (IL): The Joint Commission; 2013 Jan 1 [cited 2012 Dec 14]. Available from: https://e-dition.jcrinc.com/MainContent.aspx.

16. Format for formulary submissions. Version 3.0. Alexandria (VA): Academy of Managed Care Pharmacy; 2009.

17. Raffel MW, Barsukiewicz CK. The US Health System: Origins and Functions. Albany (NY): Delmar; 2002.

18. Balu S, O'Connor P, Vogenberg FR. Contemporary issues affecting P&T committees. Part 1: The evolution. P&T. 2004;29:709-11.

19. Worthen DB. The amazing Charles Rice and Bellevue Hospital. Pharm Pract News. 2010;37(06):[2 p.]. Available from: http://pharmacypracticenews.com/index.asp?section_id=402&show=dept&issue_id=643&article_id=15339

20. Condition of participation: pharmaceutical services. Fed Regist 1986;51:22042.

21. Millano C. Bellevue Hospital: the birthplace of formulary medicine? Pharm Pract News. 2004;31:14.

22. Plumridge RJ, Stoelwinder JU, Rucker TD. Drug and therapeutics committees: the relationships among structure, function, and effectiveness. Hosp Pharm. 1993;28:492-3, 496-8, 508.

23. World Health Organization, Management Sciences for Health. Drug and therapeutics committees—a practical guide. Geneva (Switzerland): World Health Organization, 2003.

24. Doherty EC. The JCAHO agenda for change: what changes in pharmacy and P&T activities do you need to prepare for in 1994. Hosp Formul. 1994;29:54-68.

25. The Joint Commission on Accreditation of Health care Organizations. 1995 Comprehensive accreditation manual for hospitals. Oakbrook Terrace (IL): Joint Commission on Accreditation of Healthcare Organizations; 1994.

26. Academy of Managed Care Pharmacy. Principles of a sound drug formulary system [Internet]. 2000 [cited 2004 Mar 18]. Available from: http://www.amcp.org/WorkArea/DownloadAsset.aspx?id=9280

27. Eavy GR, Swinkey NJ, Rehan A. Decentralizing the P&T committee: rationale and successes. Formulary. 2000;35:752-69.

28. Mubarak-Shaban H, Billups SJ. The pharmacy and therapeutics committee within a hospital corporation: challenges and solution. P&T. 1998;23(6):309-10, 332.

29. Herbert WJ, Mahaney LM. Consolidating P&T committees in an integrated health care system. Formulary. 1996;31:497-504.

30. Cano SB. Formularies in integrated health systems: Fallon health care system. Am J Health Syst Pharm. 1996;53:270-3.

31. Rizos AL, Levy E, Furnier J, Crowley K. Formularies in integrated health systems: Sharp HealthCare. Am J Health Syst Pharm. 1996;53:274-8.

32. Barkley GL, Krol G, Anandan JV, Isopi M. An integrated health care system's attempt to create a unified formulary. Formulary. 1997;32:60-74.

33. Jarry PD, Fish L. Insights on outpatient formulary management in a vertically integrated health care system. Formulary. 1997;32:500-14.

34. Mannebach MA, Ascione FJ, Gaither CA, Bagozzi RP, Cohen IA, Ryan ML. Activities, functions, and structure of pharmacy and therapeutics committees in large teaching hospitals. Am J Health Syst Pharm. 1999;56:622-8.

35. Balu S, O'Connor P, Vogenberg FR. Contemporary issues affecting P&T committees. Part 2: Beyond managed care. P&T. 2004;29:780-3.

36. Solow BK. P&T committees today: ensuring they bring value to your organization. Am J Pharm Benefits. 2009;1(4):189-90.

37. Teagarden JR. How many members should be on a P&T committee. P&T Society. 2003 Fall.

38. Miller WA. Making the pharmacy and therapeutics committee more effective. Curr Concepts Hosp Pharm Manage. 1986;Summer:10-5.

39. Christopherson GA. Policy for implementation of the DoD pharmacy and therapeutics committee [Internet]. Washington, DC: 1998 Mar 23 [cited 2004 Jan 23]:[4 p.]. Available from: http://www.tricare.osd.mil/policy/fy98/dptc9825.html

40. Barlas S. Role of P&T committees in Medicare: how much authority, accountability? P&T. 2004;29:678.

41. Cross M. Increased pressures change P&T Committee makeup. Managed Care. 2001:10(12):18-30.

42. The ABCs of PBMs. A discussion featuring Peter D. Fox, Ph.D, Terry S. Latanich, Chris O'Flinn, J.D. LLM, and Phonzie Brown. Washington, DC: The George Washington University. National Health Policy Forum. Issue Brief No. 749; 1999 Oct 27.

43. Lipton HL, Kreling DH, Collins T, Hertz KC. Pharmacy benefit management companies: dimensions of performance. Annu Rev Public Health. 1999;20:361-401.

44. Cross M. Do P&T committees have enough power? Managed Care. 2007;16(4):28-30.

45. Teagarden JR. Perspectives on prescription drug benefit formularies. Hosp Pharm. 2004;39:1102-25.

46. PricewaterhouseCoopers. The value of pharmacy benefit management and the national cost impact of proposed PBM legislation. Pharmaceutical Care Management Association; 2004 July.

47. Carroll J. Plans look askance at me-too medications. Managed Care. 2008;17(1):37-42.

48. Butler CD, Manchester R. The P&T committee: descriptive survey of activities and time requirements. Hosp Formul. 1986;21:89-98.

49. Chi J. When R.Ph.s talk P&T committees listen. Hosp Pharm Rep. 1994;8(5):1, 7-8.

50. Gannon K. More power to you. Pharmacists flex their muscles and exert greater influence on P&T committees. Hosp Pharm Rep. 1998;12(2):18-20.

51. Chase P, Bell J, Smith P, Fallik A. Redesign of the P&T committee around continuous quality improvement principles. P&T. 1995;20(10):25-6, 29-30, 32, 34, 37-8, 40.

52. Croft CL, Crane VS. Redesign of P&T committee functions and processes: a model. Formulary. 1998;33:1105-22.

53. Crane VS, Gonzalez ER, Hull BL. How to develop a proactive formulary system. Hosp Formul. 1994;29:700-10.

54. Poirier TI, Vorbach M, Bache T. Linking a policy on nonformulary drugs to the FDA's therapeutic–potential classification system. Am J Hosp Pharm. 1994;51:2277-8.

55. Rich DS. Pharmacies' noncompliance with 2009 Joint Commission hospital accreditation requirements. Am J Health Syst Pharm. 2009;66:e27-30.

56. Green JA, Chawla AK, Fong PA. Evaluating a restrictive formulary system by assessing nonformulary-drug requests. Am J Hosp Pharm. 1985;42:1537-41.

57. Hailemeskel B, Kelvas M. Nonformulary drug requests as a guide in formulary system management. Am J Health Syst Pharm. 1999;56:818, 820.

58. Adding drugs to the formulary: your work is never done. Hosp Pharm. 1999;34(7):828.

59. Shea BF, Churchill WW, Powell SH, Cooley TW, Maguire JH. P&T committee overview: Brigham and Women's Hospital. Pharm Pract Manag Q. 1998;17(4):76-83.

60. McCain J. P&T Committees in position to reduce medication errors. Managed Care. 2004;13(6):39-42.

61. Cunha BA. Principles of antibiotic formulary selection for P&T committees. P&T. 2003;28(6):396.

62. Empey KM, Rapp RP, Evans ME. The effect of an antimicrobial formulary change on hospital resistance patterns. Pharmacotherapy. 2002;22(1):81-7.

63. Cunha BA. Principles of antibiotic formulary selection for P&T committees. Part 1: Antimicrobial activity. P&T. 2003;28(6):397-9.

64. Cunha BA. Principles of antibiotic formulary selection for P&T committees. Part 2: Pharmacokinetics and pharmacodynamics. P&T. 2003;28(7):468-70.

65. Cunha BA. Principles of antibiotic formulary selection for P&T committees. Part 3: Antibiotic resistance. P&T. 2003;28(8):524-7.

66. Polk RE. Antimicrobial formularies: can they minimize antimicrobial resistance? Am J Health Syst Pharm. 2003;60(Suppl 1):S16-9.

67. Cunha BA. Principles of antibiotic formulary selection for P&T committees. Part 4: Antimicrobial side effects. P&T. 2003;28(9):594-6.

68. Cunha BA. Principles of antibiotic formulary selection for P&T committees. Part 5: The cost of antimicrobial therapy. P&T. 2003;28:662-5.

69. Motz JC. Influence of the P&T committee on antibiotic selection in a staff model HMO. P&T. 1998;23(8):411-8.

70. DiLiegro N, Groves AJ, Caspi A. Cost savings from an antimicrobial-monitoring program. P&T. 1998;23(8):419-24.

71. Carlson JA. Antimicrobial formulary management: meeting the challenge in a health maintenance organization. Pharmacotherapy. 1991;11(1 pt 2):32S-5S.

72. Quintiliani R, Quercia RA. How to create a therapeutics committee that is scientifically and economically sound. Formulary. 2003;38:594-602.

73. Owen RC, Shorr AF, Deschambeault AL. Antimicrobial stewardship: shepherding precious resources. Am J Health Syst Pharm. 2009;66(Suppl 4):S15-22.

74. Lesprit P, Brun-Buisson C. Hospital antibiotic stewardship. Curr Opin Infect Dis. 2008;21:344-349.

75. Drew RH. Antimicrobial stewardship programs: how to start and steer a successful program. J Manag Care Pharm. 2009;15(2)(Suppl):S18-23.

76. Chen AWJ, Khumra S, Eaton V, Kong DCM. Snapshot of antimicrobial stewardship in Australian hospitals. J Pharm Pract Res. 2010;40(1):19-25.

77. Deuster S, Roten I, Muehlebach S. Implementation of treatment guidelines to support judicious use of antibiotic therapy. J Clin Pharm Ther. 2010;35:71-8.

78. Culley CM, Carroll BA, Skledar SJ. Formulary decisions for pre-1938 medications. Am Health-Syst Pharm. 2008;65(15):1368-83.

79. Mirtallo JM. Advancement of nutrition support clinical pharmacy. Ann Pharmacother. 2007;41:869-72.

80. The Joint Commission. 2010 Provision of care, treatment and services [Internet]. The Joint Commission Web. Available from: http://www.jointcommission.org. Accessed October 21, 2010.

81. Fagan NL, Malone PM, Baltaro RJ, Malesker MA. Applying the principles of formulary management to blood banking. Transfusion 2013 Sep;53:2094-7.

82. ASHP statement on the pharmacy and therapeutics committee. Am J Hosp Pharm. 1992;49:2008-9.

83. Ventola CL. An interview series with members of the ASHP Expert Panel on Formulary Management. Part 1: Linda S. Tyler, Pharm.D. P&T. 2009;34(11):623-31.

84. Brushwood DB. Legal issues surrounding therapeutic interchange in institutional settings: an update. Formulary. 2001;36:796-804.

85. Mutnick AH, Ross MB. Formulary management at a tertiary care teaching hospital. Pharm Pract Manag Q. 1997;17(1):63-87.

86. Dore DD, Larrat EP, Vogenberg FR. Principles of epidemiology for clinical and formulary management professionals. P&T. 2006;31(4):218-26.

87. Suh D, Okpara I, Agnese WB, Toscani M. Application of pharmacoeconomics to formulary decision making in managed care organizations. Am J Managed Care. 2002;8(2):161-9.

88. Odedina FT, Sullivan J, Nash R, Clemmons CD. Use of pharmacoeconomic data in making hospital formulary decisions. Am J Health Syst Pharm. 2002;59:1441-4.

89. Pick AM, Massoomi F, Neff WJ, Danekas PL, Stoysich AM. A safety assessment tool for formulary candidates. Am J Health Syst Pharm. 2006;63:1269-72

90. Barr B. Open and closed. Pharmaceutical Representative[Internet]. 2007 May 1[cited 2008 Jul 14]:[4 p.]. Available from: http://license.icopyright.net/user/viewFreeUse .act?fuid=MTI2ODQyMg%3D%3D

91. ASHP statement on the formulary system. Am J Hosp Pharm. 1983;35:326-8.

92. ASHP technical assistance bulletin on drug formularies. Am J Hosp Pharm. 1991;48:791-3.

93. ASHP guidelines on formulary system management. Am J Hosp Pharm. 1992;49:648-52.

94. Rucker TD, Schiff G. Drug formularies: myths-in-formation. Med Care. 1990;28:928-42.

95. Tyler LS, Cole SW, May JR, Millares M, Valentino MA, Vermeulen LC Jr, Wilson AL. ASHP guidelines on the pharmacy and therapeutics committee and the formulary system. Am J Health Syst Pharm. 2008;65:1272-83.

96. Grissinger M. The truth about hospital formularies Part I. P&T. 2008;33(8):441.

97. Lehmann DF, Guharoy R, Page N, Hirschman K, Ploutz-Snyder R, Medicis J. Formulary management as a tool to improve medication use and gain physician support. Am J Health Syst Pharm. 2007;64:464-6.

98. ASHP statement on the pharmacy and therapeutics committee and the formulary system. Am J Health Syst Pharm. 2008;65:2384-6.

99. Rubino M, Hofman JM, Koseserer LJ, Swendryznski RG. ASHP guidelines on medication cost management strategies for hospitals and health systems. Am J Health Syst Pharm. 2008;65:1368-84.

100. Chi J. Hospital consultant foresees dim future for drug formularies. Drug Topics. 1999 April 19:67.

101. Horn SD, Sharkey PD, Tracy DM, Horn C, James B, Goodwin F. Intended and unintended consequences of HMO cost-containment strategies: results from the managed care outcomes project. Am J Manag Care. 1996;2:253-64.

102. Horn SD. Unintended consequences of drug formularies. Am J Health Syst Pharm. 1996;53:2204-6.

103. Goldberg RB. Managing the pharmacy benefit: the formulary system. J Manag Care Pharm. 1997;3(5):565-73.

104. Formulary effectiveness: many questions, but few clear answers. Consult Pharm. 1996;11(7):635.

105. Curtiss FR. Drug formularies provide a path to best care. Am J Health Syst Pharm. 1996;53:2201-3.

106. Formularies and generics drive up health resource use, study suggests. Am J Health Syst Pharm. 1996;53:971-5.

107. Horn SD, Sharkey PD, Phillips-Harris C. Formulary limitations and the elderly: results from the managed care outcomes project. Am J Manag Care. 1998;4:1105-13.

108. Marra F, Patrick DM, White R, Ng H, Bowie WR, Hutchinson JM. Effect of formulary policy decisions on antimicrobial drug utilization in British Columbia. J Antimicrob Chemother. 2005;55:95-101.

109. Penm J, Chaar B, Dechun J, Moles R. Formulary systems in the Western Pacific Region: exploring two Basel Statements. Am J Health Syst Pharm. 2013;70:967-79.

110. Hepler CD. Where is the evidence for formulary effectiveness. Am J Health Syst Pharm. 1997;54:95.

111. VHA formulary management process. Washington, DC: Department of Veterans Affairs, 2009.

112. Kelly WN, Rucker TD. Considerations in deciding which drugs should be in a formulary. J Pharm Pract. 1994;VII(2):51-7.

113. Corman SL, Skledar SJ, Culley CM. Evaluation of conflicting literature and application to formulary decisions. Am J Health Sys Pharm. 2007;64:182-5.

114. Shih Y-CT, Sleath BL. Health care provider knowledge of drug formulary status in ambulatory care settings. Am J Health Syst Pharm. 2004;61:2657-63.

115. Muirhead G. When formularies collide. Hospitals vs. health plans. Hosp Pharm Rep. 1994;8(10):1, 8.

116. 1999 accreditation standards address public concerns, says NCQA. Am J Health Syst Pharm. 1998;55:2221, 2225.

117. Bruzek RJ, Dullinger D. Drug formulary: the cornerstone of a managed pharmacy program. J Pharm Pract. 1992;V(2):75-81.

118. North GLT. Handling nonformulary requests for returning or transfer patients. Am J Hosp Pharm. 1994;51:2360, 2364.

119. Davis FA. Formularies: a dangerous concept for patients. Priv Pract. 1991 Sep:11-17.

120. Palmer MA, Hartman SK, Gervais S. Introducing a formulary system in long-term care facilities: initial experience. Consult Pharm. 1994;9:307-14.

121. Shulkin DJ. Enhancing the role of physicians in the cost-effective use of pharmaceuticals. Hosp Formul. 1994;29:262-73.

122. Pearce MJ, Begg EJ. A review of limited lists and formularies. Are they cost-effective? Pharmacoeconomics. 1992;1:191-202.

123. Sloan FA, Gordon GS, Cocks DL. Hospital drug formularies and use of hospital services. Med Care. 1993;31:851-67.

124. Hazlet TK, Hu T-W. Association between formulary strategies and hospital drug expenditures. Am J Hosp Pharm. 1992;49:2207-10.

125. Pickette S, Hanish L. Dealing with demands for nonformulary drugs. Am J Hosp Pharm. 1992;49:2920, 2923.

126. Corliss DA. Computer-assisted help desk for handling drug benefits. Am J Health Syst Pharm. 1997;54:1941-2, 1945.

127. NCQA draft accreditation standards for 2000 address formularies. Am J Health Syst Pharm. 1998;55:1266-7.

128. Le AG, Generali JA. From printed formularies to online formularies. Hosp Pharm. 2004;38:1003.

129. Navarro RP. Electronic formulary control. Med Interface. 1997;10(8):74-6.

130. Drug czars, electronic formulary systems increase formulary compliance. Formulary. 1997;32:171-2.

131. Ukens C. Hospital finds computer carrot can save drug dollars. Hosp Pharm Rep. 1994;8(6):20.

132. Computerized drug cost information fails to sway physician prescribing. Am J Health Syst Pharm. 1999;56:1183-4.

133. Sears EL. Development and maintenance of an online formulary for a large health system. Am J Health Syst Pharm. 2008;65:510-11-2.

134. E-prescribing applications help physicians with Vioxx recall. Pharm Pract News. 2004;31(11):67.

135. Patel B, Pichardo RV. Improve formulary adherence through effective provider engagement. Formulary. 2012;47:400-1.

136. McCaffrey S, Nightingale CH. How to develop critical paths and prepare for other formulary management changes. Hosp Formul. 1994;29:628-35.

137. Current formulary decision-making strategies and new factors influencing the process. Formulary. 1995;30:462-70.

138. Raber JH. The formulary process from a risk management perspective. Pharmacotherapy 2010;30(6 Pt 2):42S-7S.

139. Shulkin D. Reinventing the pharmacy and therapeutics committee. P&T. 2012 Nov;37(11):623-4, 649.

140. Rich DS. New JCAHO medication management standards for 2004. Am J Health Syst Pharm. 2004;61:1349-58.

141. Neumann PJ. Evidence-based and value-based formulary guidelines. 2004;23(1):124-34.
142. Murri NA, Somani S. Implementation of safety-focused pharmacy and therapeutics monographs: a new University Health System Consortium template designed to minimize medication misadventures. Hosp Pharm. 2004;39:654-60.
143. Chren M-M, Landefeld CS. Physicians' behavior and their interactions with drug companies. JAMA. 1994;271:684-9.
144. Bach PB, Saltz LB, Wittes RE. In cancer care, cost matters. New York Times. 2012 Oct 14:A25.
145. Haslé-Pham E, Arnould B, Späth H-M, Follet A, Duru G, Marquis P. Role of clinical, patient-reported outcome and medico-economic studies in the public hospital drug formulary decision-making process: results of a European survey. Health Policy. 2005; 71:205-12.
146. Ventola CL. An interview series with members of the ASHP Expert Panel on Formulary Management. Part 3: Sabrina W. Cole, Pharm.D. P&T. 2010;35(1):24-8.
147. Shrank WH. Change we can believe in: requiring better evidence for formulary coverage. Am J Pharm Benefits. 2009;Fall:134-6.
148. Asmus MJ, Hendeles L. Levalbuterol nebulizer solution: is it worth five times the cost of albuterol? Pharmacotherapy. 2000;20:123-9.
149. Desloratadine (Clarinex). Med Lett. 2002;44(W1126B):27-9.
150. Escitalopram (Lexapro) for depression. Med Lett. 2002;44(W1140A):83-4.
151. Most medications approved in the 1990s not new, but modified versions of older drugs, report states [Internet]. Menlo Park (CA): kaisernetwork.org; 2002 May 29 [cited 2004 Apr 22]. Available from: http://www.kaiserhealthnews.org/daily-reports/2002/may/29/dr00011414.aspx?referrer=search
152. Senthilkumaran K, Shatz SM, Kalies RF. Computer-based support system for formulary decisions. Am J Hosp Pharm. 1987;44:1362-6.
153. Computer tool lets P&T members assess Tx classes with their own weightings, product ratings. Formulary. 2000;35:603.
154. Janknegt R, Steenhoek A. The system of objectified judgement analysis (SOJA). A tool in rational drug selection for formulary inclusion. Drugs. 1997;53(4):550-62.
155. Janknegt R, van den Broek PJ, Kulberg BJ, Stobberingh E. Glycopeptides: drug selection by means of the SOJA method. Eur Hosp Pharm. 1997;3(4):127-35.
156. Zachry WM III, Skrepnek GH. Applying multiattribute utility technology to the formulary evaluation process. Formulary. 2002;37:199-206.
157. Jacobson SH. A web-based tool for designing vaccine formularies for childhood immunization in the United States. J Am Med Informatics Assoc. 2008;15(5):611-9.
158. Berghelli JA. Conflict of interest policy approved. P&T. 1995;20:497.
159. Alpert JS. Doctors and the drug industry: how can we handle potential conflicts of interest? Am J Med. 2005;118:88-100.
160. Ventola CL. An interview series with members of the ASHP Expert Panel on Formulary Management. Part 2: J. Russell May, Pharm.D. P&T. 2009;34(12):671-7.

161. Campbell EG. Doctors and drug companies—scrutinizing influential relationships. NEJM. 2007;357(18):1796-7.

162. Palmer MA. Developing a conflict-of-interest policy for the pharmacy and therapeutics committee. Am J Hosp Pharm. 1987;44:2012-4.

163. Fredrick DS, Maddock JR, Graman PS. Hashing out a policy on conflicts of interest for a P&T committee. Am J Health Syst Pharm. 1995;52:2791-2.

164. Campbell EG. A national survey of physician-industry relationships. NEJM. 2007; 356:1742-50.

165. Barlas S. Inspector General cautions PBMs on formulary decision making. P&T. 2003;28(6):367.

166. Trice S, Devine J, Mistry H, Moore E, Linton, A. Formulary management in the Department of Defense. J Managed Care Pharmacy. 2009;15(2):133-46.

167. JCAHO unveils medication-management standards. Am J Health Syst Pharm. 2003; 60:1400-1.

168. Cardinale V. Alternative medicine: the law, the marketplace, the formulary. Hosp Pharm Rep. 1999;13(7):15.

169. Is alternative medicine poised for hospital formularies. Drug Util Rev. 1999;15(5):65-8.

170. Brubaker ML. Setting up the herbal formulary system for an alternative medicine clinic. Am J Health Syst Pharm. 1998;55:435-6.

171. Beal FC. Herbals and homeopathic remedies as formulary items. Am J Health Syst Pharm. 1998;55:1266-7.

172. Johnson ST, Wordell CJ. Homeopathic and herbal medicine: considerations for formulary evaluation. Formulary. 1997;32:1166-73.

173. Malesker MA, Meyer RT, Kuhlenengel LJ, Galt MA, Nelson PJ. Development of an alternative medication use policy [abstract]. ASHP Midyear Clinical Meeting. 1998;33(Dec):P-406R.

174. Walker PC. Evolution of a policy disallowing the use of alternative therapies in a health system. Am J Health Syst Pharm. 2000;57:1984-90.

175. Ansani NT, Ciliberto NC, Freedy T. Hospital policies regarding herbal medicines. Am J Health Syst Pharm. 2003;60:367-70.

176. Pick AM, Massoomi F, Neff WJ, Danekas PI, Stoysich AM. A safety assessment tool for formulary candidates. Am J Health Syst Pharm. 2006;63:1269-72.

177. H-125.911 Drug formularies and therapeutic interchange [Internet]. Chicago (IL): American Medical Association; [cited 2004 Apr 23]. Available from: http://www.ama-assn.=org/apps/pf_new/pf_online?f_n=browse&doc=policyfiles/HnE/H-125.991.HTM

178. NCQA draft accreditation standards for 2000 address formularies. Am J Health Syst Pharm. 1999;56:846.

179. Chiefari DM. Effect of a closed formulary on average prescription cost in a community health center. Drug Benefit Trends. 2001;13:44-5, 52.

180. Survey reveals continued HMO shift toward closed and partially closed formularies. Formulary. 1997;32:781-2.

181. Survey finds HMOs, PBMs still moving to restricted formularies, quickly advancing in informatics. Formulary. 1998;33:622, 625.

182. Doyle JJ. The effect of comparative effectiveness research on drug development innovation: a 360° value appraisal. Comp Effectiveness Res. 2011;1:27-34.

183. Abramowitz PW. Controlling financial variables—changing prescribing patterns. Am J Hosp Pharm. 1984;41:503-15.

184. Open formularies improve oncology outcomes in capitated care system. Formulary. 1996;31:878, 881.

185. TennCare formulary restrictions hurt patient care, survey says. Formulary. 1996; 31(6):443.

186. Traynor K. Virginia passes nation's first biosimilar substitution law. Am J Health Syst Pharm. 2013 May 15;70:834-6.

187. Schachtner JM, Guharoy R, Medicis JJ, Newman N, Speizer R. Prevalence and cost savings of therapeutic interchange among U.S. hospitals. Am J Health Syst Pharm. 2002;59:529-33.

188. Bowman GK, Moleski R, Mangi RJ. Measuring the impact of a formulary decision: conversion to one quinolone agent. Formulary. 1996;31:906-14.

189. Chase SL, Peterson AM, Wordell CJ. Therapeutic-interchange program for oral histamine H_2-receptor antagonists. Am J Health Syst Pharm. 1998;55:1382-6.

190. Stoysich A, Massoomi F. Automatic interchange of the ACE inhibitors: decision-making process and initial results. Formulary. 2002;37:41-4.

191. Frighetto L, Nickoloff D, Jewesson P. Antibiotic therapeutic interchange program: six years of experience. Hosp Formul. 1995;30:92-105.

192. Vivian JC. Legal aspects of therapeutic interchange programs. US Pharm. 2003 Aug;28:58,60-2.

193. Janifer AN, Chatelain F, Goldwater SH, Mikovich G. Reengineering hospital pharmacy through therapeutic equivalency interchange while maintaining clinical outcomes. P&T. 1998;23(2):78-82, 85-8, 90-2.

194. Merli GJ, Vanscoy GJ, Rihn TL, Groce JB III, McCormick W. Applying scientific criteria to therapeutic interchange: a balanced analysis of low-molecular-weight heparins. J Thromb Thrombolysis. 2001;11(3):247-59.

195. Reich P. Therapeutic drug interchange. Med Interface. 1996;9(5):14.

196. H-125.995 Therapeutic and pharmaceutical alternatives by pharmacists [Internet]. Chicago (IL): American Medical Association; [cited 2004 Apr 23]. Available from: http://www.ama-assn.org/apps/pf_new/pf_online?f_n=browse&doc=policyfiles/HnE/H-125.995.HTM

197. American College of Physicians. Therapeutic substitution and formulary systems. Ann Intern Med. 1990;113:160-3.

198. Therapeutic interchange [Internet]. Alexandria (VA): Academy of Managed Care Pharmacy; 2012 Jun [cited 2014 Feb 17]. Available from: http://www.amcp.org/Tertiary.aspx?id=8749&terms=therapeutic%20interchange

199. American College of Clinical Pharmacy. Guidelines for therapeutic interchange. Pharmacotherapy. 1993;13(2):252-6.

200. Massoomi F. Formulary management: antibiotics and therapeutic interchange. Pharm Pract Manag Q. 1996;16(3):11-8.

201. Heiner CR. Communicating about therapeutic interchange. Am J Health Syst Pharm. 1996;53:2568-70.

202. Rosen A, Kay BG, Halecky D. Implementing a therapeutic interchange program in an institutional setting. P&T. 1995;20:711-7.

203. Kielty M. Improving the prior-authorization process to the satisfaction of customers. Am J Health Syst Pharm. 1999;56:1499-1501.

204. Carroll NV. Formularies and therapeutic interchange: the health care setting makes a difference. Am J Health Syst Pharm. 1999;56:467-72.

205. Nelson KM. Improving ambulatory care through therapeutic interchange. Am J Health Syst Pharm. 1999;56:1307.

206. D'Amore M, Masters P, Maroun C. Impact of an automatic therapeutic interchange program on discharge medication selection. Hosp Pharm. 2003;38:942-6.

207. Banahan BF III, Bonnarens JK, Bentley JP. Generic substitution of NTI drugs: issues for Formulary Committee consideration. Formulary. 1998;33:1082-96.

208. FDA comments on activities in states concerning narrow-therapeutic-index drugs. Am J Health Syst Pharm. 1998;55:686-7.

209. ASHP guidelines for selecting pharmaceutical manufacturers and suppliers. Am J Hosp Pharm. 1991;48:523-4.

210. Pummer TL, Shalaby KM, Erush SC. Ordering off the menu: assessing compliance with a nonformulary medication policy. Ann Pharmacother. 2009 July/Aug;43:1251-7.

211. Sweet BV, Stevenson JG. Pharmacy costs associated with nonformulary drug requests. Am J Health Syst Pharm. 2001;58:1746-52.

212. Tse CST, Roecker W, Benitez M, Musabji M. How to tie a drug therapy improvement program to physician credentialing. Hosp Formul. 1994;29:646-56.

213. ASHP statement on the use of medications for unlabeled uses. Am J Hosp Pharm. 1992;49:2006-8.

214. Steinberg SK. The development of a hospital pharmacy policy and procedure manual. Can J Hosp Pharm. 1980;XXXIII(6):194-5, 211.

215. Ginnow WK, King CM Jr. Revision and reorganization of a hospital pharmacy and procedure manual. Am J Hosp Pharm. 1978;35:698-704.

216. Van Dusen V, Pray WS. Issues in implementation and enforcement of hospital pharmacy policies and procedures. Hosp Pharm. 2001;36(4):398-403.

217. Piecoro JJ Jr. Development of an institutional I.V. drug delivery policy. Am J Hosp Pharm. 1987;44:2557-9.

218. Grissinger M. Eliminating problem-prone, automatic stop-order policies. P&T. 2004;29:344.

219. Galt KA. Credentialing and privileging for pharmacists. Am J Health Syst Pharm. 2004;61:661-70.

220. Galt KA. Privileging, quality improvement and accountability. Am J Health Syst Pharm. 2004;61:659.

221. Abramowitz PW, Shane R, Daigle LA, Noonan KA, Letendre DE. Pharmacist interdependent prescribing: a new model for optimizing patient outcomes. Am J Health Syst Pharm. 2012;69:1976-81.

222. Sass CM. Drug usage evaluation. J Pharm Pract. 1994;7(2):74-8.

223. Orsini MJ, Funk Orsini PA, Thorn DB, Gallina JN. An ADR surveillance program: increasing quality, number of incidence reports. Formulary. 1995;30:454-61.

224. Samore MH, Evans RS, Lassen A, Gould P, Lloyd J, Gardner RM, et al. Surveillance of medical device-related hazards and adverse events in hospitalized patients. JAMA. 2004;291:325-34.

225. Traynor K. Enforcement outdoes education at eliminating unsafe abbreviations. Am J Health Syst Pharm. 2004;61:1314, 1317, 1322.

226. Baker De. Sound-alike and look-alike drug errors. Hosp Pharm. 2002;37:225.

227. Vaida AJ, Peterson J. Common sound-alike, look-alike products. Pharm Times. 2002; 68:22-3.

228. Starr CH. When drug names spell trouble. Drug Topics. 2000;144:49-50, 53-4, 57-8.

229. Cohen M. Medication error update. Consult Pharm. 1997;12:1328-9.

230. Soulliard D, Hong M, Saubermann L. Development of a pharmacy-managed medication dictionary in a newly implemented computerized prescriber order-entry system. Am J Health Syst Pharm. 2004;61:617-22.

231. First Consulting Group. Computerized physician order entry: costs, benefits and challenges. A case study approach. Long Beach (CA): First Consulting Group; 2003.

232. FDA's counterfeit drug tasks force interim report. Washington, DC: U.S. Department of Health and Human Services; 2003 Oct [cited 2004 Mar 8]. Available from: http://www .fda.gov/oc/initiatives/counterfeit/report/interim_report.html

233. Generali JA. Counterfeit drugs: a growing concern. Hosp Pharm. 2003;38:724.

234. Young D. FDA urges adoption of anticounterfeit technologies by 2007 [Internet]. Bethesda (MD): American Society of Health-System Pharmacists; 2004 Feb 19 [cited 2004 Mar 8]. Available from: http://www.ashp.org/news/ShowArticle.cfm?cfid= 497458&CFToken=73579785&id=4194

235. Redwanski J, Seamon MJ. Impact of counterfeit drugs on the formulary decision-making process. Formulary. 2004;39:577-9, 583.

236. ASHP guidelines on managing drug product shortages. Am J Health Syst Pharm. 2001;58:1445-50.

237. Lasser KE, Allen PD, Woolhandler SJ, Himmelstein DU, Wolfe SM, Bor DH. Timing of new black box warnings and withdrawals for prescription medications. JAMA. 2002; 287:2215-20.

238. Gandey A. Propoxyphene withdrawn from US market. Medscape [Internet]. 2010 Nov 19 [cited 2010 Nov 19]:[2 p.]. Available from: http://www.medscape.com/viewarticle/732887_print

239. Fox ER, Tyler LS. Managing drug shortages: seven years' experience at one health system. Am J Health Syst Pharm. 2003;60:245-53.

240. Leady MA, Adams AL, Stumpf JL, Sweet BV. Drug shortages: an approach to managing the latest crisis. Hosp Pharm. 2003;38:748-52.

241. Schrand LM, Troester TS, Ballas ZK, Mutnick AH, Ross MB. Preparing for drug shortages: one teaching hospital's approach to the IVIG shortage. Formulary. 2001;36:52-9.

242. Huskamp HA, Deverka PA, Epstein AM, Epstein RS, McGuigan KA, Frank RG. The effect of incentive-based formularies on prescription-drug utilization and spending. NEJM. 2003;349:2224-32.

243. Thomas CP. Incentive-based formularies. NEJM. 2003;349:2186-8.

244. Crane VS, Hull BL, Hatwig CA, Teresi M, Croft CL. Presenting drug cost information to a board of directors: a case example. Formulary. 2001;36:857-64.

245. Hoffman JM, Shah ND, Vermeulen LC, Hunkler RJ, Hontz KM. Projecting future drug expenditures-2004. Am J Health Syst Pharm. 2004;61:145-58.

246. Shah ND, Vermeulen LC, Santell JP, Hunkler RJ, Hontz K. Projecting future drug expenditures—2002. Am J Health Syst Pharm. 2002;59:131-42.

247. Shah ND, Hoffman JM, Vermeulen LC, Hunkler RJ, Hontz K. Projecting future drug expenditures—2003. Am J Health Syst Pharm. 2003;60:137-49.

248. Mora MW. How P&T committees can be effective change agents: part 1. Am J Pharm Benefits. 2010;2(2):99-100.

249. Brookins L, Burnette R, De la Torre C, Dumitru D, McManus RB, Urbanski CJ, et al. Formulary and database synchronization. Am J Health Syst Pharm. 2011 Feb 1;68:204,206.

Chapter Thirteen

Drug Evaluation Monographs

Patrick M. Malone ● Nancy L. Fagan
● Mark A. Malesker ● Paul J. Nelson

Learning Objectives

After completing this chapter, the reader will be able to

- Describe and perform an evaluation of a drug product for a drug formulary.
- List the sections included in a drug evaluation monograph.
- Describe the overall highlights included in a monograph summary.
- Describe the recommendations and restrictions that are made in a monograph.
- Describe the purpose and format of a drug class review.

Key Concepts

1 The establishment and maintenance of a drug formulary requires that drugs or drug classes be objectively assessed based on scientific information (e.g., efficacy, safety, uniqueness, cost, and other appropriate items), not anecdotal prescriber experience.

2 The drug evaluation monograph provides a structured method to review the major features of a drug product.

3 A definite recommendation must be made based on need, therapeutics, side effects, cost, and other items specific to the particular agent (e.g., evidence-based treatment guidelines, dosage forms, convenience, dosage interval, inclusion on the formulary of third-party payers, hospital antibiotic resistance patterns, and potential for causing medication errors), usually in that order.

④ The recommendation must be supported by objective evidence.

⑤ The most logical decision to benefit the patient and the institution should be recommended to the pharmacy and therapeutics (P&T) committee.

⑥ While some think that cost is emphasized too much in formulary decisions, it is still an extremely important item.

⑦ Preparation of a drug evaluation monograph requires a great amount of time and effort, using many of the skills discussed throughout this text to obtain, evaluate, collate, and provide information. However, the value of having all of the issues evaluated and discussed can be invaluable in providing quality care.

Introduction

❶ *The establishment and maintenance of a* **drug formulary** *requires that drugs or drug classes be objectively assessed based on scientific information (e.g., efficacy, safety,*[1] *uniqueness, cost, and other appropriate items), not anecdotal prescriber experience.* The way to decide which drug is best for formulary addition is to rationally evaluate all aspects of the drug in relation to similar agents. In particular, it is necessary to consider need, effectiveness, risk, and cost (overall, including monitoring costs, discounts, rebates, and so forth)—often in that order. Some other issues that are evaluated include dosage forms, packaging, requirements of accrediting or quality assurance bodies, evidence-based treatment guidelines, prescriber preferences, regulatory issues, patient/nursing convenience, advertising, and consumer expectations.[2] There is increasingly more emphasis on evaluating clinical outcomes from high-quality trials, continuous quality assurance information, comparative efficacies,[3] pharmacogenomics, and quality of life.[4] Even such a factor as the public image of the institution may have an impact on the decision to add a drug to the formulary. An in-depth **drug evaluation monograph** can be prepared to assist in this process as described below.

❷ *The drug evaluation monograph provides a structured method to review the major features of a drug product.* Once a monograph is prepared, it can easily be used as a structured template or overview of a drug product. That allows for easy comparison or contrast to other products that may be used for the same indication or that are in the same product class. Commercially prepared monographs can also be obtained from several sources that can be used as is or with modifications to suit the needs of the institution. If this latter method is used, be aware that the quality of the commercial monographs may vary, even from the same publisher, and they may need extensive updating. Often, writing a new drug evaluation monograph may be easier than improving a commercial monograph.

When a pharmacy and therapeutics (P&T) committee desires to review an entire class of drugs, the drug category review is often another method used. **Drug class reviews** are often more lengthy than a single product drug evaluation monograph; however, they can also use a similar structure and format. Hospitals, health systems, and managed care organizations review an entire class of drugs on a scheduled basis, which must be at least annually, according to accreditation standards.[5] This allows an organization the opportunity to reevaluate the formulary status of products in light of new publications or trials, new products that have entered the market, or oftentimes reevaluate a drug class for possible deletion of particular products from the class. Samples of drug class reviews prepared by the Veterans Administration are available on the Internet at http://www.pbm.va.gov/clinicalguidance/drugclassreviews.asp.

Whether or not the monograph is commercial or prepared by a member from within the organization, the material should reflect the local conditions or current prescribing practices and may be sent to P&T committee members at a reasonable time before the meeting in order to allow full consideration of the information. In order to prevent drug company representatives or others from obtaining the material, however, some institutions only distribute this material for review during the meeting and then require the materials to be returned at the end of the meeting. Some institutions even number each monograph with a unique numbering system to assist in tracking the return of P&T committee documents.

Although there are recommendations concerning monograph contents,[2,6] information that may be valuable and specific to an institution, and necessary for an objective review of the product, is commonly missing.[7] An outline of a sample monograph is found in Appendix 13–1. Each of the sections of this monograph will be discussed below. An example of some of the information found in the various parts of a monograph is seen in Appendix 13–2. This sample monograph meets or exceeds the recommendations of the American Society of Health-System Pharmacists (ASHP),[6] and should serve as a good example for most circumstances. Guidelines published by the Academy of Managed Care Pharmacy (AMCP)[2,8] and The Joint Commission (TJC)[5] are also noted and discussed for situational applicability. The AMCP format is actually the standard recommended by an organization for manufacturers to submit data to managed care organizations. It is designed to restrict the marketing impact of the company in providing information and, while it has applicability as to how an institution may evaluate a drug, it also has restrictions as to the amount of information that it can cover in some areas that may make it undesirable in some cases. However, it may be very worthwhile for institutions or other organizations to request this information from the drug company, preferably, well in advance of the time it is needed. Please note, in some cases this request may require signing a nondisclosure agreement, since it may contain proprietary information.[2]

Overall, the precise monograph should be tailored to the institution, organization, patient population, clinic, and so forth. Several sections not recommended by ASHP have been added to increase the utility of the monograph for other sites of practice, including ambulatory clinics, pediatric institutions, long-term care facilities, managed care or pharmacy benefit managers, or even Medicare or Medicaid formularies. Also, in some cases, the information has been divided into multiple sections or subsections to increase clarity. This format can also be used to evaluate whole classes of drugs. In most cases, a specific drug is compared to others in the same class. The only difference in a class review is that one drug is not receiving the greatest attention; all drugs are being compared with equal attention. Comparative charts and tables are often more prevalent in drug class reviews, as they can serve as a concise method to provide an overview of comparative features for the products in a particular drug class.

Specific formats, differing somewhat from the one presented here, may be required by organizations or governments. For example, Australia (http://www.tga.gov.au/industry/pm-argpm.htm),[9] Ontario, Canada (http://www.health.gov.on.ca/english/providers/pub/drugs/dsguide/dsguide_mn.html),[10] and the United Kingdom (http://www.nice.org.uk/aboutnice/howwework/devnicetech/technologyappraisalprocessguides/technology_appraisal_process_guides.jsp)[11] have very specific published guidelines that need to be followed for a drug product to be considered for their formularies. The process recommended in this chapter appears to be common in both Canada and the United States, and has been recommended in Australia.[12] Where appropriate, features of these formats have been incorporated into the description presented in this chapter. While the format described in this chapter does provide much of the information in those government standards, with the exception of details about product manufacturing and specific pricing for the particular country, the order and amount of information is often different and the reader is referred to those standards for details.

Before discussing details about monograph preparation, it should be emphasized that the drug monograph is a powerful tool for the pharmacy to guide the rational development of a drug formulary. Although the pharmacy department or an individual pharmacist may have few, if any, votes in the ultimate adoption of a formulary agent, the monograph guides the evaluation process and is likely to be a major factor in the final decision. While monograph preparation can be very time consuming, it is extremely important and should be given proper attention. The structured evaluation process of a drug monograph, in many cases, is the only time a full, fair, and balanced review of a drug may be presented to a practitioner. Pharmacists have a unique role in the preparation of a monograph in that they view the drug product from a whole and macroeconomic view— all aspects of the drug product are objectively reviewed in a monograph, whereas, oftentimes when a prescriber is presented information about a new drug product, they may be basing their use or nonuse of the product on a single study, package insert data, pharmaceutical representative information, or some other microeconomic view of a drug product that may or may not represent the full utility of the drug product.[13,14]

In addition to FDA-regulated drug products, pharmacists need to be aware of complementary/alternative medicine use, along with the responsibilities and implications that it has for pharmacy services. These products can only be marketed as dietary substances, since the FDA does not regulate herbal products, so manufacturers and distributors cannot make specific health claims. Although there may be minimal scientific evidence regarding efficacy and safety of these products, pharmacists must provide information relating to all therapeutic agents patients are receiving, preparing a drug monograph for the P&T committee, much the same as for any FDA-approved product. This can also follow the format described in this chapter.[15]

The following sections describe the parts of the drug monograph, as shown in the appendices. Please note that skills in information retrieval (see Chapter 3), drug literature evaluation (see Chapters 4 and 5), professional writing (see Chapter 9), and areas covered in various other chapters must be employed when preparing a drug evaluation monograph.

Drug Evaluation Monograph Sections

SUMMARY PAGE

● The first page of the monograph is essentially a summary of the most important information concerning the drug, and includes a specific recommendation of the action to be taken on the product. Some P&T committees only review this first sheet; however, the remainder of the document should be prepared in order to completely evaluate a drug product and provide a record of all that was taken into consideration. The summary and recommendation could be placed at the end of the monograph, but it is probably best to keep it on the front to make it easier to refer to during the meeting.

● The format of the summary page usually begins with general institutional information. Following the name header, specific introductory information about the product is included. The generic name, trade name, and manufacturer are self-explanatory, but the classification may require some explanation. This is meant to give the readers a very quick way of classifying the agent in their head. It includes the prescription/controlled substance status, **American Hospital Formulary Service (AHFS) classification**, and FDA classification. It may also contain other classification schemes used by particular organizations, such as the Veteran's Administration. Managed care organizations may use more detail drug product identification schemes, such as those established by First DataBank (http://www.fdbhealth.com).

The AHFS classification can be found in the *AHFS Drug Information* reference book, published by the ASHP. This classification can help the reader determine where this new agent falls in therapy. Most of the time new drugs will be evaluated for possible formulary addition before they are actually placed in that book, so it will be necessary to consult the therapeutic classification table in the front of the *AHFS Drug Information* reference book or online at http://www.ahfsdruginformation.com/class/index.aspx to decide where the product fits. The classification of similar products listed in *AHFS Drug Information* can also be checked before deciding where to categorize the new product.

The FDA classification is given to nonbiologic products during the review process and is finalized when the new drug application (NDA) is approved. This classification gives some idea of the importance of the product. The classification consists of Chemical Type classification (see Table 13–1) and Therapeutic Rating classification (see Table 13–2). An FDA classification of 1P (or 1A prior to 1992) would indicate a drug that was given a priority review status by the FDA. This means that the product offered a therapeutic advance over existing products in the market, may be for a new disease state, or may represent a new drug class. The FDA generally reviews these products in an expedited manner, often not requiring as many clinical trials or a lower number of patients enrolled in the trials before the drug is approved to be on the market. In contrast, a classification of 3S (or 3C prior to 1992) is probably a me-too product, meaning that it is an additional product in a class of medications that is already on the market and is similar in many ways to the other products already marketed. These products are generally reviewed by the FDA in a standard review manner and do not receive an expedited review process. Knowing and understanding the FDA classification status of a product can assist a reviewer in preparing the drug evaluation monograph in several ways. First, if the reviewer knows that the product they are

TABLE 13–1. FDA CLASSIFICATION BY CHEMICAL TYPE*

Type	Definition
1	New molecular entity not marketed in the United States
2	New salt, ester, or other noncovalent derivative of another drug marketed in the United States
3	New formulation or dosage form of an active ingredient marketed in the United States
4	New combination of drugs already marketed in the United States
5	New manufacturer of a drug product already marketed by another company in the United States
6	New indication for a product already marketed in the United States
7	Drug that is already legally marketed without an approved NDA
	• First application since 1962 for a drug marketed prior to 1938
	• First application for DESI (Drug Efficacy Study Implementation)-related products that were first marketed between 1938 and 1962 without an NDA
	• First application for DESI-related products first marketed after 1962 without NDAs; in this case, the indications may be the same or different from the legally marketed product
8	Over-the-counter switch

*Drugs@FDA Frequently Asked Questions [Internet]. Washington, DC: Food and Drug Administration; [updated 2010 Jun 25; cited 2010 Oct 19]. Available from: http://www.fda.gov/Drugs/InformationOnDrugs/ucm075234 .htm#chemtype_reviewclass

TABLE 13–2. FDA CLASSIFICATIONS BY THERAPEUTIC POTENTIAL*

Type	Definition
P	Priority handling by FDA—before 1992 this was two categories:
	A—Major therapeutic gain
	B—Moderate therapeutic gain
S	Standard handling by FDA—before 1992 this was referred to as class C, which indicated the product offered only a minor or no therapeutic gain
O	Orphan drug

*Drugs@FDA Frequently Asked Questions [Internet]. Washington, DC: Food and Drug Administration; [updated 2010 Jun 25; cited 2010 Oct 19]. Available from: http://www.fda.gov/Drugs/InformationOnDrugs/ucm075234.htm#chemtype_reviewclass

reviewing has an FDA classification status of 1P, the reviewer will often have to compare the product to a drug outside of the class of the product they are reviewing. For example, if a new class of antibiotics was developed called ketolides, the reviewer will not have any other drugs in the class to compare the product to, and, therefore, he or she may need to search for studies or review articles of products that fall in other classes of antibiotics, such as the macrolides. Oftentimes in cases in which cancer chemotherapy medications are approved for a treatment that was previously treated by nondrug therapy, a surgical procedure or radiation therapy may be the best comparator for the product. In the case of products that are given an FDA classification status of 3S, the reviewer generally will be able to prepare a head-to-head comparison of the product to another product that is in the same drug class. For example, if a new hydroxymethylglutaryl-coenzyme A (HMG-CoA) reductase inhibitor was approved by the FDA, the reviewer would normally want to the compare the product to other HMG-CoA reductase inhibitors. Usually, when 3S or standard review products enter the market, if there are already a number of similar products available in the market, the manufacturer will conduct trials with the product compared to others in the same class. This product is generally then referred to as the comparator or gold standard product. The reviewer will want to discuss the comparator product and any other similar agents in the class. This can assist the decision makers in the P&T committee in reviewing the new product if they are already familiar with other products in the class.

● Additional product introductory information may include the product's patent exclusivity date and/or the product's patent expiration date. This information can generally be located on the FDA's Web site at http://www.accessdata.fda.gov/scripts/cder/drugsatfda/index.cfm. A particular institution may request additional or specific information that may be relevant to include in the introductory information. It is also common to provide a list of similar agents.

● The summary itself is a brief overview of the important aspects of the drug product. If there are similar products or different drugs used for the same indication, it is important to state how the drug being reviewed compares to those products. If a comparison between the agent in question and some other treatment is possible, that comparison must make up the bulk of the section, just as the comparison must be a prominent feature in every other section of the document. The summary will include information on the efficacy, safety (e.g., adverse effects and drug interactions[16]), uniqueness, cost, treatment need in the institution, inpatient versus outpatient needs, potential for inappropriate use,[17] and other factors, such as the likelihood patients would be more compliant with one agent or another[18,19] or how the therapy fits into published clinical guidelines. Information should be limited in this section to those items where a drug has a definite advantage/disadvantage or, if products are similar, where there would be concern about the possibility of a clinically significant difference. Items that are not clinically significant and not likely to be of concern should be left out of the summary to avoid distractions. In cases where the new drug under evaluation is indicated for a disease that has normally received nondrug treatment (e.g., surgery, radiation, and physical therapy), the drug should be compared to that standard treatment. It is worth pointing out that the summary should be just that—a summary of the material presented in the body of the document. Similar to the conclusion of a journal article, this is not the place to put new material or, for that matter, to provide citations; both of those items belong in the body.

❸ *Finally, a definite recommendation must be made based on need, therapeutics (including outcome data and the use of evidence-based clinical guidelines), adverse effects, cost (full pharmacoeconomic analysis, if possible), and other items specific to the particular agent (e.g., evidence-based treatment guidelines, dosage forms, convenience, dosage interval, inclusion on the formulary of third-party payers, hospital antibiotic resistance patterns, and potential for causing medication errors[20]), usually in that order.[21,22]* In hospitals, a new accreditation requirement makes it necessary to list the indications for use that the drug the P&T committee is approving; this must be a specific list, although it is okay to give a blanket authorization to FDA-approved indications in general.[23] (Note: The requirement that drugs be approved for specific indications is likely to only be practical in hospitals where there is computerized order entry and the physician has to state the indication). When making formulary recommendation as it pertains to third-party payers, consideration should also be given to the placement of the formulary agent into a multitiered copayment system where the copayment varies according to the cost of the drug and/or formulary status. The member is required to pay these varying amounts of copayment out of pocket at the time the prescription is filled. In general if the drug is a generic, the placement is at the first tier that has the lowest copayment. If the drug is a brand name drug preferred by the health plan, it is usually placed in the second tier with a higher copayment. All other brand name, nonpreferred drugs are usually placed in the third tier with the highest copayment. Drugs in the third tier, the nonpreferred agents, usually have therapeutic alternatives in either the first or second tier. Members are encouraged to talk to their prescribers about switching to the more cost-effective, therapeutic alternative drugs in the lower tiers.[24,25] Tier designation or formulary status may change, based on the discretion of the health plan and/or pharmacy benefits management (PBM), in the absence of significant new clinical evidence.[26] Quality-of-life information and patient preferences should be considered, if possible. Recommendations for third-party payers may also include a step therapy approach, quantity limits on the prescription, prior authorization, and coverage rule criteria in order for the drug to be covered. Third-party payers may require some drugs to have a prior authorization before being dispensed. Prior authorization is usually required for those drugs that are high cost and/or are likely to be used inappropriately. Examples include appetite suppressants and growth hormones. Prior authorization requires that predetermined guidelines must be met by the member before the drug can be covered by the third-party payer. As an example, the member may be required to try an established, less expensive drug therapy first. If this drug therapy proves to be ineffective or the patient is unable to tolerate the therapy, then the third-party payer may cover a newer, more expensive therapeutically equivalent drug.[27]

Recommendations should be specific to the circumstances in the institution, hospital system, third-party payer plan, and/or other organization in which it is being considered. In some cases, an institution may have a subformulary that is available for only a specific group of patients (e.g., Medicaid).[28] Recommendations to conduct drug use evaluation on the drug (see Chapter 14), clinical guidelines to be followed (see Chapter 7), how physicians are to be educated about the new drug, and other items may also be necessary. Education may range from a simple newsletter or Web page, to a specific educational program and certification required before a physician can prescribe a drug product.[29]

Some people strongly object to the presence of specific recommendations being placed in the document. This may be because they do not feel it is appropriate for them to make these decisions; however, this should not be a concern if adequate research was done in preparing the evaluation. Sometimes, they have a philosophy that an unbiased decision should be reached only through a group consensus after discussing the matter in the P&T committee meeting; however, that too should not be a concern. For one thing, the person preparing the document, who also obtains input from other appropriate individuals, is in the best situation to advance a logical recommendation. Second, without a recommendation, the discussion does not have a foundation to begin with—allowing the discussion to wander aimlessly to some conclusion that may not make optimal sense. Third, the lack of a specific recommendation allows emotion and conjecture to overcome evidence and science. The provision of a specific recommendation is one of the best opportunities for pharmacists to have a deep and wide-ranging impact on patient care, and should not be neglected.

❹ *The recommendation must be supported by objective evidence* (presented in the summary). Subjective factors that are likely to be significant from the point of view of all involved parties (i.e., physicians, pharmacists, nurses, and patients) should also be considered. Decision analysis can be used to show the best drug at the least cost (effectively this is pharmacoeconomic analysis—see Chapter 6 for details).[27,30-33] Other factors may also be considered and given weight to indicate importance (e.g., multiattribute utility theory[34]). These methods may be commonly seen in managed care.[35] They look at the possible decisions and their likely outcome, allowing a decision to be made that is likely to lead to the most desirable outcome. Meta-analysis may also find a place in the decision-making process[36]; however, it seems unlikely that most individuals evaluating products for formulary addition would have the skill or time to use that method. Tentative recommendations should be discussed with appropriate physicians and any clinical pharmacists specializing in that area of therapy before the recommendation is finalized. For example, if a cardiac medication is being evaluated, one or more cardiologists should be consulted to identify their concerns and desires. That does not mean the recommendation should necessarily be changed to what a prescriber wants. If the objective evidence supports the original recommendation, that is the one that should be made; however, it is necessary to demonstrate that the prescribers' concerns were addressed.

Overall, the items most likely to be added to the formulary include those that are unique, that serve the specific population, that are most cost-effective, and, unfortunately, those with the biggest marketing drive by the marketer. Multiple ingredient products or products that are the extended-release or other variations on the patent of a product are least likely to be added in the institutional setting.[37]

The recommendation should be whatever logical conclusion is supported by the objective evidence and the needs of the health care system, including health care staff needs, distribution concerns, drug administration, and drug availability. Whenever possible, at least in the case of recommendations prepared for an institutional pharmacy, it is best to follow the ASHP guidelines for recommendations, which would place the drug into one or a combination of the following groups[6]:

- Added for uncontrolled use by the entire medical staff.
- Added for monitored use—No restrictions placed on use, but the drug will be monitored via a quality assurance study (e.g., drug usage evaluation and medication usage evaluation) to determine appropriateness of use. This is a tie-in to the institution's quality assurance/drug usage evaluation process.[38] Note: This category does not mean that the patient is monitored, since that is necessary for every drug. It means that the quality and appropriateness of how the drug is used is monitored.
- Added with restrictions—The drug is added to the drug formulary, but there are restrictions on who may prescribe it and/or how it may be used (e.g., specific indications, certain physicians or physician groups, and certain policies to be followed).
- Conditional—Available for use by the entire medical staff for a finite period of time.
- Not added/deleted from formulary.

Note, there may be different recommendations presented for specific strengths, forms, sizes, and so forth of a drug being reviewed; however, being that specific sometimes does not result in any real benefit and may only make things more complicated to manage, with little improvement in drug therapy or decrease in costs.[39] Also, remember that, in any of the above, there is now a requirement to provide a specific list of approved indications for which the drug may be used.[5]

Most drugs should be added for uncontrolled use or, at the other extreme, not be added, simply because the three other categories cause greater work for the pharmacy or other departments. As a side point, if a recommendation to not add the drug to the formulary is approved, it is often good to require a time period before the drug can be considered again (typically 6 months) to prevent heavy political action pushing through approval of a less than desirable drug, just because the P&T committee gets tired of having it requested every month. Monitored use is occasionally needed if there is concern that a drug might be used in some inappropriate manner or has a great risk for adverse events. A limited drug usage evaluation would be conducted until it is evident that the drug is being appropriately used or not causing adverse events. One example where monitored use might be considered is an expensive biotechnology product that only has one normal dose, but multiple investigational doses, where it could be inappropriately prescribed without an investigational protocol. Also, a very toxic product might be monitored to see if adverse effects are appropriately addressed by the prescriber. As electronic drug usage evaluation becomes standard, monitoring may be used to a greater extent, but is seldom justified in systems requiring the pharmacist to manually collect data. Conditional addition to the formulary is a recommendation of last resort, simply because it is much easier to keep a drug off the formulary rather than try to delete an inappropriate drug that is being used by prescriber. This type of approval might be used when it is very difficult to clearly determine whether an agent will benefit the institution, if available data are limited at the time of the P&T meeting. If conditional approval is given, it is absolutely necessary to specify when the P&T committee will reconsider whether the drug should be retained on the formulary.

The added-with-restrictions choice deserves more explanation. Occasionally, there are drugs that should be added to a drug formulary, but are dangerous,[40] or prone to misuse or overuse. This could include agents such as antineoplastics, thrombolytics, and fourth or fifth generation cephalosporins.[41] In such cases, it may be desirable to limit the use of the drugs in some manner.[42] For example, the antineoplastics might be limited to prescriptions from oncologists or a defined group that might include a few physicians who are not oncologists (e.g., rheumatologists using methotrexate) and may be required to have written orders (i.e., verbal orders not being accepted) to eliminate errors and for dose verification. Specific antibiotics might be limited to either infectious disease physicians or to specific, culture-proven diagnoses (this could be done in conjunction with TJC requirement to approve drugs for specific indications[5]). Often antibiotics may be restricted to a specific length of therapy, after which a new order must be written or the original order will automatically be discontinued. Other restrictions could include specific floors/areas of the institution or that the physician must receive counterdetailing by the pharmacist before the drug is dispensed.[43] Relatively new methods of restriction involve formularies for managed care organizations, where there may be a cap or limitation on the price, quantity, or on how many times a patient may receive a drug (e.g., one-time use for nicotine patches to quit smoking); how much a patient may receive at one time (e.g., 3-month supply); a medication may be subject to prior authorization or precertification before the drug can be made available to a patient; there may be step therapy or medications which have to be tried and failed before a specific agent may be available for coverage for a patient; or whether the practitioners (e.g., prescribers and pharmacists) may receive financial or other incentives to cut back on the use of specific products.[44] Whenever possible, these types of restrictions should be based on objective data, such as the FDA-recommended maximum dose limitations or prescribing contraindication that can be obtained from drug usage evaluation.

Some prescribers will object to restrictions, but remember that the prescribers are given privileges to prescribe specific drugs and not rights to do anything, which allows the use of restrictions. Usually, this is not much of a problem because good prescribers realize there is a reason for the restrictions. The real problem, however, is the desire to use this category much too often in an attempt to ensure proper use of all drugs. While restrictions can be effective in changing usage of specific formulary agents,[45] every time a restricted drug is prescribed, more time and effort by the pharmacy, managed care organization, and, perhaps, the prescriber is required to ensure compliance with restrictions. At the very least, a policy and procedure, and probably appropriate forms or computer restriction methods, will need to be developed or adapted and be presented as part of the drug recommendation to the P&T committee. A cost-benefit analysis may also need to be conducted to ensure that the restriction is valid, meaning that it really does assist in curbing inappropriate prescribing or use of an agent. A drug use evaluation may also be performed to assess the usefulness of the restriction. If the results of the drug usage evaluation suggest an acceptable level of appropriate use, the P&T committee may need to reconsider the restriction placed on the product or the restriction could be costing the institution more to administer and monitor than it is saving or avoiding. Therefore, unless the computer system can eliminate much of the effort, there needs to be great restraint used when deciding to recommend that a drug be added to the drug formulary with restrictions. Oftentimes, adding with monitoring may be a viable alternative. A twist to the restrictions or monitoring types of approval is the use of critical or clinical pathways.[46,47] In this case, a drug may be approved for use in a particular manner for the treatment of a particular disease. These critical pathways may be established for several target populations or target diseases, where additional guidance of patient treatments can result in significant improvement in patient care and/or significant decreases in costs. Because a great deal of time is necessary to develop and manage these critical pathways, they will most likely only be seen in a few areas of any institution at any given time. The recommendation should state that if the drug is to be used as part of some clinical guidelines or disease state management (DSM) program.[48] The reader is referred to Chapter 7 for further information. In managed care organizations, critical pathways may be incorporated into the use parameters of a drug through prior authorization or precertification criteria. These are specific criteria that must be met, based on clinical guidelines, current medical practices, and product prescribing information before a product is deemed medically necessary for use.

While the decision to add or delete a drug from the formulary is seldom black or white, a general guideline may be helpful. If the drug is less expensive or the same price as others, and more efficacious or safer—add it to the formulary. If the drug is more expensive without added benefit, such as increased safety or effectiveness—do not add to the formulary (or delete it from the formulary if it is already on it). The problem comes when the drug is more expensive and also has more benefits. In that case, the careful analysis of the literature and weighing of the institution's needs must be carried out. This is the gray area that has no right answer, but the most appropriate decision must be found. This latter decision may also involve conditional or monitored use.

Whenever a recommendation is made to add a new agent, consideration should be given to the possibility of removing agents that will no longer be necessary or, in the case of a PBM, moving the agent to a different classification for reimbursement. This whole process can be used as a way of removing extraneous agents on the formulary; however, removal of agents can be difficult if the products are frequently prescribed. (Note: It is often worthwhile to annually review a list of products that have seen little or no use in the previous year in an attempt to remove these products from the formulary.[49]) Whether removing agents individually, or through a review of an entire therapeutic class, there needs to be adequate information presented to the P&T committee to show the product is no longer necessary. The reasons for removal may include superior agent(s) on the formulary, safety, low or no use, and/or high cost.[50] A timetable for deleting these agents from the formulary must then be developed and the prescribers must be informed when the agent will no longer be available. TJC, in their medication management standards, stated that as a requirement for accreditation, health care organizations should review medications that are available for dispensing or administration on at least an annual basis for safety and efficacy information.[5] Many managed care organizations, health systems, and individual hospitals accomplish this via the use of the drug class review on a scheduled basis. The drug classes may be placed on a schedule for review in which all classes are reviewed over the course of the year. No matter what system an institution chooses to use to delete or review agents, the use should be monitored and follow-up is necessary to ensure the formulary deletions proceed smoothly.[51] Communication of these deletions can generally appear in newsletters/e-mails/Web sites/intranet, or, if one is aware of a particular prescriber who is the only one utilizing a product, personal contact may be best to communicate the change as well as to provide information to the prescriber of alternative products.

Finally, therapeutic interchange must be considered (see Chapter 12).[52,53] If this concept is acceptable to the institution, and legal in the state, it may be appropriate that the new drug be used to substitute for a less desirable agent, or vice versa. In that case, a separate policy and procedure for handling that interchange needs to be prepared and considered at the same time. Please refer to Chapter 12 for further information on this subject. Also, there may be other policies and procedures or clinical guidelines that may need approval as part of the recommendation, including the requirement for availability and use of concomitant drug therapy (e.g., perhaps a requirement that antiemetic therapy needs to be given prophylactically prior to the administration of a new cancer chemotherapy agent).

All of the material on recommendations presented above may be confusing. ❺ However, to state it simply, *the most logical decision to benefit the patient and the institution should be recommended to the P&T committee.*

BODY OF THE MONOGRAPH

Many parts of the body of the monograph are self-explanatory from their names and will not be discussed in detail. Some specific points, however, do need to be made about the body. First, the body may not always be reviewed by the P&T committee and, even if presented, it may be covered only briefly. The body needs to be written as a means to compile the information for reference and further information. Importantly, it serves as a way of bringing all of the information together in a logical order for preparation of the summary. Some P&T committees will want to review the data presented in the body of the monograph, but all need to know that the clinical data were reviewed adequately. Other times, an abbreviated monograph may be presented to the P&T committee and the full monograph is presented to the chairman.

Second, efforts must be made to ensure that the drug in question has been adequately compared to other therapies (whether drug, surgical, radiation, or something else). The person preparing a monograph must go through each section and ask, "Have comparisons been made between this drug and the appropriate alternative therapy?" If not, there should either be a good reason for the lack of comparison or some explanation must be put in the section. Sometimes, there will be no published comparison with other drugs or therapies. For example, when anistreplase was first marketed there were only comparisons to streptokinase available, but physicians wanted to know how the drug compared to alteplase. In that case, information comparing both drugs to streptokinase was used to discern how the drugs would compare to each other. Scientifically, this leaves much to be desired, but sometimes there is no choice in the matter. Other indirect methods of comparison may also be necessary. If at all possible, studies directly comparing the drug being evaluated to the standard of therapy should be used. Also, if there are outcome studies data, that can be very important to put in the evaluation, including such hard to quantify items as quality of life.[54]

Third, every item should be addressed, even if only to state that information was not available or that it is not applicable (absorption of intravenous [IV] drugs, for example). This follows the rule that "if it was not written down, it was not done," or in this case was not reviewed.

Finally, the source of the information should be mentioned—any important statement of fact must be referenced, or must be suspected of being inaccurate. The package insert (now often available from http://www.accessdata.fda.gov/scripts/cder/drugsatfda/index.cfm for newly approved products) will serve as a basis for some of the information, particularly to define what is the FDA-approved information, but other references must be used to fill in the gaps and to back up that information. Other information can be obtained from the manufacturer, as stated in the Format for Formulary Submissions, Version 3.1 by the AMCP[2] (an example letter requesting such information is available as a part of that document), but the person preparing the monograph should also personally do an adequate literature search.

The Pharmacologic Data section is often one of the shortest. A simple one-paragraph explanation of the proposed mechanism of action and how it differs from the comparator agent(s) usually will suffice for the drug in question. More may be needed if the agent is being compared to a drug with an entirely different mechanism of action (e.g., comparing a new angiotensin-converting enzyme [ACE] inhibitor to a calcium channel blocking agent). If the agent under consideration is an antibiotic, the spectrum of activity should be discussed, which will be much longer.

The Therapeutic Indications section normally requires the most work. This section may be broken into three main subsections. The first is a brief coverage of what indications the drug has been used to treat. It is necessary to clearly indicate which uses are FDA approved, non-FDA approved but reasonably supported and likely to be seen, and those that are early in investigation. Non-FDA-approved indications or possible uses may be difficult to find for new drugs; however, a literature search may be conducted to determine if any abstracts or case reports have been published for uses that were not approved by the FDA. It is important to note these non-FDA-approved uses as they may be helpful in determining possible restrictions to place on the drug in the Recommendations section of the monograph and it will certainly be necessary to consider which, if any, of those uses will be approved for orders in an institutional pharmacy or health system. A current example is dabigatran (Pradaxa®), which is approved as an anticoagulant to manage atrial fibrillation, but because it is a relatively new alternative to warfarin, many prescribers may want to use it for investigational uses in patients in which warfarin is indicated, but not tolerated. Doses may be different in those indications. Also, this is vital when evaluating medications in a pediatric institution or various other subpopulations. Often, non-FDA-approved uses, if found to have therapeutic benefit, will be studied further and manufacturers will submit a request to the FDA to add indications for their product. So, their consideration is important when considering possible future use of the product. They can have an impact on use of an agent for an institution. If at the time the reviewer is researching the product and no off-label uses are noted, it is appropriate to note that fact in the evaluation.[55]

The second subsection will explain how the product and any comparison products fit into any published clinical guidelines. This should include methods for treatment of the condition, both pharmacologic and nonpharmacologic treatment approaches. An excellent source of these guidelines is the National Guidelines Clearinghouse (http://www.guideline .gov/). The reader may also consult Chapter 7 for further information. The use of clinical guidelines is important for a P&T committee's consideration. The inclusion of clinical guidelines allows the reader to see the product's anticipated place in therapy. If the product will be a new first-line agent, an agent should often be available for second- or third-line therapy after other agents have failed. The product's place in therapy for a particular disease or indication can play an important role in budgetary decisions when determining the usage potential of a particular product. A pharmacy department may want to increase their budget in anticipation of a new drug that will see a lot of usage for a particular condition. For example, if a new vaccine was developed to help reduce or prevent Alzheimer's disease, a nursing home or long-term care pharmacy provider may want to increase their medication budget to allow for a larger supply of the product to be on hand. However, if a product is for an indication that occurs in less than 1% of a specific gender of a particular ethnic group, the recommendation for the product may be to not add it to the formulary.

The third subsection will be abstracts of clinical studies supporting the various uses (see Chapter 9 for further information on how to prepare an abstract of a study). In the rare case where a product only has one use, data from several studies on that use should be reviewed in the monograph. If there are multiple uses, at least one well-conducted study for each FDA approved or likely to be seen indication is usually reviewed; more can be added, but may be redundant and provide no added benefit. If there are several similar studies, one may be covered in depth with a statement at the end of the paragraph that the use is supported by other studies, providing citations. If one well-conducted study for a use cannot be found, several less desirable studies may be needed to provide sufficient information. Whenever possible, clinical comparison studies should be used. When reviewing newly approved drugs, it is not unusual to find that no comparison studies have been published. In that case, a simple efficacy study should be used. In some cases, it may be necessary to use a meta-analysis, simply because the disease state is rare and a typical clinical study cannot be performed. Overall, the quality of the information needs to be evaluated, using the skills described in Chapters 4 and 5. In cases where no human trials are available, unless there are extenuating circumstances, the drug should generally not be added to a drug formulary until sufficient published information is available. An example of extenuating circumstances would be when a new drug is available for a previously untreatable illness. In that case, the philosophy of anything is better than nothing may apply. Also, products are sometimes approved on a fast track through the FDA because they treat a very serious, but relatively untreatable disease (e.g., certain cancers, Alzheimer's disease). These drugs may be approved based on a surrogate endpoint (i.e., not the ultimate desirable endpoint, such as length of life in cancer patients, but something that is more easily measured) or with an agreement that further studies be conducted. In cases like this, it may be desirable for the P&T committee to wait until further studies are conducted. Information about requirements for individual agents may be found on the FDA Web site at http://www.accessdata.fda.gov/scripts/cder/pmc/index.cfm.[56]

The information should be presented in a manner that is similar to the description of abstracts given in the Appendix 9–2 to Chapter 9, making sure all information is covered. When reviewing the clinical study, the person writing the drug evaluation monograph should point out strengths and weaknesses of the studies, along with applicability of the information to the patients that are covered by the drug formulary. This evaluation may be vital in arriving at the final recommendation. In some cases, the quality, quantity, and consistency of the literature are formally graded and given a score, in a way similar to the described evaluation of articles in Chapter 7 on evidence-based clinical guidelines, which is then used in the final evaluation of the product.[57]

A new item to consider in this section is pharmacogenomics. Pharmacogenomics has been defined as the individualization of drug therapy based on individual's genetic information.[58,59] Numerous articles have been cited showing the benefits of pharmacogenomics in potentially improving therapy and reducing adverse drug reactions.[60-62] If the genetic makeup of patients is a factor in how the medication is to be used,[63] such clinical study information should be presented in this section. In addition, where appropriate, pharmacogenomic information should be presented in other appropriate sections, such as pharmacokinetics, adverse effects, summary, and so forth. It has been postulated that by the year 2020 pharmacogenomics may become a standard of practice for many disease states and drugs. The FDA's Web site contains a table that includes genes and affected drug products.[64] The National Institutes of Health (NIH) and the FDA have announced a joint venture regarding the scientific and regulatory structure needed to support advancements in personalized medicine. Other sources of information include the Evaluation of Genomic Applications in Practice and Prevention (EGAPP) (http://www.egappreviews.org/), the International Society for Pharmacoeconomics and Outcomes Research (ISPOR) (http://www.ispor.org), and the Pharmacogenomics Knowledgebase (http://www.pharmgkb.org/). There are no specific methods for incorporation of pharmacogenomic information in a drug evaluation monograph, since the information can be limited to various areas of the evaluation, so it can be placed in the therapeutic information or other sections wherever it best fits. Quite often, if any information is available, it will be under all three subsections of the Therapeutic Information section and perhaps other places.[65]

In cases of pediatric drug use, studies may focus on adult literature and the data for pediatric literature may be available in abstracts or poster presentations only. The situation may be the same in other areas where there may not be a great deal of information on the use of the product under review. For these cases, a summary of evidence table, such as the one in Table 13–3, may be beneficial to include in the product review, which

TABLE 13–3. SUMMARY OF EVIDENCE TABLE

Summary of Evidence (Place Drug Name Here)		
Literature Type	Comments	Weight of Evidence*
Pediatric Evidence		
Efficacy		
Controlled trials		
Published reports		
Abstract		
Uncontrolled trials		
Published reports		
Abstract		
Experience reports		
Published reports		
Abstracts		
Local specialist experience		
Safety		
Published		
Abstract		
Local specialists' experience		
PK/Dosing		
Published		
Abstract		
Adult Evidence		
Efficacy		
Evaluative reviews		
Controlled trials		
Other		
Summary comments		

Ra = randomized; DB = double-blind; PC = placebo controlled; F/U = follow-up studies.
*Levels of evidence: good, fair, poor, none.
Used with permission from Linda K. Ohri, Pharm.D., MPH

should cover material whether it is positive or negative. This provides a concise overview of all the available literature, as well as a rating system for the weight of evidence that is available for a particular indication in the pediatric population. It also contains a comparative summary, in a tabular formation, of the literature and evidence available in the adult population. In cases in which published clinical trials are not available, the summary of evidence table serves to provide the P&T committee with an overview of the data available (see example in Table 13–4).

TABLE 13–4. EXAMPLE SUMMARY OF EVIDENCE TABLE

Summary of Evidence (Zonisamide [Zonegran®])		
Literature Type	**Comments**	**Weight of Evidence***
Pediatric Evidence		
Efficacy		
Controlled trials		
Published reports	2 trials; total $n = 333$ subjects; generalized and partial; intellectual disability and/or refractory	Good documentation of efficacy
Abstract		
Uncontrolled trials		
Published reports	1 review/study and 2 study reports on use for infantile spasms; total $n = \sim 109$	Good documentation for efficacy; poor for safety
Abstract	(Much of the pediatric literature is from Japan, with limited availability in English language)	Poor documentation
	14 prospective, open-label Japanese trials involving 1237 subjects were reviewed in an *Epilepsia* abstract.	Response ($\downarrow$ by >50%):
	Direct study review available for some trials.	Generalized: 47%,152/325
		Partial: 63%, 578/912
Experience reports		
Published reports	2 reports; total $n = 4$ infants with infantile spasms	Good documentation for these cases
Abstracts	8 abstracts; total $n = 135$; most were pediatric	Poor documentation of varied experience from multiple independent groups
Local specialist experience	Not indicated (NI)	
Safety		
Published	10 case/case series reports published, with extensive description of adverse events	Good documentation of ADR experience reports

continued

TABLE 13–4. EXAMPLE SUMMARY OF EVIDENCE TABLE *(Continued)*

Summary of Evidence (Zonisamide [Zonegran®])

Literature Type	Comments	Weight of Evidence*
Abstract	2 U.S. summaries of Japanese safety experience: first—4 data sources, $n = 2574$; second—14 studies, $n = 1237$. Likely overlap between 2 reports	Poor documentation; rather extensive experience
Local specialists' experience	NI	
PK/Dosing		
Published	2 reports; total $n = 194$; children and adults	Good documentation; limited data
Abstract	~6 reports; children and/or adults; drug interaction re effects on PKs	Poor documentation of limited data
Adult Evidence		
Efficacy		
Evaluative reviews	Cochrane Review of adjunctive use for refractory partial epilepsy in 3 Ra studies; total $n = 499$; 12-wk duration	Reviewer conclusions:
	An assessment of Japanese experience was compared against clinical guidelines for AED use (established by the International League Against Epilepsy); $n = 1008$ (ped $n = 403$)	Effective as adjunctive treatment for refractory partial seizures. Authors concluded that zonisamide was effective against both partial and refractory generalized seizures.
Controlled trials	Deferred review; FDA approved for adjunctive therapy of partial seizures in adults	Good documentation, based on FDA approval
Other		
Summary comments	Extensive, independent pediatric reports of efficacy in a variety of seizure types, both published and abstracts; demonstrated benefit in refractory seizure types, including infantile spasms; substantial published experience literature on a variety of adverse events, generally documenting reversibility with dosage adjustment or discontinuation. Limitations in evaluation: multiple publications representing the same subjects.	

Ra = randomized; DB = double-blind; PC = placebo controlled; F/U = follow-up studies.
*Levels of evidence: good, fair, poor, none.

Another new type of publication that may be of interest in this section is comparative effectiveness research, which helps in analyzing competing treatments for specific illnesses[3] and may be available in the FDA approval packages for as many as half of all new drug products that are approved.[66] This is different from efficacy trials in that it often consists of a great number of patients who are typical of the patients receiving the medications in normal practice (i.e., they are considered to be real-world patients and may have other confounding disease states, etc.). Often this information is developed from cohort studies, systematic reviews, observational studies, or meta-analyses, using large numbers of patients. Insurance company data may be used for obtaining information to conduct these trials and it is worth noting that these studies are much less likely to be commercially funded than normal efficacy trials.[67] While these studies are very useful for practical data and to help discover rare adverse effects, they also do suffer from the weaknesses inherent in any cohort trial or meta-analysis (see Chapter 5 for further information). They are also relatively rare in the literature, even though it is believed that they can help to obtain formulary admission for drug products[68] and are more commonly being used for formulary decisions made by national committees in countries such as Britain, Australia, and Canada.[69] They may also be used by third-party payers to determine the payment tier placement of products.[70] Overall, it is hoped that these trials will help identify overuse, misuse, and underuse of various treatments,[71] and may be seen more commonly in the future.

In preparing this section, it may also be useful to review materials that were presented to any FDA Advisory Committees, which may be found at http://www.fda.gov/AdvisoryCommittees/CommitteesMeetingMaterials/Drugs/default.htm.

Other information may also be covered in the Therapeutics section, including quality-of-life studies.

The Bioavailability/Pharmacokinetics section is similar to what would be found in most publications, but the information may be difficult to find for some new drugs. In some cases, a new dosage form may be considered in a drug evaluation. For example, when a drug is released in IV form, its use may be entirely different from the oral form, so the P&T committee might separately consider it. A change in route, however, does not necessarily mean that elimination is significantly different in the same patient population. Therefore, oral data may be more useful than no information. Whenever possible, a table comparing the drug in question to other products may be helpful.

The Dosage Form section is a good place to point out the limitations in dosage forms available for some drugs. For example, perhaps the drug in question is available only as an oral solid, but the agent it is compared to is available in oral solid, oral liquid, and injectable forms, which could be an advantage to the second agent. This section can also be used to discuss unusual preparation directions or pointing out which product would be easier, quicker, and less expensive to prepare. Additionally, this section should state if the product has any limitations on access (i.e., the product is only available from a registry or available to select facilities), distribution, supply limitations, or possible anticipated shortages.[72] This section can also cover the handling of medications that have a high risk for serious injury if misused. In addition, the

Dosage Form section should also address special provisions for the procurement, storage, ordering, dispensing, and monitoring of these high-risk agents. Medication error problems in this area are related to professional practice procedures describing product labeling and packaging, nomenclature, compounding and dispensing, education, administration, monitoring, and use. Specific recommendations are available regarding antineoplastic agents that address health care professionals, organizations, and patients.[73]

A problem often develops in presenting the information in the Known Adverse Effects/Toxicities section. Quite simply, some drugs have so many adverse effects listed that pages could be written. What should be done is to concentrate on the serious and/or common adverse effects for both the specific drug and the drug class. Whenever possible, incidence and severity should be included. An incidence comparison table listing the agent under consideration and other similar agents may be an efficient and informative method to show the material. If there are many rare, minor adverse effects, a statement to that effect can be listed at the end of the discussion. Conversely, other agents may have very little information available on adverse effects, simply because they are too new. In that case, it may be necessary to discuss adverse effects common to that class of agent, making it clear that they have not yet been seen with the new drug, but are possible. The new agent should be compared to other agents used for the same indication to determine whether there are any advantages. Keep in mind that these tables can be somewhat deceiving because older agents may have 20 years of side effect reports, whereas a number of adverse effects of the new agent may not yet be discovered.

Also, TJC now requires patient safety information to be addressed in all monographs, including sentinel event advisories.[5] It has been recommended that a list of possible safety problems be compiled. This may include concerns in such areas as ordering, transcribing, order entry, storage, order verification, compounding, dispensing, administration, and monitoring.[74] It may be good to consider **Risk Evaluation and Mitigation Strategies (REMS)** information from the FDA in this section.[75] Some drugs may be added to the formulary simply because of improved patient safety, even though that comes at an increased cost.[1] Besides the package labeling, other sources of this information can be found at:

- Institute for Safe Medication Practices (ISMP): http://www.ismp.org
- MedWatch: http://www.fda.gov/medwatch
- FDA Patient Safety News: http://www.accessdata.fda.gov/scripts/cdrh/cfdocs/psn
- United States Pharmacopeia Patient Safety Program: http://www.usp.org/

Once the list of possible safety concerns has been compiled, even a simple tally of the number of items can be helpful, but it also may be that specific items cause an overriding concern. In response, P&T committees are implementing safety focused drug mono-graphs, which include information regarding medication errors.[76]

The Patient Information section complies with the Omnibus Budget Reconciliation Act (OBRA)'90 standards for prospective drug utilization review (DUR).

The Patient Monitoring Guidelines and Patient Information sections listed are items not suggested by ASHP. These sections were originally added for use in the ambulatory environment, although they can be quite informative in any practice area.

The final section to be discussed is the cost comparison, where the product being reviewed is compared in price to other similar products. Typically, three or four medications (possibly including both trade name and generic products) are compared, although sometimes it is necessary to compare a dozen or more products or dosage forms. Preferably, a pharmacoeconomic analysis should be prepared[77] (see Chapter 6), because the seemingly more expensive agent may turn out to be less expensive, overall, as it decreases the length of hospitalization, degree of monitoring, or number of adverse events that would otherwise occur.[78,79] Such an analysis is con-sidered to be important by the majority of institutions[80] and managed care organiza-tions.[81] It may, however, take a considerable time to prepare and sometimes the assumptions made in preparing the analysis will be challenged by attendees.[82] Some-times it may even be necessary to provide a spreadsheet, which may be used during the meeting using a computer projector, to show what effect changes in assumptions may have on the economic analysis. In the case of reports prepared in the method of the AMCP guidelines, the information in this section may provide detailed abstracts of pharmacoeconomic studies, in a manner similar to that seen for clinical studies in the Therapeutics section.[2]

Often, a full pharmacoeconomic review is not practical because of lack of time or expertise, although most large hospitals do report doing a formal economic analysis of some kind for each drug reviewed for possible formulary addition.[83] With particularly expensive products, a comprehensive pharmacoeconomic analysis becomes much more necessary.[84,85] Even when a full pharmacoeconomic analysis is not practical, any pertinent information that could be used in a full analysis should be included. After all, it sometimes can be determined that the most expensive (per dose) drug product may actually be much cheaper in the long run because of increased or faster efficacy, decreased incidence of adverse effects, or lower monitoring costs.

In some cases, a simple price comparison can be prepared using just the cost of the drugs and the frequency of administration. Such a price comparison must consider that the patient may be getting medications both within an institution and after returning home, because institutional pharmacies may get considerable discounts. Therefore, both the institution's cost for the medication and the average wholesale price (AWP) price should be considered. Some medications are extremely inexpensive to the institution, making it tempting to include those agents on the formulary instead of similar therapeutic agents; however, if the AWP price is quite high, the patient may not be able to afford the product in the community, which could quickly lead to readmission into the hospital when the patient's disease is no longer being treated. In those cases, it may not be a good product to carry on the formulary. Also, the differences in package sizes and frequency of administration must be considered. In most cases, products can be compared on the cost of a typical day's therapy at a relatively normal dose; however, in some cases, a different approach may be necessary. For example, an antineoplastic agent may need to be compared with other agents based on a per cycle or per cost of therapeutic regimen basis. Another example that resulted in unusual cost comparisons in the past was Norplant® (an implantable contraceptive agent that was effective for 5 years). The cost of both the drug and the implantation procedure needed to be compared to a 5-year supply of other contraceptive agents. In cases like this, over a period of years, it may be necessary to include calculations of inflation or other factors likely to change over the time period.[86] Other costs should also be considered when possible, such as drug preparation costs, administration costs, laboratory tests, monitoring requirements, and changes of length of stay/therapy—after all, it is not a savings overall if costs are simply shifted from the pharmacy (i.e., drug price) to the laboratory (i.e., monitoring costs).[87] In the future, theranostics (also known as pharmacodiagnostics—which is defined as the analysis of a patient's genome in order to personalize medical treatment using pharmacogenomics) will be a substantial cost that needs to be included in the analysis.[88] Some pharmacies even include such items as the cost to order and hold the drug, and the cost of preparing the evaluation of the drug for the P&T committee.[89] Also, it is becoming more common to take into account some items that are more difficult to assess, such as the probability and cost of therapeutic failure in comparison to other similar agents, impact of specific drug therapy on other health care costs (a drug may be cheaper, but require an increase in the cost of other nondrug therapy for the patient), and cost of adverse drug effects.[90] Because these items may depend on the characteristics of the patients (e.g., age, socioeconomic status, and education level), the figures used are necessarily going to be uncertain. In some cases, however, they will be very important in the final formulary decisions; a drug that at first glance seems more expensive may be found to actually cost the institution less in the end.[78] Also, it is necessary to consider nondrug therapy (e.g., surgery, radiation therapy, and physical therapy) in the comparison, when they are legitimate alternatives to drug therapy. Overall, the goal is to ensure that the comparison makes sense and takes into consideration all of the relevant economic factors. ❻ *While some think that cost is emphasized too much in formulary decisions, it is still an extremely important item.* Some drugs cost thousands of dollars per dose, which can quickly deplete a pharmacy department's budget and significantly affect the economic status of an institution.

Conclusion

❼ *Preparation of a drug evaluation monograph requires a great amount of time and effort, using many of the skills discussed throughout this text to obtain, evaluate, collate, and provide information. However, the value of having all of the issues evaluated and discussed can be invaluable in providing quality care.*

Case Study 13–1

■ DRUG EVALUATION MONOGRAPH

You are a recent graduate who just completed a PGY1 residency. You have accepted a position at a local hospital medical center as a clinical pharmacist. One of your first assignments is to prepare and present a medication monograph on a new oral direct thrombin inhibitor that was just approved by the FDA. You will have 10 minutes to present at the next pharmacy and therapeutics committee meeting that will be held next week. The only piece of information that you are given is the nonformulary request to add this drug to formulary. All medications are reviewed for the outpatient pharmacy as well.

- *Having reviewed the nonformulary request, what are the steps to add this drug to the formulary?*
- *What are the essential elements of a medication monograph?*
- *What sources of information do you need to develop a complete evidence-based medication monograph.*

Case Study 13–2

Following the development of the drug evaluation monograph, you are then asked to prepare a concise high-level summary page of this medication monograph.

- *What are the elements of a high-level summary page?*
- *You are planning to use this monograph for your inpatient as well as the outpatient pharmacies. What information should be included as it relates to the outpatient dispensing of this medication?*
- *What are the different types of formulary status recommendations and how do they differ?*

Self-Assessment Questions

1. Medications or medication classes considered for a medication formulary should be objectively assessed based on:
   a. Scientific information
   b. Anecdotal prescriber experience
   c. Manufacturer information
   d. Published review
   e. All of the above

2. Pharmacists have a unique role in the preparation of a medication monograph in that:
   a. Medications are viewed from a whole and macroeconomic view
   b. Medications are viewed based on the package insert data
   c. Medications are viewed based on pharmaceutical representative information
   d. Medications are viewed from a microeconomic view

3. Manufacturers of alternative/complementary medicines prescriber cannot make specific health claims because these products are considered:
   a. Medications
   b. Dietary supplements
   c. Orphan medications

4. The summary page of a medication monograph:
   a. Provides a summary of the most important information concerning the medication
   b. Completely evaluates a medication product
   c. Provides a record of all that was taken into consideration
   d. Includes items that are not clinically significant

5. Included on the summary page is a definite recommendation primarily based on:
   a. Objective outcome data and the use of evidence-based clinical guidelines
   b. Cost
   c. Anecdotal prescriber experience
   d. Other items specific to the particular agent

6. Medications can be removed from formulary due to:
   a. Safety
   b. Cost
   c. No use
   d. All of the above

7. The body of the monograph does which of the following?
   a. Bring all the information together in a logical order
   b. Adequately compares the medication to other therapies
   c. Only address certain items
   d. Includes the source of the information
   e. a and b

8. Patient safety information is not considered essential by The Joint Commission and is not a useful part of the monograph.
   a. True
   b. False

9. Hospitals and health systems review an entire class of medications on a scheduled basis, which must be at least annually according to The Joint Commission.
   a. True
   b. False

10. A medication monograph provides a tool for the pharmacy to:
    a. Guide the rational development of a medication formulary
    b. Provide a full, fair, and balanced review of a medication
    c. View medications from a whole and macroeconomic view
    d. All of the above

11. Pharmacogenomics is the study of:
    a. Medication indications and nonapproved indications
    b. Medication cost
    c. Medication tier placement
    d. Individualized drug therapy based on an individual's genetic makeup

12. Pharmacoeconomics is primarily the study of:
    a. Medication cost
    b. Medication indications
    c. Medication adherence
    d. All of the above

13. The Therapeutic Indications section in the body of the monograph primarily contains:
    a. Indications for use both FDA- and non-FDA-approved as well as those in early investigation
    b. Product and comparison products
    c. Abstracts of clinical studies supporting the various uses
    d. Pharmacogenomic information

14. When making formulary recommendations as it pertains to third-party payers, consideration should be given to the placement of the formulary agent into a multitiered copayment system where the copayment varies according to the cost of the drug and/or formulary status.
    a. True
    b. False

15. Future medication monographs may be expected to include clinical outcomes, continuous quality assurance information, pharmacogenomics, and quality of life issues.
    a. True
    b. False

Acknowledgments

The assistance of Linda K. Ohri, PharmD, MPH, in preparation of this chapter in previous editions is acknowledged with thanks. Debra Lee, PharmD, from Alegent Creighton Health Creighton University Medical Center is acknowledged for her assistance in preparing this chapter.

REFERENCES

1. Raber JH. The formulary process from a risk management perspective. Pharmacotherapy. 2010;30(6 Pt 2):42S-7S.
2. Format for formulary submissions, version 3.1. Alexandria (VA): Academy of Managed Care Pharmacy; 2012.
3. Schumock GT, Pickard AS. Comparative effectiveness research: relevance and applications to pharmacy. Am J Health Syst Pharm. 2009;66:1278-86.
4. Wade WE, Spruill WJ, Taylor AT, Longe RL, Hawkins DW. The expanding role of pharmacy and therapeutics committees. The 1990s and beyond. Pharmacoeconomics. 1996;10(2):123-8.
5. TJC—The Joint Commission comprehensive accreditation and certification manual. Accreditation requirements for hospitals [Internet]. Oakbrook Terrace (IL): The Joint Commission; 2013 Jan 1 [cited 2012 Dec 14]. Available from: https://e-dition.jcrinc.com/MainContent.aspx
6. ASHP technical assistance bulletin on the evaluation of drugs for formularies. Am J Hosp Pharm. 1991;48:791-3.
7. Majercik PL, May JR, Longe RL, Johnson MH. Evaluation of pharmacy and therapeutics committee drug evaluation reports. Am J Hosp Pharm. 1985;42:1073-6.

8. Academy of Managed Care Pharmacy. Therapeutic interchange [Internet]. 2003 Feb [cited 2010 Nov 5]:[2 p.]. Available from: http://www.amcp.org/Tertiary.aspx?id= 8749&terms=Therapeutic%20interchange

9. Australian regulatory guidelines for prescription medicines. Woden, Australia: Australian Government, Department of Health and Ageing, Therapeutic Goods Administration; 2004.

10. Ontario guidelines for drug submission and evaluation. Toronto: Ministry of Health and Long-Term Care; 2000.

11. Technology appraisal process guides [Internet]. London: National Institute for Clinical Excellence; 2010. [cited 2010 Nov 5]. Available from: http://www.nice.org.uk/aboutnice/ howwework/devnicetech/technologyappraisalprocessguides/technology_appraisal_ process_guides.jsp

12. Duguid MJ. Evaluating new medicines for use in Australian hospitals: lessons from North America. J Pharm Pract Res. 2010;40(2):124-9.

13. Groves KE, Fanagan PS, MacKinnon NJ. Why physicians start or stop prescribing a drug: literature review and formulary implications. Formulary. 2002;37(4):186-8, 190-4.

14. Strite S, Stuart ME, Urban S. Process steps and suggestions for creating drug mono- graphs and drug class reviews in an evidence-based formulary system. Formulary. 2008; 43:135-6, 139-40, 142, 144-5.

15. Cohen KR, Cerone P, Ruggiero R. Complementary/alternative medicine use: responsibili- ties and implications for pharmacy services. P&T. 2002;27(9):440-6.

16. Chan L-N. Consider potential for drug interactions during formulary review. Am J Health Syst Pharm. 2000;57:391.

17. Schiff GD, Galanter WL, Duhig J, Koronkowski MJ, Lodolce AE, Pontikes P, et al. A pre- scription for improving drug formulary decision making. PLoS Med. 2012 May; 9(5):e1001220.

18. Feldman JA, DeTullio PL. Medication noncompliance: an issue to consider in the drug selection process. Hosp Formul. 1994;29:204-11.

19. Sesin GP. Therapeutic decision-making: a model for formulary evaluation. Drug Intell Clin Pharm. 1986;20:581-3.

20. Cohen MR. Adding drugs to the formulary: your work is never done. Hosp Pharm. 1999;34:828.

21. Hedblom EC. Pharmacoeconomic and outcomes data in the managed care formulary decision-making process. P&T. 1995;20:462-4, 468, 471-3.

22. Klink B. Formulary influences. Drug Top. 1998;142(20):72.

23. Rich DS. Pharmacies' noncompliance with 2009 Joint Commission hospital accreditation requirements. Am J Health Syst Pharm. 2009;66:e27-30.

24. Abourjaily P, Kross J, Gouveia WA. Initiatives to control drug costs associated with an independent physician association. Am J Health Syst Pharm. 2003;60:269-72.

25. Gleason PP, Gunderson BW, Gericke KR. Are incentive-based formularies inversely asso- ciated with drug utilization in managed care? Ann Pharmacother. 2005;39:339-45.

26. Reissman D. Issues in drug benefit management. Drug Benefit Trends. 2004; Dec:598-9.

27. Sroka CJ. CRS report for Congress: pharmacy benefit mangers. Washington, DC: Library of Congress; 2000.

28. Tyler LS, Cole SW, May JR, Millares M, Valentino MA, Vermeulen LC Jr, et al. ASHP guidelines on the pharmacy and therapeutics committee and the formulary system. Am J Health Syst Pharm. 2008;65:1272-83.

29. Dedrick S, Kessler JM. Formulary evaluation teams: Duke University Medical Center's approach to P&T committee reorganization. Formulary. 1999;34:47-51.

30. Kresel JJ, Hutchings HC, MacKay DN, Weinstein MC, Read JL, Taylor-Halvorsen K, et al. Application of decision analysis to drug selection for formulary addition. Hosp Formul. 1987;22:658-76.

31. Szymusiak-Mutnick B, Mutnick AH. Application of decision analysis in antibiotic formulary choices. J Pharm Technol. 1994;10:23-6.

32. Basskin L. How to use decision analysis to solve pharmacoeconomic problems. Formulary. 1997;32:619-28.

33. Kessler JM. Decision analysis in the formulary process. Am J Health Syst Pharm. 1997;54 (Suppl 1):S5-8.

34. Schumacher GE. Multiattribute evaluation in formulary decision-making as applied to calcium-channel blockers. Am J Hosp Pharm. 1991;48:301-8.

35. Barner JC, Thomas J III. Tools, information sources, and methods used in deciding on drug availability in HMOs. Am J Health Syst Pharm. 1998;55:50-6.

36. Gibaldi M. Meta-analysis. A review of its place in therapeutic decision-making. Drugs. 1993;46:805-18.

37. Gannon K. Uniqueness of a drug key to formulary inclusion. Hosp Pharm Rep. 1996;10:27.

38. Chase P, Bell J, Smith P, Fallik A. Redesign of the P&T committee around continuous quality improvement principles. P&T. 1995;20(1):25-6, 29-30, 32, 34, 37-8, 40.

39. Ain KB, Pucino F, Csako G, Wesley RA, Drass JA, Clark C. Effects of restricting levothyroxine dosage strength availability. Pharmacotherapy. 1996;16(6):1103-10.

40. Limit potential dangers by restricting problem drugs on formulary. Drug Util Rev. 1997;13(4):49-51.

41. Anassi EO, Ericsson C, Lal L, McCants E, Stewart K, Moseley C. Using a pharmaceutical restriction program to control antibiotic use. Formulary. 1995;30:711-4.

42. Berndt EM. Drug expenditures. A medical center's experience with antibiotic cost-saving measures. Drug Benefit Trends. 1997;9:32-6.

43. McCloskey WW, Johnson PN, Jeffrey LP. Cephalosporin-use restrictions in teaching hospitals. Am J Hosp Pharm. 1984;41:2359-62.

44. Goldberg RB. Managing the pharmacy benefit: the formulary system. J Manag Care Pharm. 1997;3(5):565-73.

45. Hayman JN, Sbravati EC. Controlling cephalosporin and aminoglycoside costs through pharmacy and therapeutics committee restrictions. Am J Hosp Pharm. 1985;42:1343-7.

46. McCaffrey S, Nightingale CH. The evolving health care marketplace. How to develop critical paths and prepare for other formulary management changes. Hosp Formul. 1994;29:628-35.

47. Dana WJ, McWhinney B. Managing high cost and biotech drugs: two institutions' perspectives. Hosp Formul. 1994;29:638-45.
48. Armstrong EP. Disease state management and its influence on health systems today. Drug Benefit Trends. 1996;8:18-20, 25, 29.
49. Persson EL, Miller KS, Nieman JA, Sgourakis AP, Akkerman SR. Formulary evaluation using a class review approach. Experience and results from an academic medical center. P&T. 2013 Apr;38(4):213-6.
50. Kelly WN, Rucker TD. Considerations in deciding which drugs should be in a formulary. J Pharm Pract. 1994;VII(2):51-7.
51. Lemay AP, Salzer LB, Visconti JA, Latiolais CJ. Strategies for deleting popular drugs from a hospital formulary. Am J Hosp Pharm. 1981;38:506-10.
52. Boesch D. Formularies and therapeutic substitution: gaining ground in long-term care. Consult Pharm. 1994;9:284-97.
53. Therapeutic interchange [Internet]. Alexandria (VA): Academy of Managed Care Pharmacy; 2003 Feb [cited 2010 Nov 5]:[2 p.]. Available from: http://www.amcp.org/amcp .ark?p=AA46FF1F
54. Lewis BE, Fish L. Drug approvals. Formulary decisions in managed care: the role of quality of life. Drug Benefit Trends. 1997;9:41-7.
55. ASHP statement on the use of medications for unlabeled uses. Am J Hosp Pharm. 1992;49:2006-8.
56. Marchand HC, Rose BJ, Fine AM, Kremzner ME. The U.S. Food and Drug Administration: drug information resources for formulary recommendations. J Manage Care Pharm. 2012 Nov/Dec;18(9):713-8.
57. Corman SL, Skledar SJ, Culley CM. Evaluation of conflicting literature and application to formulary decisions. Am J Health Syst Pharm. 2007 Jan 15;64:182-5.
58. Feero WG, Guttmacher AE, Collins FS. Genomic medicine—an updated primer. N Eng J Med. 2010;363:3014.
59. Hamburg MA, Collins FS. The path to personalized medicine. N Eng J Med. 2010; 363:301-4.
60. Philips KA, Veensta DL, Oren E, Lee JK, Sadee W. Potential role of pharmacogenomics in reducing adverse drug reactions: A systemic review. JAMA. 2001;286:2270-9.
61. Meyer UA. Pharmacogenetics and adverse drug reactions. Lancet. 2000;356(9242): 1667-71.
62. Empey PE. Genetic predisposition to adverse drug reaction in the intensive care unit. Crit Care Med. 2010;38(6):S106-16.
63. Morrow TJ. Implications of pharmacogenomics in the current and future treatment of asthma. J Managed Care Pharm. 2007;13(6):497-505.
64. U.S. Food and Drug Administration. Table of valid genomic biomarkers in the context of approved drug labels [Internet]. Aug 18, 2009. Available from: http://www.fda.gov/Drugs/ ScienceResearch/ResearchAreas/Pharmacogenetics/ucm083378.htm. Accessed Aug 4, 2010.
65. Poppe LB, Roederer MW. Global formulary review: how do we integrate pharmacogenomics information. Ann Pharmacotherapy. 2011 Apr;45:532-8.

66. Goldberg NH, Schneeweiss S, Kowal MK, Gagne JJ. Availability of comparative efficacy data at the time of drug approval in the United States. JAMA. 2011 May 4;305(17):1786-9.

67. Hochman M, McCormick D. Characteristics of published comparative effectiveness studies of medications. JAMA. 2010 Mar 10;303(10):951-8.

68. Brixner DI, Watkins JB. Can CER be an effective tool for change in the development and assessment of new drugs and technologies. J Manage Care Pharm. 2012 Jun; 18(5):S6-11.

69. Clement FM, Harris A, Li JJ, Yong K, Lee KM, Manns BJ. Using effectiveness and cost-effectiveness to make drug coverage decisions. A comparison of Britain, Australia, and Canada. JAMA. 2009;302(13):1437-43.

70. Doyle JJ. The effect of comparative effectiveness research on drug development innovation: a 360° value appraisal. Comp Effectiveness Res. 2011;1:27-34.

71. Comparative effectiveness research: paving the way for evidence-based decision making. Managed Care. 2011 Aug;20(7 Suppl 4):2-7.

72. Leady MA, Adams AL, Stumpf JL, Sweet BV. Drug shortages: an approach to managing the latest crisis. Hosp Pharm. 2003;38:748-52.

73. ASHP guidelines on preventing medication errors with antineoplastic agents. Am J Health Syst Pharm. 2002;59:1648-68.

74. Pick AM, Massoomi F, Neff WJ, Danekas PI, Stoysich AM. A safety assessment tool for formulary candidates. Am J Health Syst Pharm. 2006;63:1269-72.

75. Milenkovich N. Ready or not, here come the REMS. Drug Top. 2009 Oct:65.

76. Murri NA, Somani S. University HealthSystem Consortium Pharmacy Council Medication Management/Quality Improvement Committee. Implementation of safety-focused pharmacy and therapeutics monographs: a new University HealthSystem Consortium template designed to minimize medication misadventures. Hosp Pharm. 2004;39(7):653-60.

77. Sanchez LA. Pharmacoeconomics and formulary decision-making. Pharmacoeconomics. 1996;9(Suppl 1):16-25.

78. Heiligenstein JH. Reformulating our formularies to reflect real-world outcomes. Drug Benefit Trends. 1996;8:35, 42.

79. Shulkin D. Reinventing the pharmacy and therapeutics committee. P&T. 2012 Nov;37(11):623-4, 649.

80. Odedina FI, Sullivan J, Nash R, Clemmons CD. Use of pharmacoeconomic data in making hospital formulary decisions. Am J Health Syst Pharm. 2002;59:1441-4.

81. Suh D-C, Okpara JRN, Agnese WB, Toscani M. Application of pharmacoeconomics to formulary decision making in managed care organizations. Am J Manage Care. 2002;8(2): 161-9.

82. McCain J. System helps P&T committees get pharmacoeconomic data they need. Managed Care [Internet]. 2001 Apr [cited 2007 Jul 17]:[14 p.]. Available from: http://www .managedcaremag.com/archives/0104/0104.amcp.html

83. Mannebach MA, Ascione FJ, Gaither CA, Bagozzi RP, Cohen IA, Ryan ML. Activities, functions, and structure of pharmacy and therapeutics committees in large teaching hospitals. Am J Health Syst Pharm. 1999;56:622-8.

84. Shepard MD, Salzman RD. The formulary decision-making process in a health mainte-nance organisation setting. Pharmacoeconomics. 1994;5:29-38.

85. Johnson JA, Bootman JL. Pharmacoeconomic analysis in formulary decisions: an interna-tional perspective. Am J Hosp Pharm. 1994;51:2593-8.

86. Basskin L. Discounting in pharmacoeconomic analyses: when and how to do it. Formu-lary. 1996;31:1217-27.

87. Macklin R. Understanding formularies. Drug Store News Pharmacist. 1995;5:82-8.

88. Vogenberg FR, Barash CI, Pursel M. Personalized medicine. Part 1: Evolution and devel-opment into theranostics. P&T. 2010 Oct;35(1):560-2,565-7.

89. Myers CE, Pierpaoli P, Smith MA. Measurement of formulary inclusion costs. Hosp For-mul. 1981;16:951-3, 957-8, 967-8, 970-1, 975-6.

90. Crane VS, Gonzalez ER, Hull BL. How to develop a proactive formulary system. Hosp Formul. 1994;29:700-10.

14

Chapter Fourteen

Quality Improvement and the Medication Use System

David P. Nau

Learning Objectives

● *After completing this chapter, the reader will be able to*

- Explain the changing environment for quality measurement and performance reporting in health care.
- Define quality and value in the context of health care services.
- Delineate the concepts of structure, process, and outcomes for quality assessment.
- Describe a systematic method for quality improvement.
- Explain the role of performance indicators in quality improvement.
- Draft a performance indicator related to the medication use system.
- Discuss quality improvement techniques applied in drug information practice.

Key Concepts

❶ The term value has been assigned many definitions, but within health care, it usually reflects the ratio of quality and costs (value = quality/cost).

❷ Significant drivers for greater transparency in the quality and value of health care services include the federal government, employers that provide health care benefits, and accreditation organizations such as The Joint Commission (TJC).

❸ Quality improvement is prospective, continuous, team oriented, nonpunitive, systems oriented, customer focused, and data driven.

❹ A common methodology for quality improvement is known as FOCUS-PDCA (Find, Organize, Clarify, Understand, Select, Plan, Do, Check, Act).

❺ The Donabedian framework for quality assessment in health care includes the key elements of structure, process, and outcomes.

❻ Performance indicators are used to measure quality as part of the check function of quality improvement. The indicators typically focus on the process or outcomes of a care system.

❼ Performance indicators can be subdivided into sentinel (occurrence of a serious event) or aggregate categories. Aggregate indicators are further divided into continuous or rate-based indicators.

❽ Medication use evaluation is often part of an organization's overall performance improvement program that uses definitions of safe and effective use of medications to assess components of the medication use process.

❾ Performance, as demonstrated by data collected in the performance improvement process, not meeting the defined standard or threshold or falling outside the control limits (for ongoing or follow-up assessments) indicates that intervention to improve performance is necessary.

Introduction

Value-driven health care is being touted as the future model for health care in the United States.[1] ❶ *The term* **value** *has been assigned many definitions, but within health care, it usually reflects the ratio of quality and costs (value = quality/cost).* Thus, value is optimized by enhancing quality while minimizing cost. Although it was traditionally assumed that higher quality would only be possible through higher expenditures, the medical community has learned that improving the quality of care may lead to long-term control of health care costs. Health care administrators have long been attentive to measuring expenditures on care and have developed cost-accounting systems that have allowed determination of costs of procedures, drugs, and various care models. However, the health care system has only recently developed explicit measures of quality. By measuring this missing piece of the value equation, it is now possible to achieve a more balanced perspective on health system performance.

The Changing Environment for Health Care Quality

The measurement of quality within health care settings has expanded rapidly during the previous two decades. ❷ *Significant drivers for greater transparency in the quality and value of health care services include the federal government, employers that provide health care benefits, and accreditation organizations such as The Joint Commission (TJC)*. Accreditation standards for many providers have been amended to require providers to collect performance data, and many reports are now publically available on the quality of hospitals,[2] long-term care facilities,[3] health plans,[4] and prescribers.[5] Additionally, many public and private purchasers (e.g., insurance companies) of health care services have begun to demand evidence of quality and value.[6] The most notable exception to these trends has been community pharmacy, but this is starting to change.

In 2006, the Centers for Medicare & Medicaid Services (CMS) facilitated the creation of the Pharmacy Quality Alliance (PQA) to create standards for performance measurement and reporting for prescription drug plans and community pharmacies. The initial testing of these performance measures took place in 2007,[7] and several demonstration projects have been conducted to show how community pharmacies can be included in performance measurement systems.[8] Although CMS is not publicly reporting on the quality of individual pharmacies, it has included several PQA-developed quality measures within the Medicare Part D Plan ratings. As the scrutiny of prescription drug plans increases, plans are likely to begin requiring participation of their network pharmacies in quality measurement programs and to begin reporting pharmacy performance data to the public. Thus, all sectors of health care will be affected by the rapidly expanding trend of quality measurement and public reporting of performance data.

This chapter will focus on the measurement of quality in the medication use system and the use of these measures in improving the quality of medication use. The term performance will be used interchangeably with quality within this chapter, although understanding that performance can also refer to the overall value of the health care system is important.

Purpose of Measuring Quality

Quality, like value, has been defined in many different ways. Although the definitions for quality may vary, the purpose of measuring quality is to identify problems in a system (also known as opportunities for improvement) and monitor improvements in quality as systems are modified.[9] Although quality improvement is the goal of collecting performance data, the mechanisms for using performance data in achieving quality improvement may vary. For example, the performance data may be used directly by a health care organization to identify opportunities for improvement and to gauge the impact of changes in its policies or procedures.

Performance data may also be used by external entities (e.g., a regulatory or accrediting body) to determine whether a health care organization should retain its accreditation or certification. The data may also be used to determine payments to providers (e.g., pay for performance), or the data may be used by employers, governments, or the public for determining which providers to use.

When comparative data on the performance of health care providers are released to payers and patients, it is presumed that the providers in a competitive environment will improve quality to maintain market share.

Quality Improvement

Practitioners are sometimes confused when faced with the myriad of quality-related acronyms being used today, such as CQI (continuous quality improvement), QI (quality improvement), QA (quality assurance), TQM (total quality management), SPC (statistical process control), and PDCA (plan, do, check, act). Things become even murkier when many different quality-related philosophies are added—along with blurry distinctions between quality improvement, quality assurance, and quality control.

Quality improvement can generally be characterized by certain attributes, which are listed in Table 14–1. Concisely stated, ❸ *quality improvement is prospective, continuous, team oriented, nonpunitive, systems oriented, customer focused, and data driven*. Although there are a variety of methods, the quality improvement process is typically implemented via the PDCA Cycle, also called the Deming Cycle (although Deming referred to it as the Shewhart Cycle).[10,11] This cyclical process involves four key elements: Plan, Do, Check, and Act.

To apply PDCA to a new healthcare service, *Plan* would entail designing a new approach for providing the service that leads to an improvement in quality. This approach would include guidelines or procedures for how care will be provided, and also plans for how the care process will be evaluated. The *Do* step in the cycle concerns the implementation of the new plan, while *Check* refers to an objective evaluation of the plan. Once the performance of the plan has been checked, the performance data can be *Acted* upon to

TABLE 14–1. ATTRIBUTES OF CONTINUOUS QUALITY IMPROVEMENT

- **Prospective**—forward thinking; always looking for better ways to provide care
- **Continuous**—a standard element of practice rather than a one-time effort
- **Team oriented**—a collaborative effort of all employees and management; recognizes the unique and valuable knowledge of each team member
- **Nonpunitive**—employees should be rewarded for identifying problems/mistakes and not be fearful of discussing operational problems
- **Systems oriented**—focus of improvement efforts is on the process or system of care rather than the elimination of bad employees
- **Customer focused**—all team members are focused on fulfilling the needs of the customer (e.g., patient, physician, other team members)
- **Data driven**—evaluates performance based on objective data

standardize the new plan (assuming that it led to improvement) or the existing plan can be further revised and the PDCA cycle can be repeated.

❹ A common methodology for quality improvement is known as FOCUS-PDCA (Find, Organize, Clarify, Understand, Select, Plan, Do, Check, Act). It is an extension of the PDCA cycle (Figure 14–1).[8] This approach was developed by the Hospital Corporation of

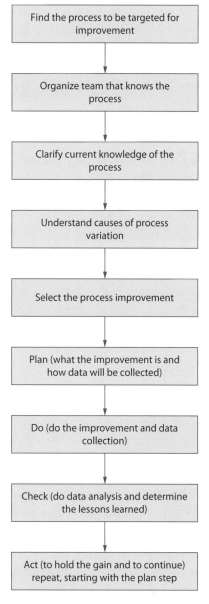

Figure 14–1. FOCUS-PDCA®.

America to facilitate quality improvement efforts in their hospitals. The first step of FOCUS-PDCA is to Find the process that will be targeted for improvement (e.g., the pharmacokinetic service referral process). The second step is to Organize a team to study the problem (e.g., pharmacists, physicians, nurses, unit clerks). Next, Clarify the team's understanding of the process (i.e., ensure that everyone has a common understanding of how the referral process is actually being carried out, perhaps through the use of a flow diagram). Then, seek to Understand the root causes of variation in performance (i.e., identify problems such as a poorly designed workflow, inadequate training, or unclear roles and determine why they occur). Finally, Select the parts of the structure or process to change. Once the target for change has been selected, a new Plan can be formulated for how the process will change and then continue the PDCA cycle through the Do, Check, and Act steps.

MEASURING QUALITY IN THE MEDICATION USE SYSTEM

One of the most challenging elements of quality improvement is measuring the quality of care. Donabedian[12] suggested that the evaluation of medical care quality could be best accomplished by subdividing care into three parts. ❺ *The Donabedian framework for quality assessment in health care includes the key elements of structure, process, and outcome.* The Donabedian framework also can be used to evaluate the quality of the medication use system.[13]

Structure refers to the characteristics of providers, the tools and resources at their disposal, and the physical or organizational settings in which they work.[12] Examples include professional licensure or certification, computer systems for tracking patient information, patient counseling areas, and human resource policies. The elements of structure create the environment for care. These structural elements may be necessary to provide optimal care, but their presence does not ensure optimal care.

Process refers to the set of activities that occur between the patient and the provider, encompassing the services and products that are provided to patients and the manner in which the services are provided. Experts often group the specific elements of care processes within two domains: technical or interpersonal. The technical domain of patient care may include gathering patient information, entering prescription information into computers, reviewing patient records, checking prescription labels, evaluating a patient's laboratory results, identifying and resolving potential drug-related problems, and answering patient questions. The interpersonal domain of patient care includes the ability of the practitioner to express empathy, listen attentively, and develop a caring relationship with the patient.[12] The process of care is often the primary focus of quality improvement efforts as practitioners strive to do what is best for patients. Care processes can be directly evaluated by using the norms or standards that exist across the health care system (e.g., what is commonly accepted as good care) or indirectly evaluated by determining their impact on outcomes.

The term **outcomes** was originally defined by Donabedian as "a change in a patient's current and future health status that can be attributed to antecedent health care."[12] Lohr also characterized outcomes in terms of the consequences of medical care for patients (death, disability, disease, discomfort, and dissatisfaction).[14] In later years, the use of this term has broadened to encompass the economic, clinical, and humanistic consequences of health care processes (ECHO model).[15] In the ECHO model, outcomes may include economic consequences (e.g., costs of care), clinical measures or endpoints (e.g., blood pressure, glycosylated hemoglobin [HgbA1c], pain, mortality—see Chapters 4 and 5), and humanistic issues (patient satisfaction or health-related quality of life). Outcomes are sometimes classified as *intermediate* or *long term*.[16] This terminology results from considering the link between process and numerous outcomes as a causal chain of events. Intermediate outcomes may occur between the health care process and long-term or ultimate outcomes. For example, providing pharmacist counseling services regarding the appropriate use of blood glucose meters (the process) will lead to better adherence to the meter (an intermediate outcome), which leads to more appropriate adjustments of medications (another intermediate outcome) that leads to better glycemic control (another intermediate outcome) that could, in turn, lead to better health-related quality of life (the long-term outcome). Thus, when evaluating the linkage of the *process* with long-term *outcomes*, identifying potential intermediate outcomes along the causal path between the process and long-term outcomes may be useful.

PERFORMANCE INDICATORS

Within the cycle for CQI, quality is often monitored through the use of **performance indicators**.[17] ❻ *Performance indicators are used to measure quality as part of the check function of quality improvement. The indicators typically focus on the process or outcomes of a care system,* although they can also focus on structure. Typically, they measure specific processes, or steps within a process, that are known to be associated with an important outcome. For example, to evaluate the process of responding to a drug information request, one could identify a few key steps within the process that can be easily measured (e.g., in what percentage of cases was the desired timeline for a response documented, or in what percentage of cases was the desired timeline met?).

Although one might think that outcomes are the ideal indicator of health care performance, they are often more difficult to measure than specific health care functions and may not always be directly, or independently, caused by the process of interest. Process indicators are useful for quality improvement when the:

- Outcome is difficult to measure.
- Outcome is far removed in time from the process (e.g., 10-year survival in cancer).

- Outcome is influenced by many factors other than the process.
- Process, by itself, is of interest (e.g., TJC says it is required to be measured for accreditation, or because it reflects an issue of social justice, such as racial inequities in receiving specific elements of care).

Therefore, if one wanted to improve the quality of care for patients with diabetes, it may be more useful to assess the appropriateness of adjustments in insulin doses than to measure the rate of hospitalizations during a 5-year period for patients in the diabetes care program. This is not to suggest that evaluating outcomes is unwise. If outcomes can be directly linked to the process and can be evaluated in a timely, efficient, and reliable manner, they become powerful tools for quality improvement.

❼ *Performance indicators are typically categorized as either sentinel or aggregate measures.*[18] **Sentinel indicators** *reflect the occurrence of a serious event that requires further investigation (e.g., adverse drug-related event, death), whereas* **aggregate indicators** *provide a summary of the frequency, or timeliness, of a process by aggregating numerous cases. Aggregate indicators are further divided into continuous or rate-based indicators.* **Continuous indicators** provide a simple count, or time estimate, related to a process (e.g., average turnaround time on medication orders), whereas **rate-based indicators** usually measure the proportion of activities, or patients, that conform to a desired standard (e.g., the proportion of stat orders that are dispensed within 15 minutes). Thus, the rate-based indicators are generally expressed as a ratio. The denominator within the ratio should be the total number of patients within the target population, while the numerator should be the number of patients who received (or failed to receive) the desired test or who achieved a specified goal. For example, if it is necessary to construct an indicator for medication errors, the numerator would be the number of medication errors within a defined time period and the denominator would be the total number of error opportunities (e.g., number of prescriptions filled) during the same time period. This facilitates the comparison of error rates over time even as prescription volume fluctuates.

Selecting and Defining an Indicator

Characteristics for an ideal indicator have been proposed by several authors and organizations.[17-19] In general, it is necessary to seek indicators that are clearly defined, quantitative, reliable, clinically meaningful, and actionable. Kerr and associates[20] also suggest using indicators where the link between process and outcome is clearly established and the link between an indicator and a potential quality improvement response is evident. Thus, the indicator provides clinically meaningful and actionable information. Indicators should be selected on the basis of their usefulness to quality improvement efforts. The indicator should help determine where potential problems are occurring within the process. For example, it may be useful to know that only 30% of patients reported that they were provided with adequate answers to their questions about medications. The way drug-related information is provided to patients can then be changed. However, knowing that only 30% of patients with diabetes had received a microalbumin test would not be as helpful if there is no control of when that test is ordered.

Providing definitions for any variables that are not intuitive will also be necessary. **Medication error** means different things to different people; therefore, if it is necessary to construct an indicator for medication errors, the staff would need to be informed what constitutes an error (see Chapter 16). It is also necessary to identify inclusion or exclusion criteria. The patients to be included within an indicator must be determined. Even for disease-specific indicators, it is necessary to decide whether to combine data for all patients with the disease or to subdivide the analyses for different types of patients with that disease. For example, it may be possible to divide patients with diabetes into at least three subgroups: Type 1, Type 2, and gestational. Other questions include the following: are people of all ages included? Are only those who attended all diabetes education sessions or anyone who completed even a portion of the program included? The answers to these questions may depend on the particular indicator. The key is to compare apples to apples. If, for example, the standard for HgbA1c testing is different for patients with gestational diabetes compared with Type 1 or Type 2 diabetes, then a person would not want to combine HgbA1C data from all these patients into a single indicator.

To judge the quality of performance from the indicator data, having a frame of reference will be necessary. Thus, current performance data can be compared with previous performance (i.e., was there an improvement over time?) or with an external criterion or standard (i.e., benchmark); both comparisons can be useful. For example, it is possible to track the proportion of patients who reached the target HgbA1C during the previous 2 years (e.g., 45% of patients last year versus 62% of patients this year). However, whether this year's result, 62% of patients reaching the target, is considered good, fair, or poor performance is less clear. To determine this, compare the success rate with that of other programs. If the latest data from surrounding health plans indicate that 60% of their enrollees with diabetes have achieved the same target for HgbA1C, the person could assert that performance is at least as good as the standard. Ideally, the goal will be to continually improve success rate, regardless of the minimal standard.

Sources for Indicator Data

Data for constructing indicators can come from numerous sources. The most common sources of performance data are (1) medical or prescription records, (2) administrative claims, (3) operations records, and (4) patient reports. Each of these sources has strengths and weaknesses. Medical records provide rich information about an individual patient; however, the aggregation of data from written documents can be very slow and labor intensive. As advances in health information technology lead to widespread adoption of electronic medical records, the use of medical records for performance review will become increasingly attractive.

Administrative claims are available in electronic format, so data across providers and across an entire patient population can be easily aggregated and analyzed. However, administrative claims lack in-depth information and may contain some inaccuracies in coding. Thus, indicators built solely on administrative claims are limited in their usefulness for problem solving.

Operations records refer to data that are collected as part of the process of care. For example, a hospital pharmacy may document the time that a medication order was received and the time that the medication was dispensed. If the pharmacy has a predetermined standard for the timeliness of medication order turnaround, then a performance indicator could be developed to show the proportion of medications that were dispensed within the designated timeframe.

Patient-reported data can also be valuable in assessing several subdomains of quality. Patient satisfaction measures are the most common way of collecting patient feedback on care. Satisfaction is an important outcome of care because patients who are dissatisfied with services are more likely to complain to external entities (e.g., regulatory agencies or employers) and are more likely to discontinue using services. Patients can also be asked questions about specific steps in the process of care to identify the source of quality deficits (e.g., were you asked if you had any questions about your medication?). The most commonly used tools for gathering patient feedback are within the Consumer Assessment of Healthcare Providers and Systems (CAHPS) family of surveys (https://cahps.ahrq.gov/).[21] CAHPS contains surveys for health systems, physicians and other facilities and clinicians. PQA has developed a CAHPS-like survey tool to gather patient feedback on ambulatory pharmacy services (http://pqaalliance.org/measures/default.asp).[22,23]

The best method for collecting performance data is to use a hybrid approach wherein several different sources of data are used to examine the same care process. This allows for a more reliable and broad-based perspective on performance. This is important because different data sources have been found to provide different estimates of the quality of care.[24,25]

The collection of performance data is good, but data are most useful when transformed into interpretable and actionable information. Several tools can help transform data into easily interpreted information. These tools include Pareto charts, bar charts, scatter diagrams, regression analyses, run charts, and control charts. Detailed information on the use of these tools can be found below and Appendix 14–1;[9,26] however, examples for a few of the tools are shown in Figures 14–2 through 14–6.

Pareto charts are vertical bar graphs with the data presented so that the bars are arranged from left to right on the horizontal axis in their order of decreasing frequency. This arrangement helps identify which problems to address in what order. By addressing the data represented in the tallest bars (e.g., the most frequently occurring problems or

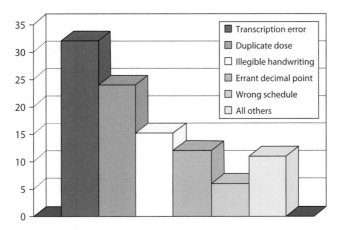

Figure 14–2. Pareto chart: factors contributing to improper dose errors.

contributing factors) efforts can be focused on areas where the most gain can be realized. Pareto charts are commonly used to identify issues to address, delineate potential causes of a problem, and monitor improvements in processes. An example of a Pareto chart is shown in Figure 14–2. This example illustrates frequently occurring factors contributing to improper dose medication errors. By looking at transcription errors as a contributing factor on which to focus quality improvement efforts, the quality improvement team will generally gain more than by tackling the smaller bars.

Bar charts and scatter diagrams are particularly useful for displaying data for sentinel events. If a pharmacy wanted to evaluate data on medication errors, a bar chart could show the distribution of errors by day of the week or by time of day (Figure 14–3).

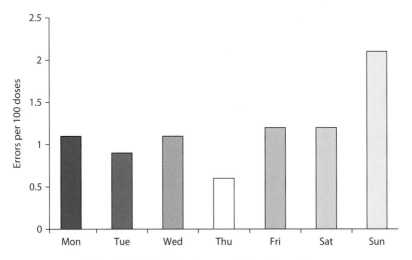

Figure 14–3. Bar chart showing percent of doses dispensed in error.

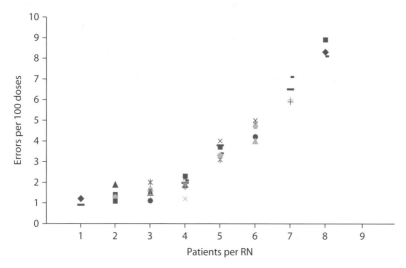

Figure 14–4. Scatter diagram to depict relationship of error rate and workload.

Displaying the rate (i.e., percent of doses dispensed in error) rather than a simple count of errors helps control for fluctuations in the workload across days of the week. This might help pinpoint whether errors were more likely to occur during particular days or shifts. If so, the staff could then investigate why the errors were higher at particular times. The frequency of errors could also be depicted on a scatter diagram. A scatter diagram illustrates the relationship of two variables. For example, a nursing home might be interested in whether the frequency of errors is related to staffing levels. A scatter diagram could be constructed wherein the number of errors was shown on the vertical (*y*) axis and the staffing level on the horizontal (*x*) axis (Figure 14–4). The data points are plotted to show the number of errors at each level of staffing.

Run charts and control charts are useful for depicting trends in rate-based indicators. Both charts illustrate the trend in a variable over time; however, the control chart also shows the extent of variation in the trend by placing control limits above and below the trend line (typically at two standard deviations from the mean). In most cases, a simple run chart will suffice for visualizing a trend. For example, if a health system wanted to examine the impact of changing the medication delivery process on the rate of missing doses of medications, the rate could be calculated for each month and trended over time (Figure 14–5).

A Stepwise Approach to Constructing a Rate-Based, Process Indicator[27]

1. **Identify an area of concern.**

   The area of concern may be identified from internal reports of quality-related problems or from external mandates (e.g., requirements for accreditation). Often, these concerns relate to areas in which errors have occurred with great frequency or in which the clinical consequences of suboptimal quality are substantial. For

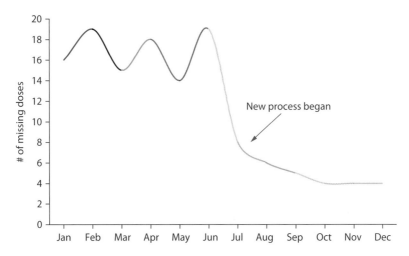

Figure 14–5. Run chart depicting rate of missing doses over time.

illustrative purposes, patient's understanding of a medication regimen will be used as the area of concern for a community pharmacy.

2. **Select the process, or segments of a process, to study.**

   The process most directly related to the area of concern should be examined, and a specific segment of the process may be selected for performance measurement. For patient's understanding of a medication regimen, the relevant process within a community pharmacy may be the dispensing process and the specific segment of the process for assessment may be patient counseling.

3. **Determine what can be measured to evaluate the process.**

   For patient counseling, it is possible to measure the frequency of patient counseling events, the accuracy of information provided to patients, or the patient's knowledge about the drug regimen. Those performing the assessment should then select the measures that are most likely to be reliable, are feasible to collect, and facilitate a valid assessment of the quality of the counseling segment of the dispensing process. In this example, the rate of patient counseling might first be selected for measurement because it should be easily and reliably collected and will provide a valid assessment of whether counseling was occurring (although it would not tell the effectiveness of counseling).

4. **Define the numerator for your indicator.**

   For an indicator, the numerator should reflect the number of times that a selected event occurred. For the patient counseling indicator, the numerator could be the number of patient counseling events within a specified time interval (e.g., 1 month). To accurately determine the number of counseling events, defining what is and what is not a counseling event is important. For example, must a counseling event involve oral communication between the patient and the pharmacist or will the provision of a written pamphlet suffice? If oral communication is required, how much communication is necessary to be considered a counseling event? Do certain elements of drug information need to be conveyed for the event to be counted? Ensuring that all employees have a clear understanding of the definition of counseling is important to reduce inaccuracies in counting the events.

5. **Define the denominator for your indicator.**

For an indicator, the denominator should represent the eligible population or the total number of opportunities in which the numerator could have occurred. For the counseling indicator, the denominator could simply be defined as the number of prescriptions dispensed in a time period (e.g., 1 month). However, it is necessary to refine this number to enhance the validity of our inferences about the quality of counseling. Should both new and refill prescriptions be included in the denominator? If the patient declines the offer to counsel, should they be included in the denominator? If the patient receives five prescriptions at one time, will they be counted as one counseling opportunity or as five counseling opportunities? Having clear inclusion and exclusion criteria will be important to the interpretability of the indicator.

6. **Determine the method for data collection.**

Numerous methods may exist for collecting data for a specific indicator. For the counseling indicator, the denominator could be derived from automated reports of new (and perhaps refill) prescriptions. If the pharmacy has a mechanism for tracking patients who were offered but declined counseling, then the prescriptions for those patients could be subtracted from the denominator. The numerator in the counseling indicator could be measured in several ways. A pharmacist could record on a notepad, or electronic record, whether he or she counseled the patient. Alternatively, the pharmacy could select a time period during which an external data collector would document the frequency of counseling. This could entail direct observation of the pharmacist–patient encounters or could entail the data collector asking the patients whether they had been offered counseling and had received counseling about their medications. In the latter approach, the patient could also be asked whether he or she understood the information they were provided. A step further would be to assess the patient's understanding, although that would take more time and, therefore, may not be possible. Each of these methods has strengths and limitations.

7. **Select tools to display the indicator data.**

After the data are collected, displaying the results in a manner that provides an efficient assessment of quality would be helpful. This can be accomplished by comparing the results with an external benchmark or by comparing the most recent results with previous results for the same provider. Currently, the only external benchmark that exists may be a regulatory requirement for counseling. For example, the state of Michigan requires pharmacists to counsel 100% of patients who receive a new prescription unless the patient meets certain exemption criteria. However, a more useful comparator may be the prior performance of the pharmacy. Thus, plotting the counseling rate on a run chart each month may eventually provide the pharmacy with insight into whether the counseling rate is improving or declining. If the rate is declining, then further investigation could reveal the potential causes of the change in performance and actions taken to improve performance.

MEDICATION USE EVALUATION

Medication use evaluation (MUE) is often included in the overall performance improvement programs within institutional settings to provide in-depth assessment of the medication use process. MUE programs should, over time, examine all aspects of medication use and require direct involvement of pharmacists.[28,29] **8** *MUE is often part of an organization's overall performance improvement program that uses definitions of safe and effective use of medications to assess components of the medication use process.* These definitions are usually described as **criteria** and are endorsed by the organization within which they are to be applied. Criteria summarize an organization's definition of appropriate or acceptable use of the medication. The manner in which medications are actually used, administered, and monitored within the organization is compared to the criteria to determine if actual practice matches the best (or at least acceptable) practice as stated with the criteria. For example, based on evidence that slowing the infusion rate of an intravenous medication reduces the risk of serious adverse events, the criteria may state that the medication should be infused over at least 60 minutes. However, when actual practice is accessed as part of an MUE, results indicate that the medication is infused over 30 minutes or less in 50% of cases and adverse effects were noted in most of these cases. These results indicate that best practice is not occurring.

Case Study 14–1

In a situation where an intravenous antibiotic was administered more rapidly than recommended, what factors could be contributing to this problem?

Endorsement of criteria is usually provided by a multidisciplinary group that includes medical staff (e.g., the pharmacy and therapeutics [P&T] committee). The goal of MUE is to provide all patients with the most rational, safe, and effective drug therapy through the assessment and improvement of specific medication use processes. MUE may focus on a specific medication (e.g., alteplase), a class of medications (e.g., thrombolytics), medications used in the management of a specific disease state or clinical setting (e.g., thrombolytics in acute myocardial infarction), medications related to a clinical event (e.g., drug therapy within the first 24 hours for patients admitted with acute myocardial infarction including aspirin, beta blockers, thrombolytics), a specific component of the medication use process (e.g., time from admission to administration of thrombolytic), or can be based on specific outcomes (e.g., vessel patency following thrombolytic administration). MUE is not designed to address if-then questions (such as if one dose is used instead of another then will outcomes be affected?), but simply determines if the actual use of a medication is consistent with the standards established within the criteria. Although MUE is no longer explicitly addressed within TJC Standards, it remains an important component of broader requirements related to performance improvement within organizations. In order to be effective, challenges such as a lack of resources or authority, politics, difficulty in identifying issues (e.g., high-use, high-risk or problematic medications or processes) or in acting on data to improve performance, and cumbersome or ineffective reporting structure or processes must be addressed. For example, unless the organization has a functional process to use the information generated by MUE to improve patient care, outcomes are unlikely to improve. If a minority of prescribers or any single group (e.g., nursing, clinical laboratory, pharmacy, respiratory therapy) can unilaterally disagree with the recommendations from an MUE and successfully block efforts to implement process improvement initiatives, efforts will fail. In order for MUE to effectively improve patient care, the organization must have a commitment to improving medication use and a committee structure that facilitates multidisciplinary collaboration and cooperation.

The Medication Use Process

In 1989, a multidisciplinary task force was organized by TJC to describe the medication use process as a component of their effort to develop tools to assess medication use. The medication use process is the outline of the steps involved in providing medications to patients (e.g., prescribing, dispensing) and what happens after the medication is administered (e.g., monitoring). The original definition of the medication use process included prescribing, dispensing, administration, monitoring, and systems and management control (see Table 14–2 for the full definition). This description serves as the basis for MUE.[30,31] Currently, systems and management control is often not included within the description of the medication use process as it applies to virtually all aspects of patient care. Medication acquisition, storage, distribution, and disposal may also be assessed if pertinent.

TABLE 14–2. DESCRIPTION OF THE MEDICATION USE PROCESS

Prescribing	Assessing the need for/selecting the correct drug
	Individualizing the therapeutic regimen
	Designing the desired therapeutic response
Dispensing	Reviewing the order for correct dose and indication for use
	Processing the order
	Compounding/preparing the drug
	Dispensing the drug in a timely manner
Administering	Administering the right medication to the right patient
	Administering the medication when indicated
	Informing the patient about the medication
	Including the patient in administration
Monitoring	Monitoring and documenting the patient's response
	Identifying and reporting adverse drug reactions
	Reevaluating the drug selection, drug regimen, frequency, and duration
Systems/management control	Collaborating and communicating among caregivers
	Reviewing and managing the patient's complete therapeutic drug regimen

It is important to note that this description outlines a process more multidisciplinary than the categories might imply. For example, while the prescribing category may imply a physician function, pharmacists are often involved as they assist in drug selection and individualization of the therapeutic regimen.

Medication Use Evaluation and The Joint Commission

The terminology used to describe MUE has changed over time and can be confusing. MUE, DUE, DUR, and **AUR (antibiotic use review)** were often used interchangeably despite being different in their approach and application (Table 14–3). Greater consistency in terminology and standards were established with an initiative called the *Agenda for Change* from TJC in 1986.[32,33] It was intended to improve standards by focusing on key functions of quality of care, monitor the performance of health care organizations using indicators, improve the relevance and quality of the survey process, and enhance the accuracy and value of TJC accreditation. Indicators are quantitative measures of an aspect of patient care and are used to screen for potential problems; indicators will be discussed in detail later in the chapter. The revised process was to focus on actual performance versus the capability to perform well. An organization could no longer hide behind having well-designed processes or policies and procedures on paper; TJC surveyors would now be looking at how processes were actually carried out. Within this initiative, TJC endorsed the concept of CQI, whereby data would be used to uncover problems and use that information to correct issues and avoid problems in the future, and included CQI within its

TABLE 14–3. ACRONYMS ASSOCIATED WITH THE EVALUATION OF MEDICATION USE

Term	Origin	Description
Drug use review (DUR)	1969 Task Force on Prescription Drugs	Retrospective evaluation to monitor medication use patterns; usually quantitative and limited to trending
	1990 Medicaid Anti-Discriminatory Drug Price and Patient Benefit Restoration Act (*Pryor II*)	Usually retrospective evaluation based on claims data; results used to direct education and reduce fraud, abuse, overuse, and inappropriate or unnecessary care
Antibiotic use review (AUR)	1978 JCAHO Standards	Retrospective evaluation of antibiotic use; usually quantitative and limited to identifying patterns of use
Drug use evaluation (DUE)	1986 JCAHO Standards	Expansion of AUR to all drugs; concurrent evaluation of prescribing and outcome only; multidisciplinary involvement
Medication use evaluation (MUE)	1992 JCAHO Standards	Expansion of DUE to include all medications and all aspects of medication use including prescribing, dispensing, administering, monitoring, and outcome

standards beginning in 1994. As part of this process, the Accreditation Manual for Hospitals (AMH) was significantly modified and much of the definition of expectations related to organization performance was deleted.[34] Multidisciplinary involvement in the evaluation of medication use was emphasized. Eventually, the standards were moved from the Medical Staff Chapter of the Accreditation Manual for Hospitals (AMH) to the Care of Patients and Performance Improvement Chapters. In 1992, the terminology was also changed from drug use evaluation to MUE to reflect that all medications and all medication-related functions are included in the standard. This change also broadened the scope to reflect TJC's expanded reach into nonacute care settings (such as clinics and intravenous infusion centers) and clarified that the process did not focus on illicit drug use. MUE standards first appeared in the 1992 AMH and were required of all institutions beginning in 1994.

Current standards focus on performance improvement, but no longer require that a specific approach be used. The organization is allowed to select, based on its characteristics and structure, a performance-improvement approach (e.g., FOCUS-PDCA, Six Sigma) that best meets their needs and that of its patients. Standards state that MUE should be a systematic, multidisciplinary process focusing on continual improvement in the medication use process and patient outcomes. The use of data for reappointment/recredentialing is still required. but the emphasis is on continuous performance improvement.

Priorities should be established based on:

- Effect on performance and improved patient outcomes
- Selected high-volume, high-risk or problem-prone processes
- Resources and organizational priorities

Evaluation of the use of high-cost medications is often a priority within organizations hoping to optimize use of available financial resources. However, in the past, many organizations based their topic selection solely on cost-saving initiatives rather than on improving the quality of medication use. As a result, this category, when stated as a sole rationale for topic selection, is no longer considered to be consistent with the goals of MUE. High-cost medications continue to be a focus of evaluation, but organizations are careful to justify the evaluation based on other criteria, such as the use of the medication being problem-prone or its importance in determining patient outcome.

The pharmacist plays a key role within the multidisciplinary MUE process. Although not always involved in specific initiatives, all pharmacists should actively identify opportunities for improvement in processes.[35] Although many pharmacists within the organization will have some role in the MUE process, those responsible for coordination and implementation of MUE initiatives are often those with drug information or performance improvement responsibilities, as well as those with specialized knowledge or experience in the component of medication use under assessment. The American Society of Health-System Pharmacists (ASHP, http://www.ashp.org) has developed guidelines for pharmacist's participation in MUE.[29] These guidelines can serve as a resource to those developing or revising an MUE program or for practitioners new to the process.

The MUE Process

The process of MUE has often been implemented through a 10-step process described by TJC in 1989.[34,36] Although this specific process is no longer mandated by TJC, it does offer a reasonable model for MUE. The 10 steps are:

1. Assign responsibility for monitoring and evaluation.
2. Delineate scope of care and service provided by the organization.
3. Identify important aspects of care and service provided by the organization.
4. Identify indicators, data sources, and collection methods to monitoring important aspects of care.
5. Establish means to trigger evaluation (e.g., trends or patterns of use, thresholds).
6. Collect and organize data.
7. Initiate evaluation of care (as indicated by triggers set in step 5).
8. Take actions to improve care and service.
9. Assess the effectiveness of actions and maintain the improvement, document improvements in care.
10. Communicate results to relevant individuals and groups.

Responsibility for the medication use evaluation function

The 10-step process begins with the organization defining which group or groups will participate in and be responsible for the evaluation of medication use. These groups oversee the process, since it has to be assumed that everyone will provide effort toward actually performing or implementing quality assurance activities. Although TJC standards no longer assign the responsibility for MUE to the P&T committee, nor do they require a P&T committee at all, the function is well suited to this group as well as to a performance/quality improvement committee. Performance improvement committees are usually multidisciplinary, but may lack medical staff participation. Their focus may be quite broad and may include oversight for a wide variety of performance improvement functions throughout the organization. Some organizations have formed an MUE subcommittee to the P&T group, while others have distributed the responsibility for MUE along patient population or product lines. Subcommittees are generally assigned responsibility for a specific set of responsibilities or information and report to the larger committee. They serve as a platform to work through the details of an issue or process and generate recommendations to the parent committee. A patient safety committee may also play a role in identification of topics, evaluation of findings, and implementation of corrective actions. The entire committee may participate in evaluations or working groups, consisting of committee members, may be established; nonmembers may be appointed to address specific issues. The size, scope, and makeup of the health care organization and its approach to performance improvement should determine the approach to be used. The participants in the group charged with overseeing MUE must have a clear understanding that the purpose is that of improving the quality of the medication use process and that each member is expected to actively participate. Newly formed groups may benefit from an overview of the organization's overall approach to quality improvement and how MUE contributes to overall goals.

Topic selection

Topic selection should be based on the mission and scope of care of the organization and should focus on high-volume, high-risk, or problem-prone medication-related processes. Topics may also focus on institutional priorities (e.g., initiation of new clinical programs or services). Several sources of information are commonly used to identify these agents and issues. They include medication error reports, adverse drug reactions (ADRs), advances in patient care modalities that involve changes in optimal pharmacotherapy, disease- or diagnosis-based length of stay or cost outliers within an organization, purchasing reports indicating a significant increase in the use of an agent (without a related shift in patient population), medications that are a key component of a process or procedure (e.g., thrombolytics, glycoprotein IIb/IIIa receptor inhibitors), etc. It is essential that the topics selected reflect the overall scope of medication use throughout the organization, including inpatients, outpatients, emergency care, and short-stay settings.

The inclusion of specific requirements within TJC's Medication Management Standards and National Patient Safety Goals related to identification and monitoring of medications described as high risk or high alert within the organization provides another mechanism to target specific medications for additional assessment. High-risk or high-alert medications are those that are most likely to result in adverse outcomes if used inappropriately or if errors are made.

Ideally, the group charged with MUE should develop an annual plan that will establish goals for new topics to be assessed and provide for follow-up on previous evaluations. Priorities should be reevaluated and the scope and breadth of recent evaluations should be assessed relative to the scope of care provided within the organization. For example, if recent MUE efforts focused primarily on issues related to antibiotic use, the plan for the upcoming year should deemphasize assessment of this class in favor of a more balanced topic selection. The planning process can identify follow-up assessments (used to assess and document that previous efforts were successful in improving performance) that remain to be performed. The failure to perform and document these follow-up evaluations is problematic in many organizations, but is a key component of the quality improvement process. Development of an annual plan also allows an opportunity to discontinue activities that are no longer useful, such as an ongoing assessment that has demonstrated sustained improvement and can now be replaced by periodic rechecks to ensure continued compliance.

Criteria, Standards, and Indicators

Criteria are statements of the activity to be measured and standards define the performance expectations. For example, criteria for the management of patients with pneumonia might state that the first dose of antibiotic must be administered within 2 hours. The standard for this criteria statement would be set at 100% if there were no acceptable exceptions to this timeframe. Criteria should be based on current best or at least accepted practice or available organization-based clinical care plans, appropriate for the target patient population(s), and be supported by current literature. Ideally, a multidisciplinary group develops the criteria. The membership of this group (e.g., prescribers, nurses, pharmacists, respiratory therapists, social workers, clinical laboratory and information systems personnel, discharge planners) should be determined by the nature of the process under evaluation. Inclusion of all involved disciplines initially will also facilitate implementation of corrective actions, if deficiencies are identified. However, criteria are most often developed by one or two of the involved disciplines and are subsequently approved by a multidisciplinary group with representation from all applicable practice groups (e.g., prescribers, pharmacists, nurses). Explicit (objective) criteria are preferred in that they are clear cut, based on specific measurable parameters, and are better suited for automation. Implicit (subjective) criteria require that a judgment be made and require appropriate clinical expertise to be effective. They are often too subjective to be consistently evaluated (i.e., different people would interpret them differently). Table 14–4 compares

TABLE 14–4. EXAMPLES OF IMPLICIT AND EXPLICIT CRITERIA STATEMENTS

Implicit Criteria Statements	Explicit Criteria Statements
Blood work ordered	Pretreatment WBC with differential ordered and completed within 48 hours prior to the initiation of therapy
Renal function assessed routinely	Serum creatinine evaluated every 3 days during therapy
Neutropenic patients	Patients with WBC <1000/mm^3

implicit and explicit criteria statements. Appendix 14–2 provides an example of criteria. It is imperative that the appropriate oversight group approves the criteria prior to initiation of data collection.

Case Study 14–2

The antibiotic that was being infused too rapidly is used to prevent surgical infections and for infections caused by gram + organisms. There is some evidence of other issues with the use of this antibiotic and an MUE is planned. The preoperative dose is given in the surgical area and the postoperative doses and treatment doses are given throughout the health system and in home care patients. Who would you invite to participate in an evaluation of the use of this antibiotic?

Criteria should be phrased in yes/no or true/false (along with *not applicable* as appropriate) formats and should avoid interpretation on the part of data collectors. They should assess important aspects in the use of the medication or therapy under evaluation and focus on aspects most closely related to outcomes of the care provided. Definition of outcome should also be established within the criteria based on the scope of care provided by the organization. For example, in a truly acute care setting, the outcome assessment of antibiotic management of pneumonia may be limited to a decrease in clinical signs and symptoms indicating a response to therapy and the ability to be discharged on an oral antibiotic(s). However, in an integrated system that includes both acute and ambulatory or long-term care, the evaluation could continue through the entire treatment course and outcome could be assessed based on cure or control of the disease state at the conclusion of therapy.

As the criteria are finalized, it is helpful to consider how opportunities for improvement identified via a criteria statement could be addressed. For example, could the computer system be used as a tool to improve prescribing, would a double check by a nurse and a pharmacist help prevent errors, or could the dispensing process be modified to improve delivery time? If the corrective action would involve participation of a group not represented in the development process, it may be wise to add them to the team at this point.

Validity should be assessed as part of the development process. Validity assessments consider how effective the criteria will be in providing the information necessary to obtain an actual comparison of what is happening to the expectations outlined in the criteria. Table 14–5 outlines several questions to test the validity of criteria or indicators.[37,38] A short pilot of data collection with an analysis of resulting information is often a good way to test the validity of criteria and its utility in assessing medication use.

Although general guidelines related to criteria are available, most texts providing example criteria are no longer published.[17,39,40] Many group purchasing organizations and other networks have systems to facilitate sharing of MUE materials (e.g., criteria, data collection forms) and methods of comparing results with those from similar organizations. The advantages to using predeveloped criteria include prior expert review and assessment, and time savings. However, criteria developed outside the organization must be adapted to the practice setting and patient population as appropriate and must be approved by the designated multidisciplinary group prior to data collection. For example, criteria intended for use in a general adult population may not be appropriate for geriatric patients without modification. Also, predeveloped criteria may include uses of a medication not applicable to certain settings or aspects of use that are not a priority for assessment

TABLE 14–5. TESTS OF THE VALIDITY OF CRITERIA OR INDICATORS

Face validity	Are they important to patient outcome?
	Do they assess a problematic area?
	Do they have some utility in improving patient care?
	Do they reflect system-wide performance?
	Are they appropriate, based on current practice standards and literature?
External validity	Have they been thoroughly reviewed by practitioners with expertise in the use of the medication?
	Are they applicable within organization?
	Has the review process clarified and improved the criteria/indicators without weakening their intent?
Feasibility of data collection and retrieval	Are they clear and not subject to interpretation?
	Are data available?
	How many cases will need to be evaluated in order to provide adequate data?
	How difficult or complex will the data collection process be?
	What benefits will be gained versus the effort for data collection?
	Will data collection methods be consistent?

within the organization. For example, criteria for the use of midazolam that address its use for conscious sedation in a setting where conscious sedation is not performed can be streamlined by eliminating criteria related to conscious sedation. Criteria related to the use of antibiotics to treat infection, when the concerns prompting the evaluation relate solely to perioperative use, should be streamlined to focus solely on perioperative use. Criteria may also be derived from guidelines for use developed or adopted within the organization. For example, the P&T committee may agree to add a medication to the formulary for specific indications and require that the use of the agent and patient outcomes be concurrently evaluated based on these guidelines. In this situation, the criteria for use of the medication would reflect the indications approved by the committee and the MUE would assess the desired outcomes as defined by the committee. Data collection would begin as the medication is first used with results reported to the P&T committee at specific intervals (e.g., quarterly) or after a defined period of time (e.g., for the first 6 months).

Case Study 14–3

Within your organization, warfarin is responsible for more adverse events than any other medication. The P&T committee wants to do an MUE to identify opportunities to reduce the number and severity of adverse effects associated with warfarin. How would you identify existing guidelines or standards for warfarin use to assist in drafting criteria for this MUE?

Performance indicators can also be used to evaluate medication use. As described previously, an indicator is a quantitative measure of an aspect of patient care that is used as a screening tool to detect potential problems in quality.[17] For example, the number of doses of flumazenil administered to reverse the effects of benzodiazepines administered in a procedure area could serve as an indicator of the appropriateness of benzodiazepine dosing in the procedure area. While the criteria used in MUE are focused and assess specific important components of medication use, indicators measure symptoms of a medication use system that could indicate that something is not working well, but there is no assurance that there really is a problem when an indicator is not met. They can serve as a tool to identify potentially problematic aspects of care, but require more focused assessment (such as an MUE) to identify the cause.

Within the MUE process, standards are used to define optimal performance and are usually set at 0% (should never happen) or 100% (should always happen). Thresholds are similar to standards but they specify that an acceptable level of compliance or performance is usually set higher than 0% or lower than 100% based on acceptable variation, standards of practice, or benchmarks.[41] Thresholds are sometimes used instead of standards to allow limited noncompliance with the criteria when the clinical impact of noncompliance is felt to be of low risk. They should not be used to avoid intervention. Thresholds are useful when the group overseeing the MUE process is most interested in addressing performance that is clearly unacceptable, while allowing some variation from best practice.

Control limits can be used when measurements continue over an extended period of time (e.g., weeks or months). Unlike standards and thresholds, they are usually not applied in the initial MUE but can be used to follow a process over time. For example, an MUE was conducted and action taken to improve the use of the medication. Control limits could be used to monitor the ongoing use of the medication to ensure that the improvement was sustained over time. Control limits define the limits of allowable or expected variation in performance (often two to three times the standard deviation from the mean initially) and may be used to assess the results on ongoing monitoring. As long as performance remains between the upper and lower control limits, action is not necessary to address the variations that occur over time. However, performance above or below the control limits is referred to as special variation and prompts assessment as to what factor(s) resulted in the special variation and should result in actions being taken to address the impact of these factors over time. For example, within an organization training medical residents, the number of pharmacists' interventions as documented on a control chart, might spike upward around July 1st, corresponding to the start date for the new residents. While the organization may have limited opportunity to stagger starting dates, specific aspects of their orientation process could be enhanced to improve initial performance. As actions are taken to address factors resulting in special variations and the overall variability are reduced, control limits should narrow.[17] An example of a control chart with limits appears in Figure 14–6.

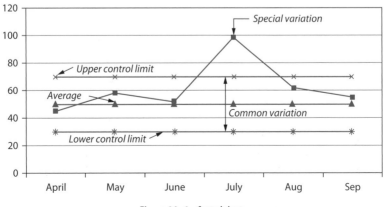

Figure 14–6. Control chart.

❾ *Performance, as demonstrated by data collected in the performance improvement process, not meeting the defined standard or threshold or falling outside the control limits (for ongoing or follow-up assessments) indicates that intervention to improve performance is necessary.* In some cases, performance outside the defined parameters may, upon review, be acceptable to the oversight group. This usually results from expectations being set too high (e.g., that the rate of adverse effects with any agent will be 0%) or when the criteria fail to include the appropriate exceptions. When this occurs, the multidisciplinary oversight group must agree that the level of performance is acceptable and that intervention is not necessary. These decisions must be clearly documented in meeting minutes or summaries of results. If this is not done, regulatory bodies may infer that the organization chose to ignore the findings of the evaluation, thus failing to meet the quality improvement requirements.

Data collection

Prior to the initiation of data collection, the multidisciplinary oversight group must approve the topic selection, criteria, patient selection process, sample size, sampling method (e.g., all consecutive patients, intermittent sampling, random sampling), evaluation timeframe, data collection method, and standards of performance.[29] It may be appropriate to distribute the approved criteria as an educational tool prior to data collection. Although this may address some performance issues prior to data collection and result in less dramatic results, it may support the ultimate goal of improving care and do so in a more expedient manner. In this situation, if there is a need to document the overall impact of an MUE effort, collection of baseline performance data, even as criteria are being finalized and approved, can provide a more accurate representation of before and after. If at any point problems are identified in the criteria or indicators or with any component of the evaluation, the issue should be brought back to the oversight group and modifications made as appropriate. Bringing necessary modifications back to the oversight group ensures that the MUE is conducted based on their guidance and approval and helps ensure their support of the results and recommendations resulting from the MUE. This step is not unusual but can often be avoided through careful preparation and review of criteria early in the MUE process.

The timing of data collection can be influenced by seasonal variations in the types of care provided (e.g., increased frequency of pneumonia in the winter months), systems issues (e.g., construction, implementation of new computer systems, initiation of new services), and personnel issues (e.g., the influx of new health professional graduates and medical house staff that occurs during the summer months, staff absences during vacation or flu seasons). Therefore, the timeframe for data collection, both in duration and time of year, should be considered in the planning process. For example, an assessment of care provided to patients with pneumonia is usually best performed during the winter months when this diagnosis is more frequent, while an assessment of the management of near-drowning may be more appropriate during the summer months. The longer the data collection period, the more likely various fluctuations in quality of care will be identified.

Retrospective data collection was used primarily in the era of AUR and DUR. This method involved reviewing the patient's medical record after discharge. It allowed data collection to be scheduled when convenient or when staff was available, but was totally dependent on documentation in the medical record. If an opportunity for improvement was identified, there was no opportunity to improve that particular patient's care; it would only help future patients.

Concurrent data collection occurs while the patient is still actively receiving the medication, but after the first dose is dispensed or administered. Data sources other than the medical record are available (e.g., staff or patient interviews) and there is an opportunity to improve patient care while the patient is receiving it. Based on complete information, results may be more complete as well as more accurate.[42] However, the need for data collection is constant and must occur within a specific timeframe, which is not always convenient. This often results in an increased number of personnel being involved in the data collection process and increased inconsistency.

Prospective evaluation occurs before the patient receives the first dose of medication and is initiated whenever an order for the medication is generated. Simple prospective evaluations can be at least partially automated and are likely to become more common. An example of this is a clinical information system that generates a warning to the pharmacist or prescriber if the dose of a drug is outside the normal limits based on a patient's organ function. Clinical judgment must also be applied in many of these settings.

In systems with computerized prescriber order entry, the system itself can drive prescribing to comply with guidelines and standards by limiting prescribing options or directing users to specific therapy. In some cases, the system can report instances where prescribers attempt to prescribe a medication outside established limits. These limits are usually developed by the P&T committee, optimally as the agent is being considered for addition to the formulary, and fall into three general categories: diagnosis, prescriber, and medication specific. Diagnosis-based limits may define the allowable indications for use or may drive the use of an agent under a specific protocol approved by the committee. Prescriber limits may restrict the use of an agent to a specific subset of prescribers (e.g., infectious disease or critical care specialists). Medication specific limits can designate approved dosage regimens (e.g., disallow intravenous push promethazine), frequency of administration (e.g., once-daily dosing of ceftriaxone), and duration of therapy (e.g., no more than 10 doses or days of therapy).

Prospective evaluations that are not automated are the most cumbersome to implement because the evaluation must occur promptly every time an order is initiated to avoid therapy delays. This requires personnel to be available to collect data and report results at all times and force immediate interaction between practitioners. This approach offers the greatest opportunity for intervention and education, but also increases the risk for potentially negative interactions with prescribers and other health professionals, and can result in therapy delays. Furthermore, it is essential that the interventions made as part of the prospective evaluation are documented in order to evaluate workload, effectiveness of the interventions, and that outcomes are assessed in some manner.

Limiting the number of data collectors or automating data collection is valuable in maintaining consistency. When multiple data collectors are involved, it becomes even more important to have clear, explicit criteria that are not subject to interpretation.

The selection of patients or cases for inclusion in the evaluation should be determined and approved by the oversight group prior to data collection. It is essential that the selection be unbiased, consistent, and representative of the care provided. Sample size should be based on the size of the patient population. It has been suggested that for frequently occurring events a sample of at least 5% of cases be used, and for events occurring less frequently that a minimum of 30 cases be assessed.[43]

Data analysis

Reports should compare actual performance with expectations defined by the standards (or thresholds or control limits) established and approved prior to data collection. Performance not meeting standards (or threshold or control limits) may be considered opportunities for improvement. The multidisciplinary oversight group does not usually conduct the actual analysis, but should be involved in interpreting the results. This group may determine that the standards were too rigorous, that unforeseen exceptions were encountered, and/or that actual performance falls within current acceptable standards of practice. Specific corrective actions should be recommended for all identified opportunities for improvement (e.g., for all criteria statements for which the standard of performance was not met) whenever possible. The need for and nature of follow-up should also be assessed based on the frequency, prevalence, and/or severity of the issue. For example, if an evaluation of the management of pneumonia identified no issues with drug selection, but did identify an unacceptable delay in time to first dose of antibiotic (e.g., more than 2 hours after admission), the follow-up evaluation could focus on the time to first dose and not assess antibiotic selection. Furthermore, if this issue was identified in patients admitted to a particular unit, then the follow-up could focus on assessing and documenting improvement in only that unit.

Computer software programs (e.g., relational databases and spreadsheets) can be very helpful in collecting data, managing data, and reporting results.[44-46] Handheld devices, bar code technology, proprietary software products, and computer systems used within the organization's clinical departments can be employed as tools to assist in patient identification, data collection and analysis, and documentation.[47]

The report to the oversight group should contain the rationale for the topic selection, team members involved in the evaluation, a description of the patient population evaluated, any selection criteria used, a copy of the criteria/indicators, discussion of the results, identification of likely causes for performance improvement opportunities identified, and recommendations for corrective action and follow-up evaluation. An example is provided in Appendix 14–3. In most settings, delineation of results on a practitioner specific basis is not appropriate at this level. The exception would be if a subset of practitioners consistently fell outside the criteria.

Interventions and corrective actions

The key to quality improvement is improving the process and outcomes, not blaming an individual or group of individuals. Steps to improve performance or avoid similar outcomes in the future fall into three categories: educational, restrictive interventions, and process changes. Educational interventions are most appropriate when knowledge deficits contribute to performance outside the criteria. They are most effective when they are directed personally, take place soon after the problem occurs, the educator is a peer or superior of the person being educated, and when the education is supported in the literature or by practice standards.[48] One-on-one or group discussion of results, letters, newsletters, and presentation via quality improvement channels are examples of educational approaches. Generally, educational interventions incorporated into ongoing processes (e.g., education screens in computer order entry systems) are more effective while one-time efforts (e.g., newsletters) may not have a sustained effect. In many situations, educational interventions are the most palatable.

Restrictive approaches may involve special ordering procedures, compliance with guidelines for use, consultation with a specialty service, or formulary restrictions. The impact of restrictive interventions often reverses when the restrictions are removed.[49,50] Restrictive interventions are perhaps most effective when used to establish appropriate practice patterns when an agent is first made available for use within the organization.

Process changes incorporate the correction into routine practice. This approach may involve changes in policy or procedures, implementation of new services, acquisition of new equipment, changes in staffing, or generation of regular notifications, etc., when practice does not appear to meet standards. As clinical information and physician order entry systems become more sophisticated, process changes can be built directly into the prescribing, dispensing, and administering processes.

Disciplinary actions against individuals are not commonly employed as an intervention; however, when individuals refuse to modify their behavior, discipline may eventually be required. Discipline may include placing limits on an individual's activities and responsibilities or termination of employment. When possible, punitive actions should be avoided, since they can result in loss of acceptance of quality improvement efforts and fear of retribution.[51,52] Generally, the concept of Just Culture is useful to consider. Greater information on Just Culture is found in Chapter 16.

Communication of MUE-related information is important and must be done carefully. Communication of the purpose of the evaluation and the significance of its outcomes should be reported to all groups involved in or impacted by the process. If a process is changed based on MUE results, the reason for the change should be explained. If, as a result of an MUE, a prescriber will be required to change the way they prescribe a medication or a nurse will no longer be able to access a medication as they had in the past, the reason for the change should be communicated along with the announcement of the change. Confidentiality of patient information (e.g., names and other identifiers) must be maintained. The identity of practitioners (physicians, pharmacists, nurses) must be revealed only in information provided for use by managers or designated peer-practitioners for assessment of personal performance.

Follow-up

Follow-up evaluation should occur within a reasonable timeframe after completion of the initial evaluation and corrective action. Follow-up is designed to assess the effectiveness of the intervention. The same criteria, standards, and sample should be used for the follow-up assessment as in the initial evaluation. Exceptions to this rule should be made if there was a problem with the initial criteria, standards, and sample; the standard of practice changes in the interim; or there is an opportunity to focus on a subset of the original data elements or patient population. For example, if issues were only found in the administration component of the use of a medication (and not in the prescribing, dispensing, or monitoring components) or only in a specific age group, follow-up evaluation could focus on these issues or populations rather than repeating the broader assessment performed initially.

MUE has been criticized as being heavy handed, nonpatient focused and for not addressing the issue of accountability for provision of care based on a unique body of knowledge. If the approach termed MUE is utilized in its true spirit, many of these challenges are addressed. MUE is a truly multidisciplinary, process-oriented approach to evaluate the quality of medication use. The process goes beyond numbers and percentages to identify opportunities for improvement and, more importantly, to improve the quality of care.

Quality in Drug Information

Quality standards for drug information practice have not been established to date and quality assessment techniques used in drug information practice vary greatly among practice sites.[53-55] Several studies have found inconsistencies in the quality of drug information practice and have called for increased emphasis on quality and the development of practice standards.[56-59] Most drug information services conduct some form of quality assessment based on the scope of service provided by that center and preestablished levels of acceptable performance. Quality assessment is usually conducted on the responses provided to drug information requests, medical literature search and evaluation processes, availability, accuracy and timeliness of drug information resources, and the quality of materials produced by the drug information service staff (e.g., monographs, newsletters, continuing education programs). Although some quality assessment processes are conducted concurrently, most assessments are done retrospectively, often by randomly sampling of drug information requests, monographs, and so forth. Furthermore, assessments may be performed via peer review or may be performed by the director of the service. Currently, no standards have been developed for this process.

Assessment of the quality of responses to drug information inquiries may include components such as timeliness, completeness and appropriateness of response, and the method of communication of the response. Additionally, aspects such as documentation of search terms, references utilized, and the availability of appropriate background or patient-specific information may also be assessed. This assessment may be carried out internally based on standards of practice at the site. This usually offers the advantage of peer review by practitioners skilled in these functions. Another method is to poll those using the service about the quality of service and response received. This approach is hampered because consumers of the response are rarely able to assess the quality or appropriateness of the search strategy utilized to formulate the response they received in lieu of performing the search themselves or being present while the search is performed. An example assessment tool appears in Appendix 14–4. Questions that are often asked in the process of assessing drug information responses include:

- Is the response correct and appropriate to the situation presented?
- Is the response provided promptly?
- Does the response completely address the question posed?
- Is the response communicated appropriately?
- Are search terms and references appropriately documented?
- Is the response clear, concise, and appropriate for the clinical situation?
- If follow-up was appropriate, was it provided?

The search process itself can be assessed by evaluation of the appropriate depth and breadth of resources used, the timeliness of the resources accessed, and the search strategy. This process can also assess documentation issues, the application of literature evaluation skills to the information, and resources used by the practitioner completing the search.

Drug information practitioners are often responsible for assessing and recommending drug information resources available within the organization. These resources may include printed references such as handbooks, textbooks, or educational materials, or electronic resources such as large search engines or Internet Web sites. This process should assess whether the appropriate information resources are available based on the scope of care provided and expertise of the practitioners and whether the resources contain accurate and timely information that can be applied in clinical situations. Available primary, secondary, and tertiary resources should be evaluated based on established standards. The explosion of medical information on the Internet has created new challenges in evaluating drug and medical information resources. Because there are currently no regulations of content on Internet sites, caution must be used when utilizing these resources to support clinical decision making. With the number of Web sites expanding faster than most practitioners can assess their content and editorial policies (if any), it has become increasingly difficult for drug information practitioners to stay abreast of those sites that offer legitimate and validated information compared to those offering only conjecture and opinion. Information obtained from other sources including manufacturer's drug information services should also be assessed. See Chapters 3, 4, and 5 for further information on assessing information.

A final component of quality relates to material produced by the drug information service. This includes newsletters, drug monographs, and guidelines developed by the service. Most measure quality related to the accuracy, timeliness, and clinical applicability of such documents. Unfortunately, more time is often spent assessing quality of grammar and writing style than is devoted to clinical content and interpretation. Once again, Chapters 4 and 5 provide further information on assessing the quality of the material itself.

Conclusion

The health care system continues to move toward greater transparency of quality as part of an overall shift toward value-driven health care. Government agencies and private purchasers of health care are demanding more evidence on quality and safety in the use of medications, and a growing number of accreditation programs are also scrutinizing performance indicators as a means for reaccreditation of organizations and providers. Thus, it is imperative that all practitioners involved in the medication use system understand how to measure and improve quality in the use of medications. Also, with the major changes to the American health care system expected over the next few years, pharmacists should be aware that this will likely be changing.

Self-Assessment Questions

1. Significant drivers of the demand for quality measurement in health care are:
   a. The U.S. Department of Health and Human Services
   b. The Joint Commission (TJC)
   c. Employers that provide health care benefits
   d. All of the above

2. The PDCA model of quality improvement stands for:
   a. Prepare, Develop, Calculate, Assess
   b. Produce, Design, Cost-control, Act
   c. Plan, Develop, Check, Assess
   d. Plan, Do, Check, Act
   e. None of the above

3. Quality improvement is a proactive technique that is focused on the entire process.
   a. True
   b. False

4. Which of the following is *not* a characteristic of continuous quality improvement?
   a. Systems oriented
   b. Data driven
   c. Team oriented
   d. Punitive
   e. a and d

5. Examples of tools used in continuous quality improvement include:
   a. Flow charts
   b. Pareto charts
   c. Scatter diagrams
   d. Control charts
   e. All of the above

6. Which of the following are common purposes for measuring quality?
   a. Identify problems within a system
   b. Monitor improvements within a system
   c. Public reporting on providers
   d. Removal of bad employees
   e. a, b, and c

7. Within the Donabedian framework for quality assessment, which of the following indicators pertain to Structure?
   a. Percent of pharmacies with a patient counseling area
   b. Percent of patients with diabetes who received an annual eye examination
   c. Death of a patient due to an adverse drug-related event
   d. Percent of patients who received counseling on medications prior to discharge
   e. a and d

8. Within the Donabedian framework for quality assessment, which of the following indicators pertain to Process?
   a. Percent of pharmacies with a patient counseling area
   b. Percent of patients who received an annual eye examination
   c. Death of a patient due to an adverse drug-related event
   d. Percent of patients who received counseling on medications prior to discharge
   e. b and d

9. Within a Donabedian framework for quality assessment, which of the following indicators pertain to Outcomes?
   a. Percent of pharmacies with a patient counseling area
   b. Percent of patients who received an annual eye examination
   c. Death of a patient due to an adverse drug-related event
   d. Percent of patients who received counseling on medications prior to discharge
   e. b and c

10. When is it useful to directly measure aspects of the process of care?
    a. Outcome is difficult to measure
    b. Outcome is far removed in time from the process
    c. Outcome is affected by many different processes
    d. All of the above
    e. None of the above since outcomes are the only valid indicator of quality

11. Within the ECHO model of outcomes assessment, the H stands for:
    a. Holistic
    b. Honorific
    c. Humanistic
    d. Humanitarian
    e. None of the above

12. The term intermediate outcome can best be defined as:
    a. A temporary status of the patient
    b. Outcomes that are measured by learned intermediaries

    c. An event that lies between the health care process and the ultimate outcome

    d. An interaction between the patient and the caregiver

13. A sentinel indicator:

    a. Reflects the occurrence of a serious event that requires further investigation

    b. Can be subdivided into rate-based or aggregate indicators

    c. Could be a death from an adverse drug-related event

    d. Is typically expressed as a percentage

    e. a and c

14. A rate-based indicator:

    a. Is typically expressed as a percentage

    b. Is a type of aggregate indicator

    c. Is typically expressed as a count of events over time

    d. Can only be used to track safety events in hospitals

    e. a and b

15. In health care, PQA:

    a. Is an acronym for Pharmacy Qualitative Assessment

    b. Is an acronym for Pharmacy Quality Alliance

    c. Has developed standards for performance measurement in pharmacy

    d. Was created by the Agency for Healthcare Research and Quality

    e. b and c

REFERENCES

1. Centers for Medicare & Medicaid Services. Roadmap for implementing value-driven health care in the traditional Medicare fee for service program [Internet]. Baltimore (MD): Centers for Medicare & Medicaid Services; 2012 Nov 25 [cited 2013 Oct 2]. Available from: http://www.cms.gov/Medicare/Quality-Initiatives-Patient-Assessment-Instruments/QualityInitiativesGenInfo/Downloads/VBPRoadmap_OEA_1-16_508.pdf

2. Medicare.gov. Hospital compare [Internet]. Baltimore (MD): Department of Health & Human Services; 2012 Nov 25 [cited 2013 Oct 2]. Available from: http://www.hospitalcompare.hhs.gov/hospital-search.aspx

3. Medicare.gov. Nursing home compare [Internet]. Baltimore (MD): Department of Health & Human Services; 2009 Jan 11 [cited 2013 Oct 2]. Available from: http://www.medicare.gov/NursingHomeCompare/search.aspx

4. Report cards [Internet]. National Committee for Quality Assurance (NCQA); 2012 Nov 25 [cited 2013 Oct 2]. Available from: http://www.ncqa.org/tabid/142/Default.aspx

5. Massachusetts Health Quality Partners [Internet]. Watertown (MA): Massachusetts Health Quality Partners; 2012 Nov 25 [cited 2013 Oct 2]. Available from: http://www.mhqp.org

6. The Leapfrog Group [Internet]. Washington (DC): The Leapfrog Group; 2012 Nov 25 [cited 2013 Oct 2]. Available from: http://www.leapfroggroup.org

7. Pillittere-Dugan D, Nau DP, McDonough K, Zakiya P. Development and testing of performance measures for pharmacy services. J Am Pharm Assoc. 2009;49:212-9.

8. Doucette WR, Conklin M, Mott DA, Newland B, Plake KS, Nau DP. Pharmacy Quality Alliance Phase I Demonstration Projects: descriptions and lessons learned. J Am Pharm Assoc. 2011;51:544-50.

9. McLaughlin CP, Kaluzny AD. Continuous quality improvement in health care. 2nd ed. Gaithersburg (MD): Aspen Publishers; 1999.

10. Deming WE. Out of the crisis. Cambridge (MA): Massachusetts Institute of Technology, Center for Advanced Engineering Study; 1986.

11. Deming WE. The new economics for industry, education, government. Cambridge (MA): Massachusetts Institute of Technology, Center for Advanced Engineering Study; 1993.

12. Donabedian A. Explorations in quality assessment and monitoring. The definition of quality and approaches to its assessment. Ann Arbor (MI): Health Administration Press; 1980:79-128.

13. Farris KB, Kirking DM. Assessing the quality of pharmaceutical care. II. Application of concepts of quality assessment from medical care. Ann Pharmacother. 1993;27:215-23.

14. Lohr KN. Outcomes measurement: concepts and questions. Inquiry. 1988;25:37-50.

15. Kozma CM, Reeder CE, Schulz RM. Economic, clinical and humanistic outcomes: a planning tool for pharmacoeconomic research. Clin Ther. 1993;15:1121-32.

16. Lipowski EE. Evaluating the outcomes of pharmaceutical care. J Am Pharm Assoc. 1996;NS36:726-34.

17. Angaran DM. Selecting, developing and evaluating indicators. Am J Hosp Pharm. 1991;48:1931-7.

18. Joint Commission on Accreditation of Healthcare Organizations. A guide to performance improvement for pharmacies. Oakbrook Terrace (IL): Joint Commission; 1997.

19. Hepler CD, Segal R. Preventing medication errors and improving drug therapy. Boca Raton (FL): CRC Press; 2003.

20. Kerr EA, Krein SL, Vijan S, et al. Avoiding pitfalls in chronic disease quality measurement: a case for the next generation of technical quality measures. Am J Manag Care. 2001;7:1033-43.

21. Agency for Healthcare Research & Quality. Consumer Assessment of Healthcare Providers & Systems (CAHPS) [Internet]. Rockville (MD): Agency for Healthcare Research & Quality; 2012 Nov 25 [cited 2013 Oct 2]. Available from: http://cahps.ahrq.gov/.

22. Blalock SJ, Keller S. Consumer Assessment of Pharmacy Quality. In: Warholak T, Nau DP, eds. Quality & safety in pharmacy practice. New York: McGraw-Hill; 2010.

23. PQA Survey of Consumer Experiences with Pharmacy Services [Internet]. Springfield (VA): Pharmacy Quality Alliance; 2012 Nov 25 [cited 2013 Oct 2]. Available from: http://pqaalliance.org/measures/survey.asp

24. Kerr EA, Smith DM, Hogan MM, et al. Comparing clinical automated, medical record, and hybrid data sources for diabetes quality measures. Jt Comm J Qual Improv. 2002;28:555-65.

25. Kerr EA, Smith DM, Hogan MM, et al. Building a better quality measure: are some patients with 'poor quality' actually getting good care? Med Care. 2003;41:1173-82.

26. Moczygemba LR, Holdford DA. Statistical process control. In: Warholak T, Nau DP, eds. Quality & safety in pharmacy practice. New York: McGraw-Hill; 2010.

27. Nau DP. Measuring pharmacy quality. J Am Pharm Assoc. 2009;49:154-63.

28. Stolar MH. Drug use review: operational definitions. Am J Hosp Pharm. 1978;35:76-8.

29. ASHP guidelines on medication-use evaluation. American Society of Health System Pharmacists. Am J Health Sys Pharm. 1996;53(16):1953-5.

30. Nadzam DM. Development of medication-use indicators by The Joint Commission on Accreditation of Healthcare Organizations. Am J Hosp Pharm. 1991;48:1925-30.

31. Cousins DD. Medication use: a systems approach to reducing errors. Chicago (IL): Joint Commission on Accreditation of Healthcare Organizations; 1998.

32. New accreditation process model for 1994 and beyond. Am J Hosp Pharm. 1993;50:1111-2, 1121.

33. Ente BH. The Joint Commission's agenda for change. Curr Concept Hosp Pharm Manag. 1989(Summer):7-14.

34. The Joint Commission on Accreditation of Hospitals. 1990 AMH. Accreditation manual for hospitals. Chicago (IL): Joint Commission on Accreditation of Hospitals; 1989.

35. Flagstad MS, Williams RB. Assuming responsibility for improving quality. Am J Hosp Pharm. 1991;48:1898.

36. Covington TR, Alexander VL. Drug use evaluation: the fundamentals. Indianapolis (IN): Eli Lilly & Co; 1991.

37. Schaff RL, Schumock GT, Nadzam DM. Development of The Joint Commission's indicators for monitoring the medication use system. Hosp Pharm. 1991;26:326-9, 350.

38. Bernstein SJ, Hilborne LH. Clinical indicators: the road to quality care? Jt Comm J Qual Improv. 1993:19(11):501-9.

39. Clark TR, Gruber J, Sey M. Revisiting drug regimen review, part III: a systematic approach. Consult Pharm. 2003;18:656-66.

40. Knapp DA. Development of criteria for drug utilization review. Clin Pharmacol Ther. 1991;50(Part 2):600-3.

41. Threshold vs. standards. QRC Advisor. 1988;5(2):5.

42. Makela EH, Davis SK, Piveral K, Miller WA, Pleasants RA, Gadsden RH Sr., et al. Effect of data collection method on results of serum digoxin concentration audit. Am J Hosp Pharm. 1988;45:126-30.

43. What is an adequate sample? QRC Advisor. 1985;1(Aug);4-5.

44. Grasela TH, Walawander CA, Kennedy, Jolson HM. Capability of hospital computer systems in performing drug-use evaluations and adverse event monitoring. Am J Hosp Pharm. 1993;50:1889-95.

45. Zarowitz BJ, Petitta A, Mlynarek M, Touchette M, Peters M, Long P, et al. Bar-code technology applied to drug-use evaluation. Am J Hosp Pharm. 1993;50:935-9.

46. Burnakis TG. Facilitating drug-use evaluation with spreadsheet software. Am J Hosp Pharm. 1989;46:84-8.

47. Libby D, Grove C, Adams M. Collaborative use of informatics among hospitals to benchmark medication use processes. Jt Comm J Qual Improv. 1997;23:626-52.

48. Soumerai SB, McLaughlin TJ, Avorn J. Improving drug prescribing in primary care: a critical analysis of the experimental literature. Milbank Quarterly. 1989;67:268-317.

49. Avorn J, Soumeri SB, Taylor W. Reduction of incorrect antibiotic prescribing through a structured educational order form. Arch Intern Med. 1991;151:1825-32.

50. Kowalsky SF, Echols RM, Peck F. Preprinted order sheet to enhance antibiotic prescribing and surveillance. Am J Hosp Pharm. 1982;39:1528-9.

51. Pierson JF, Alexander MR, Kirking DM, Solomon DK. Physician's attitudes toward drug-use evaluation interventions. Am J Hosp Pharm. 1990;47:388-90.

52. Himmelberg CJ, Pleasants RA, Weber DJ, Kessler JM, Samsa GP, Spivey JM, et al. Use of antimicrobial drugs in adults before and after removal of a restriction policy. Am J Hosp Pharm. 1991;48:1220-7.

53. Restino MS, Knodel LC. Drug information quality assurance program used to appraise students' performance. Am J Hosp Pharm. 1992;49(6):1425-9.

54. Wheeler-Usher DH, Hermann FF, Wanke LA. Problems encountered in using written criteria to assess drug information responses. Am J Hosp Pharm. 1990;47(4):795-7.

55. Moody ML. Revising a drug information center quality assurance program to conform to Joint Commission standards. Am J Hosp Pharm. 1990;47(4):792-4.

56. Smith CH, Sylvia LM. External quality assurance committee for drug information services. Am J Hosp Pharm. 1990;47(4):787-91.

57. Halbert MR, Kelly WN, Miller DE. Drug information centers: lack of generic equivalence. Drug Intell Clin Pharm. 1977;11:728-35.

58. Beard SL, Coley RM, Blunt JR. Assessing the accuracy of drug information responses from drug information centers. Ann Pharmacother. 1994;28(6):707-11.

59. Calis KA, Anderson DW, Auth DA, Mays, DA, Turcasso NM, Meyer CC, et al. Quality of pharmacotherapy consultations provided by drug information centers in the United States. Pharmacotherapy. 2002;20:830-6.

15

Chapter Fifteen

Medication Misadventures I: Adverse Drug Reactions

Zara Risoldi Cochrane ● Darren Hein ● Philip J. Gregory

Learning Objectives

After completing this chapter, the reader will be able to

- Define adverse drug reactions (ADRs).
- Discuss the impact of ADRs on health care systems and patients.
- Explain methods for determining causality and probability of an ADR.
- Identify specialty drug information resources that can be used to locate information related to ADRs.
- Classify ADRs based on type and severity.
- Explain when, where, and how to report an ADR to the United States (U.S.) Food and Drug Administration (FDA).
- Explain how to report adverse reactions related to dietary supplements and vaccines.
- Describe the use of technology in ADR monitoring and reporting.
- Use guidelines from national organizations to implement an ADR reporting program.

Key Concepts

❶ An adverse drug reaction (ADR) is any unexpected, unintended, undesired, or excessive response to a medicine.

❷ One of the first steps in establishing an ADR program is to define what each facility or organization categorizes as ADRs.

❸ Several algorithms have been published that try to incorporate information about an ADR into a more objective form.

❹ Communication is a critical component throughout the ADR monitoring process.

❺ Technology plays an important role in monitoring, identifying, and minimizing ADRs.

❻ ADR surveillance serves as a means to primarily provide early signals about possible problems.

Introduction to Adverse Drug Reactions

The terminology surrounding adverse drug reactions (ADRs) is often confusing. All adverse drug events (ADEs), ADRs, and medication errors fall under the umbrella of medication misadventures. Medication misadventure is a very broad term, referring to any iatrogenic hazard or incident associated with medications. An ADE is the next broadest term, and refers to any injury caused by a medicine. An ADE encompasses all ADRs, including allergic and idiosyncratic reactions, as well as medication errors that result in harm to a patient.[1-5] ADRs and medication errors are the most specific terms. ❶ *Adverse drug reaction refers to any unexpected, unintended, undesired, or excessive response to a medicine.* A medication error is any preventable event that has the potential to lead to inappropriate medication use or patient harm.[1] Figure 15–1 shows one way of graphically classifying these terms. Many of these concepts will be explored in greater depth later in this chapter and in Chapter 16. This chapter focuses on ADRs, highlighting the impact of ADRs, pertinent definitions and classifications, specialty drug information resources, ADR reporting systems, and future approaches to detecting and managing ADRs.

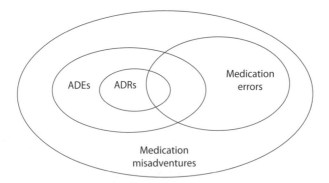

Figure 15–1. Relationship among medication misadventures, adverse drug events, medication errors, and adverse drug reactions. (*Adapted from Bates DW, et al. Relationship between medication and errors and adverse drug events. J Gen Intern Med. 1995 Apr;10(4):199-205.*)

IMPACT OF ADVERSE DRUG REACTIONS IN THE UNITED STATES

All medications, including the inactive ingredients of a product, are capable of producing adverse reactions.[6] ADRs account for about 5% to 15% of all hospital admissions, cause patients to lose confidence in their health care providers, and lead to a significant increase in morbidity and mortality.[7-13] In 2010, there were over 40,000 deaths due to drug-induced causes, landing ADRs among the 10 leading causes of death in the United States.[9]

ADRs have economic consequences as well. ADRs result in an annual cost of $5 to $7 billion to the U.S. health care system. Each hospital in the United States spends up to $5.6 million annually as a result of ADEs. After experiencing an ADR, patients spend an average of 8 to 12 days longer in the hospital, increasing the cost of their hospitalization by $16,000 to $24,000.[11]

The incidence of ADRs for hospitalized patients has been reported to be as high as 28%. Of course, ADRs do not affect hospitalized patients alone. Approximately 20% of the ambulatory population receiving medications suffers from ADRs.[10] These outpatient events do not always result in hospitalization, but certainly affect morbidity and patient quality of life. Health care professionals agree that these estimates are somewhat conservative because many ADRs go undetected, unreported, and untreated.[10] One review concluded that only 2% to 4% of all ADRs, and fewer than 10% of serious ADRs, are ever reported.[11]

Although not all adverse reactions can be prevented, a large proportion of them can; the World Health Organization (WHO) estimates that at least 60% of ADRs are preventable. Preventable ADRs may be caused by such factors as the wrong diagnosis of a patient's condition, incorrect dosing or selection of a prescription medication, interactions with other drugs including dietary supplements, and patients who do not follow the instructions for taking a medication.[14] This highlights the need for health care **practitioners** and health care facilities to engage in the process of systematically preventing and responding to ADRs. WHO terms this **pharmacovigilance**, or the process of preventing and detecting adverse effects from medications.[12]

Several agencies and professional organizations across the country have an active role in pharmacovigilance, and contribute efforts to minimize the occurrence and impact of ADRs. In addition to WHO, some of the key organizations include the FDA, The Joint Commission (TJC), and the American Society of Health-System Pharmacists (ASHP). See Table 15–1. Despite the numerous organizations involved, pharmacovigilance depends heavily on individual health care practitioners, including pharmacists, physicians, and nurses, to take measures to minimize ADRs and report events. Practitioners need to understand the potential for ADRs and be prepared to recognize and prevent such occurrences in order to minimize adverse outcomes.

Pharmacists play a vital role in the medication use process. Multiple studies have highlighted the tremendous impact individual pharmacists can have on minimizing

TABLE 15–1. ORGANIZATIONS INVOLVED IN PREVENTING ADVERSE DRUG EVENTS

Food and Drug Administration (FDA)	http://www.fda.gov
The Joint Commission (TJC)	http://www.jointcommission.org/
World Health Organization (WHO)	http://www.who.int
Institute for Safe Medication Practices (ISMP)	http://www.ismp.org
The United States Pharmacopoeia (USP)	http://www.usp.org
American Society of Health-System Pharmacists (ASHP)	http://www.ashp.org

ADRs.[15,16] In one study published in the *Journal of the American Medical Association,* pharmacists began participating in patient rounds in an intensive care unit. By implementing this measure alone, the hospital significantly reduced the incidence of ADRs and saved an estimated $270,000 per year.[13]

DEFINITIONS

After reading this chapter, the reader should be able to evaluate ADRs and, potentially, develop and implement an ADR surveillance program at their hospital, clinic, or community pharmacy. ❷ *One of the first steps in establishing an ADR program is to define what each facility or organization categorizes as ADRs.* There are many definitions for ADRs that have been described in the literature, including guidance from national and international organizations, as well as individual facilities and practitioners. Several of these definitions are presented below. Rather than getting bogged down in the differences between these many definitions, use this information for guidance when starting to evaluate ADRs and develop an ADR monitoring and reporting system. Remember that institutions, as well as clinicians, use different definitions depending on their practice needs.

WHO defines an ADR as "a response to a medicine which is noxious and unintended, and which occurs at doses normally used in man."[17] WHO additionally defines the term side effect, which is "any unintended effect of a pharmaceutical product occurring at doses normally used by a patient which is related to the pharmacological properties of the drug."[17] Note that, in clinical practice, side effect is a broad term that may be used synonymously with ADR, or may even refer to an ADE.

Defined by the FDA, an ADR is any "undesirable experience" associated with the use of a drug or medical product in a patient.[18] This definition is also fairly broad, and includes adverse events occurring from drug overdose as well as situations involving abuse. The FDA goes on to define an *unexpected* adverse reaction as one that is not listed in the current labeling for a medication as having been reported or associated with the use of the drug. This distinction is important, because unexpected ADRs are those that the FDA would like health care practitioners to report. (Reporting ADRs to the FDA will be discussed later in this chapter.) This definition focuses on reporting unusual, uncommon, or newly identified

ADRs. Although common or expected ADRs are relevant and important, they do not provide the FDA with new or additional safety information. Unexpected drug reactions may be symptomatically or pathophysiologically related to an ADR listed in the current labeling, but may differ from the labeled ADR because of greater severity or specificity. For example, a medication may have abnormal liver function listed in its labeling as an adverse reaction. A health care practitioner should still report a case of hepatic necrosis following administration of the drug, because it represents an unexpected ADR of greater severity.[19]

Edwards and Aronson propose another definition of an ADR: "An appreciably harmful or unpleasant reaction, resulting from an intervention related to the use of a medicinal product, which predicts hazard from future administration and warrants prevention or specific treatment, or alteration of the dosage regimen, or withdrawal of the product."[20] This is a very practical definition for health care practitioners, because it highlights the need to take action in order to manage the effects of the adverse reaction.

Finally, Karch and Lasagna,[21] two prominent researchers in the area of ADRs, define a drug, an ADR, and a patient drug exposure as follows:

Drug: a chemical substance or product available for an intended diagnostic, prophylactic or therapeutic purpose.

Adverse Drug Reaction: any response to a drug which is noxious and unintended and which occurs at doses used in man for prophylaxis, diagnosis or therapy, excluding therapeutic failures. (As stated by the WHO, this definition excludes intentional and accidental poisoning as well as drug abuse situations.)

Patient–Drug Exposure: a single patient receiving at least one dose of a given drug.[21]

Many institutions use Karch and Lasagna's definition because it excludes accidental poisonings as well as problems with drugs of abuse.

Remember, these definitions are intended to provide guidance and food for thought; in daily practice, the differences between these descriptions may not be relevant or clinically meaningful. What is important is that individuals find or develop a definition of ADRs that works for the needs of their pharmacy, clinic, or hospital.

Causality and Probability of Adverse Drug Reactions

One of the challenges in defining and managing ADRs is determining causality. How can it be determined whether or not a drug caused a patient's adverse reaction? Cause and effect is difficult to prove in general, and ADRs are no exception. Many investigators have dealt with this problem by developing and publishing definitions, algorithms, and questionnaires that try to determine the probability of a reaction—that is, the likelihood that an ADR was caused by a particular drug or medication. There are over 30 different published methods for assessing adverse drug reaction causality. They fall into three broad categories[22]:

1. **Expert judgment/Global introspection**: This method involves the individual assessment of the event by a health care practitioner, based on his or her clinical knowledge and experience without using any form of standardized tool.
2. **Algorithm**: This method uses specific questions to assign a weighted score that helps determine the probability of causality in a given reaction.
3. **Probabilistic**: This method uses Bayesian approaches and epidemiological data to calculate and estimate the probability of causality with advanced statistical methods.

To date, none of these attempts have been able to prove actual causality. These tools, however, are used to determine the probability that a particular drug caused an adverse event and will be described further below.

These algorithms and definitions use several important key concepts.[18,23] **Dechallenge** and **rechallenge** are often discussed. **Dechallenge** occurs when the drug is discontinued and the patient is then monitored to determine whether the ADR abates or decreases in intensity. **Rechallenge** occurs when the drug is discontinued and, after the ADR abates, the same drug is administered in an attempt to elicit the response again. Dechallenge and rechallenge are effective means for establishing a strong case that the drug was responsible for the ADR. Unfortunately, in clinical practice, a rechallenge may not be practical and may actually cause further harm to the patient. Patients who suffer a serious ADR may not be thrilled about experiencing the reaction again in the name of science. Therefore, a rechallenge may not always be practical, but a dechallenge is often essential.

Another important concept to consider is the temporal relationship between the drug and the event. Does the timeframe for development of the ADR make sense? Did the patient's exposure to the drug precede the suspected ADR? If there are previous reports of the ADR in the literature, do these reports describe a temporal relationship between the drug and the event? Case reports, specialty drug information resources, and package inserts can be helpful in noting if a drug has been known to cause a certain type of reaction in a certain timeframe in the past. Unfortunately, the literature is not likely to be helpful for rare or new ADRs, but this does not discount the fact that a reaction may have occurred.

Naranjo and colleagues[23] developed the following definitions to assist in determining the probability of a suspected ADR:

Definite ADR is a reaction that: (1) follows a reasonable temporal sequence from administration of the drug, or in which the drug level has been established in body fluids or tissue; (2) follows a known response pattern to the suspected drug; (3) is confirmed by dechallenge; and (4) could not be reasonably explained by the known characteristics of the patient's clinical state.

Conditional ADR is a reaction that: (1) follows a reasonable temporal sequence from administration of the drug; (2) does not follow a known response pattern to the suspected drug; and (3) could not be reasonably explained by the known characteristics of the patient's clinical state.

Doubtful ADR is any reaction that does not meet the criteria above.[23]

USING ALGORITHMS

❸ *Several algorithms have been published that try to incorporate information about an ADR into a more objective form.* As described above, these algorithms each use a set of specific questions to determine the likelihood that the drug was responsible for the reaction, and establish a rational and scientific approach to what previously required strictly clinical judgment. Although algorithms are helpful in offering a systematic approach to assessing the probability of ADRs, they can be very time consuming and the results vary significantly according to the interpretation of multiple observers.

In 1979, Kramer and coworkers published a questionnaire composed of 56 yes or no questions (Appendix 15–1).[24] This questionnaire includes sections about the patient's previous experience with the drug or related drugs, alternative etiologies, timing of events, drug concentrations, dechallenge, and rechallenge. Responses to each question are given a weighted value and these values are totaled. The total value then correlates to one of four categories: unlikely, possible, probable, or definite. One of the problems with the Kramer method (as well as other algorithms) is that clinicians can disagree on the weighted values because the user must make subjective judgments for some of the questions. Another problem inherent with this questionnaire is that an unexpected ADR may not score well because of lack of literature or previous experience with the ADR. If the reaction is not universally accepted or in the most recent edition of the *Physicians' Desk Reference,* the suspected reaction would score a zero in this section. This makes the method devised by Kramer and associates less useful for new medications and for unexpected or emergent ADRs. Overall, however, the questionnaire provides health care professionals with the opportunity to use a standardized tool. Hutchinson and colleagues evaluated the reproducibility and validity of the Kramer questionnaire and concluded that, although the questionnaire was cumbersome to use, the method was superior to clinical judgment alone.[25]

Naranjo and colleagues developed an alternative algorithm in 1981 (Appendix 15–2).[23] This algorithm asks 10 questions involving the following areas: temporal relationship, pattern of response, dechallenge or administration of an antagonist, rechallenge, alternative causes, placebo response, drug level in the body fluids or tissue, dose-response relationship, previous patient experience with the drug, and confirmation by any other objective evidence. Like the algorithm proposed by Kramer et al, the answer to each question is assigned a score. The score is then totaled and placed into a category from definite to doubtful. In the initial published report of this algorithm, Naranjo and colleagues tested the reproducibility and validity of the algorithm and found that their tool was a valid means of assessing ADRs. Today, the Naranjo algorithm is one of the most commonly used methods to assess adverse drug reaction causality, and has been considered a gold standard of assessing ADR causality. Compared to the method devised by Kramer et al, the Naranjo tool is much quicker to administer. However, it is not without its faults. The tool emphasizes rechallenge and dechallenge, which may pose some problems in evaluating ADRs as described previously. The Naranjo algorithm also asks about a response to placebo, which is rarely (if ever) administered in clinical practice today.

In 1982, Jones and colleagues published an algorithm that allows health care practitioners to answer a series of yes or no questions to determine the probability that an ADR occurred (Appendix 15–3).[26] The Jones algorithm asks similar questions as those used in the methods described above, but uses a dichotomous key design. Like the Naranjo algorithm, the tool developed by Jones et al is shorter and quicker to complete than Kramer's questionnaire. Unlike either Kramer or Naranjo algorithms, the Jones method does not require summation of a score. Of note, the Jones algorithm was originally designed for use in a community health setting, illustrating that the assessment of ADRs is not limited to inpatient or institutional settings only.

All of the algorithms described above possess a certain degree of observer variability. However, each can be used to help determine whether an adverse event was precipitated by a certain drug or drug–drug combination. Michel and Knodel compared the three algorithms by Kramer, Jones, and Naranjo.[27] Their study found that the Naranjo algorithm was simpler and less time consuming, and compared favorably to the 56 questions asked by Kramer. Although there was agreement between the Naranjo and Jones algorithms, the study found a higher correlation between the Naranjo algorithm and the Kramer questionnaire. The authors concluded that more data were needed to support the use of the algorithm developed by Jones and colleagues.

A modern approach to assessing the causality of ADRs is being developed by researchers at Butler University College of Pharmacy and Health Sciences.[28] Their algorithm, the Butler University Adverse Drug Reaction Causality Assessment Tool (BADCAT), has been proposed as an easy-to-use alternative to traditional methods, and aims to improve the interrater reliability of ADR assessment techniques. BADCAT comprises 11 questions that ask the health care provider to assess the temporal relationship, previous reports of the potential ADR, patient-specific factors such as co-morbidities, dechallenge, rechallenge, and so on. BADCAT is unique in that it also includes an item related to clinical judgment—that is, the clinician's professional opinion of whether or not the suspected drug caused or contributed to the patient's adverse reaction. This item is factored into the overall score, which is interpreted as either a highly likely, likely, or probable ADR. BADCAT has not yet been published in its final form, but preliminary results indicate that the tool may demonstrate higher interrater agreement than the Naranjo algorithm.

At this time, no algorithm for assessing the causality or probability of an ADR has been proven superior.[29] Therefore, it is reasonable to select a method based on factors such as availability, speed and ease of completing the tool, and clinician preference.

PROBABILISTIC METHODS

A Bayesian approach to assessing adverse reactions has been developed by Lane.[30] Using the Bayesian approach, relevant information is collected and a quantitative measure of the odds that a particular drug caused a particular event is calculated. The Bayesian approach has the potential to be an outstanding tool for predicting populations that may be at higher risk for ADRs. However, this method requires complex calculations, significant time investments to develop the model, and the involvement of a statistician.[31] Therefore, the Bayesian approach is likely not practical for implementation in individual clinics or hospitals. But WHO is using these methods to analyze data in their international drug monitoring network.[20]

In addition to the methods for assessing adverse drug reaction causality and probability discussed above, there are also tools for assessing specific types of ADRs. For example, different methods exist for assessing drug-related liver toxicity.[32]

Case Study 15–1

A patient approaches you at the community pharmacy. She explains that she began taking a dietary supplement called *ZygoControl Weight Loss* about 6 weeks ago. Every time she takes the product, she feels like her heart is racing, she becomes lightheaded, and her mouth feels dry. These symptoms last about 3 hours and then go away. She asks you if you think *ZygoControl Weight Loss* is causing these side effects. You research the product and find out that it contains high doses of caffeine and a stimulant called synephrine that is similar to ephedrine.

- *In this case, was there a dechallenge? If so, what happened when the suspected product was dechallenged?*

- *Was there a rechallenge? Is so, what happened?*
- *Was there a temporal relationship between taking this product and the reaction the patient experienced?*
- *Based on what you know about this product, is the reaction consistent with its known pharmacology?*
- *What is the likelihood of this product causing the reaction?*

SPECIALTY RESOURCES FOR ADVERSE DRUG REACTIONS

Methods used to assess the causality of ADRs, including the Kramer and Naranjo algorithms as well as the BADCAT tool, rely in part on previous documentation of the reaction occurring in response to administration of the suspected drug. For common or well-known ADRs, the prescribing information (also called the package insert) and major drug information compendia can be useful. However, for other suspected ADRs, specialty resources may be necessary.

Chapter 3 introduces ADR specialty resources, including gold standards references *Meyler's Side Effects of Drugs* and *Side Effects of Drugs Annual*. This section briefly describes a few additional specialty resources that may be useful.

FDA's MedWatch program for voluntary reporting of ADRs is discussed later in this chapter and Chapter 16. The results of this program are disseminated through a special section of the FDA Web site dedicated to ADRs and other medication safety topics (http://www.fda.gov/Safety/Medwatch). This online reference contains the FDA's latest safety alerts and recalls as well as resources for health care professionals. The site also provides monthly summaries of changes to drug labeling that the FDA has made in response to reports from health care providers and others involved in pharmacovigilance.[33] Users can sign up to receive safety alerts by e-mail, or follow FDA MedWatch on Twitter using Internet-enabled mobile devices such as smartphones or tablet computers (http://www.twitter.com/FDAMedWatch).

Because the FDA's Web site can be difficult to navigate, it is perhaps best used for current hot topics or news items related to ADRs. The search function is rudimentary, and searching MedWatch for previous reports of a suspected ADR can be challenging. An alternative solution is DrugCite (http://www.drugcite.com), an independent Web site that uses a series of algorithms to search and report on the FDA's adverse events database. Although the depth of information provided by DrugCite is minimal, the site can be used to determine whether an adverse reaction has been previously reported to MedWatch in response to a particular drug and, if so, how often.[34,35] A mobile DrugCite application is available for Android-based devices.[36]

Published case reports can also be useful in assessing and evaluating ADRs (see Chapter 5 for more information on evaluating case reports). *Reactions Weekly* is a weekly publication that indexes and abstracts ADR case reports and ADR-related news from around the world (see also Chapter 3). Because it pulls information from biomedical journals, scientific meetings, and the WHO International Drug Monitoring Programme, *Reactions Weekly* can be useful for efficiently searching the available information related to a suspected ADR.[37] *Clin-Alert* is a similar publication that summarizes reports of adverse clinical events from more than 100 key research journals, although its focus is primarily on reports of drug–drug interactions (DDIs).[38]

Classification of Adverse Drug Reactions

Various definitions and terminology have been used to classify ADRs. As discussed above, algorithms such as those developed by Naranjo, Kramer, and Jones have used the definite, probable, possible, and unlikely categories to classify ADRs by their probability. Other classification systems rank ADRs by severity or by their mechanism. When developing an ADR monitoring program, these various systems can be used to determine probability (cause and effect) and severity of ADRs and help describe and quantify data. The data may help identify severity of reactions that are occurring and which medications cause the most severe reactions. Classification systems can also help health care practitioners organize and present data, and facilitate monitoring of ADR trends and potential causative agents. These trends can be used to change prescribing habits or to alert institutions and organizations to potential problems with medications.

CLASSIFYING BY SEVERITY

Karch and Lasagna[21] developed a method of classifying ADRs by severity, from minor to severe, as defined below:

- *Minor:* No antidote, therapy or prolongation of hospitalization is required in response to the ADR.
- *Moderate:* The management of the ADR requires a change in drug therapy, specific treatment, or an increase in hospitalization by at least 1 day.
- *Severe:* The ADR is potentially life threatening, causing permanent damage, or requiring intensive medical care.
- *Lethal:* The ADR directly or indirectly contributes to the death of the patient.

The FDA and WHO also use severity to classify ADRs. According to the these organizations, an ADR is serious when it results in death, is life threatening, causes or prolongs hospitalization, causes a significant persistent disability, results in a congenital anomaly, or requires intervention to prevent permanent damage.[14,39]

CLASSIFYING BY MECHANISM

Karch and Lasagna also described various mechanisms by which ADRs occur.[21] These mechanisms are related to the pharmacologic or pharmacodynamic properties of drugs, and can be used to classify the type of reaction that occurs:

- *Idiosyncrasy:* an uncharacteristic response of a patient to a drug, usually not occurring on administration.
- *Hypersensitivity:* a reaction, not explained by the pharmacologic effects of the drug, caused by altered reactivity of the patient and generally considered to be an allergic manifestation.
- *Intolerance:* a characteristic pharmacologic effect of a drug produced by an unusually small dose, so that the usual dose tends to induce a massive overaction.
- *Drug interaction:* an unusual pharmacologic response that could not be explained by the action of a single drug, but was caused by two or more drugs.
- *Pharmacologic:* a known, inherent pharmacologic effect of a drug, directly related to dose.

Classifying the ADR by its mechanism may aid in identifying similar drugs that can be expected to cause a reaction, or may help explain patient-specific reactions to medications.

Implementing a Program

Well-designed programs that monitor and identify ADRs, as well as broadcast information to the medical community, are essential. A later section of this chapter will discuss the importance of reporting suspected ADRs to the FDA and other stakeholders. But before ADRs can be reported, a program for detecting and capturing these reactions must be implemented at a facility or institution.

Prior to implementing an ADR program, the health care facility must educate its staff on the importance and significance of the program. The pharmacy department is in an excellent position to provide this education because of its involvement in the pharmacy and therapeutics (P&T) committee, pharmacokinetic dosing, drug utilization evaluation (DUE), and drug distribution. The pharmacy department can be an excellent resource for developing an ADR program, as well as providing data about ADRs to the P&T committee.

STEPS FOR IMPLEMENTING A PROGRAM

Accrediting bodies like TJC[40] require that hospitals and health care organizations have an ADR reporting program. These programs are generally a function of the P&T committee (or other medical staff committee) and the department of pharmacy. ASHP also encourages pharmacists and health care practitioners to take an active role in monitoring adverse events. ASHP has published very specific guidelines on ADR monitoring and reporting as part of its practice standards.[41] TJC and ASHP standards can be used as a basis for starting an ADR monitoring program. In addition to the standards, the pharmacy and medical literature are rich with examples of successful programs, some of which will be reviewed in this chapter.

Steps for implementing an ADR monitoring program include the following:

1. Develop definitions and classifications of ADRs that work for the institution. The definitions and classifications in this chapter provide a good starting point for discussion.

2. Assign responsibility for the ADR program within the pharmacy and throughout other key departments. A multidisciplinary approach is an essential factor. This will improve awareness of the monitoring program and increase ADR reporting at all levels of patient care.

3. Develop a program with approval from the pharmacy department, medical staff and nursing department, as well as other appropriate areas within the facility. Cooperation is essential in initiation of a successful program.

4. Promote awareness of the program. Newsletters, e-mails, in-services, grand rounds presentations, and other educational programs are opportunities to increase awareness and garner support for the program.

5. Promote awareness of ADRs and the importance of reporting such events in order to increase patient safety. Again, newsletters, e-mails, in-services, grand rounds presentations, and other educations programs can be utilized to increase awareness of specific ADRs.

6. Establish mechanisms for screening ADRs continuously. These mechanisms should include retrospective reviews and concurrent monitoring, as well as prospective planning for high-risk groups. It is worthwhile to educate pharmacists to check for ADRs when they see orders for certain indicator drugs that are often used in treating an ADR (see Table 15–2), orders to discontinue or hold drugs, and orders to decrease the dose or frequency of a drug.[42] Also, electronic screening methods to check for laboratory tests that are indicative of ADRs (e.g., drug levels, *Clostridium difficile* toxin assays, elevated serum potassium, low white blood cell counts) can be helpful.[43] Emergency box usage is another event that may trigger investigation by the pharmacist to determine if

an ADR has occurred (e.g., use of epinephrine, diphenhydramine).[44] The previous examples highlight specific approaches to monitor for ADRs continuously. Additionally, retrospective review of indicator drug orders, laboratory tests, and/or emergency box usage may also bring to light previously unreported ADRs.

7. Develop internal forms or other mechanisms for data collection and reporting of ADRs. A quick Internet search will identify a number of ADR report forms used at specific institutions across the country. Some institutions use computer reporting, as well as hotline phone numbers.

8. Develop policies and procedures for handling ADR reports. Indicate who is responsible for sending them to the FDA.

9. Establish procedures for evaluating the causality and probability of ADRs, usually based on one of the classification systems previously discussed.

10. Routinely review ADRs for trends.

11. Develop preventive interventions. Examples of these include flagging patients who are at high risk of developing ADRs and identifying specific drugs which are likely to cause ADRs. Monitoring these patients and drugs more closely will help prevent or reduce the severity of possible ADRs.

12. Report all findings to P&T and/or other appropriate committee(s).

13. Develop strategies for decreasing the incidence of ADRs, depending on the opportunities presented by the ADRs reported. This vital step has often been ignored in the literature; however, for an ADR program to be part of the quality assurance process, it must be included wherever possible.

TABLE 15–2. ADR INDICATOR DRUGS

Antidiarrheal agents
Atropine (except preoperatively)
Dextrose 50% (IV push)
Diphenhydramine (except at bedtime)
Epinephrine (IV push)
Flumazenil
Naloxone
Potassium supplement (diuretic or digoxin patients)
Protamine
Sodium polystyrene sulfonate (patients on potassium sparing diuretics or ACE inhibitors)
Topical steroids
Vitamin K

❹ *Communication is a critical component throughout the ADR monitoring process.* To ensure that the suspected drug is not administered again, and that patients receive necessary treatment and monitoring, each ADR should be documented thoroughly in the patient's medical record. However, this action alone is not sufficient, as the information is often poorly visible and may be difficult to access. The Institute for Safe Medication Practices (ISMP) recommends that ADRs be communicated to the ADR monitoring team by documenting the reaction on a standardized order form, either in paper or electronic form, just as if prescribing drug therapy or ordering lab draws.[45] This increases visibility of the information and facilitates a timely response by all individuals involved in the patient's care. In addition, ASHP recommends that patients and their caregivers be notified when a suspected ADR has occurred.[41] Well-informed patients can help prevent ADRs from recurring in the future.[45] Finally, previously unreported or clinically important ADRs should be disseminated to the medical community by publication and/or presentation in an appropriate forum.[44]

THE ROLE OF TECHNOLOGY AND EXEMPLAR PROGRAMS

❺ *Technology plays an important role in monitoring, identifying, and minimizing ADRs.* Information systems are available that can identify and alert practitioners to potential ADRs and detect potential DDIs that may contribute to ADRs. These systems search patient records and medical data to find drug names, drug levels, or drug–lab interactions (sometimes called triggers) that frequently indicate an ADR has occurred.[46] See Chapter 24 for more information on this topic. Sophisticated systems may also search through International Classification of Diseases (ICD-9) codes, nursing notes, or outpatient medical records. For example, a medication profile that includes an angiotensin-converting enzyme inhibitor (ACE-I) and a note in the medical chart that mentions cough might trigger the ADR surveillance system. This information is then used to alert a pharmacist or prescriber who can investigate the suspected ADR and manage any adverse effects.[39]

An example of one such system was developed at Brigham and Women's Hospital. This system was programmed to detect a combination of patient-specific factors and medications that may indicate a patient who has the potential to experience an ADR. For example, patients taking medications that required renal function-based dosing and who had elevated serum creatinine were flagged as patients at risk for development of an ADR. Various other screening rules were also programmed. When compared to traditional methods of identifying ADRs, this system detected more ADRs than spontaneous reports, but fewer than retrospective chart review. Interestingly, the errors detected by the computer system were different than those detected by chart review, indicating that a combination of multiple ADR detection systems may provide the best results. As expected, using the computer system saved work time, requiring five times fewer person-hours than the chart review method.[47] In another study, a similar ADE detection system identified potential ADEs in 64 of every 1000 admissions. The prescribing physician did not recognize 44% of the ADEs detected by the system.[48]

At LDS Hospital in Salt Lake City, Utah, the Health Evaluation through Logical Processing (HELP) system monitors medical records around the clock and automatically identifies patients who may have experienced an ADR. The system does this by identifying certain flags such as stop orders, orders for antidotes, and abnormal laboratory values. The flags or signals are then reported to the pharmacy so that pharmacists can follow-up to determine if an actual adverse event has truly occurred.[43]

Because hospitals are required by accrediting bodies to have an ADR reporting system, the use of technology for identifying, reporting, and minimizing ADRs is very common in the inpatient setting. Unfortunately, this is quite different from the ambulatory care setting. In general, the reporting of ADRs and other drug-related events has experienced minimal uptake in the primary care setting. Reasons for this include busy physician schedules, high cost of implementation, and complexity of outpatient prescribing practices. Because of this, the Agency for Healthcare Research and Quality (AHRQ) recently initiated a project to develop and test a reporting system for use in ambulatory clinics nationwide. Called the Medication Error and Adverse Drug Event Reporting System (MEADERS), it was designed with input from a group of experts in patient and medication safety in the primary care setting. An intuitive electronic system was developed that allowed health care professionals to report events using both simple data entry and open text boxes in order to capture the complete story regarding each medication error or ADE. MEADERS also includes the option of sending each report to the FDA's MedWatch program.[49] ADR reports are documented via entry into an Internet-based system or a stand-alone system using Microsoft® Access™. MEADERS also includes an Internet-based report viewing system that allows users to browse reports from ambulatory setting across the country using the MedMarx[SM] database. This provides capabilities for practitioners to compare their local or organizational reports to national data.[50] Initial field testing of MEADERS involved 24 practice sites who submitted a total of 507 reports during the pilot period. Of these reports, 27% involved ADEs. While physicians maintained that time was the primary barrier to reporting medication errors and ADEs, the average time spent per report was just 4.3 minutes. In addition, only eight reports were electronically forwarded to the FDA's MedWatch program. Thus, the development team is currently adapting the nuances of the system to make reporting a seamless component of the normal work flow.[42]

AHRQ had previously concluded that the data supporting ADR monitoring and reporting programs in the outpatient setting was limited, but initiatives like MEADERS demonstrate that evidence is still emerging in this practice setting.[46] Traditionally, hospital-based pharmacists have been the health care professional to provide the greatest number of spontaneous ADR reports to the FDA.[51] However, community pharmacists are in a unique position to report on ADRs relating to nonprescription medications and dietary supplements. Community pharmacists can also report on reactions that patients are likely to detect themselves, such as ophthalmic and dermatological disorders. In fact, in countries such as the Netherlands, Japan, and Spain, the majority of ADR reports originate from community, rather than hospital, pharmacists.[51]

One of the finest examples concerning the use of information technology for ADR monitoring and reporting comes from the Department of Veterans Affairs (VA). In 2007, the VA refined its methods for collecting and reporting patient-specific ADR information. This was accomplished by developing two distinct, yet complementary, databases. The first involves patient-specific information related to ADRs. Health care providers within the VA system are responsible for entering ADR information into a specific part of the patients' electronic medical record, called the Adverse Reaction Tracking (ART) package. This locally entered ADR information is then automatically extracted to construct a national ART database. Since its inception, the ART database has received over 50,000 entries per month. The second database, the VA Adverse Drug Event Reporting System (VA ADERS), is external to the electronic medical record and requires providers to report detailed information related to specific, preselected ADRs. VA ADERS also allows for direct submission to the FDA's reporting programs MedWatch and the Vaccine Adverse Event Reporting System (VAERS), discussed later in this chapter. The impact of VA ADERS on ADR reporting is demonstrated by the number of reports generated compared to the VA's previous system (the legacy Adverse Drug Event System). In the 5 years prior to the implementation of the VA ADERS, only 21,000 ADR reports were generated. In the 3 years after the implementation of the VA ADERS, nearly 150,000 ADR reports were generated.[52]

Because DDIs may comprise as many as 59% of ADRs, computer systems that detect clinically significant interactions are also important for reducing ADRs.[53] Over the past 20 years, the integration of drug information databases with clinical information has allowed for increased screening of DDIs upon medication dispensing. As pharmacists are entering orders into patient profiles, the integrated drug information database is checking for DDIs with all concurrent medications. While these clinical decision support systems are a good first-line of defense in monitoring for DDIs, studies have suggested the interaction tools often perform at a suboptimal level, either by misclassifying the severity of specific DDIs or failing to provide sufficient evidence to support the supposed interaction. Additionally, studies have shown that clinicians override the majority of alerts, ignoring potentially important safety warnings, and may develop alert fatigue if they receive drug interaction alerts too frequently.[54] In response, Warholak and colleagues have developed a tool which allows pharmacies to evaluate the performance of their specific DDI detection system.[55]

Waller proposed a potentially significant advancement in the use of technology for reporting ADRs. With this system, information regarding ADRs would be automatically captured from the computers of health care professionals.[56] When a trigger event occurred, such as the administration of a drug antidote, reports could be generated and sent to the FDA or other regulatory bodies without any action at all from the practitioner. This proposal, while not without its challenges for implementation, has the capability to greatly reduce the underreporting of ADRs.

Due to high costs and the time required to educate health care professionals on the changes, the health care industry has traditionally lagged behind other industries in the implementation of high-end technology information systems.[57] The 2009 passage of the American Recovery and Reinvestment Act (ARRA), also known as the stimulus package, called for the development of a nationwide health record system in the United States. The ARRA both places pressure on the health care community to adopt health information technologies and provides funding to make this transition a reality.[58] If and when this national health record system is implemented, it has the potential to significantly change the way ADRs are identified and minimized.

Reporting Adverse Drug Reactions

❻ ADR surveillance serves as a means to primarily provide early signals about possible problems, according to Gerald A. Faich, MD, MPH, Former Director, Office of Epidemiology and Biostatistics, Center for Drugs and Biologics, of the FDA. He goes on to explain that "neither industry nor the FDA should consider its scientific job complete when a new drug is approved."[59] Faich is referring to the importance of **postmarketing surveillance**, or the process of continually monitoring and reviewing suspected adverse reactions associated with medications once they reach the market and are available to the public (see Chapter 22 for more about postmarketing surveillance). In order to detect an ADR that occurs once in every 10,000 patients exposed to the drug, at least 30,000 people would need to be treated with the medication.[12] Clinical trials that are required to approve a new drug may not enroll a sufficient number of patients, and often exclude special groups such as children, pregnant women, and the elderly. Due to the limited sample size and populations included in these trials, the FDA relies on postmarketing information to establish a better understanding of adverse events. In addition, the short duration of most clinical trials means that they will not detect ADRs with a delayed onset.[60] Pharmaceutical companies are required by the FDA to submit quarterly reports of all ADRs for the first 3 years that a drug is on the market, followed by annual reports thereafter, as part of the postmarketing surveillance system. However, the success of postmarketing surveillance is directly dependent on the active involvement of health care practitioners.[14] Postmarketing ADR reports from health care providers have led to changes in prescribing habits, changes to drug labeling, and the withdrawal of various drugs from the market.

REPORTING ADRS TO THE FDA

With the passage of the Kefauver–Harris Amendment of 1962, the FDA was required to maintain a Spontaneous Reporting System (SRS). The SRS allows for a relatively inexpensive monitoring system of ADRs for all drugs marketed in the United States, throughout their entire life cycle.[53,61] All health care professionals and consumers can use this program to report ADRs and participate in the postmarketing surveillance process.

In the past, however, the problem with the SRS has been the lack of voluntary reporting by the medical community. In 1988, for example, a survey demonstrated that only 57% of community-based physicians were aware of the voluntary system of reporting, which used FDA Form 1639 to allow anyone to report an adverse event through the SRS.[62] In June 1993, the FDA switched to a new program called MedWatch: The FDA Medical Products Reporting Program. With MedWatch, the FDA receives reports via mailings, phone calls, faxes, and the Internet. From 2000 to 2010, the number of reports submitted annually through MedWatch to the FDA's Adverse Event Reporting System (AERS) database grew from 266,866 to 758,890.[63]

The current MedWatch system allows health care providers to report suspected ADRs using FDA Form 3500 (Appendix 15–4), which can be submitted by mail, fax, phone, or online.[64] The MedWatch form asks for information related to the suspected ADR, the patient's relevant medical history and medication regimen, and pertinent laboratory tests, although this information does not need to be complete in order for an ADR report to be submitted. From start to finish, the FDA estimates that it takes 36 minutes to complete a MedWatch form, including gathering the patient's data, reviewing the instructions, and submitting the report.

Once submitted through the MedWatch system, ADR reports are received by a unit of the FDA called the Central Triage Unit. The Central Triage Unit screens reports and forwards them to the appropriate FDA program within 24 hours of receipt. The report becomes part of a database used by the FDA to identify signals or warnings related to drug safety that require further study or regulatory action (see the section Future Approaches to Pharmacovigilance). As a reminder, MedWatch is interested in capturing reports of serious ADRs, which the FDA defines as death, life-threatening events, hospitalization, disability, congenital anomaly, or requiring intervention to prevent permanent impairment or damage, as well as unexpected ADRs. The MedWatch program asks individuals to report an event even if they are not certain that the drug product was the cause.[65]

The MedWatch program does not overcome the traditional lack of reporting seen with voluntary systems. It is important to recall that pharmaceutical manufacturers are required to report all adverse events to the FDA, whereas individual health care practitioners do so only voluntarily. Various explanations can account for the failure of practitioners to participate in the FDA program. Hoffman elucidates several reasons that physicians do not voluntarily report ADRs, which are as follows:

1. Failure to detect the reaction due to a low level of suspicion.
2. Fear of potential legal implications.
3. Lack of training about drug therapy.
4. Uncertainty about whether the drug causes the reaction.
5. Lack of clear responsibility for reporting.
6. Paperwork and time involved.
7. No financial incentive to report.
8. Unaware of reporting procedure or little understanding of it.
9. Lack of readily available reporting forms.
10. Desire to publish the report.
11. Fear that a useful drug will be removed from the market or given a bad name.
12. Complacency and lethargy.
13. Guilty feelings because of patient harm.
14. Reaction not worth reporting.[65]

In a systematic review of available evidence, Lopez-Gonzalez and colleagues identified additional reasons why ADRs are underreported, including the beliefs that a single ADR report cannot meaningfully contribute to medical knowledge and only safe drugs are allowed on the market.[66] Another potential explanation for the lack of reporting is that medical record personnel, whose job might be to categorize and report data, are not familiar with ADRs and/or their method of documentation.[65]

Many of the reasons noted above also explain pharmacists' barriers to ADR reporting. A recent survey of Texas pharmacists investigated attitudes about voluntary reporting of serious ADEs in both community and hospital settings. While nearly 90% of respondents felt reporting could improve patient safety, 72.6% noted that the reporting process was time consuming. Furthermore, 55.5% of respondents felt the reporting process disrupted their normal workflow. Some of the pharmacists in this survey also mentioned the reporting would increase the risk of malpractice, compromise relationships with physicians, and potentially break trust with their patients.[67] Ultimately, the benefit of increased patient safety should be enough to overcome the barriers to reporting faced by health care practitioners.

Historically, consumer reporting of adverse events has provided little data to Med-Watch in comparison to the number of reports submitted by health care professionals. With the passage of the Food and Drug Administration Amendments Act (FDAAA) in 2007, however, consumer reports have been increasing. The FDAAA called for increased measures to ensure the safety of marketed drugs. In an effort to increase consumer reporting of adverse events to the FDA, the act requires direct-to-consumer advertisements of prescription drugs to include the following statement: "You are encouraged to report negative side effects of prescription drugs to the FDA. Visit http://www.fda.gov/medwatch, or call 1-800-FDA-1088."[68]

In fact, in 2006, before the FDAAA was passed, consumers reported only 127,475 adverse event reports to MedWatch. In 2010, consumers were responsible for reporting 403,746 adverse event reports, nearing the total provided by all health care providers that year.[69] While this trend is encouraging, there is still room for an increased rate of reporting by consumers. Efforts to educate the public on its role in ADR reporting could significantly impact public health.[76]

Although consumers have the option of submitting ADR reports directly to the Med-Watch program, FDA Form 3500 may be difficult for patients to navigate and complete. For example, they may not have ready access to their medical records, laboratory test results, and so on. Fortunately, a simplified, consumer-focused Form 3500B is available for patients to report ADRs to the FDA. A reporting mechanism is available for these individuals through the FDA's Consumer Complaint Coordinators. Available by telephone, these coordinators listen to consumer complaints, document the suspected problem, and follow up when needed. In the past, the FDA has recalled nonprescription products after just two or three reports of serious problems were received through the Consumer Complaint Coordinators.[70]

DIETARY SUPPLEMENT ADR REPORTING

Dietary supplements, including herbs, vitamins, minerals, and other so-called "nutraceuticals," can and do cause ADRs. Many of these products have powerful pharmacological effects and, therefore, can cause ADRs. The medical literature contains many case reports that describe ADRs related to dietary supplements. However, the exact incidence of ADRs with dietary supplements is not known. In one survey of 2743 adults, 4% who took a dietary supplement reported an adverse event in the previous 12 months.[71]

Dietary supplements are regulated much differently than pharmaceuticals. The most striking difference is that these supplements can reach pharmacies and grocery store shelves without FDA approval and without any proof of safety or effectiveness. Until recently, manufacturers of these products were not required to monitor safety of their products through postmarketing surveillance, nor were they required to share information about safety with the FDA. However, the Dietary Supplement and Nonprescription Drug Consumer Protection Act of 2006 changed this. This legislation now requires that any manufacturer, packager, or distributor of a dietary supplement whose name appears on a product label must collect and report ADR information related to their product(s). Manufacturers or marketers of dietary supplements who receive reports or information about severe adverse reactions related to their products are now required to share these reports with the FDA.[72] Retailers who sell these products may report events upstream to the manufacturer, packer, or distributor.

An interesting case related to dietary supplements and ADRs involves the herb ephedra, also known as *ma huang*. This herb was marketed as a dietary supplement and promoted primarily for weight loss and enhancing athletic performance. It received lots of negative media attention when a Minnesota football player died of heat exhaustion during a training session. It turned out that the football player was using ephedra for weight loss. Over a period of several years, there were well over 100 reports to the FDA of life-threatening ADRs linked to ephedra, including heart attacks, strokes, seizures, and death. In March 2004, the FDA banned the sale of dietary supplements containing ephedra,[73] although this ban was lifted by a judge in 2010.[74] Still, the FDA could not prove that ephedra was the cause of these numerous ADRs. Because there were no reporting standards or requirements for manufacturers to collect data on their products' safety at this time, it would be unlikely that the FDA would ever have enough data to scientifically prove causality; they had to act based on the best available evidence. The FDA's actions on ephedra will have long-lasting effects, and has ultimately set the precedent by which other cases against dietary supplements will be decided.

Currently, ADRs related to dietary supplements can be submitted through the FDA MedWatch program using the same approach that is used for prescription drugs. There are also third-party systems for collecting adverse event data such as Natural Medicines Watch. Natural Medicines Watch allows consumers or health care professionals to complete an electronic form reporting an adverse event related to any dietary supplement. This system uses a database of around 90,000 commercially available dietary supplements that allows the user to select the specific commercial product used by the patient. Since many commercially available dietary supplements contain multiple ingredients, this system may improve the reliability of adverse reaction reporting for supplements. Natural Medicines Watch is integrated with the drug information resource Natural Medicines Comprehensive Database (http://www.naturaldatabase.com), which increases its accessibility for health care practitioners. Natural Medicines Watch asks similar questions to those on the FDA MedWatch Form 3500, and all reports submitted through this system are also simultaneously shared with the FDA's MedWatch program.[75]

Just as with conventional drugs, reporting ADRs related to dietary supplements is voluntary for health care professionals. Practitioners and consumers have many options for reporting dietary supplement ADRs. As described above, they may submit them directly to the FDA, through a third-party system such as Natural Medicines Watch, or to the manufacturer or product distributor. Each of these avenues ultimately results in the information being provided to the FDA for evaluation and analysis. Within the FDA, these reports are sent to the Center for Food Safety and Applied Nutrition (CFSAN), which maintains a special group charged with evaluating these adverse events. The CFSAN Adverse Event Reporting System (CAERS) allows for a more efficient evaluation of reports specifically related to dietary supplements.[76]

Despite the availability of this reporting infrastructure, the number of adverse events submitted by health professionals is minimal. From 2007 to 2010, an average of only 440 voluntary reports related to dietary supplement ADRs were submitted to the FDA each year.[77] During the same time frame, about 790 per year were reported through mandatory mechanisms, such as manufacturer or distributor reporting. Most of these reports originate from consumers rather than health professionals.[76]

There may be a variety of reasons why few health professionals submit reports on dietary supplements to the FDA. Some of these may include:

- Patients often do not tell their providers about supplements use, or about the adverse effects they experience.
- Health professionals often do not ask about the use of dietary supplements.
- Consumers do not believe health professionals are able to answer questions about dietary supplements.
- Health professionals do not know where or how to submit reports of adverse reactions.
- There is a lack of information available to assess dietary supplement adverse reactions.
- Health care professionals may face a lack of time or support from management.
- Practitioners may have a fear of litigation.

ADRs related to dietary supplements can be assessed in much the same way as conventional drugs. However, there are some unique considerations. For example, when it comes to supplements, there is no such thing as generic equivalency. In other words, two supplement products made by different manufacturers cannot be considered equivalent. Different manufacturing practices and different extraction methods can dramatically change how a substance acts in the body, and this is especially true when it comes to herbal extracts. Because herbal extracts are made from plant material, variables such as extraction method, time of harvest, growing conditions, and so on can affect the chemical makeup of the extract. Therefore, two supplements containing Echinacea should not necessarily be considered equivalent. This may also mean that an ADR caused by one version of a supplement may not occur with another version.

VACCINE ADR REPORTING

While MedWatch accepts adverse event reports for all FDA-regulated drugs, biologics, and medical devices, as well as dietary supplements, a separate process has been established for the reporting of adverse reactions related to vaccinations. The VAERS is a post-marketing surveillance program supported by the FDA and the Centers for Disease Control and Prevention (CDC). It was established after the passage of the National Childhood Vaccine Injury Act in 1986. This act requires health care providers to report specific adverse events that follow vaccination. These events include those listed by the vaccine manufacturer as a contraindication to subsequent doses of the vaccine, as well as certain other reactions defined by the FDA and CDC. A list of these reportable reactions is available on the VAERS Web site (http://vaers.hhs.gov).[78] Around 30,000 reports are submitted to VAERS annually. Of these, approximately 13% are considered serious.[79] Similar to the MedWatch program, patients and practitioners can submit reports of adverse reactions to VAERS online, by fax, or by mail. Detailed instructions regarding this process are also available on the VAERS Web site.

Case Study 15–2

A patient approaches you at the community pharmacy. She explains that she began taking a dietary supplement called *ZygoControl Weight Loss* about 6 weeks ago. Every time she takes the product, she feels like her heart is racing, she becomes lightheaded, and her mouth feels dry. These symptoms last about 3 hours and then go away. After interviewing the patient and evaluating the available information, you decide that *ZygoControl Weight Loss* is causing these side effects.

- *As a health care professional, how can you report this suspected ADR to the FDA?*
- *Your patient decides she would like to take responsibility for reporting this ADR on her own. How can she accomplish this task?*

Future Approaches to Pharmacovigilance

The FDA has recognized that voluntary postmarketing evaluations of drug safety data alone are not sufficient to identify serious ADRs. High-profile adverse events related to drugs, such as rofecoxib (Vioxx®) and rosiglitazone (Avandia®), are prime examples of the insufficiency of the voluntary reporting system. The FDA, working with private companies and academic researchers, has developed new methodologies to get early detection signals about safety issues with medications. These latest techniques include the development of additional pharmacovigilance methods as well as the improvement of the existing SRS. For example, the FDA is using data mining approaches for a more rapid identification of potential problems. Data mining is a statistical process that attempts to find a drug-associated event that appears more often in the ADR databases than would normally be expected to occur in the general population. When a higher-than-expected event occurs, this is referred to as signal detection. Statistics are used to identify these signals using both Bayesian and non-Bayesian methods. When an association is flagged in the system, the FDA then requires a clinical review involving experts to decide if any further action is needed for these events.[80] Although data mining and signal detection cannot determine a causal relationship between a drug and an adverse reaction, it is an efficient means of identifying ADRs that may warrant further investigation by the FDA.

With these new techniques, some hospitals have investigated pharmacovigilance methods for evaluating the safety profile of drugs at their institutions. The New York Presbyterian Hospital implemented a pharmacovigilance system that involved the electronic health record and used natural language computer processing. Various statistical techniques were used to establish associations between drugs and ADRs, as well as cutoff thresholds. In the hospital's feasibility study, seven drug classes were evaluated for novel adverse events. The researchers believed that the use of a comprehensive, unstructured data-monitoring program of electronic health records was a feasible option for computerized pharmacovigilance at the local health-system level. This study demonstrates that data mining and signal detection, even at the local level, provide an effective mechanism for ADR reporting.[81]

The traditional randomized controlled clinical trial (RCT) is primarily designed to test the effectiveness of a drug or therapy, and is not usually powered to detect relevant safety information. With this in mind, it is easy to see why adverse reactions may go undetected in these trials. As discussed previously, it has been estimated that any ADR that occurs in fewer than 1 in 10,000 people will not be detected in most RCTs. Therefore, some experts have recommended the use of what is known as a large, simple trial (LST) to increase sample sizes and to monitor larger numbers of patients during clinical testing. LSTs have less stringent eligibility criteria than traditional RCTs, and subjects are typically studied for shorter periods of time. LST designs still use randomization techniques and continue to have important safety monitoring thresholds; they are not powered to determine efficacy. The larger sample sizes seen with the LST design provide more data for ADR monitoring methods such as signal detection. In addition, the larger number of subjects increases the probability of picking up adverse events that are less common.[82] However, because LSTs are of relatively short duration, they do not overcome the challenge of detecting ADRs with a long latency.

Pharmacovigilance has traditionally relied on retrospective reports of ADRs, and relatively little information is available that helps health care professionals prospectively decide whether or not to use a drug in a particular patient. Pharmacogenetics may offer a solution for identifying characteristics and risk factors that predispose an individual to an ADR.[53] Genetic variations in enzymes that metabolize and eliminate drugs can lead to a patient's increased exposure to a medication, potentially increasing their risk for adverse effects.[83] Genome-wide association studies scan for genetic markers across the DNA of many individuals to find variations that may be associated with serious ADRs.[84,85] As of 2012, 10 such studies had been published, providing evidence for specific genes associated with drug-induced hepatotoxicity, carbamazepine-related skin rash, and muscle toxicity following simvastatin administration.[85]

Conclusion

Adverse drug reactions are a serious problem in the U.S. health care system, causing significant morbidity and mortality as well as costing billions of dollars annually. The problem is undeniably widespread, with the FDA receiving over 830,000 spontaneous reports of ADRs in 2010 alone.[62] From 1998 to 2005, the number of reports documenting serious ADRs and fatal ADRs increased almost threefold. Astonishingly, during that time reports related to biological drugs grew almost 16-fold.[86] Because of documented underreporting, these numbers represent only a small fraction of the ADRs occurring annually. Recognition of the problem is an important step in developing strategies to minimize the occurrence of ADRs. Reporting of these reactions by health care professionals is vital to gauging progress and directing our efforts in medication safety and patient care.

Pharmacists and other health care practitioners play a vital role in developing, maintaining, and promoting ADR monitoring programs. Key steps in the development of these programs include identifying an institution-wide definition of ADRs, obtaining buy-in throughout the facility, establishing a mechanism to continuously screen for ADRs, and assigning responsibility for transmitting ADR reports. These programs provide valuable information about ADRs within the institution, as well as spontaneous reports of ADRs that can be forwarded to the FDA to aid in signal detection. ADR monitoring programs improve communication channels, generate additional education on adverse events, and positively impact patient care.

Technology is essential for monitoring, identifying, and minimizing ADRs, with most institutions and facilities utilizing computerized systems to screen for and alert practitioners to potential ADRs. The role of technology continues to expand as the FDA develops new approaches for signal detection and data mining. In addition, advances in pharmacogenetics may soon help practitioners proactively identify risk factors that predispose patients to an ADR, optimizing prescribing and medication management practices.

Despite the impact of ADRs and the tools available to assist in their management, ADRs remain underreported. Physicians and pharmacists report several barriers to reporting ADRs, including the time and hassle involved in reporting, as well as the beliefs that a single ADR report cannot meaningfully contribute to medical knowledge and that only safe drugs are allowed on the market. ADR monitoring programs can only be successful if health care providers believe in their potential to improve patient safety and are willing to be active participants. Therefore, future efforts should focus on strategies for overcoming barriers to ADRs reporting in order to improve medication safety–related outcomes and patient care.

Self-Assessment Questions

1. Which of the following refers to an adverse drug reaction (ADR)?
   a. Any iatrogenic hazard or incident associated with a medication
   b. Any injury caused by a medication
   c. Any preventable event that leads to inappropriate medication use or patient harm
   d. Any unexpected, unintended, undesired, or excessive response to a medication
   e. Any reaction related to the intentional or unintentional overdose of a medication

2. Adverse drug reactions account for approximately what percentage of all hospital admissions?
   a. 0.1% to 0.5%
   b. 1% to 5%
   c. 5% to 15%
   d. 15% to 25%
   e. 35%

3. Every year, adverse drug reactions cost the U.S. health care system how much?
   a. $50 to $70 million
   b. $150 million
   c. $5 to $7 billion
   d. $50 to $70 billion
   e. $150 billion

4. Which of the following reactions is *not* an example of an ADR that the FDA would like health care professionals to report?
   a. A life-threatening reaction to a drug
   b. An ADR that is not currently listed in the drug's labeling
   c. A reaction that is a more severe form of a previously-reported ADR
   d. A common or expected side effect
   e. An ADR of which the exact cause is not known

5. Which of the following definitions of an adverse drug reaction is often excluded by hospitals?
   a. Noxious reaction to a drug given at a normal dose
   b. Reactions due to drug abuse
   c. Excessive pharmacological reaction
   d. Idiosyncratic reactions
   e. None of the above

6. The first step in establishing an adverse drug reaction program at a facility is to:
   a. Determine the institution's definition of an adverse drug reaction
   b. Decide who is responsible for reporting adverse reactions to the FDA
   c. Develop an ADR reporting hotline
   d. Identify drugs most likely to cause adverse reactions
   e. Report findings of the ADR program to the P&T committee

7. Which of the following factors is *not* used to determine adverse reaction causality?
   a. Dechallenge
   b. Rechallenge
   c. Temporal relationship
   d. Patient gender
   e. Known response pattern

8. Which of the following is the most commonly used algorithm for determining adverse reaction causality?
   a. Bayesian approach
   b. Kramer method
   c. Naranjo algorithm
   d. Larch algorithm
   e. BADCAT tool

9. Which of the following sources of drug information is a specialty resource related to ADRs?
   a. DrugCite
   b. Prescribing information
   c. Physicians' Desk Reference
   d. Natural Medicines Comprehensive Database
   e. Major drug compendia

10. Who can report adverse drug reactions to the FDA's MedWatch program?
    a. Physicians
    b. Pharmacists
    c. Nurses
    d. Patients
    e. All of the above

11. Which of the following is considered a barrier to reporting an adverse drug reaction?
    a. Fear of litigation
    b. Guilt
    c. Paperwork and time involved
    d. Complacency
    e. All of the above

12. Which of the following statements about reporting adverse reactions related to dietary supplements is *true*?
    a. The FDA's MedWatch system does not accept reports related to dietary supplements.
    b. Manufacturers of dietary supplements are not required to share adverse reaction information with the FDA.
    c. Natural Medicines Watch can be used to submit dietary supplement ADR reports.
    d. There is no system for collecting adverse reaction information for dietary supplements.
    e. Dietary supplements are natural; therefore, they do not cause adverse reactions.

13. Which of the following is a job responsibility that makes pharmacists well suited to provide education on ADR programs?
    a. Involvement in P&T committee
    b. Pharmacokinetic dosing

c. Drug utilization review

d. Drug distribution activities

e. All of the above

14. Which of the following statements is/are *true* regarding the Vaccine Adverse Event Reporting System (VAERS)?

a. VAERS is a partnership between the FDA and the CDC.

b. ADRs related to vaccine administration should be reported to VAERS instead of MedWatch.

c. VAERS provides specific guidance on the kind of reactions that should be reported.

d. Over 30,000 ADR reports are reported to VAERS annually.

e. All of the above are true.

15. Which of the following best describes the role of technology in the management of ADRs?

a. Technology can help identify and alert practitioners to potential ADRs.

b. Technology eliminates the need for pharmacists to get involved in ADR management.

c. Technology systems have not proven useful in the management of ADRs.

d. Technology can only be used to report ADRs, not to aid in their detection.

e. Technology has nearly eliminated fatalities due to ADRs.

REFERENCES

1. American Society of Health-System Pharmacists. Suggested definitions and relationships among medication misadventures, medication errors, adverse drug events, and adverse drug reactions. Am J Health Syst Pharm. 1998;55:165-6.

2. Rich DS. A process for interpreting data on adverse drug events: determining optimal target levels. Clin Ther. 1998;20(Suppl C):C59-71.

3. Rich DS. The Joint Commission's revised sentinel event policy on medication errors. Hosp Pharm. 1998;33:881-5.

4. Kohn LT, Corrigan JM, Donaldson MS, eds. Institute of medicine. To err is human: building a safer health system. Washington, DC: National Academy Press; 1999 Nov 1. p. 311.

5. White TJ, Arakelian A, Rho JP. Counting the costs of drug-related adverse events. Pharmacoeconomics. 1999;15:445-58.

6. Wong YL. Adverse effect of pharmaceutical recipients in drug therapy. Ann Acad Med. 1993;22:99-102.

7. Classen DC, Pestotnik SL, Evans S, Loyd JF, Burke JP. Adverse drug events in hospitalized patients. JAMA. 1997;277:301-6.

8. Swanson KM, Landry JP, Anderson RP. Pharmacy-coordinated, multidisciplinary adverse drug reaction program. Top Hosp Pharm Manage. 1992;12:49-59.

9. Murphy SL, Jiaquan X, Kochanek KD. Deaths: Final data for 2010. Natl Vital Stat Rep. 2013;61(4):1-163.

10. Fincham JE. An overview of adverse drug reactions. Am Pharm. 1991;NS31:435-41.

11. Agency for Healthcare Research and Quality. Reducing and preventing adverse drug events to decrease hospital costs [Internet]. Rockville (MD): Agency for Healthcare Research and Quality; 2001 Mar [cited 2013 Aug 16]. Available from: http://www.ahrq .gov/research/findings/factsheets/errors-safety/aderia/.

12. Kongkaew C, Noyce PR, Ashcroft DM. Hospital admissions with adverse drug reactions: a systematic review of prospective observational studies. Ann Pharmacother. 2008: 42(7):1017-25.

13. Miguel A, Azevedo LF, Arajuo M, Pereira AC. Frequency of adverse drug reactions in hospitalized patients: a systematic review and meta-analysis. Pharmacoepidemiol Drug Saf. 2012;21(11):1139-54.

14. World Health Organization. Medicines: safety of medicines—adverse drug reactions [Internet]. Geneva (CH): World Health Organization; 2008 Oct [cited 2013 Aug 16]. Available from: http://www.who.int/mediacentre/factsheets/fs293/en/index.html

15. Lesar TS, Briceland L, Stein DS. Factors related to errors in medication prescribing. JAMA. 1997;277:312-7.

16. Leape LL, Cullen DJ, Clapp M, Burdick E, Demonaco HJ, Erickson JI, et al. Pharmacist participation on physician rounds and adverse drug events in the intensive care unit. JAMA. 1999;282:267-70.

17. Lepakhin VK. Safety of medicines—a guide to detecting and reporting adverse drug reactions—why health professionals need to take action. Geneva: World Health Organization; 2002. p. 16.

18. U.S. Food and Drug Administration. An FDA guide to drug safety terms [Internet]. Silver Spring (MD): U.S. Food and Drug Administration; 2013 Apr 12 [cited 2013 Aug 16]. Available from: http://www.fda.gov/ForConsumers/ConsumerUpdates/ucm107970.htm

19. U.S. Food and Drug Administration. Code of Federal Regulations Title 21 [Internet]. Silver Spring (MD): U.S. Food and Drug Administration; 2013 Apr 1 [cited 2013 Aug 16]. Available from: http://www.accessdata.fda.gov/scripts/cdrh/cfdocs/cfcfr/cfrsearch .cfm?fr=312.32

20. Edwards R, Aronson JK. Adverse drug reactions: definitions, diagnosis, and management. Lancet. 2000;356:1255-9.

21. Karch FE, Lasagna L. Toward the operational identification of adverse drug reactions. Clin Pharmacol Ther. 1977;21:247-54.

22. Agbabiaka TB, Savovic J, Ernst E. Methods for causality assessment of adverse drug reactions: a systematic review. Drug Safety. 2008;31:21-37.

23. Naranjo CA, Busto U, Sellers EM, et al. A method of estimating the probability of adverse drug reactions. Clin Pharmacol Ther. 1981;30:239-45.

24. Kramer MS, Leventhal JM, Hutchinson TA, Feinstein AR. An algorithm for the operational assessment of adverse drug reactions: I. Background, description, and instructions for use. JAMA. 1979;242:623-32.

25. Hutchinson TA, Leventhal JM, Kramer MS, Karch FE, Lipman AG, Feinstein AR. An algorithm for the operational assessment of adverse drug reactions: II. Demonstration of reproducibility and validity. JAMA. 1979;242:633-8.

26. Jones JK. Adverse drug reactions in the community health setting: approaches to recognizing, counseling, and reporting. Fam Comm Health. 1982;5(2):58-67.

27. Michel DJ, Knodel LC. Comparison of three algorithms used to evaluate adverse drug reactions. Am J Hosp Pharm. 1986;43:1709-14.

28. Peak AS. Butler University Adverse Drug Reaction Causality Assessment Tool (BADCAT). Paper presented at: American Society of Health-System Pharmacists Midyear Clinical Meeting; December 4, 2012; Las Vegas, NV.

29. Agababiaka TB, Savovic J, Ernst E. Methods for causality assessment of adverse drug reactions: a systematic review. Drug Saf. 2008;31(1):21-37.

30. Lane DA. The Bayesian approach to causality assessment: an introduction. Drug Info J. 1986;20:455-61.

31. Lactot KL, Naranjo CA. Comparison of the Bayesian approach and a simple algorithm for assessment of adverse drug events. Clin Pharmacol Ther. 1995;58:692-8.

32. Garcia-Cortes M, Stephens C, Fernandez-Castaner A, Andrade RJ, Spanish Group for the Study of Drug-Induced Liver Disease. Causality assessment methods in drug induced liver injury: strengths and weaknesses. J Hepatol. 2011;55(3):683-91.

33. U.S. Food and Drug Administration. Medical product safety information [Internet]. Silver Spring (MD): U.S. Food and Drug Administration; 2013 Aug 16. [cited 2013 Aug 16]. Available from: http://www.fda.gov/Safety/MedWatch/SafetyInformation/default.htm

34. DrugCite. About us [Internet]. [place unknown]: DrugCite; c2013 [cited 2013 Aug 16]. Available from: http://www.drugcite.com/about.php

35. DrugCite. Frequently asked questions [Internet]. [place unknown]: DrugCite; c2013 [cited 2013 Aug 16]. Available from: http://www.drugcite.com/faq.php

36. DrugCite. Apps and tools [Internet]. [place unknown]: DrugCite; c2013 [cited 2013 Aug 16]. Available from: http://www.drugcite.com/tools

37. Springer—International Publisher Science, Technology, Medicine. Reactions weekly: about this journal [Internet]. Berlin (DE): Springer Science+Business Media; [cited 2013 Aug 16]. Available from: http://www.springer.com/adis/journal/40278

38. SAGE Journals. Clin-Alert [Internet]. Thousand Oaks (CA): SAGE Journals; c2013 [cited 2013 Aug 16]. Available from: http://cla.sagepub.com/.

39. U.S. Food and Drug Administration. What is a serious adverse event? [Internet] Silver Spring (MD): U.S. Food and Drug Administration; [cited 2013 Aug 16]. Available from: http://www.fda.gov/medwatch/report/desk/advevnt.htm

40. The Joint Commission. Prepublication requirements [Internet]. Chicago (IL); c2013. Revisions to deeming requirements for hospitals. 2012 Dec 5 [cited 2013 Aug 13]. Available from: http://www.jointcommission.org/assets/1/18/PREPUB-12-03-2012-HAP_deeming.pdf

41. ASHP guidelines on adverse drug reaction monitoring and reporting. Am J Health Syst Pharm. 1995 Feb 15;52(4):417-9.

42. Saltiel E, Johnson E, Shane R. A team approach to adverse drug reaction surveillance: success at a tertiary care hospital. Hosp Form. 1995 Apr;30(4):226-8, 231-2.

43. Classen DC, Pestotnik SL, Evans RS, Burke JP. Computerized surveillance of adverse drug events in hospitalized patients. Qual Saf Health Care. 2005 Jun;14:221-6.

44. American Society of Consultant Pharmacists. Guidelines [Internet]. Alexandria (VA); c2013. Guidelines for detecting and reporting adverse drug reactions in long-term care environments. 1997 Jul 17 [cited 2013 Mar 6]. Available from: http://www.ascp.com/resources/policy/upload/Gui97-ADRs.pdf

45. Institute for Safe Medication Practices. Acute Care Newsletters [Internet]. Harsham (PA); c2013. Adverse drug reactions: documentation is important but communication is critical. 2000 Sep 6 [cited 2013 Mar 6] Available from: http://www.ismp.org/Newsletters/acutecare/articles/20000906.asp

46. AHRQ: Archive [Internet]. Rockville (MD); c2013. Making health care safer: a critical analysis of patient safety practices—Evidence report/technology assessment, No. 43. 2001 Jul [cited 2013 Mar 6]. Available from: http://archive.ahrq.gov/clinic/ptsafety/.

47. Jha AK, Kuperman GJ, Teich JM, et al. Identifying adverse drug events: development of a computer-based monitor and comparison with chart review and stimulated voluntary report. J Am Med Inform Assoc. 1998 May-Jun;5(3):305-14.

48. Raschke RA, Gollihare B, Wunderlich TA, et al. A computer alert system to prevent injury from adverse drug events. JAMA. 1998 Oct 28;280(15):1317-20.

49. Hickner J, Zafar A, Kuo GM, et al. Field test results of a new ambulatory care medication error and adverse drug event reporting system—MEADERS. Ann Fam Med. 2010 Nov-Dec;8(6):517-25.

50. Zafar A, Hickner J, Pace W, Tierney W. A medication error and adverse drug event reporting system for ambulatory care (MEADERS). AMIA Annu Symp Proc. 2008;6:839-43.

51. van Grootheest AC, de Jong-van den Berg LTW. The role of hospital and community pharmacists in pharmacovigilance. Res Soc Admin Pharm. 2005 Mar;1(1):126-33.

52. Emmendorfer T, Glassman PA, Moore V, Leadholm TC, Good CB, Cunningham F. Monitoring adverse drug reactions across a nationwide health care system using information technology. Am J Health Syst Pharm. 2012 Feb 15;69(4):321-8.

53. Davies E, Green C, Taylor S, Williamson P, Mottram D, Primohamed M. Adverse drug reactions in hospital in-patients: a prospective analysis of 3695 patient-episodes. PLoS ONE. 2009;4(2):e4439.

54. Issac T, Weissman JS, Davis RB, et al. Overrides of medication alerts in ambulatory care. Arch Intern Med. 2009 Feb 9;169(3):305-11.

55. Warholak TL, Hines LE, Saverno KR, Grizzle AJ, Malone DC. Assessment tool for pharmacy drug-drug interaction software. J Am Pharm Assoc (2003). 2011 May-Jun;51(3):418-24.

56. Waller P. Making the most of spontaneous adverse drug reaction reporting. Basic Clin Pharmacol Tox. 2006 Mar;98(3):320-3.

57. Felkey BG. Health system informatics. Am J Health Syst Pharm. 1997 Feb 1;54(3):274-80.

58. Webster L, Spiro RF. Health information technology: a new world for pharmacy. J Am Pharm Assoc (2003). 2010 Mar-Apr 1;50(2):e20-31.

59. Faich GA, Dreis M, Tomita D. National adverse drug reaction surveillance: 1986. Arch Intern Med. 1988 Apr;148(4):785-7.

60. Harmark L, van Grootheest AC. Pharmacovigilance: methods, recent developments and future perspectives. Eur J Clin Pharmacol. 2008 Aug;64:743-52.

61. Stang PE, Fox JL. Adverse drug events and the Freedom of Information Act: an apple in Eden. Ann Pharmcother. 1992 Feb;26(2):238-43.

62. Rogers AS, Israel E, Smith CR, et al. Physician knowledge, attitudes, and behavior related to reporting adverse drug events. Arch Intern Med. 1988 Jul;148(7):1596-600.

63. FDA: Drugs [Internet]. Silver Spring (MD); c2013. Reports received and reports entered into AERS by year. 2012 Jun 30 [cited 2013 Mar 6]. Available from: http://www.fda.gov/Drugs/GuidanceComplianceRegulatoryInformation/Surveillance/AdverseDrugEffects/ucm070434.htm

64. FDA: Safety [Internet]. Silver Spring (MD); c2013. Reporting by health professionals. 2013 Apr 18 [cited 2013 Aug 13]. Available from: http://www.fda.gov/Safety/MedWatch/HowToReport/ucm085568.htm

65. Hoffman RP. Adverse drug reaction reporting—problems and solutions. J Mich Pharm. 1989;27:400-3,407-8.

66. Lopez-Gonzalez E, Herdeiro MT, Figueiras A. Determinants of under-reporting of adverse drug reactions: a systematic review. Drug Saf. 2009;32(1):19-31.

67. Gavaza P, Brown CM, Lawson KA, Rascati KL, Wilson JP, Steinhardt M. Influence of attitudes on pharmacists' intention to report serious adverse drug events to the Food and Drug Administration. Br J Clin Pharmacol. 2011 Jul;72(1):143-52.

68. Du DT, Goldsmith J, Aikin KJ, Encinosa WE, Nardinelli C. Despite 2007 law requiring FDA hotline to be included in print drug ads, reporting of adverse events by consumers still low. Health Aff (Millwood). 2012 May;31(5):1022-9.

69. FDA: Drugs [Internet]. Silver Spring (MD); c2013. AERS reporting by healthcare providers and consumers by year. 2012 Jun 30 [cited 2013 Mar 6]. Available from: http://www.fda.gov/Drugs/GuidanceComplianceRegulatoryInformation/Surveillance/AdverseDrugEffects/ucm070456.htm

70. FDA: For Consumers [Internet]. Silver Spring (MD); c2013. FDA 101: How to use the Consumer Complaint System and MedWatch. 2009 Feb 27 [cited 2013 Mar 6]. Available from: http://www.fda.gov/ForConsumers/ConsumerUpdates/ucm049087.htm

71. Timbo BB, Ross MP, McCarthy PV, Lin CT. Dietary supplements in a nationwide survey: prevalence of use and reports of adverse events. J Am Diet Assoc. 2006;106:1966-74.

72. U.S. Food and Drug Administration. Significant amendments to the FD&C Act: Dietary Supplement and Nonprescription Drug Consumer Protection Act [Internet]. Silver Spring (MD): U.S. Food and Drug Administration; 2009 May 20. [cited 2013

Aug 16]. Available from: http://www.fda.gov/RegulatoryInformation/Legislation/FederalFoodDrugandCosmeticActFDCAct/SignificantAmendmentstotheFDCAct/ucm148035.htm

73. U.S. Government Printing Office. Federal Register Volume 69, Number 28. [Internet]. Washington, DC: U.S. Government Printing Office; 2004 Feb 11. [cited 2013 Aug 16]. Available from: http://www.gpo.gov/fdsys/pkg/FR-2004-02-11/html/04-2912.htm

74. American Botanical Council. Federal court overturns FDA ban on ephedra at low doses [Internet]. Austin (TX): American Botanical Council; c2013 [cited 2013 Aug 16]. Available from: http://cms.herbalgram.org/press/FDAephedra.html

75. Natural Medicines Comprehensive Database. Natural Medicines Watch: adverse event reporting form [Internet]. Stockton (CA): Therapeutic Research Center; c2013 [cited 2013 Aug 16]. Available from: https://naturaldatabase.therapeuticresearch.com/nd/adverseevent.aspx

76. Woo JJY. Adverse event monitoring and multivitamin-multimineral dietary supplements. Am J Clin Nutr. 2007;85:323S-4S.

77. Fabricant D. Dietary Supplement Update. Presented at: U.S. Food and Drug Administration; 2011 Jun 6; Silver Spring, MD.

78. Vaccine Adverse Event Reporting System. Information for healthcare professionals [Internet]. Rockville (MD): U.S. Department of Health and Human Services; [cited 2013 Aug 16]. Available from: http://vaers.hhs.gov/professionals/index

79. Vaccine Adverse Event Reporting System. About the VAERS program [Internet]. Rockville (MD): U.S. Department of Health and Human Services. Vaccine Adverse Event Reporting System Web site. [cited 2013 Aug 16]. Available from: http://vaers.hhs.gov/about/index

80. Van Manan RP, Fram D, DuMouchel W. Signal detection methodologies to support effective safety management. Drug Saf. 2007;6:451-64.

81. Want XY, Hripcsak G, Markatou M, Friedman C. Active computerized pharmacovigilance using natural language processing, statistics, and electronic health records: a feasibility study. J Am Med Inform Assoc. 2009;16:328-37.

82. Peto R, Collins R, Gray R. Large-scale randomized evidence: large, simple trials and overview of trials. J Clin Epidemiol. 1995;48:23-40.

83. Kacevska M, Ivanov M, Ingelman-Sundberg M. Perspectives on epigenetics and its relevance to adverse drug reactions. Clin Pharm Ther. 2011;89(6):902-7.

84. National Human Genome Research Institute. Genome-wide association studies fact sheet [Internet]. Bethesda (MD): National Institutes of Health; 2013 Jul 11. [cited 2013 Aug 16]. Available from: http://www.genome.gov/20019523

85. Daly AK. Using genome-wide association studies to identify genes important in serious adverse drug reactions. Ann Rev Pharmacol Toxicol. 2012;582:21-35.

86. Moore T, Cohen M, Furberg C. Serious adverse drug events reported to the Food and Drug Administration, 1998-2005. Arch Intern Med. 2007;167:1752-9.

SUGGESTED READINGS

1. Harmark L, van Grootheest AC. Pharmacovigilance: methods, recent developments and future perspectives. Eur J Clin Pharmacol. 2008;64:743-52.
2. Lepakhin VK. Safety of medicines—a guide to detecting and reporting adverse drug reactions—why health professionals need to take action. Geneva: World Health Organization; 2002.
3. Naranjo CA, Busto U, Sellers EM, et al. A method for estimating the probability of adverse drug reactions. Clin Pharmacol Ther. 1981;30:239-45.

16

Chapter Sixteen

Medication Misadventures II: Medication and Patient Safety

Kathryn A. Crea

Learning Objectives

After completing this chapter, the reader will be able to

- Define and compare the terms medication errors, adverse drug events, and adverse drug reactions.
- Describe methods to identify medication errors and adverse drug events.
- Discuss the role of Patient Safety Organizations (PSOs) in health care.
- Assign an event severity rating to reported errors and events.
- Discuss two methods of analyzing medication errors and adverse drug events that are utilized to develop action plans for prevention of recurrence.
- Describe examples of skill-based, rule-based, and knowledge-based errors.
- Explain a systems, approach to error.
- Compare a Just Culture with a culture of shame and blame.
- Determine strategies health care practitioners and health systems can implement to reduce medication errors.
- Reflect on the need for interprofessional education and training on quality and safety principles.

Key Concepts

❶ The terms medication error, adverse drug event, and adverse drug reaction are similar and often confused. They are interrelated, yet distinct occurrences.

❷ Several methods of identifying errors are recommended to gain a more global understanding of the risks and errors occurring within an institution.

❸ Classification of errors by type is a common method to identify common themes and causes of events.

❹ Thorough analysis of safety events through root cause analysis (RCA), **failure mode and effects analysis (FMEA)**, or other methods is a key activity to support learning from errors in an effort to prevent recurrence.

❺ Human beings (including health care professionals of all types) have a propensity to commit errors in all aspects of their lives. To err is human.

❻ Understanding the three modes of human performance (skill based, rule based, and knowledge based) is very important to understanding errors and events, and in developing appropriate strategies to reduce the risks of recurrence.

❼ Poorly designed health care systems and processes are a significant contributor to individual human error and subsequent patient harm.

❽ A Just Culture is one in which discipline is applied in a consistent manner based on the intentions of the individual and the situation in which they were placed, not on the outcome.

❾ All health professionals should be trained to deliver patient-centered care as members of an interdisciplinary team, emphasizing evidence-based practice, quality improvement approaches, and informatics.

❿ There are many resources available that identify best-practice error prevention strategies.

⓫ Researching, recognizing, and designing with human factors principles in mind is a great way to improve the safety of any process.

Introduction

Much attention has been focused on adverse outcomes in health care in the past 15 years. While pockets of research in medical errors were developing prior to 2000, the Institute of Medicine's report, *To Err Is Human: Building a Safer Health System*,[1] released in late 1999, served as a catalyst for additional research in the causes and methods to prevent adverse outcomes in health care. The mortality estimates documented in this report (an estimated 44,000 to 98,000 people die each year as a result of medical errors) were derived from two landmark studies.[1-3] The report notes that **medication errors** alone (whether occurring within or outside of the hospital) were estimated to account for over 7000 deaths annually. The majority of literature to date has focused on work in the hospital setting, as it is, for the most part, a closed and controlled environment. Other settings are less well researched, although early studies of nursing homes and ambulatory settings have shown significant opportunities for improvement. It is clear that medication safety, and the broader category of patient safety, represents a serious concern for patients and health care providers.

While many health care professionals have roles in the medication use process, which is described in depth in Chapter 24, pharmacists play a pivotal role in ensuring the safe use of medication. Pharmacist provision of accurate drug information and identification of potential medication-related adverse effects to multiple providers is of vital importance. Throughout the medication use process there are many opportunities for unexpected adverse events, including errors in prescribing, dispensing, and administering medications, idiosyncratic reactions, and other adverse effects. These events can all be described as medication misadventures.[4] All pharmacists need a sound understanding of the risks for error and the ability to identify the underlying causes of medication misadventures, as other practitioners tend to focus on other potential causes. Pharmacists are also responsible for taking steps to prevent such occurrences and minimize adverse outcomes. This usually involves collaborative work with other health care team members to ensure optimal outcomes. Pharmacists are well positioned to lead these efforts in reducing harm to patients.

Definitions: Medication Errors, Adverse Drug Events, and Adverse Drug Reactions

❶ *The terms medication error, adverse drug event, and adverse drug reaction are similar and often confused. They are interrelated, yet distinct occurrences.* The terminology surrounding medication misadventures is often confusing; there are many definitions that are very similar. The term medication misadventure is an overarching term that includes medication errors, **adverse drug events (ADEs)**, and **adverse drug reactions (ADRs)**. The American Society of Health-System Pharmacists[4-5] (ASHP) defines a **medication misadventure** as an iatrogenic hazard or incident:

- That is an inherent risk when medication therapy is indicated
- That is created through either omission or commission by the administration of a medicine or medicines during which a patient may be harmed, with effects ranging from mild discomfort to fatality
- Whose outcome may or may not be independent of the preexisting pathology or disease process
- That may be attributable to error (human or system, or both), immunologic response, or idiosyncratic response
- That is always unexpected or undesirable to the patient and the health professional

The National Coordinating Council for Medication Error Reporting and Prevention (NCCMERP), an organization composed of 24 national organizations and individual

TABLE 16–1. NATIONAL COORDINATING COUNCIL FOR MEDICATION ERROR REPORTING AND PREVENTION MEMBER ORGANIZATIONS

Founding Members

American Association of Retired Persons (AARP)

American Hospital Association (AHA)

American Medical Association (AMA)

American Nurses Association (ANA)

American Pharmacists Association (APhA)

American Society of Health-System Pharmacists (ASHP)

Food and Drug Administration (U.S. FDA)

Generic Pharmaceutical Association (GPhA)

The Joint Commission (TJC)

National Association of Boards of Pharmacy (NABP)

National Council of State Boards of Nursing (NCSBN)

Pharmaceutical Research and Manufacturers of America (PhRMA)

U.S. Pharmacopoeia (USP)

Regular Members

American Association of Homes and Services for the Aging (AAHSA)

American Society for Healthcare Risk Management (ASHRM)

American Society of Consultant Pharmacists (ASCP)

Department of Defense (DoD)

Department of Veterans Affairs (VA)

Institute for Healthcare Improvement (IHI)

Institute for Safe Medication Practices (ISMP)

National Alliance of State Pharmacy Associations (NASPA)

National Association of Chain Drug Stores (NACDS)

National Council on Patient Information and Education (NCPIE)

National Patient Safety Foundation (NPSF)

members, including the Food and Drug Administration (FDA), American Medical Association (AMA), American Pharmacists Association (APhA), United States Pharmacopoeia (USP), and several others (Table 16–1), has developed a detailed definition of what constitutes a medication error:

> "Any preventable event that may cause or lead to inappropriate medication use or patient harm while the medication is in the control of the health care professional, patient, or consumer. Such events may be related to professional practice, health care products, procedures, and systems, including prescribing; order communication; product labeling, packaging, and nomenclature; compounding; dispensing; distribution; administration; education; monitoring; and use."[6]

Key points related to medication errors include:

• Medication errors are preventable.

- Medication errors can be caused by errors in the planning (deciding what to do—which drug and/or what dose) or execution stages (completing the task that was decided on—administering the drug to the wrong patient).
- Medication errors include errors of omission (missed dose or appropriate medication not prescribed) or commission (wrong drug given).
- Medication errors may or may not cause patient harm.

Based on the NCCMERP definition, an error may occur as a result of not adequately counseling or educating a patient on proper use of medication. When, for example, a patient inappropriately uses a metered-dose inhaler for asthma and fails to receive the full amount of the medication, a medication error has occurred. The error may be secondary to a lack of education or may have occurred despite adequate counseling and education. Independent of the cause, based on the above definition, a medication error did occur.

Based on this definition, medication errors also occur when a prescriber writes an incorrect dose on a prescription pad. Even if the prescriber is called by a practitioner to clarify and change the order and the patient eventually receives an appropriately dosed medication, an error did occur in the process. An adverse outcome does not necessarily have to occur to classify an event as a medication error.

An ADE involves harm to a patient. An ADE is defined as an injury from a medicine or lack of intended medicine.[7] An ADE refers to all ADRs, including allergic or idiosyncratic reactions, as well as medication errors that result in harm to a patient. It is estimated that 3% to 5% of medication errors result in harm to a patient and can also be classified as an ADE.

An ADR is defined by the World Health Organization (WHO) as "any response that is noxious, unintended, or undesired, which occurs at doses normally used in humans for prophylaxis, diagnosis, therapy of disease, or modification of physiological function."[8]

The relationship between the terms is illustrated in Figure 16–1 (also see Chapter 15). While there are standard definitions for medication errors, there may be significant differences in the interpretation, reporting rates, and severity ranking between institutions.

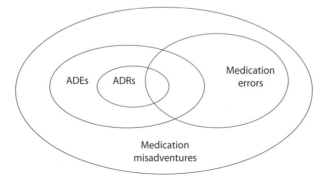

Figure 16–1. Relationship among medication misadventures, adverse drug events, medication errors, and adverse drug reactions. *(Adapted from Bates DW, et al. Relationship between medication and errors and adverse drug events. J Gen Intern Med. 1995 Apr;10(4):199-205.)*

Common questions that arise are included in Table 16–2. For example, one institution may determine that an error has occurred when a dose is not received by a patient within 30 minutes of the scheduled time, where another may permit 60 minutes before or after the scheduled administration time. Some institutions may not report an inappropriately written prescription, if that error is caught by a clinician before the medication reaches the patient. Instead, a pharmacist or nurse may report it as a professional intervention. According to most definitions, this would count as an error. These variations make it very difficult to compare data from one institution to another. Therefore, it is best for an institution to use its own data to monitor improvement.

TABLE 16–2. COMMON QUESTIONS THAT ARISE IN DEFINING MEDICATION ERRORS AND ADVERSE DRUG EVENTS

- Is it an error if it does not reach the patient?
- Is it an error if it does not cause harm?
- What constitutes minimal harm? Moderate? Severe?
- Is it an error or event if it is not clinically significant?
- Should pharmacist interventions related to inappropriate physician orders be documented and counted as prescribing errors?
- What is considered preventable?

The Impact of Errors on Patients and Health Care Systems

Patients depend on health care systems and health care professionals to help them stay healthy. As a result, patients frequently receive drug therapy with the notion that these medications will help them lead a healthier life. The initiation of drug therapy is the most common medical treatment received by patients.[9] In virtually all cases, patients and their health care providers understand that when medications are given, there are some known and some unknown risks. Patients may experience significant unexpected drug-related morbidity and mortality.

Several landmark studies have identified the risk of medication errors and ADEs in varying populations and settings. The Harvard Medical Practice Study I was a landmark study that estimated that 3.7% of hospitalized patients experience adverse events.[2] The findings and extrapolated statistics from this study along with the Harvard Medical Practice Study II served as the grounds for the statement (from *To Err Is Human*) that approximately 44,000 to 98,000 people are killed by medical error every year. Specifically related to medication errors, Bates and associates identified 6.5 ADEs per hospital admission.[7] In the nursing home setting, Gurwitz and associates[10] identified 227 ADEs per 1000 resident years. Gurwitz and associates[11] also studied the ambulatory patient population, finding 50.1 ADEs per 1000 person-years. Interestingly, preventability of all ADEs in these studies ranged from 27% to 51%, while the preventability of serious and life-threatening ADEs ranged from 42% to 72%, potentially indicating that improved processes and behaviors should be able to prevent serious harm events.

The economic impact of medication errors and ADEs is staggering and adds unnecessarily to the health care cost burden. Several important studies documented the economic burden of these events.[12-15] A landmark study in 1995 estimated that ADE-related costs were $76.6 billion annually in ambulatory patients alone.[12] Drug expenditures in ambulatory patients at that time were $80 billion per year. This means that for every $1 spent for a drug, almost $1 was also being spent due to a drug-related problem. These costs exceed the total cost of managing patients with diabetes or cardiovascular diseases.[13] A subsequent study demonstrated the cost of drug-related morbidity and mortality in the ambulatory setting exceeded $177 billion in 2000.[15]

While it was initially thought that medication misadventures were caused by individual health care practitioners, including pharmacists, physicians, and nurses, now it is clear that our health care systems and processes often are causative or contributing factors in the majority of errors and events. Efforts to decrease adverse outcomes will not be successful if these system and process-related issues are not addressed. Multiple agencies and professional organizations across the country are now contributing efforts to minimize these events (Table 16–3), which will be discussed in the section Best Practices for Error Prevention.

TABLE 16–3. ORGANIZATIONS INVOLVED IN PREVENTING ADVERSE DRUG EVENTS

Food and Drug Administration (FDA)	www.fda.gov
The Joint Commission (TJC)	www.jointcommission.org
World Health Organization (WHO)	www.who.int
Institute for Safe Medication Practices (ISMP)	www.ismp.org
The United States Pharmacopoeia (USP)	www.usp.org
American Society of Health-System Pharmacists (ASHP)	www.ashp.org
National Quality Forum (NQF)	www.qualityforum.org
Agency for Healthcare Research and Quality (AHRQ)	www.ahrq.gov
Patient Safety Network	www.psnet.ahrq.gov
Web M&M: Morbidity and Mortality Rounds on the Web	www.webmm.ahrq.gov
Institute for Healthcare Improvement (IHI)	www.ihi.org
Health Resources and Services Administrations (HRSA)	www.hrsa.gov
National Patient Safety Foundation	www.npsf.org
Centers for Medicaid and Medicare Services (CMS)	www.cms.hhs.gov
Centers for Disease Control (CDC)	www.cdc.gov
The Leapfrog Group	www.leapfroggroup.org

Identification and Reporting of Medication Errors and Adverse Drug Events

❷ *Several methods of identifying errors are recommended to gain a more global understanding of the risks and errors occurring within an institution.* It is important that a systematic approach to the identification and assessment of errors and adverse events be utilized in order to identify trends and opportunities for improvement based on events occurring at a location. This should involve several methods, and include prospective and retrospective methods of identifying errors and risks when possible. Many methods of identifying errors in health care exist, including voluntary reporting, direct observation, chart review, trigger identification, and computerized monitoring. These methods are described further here.

1. A voluntary reporting system (either paper, telephonic, or online) is the most common method of identification of errors and events. Many institutions include an anonymous option for those who do not feel comfortable providing their name and contact information. Anyone detecting or committing an error can report it without associating their name with the error. It is essentially risk free for the reporter and, therefore, it may increase the likelihood of having an error reported. While voluntary reporting is the least labor intensive method, it only identifies approximately one out of 20 errors when compared to other identification methods.[16] Therefore, it is important to include other methods of detection.

2. The direct observation method uses trained observers to watch the real-time delivery of medications. Notes from the observations are compared with physician's orders to determine if an error has occurred. Results with this method are more valid and reliable than with self-reporting, but the impact of the observer on the subject being observed and interobserver agreement has been questioned.[17,18] This method is costly, time consuming, and limited to the identification of errors that occur during the administration phase of the medication use process. It typically samples a selected time period on a selected unit, limiting the extrapolation to other time periods or patient care areas. On the positive side, errors are often identified that may never be discovered though other methods as they may go unrecognized.

3. Chart review identification of medication errors and ADEs is very labor intensive and is not generally practical outside of the research environment. Various trained staff review charts looking for particular cues or data elements that signify an error or event has occurred. This method relies on practitioners to document these

events when identified, which may lead to an underestimation of the true occurrence.

4. A modified version of manual chart review is the use of the **ADE trigger tool**. It is a tool that is promoted by the Institute for Healthcare Improvement (IHI). It is an augmented chart review method that uses automated systems to identify alerts or triggers that have been shown to efficiently identify patients with potential ADEs.[19-27] The triggers are cues that a patient may have experienced an error and/or adverse event. Example triggers include the use of reversal agents (e.g., flumazenil, naloxone, phytonadione) or abnormal lab values such as partial thromboplastin time (PTT), international normalized ratio (INR), or low blood glucose value. When these triggers are identified, it is suspected that the patient may have experienced a medication error. The patient's chart is reviewed for evidence of error and/or level of harm and data is collected and collated to determine potential common causes. For example, reviewing the charts of patients who experience hypoglycemia may reveal errors, such as incorrect insulin dosing while patients are receiving nothing by mouth in preparation for a surgical procedure. Upon review of patients requiring the use of naloxone, it may be discovered that the dosing for hydromorphone and morphine are often confused during the prescribing, administration, and monitoring phases, leading to oversedation. The advantage to using this trigger method is that these types of events are rarely reported as errors. These tools have been used in several ways—as a long-term trend and measure of ADEs and/or in a more focused scope such as triggers related to known high-risk classes of medications.[28-30] Specific information on the use of this tool is available at http://www.ihi.org.

5. Classen[20,21] and Jha[19] developed methods to identify ADEs using an electronic medical record (EMR) with text searching tools and logic-based computer rules. In Classen's model, the text within the computer charting (e.g., lab, nurses notes, physician progress notes and orders) is searched for defined conditions or cues, such as heparin-induced thrombocytopenia (HIT). When identified, a pharmacist is alerted, reviews the patient record, and relays an appropriate recommendation to the prescribing physician. This serves as a real-time intervention to prevent or mitigate harm to the patient. This seems to be an optimal model, allowing concurrent review of potential harm and intervention to prevent further error or harm. Unfortunately, while more organizations are implementing an electronic medical record, many are not capable of searching text or have not yet implemented this option.

The use of technology has presented new sources of data on potential errors. The increased use of automated distribution machines, smart pumps, computerized physician order entry (CPOE), and bar-coding technology provides rich databases. For example, every keystroke a nurse makes in programming a smart infusion pump is recorded. Once an error is identified, it is possible to download the data and review details about the error. The challenge is sorting through the massive volumes of information to derive common themes and strategies to decrease risk and optimize the technology.

The 1999 IOM report spotlighted a serious need to capture data that would help to reduce harm to patients. Congress subsequently passed The Patient Safety and Quality Improvement Act of 2005 (Patient Safety Act). The act authorized the creation of a nationwide network of **Patient Safety Organizations (PSOs)** to improve safety and quality through the collection and analysis of data on patient events.[31] The act provides a venue for institutions to report information related to errors and events with the goal of collating the information and learning the underlying risks across similar types of events.

The act provides confidentiality and privilege protection to organizations. The fear of legal action related to reported event information has prevented many organizations from voluntarily reporting errors and events to external agencies. The confidentiality protections ensure that information about an error that is provided to the authorized PSO is kept confidential. The privilege protections limit or forbid the use of protected information in criminal, civil, and other proceedings. Specifically, the information will not be subject to subpoena, discovery, or disclosure to any federal, state, or local criminal, civil, or administrative proceeding. The information may not be used in a professional disciplinary hearing, nor be admitted as evidence.

One example, the Pennsylvania Patient Safety Reporting System, has been collating error data since 2004 and publishes regular advisories with the goal of improving health care delivery systems and educating providers about safe practices. For example, in December 2009,[32] the advisory reviewed errors with neuromuscular blocking agents. In a 5-year span, 154 reports related to neuromuscular blocking agents were submitted. The advisory provides specific information related to the contributing factors (unsafe storage, look-alike drug names, similar packaging, and unlabeled syringes) that increase the risk for a fatal error. Specific risk-reduction strategies are outlined. The same errors tend to recur in facilities across the United States (U.S.). Recall the heparin errors in premature infants[33] that have occurred at least three times in different states. It is imperative that health care professionals commit to learn from others and critically self-assess the processes within their own institution to ensure their process is as safe as possible. Being a learning organization is essential to prevent errors within an organization. A learning organization is one in which the leadership supports organizational learning, creating an environment where structured processes are developed to support this. Examples include communication of performance data to the staff level, formal training in performance improvement and problem solving at the unit or department level, and active engagement of staff in local problem solving. It is recommended that hospitals, ambulatory centers, and other organizations join a PSO and commit to forwarding data related to adverse outcomes, enabling the collation of larger quantities of data, which the PSO can analyze and use to provide recommendations to member organizations. This enables local and broad scale learning from errors and events.

Classification of Error Types

❸ *Classification of errors by type is a common method to identify common themes and causes of events.* The most common way to classify errors is to identify them by type of error. For medications, this classification focuses on whether an error was related to dispensing, administering, prescribing, monitoring, or other reasons. There have been many taxonomies of errors developed by various groups, including the World Health Organization, The Joint Commission, *MEDMARX*®, and others. The ASHP previously designated categories of medication errors are listed here.[34] These are similar to those outlined by NCCMERP.

- Prescribing error
- Omission error
- Wrong time error
- Unauthorized drug error
- Improper dose error
- Wrong dosage form error
- Wrong drug preparation error
- Wrong administration technique
- Deteriorated drug error
- Monitoring error
- Compliance error
- Other medication error

As a result of the development of PSOs, a common taxonomy and language was required to enable health care providers to collect and submit standardized information related to safety events. These standard event reporting forms are called the Common Formats. The Common Formats define the standardized data elements associated with errors and events that are to be collected and reported to the PSO. The scope of Common Formats applies to all patient safety concerns including events reaching the patient (with or without harm), near-miss events that do not reach the patient, and unsafe conditions that have the potential to cause an error or event.[35] The Common Formats recently updated (V1.2) by the Agency for Healthcare Research and Quality (AHRQ) are likely to become the standard for reporting. Common Formats for Readmission and Skilled Nursing facilities are currently open for comment. The following event types have been defined for medication errors:

- Incorrect patient—An incorrect patient error occurs when a medication is given to the wrong patient, usually caused by an error in patient identification and confirmation. Two identifiers should be used to identify the patient every time a patient is given a medication. Confirming patient identification is necessary whenever a pharmacist or physician writes or enters an order or dispenses a prescription in outpatient areas.
- Incorrect medication—This error occurs when a medication is administered that was not ordered for the patient. This may occur when a patient receives a medication intended for another patient, due to inadequate patient identification, or when a nurse obtains the incorrect medication for administration, perhaps from floor stock. Barcode scanning is designed to prevent these errors and others.
- Incorrect dose (subcategories of overdose, underdose, omitted dose, extra dose, and unknown)—An incorrect dose error can occur when a prescriber orders an inappropriate dose of a medication or when the dose administered is different than what was prescribed. An omission error occurs when a patient does not receive a scheduled dose of medication. This is considered to be the second most common error in the medication use process.[36]
- Incorrect route of administration (subcategories include the intended route and the actual route). Some of the most harmful incorrect route errors have included administration of enteral tube feeding into an intravenous line or instillation of an IV medication intrathecally that is not designed to be given this route. One significant cause is the fact that these varying types of tubing fit together. Appropriate design includes different types of connectors of tubing that would not physically allow a connection to be successful.
- Incorrect timing (too early, too late, unknown)—What constitutes a wrong time error may vary considerably among organizations. In general, this type of error occurs when a dose is not administered in accordance with a predetermined administration interval. Most organizations realize that it is often impossible to be totally accurate with the administration interval and typically allow 15 to 60 minutes outside that interval. Establishing a policy to indicate what constitutes an error in this category is needed for consistent reporting and data collection.
- Incorrect rate (too fast, too slow, unknown)—This category generally applies to intravenous infusions, but can also apply to an intravenous push medication if the drug is pushed too quickly or too slowly.

- Incorrect duration—The patient receives the medication for a shorter or longer time period than prescribed. For example, a patient is prescribed a one-time dose of a medication. The pharmacist must enter the order as daily so it will show up on the medication administration record (MAR) for the nurse to administer and chart; however, he or she must remember to place "one time" in the correct field so it only appears to the nurse once to administer. If the pharmacist forgets that last step (relying on memory is a poor error prevention strategy), the medication will appear on the MAR for daily administration.
- Incorrect dosage form (e.g., extended release instead of immediate release)—A wrong dosage form error can occur when the prescriber makes an error or when a patient receives a dosage form different from that prescribed, assuming the appropriate dosage form was originally ordered.
- Incorrect strength or concentration—This is an error that can occur at several points in the medication use process, from prescribing to administration. The pharmacist may choose the wrong strength when entering the order, a pharmacy technician may select the wrong drug for dispensing, or a nurse may choose the wrong drug upon administration. The appropriate use of barcode administration of medications in the inpatient setting makes it harder to make these errors.
- Incorrect preparation (e.g., splitting tablets, compounding errors)—When medications require some type of preparation, such as reconstitution, this type of error may occur. These kinds of errors may also occur in the compounding of various intravenous admixtures and other products and can occur when nurses, pharmacists, or technicians are preparing medications.
- Expired or deteriorated product—This error occurs when a drug is administered that has expired or has deteriorated prematurely due to improper storage conditions.
- Medication that is a known allergen to the patient. These errors may occur due to lack of adequate interfaces between different computer or technology software programs.
- Medication known to be contraindicated for the patient such as a drug–drug interaction or drug–food interaction.
- Incorrect patient action (patient taking a dietary supplement that interacted with medication, whether or not he or she was told to avoid taking it)—This type of error occurs when patients use medications inappropriately. Proper patient education and follow-up may play a significant role in minimizing this type of error. This type of error may be a direct result of insufficient patient counseling from a pharmacist, a prescriber, or both. Important components in counseling include consideration of the level of health literacy of the patient and methods to gauge their understanding of their medication regimen and information provided. An adequate learning needs assessment may assist in effective counseling based on an individual patient's needs.

The second classification section of the medication Common Formats report asks at what stage the incorrect action was discovered (regardless of where or when the incorrect action originated) with the following choices:

- Purchasing
- Storing
- Prescribing
- Transcribing
- Preparing
- Dispensing
- Administering to patient (including verifying medication)
- Monitoring

Prescribing errors generally focus on inappropriate drug selection, dose, dosage form, or route of administration. Examples may include ordering duplicate therapies for a single indication, prescribing a dose that is too high or too low for a patient based on age or organ function, writing a prescription illegibly, prescribing an inappropriate dosage interval, or ordering a drug to which the patient is allergic.

In one study, the most common type of prescribing error (56.1%) was related to an inappropriate dose (either too high or too low). The second most common prescribing error was related to prescribing an agent to which the patient was allergic (14.4%). Prescribing inappropriate dosage forms was the third most common error (11.2%).[9] Other relatively common prescribing errors have included failing to monitor for side effects and serum drug levels, prescribing an inappropriate medication for a particular indication, and inappropriate duration of therapy.

Monitoring errors occur when patients are not monitored appropriately either before or after they have received a drug. For example, if a patient is placed on warfarin therapy and adequate blood tests (baseline and ongoing) are not performed to assess the patient's response, a monitoring error has occurred and has the potential to result in a life-threatening hemorrhage. The Joint Commission recognized this as a significant safety risk and developed a National Patient Safety Goal in an effort to encourage organizations to improve and standardize this process.

These types of medication errors are not mutually exclusive. Multiple types of errors may occur during a single administration of a drug and a single adverse patient outcome may be the result of more than one type of error.[34]

Additional information is gathered in the PSO reporting process. As the use of Common Formats grows, individual health care organizations will need to adopt these classifications, likely developing a standard taxonomy over time. Visit the PSO Web site for updated versions of the Common Formats at https://www.psoppc.org/web/patientsafety/commonformats

Classifying Patient Outcomes

Although the classification of errors or events frequently is based on type, most are also classified by the patient outcome related to the error or event. When an error occurs, there is not always an adverse outcome. It has been estimated that 3% to 5% of errors result in harm to patients. It is important for institutions to monitor both the types of errors that occur and the outcomes associated with them. Most reporting systems request information regarding type and outcome of a medication error.

The NCCMERP developed a medication error index that serves to categorize errors based on the severity or outcome of the error. This index is divided into four main categories and nine subcategories as follows[37]: See the index for event classification and corresponding algorithm at http://www.nccmerp.org/medErrorCatIndex.html

1. No error
   - Category A: Circumstances or events that have the capacity to cause error.

2. Error, no harm
   - Category B: An error occurred, but the medication did not reach the patient.
   - Category C: An error occurred that reached the patient, but did not cause the patient harm.
   - Category D: An error occurred that resulted in the need for increased patient monitoring, but caused no patient harm.

3. Error, harm
   - Category E: An error occurred that resulted in the need for treatment or intervention and caused temporary patient harm.
   - Category F: An error occurred that resulted in initial or prolonged hospitalization and caused temporary patient harm.
   - Category G: An error occurred that resulted in permanent patient harm.
   - Category H: An error occurred that resulted in a near-death event (e.g., anaphylaxis and cardiac arrest).

4. Error, death
   - Category I: An error occurred resulting in patient death.

Oftentimes, the initial staff member(s) reporting the error has an opportunity to indicate their interpretation of the level of harm to the patient. In follow-up, a medication safety pharmacist and the unit/department manager may investigate further details and assign a final severity classification based on the ultimate outcome to the patient.

Institutions may use information about outcomes to focus their error prevention efforts on the types of errors resulting in the most serious outcomes. It is important to remember that examining near-miss events (those that do not reach the patient) can be as valuable in preventing future errors as focusing on serious outcomes. These near-miss events are often clues to the underlying process issues that require attention before they cause harm to a patient.

National Reporting

Reporting of medication errors is important for every practitioner without regard to their practice setting. However, institutional internal reporting is often emphasized (above external reporting) because it is necessary in order to maintain the institution's accreditation status. Drug information specialists are in an ideal position to encourage the importance of medication error and ADR reporting to all health professionals, especially when they are consulted to answer questions related to potential cases. In an effort to share institutional experiences and avoid the same errors being repeated at several institutions, national reporting systems for institutions have evolved.

- *MedWatch*—This program was developed by the FDA Medical Products Reporting Program for the purpose of monitoring problems with medical products. Med-Watch monitors quality, performance, and safety of medical products, devices, and medications. This program contributes to surveillance of medication errors that may be associated with product labeling and names.[38] MedWatch collects reports about faulty products (e.g., improperly functioning devices that led to a medication error). Significant reports may result in distribution of e-mail and safety alerts to health care professionals. These announcements can also be viewed on the Internet at http://www.fda.gov/Safety/MedWatch/default.htm. Health care professionals and consumers can report ADEs and product problems by completing a MedWatch 3500 form (found on the Web site) and mailing it to the FDA, by calling 1-800-FDA-1088, or reporting online at http://www.fda.gov/Safety/MedWatch/HowToReport/ucm085568.htm
- *ISMP Medication Errors Reporting Program (MERP)*—This program provides a venue for voluntary medication error reporting to the Institute for Safe Medication Practices (ISMP). Reports can be submitted online at http://www.ismp.org/reporterrors.asp. ISMP is a federally certified Patient Safety Organization which collates errors and provides summary information across multiple cases in an effort to identify risk and support prevention strategies.

- *MEDMARX®*—This program is an anonymous, subscription-based, voluntary reporting system that enables facilities to collect and report medication error, ADE, and ADR data. This service allows subscribing organizations to report and monitor organization-specific errors online, as well as compares their error rates with other subscribing organizations of similar type. Each year the USP compiles the data, summarizes it, and presents an in-depth annual report. Information in the report includes types of medication errors, causes, contributing factors, products involved, and actions taken. More information regarding MEDMARX® can be found at http://www.usp.org/products/medMarx/. This product differs from the ISMP MERP program in that it is a fee-based service that enables comparison data within the database.

Managing an Event Reporting System

The Joint Commission and ASHP standards can be used as a basis for starting an error-reporting program. In addition to the standards, the pharmacy and medical literature contain abundant examples of successful programs. The following steps are a compilation of several of these references:

1. Develop definitions and classifications for errors and events that work for the institution. The definitions and classifications in the literature and this chapter provide a good starting point for discussion. It is anticipated that the Common Formats developed in preparation for external reporting to PSOs will eventually become the standard.
2. Assign responsibility for the program within the pharmacy and throughout other key departments. A multidisciplinary approach is an essential factor. The program needs a leader and an advocate. It also needs the involvement of nursing, physicians, quality, and risk management departments in order to function as a collaborative team to work toward improved processes.
3. Develop forms or online methods for data collection and reporting (see #1 above). Other mechanisms for reporting (hotline phone numbers) may be used as well. Electronic reporting can often be designed such that medication errors are reviewed by a medication safety pharmacist to confirm severity of the event and gather additional information as needed in order to determine whether additional analysis is appropriate. These systems can also forward events based on their severity to other appropriate parties within the institution such as risk management, quality, and safety personnel to ensure awareness of key staff and leaders. This serves as the voluntary reporting component of the program.

4. Promote awareness of the program and the importance of reporting errors and adverse events. Provide feedback to reporters and individual units that discuss their errors as well as those of others, along with steps taken to prevent them. Providing feedback is very important to ensure that those reporting feel that the identified errors are reviewed and methods to prevent recurrence are developed and implemented.

5. Develop policies and procedures for determining which errors, events, and ADRs are reported to the FDA. The responsibility for this reporting should be defined and usually resides with someone in the pharmacy department.

6. Establish mechanisms for regular screening and identification of potential medication errors and ADEs to supplement voluntary reporting. These mechanisms should include retrospective reviews, concurrent monitoring, as well as prospective planning for high-risk groups. It is worthwhile to educate clinicians to check for potential events or reactions when they see orders for certain triggers that are often used to treat an error or event (Table 16–4), orders to discontinue or hold drugs, and orders to decrease the dose or frequency of a drug.[19] Additionally, electronic screening methods to check for laboratory tests that are indicative of potential events (e.g., drug levels, *Clostridium difficile* toxin assays, elevated serum potassium, and low white blood cell counts) can be helpful.[21]

TABLE 16–4. ADVERSE DRUG EVENT TRIGGERS

Medications	Conditions
Antidiarrheal agents	PTT >100 s
Atropine (exclude preoperative use)	INR >6
Dextrose 50% (IV push)	WBC <3000
Diphenhydramine (excluding orders for sleep)	Glucose <50 mg/dL
Epinephrine (IV push)	Rising serum creatinine
Flumazenil	Clostridium difficile–positive stool
Naloxone	Digoxin level >2
Droperidol	Lidocaine level >5
Sodium polystyrene sulfonate	Gentamicin/tobramycin peak >10 or trough >2
Vitamin K	Amikacin peak >30 or trough >10
	Vancomycin level >26
	Theophylline level >20
	Oversedation, lethargy, fall, rash
	Abrupt medication stop
	Transfer to higher level of care

7. Routinely review medication errors, ADEs, and ADRs for trends. Report all findings to the pharmacy and therapeutics committee and other hospital or organization quality and safety committees. It is beneficial to present facility specific data, nationally reported errors of significance, as well as incorporate storytelling into various presentations. Oftentimes, telling a story that engages one's emotions, followed by your own data specific to the event, reinvigorates the efforts to work toward safer processes.

8. Develop strategies for decreasing the incidence of medication errors and adverse events utilizing the data collected through the various identification and reporting systems. Use caution in aggregating data by error types or other surface level classifications. The key is getting to the causes of the errors—not just the fact that the majority of errors are omitted doses. Why are the doses omitted? Is the automated dispensing cabinet filled at inappropriate intervals, is there not a clear and standardized process for delivering medications where they are easily located, or do the batteries on the computers-on-wheels drain too quickly and the doses just are not charted? Seek to discover why the doses are omitted, as these are the issues that need to be resolved.

9. Review national resources that identify errors in other organizations such as the ISMP, the FDA, and the USP. It is likely that your institution is experiencing risks similar to other institutions. Learn what risk-reduction strategies are recommended, take a close look at your own processes, and implement additional risk-reduction strategies where warranted. There is no need to repeat errors at every institution to learn what steps need to be taken for prevention.

Types of Safety Event Analysis

❹ *Thorough analysis of safety events through root cause analysis, failure mode and effects analysis (FMEA), or other methods is a key activity to support learning from errors in an effort to prevent recurrence.* Analysis of near-miss events (errors that do not reach the patient) and precursors (errors reaching the patient but causing little to no harm) can be very valuable learning experiences. These may be documented in various ways—through interventions or error-reporting systems. These are valuable when reviewed in aggregate to determine if there are common themes or causes that may warrant further investigation and process changes. It is important to remember that the causes of near misses or errors causing minimal harm are often the same errors that lead to serious harm. For example, a nurse administers a dose of cefazolin to the wrong patient. Fortunately, the patient was not allergic and there was no adverse outcome. If the same error occurs with a different drug (e.g., a high-risk drug, such as a paralytic agent), the outcome can be fatal. Precursor events (those causing little to no harm) can be an important learning experience.

Medication errors that are rated severity E through I, using the NCCMERP severity rating system, cause harm to patients, ranging from minor harm to death. Many facilities conduct an investigation on these events to better understand the causes.

The Joint Commission (TJC) is an accrediting body that is focused on continuously improving health care for the public by evaluating health care organizations (e.g., hospitals, home care organizations, nursing homes, ambulatory care providers, and clinical laboratories). The goal of TJC is to ensure each organization meets designated standards for quality and safety. A **sentinel event** is defined by TJC as "an unexpected occurrence involving death or serious physical or psychological injury, or the risk thereof. Serious injury specifically includes loss of limb or function. The phrase 'or the risk thereof' includes any process variation for which a recurrence would carry a significant chance of a serious adverse outcome."[39] The expectation is that the organization will conduct a timely, thorough, and credible **root cause analysis (RCA)** in response to a sentinel event, develop and implement an action plan to reduce the risk of recurrence, and monitor the effectiveness of the plan and its implementation. An RCA can also be conducted on events other than sentinel events, such as when a trend of similar precursor or near-miss events is identified.

The goal of the RCA is to investigate the event in such detail that the true root cause(s) of the event are identified. This requires that the team completes a thorough analysis that includes reviewing the human errors and processes that may contribute to the event. An action plan should be developed with the intent of preventing the recurrence with certainty. Risk-reduction strategies such as reeducating the department, asking staff to be more careful, and developing or editing a policy and procedure have been the norm for years. It is now recognized that these are weak action plans that are not able to prevent recurrence without some change to the processes. The concepts of mistake-proofing, standardization, and forcing functions are important considerations in the development of risk-reduction strategies. Taking an action that physically prevents something from happening is the most effective method of preventing an inadvertent action—such as requiring the foot to be placed on the brake before placing a car in reverse. Another example of a forcing function is when a computer program requires confirmation to delete a file—it prevents inadvertent deletion. An example of a fail-safe is when a garage door will not continue to close if any motion is detected that interferes with the operation of the door.

One of the key challenges in completing a quality RCA is adequate training and coordinating time for front-line staff and management team members (e.g., physicians, vice presidents) to attend the meetings. One strategy is to have predetermined times designated for team meeting use if and when an RCA is indicated. This ensures that those with busy schedules have adequate time allotted for this most vital activity. A second key in preventing recurrence is monitoring the action plan to ensure that it is implemented in a timely fashion. Measures should be defined as part of the action plan and revisited to assess the implementation and effectiveness of the action plan. Lastly, it is important to the continued development of a safety culture to be transparent within the organization (and between organizations who are a part of a system) about the lessons learned from events. Information about the event and the action plan should be shared within the facility through structured meetings and communications—all the way to the staff level. The last thing anyone wants is to restructure processes in one area of a facility and not translate the lessons learned to other applicable areas of the facility.

While RCA is a retrospective process, the use of FMEA is a prospective process that is required annually by TJC. This type of analysis involves a team that takes an issue that has been identified as a potentially risky process and examines the ways in which the process or product might fail. An FMEA can be done prior to implementation of a new process or technology in an effort to increase the awareness of how the implementation might fail, before it occurs. This allows the implementation team to take adequate steps before the new product or process is introduced to avoid failures. In an FMEA, each step of the process is outlined, the team brainstorms all the ways in which the process could fail, and defines the effect of each potential failure to the end user (often the patient). An estimation (on a 10-point scale) is made of the likelihood of the failure, the severity of the potential failure, and the probability that the failure will be detected. A criticality index is calculated and those failure modes with the highest scores are prioritized as important steps for which barriers are developed. Generally an action plan to reduce risk within the process is developed, implemented and monitored.

Case Study 16-1

At your institution, there have been many intravenous (IV) contrast dye extravasation cases. It has been determined that you will combine information from all of the known cases and conduct an aggregate root cause analysis. An aggregate RCA[40,41] provides intense scrutiny of the cases to determine what opportunities exist to decrease the rate of the extravasations.

- *What are the advantages and disadvantages of including multiple cases in the root cause analysis process?*

To Err Is Human

As long as human beings are a key component of processes such as the medication use process, errors are inevitable. Therefore, there exists a need for redundancies and incorporation of human factors principles as key elements to more reliable processes, preventing errors from reaching the patient.

When (not if) humans make errors, there are several ways to approach the event. ❺ *Human beings (including health care professionals of all types) have a propensity to commit errors in all aspects of our lives. To err is human.* Being human, health care professionals of all types have a propensity to commit errors in every area of their professional lives, including the medication use process. One approach to error management places emphasis on the individuals involved, which generally implies blame. This approach generally puts the blame on the last person touching the patient, and does not usually acknowledge other factors contributing to the error. As a result, people are urged to be more careful, pay more attention, and undergo remedial training. It also results in increased supervision and increased detail within policies and procedures. It is thought that if people are more vigilant, the number of errors will be reduced.[42] The other approach focuses on how the design of objects (e.g., smart pumps, drug names, labels for medications, connectors for IVs and tube feedings), activities, and procedures (programming a pump that is infrequently used) contributes to the actions and behaviors of individuals. This approach believes that people come to work with good intentions, are skilled and experienced, but may be led to commit errors because of the way in which the design of the system shapes their behaviors.

According to Senders,[43] "An error is a psychological event with psychological causes...." Human error is inevitable; rather a fact of life. Most human error results in little to no consequence. It occurs regardless of occupation, although the consequences vary significantly depending on the specific occupation. Therefore, an error in medicine can be fatal, as can an error in the airline industry.

To better understand why health care professionals commit errors, it is necessary to look at the cognitive processes that occur at the time of the error. Norman and Reason have written wonderful books reflecting philosophies of human error.[44-46] Humans will most likely commit errors at an unacceptable rate despite best efforts to understand and remedy the occurrence. With this in mind, it is necessary to develop systems of medication use that account for human error and have processes in place to identify and correct human error before medications reach patients.

❻ Understanding *the three modes of human performance (skill based, rule based, and knowledge based) is very important to understanding errors and events, and in developing appropriate strategies to reduce the risks of recurrence.*

- When in skill-based level of performance, humans are doing very routine tasks that are very practiced and automatic. People are very good at these tasks, as they do them all the time. In skill-based mode, a decision has been made on what the intended action is and the individuals are now in the process of executing a task. Activities such as eating or driving a car to work fit into this category. These are effortless and really unconscious activities that do not require much thought or attention. Skill-based errors are termed slips, lapses, or fumbles.[45] They are easily identified. Slips are usually associated with attention or perception failures and lapses generally involve memory failures.
  - When a person places the cereal in the refrigerator instead of the milk, this is an example of a slip. The task is something people do all the time successfully but for some reason they err. Perhaps he or she was briefly interrupted by children or the dog and unconsciously reached for the wrong container.
  - An example of a lapse might be when a person walks into a room only to say, "Now why did I come in here?"
  - If the milk is accidentally knocked over while in the process of putting it back into the refrigerator, a fumble has occurred.
- Humans perform in rule-based mode when problem solving or making decisions. Perhaps there has been a change in the situation—like an exit is closed on the usual route to work and it is necessary to choose an alternate route. The person begins to problem solve, realizing that he or she has been in this situation before. People are trained to deal with many situations, perhaps by learning a policy or procedure. It is possible to determine which rule to apply to the situation encountered. This is called an if-then scenario—if this situation, then do this action. Several scenarios can occur:
  - A wrong rule may be chosen because one misperceives the situation and applies the wrong rule.
  - If one misapplies a rule, a rule-based error occurs. It is possible to unconsciously pull the wrong pattern or rule from memory. Memory may be biased for many reasons: overgeneralization, recent occurrences (causing one to choose the first answer that comes to mind despite available evidence that would lead us to another conclusion), or other factors.
  - There is also intentional rule-based noncompliance (with defined policies and procedures) in which an individual chooses an action despite the knowledge that they should take a different action (e.g., a nurse administers a medication without checking the patient's arm band because he or she is sleeping soundly or the barcode reader is not conveniently located).[46]
- The other decision-making type is knowledge-based mode. Knowledge-based errors occur when the individual is in a situation to which he or she has never been

exposed, or has no preprogrammed rules to apply. The person has a lack of required knowledge to complete the task, or has possibly misinterpreted the problem. When in knowledge-based mode, people are much more likely to make an error than when in skill-based or rule-based mode. The best scenario is that the person recognizes that he or she is lacking the information needed and takes the time to consult with other sources (e.g., colleagues, texts, policies, or literature) to determine the next course of action. Oftentimes, humans feel pressured to proceed in the face of uncertainty, because of perceived time constraints, to avoid acknowledging lack of knowledge to complete the task, or because of overconfidence. The worst-case scenario is that an individual does not realize he or she is in knowledge-based mode, has misinterpreted the situation, and proceeds without any question. "You don't know what you don't know" is a representative phrase in this situation.

One very common type of human error is called confirmation bias. Confirmation bias refers to a type of selective thinking where individuals select what is familiar to them or what they expect to see, rather than what is actually there. A similar type of error is inattentional blindness. Inattentional blindness occurs when the person is so focused on performing the assigned task that he or she fails to see an error or change right in front of his or her eyes, which should have been plainly visible, and cannot explain the lapse. In many cases, people involved in the errors have been labeled as careless and negligent. It is human nature for people to associate items by certain characteristics, for example, color of vial, cap, or text. It is very important for the health care community to recognize the role that confirmation bias may play in medication errors and to work to develop systems with the understanding that this phenomenon exists and is part of natural human behavior. These types of accidents are common—even with intelligent, vigilant, and attentive people.[47] Attempts to combat these errors are difficult. Paying more attention is not effective. The use of barcoding has increasingly been used to avoid this phenomenon.

System Error

❼ *Poorly designed health care systems and processes are a significant contributor to individual human error and subsequent patient harm.* Interestingly enough, behind the majority of individual human errors, one or more system errors exist that contributed to the human error. Therefore, it is of utmost importance to recognize system errors and gaps when developing prevention strategies. Systems have common characteristics—these generally include technology, tools and machines, interfaces, processes, products, user interaction with the system, and people. The health care system has become, and continues to become, very complex. There are many layers and components to the health care system: individual practitioners, teams working together, policies and procedures (generally for each individual entity), regulations, devices and equipment, communications, leadership, and management. It would be optimal if all of the parts of the system were integrated and had seamless communication and coordination, but that is not the case. They are each managed separately and are likely to have their own culture, that is, common goals, values, beliefs, and behaviors. It is rare that each component of the system has similar cultures, even when speaking of departments or units within an organization, such as the patient care areas of a hospital.[42] It is clear that the development and management of systems and processes has a direct link to the actions of individuals. According to TJC's analysis of multiple sentinel events,[48] ineffective communication contributes to a significant number of adverse outcomes (60% to 70%). Optimization of systems and processes is essential to optimization of health care safety. This section discusses system failures that contribute to error that must be identified and corrected to provide safe care.

A latent failure is a weakness that is usually unconsciously built into a system or, more commonly, develops over time. When making decisions about processes, it is not uncommon that the solution to one problem actually creates a problem in another part of the system (i.e., an unanticipated consequence). One example: if bar-coding medication administration technology using computers on wheeled carts is purchased to prevent administration errors, yet there are not adequate outlets or batteries to keep the computer charged, nurses are faced with skipping the scanning step, finding another computer, or rebooting the computer. The latter two options delay the patient's medication—perhaps only 5 to 10 minutes. However, when a patient is in severe pain, the nurse has been placed in a situation where it seems better to give the medication in a timely fashion and then scan once a viable computer is found. These gaps are inevitable and usually lie relatively undetected. They may appear periodically in a near-miss event, where the error slips through several points, but is caught by one last stop-gap (a good catch). If organizations do not learn from the near misses, it is quite possible that eventually the same gaps will result in an adverse event.

When an analysis, such as an RCA is undertaken, a thorough understanding of how the system is designed (what are the defined policies and procedures) and how it actually functions (include staff in the RCA or go to the location and observe the process) is very important. When designing an action plan, include more than just actions taken with individuals (e.g., peer review, disciplinary action). A good action plan should address the gaps that were found in the system with prevention strategies to prevent the identified causes. If during a code, nursing staff pulled the wrong drug from the crash cart and it was determined that not all crash carts had the same contents and the medication labels were not readily visible, the medications were combined with other supplies, and the contents were in different drawers depending on what unit the cart was found, blaming the staff for not reading the label will not effectively prevent the next person from having similar difficulties finding the correct medication. Address the system and process issues that contributed to the human error. Appropriate to the findings of the investigation, the action plan may include standardization of the carts, with the same drugs found in the same place regardless of cart location, placement of dosing charts in the cart to avoid calculation errors, positioning of pharmacists to pull and prepare medications, or other action to address the true causes of the error.

Case Study 16–2

Discussion Question: Is it possible to eliminate all errors? Think about human nature and system design. Should the goal be no errors or no events of harm?

Case Study: A pharmacist is staffing the surgery satellite alone, entering postoperative orders for Sue Doe. She is interrupted by a nurse caring for a different postoperative patient Janie Snow from earlier in the day who has a question about her patient's orders. The pharmacist can only view one patient's profile at a time so she pulls up the computer profile to answer a question about Janie Snow. When the pharmacist returned to her original task of entering the orders for Sue Doe, she inadvertently entered them on the wrong patient. It was determined that there is a system that automatically links the scanned order page to the correct patient, but the current version of computer software does not support this process.

- *What questions would you like to ask the pharmacist involved in the error as part of an interview?*
- *Would you classify this error as human-error only, system-error only, or a combination of both and why?*

A Just Culture—Not Shame and Blame

In some instances, reporting medication errors, particularly severe or life-threatening errors, have had adverse consequences for both individuals and the organizations involved. Health care professionals have lost their jobs or voluntarily resigned from their jobs and, at times, have left their profession. Consequently, health care professionals and health systems have been reluctant to open themselves up to adverse outcomes associated with reporting medication errors.[49] For example, in one hospital there were only 36 incident reports regarding medication errors over a yearlong reporting period. At the same institution, an observational study revealed that as many as 51,200 errors were likely to have actually occurred during that same reporting period.[50]

Hindsight bias often plays a role in the way people react to an error. Hindsight bias is the inclination to see events that have occurred as being more predictable than they were before the event took place. In other words, the person should have known that this would be the outcome. It is very easy to examine the information after the event and conclude that, of course, this bad outcome was going to occur. What investigators and facilitators do not have the benefit of is the vast number of exact circumstances and choices that the individual was facing, along with their thought processes that led them to their conclusions.

In Nevada, a pharmacy was fined 2 weeks net profit for a dispensing error that resulted from understaffing.[49] A medical center in New Jersey was successfully sued for $12 million and fined by the state board of pharmacy after a medication error killed an infant.[51] In 1996, a medication error occurred in a hospital in Colorado that resulted in the death of a newborn infant. Three nurses involved in the infant's care were indicted on charges of criminally negligent homicide.[52] District attorneys in Colorado pressed criminal charges that could have resulted in three to 5 years imprisonment. A pharmacist in Ohio was indicted and jailed for a chemotherapy error resulting in the death of a young patient.[53] In these cases, there were underlying system concerns that likely contributed to the event. Without resolution of these system issues, a similar event may occur with a different clinician. Thus, the need to identify root causes to prevent recurrence.

Learning from errors, events, and near misses is vital to improvement. Despite the negative actions that have been taken against individuals and organizations in the past, the health care culture is evolving toward a culture of safety. Leaders are learning more about **Just Culture**. Just Culture is a culture in which discipline is applied in a consistent manner based on the intentions of the individual and the circumstances in which they were working—not the outcome. One must understand the circumstances (including poorly designed systems) in which errors occur before decisions related to discipline are made. If a system sets up one individual to fail, the next person in the same situation is also likely to fail in the same manner as the first. If the system is not specifically designed to avert likely human errors (no double-check of a high-risk calculation, such as chemotherapy), human errors will continue to reach patients with significant potential for harm.

Action plans to prevent recurrence of an event should be designed according to the type of error(s) made. It does not make sense to retrain someone in a procedure if they are very skilled, were distracted by a colleague, and made a skill-based error. Similarly if a knowledge-based error is identified, working to decrease distractions and interruptions will have little impact on decreasing future repeat errors with the activity. When interviewing individuals involved in errors, be sure to ask them to describe what happened and what else was going on at the time, ask them to walk through their decision-making process, and find out why they think the event occurred. Be sure to understand the options presented to them at the time.

Recall those headlines again—Child dies from medication error, Journalist dies of chemotherapy error.... The rest of the story usually involves details about what happened (on the surface) and who was fired or reprimanded. What disciplinary action should be taken in these cases, if any? It depends on the circumstances entirely. It is important to have a good understanding of exactly what happened and the "whys" behind the decisions and actions taken. If an individual did not consciously make an unsafe decision, how does discipline help one learn from mistakes? Will not staff be less willing to report and discuss them without fear of retribution? Retraining, counseling, and discipline have been hallmark actions taken to prevent error and have failed to substantially improve patient care.

The culture of blame shifted in the 1990s in the health care industry when it was recognized that the punitive nature of discipline was not the best way to encourage staff to talk about risks and errors, and assist in the process of decreasing errors. The culture then shifted to a blame-free culture in an effort to promote reporting. This culture recognized that humans will err, that most unsafe acts are slips or lapses, and that weaknesses in systems and environments contribute significantly to errors in medicine.[54]

What was not recognized at the time was that a solely blame-free culture (also termed nonpunitive) failed to attend to those few who knowingly ignore designated safety procedures and those who are unreasonably reckless or negligent. This undermines those who work hard at providing safe care.

❽ *A Just Culture is one in which discipline is applied in a consistent manner based on the intentions of the individual and the situation in which they were working—not the outcome.* A Just Culture is somewhere between the two extremes described above, with blaming individuals on one end, blame-free culture on the other end, and a Just Culture somewhere in the middle. It is unacceptable to discipline all errors regardless of their circumstances, and is just as unacceptable to be nonpunitive in the face of individuals who are intentionally ignoring safe operating principles.

The hard part is distinguishing between those who make a conscious decision to complete an unsafe action, despite knowledge that it is unsafe (i.e., at-risk behavior), and those who usually work in a safe manner and experienced a slip or lapse. The use of a substitution test has proven to be useful in these instances.[45] When dealing with a serious event and a person is implicated in an unsafe act, describe the scenario to several other individuals (at least three) of the same qualifications and experience (optimally, who are not aware of the actual incident) and ask them in the circumstances at the time, what decisions they would have made. If they would have made the same decision and completed the same actions, then blaming the individual is not likely appropriate as there is evidence that this issue has a larger scope. Another option is to observe individuals in the same situations, if possible, to determine how others behave in similar instances. This helps one determine whether the problem may lie with an individual, an expanded group (perhaps a unit or department), or is a more global problem. This also helps in the development of an action plan. There is no need to reeducate an entire department on a process, if there is only one individual that is in need of coaching.

The use of a series of questions helps determine the culpability and accountability of a person's actions and are taken from the Decision Tree for determining the Culpability of Unsafe Acts.[46] It is key that any decisions related to discipline are not made only when there is an adverse outcome. Appropriate discipline, when warranted, should be taken when unsafe behaviors are identified, regardless of the outcome.[55]

1. Were the actions as intended?
2. Was the person under the influence of unauthorized substances?
3. Did he or she knowingly violate a safe operating procedure? If so, was the procedure available, workable, intelligible, and correct? This gets at those procedures that staff feel make no sense and are not value added in their workflow. Perhaps they have a point and there is a component of system-induced error.
4. Do they pass the substitution test described above? Would others have made the same decisions and, if so, less likely to be culpable? If not, were there deficiencies in training or experience?
5. Does the individual have a history of unsafe acts? If not, again less likely to be culpable.

The use of these questions and the decision assist in determining the level of culpability of an individual. The actions in the first few questions bear more culpability than those that occur in the last several questions. Therefore, disciplinary actions are more likely to be appropriate for those acts that are intended and/or undertaken while under the influence of unauthorized substances.

There are always a few outliers within any profession—those who intentionally do not follow the processes as designed, feeling that they are immune from human error and/or believing their process is better. There is a difference between unintentional human error, at-risk behavior, and reckless behavior. Intentionally unsafe behavior is identified by the first question and is generally dealt with through disciplinary action. At-risk behavior may be amenable to coaching about the reason for the process as designed and a request to commit to better choices.

Case Study 16–3

Samuel Sneer received an overdose of a diltiazem drip and became hypotensive, requiring fluid boluses, but recovered without further effects. After further investigation, it was discovered that the nurse changed the diltiazem bag as it was nearly empty. The pump required the nurse to enter the concentration (drug in milligrams and then volume of fluid). Instead of entering the drug dose first, she mistakenly entered the fluid volume first. This is the way the concentration information appeared on the labeled bag, which was to what she was referring.

The nurse was under time pressure and was caring for more patients than the usual accepted ratio due to the flu epidemic. The pump has programmed minimum and maximum settings, but the rate was just under the maximum setting, meaning she did not receive a warning about the error. This is the first error identified for this nurse who has practiced here for over a year.

- *What system issues contributed to the error?*
- *Walk the error through the Just Culture algorithm to determine your reaction as manager of the unit (coaching, consoling, or disciplinary action).*
- *What potential system fixes can you identify?*
- *What other system fixes can you think of?*

Risk Factors for Errors and Events

The ultimate purpose for defining, classifying, analyzing, and reporting medication errors is to enable individuals and organizations to implement better systems that prevent medication errors. The ASHP has identified a multitude of risk factors associated with the occurrence of medication errors as outlined below.[34]

- Shift work—switching from days to nights or vice versa
- Inexperienced or inadequately trained staff
- Medical services with special needs (e.g., pediatrics and oncology)
- Higher number of medications per patient
- Environmental factors such as high levels of noise, poor lighting, and frequent interruptions
- High workload for staff

- Poor communication among health care providers
- Dosage form—more errors with injectable drugs
- Drug category—more errors with certain classes of drugs (e.g., antibiotics)
- Type of drug distribution systems—unit dose system is associated with fewer errors; high levels of floor stock are associated with increased errors
- Improper drug storage
- Calculations—increased errors with increased complexity and frequency of amount of calculations required
- Poor handwriting
- Verbal orders
- Lack of effective policies and procedures
- Poorly functioning oversight committees

Personal and environmental factors are thought to interact to influence cognitive function that may lead to slips. There are several factors specific to the professional involved and their working environment that may contribute to their risk of committing an error. Grasha and O'Neill[56] have outlined some of the factors that may affect cognitive processes, resulting in lapses of performance.

1. *Excessive task demand:* Many clinicians attribute their errors to this situation, complaining that their workload is so heavy and they are overloaded with tasks, making it difficult to work error free. In one survey, 68% of pharmacists rated work overload as a major contributing factor to the committal of dispensing errors.[57] Most pharmacists and experts in medication errors agree that work overload may be the most significant factor contributing to medication errors. Reevaluation of the workload distribution, with an eye for streamlining processes, may be valuable. Developing a detailed map of all of the steps required to accomplish a task is one way to discover the complexity of a task. This is called **process mapping.**

2. *Personal characteristics:* Personal factors, such as age, sensory deficits, or state of health, may contribute to performance lapses. Personal levels of stress or fatigue may also have an impact. Someone who is bored at work may be more error prone.

3. *Extraorganizational factors:* Factors, such as similar product names or packaging from pharmaceutical companies, may have an extensive impact on the commission of errors with particular drugs. In one study, look-alike or sound-alike drugs were involved in 37% of medication errors.[58] As an example, this issue is currently being addressed for the sound-alike drugs celecoxib (Celebrex®), fosphenytoin (Cerebyx®), and citalopram (Celexa®). Complex insurance plans are also extraorganizational factors that may serve to complicate the medication use process and

contribute to slips. The profession of pharmacy has been referred to as the most heavily regulated of all professions. Legal mandates for policing illegal prescriptions and other regulatory requirements are also good examples of extraorganizational factors.

4. *Work environment:* Poor working conditions may influence the rate of error committal. Poor illumination and high noise levels have been shown to affect the dispensing error rate in pharmacies.[59] Other factors in this category may include high ambient temperatures and frequent interruptions from the telephone or patients.

5. *Intraorganizational factors:* There is a significant emphasis on other factors besides the quality and safety of medication use within health care systems. Concerns related to finances, throughput, customer service, and quality of employee work life are often competing priorities and major areas of focus in many institutions. Policies and procedures demanding high output or mandating long working hours may significantly affect cognition and the ability to prevent error occurrence.

6. *Interpersonal factors:* Conflicts among coworkers or with patients may distract professionals from the tasks at hand and contribute to error commission. General interruptions from people may also fall into this category.

Some factors that may contribute to cognitive lapses and the commission of medication errors may fall into more than one of these categories. Furthermore, factors from multiple categories may occur simultaneously to contribute to error commission.

Health care professionals have indicated that other factors may also contribute to medication errors. Some of those factors are as follows:

1. *Lack of effective communication:* This factor may also fall under interpersonal factors listed above. Failure to communicate effectively among fellow employees or among health care professionals has frequently been named as contributing to medical and medication errors. For example, an error may be more likely to occur if a pharmacist chooses not to clarify physician orders, or if the pharmacist does not communicate all of the pertinent information so the physician can make an informed decision. Poor physician handwriting and verbal orders are also significant factors.[36]

2. *Failure to comply with policy:* This is a common factor in dispensing and administering drugs. In one survey, 42% to 46% of pharmacists said that failing to check drugs before dispensing was a significant factor in dispensing errors.[57] Noncompliance with policy has also been associated with drug administration errors and is the result of several factors: perceived burden of the task,

perceived risk of a bad outcome, and perceived risk of being observed. Often, nurses develop specific personal routines for administration of certain agents, which they perceive to be an improvement in the medication administration process, despite contrary policy.[36] It is important to understand the challenges that make work difficult. Ensure that processes have been designed with safety in mind.

3. *Lack of knowledge:* This is a frequently cited factor in the committal of medication errors. Mistakes, rather than slips, are typically committed as a result of inadequate knowledge. Placing inexperienced recent graduates in positions where they cannot interact with more experienced practitioners may increase medication errors. Nonspecialists covering a service that is normally staffed by a specialist may also lead to errors.[59] Nurses with less exposure to pharmacology may be more unlikely to recognize potential inconsistencies in disease state and medication usage and doses, resulting in the possibility of increased medication errors reaching the patient.[36]

4. *Lack of patient counseling:* It has been said that the last safety check prior to dispensing medication should be counseling the patient. Talking to the patient allows the pharmacist to correlate the medication and dose with the patient's condition and helps the pharmacist to detect any errors that may have occurred in the medication use process. In one study, 89% of errors committed in a community pharmacy were detected during patient counseling.[49] However, errors may occur not only from a lack of counseling, but also from providing incorrect information during patient counseling.[60] Providing incorrect information may also fall in the lack of knowledge category. One additional factor that plays a major part in understanding the patient is health care literacy. All professionals should assess the level of patient literacy to ensure that appropriate language and teaching methods are used in our interactions with the patient (see Chapter 20 for more information).

The examples provided above are a partial list of contributory factors at the level of the health care practitioner. These factors influence the occurrence of slips or performance lapses and mistakes committed by individuals. They do not address failure of a system or failure of a safety net as a whole process. The medication use process involves multiple health care professionals, nonprofessional staff, patients, and multiple physical environments. To adequately address the causes of errors, failures in the system must also be addressed. Although it is important to address the problem of individuals committing errors (e.g., increasing training if a knowledge deficit was identified and enforcing policy), adequately developed safety systems should be in place to significantly minimize the number of errors reaching patients.

Health Professions Education

Most health care professionals are trained with the thought that individuals cannot make mistakes in health care; when dealing with patients, it is unacceptable to cause an error. Students, as well as practicing professionals (e.g., physicians, nurses, pharmacists, respiratory therapists) learn little about human factors thinking, systems design, quality improvement, and reliability. They do not learn that humans err in many ways. Thus, when they do make an error in practice, many either deny the fact or are jolted into the realization that they should be more careful and develop reliable habits. Many times, the realization that they have made an error causes physicians, pharmacists, nurses, and other professionals to avoid discussion about errors—with colleagues and patients. When an error or safety event is investigated and analyzed, individuals and/or professions may point fingers at the other, some may avoid telling the whole story, some do not realize the value of the process, and many do not recognize the contribution that processes and systems play in their own errors. Many of the Institute of Medicine reports on quality and safety have referenced the need for changes in health professions education. Pertinent quotes from "To Err Is Human: Building a Safer Health System"[1] include:

> "Clinical training and education is a key mechanism for cultural change. Colleges of medicine, nursing, pharmacy, health care administration, and their related associations should build more instruction into their curriculum on patient safety and its relationship to quality improvement."
>
> "Many believe that initial exposure to patient safety should occur early in undergraduate and graduate training programs, as well as through continuing education."
>
> "The need for more opportunities for interdisciplinary training was also identified. Most care delivered today is done by teams of people, yet training often remains focused on individual responsibilities leaving practitioners inadequately prepared to enter complex settings."

Another report by the Institute of Medicine, "Crossing the Quality Chasm,"[61] identified health professions education as a priority.

Subsequently, a summit of over 150 interdisciplinary participants met in 2002 and developed recommendations for reaching this goal. The proceedings and recommendations from the summit are compiled in *Health Professions Education: A Bridge to Quality.*[62] This committee developed the following vision statement:

❾ *All health professionals should be educated to deliver patient-centered care as members of an interdisciplinary team, emphasizing evidence-based practice, quality improvement approaches, and informatics.*

The following strategies are outlined in the book:

- Develop and build consensus around a common language and core competencies.
- Integrate core competencies into oversight processes.

- Motivate and support leaders, and monitor progress of reform effort.
- Develop evidence-based curricula and teaching approaches.
- Develop faculty as teaching and learning experts.

The IHI has developed an interprofessional, international educational online community. The IHI Open School provides a mechanism by which students and their mentors in nursing, medicine, pharmacy, dentistry, health care administration, and other health care professions can interact and learn in an interdisciplinary fashion. There are online courses in quality and safety, basic and advanced certifications in quality improvement and patient safety, case studies, podcasts, videos, and feature articles. The IHI Open School program[63] is one example where online modules on quality and safety can be completed either during professional education or as a part of continuing education and learning for practitioners. See http://www.ihi.org for additional information. This is a great start to providing the types of interdisciplinary learning that will be of great value to the health care community and patients.

Best Practices for Error Prevention

❿ *There are many resources that identify best-practice error prevention strategies.* Listed here are various resources as well as strategies to ensure medication use processes are as safe as they can be. Remember to be a learning organization by constantly reviewing local and national information and taking proactive steps to prevent error. Do not wait until it happens to you.

The Institute for Safe Medication Practices publishes a "Quarterly Action Agenda" that describes known risks and errors and describes recommendations for risk-reduction strategy implementation. These can be found on the Web site at http://www.ismp.org

The Institute for Healthcare Improvement (IHI) has sponsored several campaigns (The 100,000 Lives Campaign and the 5 Million Lives Campaign) to save lives and protect patients from harm. At least half of the 12 recommended interventions within the two campaigns involve improving the safe use of medications. Pharmacists should be integrally involved in the institution team to ensure successful interventions. See Table 16–5. In addition to these two campaigns, the IHI offers many programs, conferences, IMPACT network associations, best-practice postings, the IHI Open School, and much more. Visit http://www.ihi.org for more information.

The Joint Commission's National Patient Safety Goals can serve as a guide to improving the safety of health care. Many of The Joint Commission's National Patient Safety Goals released each year are related to safe medication use and pharmacists should

TABLE 16–5. INTERVENTIONS RECOMMENDED BY THE INSTITUTE FOR HEALTHCARE IMPROVEMENT (IHI) TO SAVE LIVES AND REDUCE PATIENT INJURIES[63]

Strategies from the 100,000 Lives Campaign

- **Deploy Rapid Response Teams**...at the first sign of patient decline
- **Deliver Reliable, Evidence-Based Care for Acute Myocardial Infarction**...to prevent deaths from heart attack
- **Prevent Adverse Drug Events (ADEs)**...by implementing medication reconciliation
- **Prevent Central Line Infections**...by implementing a series of interdependent, scientifically grounded steps
- **Prevent Surgical Site Infections**...by reliably delivering the correct perioperative antibiotics at the proper time
- **Prevent Ventilator-Associated Pneumonia**...by implementing a series of interdependent, scientifically grounded steps

Strategies from the 5 Million Lives Campaign

- **Prevent Harm from High-Alert Medications**...starting with a focus on anticoagulants, sedatives, narcotics, and insulin
- **Reduce Surgical Complications**...by reliably implementing all of the changes recommended by SCIP, the Surgical Care Improvement Project (www.medqic.org/scip)
- **Prevent Pressure Ulcers**...by reliably using science-based guidelines for their prevention
- **Reduce Methicillin-Resistant** *Staphylococcus aureus* **(MRSA) Infection**...by reliably implementing scientifically proven infection control practices
- **Deliver Reliable, Evidence-Based Care for Congestive Heart Failure**...to avoid readmissions
- **Get Boards on Board**...by defining and spreading the best known leveraged processes for hospital boards of directors, so that they can become far more effective in accelerating organizational progress toward safe care

be involved in ensuring that the facility meets these goals. They are divided into the type of health care provided—hospital, home care, ambulatory care, behavioral health care, etc. There are other goals aside from those listed, some of which indirectly relate to pharmacy. These goals change frequently. A partial list includes:

- Accurately and completely reconcile medications during transitions within and across organizations (inpatient to outpatient).
- Improve the effectiveness of communication between caregivers.
  - Write down and read back verbal orders (and critical test results)—TJC safety goal sets the expectation that for all verbal orders, the receiver of the order must write the order down on the order page and then read the transcribed order back to the practitioner, who then verifies that the order has been transcribed as intended. This prevents transcription errors in which the receiver may have heard the order correctly and made an error in writing/entering the order after the conversation has ended and prevents errors in which the order was heard and transcribed incorrectly. This is also referred to as closed-loop

communication in which the giver and recipient confirm that the information provided and received is accurate.
  ◦ Designate unapproved abbreviations and monitor their use.
- Implement a standardized approach to hand-off communications, including an opportunity to ask and respond to questions.
- Improve the safety of using medications.
  ◦ Develop risk-reduction strategies around look-alike and sound-alike medications such as the use of tall man letters to draw attention to differences in similar drug names such as DAUNOrubicin and DOXOrubicin.
  ◦ Label all medications, medication containers (for example, syringes, medicine cups, basins), or other solutions on and off the sterile field.
- Reduce the likelihood of patient harm associated with the use of anticoagulant therapy.
  ◦ Includes an anticoagulation management program, approved protocols for initiation and maintenance, individualized care, appropriate baseline and ongoing lab monitoring.
  ◦ Includes notification and involvement of the dietary department, patient education, use of infusion pumps for heparin, and evaluation of anticoagulation safety.
- Implement best practices for preventing surgical site infections. Timely administration of appropriately chosen antibiotics just prior to the surgical procedure is essential to preventing surgical site infections. Most preoperative antibiotics must be given within 1 hour prior to the incision time. There are many errors that may contribute to the development of infection at the surgical site: lack of timely access to the medication, incorrect medication selection, or administration of the drug too early. At one time, the preoperative antibiotic was administered on the patient care unit before transporting the patient to the operating room; however, there are often delays in getting the patient to the operating room.

● Consult TJC Web site for the most up-to-date standards. (http://www.jointcommission.org/standards_information/npsgs.aspx)

● **The National Quality Forum (NQF)'s Safe Practices for Better Health Care** identifies 34 practices that have been demonstrated to be effective in reducing the occurrence of adverse events in health care. While there are two identified best practices identified within a chapter titled *Improving Patient Safety Through Medication Management*, many of the other Safe Practices involve medication use. The Safe Practices associated with this chapter are as follows:

- Medication reconciliation—Many adverse events are the result of patients presenting to an acute care facility such as a hospital, identifying a list of the medications that are taking at home, yet somewhere during the admission, transfer, or discharge process, these medications are inadvertently omitted or duplicate therapy occurs due to therapeutic substitution at discharge. The organization must develop a process to identify, reconcile (compare and confirm which medications are appropriate for the patient to take during the hospitalization or outpatient visit), and communicate an accurate patient medication list throughout the continuum of care (to other primary care and specialist providers).

- Pharmacist leadership structure—Pharmacy leaders should have an active role on the administrative leadership team that identifies their accountability for the performance of the medication management systems across the institution.

Other Safe Practices which relate to medication use include:

- Improving patient safety by creating and sustaining a culture of safety.
  - The elements of this safe practice include leadership structures and systems, culture measurement and intervention, teamwork training, and identification and mitigation of risks and hazards.
- Improving patient safety by facilitating information transfer and clear communication.
  - Elements of this chapter include communication of critical information, order read-back, safe adoption of CPOE, and avoiding unapproved abbreviations. Each organization must define a list of unapproved abbreviations, monitor the frequency of use, and develop strategies to reduce the use of these abbreviations. Several high-risk abbreviations have been identified (by ISMP and other organizations) such as MSO_4 and $MgSO_4$, which may be inadvertently misread and administered, causing harm to patients and U (for units), which has been misinterpreted as a zero, causing 10-fold overdoses of insulin.
- Improving patient safety through prevention of health care–associated infections.
  - This chapter includes practices around aspiration and ventilator-associated pneumonia (VAP) prevention, surgical site infection prevention, multidrug-resistant organism prevention, hand hygiene, and influenza prevention through administration of appropriate vaccines to all qualified patients. Administration of appropriate antibiotic prophylaxis in a timely manner is a key prevention strategy for surgical site infections.
- Improving patient safety through condition and site-specific practices.
  - This grouping includes perioperative myocardial infarction and ischemia prevention, venous thromboembolism prevention, anticoagulation therapy, and contrast-media-induced renal failure prevention.

Many of the practices involve medication use and pharmacy should be integrally involved in efforts to meet these goals. Visit the Web site for the latest version (http://www.qualityforum.org/Publications/2010/04/Safe_Practices_for_Better_Healthcare_-_2010_Update.aspx). These two resources combined create a great roadmap for working toward safer medication use systems.

Incorporate human factors principles into the design of processes. ⓫ *Researching, recognizing, and designing with human factors principles in mind is a great way to improve the safety of any process.* Human factors research is a developing type of research in health care, where other industries have developed strategies around human factors to successfully improve the safety (e.g., nuclear power, air travel). Some of the core principles of human factors design include the following:

- Simplify and standardize—A process that requires a policy and procedure of 10 pages is one that is much too complex.
- Reduce reliance on memory—The human mind can only hold a limited amount of things in short-term memory (four to seven items depending on what source is read). Therefore, formulating other methods of prioritization or reminders is likely to be more effective than relying on recall of individuals.
- Use constraints and forcing functions—Mistake-proofing is the use of process or design features to prevent errors or the negative impact of errors. Mistake-proofing is also known as *poka-yoke* (pronounced *pokayokay*), Japanese slang for avoiding inadvertent errors.[64] One great example is the file cabinet. Tons of papers are stored in file cabinets. An example is when one file drawer, and then a second drawer, is opened, just to find the entire cabinet falling over. If more than one file drawer is opened at a time, the center of gravity moves, causing the file cabinet to fall. Modern file cabinets are designed to avoid this type of injury, as opening one drawer locks the rest. The design forces correct behavior and only allows for proper use. It takes longer to file, but it prevents injury. Several approaches to mistake-proofing include mistake prevention, mistake detection, and reduction of the effect of user errors.
- Improve information access—Coordination and interfacing computer systems is a huge challenge, but is often the only way to ensure that all information is available to those who need it.
- Decrease reliance on vigilance—Humans will err; therefore, other mechanisms to prevent errors from reaching the patient are much more effective than asking people to be careful. They may be more vigilant for a brief time, and then revert back to previous habits.
- Increase feedback—Feedback (of actions taken and processes improved as a result of reported events) to reporters, end users, and management staff is critical

to the development of a safety culture. At times, staff report errors and never see any changes, which is discouraging and results in staff less likely to report. If there is never any perceived action taken in response to the report, no review of the reports, no activity to improve the system, or no follow-up or feedback of information back to the reporter, the staff perceives that reporting the known risks they encounter is a waste of time, and they will stop reporting. Completing a report (especially if there is no harm to a patient) takes away time from the bedside or other critical activities.

- Reduce and/or improve the reliability of handoffs—Handoffs are one of the more common points for error. Oftentimes when contacting a physician, handing off a patient to another caregiver, or during a change of shift report, only portions of the patient's pertinent history are provided. The information provided is often variable, dependent on the person handing off the information, and other factors, such as time pressure. There are often gaps when critical information (e.g., allergies, code status, pending physician response to resolve medication-related questions) is not provided, leading to errors and omissions in care.

- A structured handoff process has been incorporated as a National Patient Safety Goal by TJC as a method of reducing the likelihood that important information is not passed on to the next shift or the next caregiver. The use of SBAR as a communication tool during handoffs of patients or information is one method that has proven useful in reducing the errors introduced during the handoff of patients within or between institutions. SBAR stands for the following:
  - Situation—Describe the current situation and reason for the call.
  - Background—Provide pertinent background information (e.g., history, current medications, labs, vital signs) to the situation.
  - Assessment—Provide your assessment of the situation.
  - Recommendation/request—Provide your request or recommendation in succinct terms.

Other Principles of Error Management

- **Implement new technology and information systems—with caution.** There have been many advances in technology and information systems available within health care: bar-coding technology, smart pumps, CPOE, automated dispensing and distribution technologies, and more. These all have the potential to provide great value; however, one should undertake the implementation of these new technologies carefully. The curse of the unintended consequence is often discovered during or after implementation. Unintended consequences may occur when a new technology is implemented and a new problem develops as a result of the technology. In some cases, an FMEA is used prior to new technology implementation to brainstorm what could go wrong and develop strategies and educational tools to prevent deviations from the desired outcome. Reviewing technology from a human factors perspective early in the process is recommended. For example, placing a computer on top of an automated distribution machine provides great access to information that nursing and pharmacy staff need during the retrieval or refilling of these machines. However, if the font is so small that no one can read it, this technology may actually cause more errors by selecting the wrong patient or wrong drug. It is always recommended that the end user be involved in the selection process of these technologies, as they are the ones who interact with the products daily. They can identify potential issues very quickly.

- **Use Quality Improvement Techniques to improve safety. Develop metrics and monitor progress.** While it is not necessary to conduct a randomized controlled trial with every intervention to improve safety, it is valuable to develop measures, gather baseline data, and remeasure to show improvement. The Plan-Do-Study-Act (PDSA) cycle is one structured method to lead teams through the improvement process. This process involves a planning stage in which a problem statement and implementation strategy are developed based on gaps identified within a process (plan), the strategy is implemented (do), the results are analyzed (study), and any refinements are made to the plan (act). These cycles repeat until a reliable and efficient process is finalized. See Chapter 14 for additional information on this process. Rapid-cycle tests of change are great ways to avoid full blown implementation of a poorly designed process. Rapid-cycle testing involves identification of a new process to be considered or implemented followed by a very brief trial or pilot with just one patient, one physician's patients, or one unit. The learning from this short pilot will be used to edit the new method, allow time to try it again (often several times), gain the input and support of staff in the process, and provide valuable revisions before implementation. Once the cycles have ironed out all of the apparent problems, the process is rolled out on a broader basis.
- **Evaluate areas for environmental contributions to error.** There are numerous workplace factors that may contribute to performance lapses and medication errors. Low lighting, high levels of noise, high temperatures, and stressful work

environments are examples. Distractions and interruptions as part of the work-flow should also be evaluated and minimized.

- **Involve patients on committees such as the patient safety committee**. Place some thought into who might be chosen to join the team. Use an application process to identify the best people. Ensure that a confidentiality agreement is signed. Choose someone who will listen to other perspectives, yet provide constructive feedback into how to think from a patient's perspective. It is amazing what changes can result when involving patients and/or family members. The team will alter their thinking and priorities, becoming more patient centered.

- **Establish redundancies around high-risk processes and high-risk medication use.** As humans are susceptible to error, it is recommended that redundancy be a part of processes. This allows an error caused by a slip or lapse to be caught downstream before it reaches a patient. Independent double checks are recommended for high-risk processes and medications, such as for chemotherapy and neonatal parenteral nutrition. For maximal effectiveness, double checks should be limited to ensure they are completed appropriately. It is recommended that double checks be limited to the following[65]:
  - Situations that involve high-alert medications, such as chemotherapy (including methotrexate), insulin, opiates, and anticoagulants.
  - Complex processes (compounding, calculating doses).
  - High-risk patient populations (children and adolescents, elderly or pregnant patients; patients with severe congestive heart failure; and patients with known renal impairment or liver disease).

The average number of errors missed on a check is about 5%. In studies using simulated cart-fills, 93% to 97% of these errors were identified with an independent double check. While these numbers seem small, they add up quickly with the number of medications dispensed daily. Be sure to define exactly what is meant by an independent double check. One person should do the calculations and document the results. Then a second person, without reviewing the work of the first person, should complete the same calculations and then compare the answers for consistency. This is important to avoid confirmation bias. Recall that confirmation bias is a natural tendency to see what we think we see. When glancing at an order to confirm it for another person who has just asked, "Do you think this order says warfarin?", the chance to be biased to see warfarin in the order greatly increases. If they had just asked what the order appeared to say, there is much less chance for this bias.

Table 16–6 identifies several Web sites that remain sources of updated safe practices and updated news related to safety risks and hazards.

TABLE 16–6. ORGANIZATIONS PROMOTING BEST PRACTICES IN PATIENT AND MEDICATION SAFETY

Agency for Healthcare Research and Quality	www.ahrq.gov
AHRQ Patient Safety Network	www.psnet.ahrq.gov
American Society of Health-System Pharmacists	www.ashp.org
Centers for Disease Control and Prevention	www.cdc.gov
Institute for Healthcare Improvement	www.ihi.org
Institute for Safe Medication Practices	www.ismp.org
Massachusetts Coalition for the Prevention of Medical Errors	www.macoalition.org
National Patient Safety Foundation	www.npsf.org
National Quality Forum	www.qualityforum.org
Pathways for Medication Safety	www.medpathways.info
Patient Safety and Quality Healthcare	www.psqh.com
The Joint Commission	www.jointcommission.org
The Joint Commission International	www.jointcommissioninternational.org
The Advisory Board	www.advisory.com
United States Pharmacopeia (USP)	www.usp.org
U.S. Food and Drug Administration (FDA)	www.fda.gov

Putting It All Together

Providing safe medication use is paramount to the safety of all patients. Diligent efforts to identify errors (utilizing several methods), understand human capability and propensity to commit errors in everyday life, analyze and determine the root causes and contributing factors, and devise systems that support humans and prevent expected errors are all a part of developing a culture of safety. Involving staff on the front line when reviewing safety events and developing action plans to prevent recurrence is important. It is important not only to the development of an appropriate action plan, but also to garner support and confidence that once errors are identified, leadership is committed to improving the processes in which staff have to work every day.

Case Study 16–4

A nurse caring for a birthing mother removed a bag of bupivacaine from the automated dispensing machine prior to the arrival of the anesthesiologist in order to have everything readily available when needed. The anesthesiology department had requested a preparation checklist with other supplies and the epidural. The same patient required pro-phylactic penicillin based on Group B *Streptococcus*. Both bags of similar size were in the patient's room. The nurse administered what was thought to be the penicillin bag, but did not use the bar-coding system. The patient immediately decompensated and expired. It was discovered that the epidural bupivacaine was administered IV instead of the penicillin bag.

Upon further investigation it was identified that the bar-coding system had been imple-mented in the majority of the hospital, but was not fully implemented in the Labor and Delivery area due to several technologic and cultural issues.

1. What system or process issues can you identify?
2. Read the related article cited below to identify additional information about the case. Lead a discussion related to system errors and their impact on health care professional's behaviors and the potential impact to patients.

Smetzer J, Baker C, Byrne FD, Cohen MR. Shaping systems for better behavioral choices: lessons learned from a fatal medication error. Jt Comm J Qual Patient Saf. 2010 Apr;36(4):152-63.

- Discuss challenges with implementation of new technology.
- Discuss challenges in culture and prioritization of safety principles.
- Discuss confirmation bias and look-alike packaging.

Conclusion: Safety as a Priority

In 1998, the IOM formed the Quality of Health care in America Committee that was charged with developing a strategy to improve quality in health care. In their published report, *To Err Is Human: Building a Safer Health System,*[1] the committee highlighted what was currently known about the extent of medical errors, what contributes to medical errors, and recommendations to minimize errors and improve the quality of health care in the United States. Many of the goals set forth in this report are becom-ing closer to reality. The many other reports by the IOM have provided additional detail and insight into what is necessary to optimize the safety of the health care sys-tem in the United States.

Medication misadventures continue to be a serious problem in the U.S. health care system, both in the hospital and the ambulatory care setting. Working to provide safe care is a journey or, rather, a marathon. Changing a culture is not something that is accomplished in a few years; it may take 10 or more years. Much of that is dependent on the leadership of executives and staff. Those with a passion for safety may need to help enlighten those in higher leadership positions. Learn from others. It is an important method of preventing errors from occurring within your institution/facility. Take a close look at processes when reading a local or national headline about an error. There continues to be ongoing research aimed at increasing the safety and quality of health care. Health care will continue to be complex and require effective coordination and communication. Technology will continue to evolve. Safety truly needs to be a core value that is held by all. Teamwork and mutual respect are vital parts to success. Only through collaboration and a shared, dedicated commitment will patient safety truly become a reality.

Self-Assessment Questions

1. In an effort to improve handoffs and communication, SBAR is a recommended technique. What does SBAR stand for?
   a. Summary, background, assignment, and review
   b. Situation, background, assessment, and recommendation/request
   c. Summary, briefing, assessment, and recollection
   d. Situation, briefing, assessment, and recommendation

2. Congress passed the Patient Safety and Quality Improvement Act of 2005, from which Patient Safety Organizations (PSOs) were created. Which of the following is *not* a true statement?
   a. This act provides two types of protections: confidentiality and privilege protections.
   b. One of the goals of the PSOs is to collate and analyze data related to safety errors and events.
   c. PSOs will forward information about facility-specific reported events to The Joint Commission and the media.
   d. PSOs will require the use of Common Formats (standardized reporting and terminology) for reporting errors and events.

3. Patient A is given a dose of penicillin intended for patient B. The patient did not experience any problems as a result. The physician was notified when the error was discovered (2 hours after the dose was administered) and no further orders were given. Which of the following NCCMERP classification is most appropriate?
   a. Category A
   b. Category B
   c. Category C
   d. Category E
   e. Category F

4. Which of the following action plan items is the strongest and most likely to provide sustained reduction in risk?
   a. Reeducate the department about the error and correct process.
   b. Add detail to the very long policy and procedure, spelling out every step that needs to be taken.
   c. Talk to the people involved and ask them to be more careful.
   d. Develop a forcing function such that the human error is not possible.

5. You are an experienced nurse who was asked to float to a surgical floor. Your patient has a new patient controlled analgesia (PCA) to be started. You learned how to program a PCA pump at a training for new equipment about 10 months ago but have not had a patient on a PCA pump since that time. You make a first attempt, but decide to ask a peer for assistance. Without help, what type of human error might you have made?
   a. Skill-based error
   b. Rule-based error
   c. Knowledge-based error
   d. Interruption-based error

6. A Just Culture exists when there is a nonpunitive environment, where staff are not disciplined based on errors, to ensure people will report all errors identified.
   a. True
   b. False

7. Which of the following methods utilizes screening of patient's charts to identify clues (such as an elevated lab value or reversal agent) that a patient may have experienced a medication error or adverse drug event?
   a. ADE trigger tool
   b. Observation method
   c. Voluntary reporting method
   d. None of the above

8. Which of the following is a prospective analysis of a process to determine risk-reduction strategies?
   a. Root cause analysis (RCA)
   b. Interview people involved in previous errors
   c. Failure mode and effects analysis (FMEA)
   d. Trending of error and event reports

9. Which of the following organization(s) provides information related to prevention of medical and medication error?

CHAPTER 16. MEDICATION MISADVENTURES II: MEDICATION AND PATIENT SAFETY

a. Institute for Safe Medication Practice (ISMP)
b. National Quality Forum (NQF)
c. Institute for Healthcare Improvement (IHI)
d. The Joint Commission (TJC)
e. All of the above

10. Which of the following statements are true?
    a. All medication errors cause harm.
    b. All adverse drug events involve harm.
    c. There is no harm involved in an adverse drug reaction.
    d. All of the above are true.

11. Which of the following are gaps or failures that are designed into or develop within a system, increasing the chance that people working within the system will make an error?
    a. Latent failures
    b. Individual failures
    c. Inevitable failures
    d. Personal failures

12. Which is *not* an example of designing with human factors principles?
    a. Use constraints and forcing functions
    b. Reduce reliance on memory
    c. Simplify and standardize
    d. Reduce handoffs
    e. All of the above are examples

13. Which term refers to a type of selective thinking where individuals select out what is familiar to them or what they expect to see, rather than what is actually there?
    a. Hindsight bias
    b. Confirmation bias
    c. System failure
    d. Just Culture

14. A pharmacist is alone in the pharmacy, entering a physician order, when she receives a call about a patient. In order to answer the question, she must exit the current patient's profile to pull up another patient's profile. Once the question has been answered, she hangs up and proceeds to finish entering the order on the patient's profile (the wrong patient). Which error prevention strategy would most likely be the *least* effective at preventing a recurrence of this error?

a. Discipline the pharmacist and remind her to be more careful—do patient identification correctly on every order.

b. Purchase (or develop) technology that automatically links a physician order to the patient's profile in the pharmacy system—a forcing function.

c. Alter the practice such that there are minimal to no interruptions for pharmacists entering orders (route calls to one area and responsible staff, segregate order-entry staff to decrease interruptions).

d. All of the above will be effective and prevent the recurrence.

15. Which of the following strategies do not promote safe medication use?
    a. Requesting a double check for a high-risk medication like insulin
    b. Writing down and repeating back a telephone order
    c. Using an IV syringe to administer an oral medication
    d. Using a leading zero in writing an order for a medication dose less than 1 mg

REFERENCES

1. Institute of Medicine. To err is human: building a safer health-system. Washington, DC: National Academy Press; 1999.

2. Brennan TA, Leape LL, Laird NM, Hebert L, Localio R, Lawthers AG, et al. Incidence of adverse events and negligence in hospitalized patients: results of the Harvard Medical Practice Study I. N Engl J Med. 1991;324:370-6.

3. Leape LL, Brennan TA, Laird NM, Lawthers AG, Localio AR, Barnes BA, et al. The nature of adverse events in hospitalized patients: results of the Harvard Medical Practice Study II. N Engl J Med. 1991;324(6):377-84.

4. American Society of Health-System Pharmacists. Suggested definitions and relationships among medication misadventures, medication errors, adverse drug events, and adverse drug reactions. Am J Health Syst Pharm. 1998;55:165-6.

5. ASHP Report: Suggested definitions and relationships among medication misadventures, medication errors, adverse drug events and adverse drug reactions. Am J Health Syst Pharm. 1998;55:165-6

6. National Coordinating Council for Medication Error Reporting and Prevention. Available from: http://www.nccmerp.org

7. Bates DW, Cullen DJ, Laird N, Peterson LA, Small HD, Servi D, et al. Incidence of adverse drug events and potential adverse drug events. JAMA. 1995;274:29-34.

8. Lamy PP. Adverse drug effects. Clin Ger Med. 1990;6:293-307.

9. Lesar TS, Lomaestro BM, Pohl H. Medication-prescribing errors in a teaching hospital: a 9-year experience. Arch Intern Med. 1997;157:1569-76.

10. Gurwitz JH, Field TS, Avorn J, McCormick D, Jain S, Eckler M, et al. Incidence and preventability of adverse drug events in nursing homes. Am J Med. 2000;109:87-94.

11. Gurwitz JH, Field TS, Harrold LR, Rothschild J, Debellis K, Seger AC, et al. Incidence and preventability of adverse drug events among older persons in the ambulatory setting. JAMA. 2003;289:1107-16.

12. White TJ, Arakelian A, Rho JP. Counting the costs of drug-related adverse events. Pharmacoeconomics. 1999;15:445-58.

13. Johnson JA, Bootman JL. Drug-related morbidity and mortality. Arch Intern Med. 1995;155:1949-56.

14. Classen DC, Pestotnik SL, Evans S, Loyd JF, Burke JP. Adverse drug events in hospitalized patients. JAMA. 1997;277:301-6.

15. Ernst FR, Grizzle AJ. Drug-related morbidity and mortality: updating the cost-of-illness model. J Am Pharm Assoc. 2001;41:192-9.

16. Phillips MA. Voluntary reporting of medication errors. Am J Health Syst Pharm. 2002;59:2326-8.

17. Barker KN, Flynn EA, Pepper GA. Observation method of detecting medication errors. Am J Health Syst Pharm. 2002;59:2314-6.

18. Barker KN, Mikeal RI, Pearson RE, Illig NA, Morse ML. Medication errors in nursing homes and small hospitals. Am J Hosp Pharm. 1982;39:987-91.

19. Jha AK, Kuperman GJ, Teich JM, Leape L, Shea B, Rittenberg E, et al. Identifying adverse drug events: development of a computer-based monitor and comparison with chart review and stimulated voluntary reporting. J Am Med Inform Assoc. 1998;3:305-14.

20. Classen DC, Pestotnik SL, Evans RS, Burke JP. Description of a computerized adverse drug event monitor using a hospital information system. Hosp Pharm. 1992;27:774, 776-9, 783.

21. Classen DC, Pestotnik SL, Evans RS, Burke JP. Computerized surveillance of adverse drug events in hospital patients (published erratum appears in JAMA. 1992;267:1992). JAMA. 1991;266:2847-51.

22. Gandhi TK, Bates DW. Chapter 8: Computer adverse drug event (ADE) detection and alerts [Internet]. Available at: http://archive.ahrq.gov/clinic/ptsafety/chap8.htm

23. VHA, Inc. Monitoring adverse drug events: finding the needles in the haystack. Vol. 9. Irving (TX): VHA; 2002. VHA 2002 Research Series.

24. Raschke RA, Gollihare B, Wunderlich TA, Guidry J, Leibowitz A, Peirce, J, et al. A computer alert system to prevent injury from adverse drug events: development and evaluation in a community teaching hospital (published erratum appears in JAMA 1999;281:420J). JAMA. 1998;280:1317-20.

25. Bates DW, Evans RS, Murff H, Stetson PD, Pizziferri L, Hripcsak G. Detecting adverse events using information technology. J Am Med Inform Assoc. 2003;10:115-28.

26. Bates DW. Using information technology to screen for adverse drug events. Am J Health Syst Pharm. 2002;59:2317-9.

27. Schneider PJ. Using technology to enhance measurement of drug-use safety. Am J Health Syst Pharm. 2002;59:2330-2.

28. Rozich JD, Haraden CR, Resar RK. Adverse drug event trigger tool: a practical methodology for measuring medication related harm. Qual Saf Health Care. 2008;12:194-200.

29. Rozich JD, Resar RK. Medication safety: one organization's approach to the challenge. J Clin Outcomes Manage. 2001;8(10):27-34.

30. Crea KA, Sherrin TP, Morehead D, Snow R. Reducing adverse drug events involving high-risk medications in acute care. J Clin Outcomes Manage. 2004;11(10):640-46.

31. The Patient Safety Act and Quality Improvement Act of 2005. Public Law 109-41, 109th Congress, July 29, 2005.

32. Pennsylvania Patient Safety Authority. Vol 6(4), December 2009.

33. ISMP Newsletter. Heparin errors continue despite prior, high-profile fatal events [Internet]. Available from: http://www.ismp.org/newsletters/acutecare/articles/20080717.asp

34. American Society of Hospital Pharmacists. ASHP guidelines on preventing medication errors in hospitals. Am J Hosp Pharm. 1993;50:305-14.

35. Patient Safety Organization Privacy Protection Center (PSO PPC) [Internet]. Available from: https://www.psoppc.org/web/patientsafety

36. Pepper GA. Errors in drug administration by nurses [Internet]. ASHP Online. 1999. [cited 1999 Sep 8]:[1 screen]. Available from: http://www.ashp.org/public/proad/mederror/pep.html

37. Dunn EB, Wolfe JJ. Medication error classification and avoidance. Hosp Pharm. 1997;32:860-5.

38. MedWatch: The FDA Medical Products Reporting Program. FDA Med Bull. 1993;23:insert.

39. The Joint Commission Sentinel Event Policy and Procedure [Internet]. Available from: http://www.jointcommission.org/Sentinel_Event_Policy_and_Procedures/.

40. Using aggregate root cause analysis to improve patient safety. Jt Comm J Qual Patient Saf. 2003 Aug;29(8):434-9.

41. Using aggregate root cause analysis to reduce falls. Jt Comm J Qual Patient Saf. 2005 Jan;31(1):21-31.

42. Bogner MS. Human error in medicine. Hillsdale (NJ): Lawrence Erlbaum Associates; 1994.

43. Senders JW. Theory and analysis of typical errors in a medical setting. Hosp Pharm. 1993;28:505-8.

44. Norman DA. The design of everyday things. New York: Basic Book; 1988.

45. Reason J. Human error. Cambridge, England: Cambridge University Press; 1990.

46. Reason J. Managing the risks of organizational accidents. Burlington (VT): Ashgate; 1997.

47. ISMP Newsletter. Inattentional blindness: what captures your attention? [Internet] Available from: http://www.ismp.org/Newsletters/acutecare/articles/20090226.asp

48. The Joint Commission (TJC). (2007). Sentinel events statistics, March 31, 2007 [Internet]. Available from: http://www.jointcommission.org/SentinelEvents/Statistics/.

49. Abood RR. Errors in pharmacy practice. US Pharm. 1996;21:122-32.

50. Coleman IC. Medication errors: picking up the pieces. Drug Top. 1999;143:83-92.

51. Glut of medication errors focuses pharmacists on event reporting. Drug Util Rev. 1998:201-6.

52. Cohen MR. ISMP medication error report analysis: the mistake of blaming people and not the process. Hosp Pharm. 1997;32:1106-11.

53. ISMP Newsletter. An injustice has been done: jail time given to pharmacist who made an error [Internet]. August 21, 2009. Available from: http://www.ismp.org/pressroom/injustice-jailtime-for-pharmacist.asp

54. ISMP Newsletter: Our long journey towards safety-minded just culture. Part I: Where we've been [Internet]. Available from: http://www.ismp.org/newsletters/acutecare/articles/20060907.asp

55. GAIN Working group E, Flight Ops/ATC Ops Safety Information Sharing. A roadmap to a Just Culture: enhancing the safety environment [Internet]. Available from: http://flightsafety.org/files/just_culture.pdf.

56. Grasha AF, O'Neill M. Cognitive processes in medication errors. US Pharm. 1996;21:96-109.

57. Ukens C. Breaking the trust: exclusive survey of dispensing errors. Drug Top. 1992;136:58-69.

58. DeMichele D. Preventing medication errors. US Pharm. 1995;20:69-75.

59. Davis NM. Lack of knowledge as a cause of medication errors. Hosp Pharm. 1997;32:16-25.

60. Fitzgerald WL, Wilson DB. Medication errors: lessons in law. Drug Top. 1998;142:84-93.

61. Institute of medicine, crossing the quality chasm. Washington, DC: National Academy Press; 2001.

62. Institute of Medicine. Health professions education: a bridge to quality. Washington, DC: National Academy Press; 2003.

63. Institute for Healthcare Improvement—Open School [Internet]. Available from: http://www.ihi.org/education/ihiopenschool/Pages/default.aspx

64. Grout J. Mistake-proofing the design of health care processes. Rockville, MD, AHRQ Publication No. 07-0020, 2007.

65. Grissinger M. The virtues of independent double checks: they really are worth your time! P&T. 2006;31:9.

66. Using aggregate root cause analysis to improve patient safety. Jt Comm J Qual Patient Saf. 2003 Aug;29(8):434-39.

67. Using aggregate root cause analysis to reduce falls. Jt Comm J Qual Patient Saf. 2005 Jan;31(1):21-31.

SUGGESTED READINGS

1. Gandhi TK, Weingart SN, Borus J, Seger A, Peterson J, Burdick E, et al. Adverse drug events in ambulatory care. N Engl J Med. 2003;348:1556-64.

2. Rozich JD, Haraden CR, Resar RK. Adverse drug event trigger tool: a practical methodology for measuring medication related harm. Qual Saf Health Care. 2008;12:194-200.

3. Jha AK, Kuperman GJ, Teich JM, Leape L, Shea B, Rittenberg E, et al. Identifying adverse drug events: development of a computer-based monitor and comparison with chart review and stimulated voluntary reporting. J Am Med Inform Assoc. 1998;3:305-14.

4. Howard R, Avery A, Bissell P. Causes of preventable drug-related hospital admissions: a qualitative study. Qual Saf Health Care. 2008;17:109-16.
5. Kale A, Keohane CA, Maviglia S, Gandhi TK, Poon EG. Adverse drug events caused by serious medication administration errors. BMJ Qual Saf. 2012;21:933-8.
6. Bagian JP, Gosbee J, Lee CZ, Williams L, McKnight SD, Mannos DM. The Veterans Affairs root cause analysis system in action. Jt Comm J Qual Improv. 2002;28:531-45.
7. Smetzer J, Baker C, Byrne FD, Cohen MR. Shaping systems for better behavioral choices: lessons learned from a fatal medication error. Jt Comm J Qual Patient Saf. 2010 Apr;36(4):152-63.

17

Chapter Seventeen

Investigational Drugs

Bambi Grilley

Learning Objectives

● *After completing this chapter, the reader will be able to*

- List the major legislative acts that led to the current system of drug evaluation, approval, and regulation used in the United States (U.S.).
- List the steps in the drug approval process.
- List the components of an investigational new drug application (IND).
- Recognize the difference between a commercial IND, a treatment IND, an emergency use IND, and an individual investigator IND.
- Define orphan drug status and list the advantages of classifying a drug as an orphan drug.
- List all of the requirements (as specified by the Office of Human Research Protections [OHRP]) for an institutional review board (IRB).
- Prepare appropriate reviews of protocols for use by the IRB or other review committees when they evaluate new protocols.
- Describe the type of support that is necessary for clinical research, including (but not limited to):
  a. Ordering drug supplies for ongoing clinical trials
  b. Maintaining drug accountability records as required by the Food and Drug Administration (FDA)
  c. Preparing drug and protocol data sheets for use by health care personnel in the hospital
  d. Preparing pharmacy budgets for sponsored clinical research
  e. Aiding investigators in designing and conducting clinical trials in their institution
  f. Assisting investigators in initiating and conducting clinical trials (including emergency use INDs)

Key Concepts

1 The Food and Drug Administration (FDA) is the federal agency that decides which drugs, biologics, and medical devices are safe and effective and, therefore, can be marketed in the United States.

2 In addition to review by the FDA, research protocols are also reviewed for ethical appropriateness by IRBs.

3 The drug approval process in the United States is standardized by FDA review. It consists of preclinical testing and Phase I through IV of clinical testing.

4 The investigational new drug application (IND) is the application by the study sponsor to the FDA to begin clinical trials in humans.

5 The IND should be amended as necessary. The four types of documents used to amend the IND include:

   a. Protocol amendments
   b. Information amendments
   c. IND safety reports
   d. IND annual reports

6 After sufficient evidence is obtained regarding the drug's safety and effectiveness, the sponsor will submit a new drug application/biologics licensing application to the FDA requesting approval of the agent for marketing.

7 The FDA allows the manufacturer to charge for an investigational drug under certain conditions.

8 An orphan drug is one that is used for the treatment of a rare disease, affecting fewer than 200,000 people in the United States, or one that will not generate enough revenue to justify the cost of research and development.

9 Drug accountability records are mandated by law. They can be computerized or in paper form. Necessary components include:

   a. Transaction date
   b. Transaction type
   c. The receiving party (for patient dispensing this should include patient initials/ identifying number)
   d. The dose/number of units dispensed/received
   e. The lot number dispensed/received
   f. The initials of the person who performed the transaction

Introduction

It is estimated that $802 million is spent to get a new drug product to market in the United States.[1,2] Although there is some controversy surrounding these estimates, more recent research indicates this number may be even higher, costing on average $868 million and ranging from $500 million to more than $2 billion.[3,4] Previous data have indicated that for every 4000 products synthesized in the lab, only five will ever be tested in humans and only one of those will ever reach the market.[5] Currently the Pharmaceutical Research and Manufacturers of America (PhRMA) database is tracking 2900 new medicines in development with more than $49 billion invested in research and development (R&D) in 2011.[6] This should be compared to 35 novel drugs approved by the Food and Drug Administration (FDA) in 2012.[7] ❶ *The FDA is the federal agency that decides which drugs, biologics, and medical devices are marketed in the United States.* In fact, the FDA monitors the manufacture, import, transport, storage, and sale of $1 trillion worth of goods annually.[8] The centers of the FDA involved in regulating drugs, biologics, and medical devices used in humans are as follows:

- Center for Biologics Evaluation and Research (CBER)
- Center for Drug Evaluation and Research (CDER)
- Center for Devices and Radiological Health (CDRH)[9]

Since this book deals with drug related information, this chapter will concentrate only on the regulations associated with CBER and CDER.

Since 1940, more than a 1000 new molecular entities (NMEs) have been approved in the United States.[10] It is very important that the clinical trials upon which the FDA will base their decisions be both scientifically accurate and complete. Pharmacists can play an important role in ensuring that the clinical trials conducted at their institutions meet the goals set forth by the study sponsor, the local investigator, and ultimately the FDA.

Currently, most research conducted on investigational drugs is performed in medical schools, hospitals, and organizations specifically designed to conduct clinical research trials. In some institutions, a pharmacist will be hired specifically to handle investigational drugs. More frequently, however, this role falls to other health care providers. To successfully manage investigational drugs, this individual or team of individuals must be a bookkeeper, inventory control manager, and, most importantly, an information disseminator. Before proceeding, it is necessary to define a number of terms that will be used in this chapter.

Definitions

Biologics license application (BLA): A biologics license application is a submission that contains specific information on the manufacturing processes, chemistry, pharmacology, clinical pharmacology, and the medical effects of the biologic product. It is a request for permission to introduce, or deliver for introduction, a biologic product into interstate commerce.[11]

Clinical investigation: Any experiment in which a drug is administered or dispensed to one or more human subjects. An experiment is any use of a drug (except for the use of a marketed drug) in the course of medical practice. Although there are many other definitions, this is the FDA's definition and would seem the appropriate one to use given the nature of this topic. Please note that the FDA does not regulate the practice of medicine and prescribers are (as far as the agency is concerned) free to use any marketed drug for off-label use.[12]

Commercial IND: An IND for which the sponsor is usually either a corporate entity or one of the institutes of the National Institutes of Health (NIH). In addition, CDER may designate other INDs as commercial, if it is clear the sponsor intends the product to be commercialized at a later date.[13]

Control group: The group of test animals or humans that receive a placebo (a dosage that does not contain active medicine) or active (a dosage that does contain active medicine) treatment. For most preclinical and clinical trials, the FDA will require that this group receive placebo (commonly referred to as the placebo control). However, some studies may have an active control, which generally consists of an available (standard of care) treatment modality. An active control may, with the concurrence of the FDA, be used in studies where it would be considered unethical to use a placebo. A historical control is one in which a group of previous patients is compared to a matched set of patients receiving the new therapy. A historical control might be used in cases where the disease is consistently fatal (i.e., acquired immunodeficiency syndrome [AIDS]). (Refer to Chapter 4 for additional information on control groups.)[14]

Contract research organization (CRO): An individual or organization that assumes one or more of the obligations of the sponsor through an independent contractual agreement.[12]

Drug master file (DMF): A submission to the FDA that may be used to provide confidential detailed information about facilities, processes, or articles used in the manufacturing, processing, packaging, and storing of one or more human drugs.[15]

Drug product: The final dosage form prepared from the drug substance.[16]

Drug substance: An active ingredient that is intended to furnish pharmacological activity or other direct effect in the diagnosis, cure, mitigation, treatment, or prevention of disease or to affect the structure or any function of the human body.[16]

Food and Drug Administration (FDA): The agency of the U.S. government that is responsible for ensuring the safety and efficacy of all drugs on the market in the United States.[8]

Good clinical practice (GCP): A standard for the design, conduct, monitoring, analyses, and reporting of clinical trials that provides assurance that the results are credible and accurate, and that the rights of study subjects are protected.[17]

Institutional review board (IRB): A committee of reviewers that evaluates the ethical implications of a clinical study protocol.[18,19]

Investigational new drug: A drug, antibiotic, or biologic that is used in a clinical investigation. The label of an investigational drug must bear the statement: "Caution: New Drug—Limited by Federal (or U.S.) law to investigational use."[12]

Investigational new drug application (IND): A submission to the FDA containing chemical information, preclinical data, and a detailed description of the planned clinical trials. Thirty days after submission of this document to the FDA by the sponsor, clinical trials may be initiated in humans, unless the FDA places a clinical hold. When the FDA allows the studies to proceed, this document allows unapproved drugs to be shipped in interstate commerce.[12]

Investigator: The individual responsible for initiating the clinical trial at the study site. This individual must treat the patients, ensure that the protocol is followed, evaluate responses and adverse reactions, ensure proper conduct of the study, and solve problems as they arise.[12]

New drug application (NDA): The application to the FDA requesting approval to market a new drug for human use. The NDA contains data supporting the safety and efficacy of the drug for its intended use.[12,16]

New molecular entity (NME): A compound that can be patented and has not been previously marketed in the United States in any form.[20]

Regulatory project manager (RPM): This will be the sponsor's (see below) primary FDA contact person. Each application that is submitted is assigned a regulatory project manager (RPM). Contact information for the RPM is provided in the letter sent to the applicant acknowledging receipt of the application. If the RPM is changed during the course of the review, the applicant is notified by the new RPM.[21]

Sponsor: An organization (or individual) who takes responsibility for and initiates a clinical investigation. The sponsor may be an individual or pharmaceutical company, government agency, academic institution, private organization, or other organization.[12]

Sponsor-investigator: An individual who both initiates and conducts a clinical investigation (i.e., submits the IND and directly supervises administration of the drug as well as other investigator responsibilities).[12]

Subject: An individual who participates in a clinical investigation (either as the recipient of the investigational drug or as a member of the control group).[12]

History of Drug Development Regulation in the United States

For more than a century after the Declaration of Independence, drug products were not regulated in the United States. Available drugs were often ineffective, but some were addictive, toxic, or even lethal. During this same period, physicians were not licensed and nearly anyone could practice medicine. The public was, for the most part, responsible for using common sense when evaluating which products they would use.

The evolution of drug regulations in this country is a study in human tragedy. Crises have instigated the development of many of the laws regulating drug development, preparation, and distribution.

The first federal law developed to deal with drug quality and safety was the Import Drug Act of 1848. This law was passed after it was discovered that American troops involved in the Mexican War had been supplied with substandard imported drugs. The act provided for the inspection, detention, and destruction or reexport of imported drug shipments that failed to meet prescribed standards.

The Pure Food and Drugs Act was passed in 1906. This law required that drugs not be mislabeled or adulterated and stated that they must meet recognized standards for strength and purity. Mislabeling in this context only referred to the identity or composition of drugs (not false therapeutic claims). False therapeutic claims were prohibited with the passing of the Sherley Amendment in 1912.

In 1937, the drug sulfanilamide was released. This drug showed promise as an anti-infective agent and was prepared as an oral liquid. The vehicle used for this preparation was diethylene glycol (a sweet-tasting solvent similar to ethylene glycol, which was used as an automobile antifreeze). A total of 107 people died after taking this preparation. Within 1 year of this tragedy, the Food, Drug and Cosmetic Act of 1938 was enacted. This law required that the safety of drugs, when used in accordance with the labeled instructions, be proven through testing before they could be marketed. It was in this law that the submission of an NDA to the FDA was first described. The NDA was required to list the drug's intended uses and provide scientific evidence that the drug was safe. If after 60 days the FDA had not responded to the manufacturer regarding the NDA, the manufacturer was free to proceed with marketing of the product.

In 1951, the Durham–Humphrey Amendment was passed. This law divided pharmaceuticals into two distinct classes:

1. Over-the-counter (OTC) medications that could be safely self-administered.
2. Prescription (Rx) medications that had potentially dangerous side effects and, therefore, required expert medical supervision.

This law required the following statement be added to the labels for all prescription medications: "Caution: Federal Law prohibits dispensing without a prescription."

In 1962, another drug tragedy occurred that resulted in additional regulations. In that year, an inordinate number of pregnant women in Western Europe gave birth to children with severe deformities. These deformities were related to the use of the drug thalidomide. Although U.S. consumers were not directly affected by this tragedy, because thalidomide had not been released in the U.S. market, it was a compelling reason for the legislature to develop stronger laws regarding the testing of new drug products. The Kefauver–Harris Drug Amendment was passed the same year. This law specified that the manufacturer had to demonstrate proof of efficacy, as well as safety, prior to marketing any new drug. Additionally, this law required that drug manufacturers operate in conformity with Current Good Manufacturing Practices (CGMP). Finally, it stated that the FDA had to formally approve an NDA before the drug could be marketed.[22]

There are numerous other laws and regulations that affect drug products in the United States, but those mentioned above provide the legal foundation for the current regulation of drug products in the United States. Based on these laws, the FDA has assumed a large role in assessing the safety and efficacy of drug products prior to their distribution in the United States.

❶ *As stated, the goal of the FDA is to provide American consumers with safe and effective drugs, biologics, and devices.*[8] Extensive debate regarding the need to reform the FDA has been ongoing in the United States for years. Critics of the FDA have long claimed that the approval process for drugs in the United States is too costly and time consuming.[23,24] Interestingly, however, data show that the FDA leads the world in the first introduction of new active substances. Using data from fiscal year (FY) 2012, of the 32 novel drugs approved by the FDA and also approved in other countries, 75% of those drugs were approved by the FDA first.[7] Nevertheless, over the past two decades, the FDA and the federal government have initiated many reforms and initiatives designed to address these criticisms. Included in these reform acts are the Prescription Drug User Fee Act of 1992 (PDUFA), which was reauthorized in 1997 and 2002, and the Food and Drug Administration Modernization Act of 1997 (FDAMA). PDUFA redefined the timeframes for NDA reviews and established revenues to fund the increased demands created by the new timeframes.[20] The FDAMA, which reauthorized PDUFA in 1997, was much broader in scope and impacted not only the drug approval process, but also other aspects of the practices of pharmacy and medicine.[25] The Food and Drug Administration Amendments Act (FDAAA), which was signed into law in 2007, further expanded PDUFA to provide the FDA with additional resources to conduct timely and comprehensive reviews of new drugs in the United States.[26]

Aside from looking at review times, the FDA has also been concerned about the increasing difficulty in drug and biologic development. To attempt to address this issue, the FDA launched a new initiative in March 2004 called the Critical Path Initiative. The Critical Path Initiative is the FDA's attempt to facilitate modernization of the sciences and improve regulatory decision making. They have been working with the public, the pharmaceutical industry, other regulatory agencies, and academia to identify projects they feel are most likely to help the drug development process from test tube to bedside.[27]

Finally, the FDA has undertaken many information technology initiatives to facilitate the regulatory review process. Included in these initiatives is the development of systems allowing for electronic submission, management, and review of regulatory information.[28] Overall, the goal of the initiatives is to review priority drugs in 6 months and standard drugs within 10 months.[29] Other attempts by the FDA to increase availability of investigational drugs to patients will be discussed later in this chapter.

First initiated in response to components of FDAMA, the National Institutes of Health (NIH) developed a Web-based system that offers information about ongoing clinical trials for a wide range of diseases and conditions. The system allows potential study subjects to search for studies for particular diseases and identify treatment centers that offer enrollment into those studies. Requirements for postings have become more stringent over the past 5 years.[30] Most recently, in 2007 FDAAA required more types of trials to be registered, additional trial registration information, and submission of summary results including adverse events for certain trials.[26] The site is available at http://clinicaltrials.gov. Study sponsors are required to verify that the study is posted on the ClinicalTrials.gov Web site as part of the IND submission process through submission of a Form 3674.[31]

Increasingly, drug companies are involved in global drug development. Historically, the regulatory requirements for drug approval varied from country to country, resulting in a significant amount of time and money being spent to receive multiple approvals. For this reason, the International Conference on Harmonization (ICH) has brought together officials from Europe, the United States, and Japan to develop common guidelines for ensuring the quality, safety, and efficacy of drugs. The FDA has been very involved in the development of the ICH guidelines. The ultimate goal of these guidelines is to provide pharmaceutical firms a method to ensure simultaneous submission and rapid regulatory approval in the world's major markets. This would minimize duplication of effort, improve efficiency, and increase the quality and consistency of medical treatments available to patients worldwide.[32]

For gene therapy products, review and approval by the National Institutes of Health Office of Biotechnology Activities (NIH/OBA) and local Institutional Biosafety Committee(s) are required in addition to review and approval by the FDA and IRB (discussed below). Submission requirements for the NIH/OBA are similar to those mandated by the FDA (covered later in this chapter). The review process for gene therapy products is a separate topic that will not be further addressed in this chapter. Individuals interested in regulatory requirements of gene therapy products can refer to review articles such as

"Gene Transfer: Regulatory Issues and Their Impact on the Clinical Investigator and the GMP facility" published in *Cytotherapy* in 2003.[33]

❷ *In addition to the regulatory review of investigational drugs by the FDA, research protocols are also reviewed for ethical appropriateness by IRBs.* The formalized process for protecting human subjects began with the Nuremberg Code. This code was used to judge the human experimentation conducted by the Nazis around the middle of the twentieth century. The Nuremberg Code states that "the voluntary consent of the human subjects is absolutely essential." The code goes on to specify that the subject must have the capacity to consent, must be free from coercion, and must comprehend the risks and benefits involved in the research.[34] The Declaration of Helsinki reemphasized the above points and distinguished between therapeutic and nontherapeutic research. This document was first developed in 1964 and has been revised multiple times, most recently in 2008.[35]

The NIH, as part of the Department of Health and Human Services (DHHS), used these two documents to develop its own policies for the Protection of Human Subjects in 1966. These policies were raised to regulatory status in 1974 and established the IRB as a mechanism through which human subjects would be protected. The Belmont Report, released in 1978, further delineates the basic ethical principles underlying medical research on human subjects.[36] Title 45 Part 46 of the Code of Federal Regulations (CFR), which was released in 1981, was designed to make uniform the protection of human subjects in all federal agencies.[18] Title 21 Part 50 (approved in 1980) of the CFR sets forth guidelines for appropriate informed consent and Title 21 Part 56 (approved in 1981) of the CFR sets forth guidelines for the IRB.[19,37] Copies of these regulations can be obtained on the Internet at http://www.gpoaccess.gov/cfr/index.html

These two documents are used by the FDA and the DHHS to evaluate the ethical conduct of clinical trials in the United States. Further information regarding the role of the IRB will be presented later in this chapter.

The Drug Approval Process

❸ₐ *The drug approval process in the United States is standardized by FDA review. It consists of preclinical testing and Phase I-IV of clinical testing.* The first step in the drug approval process is preclinical testing. This testing is conducted either *in vitro* or in animals. Before filing an IND, the sponsor must have developed a pharmacologic profile of the drug, determined its acute and subacute toxicity, and have sufficient information regarding chronic toxicity to support the drug's use in humans.[38]

After the preclinical testing is completed, the sponsor will file an IND with the FDA. ❹ *The IND is the application by the study sponsor to the FDA to begin clinical trials in humans.* Most often, the sponsor is a pharmaceutical company, but occasionally an individual investigator will file an IND and serve as a sponsor-investigator. An investigator IND is submitted when a physician plans to use an approved drug for a new indication (i.e., one that is outside the package labeling) or on occasion, for an unapproved product or for an NME. The IND requirements for the sponsor-investigator are the same as those for any other sponsor. For that reason, no differentiation will be made in the following discussion of the drug approval process.

An IND is not required if the drug to be studied is marketed in the United States and all of the following requirements are met:

1. The study is not to be reported to the FDA in support of a new indication.

2. The study does not involve a different dose, route, or patient population that increases the risk to patients.

3. IRB approval and informed consent are secured.

4. The study will not be used to promote the drug's effectiveness for a new indication.

The FDA has developed a guidance document specifically to assist in determining whether or not an IND is required. However, in situations where it is unclear whether an IND is required or not, a call to the FDA is the best way to determine the appropriate way to proceed.[39]

In recent years there have been several therapeutic products developed that depend on the use of an *in vitro* companion diagnostic device (or test) for its safe and effective use. It is important to note that in this situtation, the *in vitro* device should be approved or cleared concurrently by FDA for the use indicated in the therapeutic **product labeling**. To be clear, this might require the study of the diagntic device under an **investigational device exemption (IDE)** while the therapeutic product is being studied under an IND. If the diagnostic device and therapeutic product are to be studied together to support their respective approvals (or clearance in the case of a device) both products can be studied in the same investigational study if the study has been developed and conducted in a manner that meets both IND and IDE regulations.[40] One other interesting issue related to devices is the use of a mobile app (i.e., a software application on a mobile platform such as an iPhone, Android, Windows tablet, or BlackBerry) for the diagnosis of disease, or the cure, mitigation, treatment or prevention of disease or to affect the structure of function of the body. In these situations, the mobile app can be considered to be a medical device subject to IDE regulations.[41] IDE regulations and components will not be further discussed in this chapter; however, the applicable regulations can be found in 21CFR812 and the FDA has extensive guidance regarding these products and their development.

- An IND application needs to contain the following information:

1. Cover sheet: Form 1571 (available at the FDA Web site under Forms, http://www .fda.gov/AboutFDA/ReportsManualsForms/Forms/default.htm). This form identifies the sponsor, documents that the sponsor agrees to follow appropriate regulations, and identifies any involved CRO. This is a legal document.
2. Table of contents
3. Introductory statement: States the name, structure, pharmacologic class, dosage form, and all active ingredients in the investigational drug; the objectives and planned duration of the investigation should be stated here.
4. General investigational plan: Describes the rationale, indications, and general approach for evaluating the drug, the types of trials to be conducted, the projected number of patients that will be treated, and any potential safety concerns; the purpose of this section is to give FDA reviewers a general overview of the plan to study the drug.
5. Investigator's brochure: An information packet containing all available information on the drug including its formula, pharmacologic and toxicologic effects, pharmacokinetics, and any information regarding the safety and risks associated with the drug. It is important that this brochure be kept current and comprehensive; therefore, it should be amended as necessary. The investigator's brochure may be used by the investigator or other health care professionals as a reference during the conduct of the research study.
6. Clinical protocol
   - *Objectives and purpose:* A description of the purpose of the trial (a typical Phase I objective would be to determine the maximum tolerated dose of the investigational drug, whereas a typical Phase III objective would be to compare the safety and efficacy of the investigational drug to placebo or standard therapy).
   - *Investigator data:* Provides qualifications and demographic data of the investigators involved in the clinical trial (may be presented on form 1572 (available at the FDA Web site under Forms, http://www.fda.gov/AboutFDA/ ReportsManualsForms/Forms/default.htm).
   - *Patient selection:* Describes the characteristics of patients that are eligible for enrollment in the trial and states factors that would exclude the patient.
   - *Study design:* Describes how the study will be completed; if the study is to be randomized, this will be described here with a description of the alternate therapy.
   - *Dose determination:* Describes the dose (with possible adjustments) and route of administration of the investigational drug; if retreatment or maintenance therapy of patients is allowed, it will be detailed in this section.
   - *Observations:* Describes how the objectives stated earlier in the protocol are to be assessed.

- *Clinical procedures:* Describes all laboratory tests or clinical procedures that will be used to monitor the effects of the drug in the patient; the collection of this data is intended to minimize the risk to the patients.
- *IRB approval for protocol:* Documentation of this approval is not required as part of the IND application process; however, form 1571 does state that an IRB will review and approve each study in the proposed clinical investigation before allowing initiation of those studies.

7. Chemistry, manufacturing, and control data
   - *Drug substance:* Describes the drug substance including its name, biological, physical, and chemical characteristics; the address of the manufacturer; the method of synthesis or preparation; and the analytical methods used to ensure purity, identity, and the substance's stability.
   - *Drug product:* Describes the drug product including all of its components; the address of the manufacturer; the analytical methods used to ensure identity, quality, purity, and strength of the product; and the product's stability.
   - *Composition, manufacture, and control of any placebo used in the trial:* The FDA does not require that the placebo be identical to the investigational drug; however, it wants to ensure that the lack of similarity does not jeopardize the trial.
   - *Labeling:* Copies of all labels and labeling used for the drug substance or product, and packages as it will be provided to each investigator. Labels in this context meaning the information affixed to product and used to identify the contents while labeling in this context relates to product information including prescribing information.
   - *Environmental assessment:* Presents a claim for categorical exclusion from the requirement for an environmental assessment (a statement that the amount of waste expected to reach the environment may reasonably be expected to be nontoxic).

8. Pharmacology and toxicology data
   - *Pharmacology and drug disposition:* Describes the pharmacology, mechanism of action, absorption, distribution, metabolism, and excretion of the drug in animals and *in vitro*.
   - *Toxicology:* Describes the toxicology in animals and *in vitro*.
   - A statement that all nonclinical laboratories involved in the research adhered to Good Laboratory Practice (GLP) regulations.

9. Previous human experience: Summary of human experiences, which includes data from the United States and, where applicable, foreign markets. Known safety and efficacy data should be presented (especially if the drug was withdrawn from foreign markets for reasons of safety or efficacy).

10. Additional information: Other information that would help the reviewer evaluate the proposed clinical trial should be included here. For example, if a drug has the

potential for abuse, data on the drug's dependence and abuse potential should be discussed in this section.[38]

The letter of authorization (LOA) to cross reference a drug master file, investigational new drug application, or new drug application (referred to in item nine on page one of Form 1571) is required when the investigational product (or some component of the investigational product) being used in the research is being supplied by a manufacturer other than the study sponsor. The original holder of the IND/NDA/DMF prepares the LOA. An LOA is frequently required when two companies are working together toward development of a product.[42]

● *The IND should be amended as necessary. There are four types of documents that may be used to amend the IND. They are as follows:*

1. Protocol amendments: Submitted when a sponsor wants to change a previously submitted protocol or add a new study protocol to an existing IND.[43]
2. Information amendments: Submitted when information becomes available that would not be presented using a protocol amendment, IND safety report, or annual report (example: new chemistry data).[44]
3. IND safety reports: Reports clinical and animal adverse reactions; reporting requirements depend on the nature, severity, and frequency of the experience. The following definitions are used to help evaluate adverse reactions.
   * *Suspected adverse reaction:* An adverse reaction for which there is evidence to suggest a causal relationship between the drug and the adverse event.
   * *Serious adverse event or serious suspected adverse reaction:* An event that results in any of the following outcomes: death, a life-threatening adverse drug experience, inpatient hospitalization or prolongation of existing hospitalization, a persistent or significant disability/incapacity, or a congenital anomaly/birth defect. Important medical events that may not result in death, be life-threatening, or require hospitalization may be considered a serious adverse drug experience when, based on appropriate medical judgment, they may jeopardize the patient or subject and may require medical or surgical intervention to prevent one of the outcomes listed in this definition.
   * *Unexpected adverse event or unexpected suspected adverse reaction:* An adverse reaction that is not listed in the current labeling for the drug product. This includes events that may be symptomatically and pathophysiologically related to an event listed in the labeling, but differs from the event because of greater severity or specificity.

For serious and unexpected, fatal, or life-threatening suspected adverse reactions, the sponsor is required to notify the FDA by telephone or fax within 7 calendar days after the sponsor receives the information. The sponsor must also submit a written report within 15 calendar days. For clinical and non-clinical adverse reactions that are both serious and unexpected, the sponsor must notify the FDA in writing within 15 calendar days. The written reports should describe the current adverse event and identify all previously filed safety reports concerning similar adverse events. The written report may be submitted as a narrative or as Form 3500A.[45,46]

4. Annual reports: Submitted within 60 days of the annual effective date of an IND; it should describe the progress of the investigation including information on the individual studies, summary information of the IND (summary of adverse experiences, IND safety reports, preclinical studies completed in the last year), relevant developments in foreign markets, and changes in the investigator's brochure.[47]

Each submission to a specific IND is required to be numbered sequentially (starting with 000). A total of three sets (the original and two copies) of all submissions to an IND file (whether a new IND or revisions to an existing IND) are sent to the FDA.[38]

Once submitted to the FDA, the IND will be forwarded to the appropriate review division based on the therapeutic category of the product. Examples of the different divisions include oncology products, hematology products, anti-infective products, and medical imaging products. Following submission, the IND and clinical trial will be assigned to a review team that includes:

- The project manager
- A chemistry, manufacturing, and controls (CMC) reviewer
- A nonclinical pharmacology/toxicology reviewer
- A clinical reviewer and
- Other reviewers as needed (e.g., statisticians, epidemiologists, site inspectors, patient representatives)[21]

The FDA has 30 days after receipt of an IND to respond to the sponsor. The sponsor may begin clinical trials if there is no response from the FDA within 30 days.[48] The FDA delays initiation of a new study or discontinues an ongoing study by issuing a clinical hold. Clinical holds are most often used when the FDA identifies an issue (through initial review or through later submissions) that the agency feels poses a significant risk to the subjects. After this issue has been satisfactorily resolved, the clinical hold can be removed and the investigations can be initiated or resumed.[49]

3b *There are four phases of clinical trials.* Clinical studies generally begin cautiously. As experience with the agent grows, the dose and duration of exposure to the agent may also increase. The number of patients treated at each phase of study and the duration of the studies can vary significantly depending on statistical considerations, the prevalence of patients affected by the disease, and the importance of the new drug. However, some general guidelines regarding the four phases of clinical testing are presented below.

A Phase I trial is the first use of the agent in humans. As such, these studies are usually initiated with cautious (low) doses and in a small numbers of subjects. Doses may be increased as safety is established. A Phase I study will usually treat 20 to 80 patients and last an average of 6 months to 1 year. The purpose of a Phase I trial is to determine the safety and toxicity of the agent. Frequently these trials include a pharmacokinetic portion. These trials assist in identifying the preferred route of administration and a safe dosage range. When possible, these trials are initiated in normal, healthy volunteers. This allows for evaluation of the effect of the drug on a subject who does not have any preexisting conditions. In situations in which this is not practical, such as oncology drugs, in which the drug itself can be highly toxic, these drugs are usually reserved for patients who have exhausted all conventional options.

A Phase II trial is one in which the drug is used in a small number of subjects who suffer from the disease or condition that the drug is proposed to treat. The purpose of a Phase II trial is to evaluate the efficacy of the agent. Data from the Phase I trial, *in vitro* testing, and animal testing may be used to identify which group of patients is most likely to benefit from therapy with this agent. Phase II trials usually treat between 100 and 200 patients and will average about 2 years in duration. Following Phase II trials study sponsors will frequently assess these preliminary results and predicted marketability of the product prior to initiating the larger and more expensive Phase III trials.

Phase III trials build on the experience gained during the Phase II trials. The purpose of a Phase III study is to further define the efficacy and safety of the agent. Frequently, in Phase III studies, the new agent is compared to current therapy. These trials are usually multicenter studies, generally treat from 600 to 1000 patients, and usually last about 3 years. Some of the Phase III trials will be pivotal studies and will serve as the basis for the NDA/BLA for a medicinal product's marketing approval.[50]

One interesting scientific advance in the area of drug development has been the impact of pharmacogenomics (PGx) on the field. PGx is the study of variations of DNA and RNA characteristics as related to drug response including effectiveness and adverse effects. As such, PGx can contribute to evaluation of interindividual differences in the response to drugs. The FDA is encouraging study sponsors to include PGx in early stage studies to assist in areas such as identify populations that should receive a lower or higher dose of a drug; identify potential responder populations; and identify groups at risk of serious adverse effects. An important prerequisite to use of PGx in drug development is collection and storage of DNA samples from all clinical trials. Ideally, sample collection should be collected at the time of study enrollment/at baseline in order to avoid bias related to subjects who do not complete the study. At the time of drug approval, information gained from PGx studies would be included in the product labeling to inform prescribers of the impact of a certain genotype or phenotype relative to response or adverse events. Similar approaches should be considered for proteomic (scientific analysis of proteins) and metabolomic evaluations (scientific analysis of the chemical processes involving metabolites).[51]

Case Study 17–1

Company CaCure (not a real company) has developed a drug called ALLCure. The product is approved as an intravenous product used to treat severe headaches. Dr. Smith has conducted preclinical laboratory work that indicates that when given intrahepatically the product can cause shrinkage of liver metastases.

Dr. Smith wants to try to use this ALLCure in 10 patients with cancer that is metastatic to the liver and see if the results hold true in humans.

- *Does Dr. Smith or ALLCure need approval from the FDA to transition this work into patients?*

❻ *After Phase III trials have been completed, the sponsor will submit an NDA/BLA to the FDA requesting approval of the medicinal product for marketing.* The FDA requires the completion of two well-designed, controlled clinical trials prior to submission to the FDA. However, the sponsor will include information gathered from all of the clinical trials to show that the medicinal product is safe and effective and to describe the pharmacology and pharmacokinetics of the drug. The NDA/BLA will include all preclinical data, clinical data, manufacturing methods, product quality assurance, relevant foreign clinical testing (or marketing experience), and all published reports of experience with the medicinal agent (whether sponsored by the company or not). A proposed package insert will be supplied as well.[52]

The NDA/BLA will be distributed to the same FDA review division assigned while the product was under IND status. As noted, these divisions are based on the therapeutic group of the medicinal agent. The same reviewer may be assigned to review the IND and the NDA/BLA.[21]

The speed at which the NDA will be processed is to some extent determined by the classification the drug receives during its initial review. Each agent is rated with a number–letter designation that evaluates two separate aspects of the agent. The number portion of the rating is associated with the uniqueness of the drug product (ranging from 1 for an NME to 7 for a drug that has already been marketed, but without an approved NDA/BLA—see Table 13–1). The letter portion of the rating is associated with the therapeutic potential of the medicinal agent. The P (priority review) designation is given to drugs that represent a therapeutic advance with respect to available therapy, whereas an S (standard review) is given to drugs that have little or no therapeutic gain over previously available drugs—see Table 13–2. BLA prioritization is slightly simplified but similar.[53]

During the review process, the FDA may utilize one of its prescription drug advisory committees to help review the NDA. These committees are composed of experts who provide the agency with independent, nonbinding advice and recommendations regarding the NDA. Currently the FDA has 33 advisory committees many of which are composed of various panels. Examples of such committees include the allergenic products advisory committee and the blood products advisory committee.[53,54] Within 180 days of receipt of an NDA, the FDA will review the application and send the applicant an approval letter or a complete response letter.[55] When an approval letter is sent, the drug is considered approved as of the date of the letter.[56] A complete response letter is issued to let the sponsor know that the review period for the drug is complete but that the application is not yet ready for approval. It will describe specific deficiencies and, when possible, identify recommended actions that the sponsor might take to address those deficiencies. In response to the complete response letter, the sponsor amends the NDA, withdraws the NDA, or requests a hearing with the FDA to clarify whether grounds exist for denying approval of the application.[57]

As mentioned previously in this chapter, the FDA has been under considerable criticism relative to drug review times. They have implemented many initiatives to address these criticisms. The most recent initiative implemented by the FDA is referred to as "Expanded Access to Investigational Drugs for Treatment Use." The expanded access rule clarifies exising regulations and adds new types of expanded access for treatment use. Specifically, the rule allows for investigational drugs to be used for treatment use in patients with serious or life-threatening diseases where there is no other comparable or satisfactory alternative therapy. The FDA defines immediately life-threatening conditions as those where death is likely to occur within a matter of months or in which premature death is likely without early treatment. Serious conditions are defined as those associated with morbidity that has substantial impact on day-to-day functioning.[58] The rules specify different requirements for expanded access for individual patients in emergencies; intermediate-size patient populations; and larger populations under a treatment protocol or treatment IND.[59]

The FDA must determine that in addition to the patient having a serious or immediately life-threatening disease for which there is no satisfactory alternative therapy, the potential patient benefit must outweigh the risk, and that the requested use will not interfere with clinical investigations that could support marketing approval of the expanded access use. In all cases, an expanded access submission to the FDA is required. The submission may be a new IND or a protocol amendment to an existing IND. Except as justified by emergency use guidelines further discussed below, all other regulations governing new INDs and protocol amendment including regulations regarding study initiation, adverse reaction reporting, and annual reports are identical to that described for standard INDs and described elsewhere in this chapter.[60]

For individual patients, submission requirements must include information adequate for the FDA to determine that the risk to the person from the investigational drug is not greater than the probable risk from the disease and that the patient cannot obtain the drug under another type of IND. Treatment is generally limited to a single course of therapy for a specified duration unless FDA expressly authorizes multiple courses or chronic therapy. In this type of submission, the FDA does allow for emergency procedures if the patient must be treated before a written submission can be made. In that situation, the FDA may authorize the emergency use by telephone. The sponsor must agree to submit an expanded access submission within 15 business days of the FDA's authorization of the use.[61] In addition, although the FDA must authorize emergency use of a test article (investigational drug), prospective IRB approval is not required.[62]

For intermediate patient populations there must be sufficient evidence that the drug is safe at the dose and duration proposed for treatment, and that there is at least preliminary clinical evidence of effectiveness of the drug. The sponsor must also indicate whether the drug is being developed and the patient population. If the drug is being studied in a clinical trial, the sponsor must explain why the expanded access patient population cannot be enrolled in the clinical trial and under what circumstances the sponsor would conduct a clinical trial in those patients.[63]

The treatment IND, or treatment protocol, is a way the FDA has allowed for increased accessibility of experimental drugs for widespread treatment use. The drug must be investigated in a clinical trial under an IND designed to support a marketing application for the expanded access use, or if all clinical trials have been completed, the sponsor must be actively pursuing marketing approval of the drug for the expanded access use. When the expanded access use is for an immediately life-threatening disease the available scientific evidence (usually clinical data from Phase II or Phase III trials) must provide reasonable assurance that the drug may be effective for the expanded access use and would not expose patients to significant risk.[64]

⑦ *The FDA allows for the manufacturer to charge for an investigational drug under certain conditions.* The sponsor must obtain prior written authorization from the FDA to charge for an investigational drug. In order to charge for an investigational drug, the sponsor must provide evidence that the drug has a potential clinical benefit that would provide a significant advantage over available products, demonstrate that the data to be obtained from the clinical trial would be essential to establishing that the drug is effective or safe, and demonstrate that the clinical trial could not be conducted without charging because the cost of the drug is extraordinary to the sponsor. The sponsor may only charge recovery costs for direct cost attributable to making the investigational drug, including raw materials, labor, nonreusable supplies, and equipment used to manufacture the drug or costs to acquire the drug from another manufacturer or to ship and handle the drug. In addition, for expanded access studies for intermediate-size patient populations or treatment IND/protocols a sponsor may recover the cost of monitoring the expanded access IND or protocol, complying with IND reporting requirements, and other administrative costs directly associated with the expanded access IND.[65-67]

The FDA has also attempted to expedite the review process for new drugs in three ways:

1. Priority review: CDER determines a drug will potentially provide a significant advance in medical care and sets a target to review the drug within 6 months instead of the standard 10 months.
2. Fast track review: CDER determines that a drug can treat unmet medical needs. Fast Track speeds new drug reviews, for instance, by increasing the level of communication the FDA allocates to developers and by enabling developers to use a rolling review process such that CDER can review portions of an application ahead of the submission of the full application.
3. Accelerated approval program: Allows for early approval of a drug for serious or life-threatening illness that offers a benefit over current treatments. This approval is based on a surrogate endpoint (e.g., a laboratory measure) or other clinical measure that FDA considers reasonably likely to predict clinical benefit. After this approval, the drug must undergo additional testing to confirm the benefit.[7]

After the drug has been approved, postmarketing studies may be initiated. They are conducted for the approved indication, but may evaluate different doses, the effects of extended therapy, or the drug's safety in patient populations that were not represented in premarketing clinical trials. ③c *The final phase of clinical study is referred to as Phase IV trials.* These Phase IV trials may be requested by the FDA or they may be initiated by the sponsor in an attempt to gather more data on the safety and efficacy of the drug or to identify a competitive advantage of the drug over other available therapies.[68] In some situations, the FDA may actually approve a product with restrictions limiting the facilities or physicians where the product may be used, or limiting the patient population to only those who have demonstrated certain performance on specified medical procedures.[69] Specifically, the FDA has started to utilize risk evaluation and mitigation strategies (REMS) when they determine that safety measures are needed beyond the labeling to ensure that a drug's benefits outweigh its risks. REMS can be required before or after a drug is approved. REMS are developed by drug sponsors; however, the

FDA reviews and approves them. Factors that are considered in determining the need for an REMS include:

- Size of the population likely to use the drug
- Seriousness of the disease
- Expected benefits
- Expected duration of treatment
- Seriousness of adverse events (known or potential)
- Whether the drug is an NME[50]

The REMS may include the following components: a medication guide (or patient package insert), a communication plan (for providing key information to health care providers), elements to assure safe use (ETASU), and an implementation system. Sample ETASU components include required training or certifications for health care providers, limitations on health care settings where the drug can be infused, specific laboratory results, monitoring of drug use by the patient, and enrollment of the patient in a registry. The REMS must be assessed for adequacy at least by 18 months, 3 years, and 7 years after approval.[70]

Case Study 17–2

CaCure (refer to Case Study 17–1) decided to help develop ALLCure for this indication. They successfully submitted an IND and have now completed not only Phase I and Phase II studies, but have completed two positive Phase III studies in patients with metastatic disease to the liver. The company can now apply for an NDA for this new application. Unfortunately, during the studies they became aware that some patients developed cirrhosis months or even years after treatment.

- *Assuming that the cirrhosis is related to this new route of administration, what would be an important component of the submission to the FDA as they seek licensing approval?*
- *What will be appropriate components of the REMS?*

The Orphan Drug Act

Outside of the drug development process described above, the FDA has developed an incentive program to encourage manufacturers to develop products with limited potential profit. This incentive program is known as the Orphan Drug Act and it was passed in 1983. ● This act provides incentives for manufacturers to develop orphan drugs. ❽ *An orphan drug is one used for the treatment of a rare disease, affecting fewer than 200,000 people in the United States, or one that will not generate enough revenue to justify the cost of research and development.* There are more than 6000 rare diseases impacting more than 25 million Americans. The Orphan Drug Act is administered by the FDA's Office of Orphan Products Development. The orphan drug designation provides the following incentives:

- Tax incentives: The sponsor is eligible to receive a tax credit for up to 50% of money spent on research and development of an orphan drug.
- Waive filing fees: The sponsor is eligible to file for a waiver from the application fee associated with the review of an NDA.
- Protocol assistance: If a sponsor can show that a drug is used for a rare disease, the FDA will provide assistance developing the preclinical and clinical plan for the product.
- Grants and contracts: The FDA budget may allot money for grants and contracts to be used in developing orphan drugs. The current budget allows for $14 million for development of orphan drugs. Clinical trials are awarded grants up to $200,000 per year for 3 years (Phase I studies) and up to $400,000 per year for 4 years (Phase II and III studies).
- Marketing exclusivity: The first sponsor to obtain marketing approval for a designated orphan drug is allowed 7 years of marketing exclusivity for that indication, but identical versions of the same product marketed by another manufacturer may be approved for other indications.

The Orphan Drug Act does not provide advantages for the drug approval process. Sponsors seeking approval for drugs that will be designated as orphan drugs must still provide the same safety and efficacy data as all other drugs evaluated by the FDA. Exceptions to the rules governing the number of patients that should be treated in the clinical trials may be made based on the scarcity of patients with the condition. Additionally, because in many cases there are no alternative therapies for the disease, the drug may be given a high review priority during the NDA process.[71,72]

Having discussed the federal infrastructure under which clinical research is conducted, now the approvals that need to be obtained locally before research in human subjects can be initiated will be discussed.

The Institutional Review Board

The IRB is a committee of at least five members formed to review proposed clinical trials and the progress of such studies to ensure that the rights and welfare of human subjects are protected. The IRB must contain at least one member who has specialized in a scientific area (usually this will be a physician) and at least one board member who has a specialty in a nonscientific area such as law, ethics, or religion. Additionally, the IRB must contain at least one individual who is not affiliated with the institution where the research is being conducted. Membership of the IRB varies between institutions. Common members of IRBs include physicians, pharmacists, nurses, lawyers, clergy, and laypeople. The IRB is also responsible for ensuring that the proposed clinical trial is not in conflict with the institution's research policies or philosophy. The IRB and the study sponsor will have little, if any, direct contact. The primary investigator generally acts as the liaison between these two parties. The IRB should evaluate the research proposal to ensure that the following requirements are met:

- The risks to subjects are minimal.
- The expected risk/anticipated benefit ratio must be reasonable.
- Equitable subject selection is used.
- Informed consent must be received from each participant (or his or her representative).
- Informed consent must be documented in writing.
- Data must be monitored to ensure subject safety.
- Patient confidentiality must be maintained.
- If appropriate, additional safeguards against coercion must be included in studies that include vulnerable subjects (children, prisoners, pregnant women, mentally disabled people, or economically or educationally disadvantaged persons).

A notable exception to the requirements for written informed consent, as described above, has been provided for research done in emergency circumstances involving human subjects who cannot give informed consent because of their emerging, life-threatening medical condition (for which available treatments are unproven or unsatisfactory), and where the intervention must be administered before informed consent from the subject's legally authorized representative is feasible. In these situations, the exception from informed consent requirements may proceed only after the sponsor has received prior written permission from the FDA (via IND approval) and the IRB. In this type of research, both community consultation and public disclosure must be provided for the protocol.[73]

The IRB must, at a minimum, perform annual reviews of all ongoing clinical trials and evaluate adverse experiences to ensure that the criteria listed above continue to be met.[74,75]

The IRB must maintain documentation of all IRB activities including copies of all research proposals reviewed, minutes of IRB meetings, records of continuing review activities, copies of all correspondence between the IRB and the investigators, a list of IRB members, written procedures of the IRB, and statements of significant new findings provided to subjects. This documentation and records that pertain to research should be retained for 3 years after the research is completed.[76,77]

Some institutions divide their review of proposed clinical research into two separate processes. One of these is the review of the protocol for scientific worth (scientific review), and the other is the review of the protocol for ethical considerations (IRB review). For many years, the role of the IRB and the effectiveness of the informed consent process have been questioned.[78,79] Federal officials and regulatory agencies continue to contemplate reform of the process to better meet the goals of providing study subjects with information from which they can make an educated decision regarding whether or not they wish to participate in a clinical trial. Information regarding the role the pharmacist can assume in both IRB and scientific reviews of protocols will be presented later in the chapter.

In some institutions, the IRB is also responsible for evaluating research misconduct. Research misconduct means fabrication, falsification, or plagiarism in proposing, performing, or reviewing research, or in reporting research results.[80] Research misconduct is an issue of increasing concern to study sponsors, institutions, and the government as the pressure on investigators and their associates to produce results has increased. In most institutions as the emphasis on identifying and handling research misconduct has increased, the institutions have developed separate review processes and policies to deal with the issue.

IRBs also get involved in evaluating conflict of interest (CoI). As with research misconduct, evaluation, and control of CoI is a shared responsibility for the institution, the IRB, and the investigator (and staff). Of specific concern to the IRB is whether or not financial interests may impact the protection of human subjects. The IRB should identify a mechanism for reporting such CoI, develop a mechanism for managing or eliminating such CoI, and as deemed necessary require that such conflicts be provided to potential study subjects as part of the informed consent process.[81]

Training of investigators and staff in human subject protections, GCP, and CoI is an institutional responsibility that is sometimes enforced by the IRB. Many institutions use the Collaborative Institutional Training Initiative (CITI) to provide and track such training of investigators and staff.[82]

Case Study 17–3

The FDA has mandated that before ALLCure (refer to Case Study 17–1) can be approved, further clinical trials will be required to determine the mechanism of action of developing cirrhosis and if there are clinical or genetic factors that can define the at-risk population. The lawyers at CaCure do not want the cirrhosis information provided in the consent form as the relationship between the toxicity and the drug is not yet definitely proven.

- *What is a likely IRB determination?*
- *What special issues need to be considered if children are to be included in this study to further define the risk of cirrhosis?*

• *What is required if a child reaches their legal age of majority (as defined by state law) while enrolled in this study?*

Next the role of health care professionals in clinical research will be discussed.

Role of the Health Care Professional

The health care professional can play a vital role in the clinical research process by:

- Being the primary investigator (PI) on a study
- Reporting adverse events
- Preparing the IND
- Serving on the IRB and, where applicable, on the scientific review committee
- Providing financial evaluations of investigational protocols
- Disseminating information regarding both the protocol and the investigational drug to other health care personnel
- Maintaining drug accountability records
- Ordering, maintaining and, when necessary, returning drug supplies for ongoing clinical trials
- Randomizing and, when necessary, blinding drug supplies for a clinical trial

The health care professional can serve as the PI on clinical research studies. The type of study for which an individual can serve as a PI varies based on their expertise and experience. Common types of studies for which nonphysicians serve as PIs include pharmacoeconomic, pharmacology/pharmacokinetic, quality of life, and other nontherapeutic and minimal risk trials. For some of these trials, an IRB may insist that a physician be a coinvestigator.

The health care professional can assist the investigator by reporting clinical trial adverse reactions to the FDA. A discussion of the types of adverse reactions and the applicable reporting requirements was presented in the Drug Approval Process section. Further information about the concept of adverse drug reaction reporting, including identification and classification of adverse events, can be found in Chapter 15.

The health care professional can assist in preparing the IND by following the guidelines presented earlier in this chapter. Equally important, the health care professional can assist in writing the protocol. One issue that should be considered when writing a protocol is the issue of potential drug shortages of commercially available products. Over the past 3 years, the number of drug shortages has tripled.[83] If a drug that is included in a protocol is unavailable for any portion of the study the following options are available:

1. Temporary or permanent study hold/termination
2. Drug substitution

If drug substitution is selected, there are two possible options to consider including a specific drug (as specified by the sponsor) or allowing for drug substitution by individual investigators without specification by the sponsor. While the second option may allow for better personalized clinical decision making, it is likely to yield study outcomes that are difficult to interpret. In any event, the decision about how to proceed at the time of a drug shortage will be driven by the length of time the drug is anticipated to be in short supply, the role (pivotal or not) of the drug in the study and study questions, and the rapidity at which drug substitutions need to be made. In general, drug substitutions will need to be made in the body of the protocol as an amendment; however, for a drug with therapeutic purposes where the suspected time of drug shortage may be prolonged, the treatment may need to be altered prior to approval of the amendment. This type of rapid modification of treatment is allowed for in situations where the subjects are considered to be at immediate risk of harm.[19,43] More generally, the impact of drug shortages on protocols can be avoided by only specifying drugs that are critical to study outcomes, allowing for institutional preferences in drug selection, and referencing institutional treatment standard operating procedures (SOPs) rather than specific drugs.

Preferably, health care professionals are voting members of the IRB and as such may have some control over clinical trials initiated at the institution. More important, however, is the role they may have in the scientific review of the protocol, whether this occurs as part of the scientific review board review or the IRB review. When reviewing a protocol for scientific purposes, they should help verify that the information in the protocol is complete and that it is logistically possible for the protocol to be conducted as presented. In addition, the health care professional should confirm that any potential toxicities specified in the protocol are detailed for the patient in the informed consent of the protocol.

Some roles are more specific to the training of the health care professional. Following is a description of the role of the pharmacist in clinical research.

ROLE OF THE PHARMACIST

The pharmacist should verify that the protocol or associated documents such as the investigator's brochure contain the following information:

1. The name and synonyms of the study agent
2. The chemical structure of the study agent

3. The mechanism of action of the study agent

4. The dosage range of the study agent (with appropriate rationale)

5. Animal toxicologic and pharmacologic information (when available, any known human toxicologic and pharmacologic information should also be presented)

6. How the agent will be supplied (dosage form and size)

7. The preparation guidelines for the agent (including stability and compatibility information when appropriate)

8. The storage requirements of the agent (both before and, when appropriate, after preparation)

9. The route of administration (and, if applicable, the rate of administration)

The pharmacist should also review the protocol for other potential problems (such as incompatibilities and inappropriate infusion devices). Frequently, nursing does not have an opportunity to review protocols prior to initiation and it falls to the pharmacist to ensure that the drug can be given as specified in the protocol. For complex protocols, it may be best to request secondary reviews by other specialists, such as the nurses, who will be giving the doses or the pharmacists who will be preparing the doses. The pharmacist can review the protocol for clinical and scientific issues appropriate to his or her knowledge level and experience. Those pharmacists with research experience or a strong clinical background may, and probably should, comment on the study design or scientific merit of a particular protocol.

With the central role of financial considerations in today's research environment, pharmacists can also provide valuable insight into the costs associated with clinical research. Traditionally, the study sponsors would provide the investigational drug free of charge to the hospital (and to the patient) and the patient (or the third-party payer) would be responsible for paying for all other charges associated with therapy. These charges could include hospitalization charges, laboratory tests, and examinations to name a few. Some third-party payers are reluctant to pay for such charges unless they can be considered to be standard of care. This leaves the patient, and subsequently the hospital, in a financially risky situation. More recently, some sponsors have started to implement programs for cost recovery for investigational drugs. As discussed previously, the sponsor applies to and receives approval from the FDA for a specific dollar amount that can be charged. FDA approval of this charge must be in place before cost recovery can begin.[65-67] The pharmacy will need to have procedures in place for billing properly for investigational drugs. In addition, a significant portion of costs associated with clinical research is pharmacy related (either supportive care medications or infusion devices, solutions, etc., that are used to administer the investigational drug). If, during the review process, the pharmacist can provide the investigator and the scientific review board with information regarding the potential cost of the research (at least as it relates to pharmacy charges), both the investigator and the review board can make a more educated decision regarding appropriation of resources for research purposes. When preparing an economic review of a protocol, the pharmacist should pay specific attention to the following questions:

1. Can the therapy be converted from inpatient to outpatient?
2. Can the method of infusion or the infusion device be changed to one that is more cost effective?
3. Does the treatment plan call for administration of compatible medications that could be mixed in the same container?
4. Is the supportive care adequate and not excessive (this is especially important with high-cost drugs such as antiemetics and growth factors)?
5. Does the protocol have a high risk of reimbursement denial? This can be evaluated by reviewing labeling information in the package insert, *American Hospital Formulary Service (AHFS) Drug Information,* and for oncology products, NCCN Drugs & Biologics Compendium (NCCN Compendium®). Other factors in reimbursement risk include the cost of the drug and the supportive care or tests associated with the drug. If the protocol does have a high risk of reimbursement denial, can free drug supplies offset part or all of this risk?

Following approval of the research project, the pharmacist can assist in disseminating information regarding both the protocol and the investigational agent by preparing data sheets that may be used by pharmacy and nursing personnel (and in some situations by physicians who may be unfamiliar with the research). This information can be distributed using various methods including paper, Web-based systems and the electronic medical record. The investigational agent data sheet should include the following elements:

- Agent name (synonyms)
- Therapeutic classification
- Pharmaceutical data
- Stability and storage data
- Dose preparation guidelines (where applicable)
- Usual dosage range
- Route of administration
- Known side effects and toxicities
- Mechanism of action
- Status (phase of study)
- Study chairperson
- Date effective (and dates of revision)
- References

The protocol data sheet should include the following elements:

- Protocol number (as assigned by the institution)
- Protocol title
- Agent name(s) (synonym[s])
- Protocol description
  1. Objectives
  2. Study design
     a. Registration requirements
     b. Primary location of patients
     c. Type of study
  3. Treatment course (including retreatment criteria)
- Availability
  1. Supplier
  2. Status
  3. How supplied
- Storage, stability, and compatibility
  1. Intact drug
  2. Prepared drug (for injectables this should include both reconstitution and dilution guidelines)
- Dosage range
- Dose preparation guidelines
- Administration guidelines
- Special notes
- Primary investigator
- Key study staff including the research nurse

The primary investigator and study sponsor should approve both the drug data sheet and the protocol data sheet before dissemination. This will help eliminate any potential errors and may reduce the liability the pharmacist assumes in preparing and distributing these documents.

The pharmacist can assume primary responsibility for ordering and maintaining adequate drug supplies for conducting the clinical trial. All investigational drugs should be stored in a locked area, preferably a pharmacy. Usually, ordering can be done via telephone; however, sometimes study sponsors require written drug orders. If the drug under investigation is a controlled substance, a written order will definitely be required. Shipment and receipt of the drug can vary from 1 day to several weeks (or sometimes months for very specialized drug products). The individual responsible for ordering drug must be sufficiently knowledgeable regarding the rate of patient enrollment in the protocol and subsequent drug usage to ensure that the institution does not run out of drug. The same individual(s) should also assume responsibility for returning unused drug supplies at the completion of the study. The sponsor may authorize on-site destruction of unused supplies provided this will not increase the risk to humans (or provide a risk to the environment). Many study sponsors will attempt to have the site save and return all used drug supplies as well. This is not an FDA requirement and for safety and space reasons should be discouraged.

Related to the activities above, the same individuals (or team) should assume responsibility for maintaining drug accountability records. ❾*Maintenance of such records is required by law.* Again, it is preferable to have this handled by a pharmacist. These records can be maintained manually or on a computer. The records must document all drug shipments, returns, and dispensing to patients. *At a minimum, these records should document:*

- *The date of the transaction*
- *The type of the transaction*
- *The recipient of the transaction (if this is a drug dispensing, the patient initials and an identifying number are required)*
- *The number of units being used or received (or patient dispensing this should include the actual dose the patient will receive)*
- *The lot number of the drug (if multiple lot numbers were used, each one should be documented)*
- *The initials of the individual who performed the transaction.*

An audit trail is required. The National Cancer Institute (NCI) has prepared a sample drug accountability form that may be used as a guide. It is available on the Internet at http://ctep.cancer.gov/forms/docs/agent_accountability.pdf

Computer systems that will maintain drug accountability records are available commercially. Both personal computer (PC)-based and Web-based systems exist. Some of these systems will also provide drug labels, drug and protocol information, summaries of investigational drug dispensing (useful in the preparation of productivity reports), and even monthly billing summaries to be used for posting charges to the study budget. One such Web-based system that is currently on the market is IDEA© being marketed by DDOTS, Inc.[84] Another commercially avaialable system includes Vestigo™ being marketed by the McCreadie Group.[85,86] Obviously, the development of a personalized system that meets the specific needs of the institution or pharmacy is ideal. However, this can be costly, laborious, and time consuming. If a personalized system is developed, it is important to remember that the system must be able to maintain the integrity of the records and that a clear audit trail needs to be maintained. Ultimately, the decision to computerize drug accountability records and the selection of which system to use is one that the pharmacist should make only after evaluating the needs of the institution/pharmacy and the available budget.[87]

Drug accountability records and drug supplies may be inspected at any time by the sponsor. The frequency of these inspections may vary according to the wishes of the sponsor. They may be monthly, quarterly, or annually. The FDA also has the right to inspect these records. The investigational drug pharmacist should play a key role in providing drug accountability information to either the FDA or the sponsor during an audit. If proper records are not being maintained, the sponsor or the FDA may discontinue the investigator's participation in the clinical investigation.

After the clinical trial is complete, records must be maintained at the study site for the following time periods:

- Two years after approval of the NDA *or*
- Two years after the FDA received notification that the investigation was discontinued[88]

The pharmacist should also assume primary responsibility for randomizing and, where appropriate, blinding clinical trials. These two activities assist the sponsor in reducing or eliminating the bias of the clinical trial. A randomized study is one in which patients are randomly assigned (similar to flipping a coin) to different therapies. More details regarding the statistical basis for randomized studies are included in Chapter 8 of this book. In summary, however, usually the assignment is done using a computer-generated randomization list; however, a manual list may be used as well. The randomization groups may include a number of different therapy options (e.g., a study may have four different treatment arms with an equal number of patients assigned to each arm). The number of patients assigned to the different groups may vary as well (e.g., a study may have two different treatment regimens where patients will be assigned in a 2:1 ratio to the first treatment option). The investigator should not be aware which arm the patient has been assigned to before randomization. Therefore, the involvement of a third party (such as the pharmacist) is important. A blinded study is one in which, after the patient has been randomized, the drug is masked so that at least one of the involved parties (e.g., physician, nurse, patient, or pharmacist) is not aware of what the patient is to receive. In a single-blind study, the only individual who is not aware of what the patient is receiving is the patient himself. In a double-blind study, the nurse, physician, and patient are all unaware of what the patient is receiving. The role of a pharmacist in a double-blind study is crucial and sloppy work in this area destroys a clinical investigation. A triple-blind study is one in which the drug arrives at the pharmacy already blinded. In this scenario, the patient, nurse, physician, and pharmacist are not aware of what drug the patient is to receive. Although this may seem simpler than a double-blind study, it is equally difficult because each patient has his or her own supply of medication and it is important that the supplies be dispensed appropriately. In a triple-blind study, the sponsor supplies the investigator with a mechanism for removing the blind from the patient (in case of emergency). It is critical that the pharmacist keep the master list. The protocol should state who has access to the master list and under what conditions this access should occur. If the FDA discovers that the investigator had access to this list, the study will be considered invalid.

Pharmacists should be willing and able to request reimbursement for the services they provide. Funds for these services are usually negotiated directly with the study sponsor before initiation of the protocol. The majority of pharmacies charge a base fee for each protocol initiated at the institution (these fees generally range from $1000 to $1500 per protocol). This base fee may be fixed or it may vary based on the size of the patient population, the complexity of the protocol, or the number of doses to be prepared. Some institutions also charge an annual renewal fee for ongoing clinical trials (ranging from $500 to $1000). Most pharmacies will charge a separate fee for randomizing and blinding a clinical trial. This fee can be a one-time (per study) fee or it can be a per patient fee. Some hospitals also charge dispensing fees per dose or per amount of time required to prepare a dose ($15 for oral doses up to $50 for intravenous chemotherapy). Pharmacies can also charge a monthly fee for drug storage and inventory. This fee varies based on the amount of space and type of storage (freezer, room temperature, or refrigerator) required. The pharmacist can also charge a professional fee for services that exceed the standard services provided for in the base fee. Examples of services that should be charged for separately include monitoring of patients, completing case report forms, special compounding, ordering and handling controlled substances, and completing sponsor-specific drug accountability records. These services are usually charged using an hourly rate.[89]

Conclusion

Assisting in the implementation and conduct of clinical trials can be a satisfying role for the health care professional. Clinical trials that utilize drugs, biologics, and devices in the United States are largely controlled by the FDA and local IRBs. A thorough understanding of the regulations governing those entities is extremely helpful when conducting clinical trials. The health care professional can use that knowledge to help investigators develop clinical trials, obtain and maintain proper approvals for those clinical trials, and assist in the conduct of clinical trials. Related to the conduct of clinical trials, health care professionals (and specifically pharmacists) are frequently involved in obtaining, storing, and dispensing the agents being utilized in the clinical trial. In addition, the health care professional (and specifically pharmacists) can be quite involved in providing protocol and drug information to the investigators, other study personnel, and equally importantly to the study subjects. Health care professionals can and should play an integral role in the conduct of clinical trials at their institution.

Self-Assessment Questions

1. What is the role of the FDA related to drugs, biologics, and medical devices in the United States?
   a. Evaluation of safety and efficacy
   b. Evaluation of conflict of interest
   c. Evaluation of research data
   d. Evaluation of marketability

2. What does the IRB review research protocols for?
   a. Evaluation of safety and efficacy
   b. Determining that the rights and welfare and human subjects are protected
   c. Risk benefit ratio
   d. That the consent for is written at an appropriate reading level

3. What are the FDA submissions related to drug approval in the United States?
   a. Orphan drug
   b. Phase I, II, and III
   c. IND/NDA
   d. Cost recovery

4. Which is the most common type of IND?
   a. Commercial IND
   b. Treatment IND
   c. Emergency use IND
   d. Individual investigator IND

5. What are the four types of documents used to amend an IND?
   a. Protocol amendments, product amendments, animal data, annual reports
   b. Manufacturing changes, protocol amendments, consent form changes, annual reports
   c. Protocol amendments, information amendments, IND safety reports, annual reports
   d. Protocol amendments, IND safety reports, new protocols, annual reports

6. What would be an appropriate example of an REMS and the associated requirements to mitigate those risks?
   a. Liver damage—counseling patients on signs of liver failure
   b. Serious infection—sending patients home with antibiotics
   c. Severe birth defects—requiring a negative pregnancy test prior to dispensing each dose of medication
   d. Leukemia—meeting with an oncologist prior to initiating treatment

7. What is the primary reason that the FDA developed the orphan drug program?
   a. To provide tax incentives to manufacturers
   b. To provide incentives for manufacturers to develop products with limited potential profit
   c. To provide grants to manufacturers
   d. To allow manufacturers marketing exclusivity

8. What is the most important role of the pharmacist in clinical research?
   a. Maintaining drug accountability records
   b. Reviewing protocols
   c. Disseminating protocol information
   d. Ensuring that patient dosing is accurate and compliant with the protocol

9. What does an NDA/BLA allow a sponsor to do?
   a. Market the product
   b. Charge for the product
   c. Advertise for the product
   d. Name the product

10. Who is the sponsor's primary contact at the FDA?
    a. Medical reviewer
    b. Pharmacology/toxicology reviewer
    c. Regulatory project manager
    d. CMC reviewer

11. What was the first reform initiative implemented to speed drug evaluation timeframes?
    a. Kefauver-Harris Drug Amendment
    b. FDAAA
    c. FDAMA
    d. PDUFA

12. Gene transfer products are uniquely governed by:
    a. FDA

    b. NIH/OBA

    c. IRB

    d. Scientific review committees

13. The drug data sheet should include the following elements:
    a. Dose preparation guidelines
    b. Principal investigator name
    c. Agent name
    d. All of the above
    e. Both a and c

14. The protocol data sheet should include the following elements:
    a. Dose preparation guidelines
    b. Principal investigator name
    c. Agent name
    d. All of the above
    e. Both a and c

15. The FDA regulates:
    a. Illegal drugs of abuse
    b. Practice of medicine
    c. Advertising for prescription drugs
    d. Health insurance

REFERENCES

1. Tufts Center for the Study of Drug Development. Tufts Center for the Study of Drug Development pegs cost of a new prescription medicine at $802 million [Internet]. 2000 Mar [cited 2004 Mar]. Available from: http://csdd.tufts.edu/.

2. Dickson M. The cost of new drug discovery and development. Discov Med[Internet]. 2009 Jun 20 [cited 2012 Dec]: [8p.]. Available from: http://www.discoverymedicine.com/Michael-Dickson/2009/06/20/the-cost-of-new-drug-discovery-and-development/.

3. Adams CP, Brantner VV. Estimating the cost of new drug development: is it really $802 million? Health Aff. 2006 Mar-Apr;25(2):420-8.

4. Science Based Medicine. What does a new drug cost? [Internet] 2011 Apr 4:[13p.]. Available from: http://www.sciencebasedmedicine.org/index.php/what-does-a-new-drug-cost/.

5. Tufts Center for the Study of Drug Development. How new drugs move through the development and approval process [Internet]. 2001 Nov 1 [cited 2012 Dec]:[2p.]. Available from: http://csdd.tufts.edu/.

6. PhRMA. Medicines in development [Internet]. [cited 2012 Dec]:[1p.] Available from: http://www.phrma.org/innovation/meds-in-development

7. Food and Drug Administration. FY 2012 innovative drug approvals [Internet]. 2012 Dec 10 [cited 2012 Dec]:[19p.]. Available from: http://www.fda.gov/AboutFDA/ ReportsManualsForms/Reports/ucm276385.htm

8. Food and Drug Administration. What we do: FAQs [Internet]. 2012 Jun [cited 2012 Dec]:[1p.]. Available from: http://www.fda.gov/AboutFDA/WhatWeDo/default.htm

9. Food and Drug Administration. FDA organization chart [Internet]. 2012 Nov [cited 2012 Dec]:[1p.]. Available from: http://www.fda.gov/downloads/AboutFDA/CentersOffices/ OrganizationCharts/UCM291886.pdf

10. CDER; Food and Drug Administration. Approval times for priority and standard NME's calendar years 1993–2003 [Internet]. Updated through 2012 Sep [cited 2012 Dec]:[13p.]. Available from: http://www.fda.gov/cder/rdmt/NMEapps93-03.htm

11. United States Federal Government Code of Federal Regulations [Internet]. 21CFR601.2. Updated 2012 Apr 1 [cited 2012 Dec]. Available from: http://www.gpoaccess.gov/cfr/ index.html

12. United States Federal Government Code of Federal Regulations [Internet]. 21CFR312.3. Updated 2012 Apr 1 [cited 2012 Dec]. Available from: http://www.gpoaccess.gov/cfr/ index.html

13. CDER; Food and Drug Administration. MAPP 6030.1: IND process and review procedures [Internet]. Updated 1998 May 1 [cited 2004 Sep 15]:[12p.]. Available from: http://www .fda.gov/.

14. International Conference on Harmonization (ICH). Guidance for industry: E10 choice of control group and related issues in clinical trials [Internet]. 2001 May [cited 2012 Dec]:[35p.]. Available from: http://www.fda.gov/downloads/Drugs/ GuidanceComplianceRegulatoryInformation/Guidances/UCM073139.pdf

15. United States Federal Government Code of Federal Regulations [Internet]. 21CFR314.420. Updated 2012 Apr 1 [cited 2012 Dec]. Available from: http://www.gpoaccess.gov/cfr/ index.html

16. United States Federal Government Code of Federal Regulations [Internet]. 21CFR314.3. Updated 2012 Apr 1 [cited 2012 Dec]. Available from: http://www.gpoaccess.gov/cfr/ index.html

17. International Conference for Harmonization (ICN). E6 guideline for good clinical practice [Internet]. 1996 Jun 10 [cited 2012 Dec]:[63p.]. Available from: http://www.ich.org/ fileadmin/Public_Web_Site/ICH_Products/Guidelines/Efficacy/E6_R1/Step4/E6_R1_ Guideline.pdf

18. United States Federal Government Code of Federal Regulations [Internet]. 45CFR46. Updated 2010 Jan 15 [cited 2012 Dec]. Available from: http://www.gpoaccess.gov/cfr/ index.html

19. United States Federal Government Code of Federal Regulations [Internet]. 21CFR56. Updated 2012 Apr 1 [cited 2012 Dec]. Available from: http://www.gpoaccess.gov/cfr/ index.html

20. Food and Drug Administration [Internet]. PDUFA. Updated 2009 Jun 18 [cited 2012 Dec]. Available from: http://www.fda.gov/forindustry/userfees/prescriptiondruguserfee/default.htm

21. Yager JA, Kalgren DL. Roles of regulatory project managers in the U.S. Food and Drug Administration's Center for Drug Evaluation and Research. Drug Inf J. 2000;34: 289-93.

22. Meadows M. Promoting safe and effective drugs for 100 years. FDA Consum [Internet]. 2006 Jan-Feb [cited 2012 Dec]:[8p.]. Available from: http://www.fda.gov/AboutFDA/WhatWeDo/History/CentennialofFDA/CentennialEditionofFDAConsumer/ucm093787.htm

23. Bruderle TP. Reforming the Food and Drug Administration: legislative solution or self-improvement. Am J Health Syst Pharm. 1996;53:2083-90.

24. Blum J. Drugs delayed in US as regulators struggle with new duties. Bloomberg.com [Internet]. 2008 Oct 27 [cited 2009 Jun]. Available from: http://www.bloomberg.com/apps/news?pid=newsarchive&sid=aC6L0BgriWIw#

25. Food and Drug Administration. Food and Drug Administration Modernization Act of 1997 [Internet]. Updated 2009 Jun 18 [cited 2012 Dec]. Available from: http://www.fda.gov/RegulatoryInformation/Legislation/FederalFoodDrugandCosmeticActFDCAct/SignificantAmendmentstotheFDCAct/FDAMA/default.htm

26. Food and Drug Administration. Food and Drug Administration Amendments Act of 2007 [Internet]. Updated 2011 Dec 2 [cited 2012 Dec]. Available from: http://www.fda.gov/RegulatoryInformation/Legislation/FederalFoodDrugandCosmeticActFDCAct/SignificantAmendmentstotheFDCAct/FoodandDrugAdministrationAmendmentsActof2007/default.htm

27. Food and Drug Administration. Critical path initiative [Internet]. Updated 2012 Dec 28 [cited 2012 Dec]. Available from: http://www.fda.gov/ScienceResearch/SpecialTopics/CriticalPathInitiative/ucm076689.htm

28. Food and Drug Administration. Electronic regulatory submission and review [Internet]. Updated 2012 Mar 5 [cited 2012 Dec]. Available from: http://www.fda.gov/Drugs/DevelopmentApprovalProcess/FormsSubmissionRequirements/ElectronicSubmissions/default.htm

29. Woodcock J. FDA user fee agreements: strenthening FDA and the medical products industry for the benefit of patients [Internet]. Presented to: Committee on Health, Education, Labor and Pensions United States Senate; 2012 Mar 29 [cited 2012 Dec]. Available from: http://www.fda.gov/NewsEvents/Testimony/ucm297390.htm

30. ClinicalTrials.gov [Internet]. Updated 2012 Aug [cited 2012 Dec] Available from: http://clinicaltrials.gov/ct2/about-site/history

31. Form FDA 3674: Certification of Compliance, under 42 U.S.C. § 282(j) (5) (B), with requirements of ClinicalTrials.gov data bank (42 U.S.C. § 282(j)) [Internet]. Updated 2012 Mar [cited 2012 Dec]. Available from: http://www.fda.gov/downloads/AboutFDA/ReportsManualsForms/Forms/UCM048364.pdf

32. International Conference on Harmonization. History and future of ICH [Internet]. Updated 2000 [cited 2009 Jun]. Available from: http://www.ich.org

33. Grilley B, Gee A. Gene transfer: regulatory issues and their impact on the clinical investigator and the GMP facility. Cytotherapy. 2003;5(3):197-207.

34. The Nuremberg code. Trials of war criminals before the Nuremberg military tribunals under Control Council Law No. 10, Vol. 2, pp. 181-2. Washington, DC: US Government Printing Office; 1989 Sep.

35. The World Medical Association. Declaration of Helsinki [Internet]. Updated 2008 Oct [cited 2012 Dec]. Available from: http://www.wma.net/en/30publications/10policies/b3/.

36. The Belmont report: ethical principles and guidelines for the protection of human subjects of research [Internet]. 1979 Apr 18 [cited 2012 Dec]. Available from: http://www.hhs.gov/ohrp/humansubjects/guidance/belmont.html

37. United States Federal Government Code of Federal Regulations [Internet]. 21CFR50. Updated 2012 Apr 1 [cited 2012 Dec]. Available from: http://www.gpoaccess.gov/cfr/index.html

38. United States Federal Government Code of Federal Regulations [Internet]. 21CFR312.23. Updated 2012 Apr 1 [cited 2012 Dec]. Available from: http://www.accessdata.fda.gov/scripts/cdrh/cfdocs/cfCFR/CFRSearch.cfm?fr=312.23

39. CDER/CBER; Food and Drug Administration. Guidance for industry: investigational new drug applications (INDs)—determining whether human research studies can be conducted without an IND [Internet]. 2010 Oct [cited 2012 Dec]. Available from: http://www.fda.gov/downloads/Drugs/GuidanceComplianceRegulatoryInformation/Guidances/UCM229175.pdf

40. CDER/CBER/CDRH; Food and Drug Administration. Draft guidance for industry and Food and Drug Administration staff: in vitro companion diagnostic devices [Internet]. 2011 Jul 14 [cited 2012 Dec]. Available from: http://www.fda.gov/MedicalDevices/DeviceRegulationandGuidance/GuidanceDocuments/ucm262292.htm

41. CBER/CDRH; Food and Drug Administration. Draft guidance for industry and Food and Drug Administration staff: mobile medical applications [Internet]. 2011 Jul 21 [cited 2012 Dec]. Available from: http://www.fda.gov/MedicalDevices/ProductsandMedicalProcedures/ucm255978.htm

42. CDER; Food and Drug Administration. Guideline for drug master files [Internet]. 1989 Sep [cited 2012 Dec] Available from: http://www.fda.gov/Drugs/DevelopmentApprovalProcess/FormsSubmissionRequirements/DrugMasterFilesDMFs/ucm073164.htm

43. United States Federal Government Code of Federal Regulations [Internet]. 21CFR312.30. Updated 2012 Apr 1 [cited 2012 Dec]. Available from: http://www.accessdata.fda.gov/scripts/cdrh/cfdocs/cfCFR/CFRSearch.cfm?fr=312.30

44. United States Federal Government Code of Federal Regulations [Internet]. 21CFR312.31. Updated 2012 Apr 1 [cited 2012 Dec]. Available from: http://www.accessdata.fda.gov/scripts/cdrh/cfdocs/cfCFR/CFRSearch.cfm?fr=312.31

45. United States Federal Government Code of Federal Regulations [Internet]. 21CFR312.32 Washington, DC: [updated 2008 Apr 1 cited 2009 Jun]. Available from: http://www.acc`essdata.fda.gov/scripts/cdrh/cfdocs/cfCFR/CFRSearch.cfm?fr=312.32

46. CDER/CBER; Food and Drug Administration. Guidance for industry and investigators: safety reporting requirements for INDs and BA/BE studies [Internet]. 2012 Sep [cited 2012 Dec]. Available from: http://www.fda.gov/downloads/Drugs/GuidanceComplianceRegulatoryInformation/Guidances/UCM227351.pdf

47. United States Federal Government Code of Federal Regulations [Internet]. 21CFR312.33. Updated 2012 Apr 1 [cited 2012 Dec]. Available from: http://www.accessdata.fda.gov/scripts/cdrh/cfdocs/cfCFR/CFRSearch.cfm?fr=312.33

48. United States Federal Government Code of Federal Regulations [Internet]. 21CFR312.40. Updated 2012 Apr 1 [cited 2012 Dec]. Available from: http://www.accessdata.fda.gov/scripts/cdrh/cfdocs/cfCFR/CFRSearch.cfm?fr=312.40

49. United States Federal Government Code of Federal Regulations [Internet]. 21CFR312.42. Updated 2012 Apr 1 [cited 2012 Dec]. Available from: http://www.accessdata.fda.gov/scripts/cdrh/cfdocs/cfCFR/CFRSearch.cfm?fr=312.42

50. Food and Drug Administration. The FDA's drug review process: ensuring drugs are safe and effective [Internet]. Updated 2012 May [cited 2012 Dec]. Available from: http://www.fda.gov/Drugs/ResourcesForYou/Consumers/ucm143534.htm

51. CDER/CBER/CDRH; Food and Drug Administration [Internet]. Guidance for industry: clinical pharmacogenomics: premarketing evaluation in early phase clinical studies [Internet]. 2011 Feb (cited 2012 Dec). Available from: http://www.fda.gov/downloads/Drugs/GuidanceComplianceRegulatoryInformation/Guidances/UCM243702.pdf

52. United States Federal Government Code of Federal Regulations [Internet]. 21CFR314.50 Updated 2012 Apr 1 [cited 2012 Dec]. Available from: http://www.accessdata.fda.gov/scripts/cdrh/cfdocs/cfCFR/CFRSearch.cfm?fr=314.50

53. Food and Drug Administration. How drugs are developed and approved: drug development review and definitions [Internet]. 2010 Feb 22 [cited 2012 Dec]. Available from: http://www.fda.gov/Drugs/DevelopmentApprovalProcess/HowDrugsareDevelopedand Approved/ApprovalApplications/InvestigationalNewDrugINDApplication/ ucm176522.htm

54. Food and Drug Administration [Internet]. 21CFR14: Public Hearing before a public advisory committee. Updated 2012 Apr 1 [2012 Dec]. Available from: http://www.accessdata .fda.gov/scripts/cdrh/cfdocs/cfCFR/CFRSearch.cfm?CFRPart=14&showFR= 1&subpartNode=21:1.0.1.1.10.9

55. United States Federal Government Code of Federal Regulations [Internet]. 21CFR314.100. Updated 2012 Apr 1 [cited 2012 Dec]. Available from: http://www.accessdata.fda.gov/scripts/cdrh/cfdocs/cfCFR/CFRSearch.cfm?fr=314.100

56. United States Federal Government Code of Federal Regulations [Internet]. 21CFR314.105. Updated 2012 Apr 1 [cited 2012 Dec]. Available from: http://www.accessdata.fda.gov/scripts/cdrh/cfdocs/cfCFR/CFRSearch.cfm?fr=314.105

57. United States Federal Government Code of Federal Regulations [Internet]. 21CFR314.110. Updated 2012 Apr 1 [cited 2012 Dec]. Available from: http://www.accessdata.fda.gov/scripts/cdrh/cfdocs/cfCFR/CFRSearch.cfm?fr=314.110

58. United States Federal Government Code of Federal Regulations [Internet]. 21CFR312.300. Updated 2012 Apr 1 [cited 2012 Dec]. Available from: http://www.accessdata.fda.gov/scripts/cdrh/cfdocs/cfCFR/CFRSearch.cfm?fr=312.300

59. Food and Drug Administration. Expanded access to investigational drugs for treatment use. Fed Regist. 2009 Aug 13;74(155): 40900-40945.

60. United States Federal Government Code of Federal Regulations [Internet]. 21CFR312.305. Updated 2012 Apr 1 [cited 2012 Dec]. Available from: http://www.accessdata.fda.gov/scripts/cdrh/cfdocs/cfCFR/CFRSearch.cfm?fr=312.305

61. United States Federal Government Code of Federal Regulations [Internet]. 21CFR312.310. Updated 2012 Apr 1 [cited 2012 Dec]. Available from: http://www.accessdata.fda.gov/scripts/cdrh/cfdocs/cfCFR/CFRSearch.cfm?fr=312.310

62. United States Federal Government Code of Federal Regulations [Internet]. 21CFR56.104 Washington, DC. Updated 2008 Apr 1 [cited 2012 Dec]. Available from: http://www.gpoaccess.gov/cfr/index.html

63. United States Federal Government Code of Federal Regulations [Internet]. 21CFR312.315. Updated 2012 Apr 1 [cited 2012 Dec]. Available from: http://www.accessdata.fda.gov/scripts/cdrh/cfdocs/cfCFR/CFRSearch.cfm?fr=312.315

64. United States Federal Government Code of Federal Regulations [Internet]. 21CFR312.320. Updated 2012 Apr 1 [cited 2012 Dec]. Available from: http://www.accessdata.fda.gov/scripts/cdrh/cfdocs/cfCFR/CFRSearch.cfm?fr=312.320

65. Food and Drug Administration. Charging for investigational drugs under an investigational new drug application. Fed Regist. 2009 Aug 13;74(155):40872-900.

66. United States Federal Government Code of Federal Regulations [Internet]. 21CFR312.7. Updated 2012 Apr 1 [cited 2012 Dec]. Available from: http://www.accessdata.fda.gov/scripts/cdrh/cfdocs/cfCFR/CFRSearch.cfm?fr=312.7

67. United States Federal Government Code of Federal Regulations [Internet]. 21CFR312.8. Updated 2012 Apr 1 [cited 2012 Dec]. Available from: http://www.accessdata.fda.gov/scripts/cdrh/cfdocs/cfCFR/CFRSearch.cfm?fr=312.8

68. Galson S. Office of New Drugs/Office of Drug Safety [Internet]. Presented to the House Committee on Government Reform. 2005 May 5 [cited 2012 Dec]. Available from: http://www.fda.gov/NewsEvents/Testimony/ucm113031.htm

69. United States Federal Government Code of Federal Regulations [Internet]. 21CFR314.520. Updated 2012 Apr 1 [cited 2012 Dec]. Available from: http://www.accessdata.fda.gov/scripts/cdrh/cfdocs/cfCFR/CFRSearch.cfm?fr=314.520

70. Food and Drug Administration. FDA basics webinar: a brief overview of risk evaluation and mitigation strategies (REMS) [Internet]. Updated 2012 Nov 11[cited 2012 Dec]. Available from: http://www.fda.gov/AboutFDA/Transparency/Basics/ucm325201.htm

71. United States Federal Government Code of Federal Regulations [Internet]. 21CFR316. Updated 2012 Apr 1 [cited 2012 Dec]. Available from: http://www.accessdata.fda.gov/scripts/cdrh/cfdocs/cfCFR/CFRSearch.cfm?fr=316

72. Needleman K. CDER; Presentation entitled: Overview of the Office of Orphan Products Development: Incentives for rare diseases. Food and Drug Administration [Internet].

2011 Oct 18 [cited 2012 Dec] Available from: http://www.fda.gov/downloads/Drugs/DevelopmentApprovalProcess/SmallBusinessAssistance/UCM276029.pdf

73. United States Federal Government Code of Federal Regulations [Internet]. 21CFR50.24. Updated 2012 Apr 1 [cited 2012 Dec]. Available from: http://www.accessdata.fda.gov/scripts/cdrh/cfdocs/cfCFR/CFRSearch.cfm?fr=50.24

74. United States Federal Government Code of Federal Regulations [Internet]. 45CFR46.108 Updated 2005 Jun [cited 2012 Dec]. Available from: http://www.hhs.gov/ohrp/humansubjects/guidance/45cfr46.html#46.108

75. United States Federal Government Code of Federal Regulations [Internet]. 21CFR56.109. Updated 2012 Apr 1 [cited 2012 Dec]. Available from: http://www.accessdata.fda.gov/scripts/cdrh/cfdocs/cfCFR/CFRSearch.cfm?fr=56.109

76. United States Federal Government Code of Federal Regulations [Internet]. 21CFR56.115. Updated 2012 Apr 1 [cited 2012 Dec]. Available from: http://www.accessdata.fda.gov/scripts/cdrh/cfdocs/cfCFR/CFRSearch.cfm?fr=56.115

77. United States Federal Government Code of Federal Regulations [Internet]. 45CFR46.115. Updated 2005 Jun [cited 2012 Dec]. Available from: http://www.hhs.gov/ohrp/humansubjects/guidance/45cfr46.html#46.115

78. Hochhauser M. Is "therapeutic misconception" being used to recruit subjects? ARENA Newsletter. Spring 2003;XVI:5-7.

79. Hochhauser M. "Therapeutic misconception" and "recruiting doublespeak" in the informed consent process. IRB: ethics and human research. 2002 Jan-Feb;240-1.

80. Office of Research Integrity. Definition of research misconduct [Internet]. Updated 2011 Apr 25 [cited 2012 Dec]. Available from: http://ori.dhhs.gov/misconduct/definition_misconduct.html

81. Department of Health and Human Services. Final guidance document. Financial relationships and interests in research involving human subjects: guidance for human subject protection [Internet]. 2004 May 5 [cited 2012 Dec]. Available from: http://www.hhs.gov/ohrp/archive/humansubjects/finreltn/fguid.pdf

82. Collaborative Institutional Training Initiative (CITI) Program [Internet]. [cited 2012 Dec]. Available from: https://www.citiprogram.org/rcrpage.asp

83. Stein R. Shortages of key drugs endanger patients. The Washington Post [Internet]. 2011 May 5 [cited 2012 Dec]. Available from: http://www.washingtonpost.com/national/shortages-of-key-drugs-endanger-patients/2011/04/26/AF1aJJVF_story.html

84. DDOTS, Inc. [Internet]. Cited 2012 Dec. Available from: http://www.ddots.com

85. McCreadie Group: Vestigo [Internet]. [cited 2012 Dec]. Available from: http://www.mccreadiegroup.com/vestigo/.

86. Burnham NL, Elcombe SA, Skorlinski CR, Kosanke L, Kovach JS. Computer program for handling investigational oncology drugs. Am J Hosp Pharm. 1989;46:1821-4.

87. Grilley BJ, Trissel LA, Bluml BM. Design and implementation of an electronic investigational drug accountability system. Am J Hosp Pharm. 1991;48:2816.

88. United States Federal Government Code of Federal Regulations [Internet]. 21CFR312.57. Updated 2012 Apr 1 [cited 2012 Dec]. Available from: http://www.accessdata.fda.gov/scripts/cdrh/cfdocs/cfCFR/CFRSearch.cfm?fr=312.57

89. Veteran's Medical Research Foundation Pharmacy Service [Internet]. [cited 2012 Dec]. Available from: http://www.vmrf.org/researchcenters/pharmacy-service/pharmacy.html

SUGGESTED READINGS

1. NIH/Office of Biotechnology Activities (OBA): http://osp.od.nih.gov/office-biotechnology-activities/.
2. FDA: http://www.fda.gov/.
3. FDA forms: http://www.fda.gov/opacom/morechoices/fdaforms/fdaforms.html
4. Archives of the Federal Register: http://www.archives.gov/federal-register/the-federal-register/.
5. Code of Federal Regulations: http://www.gpoaccess.gov/cfr/index.html
6. FDA Dockets Management Page: http://www.fda.gov/ohrms/dockets/default.htm
7. ICH: http://www.ich.org
8. NIH/OHRP: http://www.hhs.gov/ohrp/.
9. CenterWatch: http://centerwatch.com/.

18

Chapter Eighteen

Policy Development, Project Design, and Implementation

Stacie Krick Evans • Sabrina W. Cole

Learning Objectives

● *After completing this chapter, the reader will be able to*

- State reasons for pharmacist involvement in health system policy development.
- Describe the health system policy development process.
- List health system policies that require pharmacy involvement.
- Identify key features of projects.
- Determine strategies for effective project design and implementation.
- Define project management.
- Describe the principles of project management that are applicable to health system projects involving pharmacy.
- List skills needed to successfully manage a project.

Key Concepts

❶ Use a standardized and systematic approach to develop pharmacy department and health system policies.

❷ Recognize and use resources including, but not limited to, tertiary resources, primary literature, and colleagues with expertise in the area available to develop the content of policies.

❸ Contact other institutions and make inquiries as to their policies. If a health system is a member of a group purchasing organization (e.g., Novation®), they may have access to policies and procedures that other member organizations have created.

❹ A clear and complete description of a project is necessary prior to initiation of a project.

❺ Successful projects are those in which all members of the team actively participate.

❻ Project management is a discipline or science that is goal oriented, organized, detailed, and has built-in accountability. These characteristics make it an ideal process for use in directing health system projects.

Introduction

Pharmacists in health systems are often asked to develop **policies** that not only apply to the pharmacy department, but pertain to other parts of the health system or even the system in its entirety. Given the breadth of knowledge pharmacists possess regarding medication use, they are poised to contribute to development of policies affecting each aspect of the medication use cycle (e.g., prescribing, preparation, administration). They are also asked to participate or lead teams that are tasked with a variety of projects, such as creating a process to meet a new regulatory requirement or implementing new technology (e.g., smart pumps). These tasks are unfamiliar to many pharmacists, especially those without postgraduate residency training or exposure to management or leadership curriculum in pharmacy school. The literature available to help the pharmacist is not plentiful and is often directed toward nursing, information technology, or health information management. Much of what the pharmacist is exposed to in these areas is on the job training often by individuals who may or may not have received appropriate training themselves. The information presented here is derived from the literature and other available resources, and is designed to assist the pharmacist with policy development and projects.

Policy Development

Often pharmacists are charged with projects that result in the creation of a policy. Development and creation of policy and procedure documents for health systems require some training. Most pharmacists are not specifically trained to develop and write policies. However, there are opportunities for on-the-job training and mentoring. There are also resources available through organizations that assist in policy development, such as the Agency for Healthcare Research and Quality (AHRQ; http://www.ahrq.gov). Additionally, pharmacists are involved in professional policy development through the American Society of Health-System Pharmacists (ASHP) and state-affiliated chapters.[1] ASHP-accredited postgraduate residency training requires that residents either write or review a health system or pharmacy department policy. Other postgraduate training experiences also discuss policy development. This discussion will be limited to the role of the pharmacist in the development of health system policies.

A policy is defined as a deliberate plan or course of action designed to influence and determine decisions and actions.[1] Policies establish the minimum expectations surrounding a particular activity, outline responsibilities of those involved, and set minimum rules for documentation or communication when applicable. Policies in health systems directly or indirectly affect patient care. Those that directly affect patient care give guidance and instruction in the administration of clinical services (e.g., medication administration, wound care) and are classified as patient care policies. Those polices that indirectly affect patient care are not inherently clinical in nature, but have secondary consequences for clinical outcomes. Examples include policies relating to safety, risk management, and human resources. One example of a classification scheme for all health system policies is represented in Table 18–1. Health systems have committees that review and approve policies and procedures that affect patient care and cross into other disciplines (e.g., respiratory, laboratory, radiology). Additionally, each clinical department (e.g., pharmacy, respiratory, radiology) often has a committee that reviews and approves policies specific to their department.

Pharmacists are most often involved in department-specific and patient care polices. As expected, pharmacists are most appropriate to develop the content for policies that affect the pharmacy department. Pharmacy policies are written using the same, standardized format as a health system policy (e.g., purpose, definition) and the classification scheme (e.g., administrative, human resources) is similar. For example, a health system

TABLE 18–1. HEALTH SYSTEM POLICY SAMPLE CLASSIFICATIONS

Administrative: Policies that address organizational operations

Department specific: Policies that address an individual department or work area (e.g., pharmacy, nursing, laboratory, food, and nutrition)

Human Resources: Policies that address the work environment and staff rights

Patient Care: Policies that affect patient care directly or indirectly and cross more than one department or work area

Procurement: Policies that address purchasing issues

Safety Policies and Emergency Operations Plan

will have a policy on dress code and the pharmacy will have a dress code policy specific to particular pharmacy areas (e.g., clean room). The pharmacists responsible for writing pharmacy department policies should have expertise in the specific area. For example, the supervisor of the sterile products area may be responsible for the development of a sterile compounding policy; the pharmacy manager may develop policies that address human resource issues in the department, such as dress code, absenteeism, and training; and an infectious diseases pharmacy specialist may develop a policy on aminoglycoside and vancomycin dosing.

Other policies that pharmacists are involved with include those that directly affect patient care. These patient care policies often cross into several departments (e.g., nursing, radiology) and some are specifically related to medication use and medication management. Many of these policies are required by regulatory agencies such as The Joint Commission (TJC) and include topics such as high-alert medications; look-alike, sound-alike medications; and medication administration. The pharmacist is often asked to either lead or assist in the development of these policies. Table 18–2 includes a list of policies that are well-suited for pharmacy leadership or input. Some specific examples include policies that address the use of vasoactive medications (e.g., dopamine, norepinephrine), electrolytes, and opioids. Medication use policies benefit from the knowledge of a pharmacist and, therefore, are often written by pharmacists with review from members of the medical staff and nursing along with other departments affected by the policy. A pharmacist's insight and expertise is crucial for all health system policies that involve medications. Additionally, there are policies that indirectly affect patient care; these are not inherently clinical in nature, but have secondary consequences for clinical outcomes. Examples include policies relating to safety, admissions, and discharges. Pharmacists may or may not be involved in developing these policies.

TABLE 18–2. MEDICATION USE PATIENT CARE POLICIES

- High-alert medications
- Look-alike/sound-alike medications
- Medication administration
- Intravenous push medication administration
- Medication formulary
- Electrolyte infusions
- Investigational medications
- Medication storage and security
- Home medications
- Herbal product use

❶ *Use a standardized and systematic approach to develop department and health system policies.* The following systematic approach can be used to approach and accomplish the assignment successfully: gather background data, including the health system's requirement for formatting a policy; research the standard of care or best practice; review the published evidence using a systematic approach; query similar health systems for policies; and present the draft policy to multidisciplinary group for input and buy-in.

Gathering background data, noting the need for the policy, is the initial step. For example, determine if it is mandated by a regulatory agency (e.g., TJC) or secondary to a new procedure or process. A new policy may be needed as new technology is implemented either in the health system (e.g., smart pumps, automated dispensing cabinets) or pharmacy (e.g., bar coding). The background information can also include such things as the health system's medication error reports or outside sources such as pharmacy practice journals (e.g., American Journal of Health-System Pharmacy [AJHP]) or other publications (e.g., Institute for Safe Medication Practices [ISMP] Medication Safety Alert®).

Next, research the standard of care. In medicine, the standard of care is defined as a diagnostic or treatment process that experts agree is appropriate, accepted, and widely used. Sometimes, the standard of care is referred to as best practice. It is based on external clinical information from research, but also includes an individual's practice experiences. Interviewing physicians and others as to what the practice is in the health system is appropriate when researching the standard of care. In pharmacy, the standard of care or best practice is defined as a process or procedure that is widely accepted and routine. The standard of care or best practice can be applied to a disease state or condition and refer to practices in medicine and pharmacy. For example, the standard of care for treatment of a pulmonary embolus includes the use of a weight-based intravenous heparin infusion. Using this same example, in pharmacy, the standard of care or best practice for the treatment of a pulmonary embolus includes stocking and dispensing a commercially available, fixed-concentration heparin solution (e.g., 12,500 units/250 mL). Both of these best practices or standards of care are examples of the type of information that is included in a health system policy on anticoagulant safety. Additionally, pharmacy best practice or standard of care can be related to a pharmacy process or procedure. For example, prior to dispensing a compounded sterile product prepared by a pharmacy technician, both the technician and the pharmacist initial the product label.

A variety of resources should be used for developing policies. ❷ *Recognize and use resources including, but not limited to, **tertiary resources**, **primary literature**, and colleagues with expertise in the area available to develop the content of policies.* Tertiary resources should be used to find information on standard of care review, including those that provide general product information (e.g., AHFS® Drug Information, Micromedex®), and pharmacotherapeutic information (e.g., *Applied Therapeutics: The Clinical Use of Drugs,*

Pharmacotherapy: A Pathophysiologic Approach, Pharmacotherapy: Principles and Practice, Harrison's Principles of Internal Medicine). Next, a search of the biomedical literature is appropriate to identify the current standard of care. Suggested literature search strategies and procedures including useful search engines and databases are discussed in-depth in Chapter 3. However, the most common searchable databases include PubMed® (http://www.ncbi.nlm.nih.gov/pubmed/), CINAHL Information Systems (http://www.cinahl.com), and International Pharmaceutical Abstracts (IPA) for pharmacy-specific topics. Often health system libraries not only assist with the literature search, but are able to obtain articles that may not be part of the library's holdings. Finally, a search for **clinical practice guidelines** may be warranted. Treatment guidelines are often published in biomedical journals such as Clinical Infectious Diseases and Chest and can be found using a secondary database such as PubMed®. The National Guideline Clearinghouse (http://www.guideline.gov) indexes guidelines from many sources and may be a helpful tool to identify published guidelines. Guidelines can also be found on the Web sites of professional organizations such as the Infectious Diseases Society of America (http://www.idsociety.org), American College of Cardiology (http://www.acc.org), and ASHP (http://www.ashp.org). A comprehensive overview of clinical practice guidelines including steps to locate guidelines is included in Chapter 7.

Next, the results of the literature search are evaluated. Additionally, clinical practice guidelines and clinical practice statements are also evaluated. There are many methods available that can be used to evaluate the information depending on the type of information that is retrieved (e.g., case reports, clinical trials). See Chapters 4 and 5 for methods to evaluate primary literature and Chapter 7 for methods to evaluate clinical practice guidelines.

An evidenced-based approach can be used to evaluate the information retrieved for a patient care policy. Use of this method has been described in the nursing literature.[2] The evidence-based approach involves finding the best evidence, critically evaluating it, integrating it with clinical expertise and patient preferences, and applying the results to clinical practice.[3] Studies that are retrieved should be grouped according to their design and assigned a weight or level, much the same as is done in preparing a clinical practice guideline. If a health system is going to use an evidence-based approach for policy development, it is useful to employ a tool to complete the process of organizing the literature. The tool should be practical and useful. Currently, there is no standard or accepted tool that is recommended or routinely used. A suggested tool that can be used is presented in Figure 18–1.[4] For this tool, studies and other information that has been retrieved is assigned a ranking according to such characteristics as study design. For example, information derived from a randomized double-blind, placebo-controlled trial is assigned the highest ranking and a case study or case report the lowest.

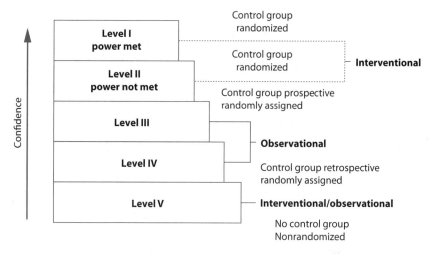

Figure 18–1. Levels of evidence. *Bryant PJ et al.*[1] *(Copyright 2009, American Society of Health-System Pharmacists.) Used with permission.*

The next step is to look to other institutions and make inquiries as to their policies. ❸ *Contact other institutions and make inquiries as to their policies. If a health system is a member of a group purchasing organization (e.g., Novation®), they may have access to policies and procedures that other member organizations have created.* Many professional organizations (e.g., ASHP, American College of Clinical Pharmacy [ACCP]) have electronic listservs for members. These listservs are often used by pharmacists for sharing information on policies and procedures. For drug information practitioners, the CAMIPR (Consortium for the Advancement of Medication Information Policy and Research) is available from the Iowa Drug Information Service.

Once the information on the background, rationale, and evidence have been gathered and summarized, a draft policy should be created and presented to policy **stakeholders** and experts for review. Most policies have several individuals responsible for writing a policy. However, there is often someone identified as the lead author. This person serves as the primary contact for comments or questions regarding the policy. Even though several individuals have written the policy, colleagues not directly involved in writing the policy may be asked to review the draft policy before it is presented to stakeholders or a committee for review. Identification of the appropriate stakeholders is crucial to creating and implementing a successful policy. A stakeholder is anyone who affects or is affected by the problem or issue addressed in the policy. Stakeholders include health system departments (e.g., nursing, pharmacy, laboratory, radiology) and their personnel. Once the stakeholders are identified, individuals, workgroups, or subcommittees that represent the stakeholders (e.g., nurse practice council, laboratory workgroup) are asked to provide comments to the primary author, who is responsible for revising the policy. At the same time, experts, those who have experience with the information contained in the policy, are asked to review the draft and provide input. After the stakeholders and experts have reviewed the draft policy, it is the lead author's responsibility to review the comments and incorporate them as necessary. Depending on the number of changes or suggestions to the draft, the policy may or may not need to be reviewed once again by the stakeholders or experts. In general, if there are major changes to the policy content (e.g., the stakeholders do not agree with the contents of the policy), a second review is warranted. However, minor changes that do not affect the purpose of the policy can be made and the policy should be presented to the pertinent health system committees.

• The content of the policy dictates what committees, subcommittees, or workgroups need to approve the policy. For instance, a health system policy that outlines the process for timely removal of health care equipment (e.g., infusion devices) that has been recalled will need review and approval from the health system's engineering and safety workgroups and committees. A policy addressing laboratory specimen collection and labeling will be reviewed and approved by clinical laboratory and nursing workgroups and committees. Finally, a policy that outlines the process for administering and monitoring hypertonic saline (e.g., 3% sodium chloride) will need review by nursing, pharmacy, and the medical staff.

• Policies may be presented and approved by the medical staff through the health system's pharmacy and therapeutics committee. At a minimum, all policies that involve the use of medications are approved by the pharmacy and therapeutics committee and the medical executive committee and/or chief of the medical staff. The structure of committees, subcommittees, and task forces in a health system is influenced by a number of factors such as regulatory agencies (e.g., TJC), practice standards particular to a geographical area, and the culture of the health system. A health system's policy-approval process may be extensive, so understanding of the process prior to developing the policy is essential. Inquiries pertaining to a health system's process for policy development (e.g., structure, format) are best directed to the regulatory or quality departments of the health system.

• The steps used for developing a policy specific to the pharmacy department are similar to those for developing a health system policy. For example, the director of pharmacy may ask the intravenous (IV) room manager to develop a policy that addresses admixture compounding for all sterile products prepared by pharmacy. The first step is to determine the justification of the policy. In this example, the United States Pharmacopeia (USP) publishes standards for preparation of sterile products, Chapter 797 Pharmaceutical Compounding—Sterile Preparations; therefore, the justification for this policy is compliance with regulatory standards and best practice. The policy ultimately affects patient safety. As the process of gathering information continues, use of professional listservs to query colleagues for any existing policies may be helpful. In this example, it is necessary to obtain and thoroughly review the most recent copy of the USP 797 chapter. Next, information gathered should be reviewed and summarized to write the policy draft. In this particular example, the amount of information needed in a policy to address the USP 797 standards is too lengthy for one policy, so separate policies may be written. Each policy contains information on one aspect of sterile compounding. For example, policies that outline environmental monitoring, personnel garb, and cleaning and disinfecting the preparation areas are reasonable. The final sets of policies are reviewed by a team of stakeholders including pharmacists, technicians, and managers/supervisors. Once these stakeholders provide their input, the policy is ready for final review and approval by pharmacy leadership.

Regardless of the type of policy (e.g., health system or department), once the policy information is reviewed and agreed upon, a structured format is used to write the policy. Most health systems have a standard format for policies including the required sections. It may be helpful to gather this information when beginning the policy-development process. Figure 18–2 contains an example of a health system policy format including the required sections of a policy. Having a standardized format for policies is important; if different departments in a health system write policies independently, this can create inconsistency and confusion for the health system. Collaboration among departments when developing policies leads to a safer environment for both staff and patients. The information that follows reviews the content of health system policy sections. It is important to note that the way in which policies are formatted will vary and is dependent on the health system.

PURPOSE STATEMENT

The purpose statement of the policy consists of one or two simple sentences explaining the reason for the policy. The purpose statement should be concise and comprehensive and is included in nearly all health system policy formats. For example, a purpose statement for a policy addressing the use of herbal products in a health system may be written as follows: "This policy establishes the position of [health system name] regarding herbal product use."

DEFINITIONS

The definitions section in the policy explains terms such as acronyms and technical or legal terms that may be unfamiliar or used with uncommon meanings. Some policy formats do not contain a definitions section and not all policies need terms defined. However, this section is helpful to the reader especially when a term has a specific meaning related to the policy. If it is necessary to provide definitions for a policy, the definitions section should start with a phrase such as, "when used in this policy, these terms have the

Type of Policy:	**PATIENT CARE**	Category:
Title:		Policy #:
		Replaces #:
Page: 1 of		Developed By:
Issue Date:		Approved By:
Revision Dates:		

I. PURPOSE: This policy	
II. DEFINITIONS: When used in this policy these terms have the following meanings:	
III. POLICY: It is the policy of	
IV. PROCEDURE: A. B.	
V. DOCUMENTATION:	
VI. REFERENCES:	
VII. ATTACHMENTS:	

Figure 18–2. Policy template for a patient care policy.

following meanings." For example, using the previous herbal product use policy example, the definitions section includes the term herbal product so that the reader is clear as to what products are included in the policy. Another example is a pharmacy policy on pharmaceutical deterioration that contains not only a definition for expiration date/time, but also states in this policy expiration date/time may be used interchangeably with the term, beyond-use date.

POLICY STATEMENT

The next step is the policy statement, which is a succinct statement of the health system's position regarding the subject matter. The policy statement is usually only one sentence, but it can be divided into subpoints if there are multiple objectives to the policy. For example, using the herbal product policy as the example, the policy statement reads, "It is the policy of the [health system name] that: A. [The health system name] does not support the use of herbal products in the acute care setting; B. The pharmacy shall not supply herbal products; C. [The health system name] employees shall not administer nonformulary herbal products to patients."

PROCEDURE

The procedure section contains a description of the steps taken to accomplish the purpose of the policy statement. This section is as detailed as possible, while allowing flexibility to individual department's operational needs. It is important to remember that the policy needs to be doable within the organization and, therefore, be written in a manner so that all may comply. Using the same herbal product use policy example, the procedure statements are clearly written to delineate nursing and prescriber responsibilities. For example, the procedure statements for nursing state that the nurse is to collect information from the patient on home herbal product use and how to document that information. It does not state when in the admission process this is to be completed, so this process can be fit into the workflow on the particular patient care unit. Additionally, the nurse is given clear instructions on how to explain to the patient and family why herbal medications are not allowed in the health system. Each procedure statement is detailed, however, not too restrictive that it interferes with current processes on the patient care unit.

DOCUMENTATION

The documentation section of the policy follows the procedure statement and contains information on what needs to be documented in the medical record or elsewhere. Usually documentation statements are written using the following statement: as appropriate in the medical record. However, there are some policies that require documentation specific to the content of the policy. For example, a pharmacy department policy on staff education may require that attendance at educational sessions be documented on a department-specific roster attached to the policy.

REFERENCES

Finally, policies are appropriately referenced. A list of related policies and professional, legal, and/or regulatory authorities is included in the references section of the policy along with any references from the literature. A health system policy on look-alike, sound-alike medications contains references such as TJC's *Comprehensive Accreditation Manual for Hospitals: The Official Handbook*, ISMP's List of Confused Drug Names, and other health system policies. Referencing another policy is done when a procedure contained in the policy is explained or contained in another policy. For example, a policy on look-alike, sound-alike medications contains information on storing look-alike products separately in order to avoid selecting the incorrect medication. Therefore, the health system's policy on medication storage is listed as a reference. Additionally, if information for a policy is obtained from tertiary resources, clinical practice guidelines, and journal articles, these resources are included in the reference section of the policy.

Policies are designed to equip both the health system and the employee with a means to ensure compliance with relevant rules and regulations. All policies must be in compliance with applicable laws and standards of regulatory accrediting agencies including, but not limited to, TJC and state licensing boards (e.g., board of pharmacy, board of nursing). A health system will have established standards for policy review, usually every 2 to 3 years and/or as required by changes in processes.

Finally, the policy development process can take several weeks to months for completion. Usually, pharmacy policies can be developed more quickly as there are fewer departments affected and, thus, fewer stakeholders who must review the policy. The most time-consuming process when developing a health system policy is trying to reach consensus among all stakeholders and experts. Initially, when asked to develop a health system policy, identification of others who will be affected by the policy (e.g., nursing, medicine) and recruitment of key nurses and physicians with whom to collaborate and ask for assistance will help facilitate the process.

Project Design

A project is defined as a temporary endeavor undertaken to produce a product or service.[5] Health system projects are diverse and can range from simple projects, such as implementation of a standard end-of-shift report, to a health system wide project, such as implementation of the **National Patient Safety Goal (NPSG)** for medication reconciliation. Projects can also include the development and implementation of a policy discussed in the previous section of this chapter. Often projects in health systems are initiated to provide a solution to an identified problem, for example, medication-dispensing errors originating from poor communication among pharmacy staff at change of shift. In this example, the solution was to create a standardized change of shift procedure, which then became a pharmacy department project. Additionally, projects may arise secondary to regulatory requirements (e.g., TJC Medication Management standards or National Patient Safety Goals).

Projects that involve or are led by pharmacists include those that impact the pharmacy only, the pharmacy and other departments (e.g., nursing, radiology), or the entire health system. Projects may affect pharmacists alone or other health care professionals (e.g., nurses, physicians, radiology technologists, laboratory technologists). Projects are unique and often involve creation of a new product or service, therefore, involve uncertainty and change. Because of this, projects may be challenging to complete and implement. Regardless, all projects have similar characteristics by definition. They have a beginning and an end, and, therefore, are temporary. The project should have a clear description and scope. The project cycle includes definition, development, implementation, and closeout.[5] Each of the steps in the project cycle will be presented.

PROJECT DEFINITION

Projects can be an original idea or assigned by supervisors or managers. They can also be assigned as part of a workgroup or committee. Regardless of who assigns the project, when it is assigned and prior to the initiation of the project, careful attention must be focused on defining it. If the project is assigned as part of a workgroup or subcommittee, it may already be defined by that individual or group who assigned the project. For example, a patient education subcommittee may assign a project to a pharmacist that requires creation of a comprehensive list of all materials used by health care professionals (e.g., nurses, pharmacists) to teach patients about medications. ❹ *A clear and complete description of a project is necessary prior to initiation of a project.* It is important to note that the pharmacist, the project lead in the example above, must have a clear vision or idea of the project outcome or goal before starting the project. In other words, the project should be begun with the end in mind. Is the project outcome to identify outdated patient education materials, update a list of available educational materials, or decide what patient education resources are to be kept or discarded? It may appear as if the patient education subcommittee has clearly defined the project to the pharmacist, and thus the outcome is clear. However, if the project lead, the pharmacist in this example, does not have a clear definition of the project, it is important to seek further clarification or direction from the person who assigned the project. With this same example, does the project include patient medication education tools that are available electronically and in paper format? Does it include educational tools produced by pharmaceutical companies?

PROJECT DESCRIPTION

After the project has been clarified, the project lead or manager develops a project description or statement. The project description explains the scope of the project. A clear and concise project description is very important as it assists with keeping the project team focused and on task. An example of a project statement for the following project, revision of the health system's patient education system is, "to establish a centralized, integrated,

I.	Project Title—brief and unique
II.	Team, department, or unit conducting the project
III.	Purpose statement—concise and clear; use an action verb in the beginning of the statement
IV.	Key personnel assigned to the project—project manager's name is listed first
V.	Methodology and milestones

Figure 18–3. Project description outline.

state-of-the-art patient education system that will further the corporate mission and strengthen the hospital image as the caregiver of choice."[6] This is an example of a project statement that accurately and concisely describes the project and coincides with the organization's mission statement. Project descriptions are more detailed and usually include the following sections: project title, unit (e.g., team conducting the project), and purpose statement. The purpose statement is concise and clear and provides the overall objective of the project. It may contain a sentence stating what the project is not addressing, as this may help the project team stay focused. Other sections of the project description include terms of reference (i.e., those key personnel assigned to the project), and methodology and milestones.[7] Regardless of what format is chosen, a project description or statement is an important tool for the members of the team, including the project lead, as it helps with communication and keeps team members aligned with the goal of the project. Figure 18–3 contains an example of a project description that can be used for health system projects.

Once the project is defined and a project description or statement is complete, a summary of the information is presented to gain the support of key stakeholders and others. This is especially true when the project affects other health care professionals, patients, or a budget. For example, the purchasing department requests that the pharmacy department purchase and replace the current intravenous immunoglobulin (IGIV) product with another that is more cost effective. This product change affects not only the pharmacy department, but also physicians, nurses, and patients. A pharmacist is asked to lead this project and begins with writing a project description. Once completed, the pharmacist identifies key stakeholders including physicians, nurses, and other pharmacists. The project is presented to pharmacists in the department with IGIV experience including those who prepare and dispense IGIV. These pharmacists assist the project leader by reviewing the new product and providing input as to the feasibility of changing IGIV products. Presentations are then developed for physicians focusing on the therapeutic equivalency of the current IGIV product and the new IGIV product. In this case, a comparison table is something that can be created to highlight both of the products. Next, the new IGIV product is reviewed with key nurse leaders (e.g., nurse educators, nurse managers) and their recommendations for introduction of the new product are discussed (e.g., pharmacist- or nurse-led education). To proceed without nursing input may make implementation problematic and jeopardize future joint nursing and pharmacy projects. Finally, the information services department must be consulted to review how the product is to be listed in the clinical information system (e.g., special instructions, infusion rates, alerts).

For projects that need approval and support of many key stakeholders and others in the health system (e.g., administration) prior to initiation, several customized presentations of the project may be needed. This may be accomplished in different venues ranging from informal discussions (e.g., focus groups) to formal presentations. Projects that impact the health system on many levels (e.g., nursing, pharmacy, medical staff) necessitate a more formal presentation to the groups most affected by the project. When preparing these communications, it is important to know the audience and develop the presentation accordingly. For example, TJC developed a NPSG that directs a health system to have a process that accurately and completely reconciles medications across the continuum of care. In other words, the health system must have a process in place as the patient enters the health system (either as an inpatient or outpatient) to collect a list of medications that the patient uses. The list is reviewed by the physician prior to initiation of any new medication. Additionally, the prescriber selects what medications from the list are to be continued. This process of medication reconciliation continues as the patient is transferred to a different level of care (e.g., from the intensive care unit to an intermediate care unit) or to another facility within the health system (e.g., a rehabilitation unit). Finally, the medications are reviewed prior to patient discharge from the health system. A list of the medications the patient is to continue at home or in another facility (e.g., a skilled nursing facility) is prepared and given to the patient and the next health care provider. At many health systems, the task of developing a process that addresses this NPSG is assigned to pharmacy and nursing. Because this is a health system project affecting many different departments, presentations to several groups of key stakeholders are required. Additionally, because this project involves many health care professionals including physicians and other prescribers, pharmacists, and nurses, several presentations are developed. It is important to prepare these presentations with an understanding of the audience and customize them accordingly. One presentation is developed for health system leadership (e.g., managers, administrators) and another for the staff (e.g., nursing and pharmacy). The health system leadership or administration is more interested in learning how the proposed medication reconciliation process can improve patient safety and achieve compliance with TJC accreditation. However, the staff is interested in hearing how performing medication reconciliation will enhance their efficiency and improve patient safety. Managers may be interested in how to educate and motivate staff to carry out the medication reconciliation process. The presentations given to the different groups are not meant to be a comprehensive review of the complete project, but provide enough information to gain approval and support from key stakeholders; the presentations focus on important points for the particular stakeholders. Such presentations can serve to motivate, and often project team members are chosen from these initial sessions. See Chapter 9 for additional information on making presentations.

PROJECT DEVELOPMENT

● The next step after support has been gained for the project is to select the project team. In the medication reconciliation example previously mentioned, members of the project team can be identified from the various meetings used to introduce the project. For all projects, large or small, project team members from several different groups including those who will be affected by the project (e.g., staff pharmacists, nurses) and those with particular skills and expertise (e.g., clinical pharmacy specialists, clinical nurse specialists, physicians) should be identified. Remember, others, such as managers, directors, and administrators, are also needed as project team members. Many projects thought to only affect a pharmacy department additionally impact other departments such as nursing, respiratory care, laboratory, and food and nutrition. Having project team members with diverse backgrounds and experiences is crucial to team success.

● Effective team leadership is challenging, and often project leaders have responsibility for completion of the work, but little authority over the team members. At times the project leader may even be subordinate to a project team member(s). However, project leaders can create effective teams by actively managing expectations. A clear and compelling picture of each task's place in the project should be communicated. Project staff should be informed of their roles and responsibilities and held accountable. The project leader plays a supportive and facilitating role rather than a directive role as the project lead. Project ownership and team development can be fostered by keeping members informed and involving team members in discussions during team meetings.[8] Effective and successful project leaders or project managers create an environment of shared responsibility. Examples of key project management leadership skills are outlined in Table 18–3. Flexibility is a critical leadership skill and different leadership styles are needed depending on the type of project and the qualifications and experience of the project team members.[7] For example, the project leader may need to use a more direct style when working with a newly licensed pharmacist, whereas a seasoned pharmacist may need less direction and a hands-off approach could prove more effective.

● Once the team is assembled, there are several methods that the project lead can use to identify the tasks that must be accomplished in order to complete the project. One method is to have the project lead develop a task schedule, which is a relatively simple process and does not require the use of project management software.[9] The tasks are listed on a sheet of paper divided into sections (Figure 18–4a). One column prioritizes tasks, another one lists the actual task, and the last two columns are to list who or what

TABLE 18–3. RECOMMENDED LEADERSHIP SKILLS FOR PROJECT MANAGERS

Ability to work with a variety of team members with different:

- Backgrounds (e.g., new employees, long-term employees)
- Disciplines (e.g., nurses, physicians, radiology technologists, laboratory technologists, nutritionists)
- Knowledge level (e.g., new graduates and nonlicensed personnel)

Ability to translate or bridge the gap among the different team members:

- Limit the use of technical jargon

Provide a clear vision, alternative solution, and plan when needed.

Build trust and respect among team members:

- Make team members decision makers especially in their specialty areas

Manage conflict or emotional responses:

- Be prepared and focus on the facts without blame or emotion

Influential:

- Build and maintain strong professional relationships with members of the health care team, including key stakeholders in specialty areas

resources are needed and the timeframe for completion. Using a task schedule allows the project lead to identify all the tasks, prioritize them, and assign the tasks to the appropriate person or persons along with a timeframe for completion. Figure 18–4b depicts a task schedule for creating patient education materials for warfarin, an oral anticoagulant. There are other methods that can be used to develop the project and they utilize two key project management tools: the work breakdown structure (WBS) and **Gantt chart**. These tools are part of project management software packages. Project management and how it can be applied to health care–related projects will be discussed later in the chapter. The

Priority	Task	Person responsible	Completion time

Figure 18–4a. Task structure outline.

Priority	Task	Person responsible	Completion time
1	List the requirements for warfarin patient education as stated in TJC* NPSG^ .03.05.01	Pharmacist team member	1 week
2	Gather the current health-system patient education booklet	Nurse team member	1 week
3	Review and edit the general information in the booklet (e.g., INR measurement, follow-up appointments, when to contact 911 or physician office, etc.)	Nurse team member	2 weeks
4	Review and edit the drug interaction information	Pharmacist team member	2 weeks
5	Review and edit the dietary information	Pharmacist and dietician team members	2 weeks
6	Present first draft to team for review	Team	4 weeks
7	Incorporate comments and present to team	Team leader	2 weeks
8	Present edited draft to team for comments	Team leader	1 week
9	Deliver final copy to printer	Team leader/printer	4 weeks
10	Proof the final copy	Team leader	2 weeks
11	Place the final copy on the health-system intranet	Printer and IS team	4 weeks
12	Notify clinical staff (nurses and pharmacists)	Nurse and pharmacist team members	

*The Joint Commission.
^National Patient Safety Goal.

Figure 18–4b. Task structure—Project: warfarin patient education booklet.

WBS is a tool that takes a defined project and groups the project's discrete work elements in a way that helps organize and define the total work scope of the project.[10] It is simply a list of all the individual tasks that must be completed in order to achieve the objective in mind. The WBS structure is a critical first step because it provides a framework for organizing and managing the approved project scope, helps to ensure that all the work has been defined, and sets the structure for planning and scheduling information. The WBS will also help each team member understand all of the project's tasks and how they relate to the project outcome. The concept of the WBS is similar to the task schedule described previously, but the WBS can be completed with the help of project management software such as Microsoft® Office Project.

The advantage of using the WBS is that with the help of project management software, it can be converted into a Gantt chart. A Gantt chart is a project management tool used to plan and monitor elements of a project. A Gantt chart takes the task identified in the WBS and represents these as elements of a bar chart.[8] This tool is not commonly used in pharmacy; however, its use in other health care disciplines (e.g., nursing) has been described.[8] The Gantt chart also guides the execution of the project and serves as a timeline. In the past, Gantt charts were drawn by hand; however, software programs, such as Microsoft® Office Project can be used to complete a WBS and Gantt chart. A Gantt chart can also be created using Microsoft® Word or Excel®. A very basic and simple example of a Gantt chart that outlines a project related to TJC NPSG on anticoagulant safety and staff education is described. In order to be in compliance with this NPSG, the health system provides staff education on the safe use of anticoagulants. In this example, a health system taskforce assigned this project to two nurses and one pharmacist. Figure 18–5 is the Gantt chart, created using Excel®, developed for this project. Notice the Gantt chart is a visual representation of the project and places each of the elements of a project clearly on a timeline; this is an example of what can be distributed at the first team meeting. Project meetings should be organized and efficient, including a meeting agenda with an assigned recording secretary to document the progress of the group.

Regardless of what tool is used to identify tasks (e.g., task schedule, WBS), one of the most effective ways to develop project tasks is to bring the project team together for a brainstorming session during which the project lead presents the project and asks the team to identify the tasks that need to be accomplished in order to complete the project. ❺ *Successful projects are those in which all members of the team actively participate.* Unequal participation in project teams frustrates team members, other health care staff and managers, and can jeopardize successful completion of projects. Since the entire

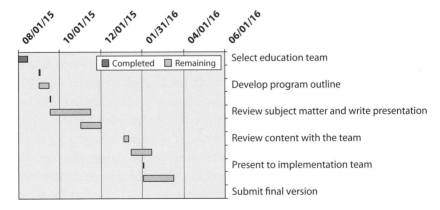

Figure 18–5. Gantt chart for a sample project using Excel® software.
Project title: Staff education for safe use of anticoagulants.

team participates in the development of the task schedule and takes ownership in completing the tasks, using this approach fosters cooperative learning and management skills development.[7] It is not necessary to prioritize the tasks until all of them have been identified. When prioritizing tasks, all team members should be encouraged to participate. The likelihood that all tasks will be completed and the project outcome will be a success is increased since all team members have an active role in task identification and prioritization.

Communication is vital to the success of the team. Regular meetings, including a project kick-off meeting, will help set an expectation of regular communication. Follow-up meetings should be concise and include regular updates and use of the Gantt chart to track progress. Showing project team members their accomplishments and progress to project completion will motivate team members to stay on track up to implementation and project completion. If a Gantt chart is not used, a task schedule should be updated regularly before every meeting. Team members can then see how the project is progressing. Strike through those tasks as they are completed again to show the team that progress is occurring. It is also possible to use other software that facilitates group work, such as Microsoft® SharePoint, which can create a work area with a library of documents, calendar, and centralized, dynamic task list.

Project Implementation

If a project has been well organized and managed appropriately, implementation should be successful. Once project details have been finalized, the team should create an implementation packet. The packet focuses on how the project will be implemented rather than development. A complete implementation packet contains the following: background and rationale for the project, pertinent policies and procedures, educational materials that are created for the specific disciplines involved, and an effective date. In the previous example of a medication reconciliation process, the project implementation phase must be complete in order for the process to be used correctly and thus improve patient safety. The rationale for why this process is being introduced into the health system must be clear. For example, the rationale can include a review of health system medication errors related to a lack of reconciliation and any other local or national medication error data (e.g., ISMP reports). A patient care policy outlining the procedure for the nursing, pharmacy, and medical staff must be developed, reviewed, and approved by the appropriate committees (e.g., pharmacy and therapeutics) prior to introducing the medication reconciliation process. In this example, an education plan is completed prior to introduction of the program to the patient care unit.

Project Closeout

Once the project has been completed successfully, the next step is an evaluation of the project.[9] Often, teams are so thankful that a project is completed that they fail to reflect on the project. The team should meet to discuss whether project goals were met and if the project was to be done again and which processes or steps would be modified for future projects.

Project Management

❻ *Project management is a discipline or science that is goal oriented, organized, detailed, and has built-in accountability. These characteristics make it an ideal process for use in directing health system projects.* This discipline combines concepts from a variety of fields, including engineering and construction.[11] It focuses on organizing and managing resources so that the project can be completed within a given time period. Using a project management approach offers much strength. Its strong goal orientation, detailed planning, and accountability help ensure the successful completion of projects. The task schedule, WBS, and Gantt chart previously described are project management tools to facilitate the process.

Project management has been applied to large-scale projects (e.g., data systems implementation, large construction projects) in a number of industries other than health care. In health care, the project management methodology has been traditionally associated with information technology (IT) projects (e.g., implementation of a clinical information system). Project management has also been utilized by the pharmaceutical industry to develop new drugs. Additionally, project management techniques have been used to provide care for inpatients[12] and develop patient education materials,[6] and have been suggested as a means to provide health care services and reduce costs with the physician serving as the project manager.[13] However, the principles of project management can be applied to many other and different pharmacy-related projects both large and small. Actually, project management principles have been recommended for use in practice-based research (e.g., residency research projects).[11] Some other pharmacy projects that can utilize the project management process include the implementation of a continuing education lecture series or opening an operating room satellite pharmacy. These projects affect not only personnel but budgets, so they are well suited for a project manager.

There are a number of tools and processes that need to be in place in order for a project management approach to be used successfully in the pharmacy department.

Merely purchasing project management tools, such as software, without the necessary staff training and development will not create a project-management-savvy department and will not help the pharmacist become an effective project manager. The pharmacy department, including administration and the pharmacy staff (those that lead projects and participate in teams), must be committed to using a project management approach and adopt project management principles as part of their culture. Additionally, senior management must be committed to project management, otherwise staff may not make an effort to use project planning tools effectively.[7] If a department decides to embrace project management, training of the pharmacists is critical. As mentioned, project management tools and techniques along with leadership skills are used to effectively manage projects. Pharmacists may have some of the basic leadership skills; however, this skill set may need to be enhanced because of challenges based on time constraints and interpersonal conflicts that may arise among project team members. Additionally, training on the use of various software tools and other techniques used in project management is essential. There are a variety of organizations and universities that offer project management training. A proposed training program for nursing is described[7] that includes a train-the-trainer format encompassing 3 to 5 days of education. Course content includes a discussion of the tools used in project management and essential leadership skills. The Project Management Institute (http://www.pmi.org), a nonprofit professional organization for project management professionals, offers useful resources such as journals, textbooks, and educational conferences. Professionals can also become certified or credentialed in various project management areas. Professional pharmacy associations (e.g., ASHP, ACCP) offer leadership conferences and seminars that provide education on leadership styles in addition to project management.[14] Health systems that have embraced project management may also offer classes or training. These classes are often coordinated in the organization development department of human resources.

Pharmacists who assume health system leadership roles in designing, implementing, and evaluating programs that affect patient care can serve as project managers. In order to be effective project managers, pharmacists must possess management and leadership abilities and skills. A flexible leadership style is essential in order to benefit from the talents, skills sets, and ideas of each member of the team. Leaders who are flexible encourage and acknowledge input from all team members and empower members to carry out the assigned task. Management skills not only include product and technical knowledge, but knowledge of project management activities and tools. The pharmacist managing the project must be able to define the project and scope, gain approval and support from key stakeholders, establish a team, develop a timeline providing regular updates, allocate resources (e.g., time), direct project activities, manage problems, and ensure quality control. This is a complex task, but there are resources (e.g., textbooks, seminars) available to assist the pharmacist in successful completion of a project.

Conclusion

Today's health system pharmacist is recognized as not only a valuable member of the health care team, but someone who has an important role in the success of a health system. Pharmacists, with their expertise in pharmacotherapy and medication safety, are uniquely situated to be involved in and lead policy development. They also have skills that allow them to be active participants and leaders on project teams. The tools that pharmacists use for these activities are gradually being introduced via the health care literature and professional societies. This skill set should be taught early in the educational process for pharmacists, with a specific recommendation from the Center for the Advancement of Pharmacy Education to engage pharmacy students in the development of professional documents that are relevant to needs of various organizations, specifically formulary monographs and policy development.[15] This may be accomplished in the drug information curriculum. Pharmacists with additional training in drug information are often involved with policy development and project implementation given their involvement with formulary management. Additionally, a pharmacist with a strong drug information skill set is an ideal candidate to participate in policy development since it requires thorough and accurate analysis of evidence-based medicine and quality improvement initiatives. For more in-depth training, professional certificate programs or a Master of Business Administration (MBA) program may be of interest. The information contained in this chapter is designed to assist the pharmacist in policy development and project design and implementation.

Case Study 18-1

As a clinical pharmacist in the ambulatory care clinic of a large academic medical center, you participate in formulary management to support the efforts of the pharmacy department and the health system to provide safe, effective, and cost-effective medications for use within the system. Currently, atorvastatin, an HMG-CoA reductase inhibitor, is the formulary agent in this class. Nonformulary usage reports indicate significant dispensing of simvastatin and rosuvastatin as well. You are asked to develop an automatic therapeutic interchange policy for the health system to decrease the amount of nonformulary prescribing of these agents.

- *List the steps used to approach this assignment.*
- *Discuss the resources used when gathering background information.*
- *Explain the process to summarize the information collected for development of the policy.*
- *Define stakeholder and identify key stakeholders for this policy.*

Self-Assessment Questions

1. The following health system policies require a pharmacist's participation, *except*:
   a. Herbal product use
   b. High-alert medications
   c. Medical resident supervision
   d. Electrolyte infusions
   e. Drug shortages

2. When gathering information for inclusion in a health system policy, what is the initial step?
   a. Conduct a literature search using CINAHL information systems.
   b. Ask for a meeting with the director of pharmacy.
   c. Contact colleagues who work at other health systems.
   d. Gather background information including the justification of the policy.
   e. Conduct a literature search using PubMed®.

3. Prior to starting a project, a tool that is recommended to use for defining the project is:
   a. Project description
   b. Procedure
   c. Work breakdown structure (WBS)
   d. Gantt chart
   e. Policy

4. Select the skills needed to be an effective project manager.
   a. Technical knowledge of the project components
   b. Ability to work with a multidisciplinary team
   c. Capacity to manage conflicts or emotional responses from project team members
   d. Organizational and time management
   e. All of the above

5. The components of the project cycle are:
   a. Project definition, development, implementation, and closeout
   b. Project development, justification, implementation, and review
   c. Project strengths, weaknesses, opportunities, and threats
   d. Project identification, justification, implementation, and closeout
   e. Project deliberation, strengths, weaknesses, and review

6. Which of the following provides specific guidance on how to perform a given task?
   a. Policy
   b. Procedure
   c. Project description
   d. Purpose statement
   e. Project activities

7. Which of the following resources should be used to research the standard of care before engaging in writing a policy?
   a. Tertiary references
   b. Clinical treatment guidelines
   c. Primary literature
   d. Colleagues and coworkers
   e. All of the above

8. Which of the following has the strongest level of evidence?
   a. Tertiary resources
   b. Randomized controlled trial
   c. Case series
   d. Cohort study
   e. Systematic review

9. Which of the following is/are a type(s) of health system policy classification?
   a. Patient care
   b. Procurement
   c. Administrative
   d. Human resource
   e. All of the above

10. Additional resources to build a skill set in policy development and/or project design include:
    a. Professional pharmacy organization programs
    b. Business programs (e.g., MBA program)
    c. Tertiary references (e.g., textbooks)
    d. Agency for Healthcare Research and Quality (AHRQ)
    e. All of the above

11. At what phase should a policy *first* be presented to key stakeholders for review and consideration?
    a. Brainstorming phase
    b. Following policy approval

    c. Draft phase

    d. At the time of approval

    e. It is not necessary at any phase

12. A purpose statement of the policy is a step-by-step description of how the issue addressed in the policy should be managed.

    a. True

    b. False

13. When establishing the standard of care prior to policy development, it is appropriate to interview physicians to understand current practice in the health system.

    a. True

    b. False

14. Project descriptions include the following:

    a. Project title

    b. Team members

    c. Purpose statement

    d. Methodology

    e. All of the above

15. A project implementation packet should include the following, *except:*

    a. Background

    b. Rationale

    c. Barriers to implementation

    d. Policies and procedures

    e. Effective date

REFERENCES

1. Allcock NM. Getting involved in professional policy development. Am J Health Syst Pharm. 2007;64:1144-6.
2. Oman KS, Duran C, Fink R. Evidence-based policy and procedures. JONA. 2008;38(1):47-51.
3. Sackett DI, Rosenberg WM, Gray JA, Haynes RB, Richardson WS. Evidence-based medicine: what it is and what it isn't. BMJ. 1996;312(7023):71-2.
4. Stetler CB, Brunell M, Giuliano KK, Morsi D, Prince L, Newell-Stokes V. Evidence-based practice and the role of nursing leadership. JONA. 1998;28(7):45-53.
5. Doll BA. Project management 101. Skills for leading and working in teams, Part 1. JAHIMA. 2005 Jan;76(1):50.
6. Patyk M, Gaynor S, Verdin J. Patient education resource assessment: project management. J Nurs Care Qual. 2000;14(2):14-20.

7. Loo R. Project management: a core competency for professional nurses and nurse managers. J Nurse Staff Dev. 2003;19(4):187-93.

8. Doll BA. Project management 101. Skills for leading and working in teams, Part 4. J AHIMA. 2005 Apr;76(4):48, 50.

9. Berry R. Project management for nurses. J Intraven Nurs. 1994;17(1):28-34.

10. Shirey MR. Project management tools for leaders and entrepreneurs. Clin Nurse Spec. 2008;22(3)129-31.

11. Weber RJ, Corbaugh DJ. Developing and executing an effective research plan. Am J Health-Syst Pharm. 2008;65:2058-65.

12. Kaufman DS. Using project management methodology to plan and track inpatient care. Jt Comm J Qual Patient Saf. 2005;31(8):463-8.

13. Sa Couto J. Project management can help to reduce costs and improve quality in health care services. J Eval Clin Pract. 2008;14:48-52.

14. American Society of Health-System Pharmacists. Proceedings of the ASHP 2007 Conference for Leaders in Health-System Pharmacy. Am J Health Syst Pharm. 2008;65:e19-22.

15. Medina MS, Plaza CM, Stowe CD, Robinson ET, DeLander G, Beck DE, et al. Center for the Advancement of Pharmacy Education (CAPE) Educational Outcomes 2013. Am J Pharm Educ. 2013;77(8):Article 162.

SUGGESTED READING

Fortier CR, Mitchell SH. Pharmacists' role in managing medication use projects. In: Fox BI, Thrower MR, Felkey BG, eds. Building core competencies in pharmacy informatics. Washington, DC: American Pharmacists Association; 2010.

19

Chapter Nineteen

Drug Information in Ambulatory Care

Debra L. Parker

Learning Objectives

After completing this chapter, the reader will be able to

- Describe the importance of drug information provided by the health care professional in the ambulatory care setting.
- Discuss the importance of access to up-to-date formulary information in the provision of care in the ambulatory setting.
- Identify sources with links to full-text evidence-based practice guidelines.
- Describe desired characteristics of drug information resources specific to the ambulatory environment.
- Describe reputable drug information sources geared toward the health care professional that are also useful in providing drug information to patients.
- List ways that practitioners may address concerns regarding access to information.
- Discuss importance of providing drug information regarding disposal of unused, unwanted, or expired medications and immunizations.
- Identify resources providing quality-assurance indicators for optimal provision of ambulatory care.

Key Concepts

① The clinician in the ambulatory care setting routinely utilizes multiple drug information skills on a daily basis to not only provide drug information to patients and other health care providers, but to function competently and efficiently within this practice setting.

② The ambulatory care practitioner is the person with the greatest opportunity to fill the role of medication information provider and interpreter to the lay public.

❸ Knowledge of formulary status of medications is only one part of the prescription decision-making process. Whenever they exist, evidence-based clinical practice guidelines should guide prescriptive decision making.

❹ Ambulatory practitioners have the responsibility to remain up-to-date regarding current practice guidelines.

❺ Increasingly more medical literature, including tertiary references, is being provided in the electronic or Internet-based format, and such databases are attractive to utilize in ambulatory care for multiple reasons.

❻ Ambulatory care clinicians bear a responsibility to educate patients on the proper disposal of unused and unwanted medications and should, therefore, be aware of pertinent sites for information.

❼ While ambulatory clinicians (in particular, pharmacists) typically recommend and/or dispense most medications, immunizations are medications that are administered in the ambulatory care setting. Those practitioners immunizing in this setting have the obligation to not only provide these services safely, but to serve as immediate sources of information (i.e., drug information) regarding the medications they are administering.

❽ Health care professionals involved in the provision of care in the ambulatory care setting should familiarize themselves with the pertinent established quality measures.

Introduction

This textbook covers a long list of drug information topics and skills, although not every clinician will use all of these skills on a daily basis. **❶** *The clinician in the ambulatory care setting routinely utilizes multiple drug information skills on a daily basis to not only provide drug information to patients and other health care providers, but to function competently and efficiently within this practice setting.*

The ambulatory care practitioner is required to use a variety of drug information skills and resources during routine encounters with patients to provide information at a personalized and appropriate level. Before doing so, the practitioner must know where to look for appropriate information, and how to interpret and practically apply this information to a specific patient or population. This is where many practitioners may be challenged.

This chapter discusses the resources and skills commonly needed by the ambulatory care provider in order to provide appropriate drug information. Topics covered will include (a) commonly used references for prescription formularies and for obtaining evidence-based guidelines, (b) desired characteristics of drug information resources and examples of those particularly useful to the ambulatory care clinician, (c) information resources pertinent to the current trends in ambulatory care, such as the proper disposal of unused or unwanted or expired medications, (d) preventive health information (specifically regarding immunizations), and (e) quality-assurance measures in ambulatory care.

Ambulatory care encompasses a variety of settings. For example, an ambulatory care practitioner may be a clinician who practices in a community pharmacy (including persons in medication-dispensing roles), a community-based clinic or office, an outpatient setting of an institutional care facility, or someone who provides on-site services within an employer-provided wellness and disease management program. As such, the case scenarios within this chapter include scenarios where the provider is in a medication-dispensing role as well as where the provider is in a nondispensing role.

Why Focus on Drug Information Specifically in the Ambulatory Care Setting?

Although the provision of health care takes place in a variety of settings, ranging from hospital and long-term care facilities to patients' homes, the emphasis in today's patient care environment is to provide as much health care as possible in the outpatient, ambulatory setting. This may or may not be a setting that dispenses medications. It is also commonly recognized that patients are increasingly technologically savvy and utilize the Internet and news media to provide self-care in the outpatient setting. The quality of the medical and drug information patients obtain themselves varies widely, depending on the source (see Chapters 4 and 5 for drug literature evaluation); however, even when quality information is obtained by a patient or family member, someone with clinical expertise and drug information training is necessary to explain medical information and to provide guidance in the decision-making process.

Finally, with increasing numbers of team-based patient care models such as **patient-centered medical homes (PCMHs)** being established across the country, the provision of accurate, comprehensive drug information in the ambulatory setting is growing exponentially, as it is crucial to (a) researching appropriate medical treatment, especially of chronic conditions, (b) bridging the gap between data provided from health information technology and how to most effectively use these data to treat patients on an individual and population-based basis, and (c) educating patients regarding their treatment.

Providing Drug Information in the Ambulatory Setting

"I CAN JUST GOOGLE® IT MYSELF"

Given the name of a medication, the average lay person may well be able to Google® the name of the drug, and would very likely find general information regarding its use and side effects. Blogs regarding the experiences of other people with that particular medication may also be easily found, as well as anecdotal comments about the drug and the condition being treated, including outdated information. The average patient is, in fact, able to access a plethora of information via Web sites and blogs; however, the reliability, accuracy, and timeliness of this information can vary widely, as discussed in Chapter 3. While some of these sources of drug information may be reputable, they are impersonal and can only offer general information to the reader. Such sites typically advise patients to talk with their practitioners for specific personal questions.

WHAT SHOULD THE PUBLIC (OR OTHER HEALTH CARE PROVIDERS) KNOW ABOUT UTILIZING CLINICIANS TRAINED IN DRUG INFORMATION VERSUS PERFORMING THEIR OWN SEARCHES?

Health care providers fill an important role in the provision, interpretation, perspective on clinical application, and, perhaps most importantly, providing patient-specific application of drug information that is often targeted toward the layperson by the media. While there is an ever-increasing trend toward patient empowerment, self-care, and self-education, the lay public is often unaware that the health care provider has access not only to the same Web sites as the patient, but also to professional literature and databases (see Chapter 3) that expand and often provide critical analysis of the information the public accesses. The lay person is unable to access and/or interpret such information. Depending on their clinical training, even certain health care providers may also lack knowledge regarding available resources and how to best interpret health information data.

Although in some cases, individuals may be able to personally access secondary or even primary literature, interpreting this information and putting it into context with their personal health conditions as well as with current evidence-based guidelines (see Chapter 7) require a health care professional trained in drug information. Interpreting and evaluating primary literature (see Chapters 4 and 5) as well as locating and interpreting evidence-based guidelines are skills that require training and practice. These activities call for an individual trained in drug evaluation and with expertise in these areas (see Chapters 3, 4, 5, 7, and 8).

❷ *The ambulatory care practitioner is the person with the greatest opportunity to fill the role of medication information provider and interpreter to the lay public.* The definition of the ambulatory care practitioner is changing, with a growing number of health care settings (e.g., particular PCMHs) lending themselves to providing streamlined, comprehensive outpatient care. Any medical care delivered on an outpatient basis is considered ambulatory care. For example, an ambulatory care practitioner may be a clinician who practices in a community pharmacy (including persons in medication-dispensing roles), a community-based clinic or office, an outpatient setting of an institutional care facility, or someone who provides on-site services within an employer-provided wellness and disease management program.

Although proficiently providing drug information is a skill which requires training and practice, often the biggest challenge for ambulatory care practitioners is not providing the needed drug information skills proficiently, but convincing the public that they offer a unique skill in drug information beyond the Internet.

Unfortunately, many practitioners place too little emphasis on the need for their involvement in interpretation of drug information, assuming that other health care professionals and even the public itself, with adequate access to information databases, can research and answer their own questions. In 2001, it was reported that in 1 year, approximately nine million hospital admissions and over 18 million emergency room visits in the United States (U.S.) were caused by incorrect use of medications.[1] Although these data were published several years ago, this is an issue that has not resolved. Consider a study conducted in Vancouver, Canada, published in 2008, which reported pharmaceuticals were the cause of 12% of emergency room visits and resulted in significantly longer length of stays for those patients admitted.[2] In a 2011 study published by Budnitz and associates, of over 100,000 medication-related emergency room visits, only 1.2% of medication-related emergency room visits were attributed to what were classified as high-risk medications.[3] Finally, according to a 2012 update from the Centers for Disease Control and Prevention (CDC), over 700,000 emergency room visits are made in the United States every year as a result of what are often preventable adverse drug events.[4] The circumstances behind these statistics are certainly multifactorial, and may include nonadherence or misuse of medications, lack of communication between patients and health care providers, and clinically inappropriate prescribing patterns. Paramount to correcting each of these factors is the research, interpretation and communication of drug-related information to all parties.

In today's environment, with direct-to-consumer advertising (see Chapter 23) and increasing numbers of nonprescription medications that were formerly available only by prescription, the decision to use a medication is not made solely by prescribers, but also by patients themselves. It is evident that all decision makers need guidance. Who guides these decision makers? Unfortunately, the answer is often no one.

There is certainly not a lack of available drug information, nor is there, for many individuals, a lack of accessibility. What is lacking, however, is the provision of quality drug information provided by a practitioner trained to do so for not only patients, but for other health care providers.

The emphasis placed on drug information in the curricula for different types of health care professionals vary widely; however, it can be said that pharmacists are the health care professionals with the greatest amount of time devoted to this topic in their professional training. As such, this profession bears the responsibility to educate both the public and fellow health care providers. Examples of this type of education in the ambulatory setting may include (a) whenever possible, ensuring that biased sources such as pharmaceutical salespersons are not the main source of new product education for prescribers, (b) leading or facilitating discussions with prescribers regarding newly published studies, meta-analyses, and clinical guidelines, with emphasis on an understanding of limitations of these publications and how they apply specifically to those prescribers' patient populations, (c) researching and answering drug information questions (which may or may not be patient-specific), (d) writing newsletters regarding topics pertinent in the media, and/or in the condition-specific clinic(s) in which the pharmacist works, (e) "debunking" misperceptions that may arise from direct-to-consumer advertising regarding exaggerated efficacy or risk associated with treatments, (f) providing basic statistical training including terms such as relative risk versus actual risk of treatments, and how to determine them. In addition, it is worth mentioning that in order to provide patient-specific drug information, complete medication profiles must be obtained, and this often involves communication between not only outpatient/ambulatory care clinics, but one or more pharmacies to get the full picture regarding all pertinent medical conditions and medications. Regardless of which method(s) are used to educate fellow clinicians, it is vital that pharmacists are prepared to explain the vital role they play in assisting others to understand and use medications in the safest and most effective way possible.

In today's busy society, the case for the pharmacist (and subsequent pharmacist-provided drug information) needs to be concise and to the point. Until that case is made to the public and other payers for health care, including both employers and legislators, it is likely that pharmaceuticals will continue to have the unintended effect of increasing, rather than decreasing morbidity and mortality, and contributing to rising health care expenditures.

The following section discusses resources integral to the provision of drug information in ambulatory care.

Drug Information Responsibilities in Ambulatory Care

Integral drug information-related responsibilities of the ambulatory care clinician are many. Several key responsibilities include (1) assisting prescribers and consumers to find the most cost-effective drug to treat a given condition, (2) ensuring a prescribed medication is appropriate and follows current treatment guidelines, (3) ensuring a patient's understanding of the appropriate use of their medications (see Chapter 20), (4) guiding others regarding the proper disposal of unused or unwanted medications, (5) delivering preventive health information, and (6) incorporating quality-assurance indicators into daily practice.

Practitioners who may not be the initial prescribers of medications (e.g., those who work under consult agreement, collaborative practice agreement, or who work with supervisory physicians or collaborating physicians) must be familiar with this information. Regardless of the U.S. state in which a clinician practices, and regardless of health care provider degree (e.g., PharmD, Physician Assistant, Nurse Practitioner), sound recommendations regarding modifications in drug therapy, drug therapy renewal, and initial drug therapy recommendations all hinge upon a solid understanding of drug formularies, appropriate practice guidelines, and drug information database considerations.

DRUG FORMULARY INFORMATION

Key to assisting prescribers and consumers in finding the most cost-effective treatment is familiarity with drug **formularies**. Whether a clinician is prescribing or filling a prescription order, formulary restrictions increasingly influence **medication usage patterns**.

A formulary is a list of medications that are approved to be paid for or provided at a discounted rate through prescription insurance plans. It is important to note that even if a medication is not included on a formulary (i.e., is considered "nonformulary"), or is not listed as a preferred option by the payer for a patient's prescription drugs, the prescriber is *not* bound to this when deciding whether to prescribe that medication and nothing prohibits the pharmacist from filling an appropriate medication for a patient, *regardless* of its formulary status.

Additionally, there are some medications that, while on formulary, may require prior authorization from the insurance company before it will be paid for. That does not mean it cannot be dispensed—it only means that if the patient wants the insurance company to pay for the medication, additional information must be provided in advance regarding the medical need. The pharmacist plays an integral role in working with the prescriber on a patient's behalf to obtain an insurance company's authorization to fill a prescription for such a medication.

What formulary status ultimately affects is the amount the patient will personally pay for a medication. Several useful tools exist to assist in determining formulary restrictions and then making decisions as to risks versus benefits of abiding by these restrictions.

Center for Medicaid and Medicare Services

The Center for Medicaid and Medicare Services (CMS) is a government agency within the U.S. Department of Health and Human Services that is responsible for the administration of this country's Medicare and Medicaid services, through which medical and prescription benefits are derived for select components of the populations, traditionally for the poor, elderly, and disabled. Historically, private insurances have modeled reimbursement structures for medical and medicine-related costs after the CMS model. Current health care reform in the United States is anticipated to result in increasing numbers of persons who were either uninsured or underinsured (without adequate prescription insurance to cover medical-related costs) to now being insured through either Medicaid or other government mandated programs. In other words, the landscape of prescription coverage will change, and many patients' prescription constraints will shift from those related to personal finance to those related to formulary restrictions.

In addition, it remains a fact that the largest proportion of the population taking prescription medications are already Medicare recipients. These persons' drug coverage is provided through a component of Medicare called Medicare Part D. Through this program, various insurances provide government-funded prescription coverage for Medicare recipients. Each insurance company has a different formulary, or list of drugs that are provided at a reduced price to Medicare recipients. As such, understanding formularies and their restrictions, as well as the ability to access to Medicare drug plan (i.e., Medicare Part D) formulary information is paramount. Although many patients may select their own Medicare drug provider and plan, others often look to their pharmacist to assist them in this decision. Drug plan selection is done largely online and is based on a patient's prescription profile as well as geographic location. A pharmacist is an ideal person to assist with this process as this is the provider likely to be most familiar with various drug classes listed on drug plan formularies as well as acceptable over-the-counter and generic alternatives to specific medications. Information to guide selection is available at http://www.medicare.gov and clicking on the link to "Find health and drug plans," https://www.medicare.gov/find-a-plan/questions/home.aspx. Users choose their state of residence and enter their prescription drug profile (i.e., the list of prescriptions the patient takes). The program will then provide a list of Medicare Part D plans that include some or all of the medications the patient takes, as well as information regarding the status of each drug in a particular plan, and the number of pharmacies that participate with a plan in a given state. Users, including prescribers, can also download complete formularies, as well as appeals and exceptions forms. These are forms that may be completed, usually by the prescriber on behalf of the patient asking for consideration of payment for a drug due to extenuative circumstances or a situation specific to that patient. This Web site can be used by patients alone or may be used by a provider on behalf of the patient. Additionally, it is useful for the provider needing to complete necessary forms for patients requiring a medication not covered on their formulary plan. Finally, although not required to prescribe for medications on a patient's specific drug plan, providers may use the site to determine if a drug will be paid for, and if not, if there are acceptable therapeutic alternatives that will be covered.

An additional method for obtaining formulary information via the Internet is by typing the name of the prescription insurance provider+formulary+the calendar year you desire (e.g., 2015) in the Internet search engine (e.g., Google®, Bing™). Most prescription insurance providers will have Web pages that include a full formulary guide, a list of covered medications listed by drug or by drug class, **medications tier status** in which participants are subject to varying levels of copayment options for a given drug (depending on its formulary status) links to suggested alternatives to a medication if it is not covered, and links for forms necessary for prior approval, appeals, and exceptions. An advantage to using these Web sites is immediate access to information and necessary forms. Each prescription insurance provider, however, will have a different Web page design and there is often not consistency as to where the user will find information.

Epocrates®

Many clinicians may be familiar with Epocrates®, Inc., software programs (http://www.epocrates.com/). Epocrates®, Inc., markets programs with a variety of content areas including calculations, continuing medical education, diagnostics, a medical dictionary, disease state information, drugs, pill identification, medical news, and tables. These content areas are bundled into various data packages, some of which are free. All Epocrates® programs, including those that are available at no cost, include both national and regional formulary information, including Medicare Part D. Users can access formulary status and restrictions for over 3300 brand and generic medications. Users of these programs select the formulary or formularies they desire to include in their searches. Epocrates®, Inc., updates formulary information at least once per week.[5]

Epocrates® accounts may be established on the Internet, but for those practitioners who work without Internet access; these programs are downloadable to handheld electronic devices (e.g., iPhone/iPad and Android). This program may prove the most practical solution for providers who require timely formulary information and who operate without full Internet access. It is strongly recommended, however, in light of increasing amounts of current drug information available exclusively online, or for which online access provides regularly updated information not otherwise available, that all providers of drug information and direct patient care insist on Internet access in order to ethically and competently perform their responsibilities.

Electronic Prescribing (e-Prescribing) Platforms

Clinicians with prescribing privileges should also note that electronic prescribing (e-prescribing) platforms provide drug and formulary information at the point of care. In a 2008 study conducted by the Agency for Healthcare Research and Quality (AHRQ) and published in the Archives of Internal Medicine, prescribers utilizing e-prescribing platforms with **formulary decision supports (FDS)** were significantly more likely to prescribe tier 1 (least expensive) medications, with resulting significant potential cost savings.[6] Chang and associates evaluated over 21,000 prescriptions for just over 1 year, and reported in 2010 that generic drug use was 6% higher, formulary drug use was 3% higher, and cost savings for the payer and prescription drug member was over 17% higher for those prescriptions electronically prescribed.[7]

Lexicomp®

Finally, as outlined later in this chapter, Lexicomp® online drug information, http://lexi .com, also contains useful formulary information.

It is important to note, however, that ❸ *knowledge of formulary status of medications is only one part of the prescription decision-making process. Whenever they exist, evidence-based clinical practice guidelines should guide prescriptive decision making.*

CURRENT PRACTICE GUIDELINE INFORMATION

It is beyond the scope of this chapter to discuss in depth the development and the interpretation of evidence-based clinical practice guideline recommendations (see Chapter 7). It is important to note, however, that ❹ *ambulatory practitioners have the responsibility to remain up-to-date regarding current practice guidelines.* No individual can be expected to know the current treatment guidelines for every condition; however, clinicians can and should be expected to be able to retrieve this information quickly and efficiently. The following outlines several sources for such retrieval.

Perhaps most useful to the ambulatory care clinician may be the databases that include mobile applications. The Centers for Disease Control and Prevention Web site includes free mobile apps (compatible with iPhone/iPad, Android, and Microsoft Windows 8) for a variety of medical conditions, available at http://www.cdc.gov/mobile/mobileapp.html.

Clinicians searching for current practice guidelines may also wish to visit the National Guideline Clearinghouse (NGC), http://www.guideline.gov. This compilation of evidence-based clinical practice guidelines is a project of the American Health Insurance Plan (AHIP) and the AHRQ, and is a public resource for evidence-based clinical practice guidelines. The NGC includes links to full-text current treatment guidelines, guidelines in process, as well as archived guidelines. Side-by-side comparison of two or more treatment guidelines for a given condition is also available. Users may search this site by disease/ condition, treatment/intervention, or organization.[8] If Internet or wireless Internet access (depending on practice location) is not readily available, users can download guidelines, often at no cost, in HTML format to their personal handheld devices for quick reference. Clinicians in this situation may wish to consider downloading treatment guidelines they most commonly refer to in their particular practice, checking regularly for updates. For example, a general practitioner may wish to download the current American Diabetes Association (ADA) guidelines, the current American College of Cardiology and American Heart Association guideline for the treatment of hypercholesterolemia, and the current Joint National Committee (JNC) guidelines for the treatment of hypertension. Clinicians who may work primarily with a specialized population may wish to tailor downloads to those pertinent to their area of practice. The NCG Web site also provides links to the Web sites of various guideline developers (e.g., American Academy of Dermatology, American Academy of Family Physicians, etc.) for those that have mobile-device-friendly formats of their guidelines.

The Iowa Drug Information Service (IDIS) database also provides an efficient method for locating treatment guidelines.[9] Users may narrow the type of journal article the database retrieves by utilizing the descriptor *practice guidelines*, and then typing the disease state they are researching in the appropriate text box. Users have online full-text access to articles published after 1988. This database requires a subscription, however, and is *not* freely available to the public.

Many additional search engines and Internet sites, including sites for the organizations such as the American Heart Association and the American Diabetes Association include links to current full-text, pertinent practice guidelines. Those sites that may be particularly useful to the ambulatory care practitioner because they (a) are available without a subscription and (b) provide links to full-text guidelines for a large number of medical conditions include Health Services Technology Assessment Texts (HSTAT), http://www.ncbi.nlm.nih.gov/books/NBK16710/; the Turning Research Into Practice (TRIP) Database, http://www.tripdatabase.com//; and PubMed®, http://www.pubmed.com; PubMed does allow the user to establish (for free) a user account and allow the viewer to filter searches to include review articles (which may include clinical practice guidelines). Some, but not all, search results within PubMed® provide links to full-text articles. Those that do not provide full-text article links provide full citations.[10]

The American Society of Health-Systems Pharmacists (ASHP) also provides links to what it has deemed Best Practice policies and treatment guidelines (http://www.ashp .org/bestpractices). The American Pharmacists Association (APhA), while it does not endorse guidelines as ASHP does, also provides links from its Web site to select practice guidelines (http://www.pharmacist.com).

This list is not all inclusive. For example, MEDLINE® (which is partially available via PubMed), EMBASE, and the Cochrane Database of Systematic Reviews indexing systems are excellent resources for retrieving clinical practice guidelines; however, they require subscriptions and familiarity with the search techniques in order to yield optimal results. The reader should refer to Chapters 3 and 7 for a more detailed description of each of these, as well as other databases that may be utilized when searching for clinical practice guidelines. Of note, the most effective search term may be *practice guideline* in the publication-type field of various search pages. An additional useful search term may be *treatment guideline*.

Case Study 19–1

Consider the following scenario:

Sue Granger, PharmD, is working in an outpatient anticoagulation clinic, when TH, a Hispanic woman in her mid-30s who takes warfarin for a mechanical heart valve, stops by to report a new medication and to confirm it is "okay" to take with her warfarin. TH says, "My doctor says I can just take it as needed, but I'm always nervous about any new medication! I just filled the prescription and it was really expensive—they told me it 'wasn't on formulary,' whatever that means. I wish there was something I could do instead of taking this medication." After some discussion, Sue discovers that TH has been experiencing a burning feeling in her chest for the last month, saw her family doctor today, and was told it was "just heartburn."

- *In addition to asking Sue to check for a drug interaction between warfarin and esomeprazole, what drug information questions has TH either requested or implied she needs to know?*
- *How might Sue begin to answer each of these questions?*

The patient (TH) requires the ambulatory care pharmacist to assist with several drug information queries. Before leaving the clinic, TH now asks for any information available (in addition to the leaflet stapled to the prescription bag she got at the pharmacy) regarding her new prescription and what to expect with gastroesophageal reflux disease (GERD). TH further requests that, if possible, she would like information in Spanish, as it is easier for her to read health-related information in her first language.

- *What resource database(s) could Sue refer to with patient information written at an appropriate level? Are there databases that are useful for traditional drug information geared toward the health care professional and that also have information geared toward patient education?*

- *Do any of these databases provide patient information in multiple languages?*

DESIRED CHARACTERISTICS OF DRUG INFORMATION RESOURCES IN THE AMBULATORY SETTING

⑤ *Increasingly more medical literature, including tertiary references, is being provided in the electronic or Internet-based format, and such databases are attractive to utilize in ambulatory care for multiple reasons.*

- Electronic databases are easily accessible, which is of utmost importance, as ambulatory care may take place in clinics or pharmacies that are part of the same health system, but located in multiple locations.
- Electronic databases tend to be updated more easily and frequently, with new drug updates and pertinent changes in patient and disease management versus print copies of drug information that may outdate quickly.
- Electronic drug information databases are more quickly and easily searched for specific topics pertinent to a given patient, and often utilize hyperlinks or search functions. Recall that, as reviewed in Chapter 3, regardless of the format (electronic versus print), patient education materials should contain language that is directed either toward the patient, parent, or caregiver, and be written at an appropriate reading level. It is recommended that databases specify the reading level of patient education material.

Examples of particularly useful databases are provided below.

A REVIEW OF SELECTED DRUG INFORMATION RESOURCES FOR THE AMBULATORY CLINICIAN

Many of the following tertiary resources are also mentioned in Chapter 3, however, rather than focusing solely on the appropriate resource for a specific drug information request, the following is a brief overview of selected resources that (a) are available electronically, (b) are primarily geared toward the health care professional and are also particularly useful to the ambulatory care practitioner, (c) provide in-depth drug and alternative product monographs, and (d) provide useful patient-oriented material.

Clinical Pharmacology®

Gold Standard, http://www.clinicalpharmacology.com. This database includes MedCounselor® Consumer Drug Information Sheets that are available in both

English and Spanish, and includes the date of last revision of any given patient education sheet. MedCounselor® Sheets are available via hyperlinks from drug monographs or by searching by drug product under a patient education tab within the site. This product includes patient education materials written at a sixth- to eighth-grade reading level regarding prescription, nonprescription, and some herbal medications.

- In addition to this information geared toward the consumer, this database also includes clinical calculators, manufacturer contact information, normal laboratory reference values, drug class overviews, clinical comparison reports, and convenience charts (e.g., meds that should not be split, that interact with grapefruit juice, etc.). Information on complementary and alternative medicine (CAM) is also found in this database. This may of particular value in the ambulatory setting as these patients are most likely to be concurrently taking or inquiring about CAM in addition to their prescription medications.

Drug Facts and Comparisons®

- Wolters Kluwer Health, Inc., http://www.factsandcomparisons.com. The electronic version of this database, utilizes MedFacts Patient Information®, which provides customizable patient information in both English and Spanish for over 4000 brand and generic drugs, and includes some herbal medication patient education materials. The reading level is written at the eighth-grade level or below, with the date of last issue clearly provided on each education sheet.

- In addition, the ambulatory care clinician can find within this database clinical calculators, comparative data tables, and comparative efficacy tables within drug classes, a "don't crush/chew" list of medications, a drug identifier tool, drug interactions tool, immunization schedules, and even information regarding patient assistance programs for those patients experiencing difficulty affording their medication(s). Additional information on pregnancy and lactation with medications, natural medicines, and toxicology treatment guidelines (e.g., for overdose treatment or for reversal of effects of medications) is also available within this database.

    Apps from this database are available for the iPhone/iPad as well as Android devices.

Lexicomp® Online

- Available as an online subscription through Lexicomp, http://www.lexi.com, Lexicomp® Online incorporates an Internet-based platform to provide not only the electronic version of information found in Lexicomp's *Drug Information Handbook*, but, depending on the subscription purchased, may also include information from AHFS® Drug Information reference, and prescription drug plans including information regarding pricing, formulary status, and prior authorization status. Of particular interest to the ambulatory clinician, this resource includes links within drug monographs to Patient Education Modules (PEM).

• PEM deliver patient-specific education regarding a particular medication or a disease, condition, or procedure. Condition and procedure information is available in either English or Spanish, with medication leaflets available in up to 19 different languages. PEM are also available for select natural products. Patient information is written at a fifth- to sixth-grade reading level, and may be personalized and printed for distribution to the patient.[11] The practitioner specifies whether a PEM is for an adult or pediatric patient, with pediatric information written toward the parent or caregiver.

• The Lexicomp platform is also available for handheld apps (e.g., on the iPhone/iPad, Android, Blackberry).

Micromedex® Healthcare Series' Detailed Drug Information for the Consumer™

• Available as an online subscription through Truven Health Analytics, http://www.micromedex.com, the Micromedex Patient Connect Suite® includes educational resources written at third- to seventh-grade reading level in up to 15 languages and that may be delivered in multiple media formats (e.g., written, video, interactive tools, a 3D avatar, and more). This suite of resources is intended for use by not only retail and hospital pharmacists, physicians, and nurses, but also patient education program coordinators.[12]

• Separate tabs contain information within this database regarding drug interactions, drug identification, calculators, and toxicology/drug effect reversal. The toxicology section may be of particular interest to clinicians in ambulatory setting who work with high-risk medications such as anticoagulants (e.g., warfarin) or insulin products.

CareNotes™ System

• Also available via a subscription, by Truven Health Analytics, http://www.micromedex.com, the CareNotes® System enables the clinician to provide customizable patient education documents (in 15 different languages, confirmed to be written at a sixth- to eighth-grade reading level in English and Spanish). These documents may address general health condition information, preprocedure or presurgical information, and information regarding inpatient and discharge care for patients, laboratory test information, and a section titled DrugNotes, which includes patient-directed drug information for both prescription and nonprescription medications.[13]

• In addition, of use to the ambulatory care provider in particular, this database includes drug identification, toxicology management, drug comparison tables, clinical calculators, and even pricing and manufacturing information in medical devices and select diagnostic equipment (e.g., blood glucose monitors).

• Apps from this database are compatible with iPhone/iPad and Android devices, but not with Palm and Pocket PC/Windows Mobile Classic platforms.

- **Natural Medicines Comprehensive Database®, Pharmacist's Letter®, and Prescriber's Letter®**

  All published by Therapeutic Research Center, subscriptions to each of these publications are available electronically, may be downloaded to electronic handheld devices, and may be of great value, especially in the ambulatory care setting.

The Natural Medicines Comprehensive Database®

- The Natural Medicines Comprehensive Database® (NMCD), http://naturaldatabase. therapeuticresearch.com (subscription required), provides evidence-based information regarding complementary, alternative, integrative medicine, and natural medicines. The database provides full monographs with evidence-based ratings, safety ratings, and interaction ratings based on currently available literature. NMCD includes a useful natural product/drug interaction checker and patient handouts written in both English and Spanish.[14]

- Of use to the ambulatory clinician, enabling frank discussion of the risk versus benefit of complementary or natural medicines is an "efficacy" rating, which rates each natural medication on the likelihood of its being effective for a given condition, coined the NMBER™+ (Natural Medicines Brand Evidence-based Rating). Information regarding perioperative use of natural medications is also available.

Pharmacist's Letter® and Prescriber's Letter®

- Pharmacist's Letter®, http://pharmacistsletter.com, and Prescriber's Letter, http://prescribersletter.com (subscription required), provide detailed information regarding traditional prescription and nonprescription medication, including full monographs with evidence-based ratings, safety rating, and interactions based on currently available literature. The main difference between these two databases is the target audience. These publications cover new developments in drug therapy and trends in pharmacy practice, concise updates, and advice regarding current therapeutic issues with links to a detail document with a more in-depth explanation of the topic. These publications also include very useful comprehensive disease-, medication-, and practice-related charts. For example, ambulatory care clinicians may find comparison charts for statins, insulin products, injectable anticoagulants, anticipated availability of first-time generics, etc. Links for treatment guidelines for a variety of commonly treated conditions are also available (e.g., cardiology, diabetes, gastroenterological conditions, asthma, COPD). A "Rumor vs. Truth" section may also be of use for quick reference when fielding questions from the public on misstated facts or exaggerated efficacy claims in the media, for example.

  Apps from this database are available for the iPhone/iPad as well as Android devices.

Drug Information Web Sites

- Particularly useful Web sites include those of the (a) Food and Drug Administration (FDA), http://www.fda.gov, as it provides recent drug-related news, drug approvals, recalls and safety warnings, therapeutic equivalency codes, and MedWatch adverse event reporting data; (b) Centers for Disease Control and Prevention (CDC), http://www.cdc.gov, as it provides useful information regarding infectious disease treatment and prevention, immunization information, treatment guidelines for infectious disease, and even traveler's health information, some of which may be available in more than one language; and (c) Medscape, http://www.medscape.com, which provides free access to continuing education, select health-related journals, evidence-based information, and pertinent review articles.

ACCESS CONSIDERATIONS

- For the reasons outlined above, the electronic version of each of these databases and publications is the preferred format. Whenever possible, databases that are available for downloading to a smart phone or alternate handheld device are included; however, even these will require intermittent Internet access for synchronizing and updating information. Responsible provision of up-to-date drug information requires Internet access. Health care providers and employers should ensure that this is available to those providing medical information to others.

- Practitioners may also note that by partnering with colleges of pharmacy or medicine to provide experiential education to students, they may expand their access to drug information databases to which the college subscribes, depending on subscription limitations.

- Drug information centers, also referred to as medication information centers, may be a viable source of information, particularly when in-depth research of a topic is not feasible due to either a lack of access to appropriate databases, paucity of individuals trained in drug information, or lack of time.

PATIENT EDUCATION

The preceding sections (e.g., practice guidelines, desired characteristics of databases, and other drug information resources) address the role of the ambulatory care provider in researching appropriate medical treatment and using this data to treat patients on an individual basis. This section focuses on yet another important aspect to ambulatory drug information: educating patients on the appropriate use of their medications. Certainly documents generated from the databases outlined above, manufacturer-provided patient information leaflets, and direct patient counseling at the pharmacy, all serve to educate patients on intended use(s), cautions, possible side effects, and required monitoring for each medication, but this is not enough. Ambulatory care clinicians fill an important role in educating patients regarding the proper administration of certain medications (e.g., insulin, inhalers, injectable anticoagulants), the management of adverse reactions (e.g., hypoglycemia, bleeding), and dosing adjustments that may be required such as during perioperative periods or during periods of illness. While most of this information may be found within the individual drug information databases (e.g., how to reverse the effects of hypoglycemia caused by excess insulin or how to reverse the effects of warfarin), it is not always included in patient education materials, and must be taught to the patient. Additionally, for those medications that require specific administration technique, providing patients with written instructions is not enough.

Hands-on demonstration and teach-back communication are vital to ensuring medications are used optimally. Manufacturers of drug products that require special administration typically provide patient handouts for this purpose. The Centers for Disease Control Web site (http://cdc.gov) also has useful videos as well as tutorial sheets (e.g., asthma inhaler use, how to check blood glucose), which may be modified or used "as is." Finally, for the condition of interest, there are often topic-specific patient education materials available from a national Web site for the disorder being treated. For example, the American Diabetes Association (http://www.diabetes.org/) Web site includes links for recognizing and treating hypoglycemia, testing blood glucose, and "sick-day" management. Information obtained from any of these places, however, must be explained, tailored to the patient and the situation, and even demonstrated (e.g., glucose monitor, insulin pen); ambulatory clinicians fill an important in the provision of this type of drug information.

Patient Disposal of Unused Medications

While health care providers may know that they cannot legally accept medications that have previously been dispensed, they must also be able to take the next step and provide drug information to the inquirer regarding the legal, safe, and appropriate disposal of these medications.

More often than in any other setting, ambulatory care practitioners are asked about disposal of unused or unwanted medications. While there no specific laws regarding personal disposal of medications by patients, disposal of unused or unwanted pharmaceuticals (both prescription and nonprescription) is becoming an emerging and complex environmental issue. In a 2006 survey published in the *Journal of the American Board of Family Medicine*, of 301 patients surveyed at an outpatient pharmacy, 50% reported storing unused or expired medication and another 50% report they have flushed such medications down the toilet. Less than 20% of respondents reported having been counseled by a health care provider about the appropriate means of medication disposal.[15] Drug information is often considered (among other things) the provision of information to patients or health care providers about safe and appropriate use about medications, but it also includes serving as a resource for information about the proper storage and disposal of medications when they are not in use. ❻ *Ambulatory care clinicians bear a responsibility to educate patients on the proper disposal of unused and unwanted medications and should, therefore, be aware of pertinent sites for finding this information.* The Pharmaceutical Research and Manufacturers of America (PhRMA), the American Pharmacists Association (APhA), and the U.S. Fish and Wildlife Service (FWS) have joined forces to educate the public on the importance of appropriate medication disposal via the SMARxT DISPOSAL™ campaign, http://www. smarxtdisposal.net/. Their key message to consumers: do not flush medications down the toilet and do not pour them down a sink or drain. The campaign actively promotes people to participate in medication take-back collection days, and provides a hyperlink to the U.S. Department of Justice and Drug Enforcement Administration's Web page regarding the national drug take-back initiative.[16]

The FDA, http://www.fda.gov, provides consumer health information regarding the disposal of unused medicines, and has worked with the White House Office of National Drug Control Policy (ONDCP) to develop consumer guidance regarding this topic. Documents developed by these organizations are available online at the FDA and ONDCP Web sites.[17,18] In addition, disposal information for some, but not all, medications may be found in DailyMed, http://dailymed.nlm.nih.gov/dailymed/about.cfm, by searching within monographs in one or more of the following fields: Information for Patients and Caregivers, Patient Information, Patient Counseling Information, Safety and Handling Instructions, or Medication Guide.

Additional useful online resources with information on the safe disposal of medications include those of the Pharmacist's Letter, http://www.pharmacistsletter.com, and the Institute for Safe Medical Practice (ISMP), http://www.ismp.org. Finally, the Community Medical Foundation for Patient Safety, http://www.communityofcompetence.com, has developed a very useful document, the National Directory of Drug Take-Back and Disposal Programs. The first edition, published in 2008, detailed the rationale, federal laws, state laws, published resources, useful Web sites, and practice guidelines for handling unused and expired medications. The second edition, published in 2011, listed just under 500 drug take-back programs, including locations and contact information for each and was available for purchase through the Community Medical Foundation for Patient Safety.[19] Local and state drug take-back initiative sites may be listed on a case-by-case basis online; however, one site attempts to centralize drug take-back information on a national basis. The Product Stewardship Institute (PSI) addresses appropriate disposal of multiple types of products, including pharmaceuticals, and visitors to the PSI Web site may research take-back efforts and activities on a state-by-state basis.[20]

There are a select few medications for which flushing medications down the toilet is the FDA-recommended method of disposal. For these medications, the sentiment of FDA officials is that in order to best protect persons and animals that could inappropriately use these medications, prompt flushing of unused or unwanted medication down the toilet is the preferred method of disposal. The drugs are listed in Table 19–1.[21]

TABLE 19–1. MEDICATIONS FOR WHICH FLUSHING DOWN THE TOILET REMAINS THE FDA-RECOMMENDED METHOD OF DISPOSAL[21]

Medicine	Active Ingredient
Abstral, tablets (sublingual)	Fentanyl
Actiq, oral transmucosal lozenge*	Fentanyl citrate
Avinza, capsule (extended release)	Morphine sulfate
Daytrana, transmdermal patch system	Methylphenidate
Demerol, tablets*	Meperidine hydrochloride
Demerol, oral solution*	Meperidine hydrochloride
Diastat/Diastat AcuDial, rectal gel	Diazepam
Dilaudid, tablets*	Hydromorphone hydrochloride
Dilaudid, oral liquid*	Hydromorphone hydrochloride
Dolophine hydrochloride, tablets*	Methadone hydrochloride
Duragesic, patch (extended release)*	Fentanyl
Embeda, capsule (extended release)	Morphine sulfate; naltrexone hydrochloride
Exalgo, tablets (extended release)	Hydromorphone hydrochloride
Fentora, tablets (buccal)	Fentanyl citrate
Kadian, capsules (extended release)	Morphine sulfate
Methadone hydrochloride, oral solution*	Methadone hydrochloride
Methadose, tablets*	Methadone hydrochloride
Morphine sulfate, tablets (immediate release)*	Morphine sulfate
Morphine sulfate, oral solution*	Morphine sulfate
MS Contin, tablets (extended release)*	Morphine sulfate
Nucynta ER, tablets (extended release)	Tapentadol
Onsolis, soluble film (buccal)	Fentanyl citrate
Opana, tablets (immediate release)	Oxymorphone hydrochloride
Opana ER, tablets (extended release)	Oxymorphone hydrochloride
Oxecta, tablets (immediate release)	Oxycodone hydrochloride
Oxycodone hydrochloride, capsules	Oxycodone hydrochloride
Oxycodone hydrochloride, oral solution	Oxycodone hydrochloride
Oxycontin, tablets (extended release)*	Oxycodone hydrochloride
Percocet, tablets*	Acetaminophen; oxycodone hydrochloride
Percodan, tablets*	Aspirin; oxycodone hydrochloride
Xyrem, oral solution	Sodium oxybate

*These medications have a generic version or are only available as a generic.
Note: Updated in Feb 2013.

Case Study 19-2

Sara P., who works in a busy endocrinology clinic, is approached by the widower of a former patient of the diabetes clinic. The man is carrying a grocery bag which appears to be full of prescription bottles, insulin pens, and vials. "Can you take these, and perhaps use them for someone who could use them? My wife passed away last month, and I probably have hundreds of dollars' worth of medication in this bag! If you can't use them, can you tell me where I should take them?"

- *Where can unused, unwanted, or expired medications be taken?*
- *If a patient wishes to dispose of medications, are there any associated legal requirements or guidelines?*

DRUG REPOSITORY PROGRAMS

Drug repository programs (which allow nursing homes, long-term care pharmacies, and wholesalers to donate unused medication for redistribution to those patients who meet prespecified criteria) may exist in certain states. While patients understandably may be reluctant to throw away their personal unused or unwanted medications, these medications, once dispensed and in patients' homes, are not eligible for donation to drug repository programs, as these drugs have left the custody and controlled environment of a pharmacy or institution. Practitioners should refer to their respective state's Board of Pharmacy Web site for information regarding drug repository programs.

Providing Immunization Information

Formerly provided primarily in the traditional clinician's office or in county or city health departments, immunizations are increasingly being delivered by pharmacists and other health care providers in ambulatory care settings, including pharmacies and retail groceries. ❼ *While ambulatory clinicians (in particular, pharmacists) typically recommend and/ or dispense most medications, immunizations are medications that are administered in the ambulatory care setting. Those practitioners immunizing in this setting have the obligation to not only provide these services safely, but to serve as immediate sources of information (i.e., drug information) regarding the medications they are administering.*

SOURCES OF IMMUNIZATION INFORMATION

Centers for Disease Control and Prevention

While multiple texts exist regarding immunization and vaccine-preventable disease, the Department of Health and Human Services Centers for Disease Control and Prevention Web site, http://www.cdc.gov, provides the most comprehensive, regularly updated information regarding immunizations. Links are available from the CDC Web page titled Vaccines and Immunizations, http://www.cdc.gov/vaccines, for both the health care provider and patients, that provide up-to-date information regarding vaccine-preventable disease, as well as safety, adverse events, administration schedule, and dosing recommendations for immunizations. Also available from this site are Vaccine Information Statements (VISs), which must be distributed with their respective immunizations.

Epidemiology and Prevention of Vaccine-Preventable Disease

This textbook, commonly referred to as the Pink Book, is published annually by the National Center for Immunization and Respiratory Diseases (part of CDC) (http://www .cdc.gov/vaccines/pubs/pinkbook/index.html).[22] It provides physicians, nurses, nurse practitioners, physician assistants, and pharmacists with comprehensive information regarding the vaccine-preventable diseases. The textbook is available for purchase in print; however, PDFs of each chapter are available fully formatted for download from the CDC Web site. While this text does not provide vaccine specific information, it provides detailed information regarding respective vaccine-preventable disease, including epidemiology, prevalence, and prevention recommendations.

Immunization Training for the Pharmacist

The prerequisites for pharmacists to administer immunizations vary from state to state, and pharmacists are advised to refer to their state's laws and confer with their state board of pharmacy regarding specific questions; however, in each state that allows for pharmacist-administered vaccines, a training program approved by the state pharmacy board is required. The most widely recognized training program, Pharmacy-Based Immunization Delivery, is offered nationally by the American Pharmacists Association, http://www.pharmacist.com. Other programs do exist that may be recognized nationally or within specific states only. Pharmacists may wish to inquire with their specific state board of pharmacy regarding recognized and approved training programs. Regardless of the training program initially utilized, it is expected that pharmacists, as well as all other providers of health care, maintain and document appropriate continuing education for the immunizations and the associated drug information they deliver.

Quality Assurance Considerations in Ambulatory Care

This chapter has thus far covered a variety of drug information topics pertinent to ambulatory care practice and the case has been made that efficiently accessing and interpreting a variety of types of information is necessary for functional competence in ambulatory care. A final drug information consideration for safe and competent function in the ambulatory setting is quality-assurance.

While facilities that are under the umbrella of a health care facility generally consider the standards set forth by The Joint Commission (TJC) (see Chapter 14) as a primary source of quality-assurance guidelines, several other organizations provide quality-assurance guidelines that may be applied to a variety of care settings, and will be discussed in the following paragraphs.

Via a variety of initiatives, including the **Accountable Care Organizations (ACOs)** model, The Department of Health and Human Services Centers for Medicaid and Medicare Services (CMS) has specified 33 required **quality measures** that are evaluated in order to determine payment structure for patient care networks, which are inclusive of ambulatory care settings. The quality measures themselves are standards set forth that evaluate efficiency (or resource use), structure, process, intermediate outcome, long-term outcome, and patient centeredness (which includes patient reports of satisfaction).[23]

The Department of Health and Human Services Center for Medicaid and Medicare Services (CMS) has also contracted with Florida Medical Quality Assurance, Inc. (FMQAI) in a project particularly pertinent to quality-assurance in the ambulatory care setting. The project, Medication Measure Special Innovation Project, is tasked with maintaining the current 33 quality measures and expanding them to include new measures focused on medication-related patient safety (e.g., detecting/preventing medication errors, adverse drug reactions). The project specifically includes a portfolio of six National Quality Forum (NQF)-endorsed measures for the ambulatory care setting, including measures related to patient adherence to specific medication classes, adherence to regular monitoring for warfarin (both routine and when on antibiotics), and adherence of patients with schizophrenia to antipsychotic therapy.

❽ *Health care professionals involved in the provision of care in the ambulatory care setting should familiarize themselves with the pertinent established quality measures.*

The Patient Safety and Clinical Pharmacy Services (PSPC) Collaborative is one of the newest nation-wide initiatives to improve quality of care. Launched in 2008, PSPC is sponsored by the U.S. Health Resources and Service Administration (HRSA). The initiative focuses on cutting medication-related patient errors and improving the quality of health care in the United States by incorporating clinical pharmacy services into the provision of primary care. Each of the participating organizations in this initiative is focused on incorporating evidence-based clinical pharmacy services into the care of patients with chronic diseases. More information about the PSPC may be found at http://www.hrsa.gov/publichealth/clinical/patientsafety/index.html.[24]

Ensuring patient safety is a crucial component of quality care, and the ISMP is an important resource for health care providers in any setting. The ISMP publishes four distinct newsletters, each geared toward practitioners in a different health care setting. The ISMP Medication Safety Alert! Community/Ambulatory Care edition is targeted toward pharmacists, pharmacy technicians, nurses, physicians, and other community health professionals. This newsletter is sent monthly as an e-mail, and provides up-to-date information about medication-related errors, adverse drug reactions, and their implications for community practice sites. Finally, the newsletter includes recommendations on how to improve medication safety within the community setting (http://www.ismp.org/Newsletters/default.asp). A subscription to this newsletter is recommended for all ambulatory care providers (ISMP Medication Safety Alert! Community/Ambulatory Care edition). More information regarding ISMP as well as its newsletters can be found at http://www.ismp.org/.[25]

Finally, the tracking, reporting, and prevention of not only medication errors, but of near misses, is paramount to assuring quality in any health care setting, including ambulatory care. ISMP is one organization dedicated to this task. The reader should refer to Chapter 16 for a complete discussion on organizations and programs devoted to assuring quality by reporting and prevention of medication errors.

The American Pharmacists Association Web site, http://www.pharmacist.com, has a Patient Safety and Quality Assurance page that provides links to AHRQ, ISMP, the National Patient Safety Foundation (NPSF), the United States Pharmacopeia (USP) Medication Errors Reporting Form, and the PSPC Collaborative.

Case Study 19–3

Kyle, a recent graduate from a college of pharmacy, is working in a private practice ambulatory care clinic where, in addition to dispensing responsibilities, he provides medication recommendations to prescribers and counsels patients regarding disease state management. The manager of the clinic approaches Kyle and asks him to become involved in measuring quality-assurance indicators for all health care providers in the clinic, including patient satisfaction with the care that has been provided.

- *What type of quality-assurance indicators/metrics are utilized by outside organizations?*
- *Is patient satisfaction with care a recognized quality indicator?*
- *Are there published guidelines for quality indicators in ambulatory care?*

Conclusion

As health professionals committed to optimal patient care, the provision of drug information goes far beyond providing patient information leaflets with medications. Application of drug information is performed routinely in the ambulatory care setting in a variety of manners, and it is in this setting that the clinician pulls it all together and takes the most important step—imparting this information not only to patients and their caregivers, but to other health care providers in a understandable, personalized, and practical format that will serve to improve health care.

Self-Assessment Questions

1. All of the following statements support the need for the skilled provision of drug information in ambulatory care *except*:
   a. There is not a consistent level of education in the curricula of various health care fields.
   b. There is a lack of high-quality drug information freely available to the public.
   c. The ambulatory care clinician is able to access databases that may not be available to the public.
   d. A significant number of emergency room visits and hospital admissions every year are attributed to pharmaceuticals.

2. Which of the following statements is true regarding prescription formularies?
   a. Prescription insurance providers often require cardholder identification information in order to gain full access to formulary information.
   b. Clinician use of electronic prescribing has not been shown to affect the likelihood of prescribing tier 1 medications.
   c. Software programs such as Lexicomp® and Epocrates® include formulary information that can be downloaded to a handheld electronic device.

    d. Medicare Part D participants cannot perform side-by-side comparisons of prescription plans that are available to them and that cover some or all of their medications.

3. Evidence-based clinical practice guidelines are:
    a. Used solely by practitioners who develop formularies.
    b. Accessible without a fee only to practitioners who are members of the organization that developed a given set of guidelines.
    c. Typically too large to download to most handheld devices.
    d. Freely available in full text from a variety of government and public Internet sites.

4. All of the following support the desirability of electronic drug information resources in the ambulatory setting *except*:
    a. Ambulatory care may be provided in multiple sites by the same organization.
    b. Internet access is available to all clinicians.
    c. Updates to information are more readily performed.
    d. Electronic databases are conducive to faster and more efficient searches.

5. Which of the following databases provides patient information in languages other than English?
    a. Clinical Pharmacology
    b. Drug Facts and Comparisons
    c. Lexicomp® Online
    d. All of the above

6. The Pharmacist's Letter Web site provides all of the following except:
    a. Comparison tables for drug classes
    b. Links to medication error reporting databases
    c. Developments in drug therapy
    d. Downloadable documents for handheld devices

7. Which of the following are potential options to increase access to drug information when resources are limited?
    a. Encourage employers to ensure Internet access is available to all those providing medical information to others.
    b. Consider partnering resources with a local college of medicine or pharmacy.
    c. Utilize the services of a drug information center.
    d. All of the above

8. Which of the following is considered by the Food and Drug Administration (FDA) to be an *appropriate* method for the disposal of unwanted medication?

  a. Flushing unused liquid medications
  b. Mixing medications with cat litter
  c. Burning with other trash
  d. Using a community dumpster

9. Which of the following organizations has/have been involved in the development of the SMARxT DISPOSAL™ campaign:
  a. American Pharmacists Association (APhA)
  b. Pharmaceutical Research and Manufacturers of America (PhRMA)
  c. U.S. Fish & Wildlife Service (FWS)
  d. a and c
  e. a, b, and c

10. Which of the following statements is false?
  a. Immunizations are not considered medications.
  b. Immunizations may be administered by pharmacists.
  c. Immunizations must be accompanied by a vaccine information statement (VIS) upon administration.
  d. Immunizations are becoming increasing available in variety of community settings including grocery store stores and pharmacies.

11. Which of the following organizations utilizes reports which include quality indicators as rated by consumers of health care?
  a. Institute for Safe Medical Practice (ISMP)
  b. Centers for Medicare and Medicaid Services (CMS)
  c. Patient Safety Clinical Pharmacy Services (PSPC)
  d. SMARxT DISPOSAL™

12. The Patient Safety and Clinical Pharmacy Services (PSPC) collaborative focuses on:
  a. Safe disposal of unwanted and expired medications
  b. Providing the community with up-to-date immunization information
  c. Cutting medication-related patient errors by incorporating clinical pharmacy services into primary care provision
  d. Creating patient education documents that are written at an appropriate reading level for the target audience

13. Which of the following is *not* a Centers for Medicare and Medicaid Services (CMS) quality measures?
  a. Patient perception of quality of care
  b. Family perception of quality of care

  c. Patient clinical outcome

  d. Efficient use of resources

14. Which of the following publishes a monthly newsletter regarding medication safety targeted at pharmacists, pharmacy technicians, and other community health care professionals?

  a. American Pharmacists Association (APhA)

  b. American Health-Systems Pharmacists (ASHP)

  c. Centers for Disease Control and Prevention (CDC)

  d. Institute for Safe Medication Practice (ISMP)

15. Which of the following organizations has a publication which details the rationale, federal laws, state laws, published resources, useful Web sites, and practice guidelines for handling unused and expired medications?

  a. Community Medical Foundation for Patient Safety

  b. Agency for Healthcare Research and Quality (AHRQ)

  c. American Pharmacists Association (APhA)

  d. Food and Drug Administration (FDA)

REFERENCES

1. Ernst FR, Grizzle AJ. Drug-related morbidity and mortality: updating the cost of illness model. J Am Pharm Assoc. 2001;41:192-199.

2. Zed PJ, Abu-Laban RB, Balen RM, Loewen PS, Hohl CM, Brubacher JR, et al. Incidence, severity and preventability of medication-related visits to the emergency department: a prospective study. Can Med Assoc J. 2008;178(12):1563-9.

3. Budnitz DS, Lovegrove MC, Sehhab N, Richards CL. Emergency hospitalizations for adverse drug events in older Americans. NEJM. 2011;365:21.

4. Centers for Disease Control and Prevention. Medication safety program [Internet]. [updated 2012 Aug 12; cited 2013 Jun 03]. Available from: http://www.cdc.gov/medicationsafety/.

5. Epocrates®. San Mateo (CA): Epocrates, Inc. 2011 [cited 2013 Jun 3]. Available from: http://www.epocrates.com./products/comparison_table.html

6. Fischer MA, Vogeli C, Stedman M, Ferris T, Brookhart A, Weissman JS. Effect of electronic prescribing with formulary decision support on medication use and cost. Arch Intern Med. 2008;168(22):2433-9.

7. Chang C, Nguyen N, Smith A, Huynh D. Impact of electronic prescribing on outpatient prescription drug use and adherence in a network-model health plan. Presented at: Academy of Managed Care Pharmacy 22nd Annual Meeting and Showcase; April 9–10, 2010; San Diego (CA). Available from: http://dbt.consultantlive.com/display/article/1145628/1582622

8. National Guideline Clearinghouse (NGC) [homepage on the Internet]. Rockville (MD): Agency for Healthcare Research and Quality. Rockville (MD); [updated 2012 Sep 7; cited 2013 Jun 3]. Available from: http://www.ahrq.gov/about/index.html

9. Iowa Drug Information Service [database on the Internet]. Iowa City (IA). [cited 2013 Jun 3]. Available from: http://www.uiowa.edu/~idis/.

10. National Center for Biotechnology Information, U.S. National Library of Medicine, National Institutes of Health. PubMed.gov [Internet]. [cited 2013 Jun 3]. Available from: http://www.ncbi.nlm.nih.gov/pubmed/.

11. Lexicomp® ONLINE User Guide [Internet]. Lexicomp, Inc. Hudson (OH); [cited 2013 Jun 3]. Available from: http://online.lexi.com

12. Micromedex® Consumer Health Information [Internet]. Ann Arbor (MI): Truven Health Analytics Inc.; [cited 2013 Jun 3]. Available from: http://www.truvenhealth.com/Your-Healthcare-Focus/Hospital-Patient-Care-Decisions/Consumer-Engagement

13. The Carenotes® System [Internet]. Ann Arbor (MI): Truven Health Analytics, Inc.; [cited 2013 Jun 3]. Available from: http://www.truvenhealth.com/Your-Healthcare-Focus/Hospital-Patient-Care-Decisions/Micromedex-Patient-Connect-Suite

14. Natural Medicines Comprehensive Database. Therapeutic Research [Internet]. Stockton (CA). [cited 2013 Jun 3]. Available from: http://naturaldatabase.com

15. Seehusen D, Edwards J. Patient practices and beliefs concerning disposal of medications. J Am Board Fam Med. 2006;19(6):542-7.

16. SMARxT disposal. A prescription for a healthy planet [Internet]. [cited 2013 Jun 3]. Available from: http://www.smarxtdisposal.net

17. FDA Consumer Health Information. How to dispose of unused medications [Internet]. [updated 2011 Apr; cited 2013 Jun 3]. Available from: http://www.fda.gov/downloads/Drugs/ResourcesForYou/Consumers/BuyingUsingMedicineSafely/UnderstandingOver-the-CounterMedicines/ucm107163.pdf

18. Disposal of unused medications: what you should know [Internet]. [cited 2013 Jun 3]. Available from: http://www.fda.gov/Drugs/ResourcesForYou/Consumers/BuyingUsingMedicineSafely/EnsuringSafeUseofMedicine/SafeDisposalofMedicines/ucm186187.htm

19. Communities now have a resource to get rid of unused and expired medicines from home [Internet]. News Release. [updated 2011 Sep 16; cited 2013 Jun 03]. Available from: http://www.comofcom.com/News%20Release_National%20Directory%20091611.pdf

20. Product Stewardship Institute. The drug take-back network [Internet]. [cited 2013 Jun 3]. Available from: http://www.takebacknetwork.com/local_efforts.html

21. Food and Drug Administration. Medicines recommended for disposal by flushing. Listed by medicine and active ingredient [Internet]. [updated 2013 Feb; cited 2013 Jun 03]. Available from: http://www.fda.gov/downloads/Drugs/ResourcesForYou/Consumers/BuyingUsingMedicineSafely/EnsuringSafeUseofMedicine/SafeDisposalof Medicines/UCM337803.pdf

22. Centers for Disease Control and Prevention. Epidemiology and prevention of vaccine-preventable diseases [Internet]. Atkinson W, Wolfe S, Hamborsky J, eds. 12th ed., second printing. Washington, DC: Public Health Foundation, 2012. [cited 2013 Jun 3]. Available from: http://www.cdc.gov/vaccines/pubs/pinkbook/index.html

23. Centers for Medicaid and Medicare Services. Quality measures for performance standards [Internet]. [updated 2013 May 23; cited 2013 Jun 4]. Available from: http://www.cms.gov/Medicare/Medicare-Fee-for-Service-Payment/sharedsavingsprogram/Quality_Measures_Standards.html

24. United States Health Resources and Service Administration. Patient safety and clinical practice services collaborative (PSPC) [Internet]. [updated 2012 Oct; cited 2013 Jun 3]. Available from: http://www.hrsa.gov/publichealth/clinical/patientsafety/pspcoverview.pdf

25. ISMP Medication Safety Alert®! Newsletters [Internet]. Institute for Safe Medical Practice. [cited 2013 Jun 03]. Available from: http://www.ismp.org/Newsletters/default.asp

SUGGESTED READINGS

1. Budnitz D. CDC expert commentary: what to tell your patients about medication safety [Internet]. 2010 Sep 27 [cited 2013 Jun 03]. Available from: http://www.medscape.com/viewarticle/728220

2. United States Environmental Protection Agency. Pharmaceuticals and personal care products (PPCPs) [Internet]. 2010 Oct 27 [cited 2013 Jun 03]. Available from: http://www.epa.gov/ppcp/faq.html

3. Centers for Medicare and Medicaid Services. Accountable care organizations (ACO) [Internet]. [updated 2013 Mar 22; cited 2013 Jun 03]. Available from: http://www.cms.gov/Medicare/Medicare-Fee-for-Service-Payment/ACO/index.html

Chapter Twenty

Drug Information and Contemporary Community Pharmacy Practice

Morgan L. Sperry • Heather A. Pace

Learning Objectives

After completing this chapter, the reader will be able to

- Discuss limitations of the current approaches pharmacists use to deliver drug information to their patients.
- Compare and contrast patient education and consumer health information (CHI) as drug information sources for patients.
- Define Web 2.0 and social networking and describe how patients use these tools as a drug information source.
- Discuss mobile health information technology and its impact on how consumers are obtaining information.
- Describe the model for drug information services delivered by community pharmacists.
- Design three strategies using electronic media to assist patients in receiving and applying high-quality drug information.
- List seven characteristics of a high-quality health literate Internet site.
- Define information therapy in the context of a pharmacist delivered drug information service.

Key Concepts

❶ The trend for patients to obtain their health information from sources disconnected from health care professionals is not going away and it has shifted relationships between patients and their traditional touchstones in health care, namely physicians, nurses, and pharmacists.

② Answering drug information questions is a routine part of a pharmacist's day, but it is too often a passive process that hinges upon the patient's initiative to ask the important questions regarding their health.

③ Patient education delivers written or verbal drug information through a planned activity initiated by a health care provider. The goal is to change patient behavior, improve adherence, and ultimately improve health.

④ Consumer health information (CHI) is actively sought by the patient in response to their need for more information about their health. Importantly, CHI is not individualized for a specific patient.

⑤ Social media sites allow patients to create content and share information about their health on the Internet.

⑥ Wisdom of crowds is a belief that when patients share information about their common conditions through social networking, their collective wisdom is more beneficial than the expert opinion of just one individual.

⑦ The use of mobile technology to obtain consumer health information has experienced a sharp increase within the last few years and continues to skyrocket.

⑧ Pharmacists should discuss with their patients why they remain an important source of drug information. Patients should be encouraged not to see CHI as a replacement for actual interaction with a health care provider, but as an extension of care and a way to improve communication.

⑨ Patients often have difficulty finding appropriate information in response to their specific health concerns on the Internet.

⑩ Once patients identify or are given quality health information, they still may face barriers in being able to use it to improve their health.

⑪ Information therapy elevates the term drug information from a passive sounding process to an active component of treatment plans by recognizing that accurate and complete drug information proactively relayed to patients is much more effective than just assuming it will be sought out.

Introduction

Pharmacists' roles and responsibilities continue to evolve in response to changing pharmacy practice acts and a dynamic health care environment. One constant is the pharmacist's key function as a provider of quality, evidence-based drug information. However, pharmacists are not the only source of drug information. The Internet has made information from sources other than health professionals more readily available and Web sites devoted to health information are accessible to anyone on the Web. The move toward patient-centered care and consumerism increases the desire for patients to be in control of their health care and be an active part of the decision-making process. ❶ *The trend for patients to obtain their health information from sources disconnected from health care professionals is not going away and it has shifted relationships between patients and their traditional touchstones in health care, namely physicians, nurses, and pharmacists.*[1] Recent surveys suggest 60% to 80% of American consumers use the Internet to search for some type of health or wellness information.[2] The pharmacist's role as drug information expert may also be changing in the eyes of the patient. In 2010, 29% of patients reported not using health care professionals, including pharmacists, as a source to locate or access health information.[2]

Pharmacy practice is moving away from its emphasis on the hands-on drug distribution model toward an emphasis on system management and patient care services.[3,4] It is important for pharmacists to enhance patient care services because of significant expenditures seen with unresolved drug-related problems. Nonadherence to medication therapy was estimated to cost $300 billion annually in direct and indirect costs in 2011 by the National Council on Patient Information and Education.[5] A key strategy to improve adherence is to improve patients' understanding of their disease and its management and include their needs in the treatment planning. Both strategies require individualized care that is not available from the World Wide Web and other information sources. Pharmacists can remain a valuable drug information source for patients because they are one of the most accessible health care practitioners. Pharmacists can help patients customize information they find on the Internet and from other such sources. The danger right now for pharmacists is that if they do not step up and add drug information services beyond what a patient can find on their own, as well as develop patient demand for these services, they will become less relevant. Project Destiny, an initiative between the National Association of Chain Drug Stores (NACDS), American Pharmacists Association (APhA), and the National Community Pharmacists Association (NCPA) introduced in 2008, encourages pharmacists to "embrace community pharmacy health care beyond dispensing" and identifies a number of significant unmet needs for improved medication therapy management, including **health product information** and derivative services. Pharmacists are well positioned to address these needs as they are medication experts and trusted professionals. In this model, patients will view pharmacists as a key medication advisor. For example, patients see results from clinical research on the news or through the Internet. They may not understand how these results relate directly to them and may reconsider continuing their medication. Pharmacists, with their understanding of both the literature and the patient's medical history, can help the patient understand whether these new findings are relevant to their individual situation.

According to a 2012 survey, 94% of patients select a specific pharmacy based on location and convenience. When price is not a factor, accuracy and trust provided by the pharmacists were cited as a reason for going to a pharmacy only 9% and 4% of the time, respectively. These results further support the need to develop consumer demand for patient care services.[6] The purpose of this chapter is to shed light on how increased patient demand for autonomy and responsibility over their own health care and use of information sources beyond health professionals impacts community pharmacy. Additionally, new models for community pharmacists delivering drug information will be addressed.

Pharmacists as Drug Information Providers in the Community Setting

Pharmacists are required by Omnibus Budget Reconciliation Act of 1990 (OBRA'90) to deliver patient counseling when they dispense a Medicaid prescription.[7] Individual states can and sometimes do mandate that counseling be extended to all patients, irrespective of their insurance. Some pharmacists are very diligent in providing important information to their patients when they pick up a prescription, while others only give information if specifically asked. Patients may be asked by pharmacy staff to electronically sign to decline counseling without being asked whether they want it or not. Some patients do not even know what they are signing. ❷ *Answering drug information questions is a routine part of a pharmacist's day, but it is too often a passive process that hinges upon the patient's initiative to ask the important questions regarding their health.* A variety of reasons make patients reluctant to use their pharmacist as a primary health information resource. Although the most accessible health care professional to patients, pharmacists often may appear too busy and unavailable within the sometimes hectic pharmacy. Technicians or cashiers may be the only staff who speaks directly to the patient. Simply asking whether or not a patient has questions is the wrong way to initiate counseling. Patients may not be sure what they need to know in the first place, or feel embarrassed or ashamed to admit their lack of knowledge. In some cases, patients are unaware they should be asking questions. Some simply do not understand the importance of pharmacotherapy to their long-term health and well-being and are not vested in learning about the appropriate medication use.

Patient leaflets are just one example why patients may not seek out their pharmacist as a primary health information resource. Instead of direct patient communication, patient leaflets are commonly stapled to the prescription as a substitute for actual **patient education**. In fact, a survey of community pharmacies found that while 89% of patients received leaflets from their pharmacy, only 5% were given verbal explanation along with it and only 8% of the time did the pharmacist emphasize the important content found within the leaflet.[8] Sixty-six percent of patients were given the document without any further information at all, making it hard for them to establish key points to be taken away from the leaflet. Additionally, many of these leaflets do not adhere to the qualities of good **health literacy**, making them hard for patients to use as a source of health information. Additional information on the importance of good health literacy will be discussed later in the chapter.

Some pharmacies have developed Web sites to direct patients to quality drug information and offer an additional path for patients to ask questions. Many large chain pharmacies and mail-order pharmacies have begun to post answers to the most frequently asked drug information questions for their consumers on their Web sites and some allow for even more interaction online by giving patients the opportunity to ask their questions to a pharmacist. In addition, these Web sites also provide general information regarding medications in the form of patient leaflets. It is important to note that while these pharmacies are headed in the right direction in terms of giving patients more readily available access to quality health information online; these Web sites still have many limitations. Patients enrolled in disease state management and medication therapy management (MTM) programs require the pharmacist to be engaged in focused and directed patient education as part of a comprehensive treatment plan; something that cannot be done by passive answering of questions or interfacing with a Web site alone.

Current Patient Sources of Drug Information

The practice of drug information continues to evolve along with the profession. Drug information can be as simple as obtaining information from references, or an interactive experience between a specific patient and the pharmacist.[9] Drug information can be as active as counseling a patient on all of his or her medications and disease states or as passive as a pharmacy technician dispensing a medication leaflet with a prescription. Regardless of how drug information is delivered, patients are in need of a more connected experience when receiving drug information, not only from health care professionals, but also from peers.

PATIENT EDUCATION VERSUS CONSUMER HEALTH INFORMATION

Patient education and **consumer health information (CHI)** are two distinct ways patients get information about medications, although the two may merge when pharmacists truly engage their patients. ❸ *Patient education delivers written or verbal drug information through a planned activity initiated by a health care provider. The goal is to change patient behavior, improve adherence, and ultimately improve health.*[10] Pharmacist-driven patient education formats include brief counseling when a patient picks up their medication, more comprehensive education as a part of medication therapy management, point-of-care testing (e.g., blood glucose or cholesterol testing), and health screenings. Patient education can be delivered face-to-face or through a variety of technologies, including the telephone, e-mail, and Webcams. The key is that pharmacists interact with individual patients to customize the information to their specific situation.

❹ *CHI is actively sought by the patient in response to their need for more information about their health. Importantly, CHI is not individualized for a specific patient.* Unlike patient education, which is initiated by the pharmacist, CHI is completely patient driven and has evolved out of the patient's need to be their own advocate. CHI has long been available to patients, but the Internet accelerated both the access to and the volume of information; the choices are endless for patients seeking their own information. In 2011, searching for health information online became the third most common activity among Internet users.[11]

For either patient education or CHI to be of any value to the patient, it is crucial that evidence presented to the patient be of high quality and strength. Controlling quality during a patient education encounter is easier because the health care professional filters information distributed to patients. In contrast, the quality and reliability of consumer health information is variable.[12] CHI may be of excellent quality and beneficial to the patient, or it may be of high quality but dangerous because it lacks relevance to their situation, be incomplete, or simply be wrong. Table 20–1 lists examples of popular consumer health information sites.

SOCIAL MEDIA—A NEW FORM OF CONSUMER HEALTH INFORMATION

Patients have long used friends, family, coworkers, and support groups as sources of medical information. The Internet adds to these traditional sources through **social media**, as described in Table 20–2.[1] ❺ *Social media sites allow patients to create content and share information about their health on the Internet.* Web **2.0** is an important concept in understanding the power of the social media. Web 2.0 is not new software but a different strategy to use the Web. The Web goes beyond being a search engine and a source of information to include a platform to create, share, and collaborate in developing new knowledge. Social networking is the phenomenon of online communities in which people share interests and/or activities with one another and is an outgrowth of Web 2.0. With respect to CHI, patients no longer just read about their health information online, but can have an active role controlling content, creating new information, and sharing their experiences with others. For example, PatientsLikeMe® (http://www.patientslikeme.com/) is a privately funded company founded in 2004 with the purpose of creating a community of patients with neurological, neuroendocrine, psychiatric, and immune conditions. Site

TABLE 20–1. EXAMPLES OF POPULAR CONSUMER HEALTH INFORMATION AND SOCIAL MEDIA SITES[13-19]

Consumer Health Platform	Description
Angie's List® (http://www.angieslist.com)	Web site tailored to help consumers find high quality, unbiased reviews, and recommendations on a variety of services including contractors, service companies, home repair, and health care providers. Allows patients to seek perspectives and opinions from fellow patients who have previously seen certain health care providers in their area. Angie's List maintains that both patient members and health care providers benefit from feedback given. Consumers may choose from several different membership options which include monthly and annual payment plans.
Consumer Reports® (http://www.consumerreportshealth.org)	Requiring a monthly or annual subscription, this online resource provides patients with information and unbiased ratings on topics such as healthy living, conditions and treatments, physicians, insurance companies, natural health, and prescription drugs. Health expert blogs are also provided for subscribers on an array of health topics. The Best Buy Drugs feature of this Web site was created in 2004 to help patients compare brand prescription drugs against generics and provide consumers with the best medicine to treat their disease state for their money.
Healthfinder (http://www.healthfinder.gov)	A site operated by the Department of Health and Human Services that serves as a gateway to consumer information. The major goal of this site is to improve consumer access to health information via government agencies, their partner organizations, and other trustworthy sources that serve the public interest.
Microsoft HealthVault (http://www.healthvault.com)	Offers patients a way to store their personal or family's health information all in one location. Patients are then given the option to make their health information accessible to personal health care providers. HealthVault works with physicians, pharmacies, insurance providers, hospitals, and employers to ensure ease of adding information electronically to the HealthVault record. The site is also compatible with certain health devices such as blood pressure monitors and heart rate monitors, allowing patients to upload important health data and readings straight to their HealthVault. The goal of this Web site is to provide the consumer with a more complete picture of their overall health and giving them an opportunity to make the best informed decision.
PatientsLikeMe® (http://www.patientslikeme.com)	Privately funded social media site that was founded in 2004 with the intent of positively impacting patients diagnosed with life-changing diseases. This site primarily focuses on neurological, neuroendocrine, psychiatric, and immune conditions and is geared toward developing a new system of health care created by patients for patients. Through an online community of physicians, organizations, and patients, patients are encouraged to share information about their disease states, treatments, and overall experiences. The hope is that through this online platform patients will feel more connected to others going through similar circumstances as well as empowered and in more control of their disease state.

continued

TABLE 20–1. EXAMPLES OF POPULAR CONSUMER HEALTH INFORMATION AND SOCIAL MEDIA SITES[13-19] (*Continued*)

Consumer Health Platform	Description
Everyday Health® (http://www.everydayhealth.com)	Consumer-centric health company founded to empower and encourage patients to put themselves at the center of their health care. Claims to be a site for comprehensive health and medical information. Free to consumers, the site gears information toward the person they consider the family's chief medical officer (CMO) women or other caregivers. Blogs, forums, and online communities are available so patients can talk to people just like them.
WebMD® (http://www.webmd.com)	Health Web site allowing patients to obtain their health information via a variety of different ways. Health information is available on a wealth of different topics such as drugs and treatments, disease states, and prevention. Online communities for patients seeking support or desiring to share their experiences are also set up in the form of blogs, video, and message boards. Additionally patients have access to slide shows, newsletters, FDA consumer updates, symptom checkers, drug identifiers, and ask the expert feature. WebMD® has established an Independent Medical Review Board to ensure all health information made available to the public is accurate and timely.

TABLE 20–2. SOCIAL MEDIA DEFINITIONS AND PLATFORMS USED TO OBTAIN HEALTH INFORMATION[1]

Social Media	Definition	Platform Examples	URLs
Wikis	Allows user editing and adding of content via a collaborative Web site	Wikipedia	http://www.wikipedia.org
		FluWikie	http://www.fluwikie.com
Social networks	A Web site where those with special interests in common can connect and share with one another	Angie's List®	http://www.angieslist.com
		PatientsLikeMe®	http://www.patientslikeme.com
		OrganizedWisdom®	http://www.organizedwisdom.com
		Everyday Health®	http://www.everydayhealth.com
		Facebook	http://www.facebook.com
		MySpace	http://www.myspace.com
Blogs	An online diary; one can log their personal thoughts on various topics and post to a Web page	WebMD®	http://www.webmd.com
		Mayo Clinic	http://www.mayoclinic.com/health/blogs/BlogIndex
Online forums	Thoughts and ideas are shared and open discussion takes place via various mediums such as a Web site, newspaper, or radio	Everyday Health®	http://www.everydayhealth.com
		Google Health	http://groups.google.com
		Yahoo! Groups	http://groups.yahoo.com
Video-sharing	A medium where information, ideas, and opinions can be shared via videos accessible to many	YouTube	http://www.youtube.com

content is posted by actual patients and includes what treatments they have tried, what works and what does not work for them, and what side effects they experience. Discussions often include the quality of the care delivered by their providers.

❻ *Wisdom of crowds is a belief that when patients share information about their common conditions through social networking, their collective wisdom is more beneficial than the expert opinion of just one individual.* Patients do not completely resist the advice of health professionals, but are just not as willing to rely on a single expert opinion for their information.[1] Health information received via social media is greatly valued by many consumers, especially the "net generation" as described by Don Tapscott in *Grown Up Digital.*[20] This "net generation" made up of consumers born in the early 1980s or after, have grown up online and prefer to engage and collaborate via technology. Extremely used to the digital world, they often trust a search engine on the Internet to provide answers or an online peer review over an expert. Opinions, stories, successes and failures, treatment options, and adverse effects are just some of what this "net generation" of patients share in the social media. This feeling of camaraderie and support obtained via networks is something patients feel they cannot attain from most health care professionals. Some patients may even have reservations when it comes to trusting their health care professional. According to the Edelman Trust Barometer conducted in 2012, people are inclined more than ever to trust social media (consists of social networking sites, content-sharing sites, and blogs) as a source for information.[21] In fact, one in five adult Internet users state they have gone online to connect with other people who have health conditions similar to themselves.[22] The concern is that posts made by patients are a reflection of their unique experience and may be incorrect or inappropriate for another individual. It is imperative patients keep in mind the wealth of information retrieved from peers should be used only to supplement the wealth of information provided by practitioners and that the Internet does not replace health care professionals.[22]

Most social media outlets that give consumers the ability to post opinions, recommendations, and health information state that they are not a substitute for advice of a qualified health professional. While the provision of these disclaimers can be a sign of a quality site, unfortunately, they are not always posted in the most visible place for many consumers on these Web sites, nor do consumers often heed these disclaimers' warning.

Case Study 20-1

You are the only pharmacist on duty at a local community pharmacy. You are short staffed, the phone is ringing, and you have 50+ prescriptions yet to verify. You are doing your best to make the wait as short as possible. In the midst of all this, one of your regular patients comes up to the counter and announces that she will no longer be taking her antidepressant. She describes how lately she has been feeling strange and feels fairly certain it is due to the antidepressant. She then explains to you how she has recently gone online to find more information about the specific medication she is taking. "You wouldn't believe all the good information that is out there," she says, "I was able to talk to other patients and they were so helpful!" She then goes on to talk about the many patient testimonials she read telling her to discontinue her medication.

The patient seems adamant that she is going to stop taking her antidepressant. As a pharmacist, this concerns you. The pharmacy technician calls you to resume verifying prescriptions because the pharmacy is quickly getting out of control.

- *Do you take the time to counsel this patient or do you get back to filling prescriptions before patients start complaining about the wait time?*
- *If you decide to counsel this patient, how would you educate her on the appropriate use of online resources to find health information?*
- *After counseling your patient, she still is determined to stop her antidepressant. What is the most important advice you can give her at this point?*

MOBILE HEALTH—THE DAWN OF THE SMARTPHONE AND OTHER MOBILE DEVICES

Cell phones have made obtaining health information via mobile software applications that much easier. In 2012, a total of 85% of U.S. adults carry a cell phone,[23] 31% of which have accessed health information with their cell phones, a statistic that has increased 14% from 2010. Of the 85% of cell phone users, 53% of these are a **smartphone** user, which means retrieving health information is as simple as the touch of a fingertip. One in five smartphone owners report downloading at least one health application software (apps) to their phone, with exercise, weight, and diet applications being among the most popular. According to ABI research, by 2016 the market for mobile health apps is predicted to quadruple to $400 million with worldwide sales of smartphones anticipated to hit 1.5 billion units.[24] This increasing trend toward smartphone use means that U.S. adults are not only going on the Internet to find health information but are tracking and managing their own health data. This so-called mobile health era is yet another facet of technology pharmacists must adapt to and understand to better serve their patients. Table 20–3 introduces just a few of the smartphone applications making up this almost half a billion dollar industry.

The idea that health care professionals could start medically prescribing **health applications** for their patients is a concept that is gaining momentum. Many of these health applications do not just track health data but function as mobile devices allowing patients

TABLE 20–3. EXAMPLES OF POPULAR MOBILE HEALTH AND FITNESS APPLICATIONS[25-34]

Health and Fitness Applications	Description	Smartphone Availability	Fee
GlucoseBuddy	An application designed for diabetic users who can monitor blood glucose levels, record when they take medication, and track food intake and physical activity.	iPhone, iPod touch, and iPad	Free
iTriage®	iTriage was created by two emergency room physicians that wanted to help users more easily determine what medical condition they might have and where the best place to go for treatment is located.	iPhone and Android	Free
Lose It!	Users looking to lose weight download this app in order to set daily calorie goals, track physical activity, find new exercises, and search for new health conscious recipes. Progress reports are also available for the consumer as well as the ability to share accomplishments via social media.	iPhone, iPod touch, and iPad	Free
MapMyRun	This app not only tracks the runners' exact path, but also records other aspects of a workout like speed, distance, pace, and calories burned. The runner can also share their run data via social media. Versions also exist for walking, hiking, biking, and triathlons.	iPhone, Android, iPad, and Windows	Free—lite version Paid—full version
MyFitnessPal	A popular app that gives users the ability to track their daily activity and food intake. Another feature making this a unique download is the searchable food database providing nutritional information on over two million items. The app even comes with a bar code scanner so users can easily upload nutritional data anywhere. Users can also get support from friends with similar health goals and track each other's progress.	iPhone, iPod touch, iPad, BlackBerry, Android, and Windows	Free
MyPlate	A calorie tracker app developed by LiveStrong.com that gives users access to largest database of nutritional information on food and restaurant items. It provides personalized daily calorie and water intake goals as well as allows the user to update others of their progress via social media.	iPhone, Android, iPad, BlackBerry, and Windows	Free—lite version Paid—full version

continued

TABLE 20–3. EXAMPLES OF POPULAR MOBILE HEALTH AND FITNESS APPLICATIONS[25-34] (*Continued*)

Health and Fitness Applications	Description	Smartphone Availability	Fee
MyQuitCoach	This app put out by Livestrong.com helps smokers quit the habit gradually or right away. Users trying to quit can track their progress and will receive motivational tips and inspirational messages to help them remain strong.	iPhone, iPod touch, iPad	Free—lite version Paid—full version
RunKeeper	Developed for the runner, this app tracks the progress of a workout and the global positioning system (GPS) lets users know where they are running, how fast they are going, and how many calories they have burned. Similar to MapMyRun, this app allows users to share statistics via social media. Other versions track activities like walking and cycling.	iPhone, iPod touch, iPad, Windows, and Android	Free
WebMD®	Few users are unfamiliar with WebMD® and all it has to offer. This mobile app provides much of the same information found online such as popular symptom checker. It also provides first aid information that is available without a wireless connection in emergency instances where Internet access is unavailable. WebMD® Pain Coach and WebMD® Baby are also available.	iPhone, iPad, and Android	Free
ZocDoc	An application developed to provide users a way to peruse reviews of local doctors and dentists while also conveniently booking appointments.	iPhone, iPod touch, iPad, Android, and BlackBerry	Free

to manage various disease states. For example, WellDoc is one of the first health care companies to gain Food and Drug Administration (FDA) approval for their smartphone health application as a medical device. This device gathers data on meals, carbohydrates, blood sugar levels, insulin doses, exercise, and medication about specific patients. The application, DiabetesManager, then advises the patient on how to treat episodes of low blood sugar. It can also send medical data and clinical recommendations to the health care provider. The number of health applications being developed to function as medical devices are increasing and more are entering the market on a daily basis. This trend has created a need for guidelines regarding the regulation required for health applications and clarification of the role of the FDA in the approval process. Currently, developers of

TABLE 20–4. AREAS OF EVALUATION FOR CONSUMER HEALTH MOBILE APPLICATIONS[36]

Areas of Evaluation	Questions to Consider
Credibility of app	Are credentials of app suitable?
	Are authors/publishers clearly listed?
	Are there advertisements?
	Is the organization that developed the app reputable?
	Are there disclaimers of content?
Accuracy of information	Is it peer reviewed?
	Is the information current and/or frequently updated?
	Are recent and reputable guidelines used to support recommendations made?
	Are references cited?
Evidence-based medicine	Are recommendations evidence based?
	Do recommendations target a specific audience or are they general in nature?
	Are opinion statements clearly marked?
	Are users directed to a health care professional before making changes to health care routine?
Ease-of-use	Does the app fit to the screen?
	Is the setup of the app well designed and organized?
	Is the app easily navigated?
	Does the app have a search function?
	Is there a main menu that helps clearly lay content out?
Health literacy	Is medical jargon used easy for the lay reader to understand?
	Is font and setup of app easy to read?
	Does app gear information for the consumer?

heath care applications are providing a laundry list of disclaimers to accompany their product to avoid FDA clearance and the requirement of medical device application.[35] As health care continues to shift into this new era of health information exchange, the role of the practitioner will also evolve and transform. Considerations for evaluation of mobile health applications are presented in Table 20–4.

❼ *The use of mobile technology to obtain consumer health information has experienced a sharp increase within the last few years and continues to skyrocket.*

Case Study 20–2

As you are giving a patient his annual flu shot he brings up the fact that he has recently downloaded the most amazing app for his smartphone that allows him to more easily manage his diabetes. He shares that the app does things like track his blood glucose levels, food intake, and physical activity. The app also adjusts his insulin dose based on his specific data. He swears by the app and is convinced his diabetes is better controlled and that he has never felt better. He also states that he suffers from fewer hypoglycemic episodes than he previously used to experience. You are unfamiliar with the app he is talking about.

• *What initial follow-up questions do you have for this patient?*
• *What guidance do you have for this patient navigating the mobile health arena?*

Case Study 20–3

During the patient's follow up visit with his physician, he is sure to mention the diabetes application that he has been using, following his discussion with you (refer to Case Study 20–2). The physician is unsure what process he should be using to evaluate this application for his patient. He has contacted and asked for you to provide some guidelines to help him evaluate this application as well as other applications his patients are using to manage various disease states.

• *What suggestions do you have to help the physician in evaluating mobile health applications?*

A New Model of Drug Information in the Community Pharmacy

According to a 2011 Pew Internet report, even with the explosion of online and mobile CHI opportunities a majority of people still turn to a health care professional before using the Internet to find information. For the meantime, it appears patients still view the Internet's role as supplemental and are looking at health care professionals to guide them in their search.[2] Patients need to know the differences between patient education and CHI. However, pharmacists should anticipate this trend to shift and expect patients may likely seek health information before talking to their health care provider. This can be a dangerous practice as many patients are ill equipped to find and understand all the information they need to address their health care situation. Pharmacists have an option to either ignore the fact that patients can seek health information elsewhere, or embrace the opportunity to collaborate with their patients as they seek and use information to improve their health and quality of life. As part of the screening process, pharmacists should ask their patients where they get health information and what their preferred method is to obtain such information. The answer to these simple questions can open the door to more specific education about how the patient can obtain useful, quality health information. Pharmacists must become familiar with the range of consumer health information sources and how and why their patients use them. ❽ *Pharmacists should discuss with their patients why they remain an important source of drug information. Patients can be encouraged not to see CHI as a replacement for actual interaction with a health care provider, but as an extension of care and a way to improve communication.* Pharmacists can direct patients to quality CHI sites tailored to their situation and teach them how to seek information from the Web. This skill is important as 75% of patients report that they do not consistently check the source of information they find on the Web.[37] In addition, 52% of patients report believing that almost all or most health information they see online is credible.[38] Pharmacists may consider developing a list of online resources that have their seal of approval as providing high-quality information. Pharmacist-recommended Web sites can be shared in a variety of different ways ranging from pamphlets, bulletin boards, and space provided on the pharmacy Web site. Such a service is something relatively easy and quick to do and goes a long way to helping patients avoid low-quality or risky information. When providing resources, it is imperative they are monitored and updated on a consistent basis; otherwise, potential exists for these same resources to become yet another avenue that low-quality CHI reaches patients. Patients will also need tips on how to navigate the range of information sources as well as how to decide what information is relevant to their individual situation. Not only does this include aiding the navigation of health information found on the Web, but also in other resources, such as brochures and patient leaflets given out with prescriptions. The success of a Web site in delivering meaningful information is heavily reliant on the consumers' ability to identify, interpret, and apply information that is relevant to their situation. If the patient does not understand their health condition, they may use the wrong information for their situation, even if it is of good quality. A 2008 study in the Journal of the American Medical Informatics Association gave patients a scenario describing angina symptoms, but not the actual diagnosis. They used MedlinePlus® to find information on the condition. The authors found that searches yielded information leading patients to draw incorrect conclusions 70% of the time. The authors concluded that patients and/or family and friends of patients searching the Web for information without a diagnosis most likely are confronted with a wealth of information and are unable to sift through what is relevant versus irrelevant.[39]

❾ *Patients often have difficulty finding appropriate information in response to their specific health concerns on the Internet.*

Additionally, pharmacists may offer classes to teach patients how to use CHI to their advantage. Patients can be taught about the Health On the Net Foundation (HON). This nonprofit, nongovernmental organization's mission is to assess and stringently review those Internet sites out there offering health information. Sites passing inspection receive HON certification and are given the HON symbol to place on a visible area of their Web site for patients to see, giving assurance the Web site provides reliable and appropriate information. Unfortunately, as the number of health Internet sites increase, there are more and more places patients will find their health information and many may not have the HON seal of approval. The FDA and the Agency for Healthcare Research and Quality (AHRQ) have also developed checklists for both consumers and health care professionals to determine quality of health information.[40,41] Furthermore, patients can be referred to the National Library of Medicine's tutorial through MedlinePlus. It is specifically dedicated to giving patients instruction on how to evaluate health information they find on the Web and is located at http://www.nlm.nih.gov/medlineplus/webeval/webeval.html.[42]

Moreover, pharmacists can function as rumor control for misinformation on the Internet, mainstream media, or from family and friends. A paper by IBM Global Business Services entitled "Healthcare 2015 and Care Delivery: Delivery Models Refined, Competencies Defined" discussed the need for health coaches who support citizens in their lifestyle decisions and proactively help them understand the risks and outcomes of their choices.[38] Providing quality drug information is clearly a role for a health coach.

EVALUATING THE QUALITY OF HEALTH INTERNET WEB SITES

Questions have been raised about current standards for evaluating the quality of health and medical information on the Internet; many health care professionals feel proxy measures for evaluating the quality of such Web sites are less than ideal. One study suggests that even sites certified with the HON code may be questionable with little correlation between certification and accuracy or completeness of information.[12] Table 20–5 is an example of the aforementioned current standards in health Internet evaluation.

Much focus is put on structural design of a Web site, who the site sponsor (e.g., government, nonprofit, academic institution), and whether or not the site lists its sources; but little emphasis is placed on actual content made available to consumers. When actual health information content has been reviewed in terms of a specific disease state across many different Web sites, Web site sponsorship has been a very poor predictor of quality.[43] In fact, most health information available on the Internet is not monitored for quality or accuracy. According to the Federal Trade Commission, health care professionals review only about 50% of the health and medical content on Web sites.[44] This suggests there is no real efficient and effective method in place to evaluate the quality of health

TABLE 20–5. EXAMPLE OF CURRENT STANDARDS USED TO EVALUATE THE QUALITY OF HEALTH INFORMATION ON THE INTERNET[40]

Considerations When Determining Whether or Not Health Information on the Internet Is Reliable
Who is responsible for the Web site? Does the Web site provide this information? Is the sponsor a government agency, medical school, or reliable health-related organization?
Is the only purpose of the Web site to provide information or is the Web site trying to sell something?
If the Web site inquires about personal information, does it offer a reason why and give an explanation about what it will do with that information once collected?
Is health information provided on the Web site backed up with evidence? Are there references to support recommendations being made, etc.?
Does the Web site give the source of their health information? If so, is that source credible? Does the Web site provide explanation about whether or not health information is reviewed and by whom?
Is health information provided in an unbiased and objective manner? Is material written in a way that would be understandable to most patients no matter their health literacy level?
Does health information on the Web site get updated regularly? Is material provided current?
Does health information on the Web site seem reasonable and credible overall?
Is information provided by the site to allow visitors to contact Web site owners with feedback, problems, and questions?

information online. The only real way is for the pharmacist to individually review each Web site or resource and evaluate health information content provided before they recommend them to patients. Sites devoted to a particular disease state tend to be much more complete and more accurate than sites that attempt to cover multiple health topics, but there are still no guarantees. Strict regulation of health content on the Internet is improbable, but health care providers can attempt to help patients by selecting and evaluating a handful of sites to recommend for patients.[43]

HEALTH LITERACY—FINAL KEY TO THE PATIENT'S SUCCESSFUL USE OF INFORMATION

⑩ *Once patients identify or are given quality health information, they still may face barriers in being able to use it to improve their health.* Health literacy is the capability of patients to read or hear health information, understand it, and then act on health information.[45] The Institute of Medicine estimates that nearly 90 million adults lack the ability to use the U.S. health system sufficiently due to their poor literacy skills. Patients with poor health literacy may have trouble recognizing when health information is even needed, identifying or getting a hold of health information resources, determining the quality of health information resources or acknowledging that quality is even an problem, and even more so analyzing and understanding information found. Pharmacists must consider a patient's health literacy when they provide information and education to their patients. Studies show that most health-related materials whether on the Web or given out in the pharmacy surpass

TABLE 20–6. GUIDELINES FOR HIGH-QUALITY HEALTH LITERATE INTERNET SITES[47]

• Designed for old hardware and software	• Link clearly defined
• Simple home page	• Printer-friendly option
• Information prioritized	• Audio option
• Minimal text per screen	• Site map easy to find
• Navigation simple and consistent	• Contact information easy to find
• Searching simplified	• Content uses other principles of health literacy
• Scrolling need minimized	

most U.S. adults' average reading ability.[46] Table 20–6 describes the qualities of health literate Web sites and can be used as a screen for pharmacists as they identify Web sites for their patients. Visit Pfizer Clear Health Communication at http://www.pfizerhealthliteracy.com/ for additional detail about health literacy standards and the role health care professionals can play in helping their patients.

INFORMATION THERAPY

The term **information therapy** has recently appeared as an organizing principle for a new model of drug information. In 2009, the Argus Commission, a committee of past presidents of the American Association of Colleges of Pharmacy (AACP) who offer analysis on contemporary education issues in pharmacy, included information therapy, a term coined by the Center for Information Therapy, as a new way to think about the pharmacist's role in patient care. The Argus Commission recognized that health care is in the midst of a knowledge technology revolution in which the availability of health information is accelerating at an extraordinary rate. They raised questions about the pharmacist's role in this revolution.[48] Information therapy provides the patient with evidence-based patient education and/or medical information at just the right time to most effectively assist the patient in making a specific health decision or change in their behavior.[12,49] Although an initial counseling session can be very effective for patients, oftentimes, reminders or reiteration of concepts will do more to help the patient if provided at a later time in the form of an information prescription. Information prescriptions are delivered to patients via technology when certain key points between a health care professional and patients need to be reemphasized, a very exciting and practical approach to patient education for community pharmacists. For example, every counseling session could include a follow-up information prescription given at just the right time to effectively reinforce any important late onset adverse drug reactions (ADRs), adherence strategies, or administration techniques. Adherence to preventative health measures could be improved with information prescriptions if patients receive reminders to seek care individualized to their health status. Pharmacy-based examples include flu shots for those at high risk or a bone mineral density measure for postmenopausal women. These reminders, along with simply written evidence-based information on why the procedure is important, increase awareness and demand for important pharmacy-delivered preventative services.[50] ⓫ *Information therapy elevates the term drug information from a passive sounding process to an active component of treatment plans by recognizing that accurate and complete drug information proactively relayed to patients is much more effective than just assuming it will be sought out.* Information therapy encompasses both the patient and the health care professional, asking both to work together in making the best possible health care decision for the patient. From asking more useful questions of physicians and other health care providers to more effectively managing conditions and participating in their own treatment, information therapy may help patients have more control over their lives in terms of their health.

PHARMACISTS' PAYMENT FOR PROGRESSIVE DRUG INFORMATION SERVICES

In order for pharmacists to evolve into progressive drug information practitioners, a sustainable business model that includes reimbursement must be designed. The need for reimbursement is key in light of declining revenues from the dispensing operation. MTM is reimbursable through Medicare Part D and according to MTM program requirements optimum therapeutic outcomes must be ensured for patients through improved medication use and adverse event risk reduction.[51] Effective patient education can play a big role in helping MTM participants meet these specified requirements. Pharmacists should include the strategies described in this chapter in their MTM patient education approaches to begin to get reimbursed for these services. Additionally, some patients are willing to pay directly for care that they cannot receive from other sources. Initiatives such as Project Destiny and the Joint Commission of Pharmacy Practitioner's (JCPP's) Pharmacy 2015 Vision understand the key role reimbursement plays in the sustainability of new practice models and they incorporated financial models for how pharmacists can get paid for these services into their strategic plans.[3,4] The business case for reimbursement cannot rest solely on financial models alone though; it is imperative that establishment of patient and consumer demand for these services are also built into business plans and future visions for pharmacy practice.

Conclusion

A brand new frontier exists for both patients and pharmacists when it comes to obtaining and using health information. It is vital that pharmacists be positioned to be an integral part of patients' approach to gaining an understanding of their health. As traditional pharmacist roles change, new opportunities to get involved in managing patients' health care are presenting themselves. A lot is at stake if pharmacists do not move toward these new roles as someone else will step in and take over this responsibility. It has been the responsibility of pharmacists for decades to educate and provide patients with quality drug information. In the end, it is up to pharmacists to design this new role and demonstrate value to the patient so that they continue to be used as a key ally in providing patient care.

Self-Assessment Questions

1. Which of the following are limitations a pharmacist faces when delivering drug information to their patients?
   a. Lack of readability of most patient leaflets given with prescription.
   b. Pharmacists appear too busy and unavailable.
   c. Counseling has become a passive process where patient education is only given if requested.
   d. Pharmacists lack of understanding in regards to patient's desire to take control of their own health.
   e. All of the above.

2. Patient education is best described by the following:
   a. Delivered by health care professional verbally only
   b. Occurs with the pickup of new prescriptions only
   c. Unplanned activity
   d. b and c only
   e. None of the above

3. Consumer Health Information (CHI) is best described by the following:
   a. Tailored to a patient's specific situation
   b. Actively sought by patients
   c. Created in response to patients need for more information about their health
   d. b and c only
   e. None of the above

4. Which of the following site(s) is considered a social media or social networking site?
   a. WebMD®
   b. Facts and Comparisons®
   c. Everyday Health®
   d. a and b only
   e. a and c only

5. Through social media sites patients share a wealth of personal information regarding their disease states and conditions. Examples of personal information shared includes all of the following *except*:
   a. Treatment successes
   b. Treatment failures
   c. Adverse effects
   d. Opinions
   e. None of the above

6. All of the following are reasons why some patients prefer the collective wisdom of a group over the advice of an expert individual *except* for:
   a. Patients are provided with a feeling of camaraderie and support.
   b. Patients may not trust their health care professional.
   c. Patients are more inclined to trust a person like them.
   d. Patients are not as willing to rely on a single expert for their information.
   e. None of the above.

7. Which of the following is *not* a useful strategy for community pharmacists to employ when helping patients to empower themselves and effectively use consumer health information (CHI)?
   a. Ask patients where else they get health information besides their health care professional.
   b. Encourage patients to quit seeking information online regardless of the source.
   c. Become familiar with the range of CHI resources available.
   d. Develop a list of smartphone health applications that are pharmacist recommended.
   e. Discuss with patients why pharmacists still remain an important DI source.

8. Which of the following are characteristics of a high-quality health literate Internet site?
   a. Simple home page
   b. Navigation simple and consistent
   c. Contact information easy to find
   d. a and b only
   e. All of the above

9. Which of the following questions are considered standard for evaluating the quality of a consumer health information site?
   a. If the Web site inquires about personal information, does it offer a reason why and give an explanation about what it will do with that information once collected?

b. Does health information on the Web site get updated regularly?

c. Does the Web site require you to sign in with a username and password in order to access health information?

d. a and b only

e. All of the above

10. Which mobile health and fitness application provides its users with motivational tips, inspiration, and advice on how to quit smoking?

a. MyPlate

b. MyQuitCoach

c. MyFitnessPal

d. Lose It!

e. ZocDoc

11. LiveStrong developed which of the following mobile health and fitness application(s)?

a. MyPlate

b. MyQuitCoach

c. MyFitnessPal

d. a and b only

e. b and c only

12. Which mobile health and fitness application provides its users with the ability to scan the bar codes of their favorite foods to more easily upload nutrition information?

a. Myplate

b. MyQuitCoach

c. MyFitnessPal

d. Lose It!

e. GlucoseBuddy

13. Which type of social media is best defined as "a Web site where those with special interests in common can connect and share with one another?"

a. Wiki

b. Blog

c. Social network

d. b and c only

e. None of the above

14. Which of the following are issues patients with poor health literacy may face?

a. Trouble recognizing when health information is needed

b. Trouble identifying or getting a hold of health information resources

c. Trouble analyzing and understanding information found

 d. a and b only
 e. All of the above

15. Information therapy can best be described as a/an:
   a. Passive process providing patients with evidence-based drug information at just the right time to most effectively assist the patient
   b. Passive process providing health care professionals with evidence-based drug information at just the right time to most effectively assist the patient
   c. Active process providing health care professionals with evidence-based drug information at just the right time to most effectively assist the patient
   d. Active process providing patients with evidence-based drug information at just the right time to most effectively assist the patient
   e. None of the above

REFERENCES

1. California HealthCare Foundation. The wisdom of patients: health care meets online social media [Internet]. Oakland (CA): California HealthCare Foundation; c2009, 2008 Apr [cited 2009 Nov 10]. Available from: http://www.chcf.org/.
2. Fox S. The social life of health information [Internet]. Washington, DC: Pew Research Center's Internet & American Life Project; 2011 May [cited 2012 Dec 20]:[19 p.]. Available from: http://pewinternet.org/Reports/2011/Social-Life-of-Health-Info.aspx
3. National Community Pharmacists Association. American Pharmacists Association, National Association of Chain Drug Stores, National Community Pharmacists Association. Project Destiny executive summary [Internet]. 2008 Feb [cited 2013 Jul 14]:[5 p.]. Available from: http://www.ncpanet.org/pdf/projectdestinyexecsummary.pdf
4. National Alliance of State Pharmacy Associations. Joint Commission of Pharmacy Practitioners. Executive summary: an action plan for implementation of the JCPP future vision of pharmacy practice [Internet]. 2007 Nov [updated 2008 Jan; cited 2013 Jul 14]:[19 p.]. Available from: http://www.naspa.us/documents/jcpp/Executive%20Summary.pdf
5. Bullman R. Recognizing the full benefits of medication [Internet]. New York: Media Planet; 2011 Mar [cited 2012 Dec 20]:[10 p.]. Available from: http://www.talkaboutrx.org/assocdocs/TASK/531/MedicationNonAdherenceFINALREPORT.pdf
6. Eder R. How consumers choose a primary pharmacy [Internet]. [updated 16 Apr 2012; cited 20 Dec 2012]. Available from: http://www.drugstorenews.com/article/how-consumers-choose-primary-pharmacy
7. Omnibus Budget Reconciliation Act of 1990, Pub. L. 101-508, 104 Stat.1388 (Nov 5, 1990).
8. Svarstad BL, Bultman DC, Mount JK. Patient counseling provided in community pharmacies: effects of state regulation, pharmacist age, and busyness. J Am Pharm Assoc. 2004;44(1):22-9.
9. Malone PM, Kier KL, Stanovich JE. Drug information: a guide for pharmacists. 4th ed. New York: McGraw-Hill; 2011.
10. Massengale L. Resources for Quality Health Information Online. Proceedings of the 119th Annual Meeting of the American Association of Colleges of Pharmacy. 2008 July 19-23; Chicago, IL.

11. Fox S. Health Topics [Internet]. Washington, DC: Pew Research Center's Internet & American Life Project; 2011 Feb [cited 2012 Dec 20]:[24 p.]. Available from: http://pewinternet.org/Reports/2011/HealthTopics.aspx

12. Felkey BG, Fox BI, Thrower MR. Health care informatics: a skills-based resource. Washington, DC: American Pharmacists Association; 2006.

13. Angie's List. [Internet]. Indianapolis (IN): Angie's List; c1995-2012 [cited 2012 Dec 12]. Available from: http://www.angieslist.com/.

14. Consumer Reports Health [Internet]; c2004-2012 [cited 2012 Dec 12]. Available from: http://www.consumerreportshealth.org/.

15. Healthfinder [Internet]; c2012 [cited 2012 Dec 18]. Available from: http://www.healthfinder.gov/.

16. Microsoft HealthVault [Internet]; c2013 [cited 2013 Jun 12]. Available from: https://www.healthvault.com/us/en

17. PatientsLikeMe [Internet]; c2005-2012 [cited 2012 Dec 12]. Available from: http://www.patientslikeme.com/.

18. Everyday Health Group, LLC [Internet]; c2012 [cited 2012 Dec 12]. Available from: http://www.everydayhealth.com/.

19. WebMD [Internet]; c2005-2012 [cited 2012 Dec 12]. Available from: http://www.webmd.com/.

20. Tapscott D. Grown up digital: how the net generation is changing your world. New York: McGraw-Hill; 2009.

21. Edelman. 2008 Edelman Trust Barometer [Internet]. 2008 Jan 22 [cited 2009 Nov 10]. Available from: http://www.edelman.com/trust/2008/.

22. Fox S. Medicine 2.0: Peer-to-peer healthcare [Internet]. Washington, DC: Pew Research Center's Internet & American Life Project; 2011 Sep [cited 2012 Dec 20]. 10 p. Available from: http://www.pewinternet.org/Reports/2011/Medicine-20.aspx

23. Fox S, Duggan M. Mobile Health 2012 [Internet]. Washington, DC: Pew Research Center's Internet & American Life Project; 2012 Nov [cited 2012 Dec 20]. 13 p. Available from: http://pewinternet.org/Reports/2012/Mobile-Health.aspx

24. Savitz E, Newell D. 5 Ways Mobile Apps Will Transform Healthcare [Internet]. New York City: PARS International Corporation; 2012 Jun [cited 2012 Dec 20]: [about 9 paragraphs]. Available from: http://www.forbes.com/sites/ciocentral/2012/06/04/5-ways-mobile-apps-will-transform-healthcare/.

25. GlucoseBuddy [Internet]; c2011-2012 [cited 2012 Dec 18]. Available from: http://www.glucosebuddy.com/.

26. iTriage [Internet]; c2008-2012 [cited 2012 Dec 18]. Available from: https://www.itriagehealth.com/.

27. Lose It! [Internet]; c2008-2012 [cited 2012 Dec 12]. Available from: http://www.loseit.com/.

28. MapMyRun [Internet]; c2005-2012 [cited 2012 Dec 18]. Available from: http://www.mapmyrun.com/.

29. MyFitnessPal [Internet]; c2005-2012 [cited 2012 Dec 18]. Available from: http://www.myfitnesspal.com/.

30. MyPlate [Internet]; c2011-2012 [cited 2012 Dec 18]. Available from: http://www.livestrong.com/calorie-counter-mobile/.

31. MyQuitCoach [Internet]; c2012 [cited 2012 Dec 18]. Available from: http://www.livestrong.com/quit-smoking-app/.

32. RunKeeper [Internet]; c2012 [cited 2012 Dec 18]. Available from: http://runkeeper.com/.

33. WebMD [Internet]; c2005-2012 [cited 2012 Dec 18] Available from: http://www.webmd.com/mobile

34. ZocDoc [Internet]; c2012 [cited 2012 Dec 18]. Available from: http://www.zocdoc.com/.

35. Brustein J. Coming next: using and app as prescribed. New York Times (New York ed.). 2012 Aug 20:Sect. B:1.

36. Pope A, Bryant P, Pace H, Sperry M. Evaluation and ranking of consumer health and drug information smart phone applications. Poster session presented at: American Society of Health System Pharmacists Midyear Meeting; 2011 Dec 4-8; New Orleans, LA.

37. Centers for Disease Control and Prevention [Internet]. Atlanta (GA): National Center for Health Marketing. Online health information seekers: eHealth marketing; 2007 Dec 5 [cited 2009 Nov 1]. Available from: http://www.cdc.gov/healthmarketing/ehm/databriefs/healthseekers.pdf

38. Adams J, Bakalar R, Boroch M, Knecht K, Mounib EL, Stuart N. Healthcare 2015 and care delivery: delivery models refined, competencies defined [Internet]. Somers (NY): IBM Institute for Business Value; 2008:[2 p.]. Available from: http://www-03.ibm.com/industries/ca/en/healthcare/files/hc2015_full_report_ver2.pdf

39. Keselman A, Browne AC, Kaufman DR. Consumer health information seeking as hypothesis testing. J Am Med Inform Assoc. 2008;15(4):484-95.

40. U.S. Food and Drug Administration. How to evaluate health information on the internet: Information for consumers [Internet]. Silver Spring (MD): U.S. Health and Human Services; 2010 Mar 9. [cited 2013 Jun 28]. Available from: http://www.fda.gov/Drugs/ResourcesForYou/Consumers/BuyingUsingMedicineSafely/BuyingMedicinesOvertheInternet/ucm202863.htm#resources

41. Agency for Healthcare Research and Quality. Assessing the quality of Internet health information [Internet]. Rockville (MD): U.S. Health and Human Services; 1999 Jun. [cited 2013 Jun 28]. Available from: http://www.ahrq.gov/research/data/infoqual.html

42. Medline Plus. Evaluating Internet health information: a tutorial from the national library of medicine [Internet]. Bethesda (MD): National Library of Medicine; 2007 [cited 2009 Jan 12]. Available from: http://www.nlm.nih.gov/medlineplus/webeval/webeval.html/.

43. Center for Information Therapy. Seidman J, Steinwachs D, Rubin HR. The mysterious maze of the World Wide Web: what makes Internet health information high quality [Internet]. Bethesda (MD): Center for Information Therapy, Inc.; 2004 July 6 [cited 2009 Jan 13]. Available from: http://www.ixcenter.org/publications/documents/e0035.pdf

44. Fox S, Rainie L. The online healthcare revolution: how the web helps Americans take better care of themselves [Internet]. Washington, DC: Pew Research Center's Internet and American Life Project; 2000 Nov [cited 2012 Dec 20]:[19 p.] Available from: http://www.pewinternet.org/Reports/2000/The-Online-Health-Care-Revolution.aspx

45. Kutner M, Greenberg E, Jin Y, Paulsen C. The health literacy of America's adults: results from the 2003 national assessment of adult literacy. Washington, DC: National Center for Education Statistics; 2003. Report No.: NCES 2006-483. Supported by the U.S. Department of Education.

46. Nielsen-Bohlman L, Panzer AM, Kindig DA. Health literacy: a prescription to end confusion, Committee on Health Literacy, Board on Neuroscience and Behavioral Health. Institute of Medicine. Washington, DC: The National Academies Press; 2004:[41p.]. Available from: http://hospitals.unm.edu/health_literacy/pdfs/HealthLiteracyExecutiveSummary.pdf

47. Agency for Healthcare Research and Quality. Accessible health information technology (IT) for populations with limited literacy: a guide for developers and purchasers of health IT. 2007 Oct [cited 2013 Jan 15]. Available from: http://healthit.ahrq.gov/sites/default/files/docs/page/LiteracyGuide_0.pdf

48. Wells BG, Beck DE, Draugalis JR, Kerr RA, Maine LL, Plaza CM, Speedie MK. Report of the 2007–2008 Argus Commission: what future awaits beyond pharmaceutical care? Am J Pharm Educ. 2008 Nov 15;72(Supp):S08.

49. Center for Information Therapy [Internet]. Bethesda (MD): Center for Information Therapy, Inc.; c2006 [cited 2009 Jan 12]. Available from: http://www.ixcenter.org/.

50. Center for Information Therapy [Internet]. Bethesda (MD): Center for Information Therapy, Inc. Kemper DW. The business case for information therapy in hospitals; 2006 [cited 2009 Jan 12]. Available from: http://www.ixcenter.org/publications/documents/e0678.pdf

51. Centers for Medicare and Medicaid Service. Requirements for medication therapy management programs [Internet]. Baltimore (MD); 2013 Apr 10. [cited 2013 Jun 28]. Available from: http://www.cms.gov/Medicare/Prescription-Drug-Coverage/PrescriptionDrugCovContra/MTM.html

SUGGESTED READINGS

Suggested Readings and Web Sites for Additional Information

Healthwise® Information Therapy	http://www.healthwise.org/insights/information-therapy.aspx
Pew Internet—Chronic Disease and the Internet	http://pewinternet.org/Reports/2010/Chronic-Disease.aspx
MedlinePlus®—Evaluating Health Information	http://www.nlm.nih.gov/medlineplus/evaluatinghealthinformation.html
MedlinePlus®—Guide to Healthy Web Surfing	http://www.nlm.nih.gov/medlineplus/healthywebsurfing.html
Consumer and Patient Health Information Section (CAPHIS)	http://caphis.mlanet.org/
Pfizer Clear Health Communication Initiative	http://www.pfizerhealthliteracy.com
National Institutes of Health—Mobile (mHealth) Health Information and Resources	http://www.fic.nih.gov/ResearchTopics/Pages/MobileHealth.aspx

21

Chapter Twenty-One

Drug Information Education and Training

Michelle W. McCarthy

Learning Objectives

After completing this chapter, the reader will be able to

- Determine fundamental drug information skills for all pharmacy students.
- Identify settings in which student drug information skills can be developed and refined.
- Define the recommended training path for drug information specialists.
- Describe job responsibilities of contemporary drug information specialists.
- Formulate a strategy by which interested candidates can learn about available drug information residencies and fellowships.

Key Concepts

1. Information retrieval, evaluation, and application skills represent a significant component of the core skill set each pharmacist must possess.

2. Drug information skills are core concepts that must be incorporated in pharmacy curricula.

3. The majority of foundational skill development should occur prior to student participation in advanced pharmacy practice experiences (APPEs).

4. Drug information rotations may also occur in nontraditional settings (e.g., pharmaceutical industry, managed care, group purchasing organization), a reflection of the expanding role of drug information in contemporary pharmacy practice.

5. Activities identified by the Accreditation Council for Pharmaceutical Education (ACPE) in which students should engage to foster their skill development range from responding

to drug information requests to preparing materials for consideration by a pharmacy and therapeutics committee.

⑥ Pharmacy residency training standards include core drug information retrieval and evaluation skills for both postgraduate year one (PGY1) and postgraduate year two (PGY2) programs.

⑦ Consistent with the profession-wide model for specialist training, the preferred training model for a drug information specialist is a PGY1 residency program, followed by completion of a PGY2 residency in drug information.

⑧ The American Society of Health-System Pharmacists (ASHP), the organization charged with accrediting pharmacy residency programs, has developed outcomes, goals, and objectives that must be incorporated into ASHP-accredited PGY2 residency programs.

⑨ PGY2 programs in drug information are not limited to health systems, as programs exist in academic, pharmaceutical industry, and managed care settings.

⑩ Fellowship programs build research skills beyond those provided during residency training programs.

Introduction

❶ *Information retrieval, evaluation, and application skills represent a significant component of the core skill set each pharmacist must possess.* Combined with other practice responsibilities that have traditionally been linked to the practice of drug information (e.g., medication use policy), developing and maintaining practitioners with expertise in such activities is critically important. This chapter will focus on key models of education and training for all pharmacists, as well as those specializing in drug information practice.

Foundation Skill Development

Building basic drug information skills, a signature feature of early doctor of pharmacy degree programs, remains an essential component of contemporary entry-level doctor of pharmacy education.[1-3] Skills are developed by both didactic and experiential methods. Didactic drug information education is provided through stand-alone courses as well as being integrated within other courses or throughout the professional curriculum.

❷ *Drug information skills are core concepts that must be incorporated in pharmacy curricula.* Pharmacy curricula must be designed to prepare program graduates with entry-level professional competencies to ensure optimal medication therapy outcomes and patient safety in any pharmacy practice setting and incorporate core drug information skills. To meet the profession's broader needs, the scope of drug information practice has evolved beyond a focus on literature retrieval, evaluation, and application to specific organizational needs and patient care situations such as therapeutic policy management, oversight of safe medication practices including information systems, and promotion of health and wellness.[4] The accreditation standards for professional degree programs include the broad set of related concepts that must be taught and evaluated (e.g., professional communication, practice management, biostatistics).[2] Those that are readily identifiable as connected to drug information are broadly categorized as drug information, literature and research design evaluation (see Chapters 4 and 5), biostatistics (see Chapter 8), economics/pharmacoeconomics (see Chapter 6), pharmacoepidemiology, pharmacogenomics, and medication safety (see Chapter 16). However, a number of foundational elements relevant to drug information practice are integrated into other categories of the Accreditation Council for Pharmacy Education (ACPE) accreditation standards.[2] Those elements include:

- Interpretation of drug screens (e.g., urine toxicology)
- Pharmacist's role in poison control centers
- Dietary Health Supplement and Education Act and impact on regulation of dietary supplements and herbal products
- Drug-herbal interaction
- Indigent care programs
- Incidence of and problems associated with drug overuse, underuse, and misuse in the health care system
- Tools, including informatics, needed to assess and address change, increase competitiveness, improve quality, and optimize patient services
- Managing and improving the medication use process
- Ethical issues related to the development, promotion, sales, prescription, and use of drugs
- Conflict of interest
- Effective verbal and written interpersonal communication
- Health literacy
- Use of data in continuous quality improvement initiatives
- Systematic processing of data, information, and knowledge in health care
- Identifying pharmacotherapeutic knowledge gaps in the professional literature
- Evidence-based practice and decisions
- Assurance of safety in the medication use process
- Medication error identification and prevention programs
- Identification and prevention of drug toxicity

- Role of automation and technology in workload efficiency and patient safety
- Continuous quality improvement programs
- Evaluation of clinical trials that validate treatment usefulness

The American College of Clinical Pharmacy (ACCP) Drug Information Practice and Research Network (PRN) published an opinion paper to ensure that drug information education and practice is designed to meet the needs of the changing health care environment. This paper recommended core specific drug information concepts that should be formally taught and evaluated in all colleges of pharmacy (see Table 21–1).[4] Other topic areas closely aligned with drug information practice include alternative medicine, adverse drug event (medication misadventure) surveillance, drug shortage management and mitigation, safety monitoring during clinical trials, risk evaluation mitigation strategies (REMS), and managing investigational drug services.

A number of pedagogical approaches may be used to build drug information associated skills in the didactic setting. A 2012 survey conducted by the ACCP Drug Information PRN summarized the methods by which colleges of pharmacy include drug information, literature evaluation, and biostatics content into the curricula. Survey responses represented 50% of the pharmacy schools listed in the American Association of Colleges of Pharmacy (AACP) online directory. Instructional methodology used included didactic lectures, small group learning, Internet-based learning, and other formats. Survey respondents indicated using online course management programs, audience response systems, YouTube, online blogs, tweets, and wikis to teach drug information, literature evaluation, and biostatistics content.[5] The availability of instructional technologies and focus on active learning components in the professional program provide many opportunities for instructors to engage learners through incorporation of practical, practice-oriented scenarios.

❸ *The majority of foundational skill development should occur prior to student participation in advanced pharmacy practice experiences (APPEs)*. Integration of practice-related activities in the introductory pharmacy practice experiences (IPPEs) are also important activities supported by the ACPE.[2] Once a student reaches the final year in the professional curriculum, he or she can benefit greatly from a practice experience devoted to drug information practice. Having the opportunity to provide responses to drug information requests following completion of didactic coursework and complete other drug-information-related projects (e.g., medication use evaluation, formulary class review or monograph, evaluation of adverse drug events) provides students even greater opportunities to apply pharmacotherapeutic, pharmacokinetic, legal, and ethical principles to their approach to providing drug information. Drug information historically was a required learning experience for each doctor of the pharmacy student. The growth in the number of colleges of pharmacy and pharmacy student population and reductions in the number of formal drug

TABLE 21–1. ESSENTIAL DRUG INFORMATION CONCEPTS FOR PROFESSIONAL DEGREE CURRICULA[3]

- Applying medical information to specific patient situations
- Counterdetailing and appropriate interactions with the pharmaceutical industry
- Creating effective and efficient literature searching strategies
- Critically evaluating marketing and promotional materials and advertisements
- Critically evaluating medical literature
- Describing the process of drug regulation in the United States
- Distinguishing statistical versus clinical significance
- Discerning and communicating appropriate health information for patient education
- Evaluating drug use policies and procedures
- Identifying, evaluating, and utilizing key print (text) sources of medical information
- Identifying, managing, reporting, and preventing adverse drug events
- Incorporating principles and practices of evidence-based medicine (EBM) into pharmaceutical care
- Locating and critically evaluating medical information on the Internet
- Preparing, presenting, and participating in journal clubs
- Providing verbal and written responses to drug information requests
- Summarizing basic biostatistics and research design methods
- Understanding the creation, maintenance, and management of a drug formulary
- Using electronic medical information databases and other technologically enhanced references and resources in an effective and efficient manner to advance pharmaceutical care

information centers has resulted in an inadequate number of teaching sites to support a required drug information APPE for every student.[6] While some colleges have developed their own formalized centers, others provide only elective drug information advanced practice experiences.[1,6] ❹ *Drug information rotations may also occur in nontraditional settings (e.g., pharmaceutical industry, managed care, group purchasing organization), a reflection of the expanding role of drug information in contemporary pharmacy practice.*

❺ *Activities identified by ACPE in which students should engage to foster their skill development range from responding to drug information requests to preparing materials for consideration by a pharmacy and therapeutics committee.* Table 21–2 provides a comprehensive list of suggested drug information skill building activities to incorporate into APPEs.[2] Students require adequate supervision and oversight to ensure the quality of service they provide, as well as to provide them valuable feedback to subsequently improve their performance. Sites often realize that incorporation of students into the practice site may expand the capacity of services provided, including responding to more drug information requests, preparing analyses of drug policy issues for consideration by the pharmacy and therapeutics committee, and conducting medication use evaluations or adverse drug reaction surveillance. Other APPE experiences beyond those labeled as drug information (e.g., pharmacy management, informatics, and medication safety) also provide opportunities that are beneficial to building skills in drug information.

TABLE 21–2. SUGGESTED DRUG INFORMATION ACTIVITIES FOR INCORPORATION IN ADVANCED PHARMACY PRACTICE EXPERIENCES[2]

- Identifying and reporting medication errors and adverse drug reactions
- Providing patient education to a diverse patient population
- Educating the public and health care professionals regarding medical conditions, wellness, dietary supplements, durable medical equipment, and medical and drug devices
- Retrieving, evaluating, managing, and using clinical and scientific publications in the decision-making process
- Accessing, evaluating, and applying information to promote optimal health care
- Participating in discussions and assignments regarding compliance with accreditation, legal, regulatory/legislative, and safety requirements
- Participating in discussions and assignments regarding the drug approval process and the role of key organizations in public safety and standards setting
- Participating in discussions and assignments concerning key health care policy matters that may affect pharmacy
- Working with the technology used in pharmacy practice
- Managing the medication use system and applying the systems approach to medication safety
- Participating in the pharmacy's quality improvement program
- Conducting a drug use review
- Managing the use of investigational drug products
- Participating in the health system's formulary process
- Participating in therapeutic protocol development
- Performing prospective and retrospective financial and clinical outcomes analyses to support formulary recommendations and therapeutic guideline development

Specialized Skill Development

Drug information skills are a core skill set for all pharmacists, regardless of their practice setting, area of therapeutic focus, or declared area of specialty. ❻ *Pharmacy residency training standards include core drug information retrieval and evaluation skills for both postgraduate year one (PGY1) and postgraduate year two (PGY2) programs.*[7,8] As early as 1966, the need for pharmacists with specialized skills in drug information was documented.[9] The focus of doctor of pharmacy degree programs has evolved to the current model of postgraduate training, specifically through residency programs, to train drug information specialists. ❼ *Consistent with the profession-wide model for specialist training, the preferred training model for a drug information specialist is a PGY1 residency program, followed by completion of a PGY2 residency in drug information.* This training model is also supported by drug information specialist members of ACCP.[4]

Although there is long-standing recognition regarding the importance of advanced training, one survey identified that 40% of drug information pharmacists have completed such training and the remaining 60% developed skill in their position responsibilities through on-the-job training.[10] This may reflect an imbalance in pharmacists with advanced trained and available job openings. A relative lack of popularity or desirability of the specialty to students and new trainees, or pressures on employers to fill positions with applicants who lack the desired formal training, may have contributed to this imbalance; no formal assessment of these or other factors has been conducted. One theory for the decreasing numbers of available PGY2 drug information residency programs is the misconception regarding the activities of drug information residents and specialists. Drug information is evolving from merely providing responses to drug information queries to serving as organizational leaders in medication use policy and safety.[11,12] The number of available positions for individuals with advanced training in drug information often exceeds the number of candidates who have completed advanced training. This imbalance is cause for concern and may result in a shortage of qualified candidates to meet the drug information needs of the changing health care environment.[4,11]

A 2006 survey of United States (U.S.) pharmacists with presumed drug information practices was conducted to determine the perceptions regarding drug information practice and training.[10] The survey was sent to members of the ACCP DI PRN, participants of a drug information practice listserv, and pharmacists employed by drug information centers; because of this methodology, the sample may not reflect all pharmacists with drug information responsibilities. The most common job responsibilities of those surveyed were instructing pharmacy students and staff (64%), maintaining formal drug information center operations (63%), responding to drug information queries (59%), conducting original research (53%), providing pharmacy and therapeutics committee support (46%), providing medication safety support, publishing pharmacy-related newsletters (38%), and developing medication use policy (35%). Respondents generally felt prepared to undertake their responsibilities in relation to the extent of postgraduate training they received. However, areas in which pharmacists felt less prepared included information systems support (41%), pharmacoeconomic evaluations (32%), and clinical outcomes research (19%). Approximately 80% of those who had completed postgraduate training felt adequately prepared overall for their job roles. Preparing for practice changes and innovations is a focus of residency training, and perhaps was reflected in the greater sense of preparedness reported by residency-trained pharmacists.[10] A 2011 survey of pharmacy residents and fellows identified that a new motivator of pharmacy students to pursue residency and **fellowship** training is that these additional training programs are prerequisites for certain jobs.[13]

❽ *The American Society of Health-System Pharmacists (ASHP), the organization charged with accrediting pharmacy residency programs, has developed outcomes, goals, and objectives that must be incorporated into ASHP-accredited PGY2 residency programs.*[7] Required outcomes of PGY2 drug information residencies are to demonstrate excellence in the provision of education, training, and evidence-based information for health care professionals and health care professionals in training; contribute to the management of the organization's medication use policies processes; exercise leadership and practice management skills; conduct drug-information-practice-related projects; and contribute to the management of the organization's budget. There are additional outcomes suggested for those residencies conducted in formal drug information centers and hospitals or health systems. PGY2 drug information residencies are designed to "transition PGY1 residency graduates from generalist practice to a specialized role as an organizational leader in the development of safe and effective medication use policies and/or processes and in the expert analysis of medication-related information."[7] As noted in the 2006 survey, contemporary drug information specialists should be prepared to utilize technology and advance population-based approaches (e.g., data mining, pharmacoepidemiology, pharmacovigilance) to support a safe and effective medication use process.[10] These tools and approaches may include information systems support, clinical outcomes research, pharmacoeconomic evaluations, and other such techniques are also consistent with the Institute of Medicine's (IOM) focus on evidence-based medicine, technology, and quality assurance as core competencies for health care practitioners.[14]

❾ *PGY2 programs in drug information are not limited to health systems, as programs exist in academic, pharmaceutical industry, and managed care settings.* The ASHP required outcomes, goals, and objectives of PGY2 drug information residency programs provide opportunity for development of an advanced skill set that can be applied to many practice settings. Residency graduates who are actively engaged in the practice environment of their training program and then become employed in the same type of practice environment should be well equipped to effectively contribute to the drug information needs of their new organization, and the time to effectively transition from resident to independent practitioner may be shortened. For example, a graduate of an ASHP-accredited PGY2 drug information residency in an academic medical center would likely be a highly desirable candidate for drug information specialist positions within other hospitals and health systems. However, the skills afforded by advanced drug information training in any setting are transferable and beneficial to other settings since having a greater understanding of the operations of an alternate setting may improve decision making in the new environment. For example, training in pharmaceutical industry can better inform a pharmacist of the Food and Drug Administration (FDA) about regulations and internal policies that may shape the manner in which a manufacturer can provide information about an investigational drug or suspected adverse effects of a marketed drug.

❿ *Fellowship programs build research skills beyond those provided during residency training programs.* These fellowships have focus in a number of subspecialty areas including evidence-based practice, medical communications, medication use policy, medication safety, pharmacoepidemiology, and pharmacoeconomics. As with therapeutic specialties, fellowship training in drug information should focus on expanding the fellow's research abilities. There are no accreditation standards for fellowship programs, so their structure, duration, and delivery are guided by the program director.[15] Given the growing complexity and cost of health care, the need for practice-focused researchers has grown more vital. Drug information fellowships that focus on research skills in pharmacoepidemiology, pharmacoeconomics, and comparative effectiveness, or the role of informatics to support a safe and effective medication use system, would be well suited to fill this need.[4,10,13]

Pursuing Specialty Training

Identifying potential residency or fellowship programs that may meet an individual's training needs should begin with a search of available training directories such as the ASHP online residency directory and the ACCP Directory of Residencies and Fellowships.[15,16] Different factors may be important to individual applicants as they evaluate available programs. Beyond traditional drug information activities like responding to queries and providing formulary management, factors that may be important to individual candidates include the ability to gain experience working with students or PGY1 residents, performing contract work, extensive opportunities to manage drug policy across a health system, and intensive training in medical writing. Regardless of the special features or characteristics, there should be opportunities that will prepare the individual for the type of practice they envision. In addition to being prepared for a position as a drug information specialist, graduates of PGY2 drug information residencies may pursue positions in medication safety (see Chapter 16), regulatory/quality pharmacists (see Chapter 22), drug policy (see Chapter 18), and medical writing (see Chapter 9). Settings in which positions may be available include hospitals and health systems, managed care organizations, government organizations, pharmaceutical industry, and academia. A directory of accredited or accreditation-pending residency programs can easily be accessed from the ASHP Online Residency Directory (http://accred.ashp.org/aps/pages/directory/residencyProgramSearch.aspx).[16] In addition to employment (e.g., salary, benefits) and contact (e.g., program director) information, each program's listing includes a description of the practice site, key program features, application information, and a hyperlink to the provider's Web site. More detailed information such as schedules, learning experience descriptions, and accomplishments of program graduates may be found on the Web sites of the individual programs. Residency programs, including those that are not accredited, may also be identified through a review of the Directory of Residencies, Fellowships, and Graduate Programs hosted on the ACCP Web site (http://www.accp.com/resandfel/).[15] This directory is also the primary catalog of possible fellowship options. Fellowship programs may be identified by searching drug information as well as the heading of the research focus (e.g., pharmacoeconomics, pharmacoepidemiology, outcomes research, medication safety). The program listings also provide descriptions of secondary specialty, which include evidence-based medicine or practice, medical communications, and medication use policy. These secondary specialty descriptions may continue to evolve as program's morph to meet the demands of the changing health care environment.

Case Study 21–1

As the coordinator of experiential education at a college of pharmacy, you are responsible for assessing rotation sites. You are working with a number of new sites encouraging them to offer elective advanced pharmacy practice experiences (APPEs) in drug information. Some sites are hesitant to agree to this as they do not have a formal drug information service.

- *In which of the following sites could an elective drug information APPE be offered?*
  - *Community hospital without DI service*
  - *Academic medical center with DI service*
  - *Consultant pharmacist company*
  - *All of the above*
  - *None of the above*

- *What types of activities could students enrolled in the drug information elective APPE complete during their rotation?*
  - *Drug monograph for pharmacy and therapeutics committee*
  - *Medication use evaluation of a high risk agent*
  - *Departmental newsletter article summarizing recent medication errors*
  - *All of the above*
  - *None of the above*

Conclusion

All pharmacists, regardless of practice setting, require drug information skills in order to provide evidence-based patient-centered care and appropriately support other health care professionals. Equipping pharmacists with those skills begins in professional degree programs, continues into residency training, and may extend into fellowship programs.

Additionally, pharmacists may continue to expand drug information skill development throughout their careers by involvement in continuing professional development and on-the-job training. Each of these important elements of education and training should continue to evolve to meet contemporary practice and research needs and to prepare future practitioners to provide innovative services grounded in principles of evidence-based medicine.

Self-Assessment Questions

1. As a faculty member at a new college of pharmacy, you have been asked to assist your colleagues in integrating drug information concepts into their coursework. Which pharmacotherapeutic content area is suitable for integration with drug information skill development?
   a. Cardiology
   b. Neurology
   c. Pediatrics
   d. All of the above
   e. None of the above

2. A drug information advanced pharmacy practice experience (APPE) can be conducted in which of the following settings?
   a. College-based drug information center
   b. Hospital or health-system-based drug information center
   c. State Medicaid formulary management group
   d. All of the above
   e. None of the above

3. In which settings are PGY2 drug information residencies and fellowships offered?
   a. Hospital, college of pharmacy
   b. Hospital, college of pharmacy, managed care
   c. Hospital, college of pharmacy, managed care, industry, and medical communications company
   d. None of the above

4. The organization responsible for conducting the accreditation process for drug information residencies is:
   a. American Society of Health-System Pharmacists (ASHP)
   b. American College of Clinical Pharmacy (ACCP)
   c. Accreditation Council for Pharmacy Education (ACPE)

d. All of the above

e. None of the above

5. In which APPE(s) can a student continue to develop his/her ability to evaluate the biomedical literature?

a. Internal medicine

b. Pediatrics

c. Hospital pharmacy

d. All of the above

e. None of the above

6. The preferred credentials for a drug information specialist practicing in a drug information center are:

a. Pharmacy degree

b. Pharmacy degree + postgraduate year one pharmacy residency

c. Pharmacy degree + pharmacoeconomics fellowship

d. All of the above

e. None of the above

7. What role(s) can postgraduate year two (PGY2) drug information residents play in the education of health care professionals and heath care professionals in training?

a. Provide an in-service to respiratory therapists regarding a new medication

b. Provide classroom instruction about literature evaluation skills to doctor of pharmacy students

c. Prepare a newsletter article summarizing recently released therapeutic guidelines for distribution throughout the organization

d. All of the above

e. None of the above

8. What activities support the required outcomes, goals, and objectives of ASHP-accredited PGY2 drug information residencies?

a. Develop therapeutic guidelines for high-cost agents used within an organization

b. Peer review of a paper submitted for publication

c. Completion of a pharmacoeconomic analysis to support a medication use policy or process

d. All of the above

e. None of the above

9. During your college's review of its professional degree program, a committee member recommends to eliminate a course entitled "Drug Information Skill

Development." When asked to justify the recommendation, the faculty member replies, "The accreditation standards don't require a drug information course." What is a factual response to the statement?

a. The standards *do not* prescribe specific concepts that must be taught in professional degree curricula.

b. The standards *do* require the inclusion of concepts directly categorized as drug information, in addition to related concepts.

c. Drug information concepts *are* required to be taught only during advanced pharmacy practice experiences (APPEs).

d. All of the above.

e. None of the above.

10. In which activity can you engage college of pharmacy students enrolled in a drug information course to demonstrate the broad applicability of drug information skills, using an example from the popular media?

a. Critiquing the accuracy of a local television news reporter's segment about a newly approved prescription drug

b. Crafting a letter to the editor describing the role pharmacists play in preventing medication errors, in response to an article about the national impact of medication errors published in the local newspaper

c. Evaluating a front page article from the New York Times regarding a drug study

d. All of the above

e. None of the above

11. What types of skill-building activities can be assigned to students enrolled in a drug information course within a college of pharmacy?

a. Drug information requests that have been posed to the college's drug information center

b. Journal club presentation

c. Drug monograph

d. All of the above

e. None of the above

12. Analyzing the contents of a direct-to-consumer advertisement for a newly approved prescription drug is an activity that can illustrate which drug-information-related concept to students?

a. Regulation of dietary supplements and herbal products

b. Incidence of drug overuse, underuse, and misuse in the U.S. health care system

   c. Ethical issues related to the promotion of drugs
   d. All of the above
   e. None of the above

13. What types of positions may individuals completing an ASHP-accredited PGY2 drug information residency pursue?
   a. Drug information specialist in hospital/health system
   b. Editor at medical communications company
   c. Medication safety pharmacist
   d. All of the above
   e. None of the above

14. Drug information and associated fellowships may be desired by individuals interested in the following:
   a. Extensive-research-related activities
   b. Pharmacoeconomics
   c. Pharmacoepidemiology
   d. All of the above
   e. None of the above

15. Where would you be able to determine the employment paths graduates of Postgraduate Year Two (PGY2) drug information residencies have pursued over the last 5 years.
   a. The individual training program's Web site
   b. The ACCP Online Residency Directory
   c. The ASHP Online Residency Directory
   d. All of the above
   e. None of the above

Acknowledgments

The author acknowledges Kelly M. Smith, PharmD, BCPS, FASHP, FCCP, who wrote this chapter in the previous edition.

REFERENCES
1. Wang F, Troutman WG, Seo T, Peak A. Rosenberg JM. Drug information education in doctor of pharmacy programs. Am J Pharm Educ. 2006;70:1-7.
2. Accreditation Council for Pharmacy Education. Accreditation standards and guidelines for the professional program in pharmacy leading to the doctor of pharmacy degree

version 2.0 [Internet]. Chicago: 2011 [cited 2012 Nov 29]. Available from: https://acpe-accredit.org/pdf/FinalS2007Guidelines2.0.pdf

3. Medina MS, Plaza CM, Stowe CD, Robinson ET, DeLander G, Beck DE, et al. Center for the Advancement of Pharmacy Education (CAPE) Educational Outcomes 2013. Am J Pharm Educ. 2013. Available from: http://www.aacp.org/Documents/CAPEoutcomes071213.pdf

4. Bernknopf AC, Karpinski JP, McKeever AL, Peak AS, Smith KM, Smith WD, et al. Drug information: from education to practice. Pharmacotherapy. 2009 Mar;29(3):331-46.

5. Phillips JA, Gabay MP, Ficzere C, Ward KE. Curriculum and instructional methods for drug information, literature evaluation, and biostatistics: survey of US pharmacy schools. Ann Pharmacother. 2012;46:793-801.

6. Cole SW, Berensen NM. Comparison of drug information practice curriculum components in US colleges of pharmacy. Am J Pharm Educ. 2005;69:240-4.

7. American Society of Health-System Pharmacists. Educational outcomes, goals, and objectives for postgraduate year two (PGY2) pharmacy residencies in drug information [Internet]. [cited 2013 Jan 14]. Available from: http://www.ashp.org/DocLibrary/Accreditation/Regulations-Standards/RTPObjDrugInformationMarch2008.aspx

8. American Society of Health-System Pharmacists. Educational outcomes, goals, and objectives for postgraduate year one (PGY1) pharmacy residencies [Internet]. [cited 2013 Jan 14]. Available from: http://www.ashp.org/DocLibrary/Accreditation/Regulations-Standards/RTPPGY1GoalsObjectives.aspx

9. Walton CA. Education and training of the drug information specialist. Drug Intell. 1967;1:132-7.

10. Gettig JP, Jordan JK, Sheehan AH. A survey of current perceptions of drug information practice and training. Hosp Pharm. 2009;44:325-31.

11. Vanscoy GJ, Gajewski LK, Tyler LS, Gora-Harper ML, Grant KL, May JR. The future of medication information practice: a consensus. Ann Pharmacother. 1996;30:876-81.

12. American Society of Health-System Pharmacists. ASHP guidelines on the provision of medication information by pharmacists. Am J Health-Syst Pharm. 1996;53:1843-5.

13. McCarthy BC, Weber LM. Update on factors motivating pharmacy students to pursue residency and fellowship training. Am J Health-Syst Pharm. 2013;70:1397-403.

14. Institute of Medicine: executive summary. In: Greiner AC, Knebel E, eds. Health professions education: a bridge to quality. Washington, DC: National Academy Press; 2003. p. 1-18.

15. American College of Clinical Pharmacy Directory of Residencies, Fellowships and Graduate Programs [Internet]. Lenexa: American College of Clinical Pharmacy; c2013 [cited 2013 Aug 25]. Available from: http://www.accp.com/resandfel/index.aspx

16. American Society of Health-System Pharmacists Online Residency Directory [Internet]. Bethesda (MD): American Society of Health-System Pharmacists; c2013 [cited 2013 Aug 25]. Available from: http://accred.ashp.org/aps/pages/directory/residencyProgramSearch.aspx

SUGGESTED READINGS

1. Accreditation Council for Pharmacy Education. Accreditation standards and guidelines for the professional program in pharmacy leading to the doctor of pharmacy degree version 2.0 [Internet]. Chicago, IL. 2011 [cited 2012 Nov 29]. Available from: https://acpe-accredit.org/pdf/FinalS2007Guidelines2.0.pdf

2. Bernknopf AC, Karpinski JP, McKeever AL, Peak AS, Smith KM, Smith WD, et al. Drug information: from education to practice. Pharmacotherapy. 2009 Mar;29(3):331-46.

3. Cole SW, Berensen NM. Comparison of drug information practice curriculum components in U.S. colleges of pharmacy. Am J Pharm Educ. 2005;69:240-4.

4. Phillips JA, Gabay MP, Ficzere C, Ward KE. Curriculum and instructional methods for drug information, literature evaluation, and biostatistics: survey of US pharmacy schools. Ann Pharmacother. 2012; 46:793-801.

5. Gettig JP, Jordan JK, Sheehan AH. A survey of current perceptions of drug information practice and training. Hosp Pharm. 2009;44:325-31.

6. American Society of Health-System Pharmacists. Educational outcomes, goals, and objectives for postgraduate year two (PGY2) pharmacy residencies in drug information [Internet]. Bethesda (MD): ASHP Commission on Credentialing; 2008 [cited 2013 Jan 14]. Available from: http://www.ashp.org/DocLibrary/Accreditation/Regulations-Standards/RTPObjDrugInformationMarch2008.aspx

22

Chapter Twenty-Two

Pharmaceutical Industry and Regulatory Agency Drug Information*

Jean E. Cunningham • Lindsay E. Davison

Learning Objectives

After completing this chapter, the reader will be able to

- Design an organization chart for a pharmaceutical company.
- Discuss opportunities for health care professionals (HPs) within the pharmaceutical industry.
- Describe how HPs are regulated in the pharmaceutical industry.
- Determine acceptable interactions between pharmaceutical companies and practitioners.
- List the components of a standard response and personalized letter.
- Explain the importance of collecting adverse event information.
- Identify pharmaceutical industry–associated organizations.
- Recommend methods for communicating safety information to consumers.
- Describe the role of the Division of Drug Information (DDI) at the Food and Drug Administration (FDA).
- List the main differences between the DDI and a typical drug information center.
- Illustrate the different types of drug information services provided by the FDA.
- Identify factors that guide selection of a specific FDA-sponsored resource or Web site.
- Discuss student and professional opportunities within the FDA.

---

* The views expressed in this chapter do not necessarily represent the views of the Food and Drug Administration or the United States.

Key Concepts

① Pharmaceutical companies' scientific or medical divisions are staffed with highly trained health care professionals (HPs) working in a multitude of specialized fields.

② Medical information specialists respond to inquiries, provide training, and draft materials for a variety of internal and external audiences.

③ Pharmaceutical companies are regulated both externally by the FDA and internally by standard operating procedures (SOPs).

④ The FDA's draft Guidance for Industry "Responding to Unsolicited Requests for Off-Label Information About Prescription Drugs and Medical Devices" describes the FDA's current thinking about how manufacturers and distributors of prescription human drug products can respond to unsolicited requests for information about unapproved indications (off-label information) related to their FDA-approved or cleared products.

⑤ Unsolicited requests are those initiated by persons or entities that are completely independent of the relevant firm.

⑥ The FDA considers requests for off-label information that are prompted in any way by a manufacturer or its representatives to be solicited.

⑦ Interactions between pharmaceutical companies and HPs are defined, but not regulated, by a code of conduct established by the Pharmaceutical Research and Manufacturers of America (PhRMA) through the revised version of the *Code on Interactions with Health Care Professionals*.

⑧ Clinical response letters are written correspondence that contains company-approved content in response to an unsolicited request for medical information.

⑨ Patient variability, clinician experience, and previously unaddressed questions require personalized responses that cannot be fulfilled with a standard response letter.

⑩ Adverse drug experiences, or adverse events, are required to be reported to the FDA by pharmaceutical companies.

⑪ The mission of the FDA is to protect "the public health by assuring the safety, efficacy, and security of human and veterinary drugs, biological products, medical devices, our nation's food supply, cosmetics, and products that emit radiation."

⑫ Timely communication of important drug safety information provides HPs, patients, consumers, and other interested persons with access to the most current information concerning the potential risks and benefits of a marketed drug, helping them to make more informed treatment choices.

⑬ The FDA uses various tools and methods to communicate drug safety information to the public.

⑭ The mission of the Division of Drug Information (DDI) is to optimize the Center for Drug Evaluation and Research's (CDER) educational and communication efforts to the global community. The DDI supports the FDA's mission to promote and protect public health.

⑮ The DDI has built effective internal and external interactions to provide timely, accurate, and useful information through both traditional and social media channels.

⑯ In addition to dedicated drug safety communication (DSC) channels, the DDI has several proactive and innovative tools to communicate information about human drug products to the public.

⑰ The FDA offers many opportunities for health professional students. One of the most popular programs is the FDA Pharmacy Student Experiential Program. Student opportunities are also available within the United States Public Health Service (USPHS) Commissioned Corps.

Introduction

There are many roles available to health care professionals (HPs) within the pharmaceutical industry and regulatory agencies focused on public health. In industry, these roles span medical education, publications, marketing, medical information, and more. In public health agencies, the roles are usually separate functions supporting the organizational mission statement and generally pertain to protecting the health of all Americans and providing essential human services, especially for those who are least able to help themselves. Job titles and descriptions may vary slightly from company to company or agency to agency, but the importance of HPs within each area is constant across organizations.

Throughout this chapter the reader will become familiar with the organization of a pharmaceutical company, professional mentoring relationships, industry's regulated interactions with outside HPs, fulfillment of a medical information request and responses to unsolicited inquiries, the many roles and career paths available to HPs in industry, and the importance and requirements of adverse event reporting and **postmarketing surveillance**. Information surrounding the role of medical information within a regulatory agency, specifically the Food and Drug Administration (FDA), will then be presented. At the end, the reader should have a general knowledge of the roles and responsibilities of HPs employed in the pharmaceutical industry and FDA, the expectations practitioners receiving medical information from a pharmaceutical company or regulatory agency may have, and how to pursue opportunities and careers within the pharmaceutical industry or a regulatory agency with a public health mission.

Opportunities for Health Professionals Within Industry

❶ *Pharmaceutical companies' scientific or medical divisions are staffed with highly trained* ● *HPs working in a multitude of specialized fields* (see Figure 22–1).[1] The following section will highlight specific opportunities within the pharmaceutical industry for HPs.

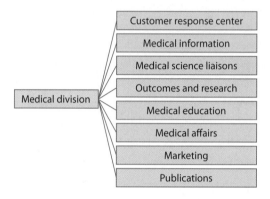

Figure 22–1. Organization of pharmaceutical companies' medical division.[1]

CUSTOMER RESPONSE CENTER

Customer response center representatives are the first-line response team for unsolicited requests* for medical information. HPs in this setting are well trained for customer response center representative positions. Customer response center HPs are faced with a variety of responsibilities as the first line of communication with patients and providers. Responsibilities include capturing adverse events (AEs) that are reported and triaging nonmedical and medical information requests (MIRs). Customer response center HPs are provided with a variety of tools, including, but not limited to, product labeling (or package inserts), response letters, question and answer (Q&A) documents, and clinical topic overviews, typically drafted by peers in the medical information division to assist in answering unsolicited requests for product information. A guidance document, published by the FDA, regarding responding to unsolicited requests, also offers industry the FDA's current thinking on this topic.[2] Customer response center staff use product labeling, response letters, and literature searches to assist them in responding to MIRs. HPs serving in this capacity must have excellent verbal communication skills and are highly trained in effectively searching for information. Some MIRs may require additional

---

* Unsolicited requests must be created by the requester free from prompting by the pharmaceutical company or its representatives.

research or analysis resulting in the customer response center HPs escalating the inquiry to a medical information specialist for further investigation.

MEDICAL INFORMATION

❷ *Medical information specialists respond to inquiries, provide training, and draft materials for a variety of internal and external audiences.* Medical information specialists are HPs who respond to unsolicited MIRs, write and update response letters, conduct scientific analysis of medical literature topics, review promotional materials, develop Academy of Managed Care Pharmacy (AMCP)-formatted dossiers for formulary consideration, and train company staff (e.g., sales force, peers, account managers, and others [see Figure 22–2]).[3,4]

Medical information specialists also respond to MIRs that are escalated to them by customer response center representatives. Escalation, or the transfer of MIRs, occur frequently when the customer response center representatives do not have the resources necessary to formulate a response. Frequently, escalations involve questions about off-label use. This will be discussed later in the section entitled Regulation of Health Care Professionals in Industry. Medical information specialists may have access to additional resources, such as comprehensive reports from clinical trials, information provided to study investigators, marketing materials, posters and abstracts, and contacts in other departments, which makes them invaluable resources for analyzing and synthesizing information.

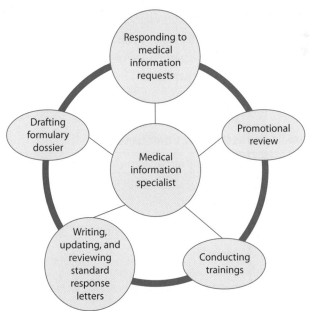

Figure 22–2. Responsibilities of medical information specialists.[2]

MEDICAL SCIENCE LIAISONS

Medical science liaisons (MSLs) originated as a highly specialized customer response center representative. An MSL supports, and is supported by, the scientific affairs and medical information team. MSLs have a close working relationship with **key opinion leaders** and are expected to engage in clinical conversations ranging from broad clinical guidelines to patient-specific care (Table 22–1).[5] MSLs are expected to attend national meetings and provide comprehensive clinical presentations. MSLs may focus on one product or therapeutic area, so there may be overlapping MSLs working for the same company in one location, supporting different products and specialty areas, or vice versa, there may be one MSL in a remote location responsible for multiple products and therapeutic areas.

OUTCOMES RESEARCH

Outcomes research specialists are known in some companies as field-based outcomes liaisons or FBOLs. This position is similar to that of an MSL, except the focus of FBOLs may be to demonstrate the value of a product to managed care organizations, pharmacy benefit managers (PBMs), or other HPs in similar decision-making roles through the generation of outcomes data. Outcomes data typically provides studies focused on identifying, measuring, and evaluating the end result of a health care service or treatment. For example, a company that is marketing an antiplatelet medication might request that their FBOLs demonstrate to customers the value of the product through quality-life years gained or may request that the FBOLs create a risk stratification tool (e.g., stratification of risk for patients with cardiovascular disease) to assist clinicians in determining appropriate therapy options for their patients.

TABLE 22–1. **RESPONSIBILITIES OF MEDICAL SCIENCE LIAISONS**[5]

Responsibilities of medical science liaisons may include the following:
Building and maintaining relationships with key opinion leaders
Recruiting interested investigators for clinical trial research
Supporting advisory boards
Assisting with company projects
Providing peer-to-peer exchange of information
Presenting at meetings with formulary decision makers
Conducting training sessions for branded product speakers, medical residents, and/or sales representatives
Performing and overseeing clinical trial and health outcomes research
Providing continuing education and branded product presentations

MEDICAL EDUCATION

HPs in medical education evaluate funding requests for continuing medical education (CME), continuing education (CE), and other programs submitted by qualified organizations. Grants are reviewed by medical education to ensure the program outlined in the grant addresses specific needs of clinicians in clinical practice and is consistent with the company's educational goals and objectives for a specific therapeutic area.[1] CME and CE programs must meet standards set by the corresponding accrediting body for the audience and should follow guidance documents published by the FDA.[6,7]

MEDICAL AFFAIRS

Medical affairs HPs typically oversee phase IV clinical trial programs and may also be involved with preclinical studies through phase IV or postmarketing studies. These HPs are primarily conducting research on marketed pharmaceuticals in areas of high therapeutic demands or information need. Medical affairs HPs play a key role in shaping the direction of future clinical development including where to focus resources on specific disease states, what drug candidates to support in human clinical studies, and what marketed drugs to develop with new indications or to study through the investigator-initiated study process. In addition, medical affairs staff is involved in a variety of tasks with peers in medical information, marketing, and with key opinion leaders in the field. These tasks include reviewing promotional and marketing materials, supporting phase IV clinical trial sites and maintaining communication with trial investigators, reviewing product labeling, formulary dossiers, training materials for promotional and education purposes, and developing and presenting original research in the form of posters, abstracts, and manuscripts. Medical affairs HPs are responsible for reviewing these materials for accuracy of medical information and to ensure that the final products (e.g., promotional materials, package inserts) are unbiased, fair balanced, and not misleading.[1]

MARKETING

HPs in the marketing division of a pharmaceutical company are responsible for developing the branded messages for a product. See Chapter 23 for further information on pharmaceutical marketing. The tag lines and main selling points seen in journal advertisements, on Web pages, and on printed materials are created by the marketing division. It is important for HPs in marketing to understand the clinical practice environment of their peers so they can provide useful, valuable tools and materials. Marketing drafts a plethora of promotional materials from journal and television advertisements to functional educational tools such as dose conversion guides. All of these materials are then reviewed by peers in medical information and medical affairs, and other internal business partners in regulatory and legal.[1]

PUBLICATIONS

The team of HPs in the publications department has the important task of ensuring the appropriate information reaches the appropriate audience. For example, a company coming to market with a new blood pressure medication would want its publications department to create a plan that would publish trial data (preclinical through *post hoc* and review data) concurrently with major meetings of prescribers treating blood pressure. The publications department ensures that reprints of posters, abstracts, and manuscripts are readily available for dissemination to HPs in the field. HPs in this department are also responsible for reviewing the final content of publications and drafting comments if necessary, often through a partnered review process with medical affairs and medical information, to make certain accurate information is available for practitioners in clinical practice.[1]

As outlined in this section, HPs have many varied opportunities within the industry. Each of the functions described previously abide by a set of rules and regulations. Understanding and complying with these rules and regulations help ensure the success of industry-employed HPs.

Regulation of Health Care Professionals in Industry

❸ *Pharmaceutical companies are regulated both externally by the FDA and internally by standard operating procedures (SOPs).*[8,9] To help internal staff understand the regulations governing their department's duties and establish an efficient methodological approach to the business, SOPs are developed internally by the company.[2,3] While practitioners in clinical practice may not be governed by the same regulations as industry, having a basic understanding of company's regulations will help align the external clinicians' expectations with what can be provided by internal industry HPs.

CODE OF FEDERAL REGULATIONS

The Code of Federal Regulations (CFR) Title 21 regulates the United States (U.S.) pharmaceutical industry throughout the life cycle of a product, from before the investigational new drug application (pre-IND) through phase IV clinical trials, including postmarketing data collection.[6,7,10–14] HPs working for a U.S. pharmaceutical company must achieve a thorough understanding of these regulations to ensure compliance with the regulations that pertain to their daily duties.

FDA GUIDANCE DOCUMENTS

FDA guidance documents represent the FDA's current thinking on a topic. Guidance documents do not create or confer any rights for or on any person and do not operate to bind the FDA or public. Guidance documents are very useful because they expand upon the regulations. ❹ *The FDA's draft Guidance for Industry, "Responding to Unsolicited Requests for Off-Label Information About Prescription Drugs and Medical Devices," describes the FDA's current thinking about how manufacturers and distributors of prescription human drug products can respond to unsolicited requests for information about unapproved indications (off-label information) related to their FDA-approved or cleared products.* An important portion of this guidance document for pharmaceutical companies is the discussion of unsolicited requests that are encountered through emerging electronic media. First though, several important definitions are provided with examples.

UNSOLICITED REQUESTS

❺ *Unsolicited requests are those initiated by persons or entities that are completely independent of the relevant firm.* (This may include many HPs, health care organizations, members of the academic community, and formulary committees, as well as consumers such as patients and caregivers.) Requests that are prompted in any way by a manufacturer or its representatives are not unsolicited requests.

Two Types of Unsolicited Requests
Nonpublic unsolicited requests
A **nonpublic unsolicited request** is an unsolicited request that is directed privately to a firm using a one-on-one communication approach. For example: An individual calls or e-mails the medical information staff at a firm seeking information about an off-label use. In this case, neither the request nor the response would be visible to the public.

Public unsolicited requests
A **public unsolicited request** is an unsolicited request made in a public form, whether directed to a firm specifically or to a forum at large. For example: During a live presentation, an individual asks a question, directed to a firm's representative but heard by other attendees, regarding off-label use of a specific product. This request is a public request. Similarly, a response by the firm that is conveyed to the same audience as the original question would be considered a public response. Another example is if an individual posts a question about off-label use of a specific product on a firm-controlled Web site (or a third-party discussion forum), that is visible to a broad audience. The request could be directed to a firm specifically or posed to users of a discussion forum at large. This request

is a public online request. Similarly, a response by the firm that is visible to the same audience as the original question would be considered a public online response.

SOLICITED REQUESTS

❻ *The FDA considers requests for off-label information that are prompted in any way by a manufacturer or its representatives to be solicited.* Such solicited requests may be considered evidence of a firm's intent that a drug be used for a use other than that specifically approved by the FDA. For example, if a firm announces results of a study via a microblogging service (e.g., Twitter) and suggests that an off-label use of its product is safe and effective, any comments and requests received as a result of the original message about the off-label use would be considered solicited requests.

The FDA has long taken the position that firms can respond to unsolicited requests for information about FDA-regulated medical products by providing truthful, balanced, nonmisleading, and nonpromotional scientific or medical information that is responsive to the specific request, even if responding to the request requires a firm to provide information on unapproved indications or conditions of use.

STANDARD OPERATING PROCEDURES

SOPs provide additional guidance to employees, supplementing regulations from federal and state government agencies. SOPs allow a company to digest federal regulations, making them applicable to employees and their everyday job functions.[15] The pharmaceutical industry employs HPs and lawyers in regulatory affairs to ensure SOPs are up-to-date and provide employees proper guidance for complying with all applicable regulations.

Case Study 22–1

■ DRUG A®

The pharmaceutical company, Awesome Drug R Us, Inc., is planning to file a new drug application (NDA) for DRUG A®, their new medication to treat moderate to severe hiccups. Awesome Drugs R Us, Inc., is a small start-up company and has never launched a marketed product prior to DRUG A®. The company currently employs a small number of HPs in medical affairs and marketing. Awesome Drug R Us, Inc., received a priority review (a drug product with priority review designation is one where the FDA's goal is to take action on the application within six months, rather than 10 months in a standard review, although it is not a requirement to do so) for DRUG A® and is expecting a review action in 6 months following the NDA filing.

- *What internal documents should Awesome Drugs R Us, Inc., prepare so their employees are aware of the regulations governing their job functions?*
- *What external regulations should Awesome Drugs R Us, Inc., include in education for their staff?*
- *Discuss the job responsibilities in the current departments at Awesome Drugs R Us, Inc.*

- *What are some other departments Awesome Drugs R Us, Inc., should consider developing in the future? What are some of the job responsibilities of these departments?*

Pharmaceutical Research and Manufacturers of America and the Code on Interactions with Health Care Professionals

HPs within the pharmaceutical industry hold themselves to a high standard when it comes to providing accurate, concise, and timely information. ❼ *Interactions between pharmaceutical companies and HPs are defined, but not regulated, by a code of conduct established by* **Pharmaceutical Research and Manufacturers of America (PhRMA)** *through the revised version of the Code on Interactions with Health Care Professionals.*[16] The prior edition, from 2002, addressed primarily products being marketed and activities prior to the launch of a medication. The updated version released in January 2009 includes more specific guidance regarding the interactions between pharmaceutical industry representatives and HPs. The goal of these regulations is to provide transparency to HPs and patients alike as to the motives and channels through which industry conducts business with external customers and business partners.[17]

Case Study 22–2

Use information from Case Study 22–1.

- *What department(s) would review grants for educational programming for DRUG A®?*
- *What department(s) may be involved in approving marketing materials for DRUG A®?*

Fulfillment of Medical Information Requests

HPs and patients may contact a pharmaceutical company with questions regarding a medication when an answer is not readily available. A typical process for responding to these questions is described in Figure 22–3.

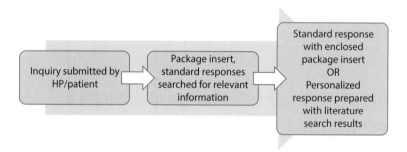

Figure 22–3. Medical information request receipt and fulfillment process.

RESPONSE LETTERS

❽ *Clinical response letters are written correspondence in response to unsolicited requests for medical information.* The use of evidence-based medicine in response letters allows consumers and HPs to be confident they are receiving fair-balanced, unbiased, and not misleading information.[18] Response letters are usually created according to a template for consistency (see Table 22–2) and drafted in anticipation of, or in response to, frequently asked questions.[10] Solvay Pharmaceuticals determined that prior to the launch of a product, response letters took four to 8 hours each to create. The time spent by Solvay's staff to create a response letter following launch significantly increased, taking 4 to 7 days to create. This was directly related to the increased workload and the continuous arrival of new MIRs.[19] Once a product is available on the market, the number and complexity of MIRs is likely to increase. This increases HP's total workload and, therefore, increases the time it takes to complete individual tasks, such as creating response letters. Because of this, the time to create a response letter and respond to an MIR may differ from Solvay's results.

Pharmaceutical companies' response letters are created from source documents in response to frequently asked questions and are peer reviewed internally.[20] Standard response letters developed by companies may be either proactive or reactive. For example, if the evening news reports that a marketed drug, similar to Drug A® causes yellow stripes to appear on patients' skin, the company that makes the competitor to Drug A® should react

TABLE 22–2. COMPONENTS OF A STANDARD RESPONSE LETTER[21]

Opening
Indication(s)
Disclaimer
Body
Closing
Adverse Event Reporting
Signature and Contact Information
Enclosure(s)
References

immediately by developing a response letter to address questions from HPs and patients on this adverse event (i.e., reactive). In another example, the sponsor of Drug A®, may wish to proactively develop a response letter in anticipation that the likelihood of experiencing yellow stripes with Drug A will be frequently asked, based on the report of this reaction with the competing similar drug. Using the example above, the company that manufacturers Drug A® may need more than 1 day to prepare a complete, concise response and, thus, in the meantime may tell customers they are currently researching the issue in question. When this response is provided, the requestor should expect a complete response to be delivered in a timely manner (see Appendix 22–1 for an example of a response letter).

UNIQUE RESPONSES FOR NONFREQUENTLY ASKED QUESTIONS

❾ *Patient variability, clinician experience, and previously unaddressed questions require personalized responses that cannot be fulfilled with a standard response letter.* HPs in the customer response center and medical information department then use their literature search and evaluation skills to determine if relevant information has been published or is available through internal company data (also known as data on file) that addresses the inquiry.[20] If no information is found, the requestor is contacted with the results and a statement that the company cannot provide any information. If relevant publications are found, a response is drafted that includes the citations or reprints (when copyright allows) of the information and this is provided to the requestor along with a verbal conversation (if possible) to discuss the findings and applicability to the requestor's situation.[22] Requestors expect their inquiry to be addressed in a timely manner and often prefer a verbal answer, allowing for a peer-to-peer discussion and the option to request written information.[23] All MIRs are valuable and provide timely information to the company regarding the current state of their product in clinical practice. MIRs are typically compiled and analyzed periodically to identify trends and patterns. These trends are published internally in the form of periodic reports; this may signal to a company that a response letter is needed on a particular topic that is reported frequently, identify new educational gaps, or lead to the development of new product formulations. Periodic reports may alternatively signal to a company that previous "hot topics," or frequently asked questions, are no longer of interest to practitioners in clinical practice; often times identifying new areas of interest that practitioners need to have addressed.

Case Study 22–3

DRUG A® received marketing approval by the FDA and has quickly become very successful. Awesome Drugs R Us, Inc., has expanded the number of HPs on staff and now employs clinicians in multiple departments within the medical division. Due to the media coverage of DRUG A®'s success, other companies are investigating similar compounds. One company has manufactured the product STRIPES™ for the treatment of mild to moderate hiccups in another country for many years and is looking to enter the U.S. market. It is suspected that STRIPES™ will have a **Risk Evaluation and Mitigation Strategy (REMS)** (see description later in chapter) It is suspected that STRIPES™ will have a REMS approved by the FDA along with a restricted distribution program because it the drug is well known to occasionally cause yellow stripes to appear on the skin.

- *What should Awesome Drug R Us, Inc., do to prepare for inquiries regarding product comparisons to STRIPES™ and other investigational compounds?*
- *What questions should Awesome Drugs R Us, Inc., anticipate receiving due to their similar indication to STRIPES™?*

Adverse Event Reporting

FDA approval of a medication does not denote complete safety of the product. It is important to keep in mind that any medicine capable of curing or treating a disease may also have the potential for serious adverse events. An adverse drug experience is defined by the CFR Title 21, Section 314.80—Postmarketing reporting of adverse drug experiences as, "Any adverse event associated with the use of a drug in humans, whether or not considered drug related, including the following: an adverse event occurring in the course of the use of a drug product in professional practice; an adverse event occurring from drug overdose whether accidental or intentional; an adverse event occurring from drug abuse; an adverse event occurring from drug withdrawal; and any failure of expected pharmacological action."[24] ⑩ *Adverse drug experiences, or adverse events, are required to be reported to the FDA by pharmaceutical companies.* It is the charge of the pharmaceutical company to monitor these risks once the drug is on the market, also known as the postmarketing phase of the drug's life cycle.[24,25]

Pharmaceutical companies learn of adverse events in a variety of ways, including postmarketing trials, publications, customer calls, physician reports, social media sites, blogs, and in some cases, even by being in close proximity to a personal conversation. The reporting process may vary from company to company so long as the information required by the FDA is reported with each adverse event through completion of FDA Form 3500A. FDA Form 3500A differs from voluntary FDA Form 3500 and FDA Form 3500B, which are intended for HPs and consumers, respectively. FDA Form 3500A requests such information as patient demographics, medication identifiers, and a description of the adverse event.[26]

Case Study 22–4

Use information from Case Study 22-3.

The company that manufactures DRUG A® begins receiving reports of patients noting yellow stripes on their skin.

- *How will Awesome Drugs R Us, Inc., document patient reports of yellow stripes?*
- *Does Awesome Drugs R Us, Inc., need to send the reports of yellow stripes to any additional agency or organization?*

Staying Connected with the Pharmaceutical Industry

Pharmaceutical companies are dynamic entities that are constantly evolving. In today's media it is possible to stay up-to-date with new information from industry including drug approvals, publications, and presentations, as well as safety alerts and labeling changes. The Drug Information Association (DIA) and other industry-associated organizations (see Table 22-3) are resources for pharmaceutical company information. HPs in clinical practice should familiarize themselves with these reliable sources for

TABLE 22–3. PHARMACEUTICAL INDUSTRY ORGANIZATIONS

Organization	Web Site
American Association of Pharmaceutical Scientists (AAPS)	http://www.aaps.org/default.aspx
Association of Clinical Research Professionals (ACRP)	http://www.acrpnet.org/default.aspx
Drug Information Association (DIA)	http://www.diahome.org/DIAHome/Home.aspx
Generic Pharmaceutical Association (GPhA)	http://www.gphaonline.org/
Health Industry Representatives Association (HIRA)	http://www.hira.org
Institute for Safe Medication Practices (ISMP)	http://www.ismp.org/
National Association of Pharmaceutical Representatives (NAPRx®)	http://www.napsronline.org/
Pharmaceutical Research and Manufacturers of America (PhRMA)	http://www.phrma.org/
Regulatory Affairs Professionals Society (RAPS)	http://www.raps.org/

industry news so that they can share current industry information with their patients and other clinicians.

Anatomy of Federal Agencies

The Department of Health and Human Services (HHS) is the U.S. government's principal Agency for protecting the health of all Americans and providing essential human services, especially for those who are least able to help themselves. HHS is headed by the Secretary who is the chief managing officer for the HHS family of agencies, including 11 operating divisions, 10 regional offices, as well as the Office of the Secretary.[11,27] Table 22–4 describes each agency and office and provides the mission statement for each. This

TABLE 22–4. LIST OF HEALTH AND HUMAN SERVICES AGENCIES AND OFFICES

Agency or Office	Purpose
Office of the Secretary (OS)	"To help provide the building blocks that Americans need to live healthy, successful lives"
Administration for Children and Families (ACF)	"...to provide family assistance (welfare), child support, child care, Head Start, child welfare, and other programs relating to children and families."
Administration on Aging (AoA)	"...to develop a comprehensive, coordinated and cost-effective system of home and community-based services that helps elderly individuals maintain their health and independence in their homes and communities."

Continued

TABLE 22–4. LIST OF HEALTH AND HUMAN SERVICES AGENCIES AND OFFICES *(Continued)*

Agency or Office	Purpose
Agency for Healthcare Research and Quality (AHRQ)	"…to improve the quality, safety, efficiency, and effectiveness of health care for all Americans. Information from AHRQ's research helps people make more informed decisions and improve the quality of health care services."
Agency for Toxic Substances and Disease (ATSDR)	"… serves the public by using the best science, taking responsive public health actions, and providing trusted health information to prevent harmful exposures and diseases related to toxic substances."
Centers for Disease Control and Prevention (CDC)	"…to collaborate to create the expertise, information, and tools that people and communities need to protect their health—through health promotion, prevention of disease, injury and disability, and preparedness for new health threats."
Centers for Medicare and Medicaid Services (CMS)	"… to ensure effective, up-to-date health care coverage and to promote quality care for beneficiaries."
Food and Drug Administration (FDA)	…to protect "the public health by assuring the safety, efficacy, and security of human and veterinary drugs, biological products, medical devices, our nation's food supply, cosmetics, and products that emit radiation."
Health Resources and Services Administration (HRSA)	"…to improve health and achieve health equity through access to quality services, a skilled health workforce and innovative programs."
Indian Health Service (IHS)	"…to raise the physical, mental, social, and spiritual health of American Indians and Alaska Natives to the highest level."
National Institutes of Health (NIH)	"…to seek fundamental knowledge about the nature and behavior of living systems and the application of that knowledge to enhance health, lengthen life, and reduce the burdens of illness and disability."
Office of Inspector General (OIG)	"…to protect the integrity of Department of Health and Human Services (HHS) programs, as well as the health and welfare of the beneficiaries of those programs."
Substance Abuse and Mental Health Services Administration (SAMHSA)	"…to reduce the impact of substance abuse and mental illness on America's communities."

illustrates how HHS programmatic areas each have their own goals and objectives. The composition of each agency or office under HHS varies. Ultimately, a common theme can be applied to these agencies. HHS creates agencies to address specific areas of public health. Each organization is further divided into groups depending on the roles and responsibilities assigned to the agency. These agencies are further divided into centers supporting the role assigned to the agencies. In the United States, there is a center or office available to provide some regulatory guidance on most, if not all, areas of public health.

MISSION OF A FEDERAL AGENCY IN THE DEPARTMENT OF HEALTH AND HUMAN SERVICES

⓫ *The mission of the FDA is to protect "the public health by assuring the safety, efficacy, and security of human and veterinary drugs, biological products, medical devices, our nation's food supply, cosmetics, and products that emit radiation."*[12] The FDA consists of nine centers and offices. Figure 22–4 shows the FDA's organization chart. The Center for Drug Evaluation and Research (CDER) is of particular interest to pharmacists and other HPs because of the Center's responsibility for ensuring that drug products are of high quality, and are safe and effective for their intended use.[24] CDER provides the public with access to accurate, science-based information needed to evaluate the risks and benefits of human drugs and strives to provide easily retrievable information about human drugs through the FDA Web site, www.fda.gov.

COMMUNICATION OF DRUG SAFETY INFORMATION

⓬ *Timely communication of important drug safety information provides HPs, patients, consumers, and other interested persons with access to the most current information concerning the potential risks and benefits of a marketed drug, helping them to make more informed treatment choices.*[28] The FDA's safety assessment of medicines does not diminish after drugs are approved for marketing.[15] Although the premarket phase of study is very intensive, much work still remains to monitor approved drugs over time. Once a drug is approved and marketed, the FDA often gains additional information as the drug is used and studied in broader and more diverse populations. Such information helps provide a better picture of a drug's benefits, risks, and enables FDA to give HPs and patients the latest information on potential or newly identified risks, and strengthens FDA's ability to safeguard patients against unacceptable risks.

SAFETY COMMUNICATION TOOLS

The FDA has created effective and ongoing relationships with a wide array of trade and professional associations, patient advocacy and consumer groups, safety organizations, media, and other entities. When drug safety issues arise, the FDA contacts these groups and works with them to communicate the safety issue to their constituencies. ⓭ *The FDA uses various tools and methods to communicate drug safety information to the public.*

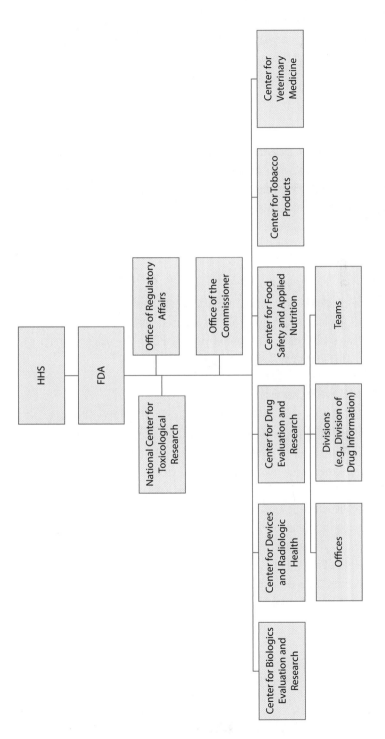

Figure 22–4. Organization of centers and offices within the FDA. Fall 2013. FDA = Food and Drug Administration. (This figure represents an overview of how FDA is organized. Every Center and Office at FDA has their own organization chart.)

Important tools used in this effort include, but are not limited to, FDA-approved prescribing information (i.e., drug labeling) and a postmarket communication tool called a *Drug Safety Communication* (DSC), along with other important tools and methods used to communicate drug safety information to the public.

LABELING UPDATES

The drug labeling, or written material that accompanies drug products, is the most complete single source of information on the drug. A change to the drug label may have tangible benefit in expanding the education of risks, benefits, and optimal usage of marketed drugs.

Over time, new information often emerges about a product, such as:

- Side effects
- Dosing
- New indications

This new information is added by the manufacturer to the drug's label so consumers and HPs have all the information necessary for safe and effective use of the drug. All changes to a drug's label must be approved by the FDA. The manufacturer sends proposed changes to the FDA for review and, revision if necessary.

Risk Evaluation and Mitigation Strategies

The creation of Risk Evaluation and Mitigation Strategies (REMS) is one of the many methods of communicating safety information to patients and practitioners beyond the traditional labeling.[13] REMS were enacted on September 27, 2007, as part of the FDA Amendments Act (FDAAA). A REMS provides information regarding the risks of a specific medication in an effort to ensure the benefits will outweigh the risks for a potential patient, mitigating the likelihood of a negative outcome with the product's use. Following the enactment of FDAAA, REMS programs may be requested by the FDA for a particular drug as part of the NDA process. A REMS may also be submitted voluntarily as part of the NDA prior to receiving a request from the FDA. Finally, a REMS may be requested by the FDA after a drug receives approval. (See Figure 22–5.) General REMS program requirements are outlined by the FDA, subject to the FDA's approval, and enforceable through penalties.[13]

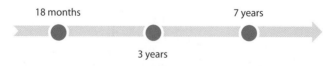

Figure 22–5. Timeline of REMS evaluation following approval.[13]

Prior to the codification of REMS, **risk minimization action plans (RiskMAPs)** were established. RiskMAPs are safety plans that are designed to achieve prespecified goals and objectives[17] to minimize known safety risks of a medication while concomitantly maintaining the benefits. RiskMAPs can employ one or more tools to achieve its set goals and objectives (see Table 22–5 for more detail). Some drug and biological products that previously were approved and/or licensed with RiskMAPs are now deemed to have a REMS.[29]

Medication Guides and Patient Package Inserts

Medication Guides and patient package inserts (PPI) are other examples of safety measures required by the FDA prior to 2007.[10,13] Medication Guides are paper handouts issued with certain prescription medications to address safety concerns specific to that drug or drug class in an effort to reduce adverse events.[30] All Medication Guides are subject to the requirements of 21 CFR 208, which means for HPs that the medication guide must be provided directly to the patient or their agent when the drug product is dispensed, unless an exemption applies.[21] Alternatively, PPIs are required to be issued

TABLE 22–5. METHODS OTHER THAN A DSC FOR COMMUNICATING SAFETY INFORMATION TO CONSUMERS[10,13]

Medication Guides	Medication Guides may be required: • If patient labeling could mitigate serious adverse events • If the product has serious adverse events relative to benefits that may cause patients to reconsider their use of the product • If patient adherence can seriously alter the drug's effectiveness
Patient Package Inserts (PPIs)	PPIs may be required if the FDA believes the package insert will help mitigate a serious risk. Usually a medication guide or PPI exists for a product, not both.
Communication Plan	A communication plan may be requested in which a company submits their plan to educate practitioners about their strategy for minimizing risk/maintaining benefit as outlined in their REMS.
Elements to Assure Safe Use (ETASU)	In certain cases, if these previously described measures are not sufficient to mitigate the risks associated with the medication, additional ETASU may be implemented. ETASU include specific goals to minimize serious risk. If a REMS program includes ETASU, the REMS must also include a specific implementation plan and education for the patient to be able to monitor and evaluate the risks of the medication and to recommend improvementsto the ETASU.

with oral contraceptive products to satisfy the requirement that patients using these products are fully informed of all the potential risks and benefits.[11] Manufacturers of oral contraceptives may request informal guidance from the FDA to help them create a PPI.

Drug Safety Communications

A Drug Safety Communication (DSC) is a specific tool used by the FDA to communicate to the public important information about safety issues, including emerging safety information, about marketed drugs.[20] DSCs are standardized electronic communications posted on the FDA Web site. Written clearly, DSCs are targeted to both HPs and patients. DSCs generally communicate the following information:

- A summary of the safety issue and the nature of the risk being communicated
- The established benefit or benefits of the drug being discussed
- Recommended actions for HPs and patients, when appropriate
- A summary of the data reviewed or being reviewed by the FDA

The DSC is the FDA's primary safety communication tool for important postmarket drug safety issues. In the past, safety communications were issued by the FDA in a variety of formats. They were issued under different titles and targeted to different audiences. Safety communications have been issued under the titles *Early Communications about Ongoing Safety Reviews, Public Health Advisory, Patient Information Sheet, Healthcare Professional Sheet,* and *Alerts on Patient Information and Healthcare Professional Sheets.* In early 2010, the FDA began using a single communication tool—the *Drug Safety Communication.*

It is important to note that while a DSC communicates important safety issues about marketed drugs, it is not a crisis communication document. If a drug product is defective or tainted, or poses some other form of immediate danger, the FDA uses other communication tools, such as *Public Health Alerts*, press releases, stakeholder calls, and media briefings, to inform the public rapidly.

Case Study 22–5

DRUG A® and STRIPES™ are found to have a high incidence of causing yellow stripes on the skin. The FDA believes this adverse event warrants additional communication to patients regarding safety information.

- *What are some examples of ways safety information is communicated to patients?*

Case Study 22–6

The manufacturer of SPOTS™, a drug with a similar mechanism of action to DRUG A® and STRIPES™, is preparing its NDA for submission to the FDA for approval to market their product for the treatment of mild to severe hiccups.

- *What might SPOTS™ manufacturer want to submit voluntarily with its NDA package given the known risks associated with DRUG A® and STRIPES™?*

Division of Drug Information at the FDA

The focal point at the FDA for public inquiries related to human drugs is the Division of Drug Information (DDI). ⓮ *The mission of the DDI is to optimize CDER's educational and communication efforts to our global community. The DDI supports the FDA's mission to promote and protect public health.*[31] The DDI is staffed with a team of pharmacists and other HPs. They provide expert advice and guidance on a broad range of CDER activities. This requires the DDI's staff to have an extensive knowledge of human drug products and the regulations guiding drug development and marketing. The role of the DDI is unique from hospital and academic-based drug information centers because it serves the general public domestically and internationally through direct contact via phone, letter, and e-mail. The DDI also works internally to support the center by collaborating with experts throughout the center to effectively communicate important and emerging topics.

The division has several unique characteristics that differentiate it from a more traditional drug information centers. First, the DDI has a unique visitor (customer) makeup. Visitors include the United States and international regulated industry, consumers, HPs, insurance companies, academia, law enforcement, attorneys, and other government agencies. The majority of requests received from U.S. visitors are from consumers, followed by industry and HPs. Industry and small businesses make up most of international requests.

It is not uncommon for the DDI to prepare responses for a wide variety of requestors (Table 22–6). The preponderance of the information used by the DDI to answer drug information queries comes directly from the FDA's Web site. The DDI's staff are highly trained experts in drug information and retrieval. In fact, DDI's drug information specialists are able to answer most inquiries without further consult by using their knowledge of FDA's available public resources. Sometimes, an inquiry cannot be addressed using readily available information. In that case, the DDI's specialists work with subject matter experts across the center to find information suitable to answer the inquiry.

TABLE 22–6. DDI REQUESTORS

Consumers	Consultants
Health Professionals	Attorneys
Academia	Insurance Providers
Federal/State Agencies	Special Interest Groups
Investment Brokers	Law Enforcement
Clinical Investigators	International Government Agencies
Correctional Facilities	Students
Small Businesses	Others
Industry	

DDI SERVES CDER AND PUBLIC HEALTH

Drug information services provided by the DDI fit generally into one of three categories: correspondence, dissemination, and other (Table 22–7). Correspondence represents a majority of direct contact provided by the DDI. In an average month, the DDI responds to 2000 e-mails, 6000 telephone calls, and over 100 letters. The most common inquiries are related to regulatory issues, such as the drug review and approval process (Table 22–8). Many times the same question will be asked in a different way by a different requestor. For example, a consumer might call FDA asking for more information about a DSC. The same question might be addressed by an HP wanting to know the impact on clinical practice and possible labeling changes.

TABLE 22–7. DRUG INFORMATION SERVICES PROVIDED BY THE DDI

CORRESPONDENCE
- Phone calls
  - Drug Information 1-855-543-DRUG (3784)
  - MedWatch Adverse Event Reporting (1-800-FDA-1088)
  - CDER Small Business and Industry Assistance and GDUFA (1-866-405-5367)
- E-mails
  - Drug Information and MedWatch (DrugInfo@fda.hhs.gov)
  - CDER Small Business and Industry Assistance (CDERSBIA@fda.hhs.gov)
  - Generic Drug User Fee Amendments (GDUFA) (AskGDUFA@fda.hhs.gov)
  - Global Alliance of Drug Information Specialists (GADIS) (GADIS@fda.hhs.gov)
- Mail

Division of Drug Information (CDER) or CDER Small Business and Industry Assistance

Office of Communications

10001 New Hampshire Avenue

Hillandale Building, 4th Floor

Silver Spring, MD 20993

Continued

TABLE 22–7. DRUG INFORMATION SERVICES PROVIDED BY THE DDI *(Continued)*

DISSEMINATION
- DDI Web site
- Listservs: DDI, CDER Small Business and Industry Assistance (http://www.fda.gov/aboutddi), GADIS
- Twitter @FDA_Drug_Info
- Publications, Posters, Presentations
- Exhibits
- Student Webinars
- CDERLearn
- CE Courses
- CDER Small Business Workshops and Webinars
- CDER Trade Press

OTHER
- Imprint Identification
- International Visitors
- FDA Pharmacy Student Experiential Program
- Regulatory Pharmaceutical Fellowship
- Global Alliance of Drug Information Specialists (GADIS)
- Public Affairs Specialists (PASes) and Public Affairs Liaisons (PALs)

TABLE 22–8. CLASSIFICATION OF COMMON DDI INQUIRIES

Drug review process
Generic drugs
Specific drug safety issues
Investigational new drugs
New drug approvals
Importation of drugs
Adverse reactions
Nonprescription drugs
Drug identification
Recalls and shortages

FDA DRUG INFORMATION RESOURCES

⓯ *The DDI has built effective internal and external interactions to provide timely, accurate, and useful information through both traditional and social media channels.* Table 22–9 lists commonly used FDA Web sites and the intended purpose of each page. In order to select the most appropriate FDA sponsored resource/Web site, practitioners should have a basic understanding of what Web sites are available and what information is provided. Table 22–9 provides a brief overview of these Web sites. Practitioners are strongly encouraged to visit and explore these Web sites to become familiar with what is offered.

TABLE 22–9. FDA-SPONSORED DRUG INFORMATION LINKS

Web site	Purpose
www.fda.gov/aboutddi	Division of Drug Information (DDI) Homepage.
	Provides background, mission, and purpose of the DDI.
	Also maintains several helpful links for finding information relating to:
	• Student and fellowship opportunities
	• Small Business and Industry Assistance
	• CE programs, Webinars, trainings, audio podcasts, videos, Twitter and listserv
	• Drug identification
www.fda.gov/drugs	CDER Homepage.
	DDI's first resource for responding to questions from the public and where most questions pertaining to regulations can be answered.
	Site maintains sections dedicated to the following topics:
	• Drug approvals and databases
	• Drug safety and availability
	• Drug development and approval process
	• Guidance documents, compliance, and regulatory information
	• Drug science and research
	• Consumer, health professional, and industry resources
	• Recalls and alerts
	• Approvals and clearances
http://www.fda.gov/Drugs/DrugSafety/ PostmarketDrugSafetyInformationfor PatientsandProviders/default.htm	Index to drug-specific Information.
	This page provides a list of drugs that have been the subject postmarketing drug safety communication efforts.
http://www.fda.gov/AboutFDA/ContactFDA/ StayInformed/GetEmailUpdates/default.htm	E-mail Updates Homepage.
	This page allows users to sign up for the FDA e-mail alert service that distributes important FDA news and information as it is available.
www.fda.gov/drugsatfda	Drugs@FDA Homepage.
	Searchable FDA database containing official information about FDA-approved brand and generic drugs and therapeutic biological products. This database also contains:
	• Labels for approved drug products
	• Consumer information for drugs approved after 1998
	• Approval history for drug products (including FDA review documents)

Continued

TABLE 22–9.   FDA-SPONSORED DRUG INFORMATION LINKS *(Continued)*

Web site	Purpose
http://www.accessdata.fda.gov/scripts/cder/ob/default.cfm	Orange Book: Approved Drug Products with Therapeutic Equivalence Evaluations Homepage.
	Free electronic access to the Orange Book: Approved Drug Products with Therapeutic Equivalence Evaluations.
	Can search by active ingredient, proprietary name, patent, applicant holder, or application number.
www.fda.gov/cder/ndc	National Drug Code Directory Homepage
	Searchable list of universal product identifier for human drugs. Old and new NDC Directories available; background page provides overview of differences between the two databases.
http://www.fda.gov/Training/ForHealthProfessionals/default.htm	CDERLearn Homepage.
	Web page for CDER-sponsored educational tutorials, some of which have CE credit available.
www.fda.gov/MedWatch	MedWatch Homepage.
	Homepage for the FDA's safety information and adverse event reporting program.
	Contains a searchable list of safety labeling changes and updated safety information. Also, it contains links to online and downloadable forms to report serious problems to the FDA.
http://www.fda.gov/DrugSafetyPodcasts	Drug Safety Podcasts Homepage.
	Podcasts broadcast in conjunction with the release of new Drug Safety Communications. Also available on iTunes under Drug Safety Podcasts.
www.fda.gov/DrugInfoRounds	FDA Drug Info Rounds.
	Series of training videos for practicing clinical and community pharmacists. Also available on YouTube.
www.fda.gov/smallbusinessdrugs	CDER's Small Business Assistance Program.
	The purpose of this website is to support CDER's Small Business and Industry Assistance (SBIA) Program's mission of promoting productive interaction with regulated domestic and international small pharmaceutical business and industry by providing timely and accurate information relating to development and regulation of human drug products.
www.fda.gov/gadis	Global Alliance of Drug Information Specialists: A Partnership among Pharmacists for the Advancement of Public Health.
	GADIS provides a network among drug information pharmacists and the FDA to support collaborative strategies on critical trends and transformations for addressing FDA regulatory actions.

⓰ *In addition to dedicated DSC channels, the DDI has several proactive and innovative tools to communicate information about human drug products to the public.* Information is disseminated through DDI's listservs, RSS feeds, CDERLearn continuing education (CE) programs, videos, Twitter, radio, and audio podcasts. All of these examples represent new ways to promote the safe and effective use of human drug products.

CDER SMALL BUSINESS AND INDUSTRY ASSISTANCE

Most DI centers would not have a component that serves industry, which is a unique characteristic of this federal DI center. The DDI is the home of CDER's Industry and Small Business Assistance Program and interacts with regulated industry by assisting domestic and international industry seeking timely and accurate information relating to development and regulation of human drug products. SBIA outreach activities include a series of online Webinars and live workshops held around the United States. Inquiries are received, triaged to subject matter experts if necessary, and responses are coordinated from the CDERSBIA@fda.hhs.gov e-mail account. Additional key elements of the industry assistance program are monthly Webinars and CDERLearn CE programs. These are methods by which the FDA educates specific audiences about the safe use of medicine, drug regulatory process, vital role HPs play to assist FDA in fulfilling its duties, and many other important issues with the added benefit of CE credit for pharmacists, physicians, and nurses, many of whom work in industry.

CDER TRADE PRESS

An additional team within the DDI, the CDER Trade Press team, provides members of the trade press with accurate and timely information regarding CDER policies, programs, and initiatives. In addition to facilitating interactions between trade press and FDA subject matter experts, CDER Trade Press also alerts FDA leadership and staff to relevant FDA coverage in the trade media. Relationships with members of the trade press are fostered, and maintained by this unique team of practitioners. The CDER Trade Press team provides general and ongoing assistance to the FDA's Field Office Public Affairs Specialists (PASes) and Public Affairs Liaisons (PALs).

SOCIAL MEDIA OUTREACH

The DDI uses social media to reach audiences that prefer to receive the latest drug information in a variety of media formats. The DDI tweets the latest drug information and may be followed on Twitter @FDA_Drug_Info. FDA Drug Info Rounds is a series of training videos for practicing clinical and community pharmacists written and casted by DDI pharmacists. These videos may be viewed on the FDA's Web site and YouTube. Audio podcasts are broadcast in conjunction with the release of each new DSC. If interested, a person may find and subscribe to the FDA's Drug Safety Podcasts on iTunes and the FDA's Web site RSS feed.

GLOBAL ALLIANCE OF DRUG INFORMATION SPECIALISTS (GADIS)

DDI networks with fellow drug information specialists around the world through the Global Alliance of Drug Information Specialists (GADIS). GADIS advances public health by promoting partnerships among drug information pharmacists in academia, hospitals, and federal government. GADIS establishes a community among DI specialists to support collaborative strategies, a forum for the exchange of evidence-based best practices, and an opportunity to gain insights and feedback from peers to support collaborative strategies on critical trends and transformations for addressing FDA regulatory actions. GADIS offers online Webinars with speakers from within the FDA, and external experts on topics such as the implementation of REMS programs. GADIS also provides a monthly News & Notes service to its members. GADIS News & Notes highlights important FDA information to drug information specialists that occurred over the prior calendar month.

Case Study 22–7

FDA announced a final rule to amend regulations (21 CFR 2.125) on the use of ozone-depleting substances (ODSs) in medical products. This rule established December 31, 2008, as the date by which production and sale of single ingredient albuterol chlorofluorocarbon (CFC) metered-dose inhalers (MDIs) had to stop, by removing the essential use designation for albuterol MDIs under 2.125. Many consumers contacted the DDI with questions and concerns regarding the discontinuation of single ingredient albuterol CFC MDIs.

- *Since the rules stated that production had to stop by December 31, 2008, a pharmacist wanted to know if he can dispense the remaining CFC MDIs he has in stock after December 31, 2008, until he runs out. Can he do this? What information can you find on the FDA's Web site to support your answer?*
- *A pharmacist wanted to know if they can automatically switch patients from an albuterol CFC to an HFA inhaler. Can they do this? What rules and regulations support your answer?*

- *A patient was complaining that the new HFA inhalers do not work for them and they cannot feel any effect after using the inhaler. What do you tell them? Where can you refer them to report this problem?*
- *An advocacy group comprised of asthmatic patients who only paid a $10.00 copay for the CFC inhaler sent hundreds of letters to the FDA regarding the new copays averaging $125.00 for the HFA inhalers. What type of response does FDA have regarding the price of medications? What authority does FDA have over the pricing of medications? Based on the information you find, do you feel it is right that the FDA can mandate changes to consumers that will impact the price of medications?*
- *A mother of an asthmatic child called FDA suggesting that the government cares more about the ozone than the health of her child. What potential responses can you develop that supports both arguments?*

Opportunities Within FDA

There are several opportunities for both current and future HPs within the FDA.

FOR THE STUDENT

⑰ *The FDA offers many opportunities for health professional students. One of the most popular programs is the FDA Pharmacy Student Experiential Program.[32] Student opportunities are also available within the United States Public Health Service (USPHS) Commissioned Corps.[13]* The experiential program provides an opportunity for students to gain experience working in various divisions within the FDA. Depending on where the student is placed, he or she will have the chance to learn about the FDA's multidisciplinary processes for addressing public health issues involving drugs, biologics, or medical devices. Pharmacy students who complete the FDA Pharmacy Student Experiential Program gain unique experience in regulatory affairs, which proves beneficial to their future careers.

The Commissioned Corps created the Commissioned Corps Officer Student Training and Extern Program (COSTEP) for students studying in the health professions field. There are two programs: the Junior COSTEP and Senior COSTEP. Students in selected health fields can apply to the Junior COSTEP program if they have completed at least one to 2 years of their professional program. The Junior COSTEP program takes place during school breaks and most assignments last anywhere from 1 to 4 months. There is no obligation to commit or work for the Commissioned Corps after graduation as this opportunity is focused on allowing students to experience the program before joining. One major benefit for those students enrolled in the COSTEP programs is the diverse opportunities available after completion of the program. Some have gone on to provide clinical services in the Indian Health Service, work in labs at the National Institutes of Health, provide care to patients in the Bureau of Prisons, or join agencies within the FDA or Centers for Disease Control, just to name a few. For those students who wish to find out more information or apply, they are encouraged to visit the U.S. Public Health Service Web site at http://www.usphs.gov/student/.

FOR THE PHARMACY GRADUATE

Postgraduate opportunities for students are also available with the FDA. One opportunity is the Regulatory Pharmaceutical Fellowship.[14] The purpose of this fellowship is to develop candidates with advanced experience in the medical and regulatory aspects of drug information dissemination, drug safety, or drug marketing and advertising. The program exposes fellows to three areas of regulatory pharmaceutical experience: FDA, academia, and pharmaceutical industry.

Only a few of the potential opportunities for health professional students are described in this chapter. There are several opportunities for students interested in regulatory affairs beyond what is described here, and students are encouraged to research and contact those programs directly for further information.

FOR THE PROFESSIONAL

Due to new legislation, CDER has an ongoing need to recruit qualified HPs in order to carry on the mission of the FDA. HPs have several opportunities to serve either as civil service or join the U.S. Commissioned Corps. Physicians are needed to help evaluate submitted clinical trial data of new drugs for safety and efficacy. Pharmacists are needed for a variety of duties including reviewing, evaluating, and recommending approval (or nonapproval) of new and generic drugs. Scientists evaluate the technical portions of applications such as INDs and NDAs. Mathematical statisticians and computer specialists are hired for statistical and technical support of human drug product reviews. Consumer safety officers are vital to managing and monitoring regulatory teams in certain divisions. The consumer safety officer is sometimes referred to as a project manager or division liaison and often these roles are filled with biologists, chemists, pharmacists, nurses, physicians, engineers, and others. The team of HPs working at the FDA is diverse and so are the opportunities to help fulfill the mission of assuring the quality, safety, and efficacy of drugs available to the American public.

Conclusion

Pharmaceutical companies and regulatory agencies provide many services to and have many opportunities for HPs. Pharmaceutical companies' scientific or medical divisions are filled with highly trained HPs working in a variety of specialized fields in order to provide medical information and support for various brands marketed by the company. Efforts are currently ongoing to make the pharmaceutical industry more transparent in the way they conduct the business of drug development and product marketing. Regulatory agencies are also focusing on ways to be more transparent, and monitor and improve the communication of the benefit/risk equation to the general public. The DDI offers traditional and social media channels to those seeking regulatory drug information. Most pharmaceutical companies have detailed and structured processes for responding to clinician's questions. The DDI uses effective internal and external interactions to provide timely, accurate, and useful responses to individual inquiries. An informed HP is a professional who is aware of the valuable information available from industry and FDA, can effectively communicate safety and risk information, and dedicates their career to positively impacting public health.

Self-Assessment Questions

1. Which of the following is a department within the medical division of a company that employs HPs?
   a. Research and Development
   b. Medical Information
   c. Epidemiology
   d. Biometrics

2. Which of the following best describes an appropriate lifecycle of a medical information request?
   a. Inquiry solicited by representative, standard response letter verbally communicated
   b. Inquiry solicited by representative, package insert information verbally communicated

   c. Inquiry submitted by practitioner, package insert information verbally communicated

   d. Inquiry submitted by representative, opinion of industry health professional verbally communicated

3. Identify which of the following is *not* a typical component of a standard response letter.
   a. Outline
   b. Opening
   c. Signature
   d. Closing

4. Which of the following departments may be involved in approving a standard response letter?
   a. Medical Publications
   b. Marketing
   c. Medical Information
   d. Metrics

5. HPs are regulated in industry in which of the following ways?
   a. Externally by the Food and Drug Administration
   b. Externally by Food and Drug Administration Amendments Act
   c. Internally by standard operating procedures
   d. All of the above

6. Identify which interaction between the pharmaceutical industry and HPs is unacceptable according to PhRMA's *Code on Interactions with Health Care Professionals.*
   a. An industry representative stops by a clinician's office to invite them to an upcoming industry-sponsored continuing medical education event.
   b. An industry representative makes an appointment with a practitioner to discuss a newly approved indication for BESTDRUGEVER®.
   c. An industry representative drops off a basket of BESTDRUGEVER® pens, mugs, and coffee to a health professional's office.
   d. An industry representative refers a health professional to contact their medical information department to discuss an off-label use.

7. What is the purpose of the FDA mandating the pharmaceutical industry collect adverse event information?
   a. The FDA wants to ensure the pharmaceutical industry captures all postmarketing adverse effects (AEs).

b. The FDA wants to ensure the pharmaceutical industry professionals are busy at their desks.

c. The FDA wants to ensure the pharmaceutical industry is burdened by AE paperwork.

d. The FDA wants to ensure the pharmaceutical industry captures all bad doctors causing AEs.

8. Which of the following is *not* a valid method for communicating safety information to consumers?

a. Elements to Assure Safe Use

b. Risk minimization action plans

c. Risk mitigation and evaluation strategies

d. Risk minimization television ads

9. Identify which of the following is an organization associated with the pharmacy industry.

a. American Pharmaceutical Association

b. Drug Information Association

c. American Medical Association

d. Parenteral Drug Association

10. The role of the Division of Drug Information (DDI) at the Food and Drug Administration (FDA) is best described by which of the following?

a. CDER's last option for unanswered general inquiries regarding regulations and human drug products.

b. The division exists as a traditional drug information center responding to calls and questions from the general consumer.

c. CDER's focal point for public inquiries regarding human drug products.

d. The division supports the FDA's mission to promote and protect public health by building effective internal and external interactions to provide timely, accurate, and useful information through both traditional and social media channels.

e. b and d.

11. Which of the following is *not* a main difference between the DDI and a typical drug information center?

a. Visitors

b. Resources used

c. Role of the Division

d. None of the above

e. All of the above

12. An FDA Consumer Safety Officer prepares a podcast updating HPs about a new safety concern with a marketed human drug product. This activity would best be categorized by which of the following?
    a. Correspondence of information by the FDA
    b. Dissemination of information by the FDA
    c. Development of a standard response
    d. Reactive responses by the FDA
    e. Other

13. An international manufacturer e-mails DDI with questions regarding the regulatory pathway for marketing an all-natural toothpaste in the United States. When the DDI responds, this activity would best be categorized by which of the following?
    a. Correspondence of information by the FDA
    b. Dissemination of information by the FDA
    c. Development of a standard response
    d. Reactive responses by the FDA
    e. Other

14. A researcher contacts the DDI about the preinvestigational new drug application (pre-IND) consultation program and how to get started. Which Web site would be the best place to refer the requestor for this information?
    a. CDER homepage
    b. Drugs@FDA database
    c. Electronic Orange Book
    d. National Drug Code Directory online
    e. CDER Small Business and Industry Assistance homepage

15. Which of the following is *not* a student opportunity within the FDA?
    a. Junior COSTEP Program
    b. Senior COSTEP Program
    c. FDA Pharmacy Student Experiential Program
    d. FDA/CDER Academic Collaboration Program
    e. Commissioned Corps Officer Student Training and Extern Program

REFERENCES

1. Cadogan AA, Fung SM. The changing roles of medical communications professionals: evolution of the core curriculum. Drug Inf J. 2009 Nov;43(6):673-84.
2. U.S. Food and Drug Administration. FDA guidance for industry: responding to unsolicited requests for off-label information about prescription drugs and medical devices. Draft

Guidance [Internet]. Silver Spring (MD): U.S. Department of Health and Human Services; c2011 [cited 2013 Jun 13]: [15 screens]. Available from: http://www.fda.gov/downloads/Drugs/GuidanceComplianceRegulatoryInformation/Guidances/UCM285145.pdf

3. Soares SC, March C. Metrics implementation in an industry-based medical information department and comparison to metrics tracked within other industry-based medical information departments. Drug Inf J. 2008 Mar;42(2):175-82.

4. Academy of Managed Care Pharmacy (AMCP). The AMCP format for formulary submissions Version 3.0 [Internet]. Alexandria (VA): Academy of Managed Care Pharmacy; c2013, 2010 Jan [cited 2013 Jun 13]: [about 32 screens]. Available from: http://www.amcp.org/data/jmcp/1007_121%2019%2009(3).pdf

5. Marrone CM, Bass JL, Klinger CJ. Survey of medical liaison practices across the pharmaceutical industry. Drug Inf J. 2007 Jul;41(4):457-70.

6. Department of Health and Human Services (U.S.). FDA guidance for industry: industry-supported scientific and educational activities. Final rules. Fed Regist. 1997 Nov;62(232):64093.

7. ACCME standards for commercial support: standards to ensure the independence of CME activities. Chicago (IL): Accreditation Council for Continuing Medical Education (U.S.); 2007. p. 3.

8. Electronic records; electronic signatures, 21 C.F.R. Sect. 11 (2009).

9. Gough J, Hamrell M. Standard operating procedures (SOPs): how companies can determine which documents they must put in place. Drug Inf J. 2010 Jan;44(1):49-54.

10. Gazo A, Wyble C, Schiappacasse H, Petses J, Toscano M, El-Toukhy N, et al. Mega mergers: a systematic approach to the integration of two medical information departments. Drug Inf J. 2008 Mar;42(2):183-91.

11. U.S. Department of Health and Human Services. About HHS [Internet]. Washington, DC: U.S. Department of Health and Human Services; c2010 [cited 2010 May 1]:[about 1 screen]. Available from: http://www.hhs.gov/about/index.html

12. U.S. Food and Drug Administration.What we do [Internet]. Silver Spring (MD): U.S. Department of Health and Human Services; c2010, 2009 May 22 [cited 2010 May 1]:[about 1 screen]. Available from: http://www.fda.gov/AboutFDA/WhatWeDo/default.htm

13. U.S. Public Health Service Commissioned Corps. Student opportunities [Internet]. Rockville (MD): U.S. Department of Health and Human Services; c2010, 2010 Jan 4 [cited 2010 May 3]:[about 4 screens]. Available from: http://www.usphs.gov/student/.

14. U.S. Food and Drug Administration. Regulatory Pharmaceutical Fellowship [Internet]. Silver Spring (MD): U.S. Department of Health and Human Services; c2010, 2009 Nov 3 [cited 2010 May 3]:[about 2 screens]. Available from: http://www.fda.gov/aboutfda/centersoffices/officeofmedicalproductsandtobacco/cder/ucm188804.htm

15. U.S. Food and Drug Administration. FDA Basics. How does FDA monitor safety after drugs are approved and marketed? [Internet]. Silver Spring (MD): U.S. Department of Health and Human Services; c2009 [cited 2013 Sept 4]:[1 screen]. Available from: http://www.fda.gov/AboutFDA/Transparency/Basics/ucm305058.htm

16. Pharmaceutical Researchers and Manufacturers of America (PhRMA). Code on interactions with healthcare professionals [Internet]. Washington, DC: Pharmaceutical Researchers and Manufacturers of America; c2010 2009 Jan [cited 2010 Mar 10]:[about 3 screens]. Available from: http://www.phrma.org/code_on_interactions_with_healthcare_professionals

17. U.S. Food and Drug Administration. FDA guidance for industry: development and use of risk minimization action plans [Internet]. Silver Spring (MD): U.S. Department of Health and Human Services; c2010; [cited 2010 Sep 15]:[27 screens]. Available from: http://www.fda.gov/downloads/RegulatoryInformation/Guidances/UCM126830.pdf

18. Bryant PJ, Steinberg MJ, Marrone CM. A practical approach to evidence-based medicine for the medical communications professional. Drug Inf J. 2009 Nov;43(6):663-72.

19. Donald T, Marsh C, Ashworth L. An assessment of preparation methods and personnel requirements in a medical information department during product launch. Drug Inf J. 2007 Mar;41(2):241-49.

20. U.S. Food and Drug Administration. FDA guidance: drug safety information—FDA's communication to the public [Internet]. Silver Spring (MD): U.S. Department of Health and Human Services; c2012. [cited 2013 Nov 27]:[17 screens]. Available from: http://www.fda.gov/downloads/Drugs/GuidanceComplianceRegulatoryInformation/Guidances/UCM295217.pdf

21. U.S. Food and Drug Administration. FDA guidance for industry: Medication Guides—distribution requirements and inclusion in risk evaluation and mitigation strategies (REMS) [Internet]. Silver Spring (MD): U.S. Department of Health and Human Services; c2011 [cited 2013 Apr 9];[12 screens]. Available from: http://www.fda.gov/downloads/Drugs/GuidanceComplianceRegulatoryInformation/Guidances/ucm244570.pdf

22. Black P, March C, Ashworth L. Assessment of customer satisfaction with verbal responses provided by a pharmaceutical company's third-party medical information call center. Drug Inf J. 2009 May;43(3):263-71.

23. Fett R, Bruns K, Lischka-Wittmann S. Results of a qualitative market research study evaluating the quality of medical letters. Drug Inf J. 2009 Nov;43(6):697-703.

24. U.S. Food and Drug Administration. A conversation about the FDA and drug regulation with Janet Woodcock, M.D., Deputy FDA Commissioner for Operations [Internet]. Silver Spring (MD): U.S. Department of Health and Human Services; c2011; [cited 2013 Sep 4]; [3 screens]. Available from: http://www.fda.gov/Drugs/ResourcesForYou/Consumers/ucm143467.htm

25. U.S. Food and Drug Administration. FDA guidance for industry: format and content of proposed risk evaluation and mitigation strategies (REMS): REMS assessments, and proposed REMS modifications. Draft Guidance [Internet]. Silver Spring (MD): U.S. Department of Health and Human Services; c2010 [cited 2010 Mar 9]:[38 screens]. Available from: http://www.fda.gov/downloads/Drugs/GuidanceComplianceRegulatoryInformation/Guidances/UCM184128.pdf

26. U.S. Food and Drug Administration. MedWatch Form FDA 3500A [Internet]. Silver Spring (MD): U.S. Department of Health and Human Services; c2010 [cited 2010 Mar 4]:

[2 screens]. Available from: http://www.fda.gov/Safety/MedWatch/HowToReport/DownloadForms/ucm149238.htm

27. U.S. Department of Health and Human Services. About HHS [Internet]. Washington, DC: U.S. Department of Health and Human Services; c2010 [cited 2010 May 1]:[about 1 screen]. Available from: http://www.hhs.gov/about/.

28. U.S. Food and Drug Administration. FDA guidance: drug safety information—FDA's communication to the public [Internet]. Silver Spring (MD): U.S. Department of Health and Human Services; c2012; [cited 2013 Sep 4]: [17 screens]. Available from: http://www.fda.gov/downloads/Drugs/GuidanceComplianceRegulatoryInformation/Guidances/UCM295217.pdf

29. Federal Register. [Docket no. FDA-2008-N-0174] Identification of drug biological products deemed to have risk evaluation and mitigation strategies for purposes of the food and drug administration amendments act of 2007 [Internet]. Silver Spring (MD): U.S. Department of Health and Human Services; c2008 [cited 2013 Nov 13]:[2 screens]. Available from: http://www.fda.gov/OHRMS/DOCKETS/98fr/E8-6201.pdf

30. U.S. Food and Drug Administration. Medication Guides [Internet]. Silver Spring (MD): U.S. Department of Health and Human Services; c2010 [cited 2010 Sep 15]:[1 screen]. Available from: http://www.fda.gov/Drugs/DrugSafety/UCM085729

31. U.S. Food and Drug Administration [Internet]. Silver Spring (MD): U.S. Department of Health and Human Services; c2010. Division of Drug Information; 2009 Nov 3 [cited 2010 May 1]; [about 3 screens]. Available from: http://www.fda.gov/AboutFDA/CentersOffices/OfficeofMedicalProductsandTobacco/CDER/ucm075128.htm

32. U.S. Food and Drug Administration. FDA Pharmacy Student Experiential Program [Internet]. Silver Spring (MD): U.S. Department of Health and Human Services; c2010, 2010 Mar 23 [cited 2010 May 3]; [about 3 screens]. Available from: http://www.fda.gov/AboutFDA/WorkingatFDA/FellowshipInternshipGraduateFacultyPrograms/PharmacyStudentExperientialProgramCDER/default.htm

SUGGESTED READINGS

1. Drug Safety Communications—http://www.fda.gov/Drugs/DrugSafety/ucm199082.htm
2. Guidance for Industry "Format and Content of Proposed Risk Evaluation and Mitigation Strategies (REMS), REMS Assessments, and Proposed REMS Modifications"—http://www.fda.gov/downloads/Drugs/GuidanceComplianceRegulatoryInformation/Guidances/UCM184128.pdf
3. Guidance "Medication Guides—Distribution Requirements and Inclusion in Risk Evaluation and Mitigation Strategies (REMS)"—http://www.fda.gov/downloads/Drugs/GuidanceComplianceRegulatoryInformation/Guidances/ucm244570.pdf
4. Guidance for Industry "Post-marketing Safety Reporting for Human Drug and Biological Products Including Vaccines"—http://www.fda.gov/downloads/BiologicsBloodVaccines/GuidanceComplianceRegulatoryInformation/Guidances/Vaccines/ucm092257.pdf

5. Guidance for Industry Public Availability of "Labeling Changes" in "Changes Being Effected" Supplements—http://www.fda.gov/downloads/Drugs/GuidanceCompliancRegulatory Information/Guidances/ucm075091.pdf

6. Guidance "Drug Safety Information—FDA's Communication to the Public"— http://www.fda.gov/downloads/Drugs/GuidanceComplianceRegulatoryInformation/Guidances/UCM295217.pdf

7. Guidance for Industry "Expanded Access to Investigational Drugs for Treatment Use—Qs & As—http://www.fda.gov/downloads/Drugs/GuidanceComplianceRegulatoryInformation/Guidances/UCM351261.pdf

8. Guidance for Industry "Self-Identification of Generic Drug Facilities, Sites, and Organizations"—http://www.fda.gov/Drugs/GuidanceComplianceRegulatoryInformation/Guidances/ucm316721.htm

9. Guidance for Industry "Generic Drug User Fee Amendments of 2012: Questions and Answers"—http://www.fda.gov/downloads/Drugs/GuidanceComplianceRegulatoryInformation/Guidances/UCM316671.pdf

10. Cunningham JE, Sheehan AH. Proposed guidelines for uniformity of postgraduate industry-affiliated fellowships. Am J Pharm Educ. 2009 Aug 28;73(5):93.

23

Chapter Twenty-Three

Assessing Drug Promotions

Robert D. Beckett • Genevieve Lynn Ness

Learning Objectives

After completing this chapter, the reader will be able to

- Define drug promotions.
- List World Health Organization (WHO) recommendations for appropriate drug promotions.
- Describe the role of the Food and Drug Administration (FDA) Office of Prescription Drug Promotion (OPDP).
- Determine whether a piece of direct-to-consumer advertising (DTCA) has been cited in FDA warning letters to companies.
- Describe the allowed content for a specific type of DTCA.
- Evaluate a given piece of DTCA based on FDA and Pharmaceutical Research and Manufacturers of America (PhRMA) guidelines.
- Report a drug promotion concern using the Bad Ad program.
- Evaluate the appropriateness of a piece of drug promotion designed for a health care professional.
- List system and individual strategies that may be used to combat proliferation of misinformation in drug promotions.
- Identify logical fallacies used in drug promotion, when given an interaction with a pharmaceutical industry representative.
- Describe the goals and design of academic detailing programs.
- Describe the clinical, economic, and humanistic effects of academic detailing.

Key Concepts

❶ Drug promotion is defined by the World Health Organization (WHO) as material or information provided by drug manufacturers with the ultimate goal of increasing prescribing or purchasing of medications.

❷ The FDA currently recognizes and outlines appropriate content for three types of direct-to-consumer advertising (DTCA): help-seeking ads, reminder ads, and product claim ads.

❸ The following information should be considered when validating appropriateness of DTCA: balance of risk and benefit information and inclusion of a brief summary of the risks listed in the labeling, a statement encouraging patients to seek information from their physicians, and references to other sources to find the full prescribing information.

❹ Drug promotion to health care professionals makes up the majority of drug promotions activity in terms of financial expenditure on the part of the pharmaceutical industry; this information can be effective in eliciting changes in prescribing behavior.

❺ All health care professionals, including pharmacists, should arm themselves using strategies of information mastery and vigilance for flawed reasoning when interacting with pharmaceutical sales representatives.

❻ Health care professionals are encouraged to report drug promotion violations to the FDA's Bad Ad program.

❼ Academic detailing programs, often led by pharmacists, are designed to combat pharmaceutical industry detailing by providing evidence-based information in the form of one-on-one or small group interactions between a clinician and prescribers.

Introduction

❶ *Drug promotion is defined by the World Health Organization (WHO) as material or information provided by drug manufacturers with the ultimate goal of increasing prescribing or purchasing of medications.* Every year, the pharmaceutical industry spends billions of dollars advertising their medications to the public and to health care professionals.[1-11] In 2012, about $27 billion was spent on drug promotion in the United States (U.S.) alone.[12] The channels companies use to promote their products include medical journals, newspapers, radio, television, magazines, Web sites, social media, search engine marketing, distributed promotional materials, billboards, direct mailings, medication samples, and sales representatives.[2,7,10,13-15]

Health care professionals and consumers may not recognize the impact drug promotion can have on individual behavior.[7] The literature has reported increased prescribing patterns, rapid implementation of new medications, and an increase in inappropriate prescribing among physicians who utilize promotional materials to obtain drug information.[7] The effect of medication promotion on overall public health remains uncertain. WHO suggests clinical trials be conducted to assess the correlation of drug promotion with inappropriate prescribing and the occurrence of adverse events, to identify the public health outcomes of drug promotion.[7] For these reasons, health care professionals must be prepared to critically interpret and evaluate verbal and written drug promotions. In particular, pharmacists play an important role as an interpreter of drug advertisements to their patients. The following section describes the full scope of drug promotion according to WHO.

WHO Ethical Criteria for Medicinal Drug Promotion

In 1988, the WHO published criteria for the ethical promotion of medications.[16] The guidelines state the promotion of drugs should comply with the national standards established by the country where the drugs are being promoted. These guidelines apply to both domestic and exported drug products. Overall, information presented for the purposes of promotion should be balanced, accurate, and current.

Advertisements targeted specifically to health care professionals should follow the approved product labeling and all writing should be clear and readable.[16] A scientific summary is required when product claims are made within an advertisement directed at health care professionals. These advertisements should include generic name, brand name, amount of active ingredient per dosage form, other ingredients that can lead to allergies or adverse effects, indications, dosage form, adverse reactions, warnings and precautions, contraindications, drug interactions, additional notable interactions, manufacturer/distributor name and address, and scientific literature references. Detailed information about the scientific properties of a medication should be made available to health care professionals as appropriate.

The WHO criteria also provide information about direct-to-consumer advertising (DTCA).[16] According to the WHO, DTCA should assist consumers in making decisions about nonprescription medications; however, the use of DTCA for prescription medications is not recommended. Scientific evidence must support all factual information provided. DTCA should not use fearful language or tactics and only information available in the approved labeling should be used, including the following: generic name, brand name, indications, major warnings and precautions, contraindications, and manufacturer/distributor name and address.

The WHO also outlines guidelines for pharmaceutical representatives.[16] These personnel should be properly trained and retain adequate technical and medical knowledge. The information presented should only discuss the material from the approved labeling. The pharmaceutical industry is responsible for the statements made by their sales representatives and the salary of those representatives should not be influenced by the number of prescriptions written for the product they are promoting. The WHO recognizes that free samples of prescription medications can be given to prescribers in small quantities on request.

The WHO guidelines outline the proper features of drug promotion that are required to produce beneficial and accurate materials. These criteria provide the basis of drug promotion regulations and evaluative strategies, which will be discussed in more detail later in this chapter.

Direct-to-Consumer Advertising

The U.S. FDA defines DTCA as any advertisement created by a pharmaceutical company to promote products to a general audience.[15] The goal of such advertising is to encourage patients to discuss a medication with their prescribers, ultimately leading to a prescription.[9]

There are many methods pharmaceutical companies use to present DTCA to patients. The two most well known are print, through magazines or newspapers, and broadcast through television. The Pharmaceutical Research and Manufacturers of America (PhRMA) defines direct-to-consumer print advertisements as "space that is bought by a company in newspaper or magazine publications targeted to patients or consumers, or a direct mail communication paid for and disseminated by a company to patients or consumers, for the purpose of presenting information about one or more of the company's medicines."[17] The PhRMA also defines direct-to-consumer television advertisements as, "portion of television air time on broadcast or cable television that is bought by a company for the purpose of presenting information about one or more of the company's medicines."[17]

DTCA has been known to increase prescription drug profit for the pharmaceutical industry.[18] Specifically, for each dollar spent on DTCA the company makes about $4.20 in sales.[9,18] One study, assessing data from 1992 to 1997, found that 32 extra diagnoses and 41 additional prescriptions for statin medications were prescribed for every $1000 spent on DTCA.[6] In 2002, the U.S. General Accounting Office (GAO) projected that each year eight million Americans requested and received prescriptions due to DTCA.[6] A 2009 study found that there were an additional one million physician visits and 397,025 added Irritable Bowel Syndrome (IBS) diagnoses after the promotion of tegaserod (Zelnorm®).[18] In addition, 1796 prescriptions were written for every $1 million spent on tegaserod DTCA (1041-2529, 95% confidence interval).[6,18]

Based on these reports, it is not surprising that between 1996 and 2005 spending on DTCA increased from $985 million to about $4 billion.[2-4] DTCA spending peaked at $5.4 billion in 2006, and spending decreased to $4.8 and $4.3 billion in 2007 and 2010, respectively.[2,8,10,11] These recent spending decreases could be due to loss of patent on highly advertised medications, fewer products being brought to the market, an increase in consumer doubt, and budget cuts due to the recent recession.[2] Some of the most highly marketed products in the United States in 2009 included atorvastatin (Lipitor®) at $247.1 million and tadalafil (Cialis®) at $179.2 million.[2] From January 2007 to March 2011, the highest DTCA marketed products were atorvastatin (Lipitor®) at $917.70 million, duloxetine (Cymbalta®) at $820.50 million, and fluticasone/salmeterol (Advair®) at $766.3 million.[6]

Today, most of the DTCA spending is allotted for television advertisements, which results in the average American watching about 16 hours of televised drug advertisements per year.[6,10] Interestingly, smoking cessation products, impotence medications, and antidepressant television ads have the highest changing channel rates among viewing audiences.[2] The ads that retain most of the television audience through the commercial include overactive bladder treatments and osteoporosis medications.[2]

TYPES OF DTCA

❷ *The FDA currently recognizes and outlines appropriate content for three types of DTCA: help-seeking advertisements, reminder advertisements, and product claim advertisements.* The following describes each of these types of advertisements, including evaluative criteria, in detail.[15]

• Help-seeking advertisements do not recommend a particular medication but provide information about a disease state or condition.[6,10,15,18,19] The advertisement can describe particular symptoms, point patients to discuss their symptoms with their physicians, and offer a phone number for more information about the disease state.[19,20] These advertisements are regulated by the Federal Trade Commission (FTC) since a specific drug product is not mentioned.[19,20]

• Reminder advertisements do not describe the indication of a medication but do present the brand name.[6,10,15,18,21] These particular advertisements are created with the assumption that patients are already familiar with the drug's indication.[19] Risk information is not included in these advertisements and, therefore, reminder advertisements of drugs with boxed warnings are illegal.[6,10,19,22] Any information or even implied information (through images or text) about a product's benefits or risks is not permitted in reminder advertisements.[19] For example, a medication for osteoporosis would not have an image of bones in the reminder advertisement as this implies the product's indication.[19]

● Product claim advertisements require more detail and should contain the drug name, the indication, as well as a balance between the risks and benefits associated with the product.[6,10,15,18,19,21] Specifically, printed product claim advertisements should include a brief summary that provides details about all of the risk information listed in the FDA-approved labeling.[10,19] Printed advertisements must also include a reference to the FDA MedWatch program for patients to report side effects to the medication.[19] Product claim advertisements that are broadcasted either by television, radio, or phone are not required to include the brief summary of risk information.[2,15,19] Instead, television advertisements are required to contain a major statement of the main risks associated with the product, which can be presented verbally.[8,10,19,21,23] In addition, when broadcast advertisements do not include all risk information listed in the labeling, the advertisement is expected to provide resources patients can consult to obtain the full prescribing information.[19] For example, the advertisement can refer a patient to consult with their health care professional, call a toll-free number, visit the product Web site, or refer to a printed advertisement that contains more detailed information.[15,19,23] This is known as the adequate provision requirement.[3,10,19] Information DTCAs are not required to include is listed in Table 23–1.[24]

Tone and themes of DTCA can vary.[21,23] Many advertisements only portray characters after successfully taking the product; similarly, advertisements tend to portray the product as a facilitator of healthy or recreational activities.[21] Most advertisements rely on emotional, rather than logical appeals; these emotional appeals could be positive, negative, or both. One study used content analysis to describe major themes present in advertisements, finding that promotion, prevention, individualism, collectivism, cheerfulness, quiescence, dejection, agitation, fear, and affection were all prevalent.[23]

TABLE 23–1. INFORMATION NOT REQUIRED FOR INCLUSION IN DTCA[24]

- Cost information
- Generic availability
- Availability of similar drugs that have the same indication with less adverse effects
- Whether lifestyle changes could help the condition (this is only required if it is listed in the prescribing information for the product)
- Incidence of the disease that the medication treats
- Mechanism of action
- Onset of action (if the product states that it works quickly it must define the meaning of quickly)
- How many people have experienced benefit from the drug

DTCA LEGISLATION

Currently, among developed countries, DTCA is only permitted in the United States and New Zealand.[6,10,15,18,21] New Zealand relies on self-regulation of DTCA by the pharmaceutical companies; however, in the United States the FDA is responsible for overseeing DTCA.[6]

The FDA's authority over prescription drug advertising targeted to health care professionals was established in 1962 by the Kefauver-Harris Amendment.[3,10,25] Shortly after, in 1969, the FDA released regulations requiring drug advertisements to be accurate and not misleading; contain a brief summary of indications, adverse effects, warnings, and contraindications; be **fair balanced**; and include only factual information about the product's advertised uses.[7,10,23,26,27] Television advertisements were also required to contain the brief summary, which made these ads too lengthy for broadcast.[2]

The FDA first allowed companies to promote their products directly to consumers in 1985.[3,10,11] In 1997, the FDA released a draft guidance that stated television advertisements no longer required the brief summary; however, the guidance did require a major statement of the main safety risks and referral to a source for detailed information about the product.[1,2,8,10,15,23] This guidance was finalized in 1999.[3,10] In addition, printed product claim advertisements were required to include the entire prescribing information prior to the release of 2004 regulations stating that only a simplified brief summary is required.[10] However, patient mailings, brochures, and other drug company materials that promote a drug product still require the full FDA-approved prescribing information if any such materials mention the benefits of the medication.[19] In 2007, the Food and Drug Administration Amendments Act (FDAAA) required the MedWatch reporting statement to be added to all printed advertisements, which states: "You are encouraged to report negative side effects of prescription drugs to the FDA. Visit MedWatch, or call 1-800-FDA-1088."[19,28] Today, prescription drug advertising regulations can be found in title 21, volume 4, part 202 of the Code of Federal Regulations (CFR).[27]

To ensure that DTCAs are following FDA guidelines and to protect consumers from false information, the FDA maintains a surveillance and enforcement program through their Office of Prescription Drug Promotion (OPDP) division.[15] It is important to remember that the FDA has the authority only over prescription medication DTCA.[24] Nonprescription DTCA and help-seeking ads are regulated by the FTC.[19,20,24] In addition, the FDA does not require pharmaceutical companies to submit DTCA prior to its distribution or being aired.[24] However, the FDA does require advertisements be submitted for review as soon as they are released to the public.[6,9,24]

If the FDA discovers that a DTCA is not in compliance with the set of laws in place, warning letters can be issued to the pharmaceutical company, requesting the removal of the advertisement and to address the material that violates the law.[9,24] These letters are publically available on the FDA's Warning Letters Web site.[24,29] If the advertisement has created a severe threat on public health, the FDA can also request the company to correct the advertisement and publish or broadcast the corrected version.[24] In rare cases, the FDA may bring criminal charges against the company in court and seize the company's drug supply.[24] The FDA does not have authority to levy fines on pharmaceutical companies for DTCA violations.[9]

Recently there has been a decrease in the number of DTCA regulatory actions by the FDA.[10] Critics say this could be the result of decreased FDA supervision or, in contrast, could be due to better compliance with DTCA laws.[10] Another added factor is that all warning letters must be reviewed and approved by the FDA's Office of Chief Counsel, which was mandated by the Secretary of Health and Human Services (HHS) in 2002.[10] This action alone may have resulted in a decline in the number of promotional-related warning letters issued between 2001 and 2002, 68 and 28, respectively.[10] In addition, the FDA has limited staff to review DTCA.[10] Fewer than six FDA employees were assigned to review more than 15,000 brochures and DTCA in 2006.[10] Since then, the OPDP staff has increased to accommodate the growing number of advertisements to review.

There is still a need for FDA guidelines in regard to online promotion of prescription medications.[10] After warning letters issued from the FDA in 2009 stating that online search engine results need to include risk information since the drug name and indication is mentioned, the pharmaceutical companies now only include either the name of the drug or the indication in search engine links.[10]

Since studies have reported a lack of consumer awareness of the FDA role in DTCA oversight, it is vital for health care professionals to monitor and evaluate DTCA.[6,10]

PhRMA GUIDING PRINCIPLES FOR DTCA

With the increasing role of DTCA in health care, the PhRMA established guiding principles for DTCA of prescription medications.[17] These principles are voluntary, but do serve as guidance for pharmaceutical companies to create accurate, educational, and encouraging DTCAs that follow FDA regulations.[17] See Table 23–2 for an overview of the PhRMA principles. A commitment to follow the PhRMA guiding principles and completion of an annual certification entitles the company to be identifiable as a signatory company and be recognized by PhRMA online.[17]

SUPPORT OF DTCA

Supporters of DTCA believe these advertisements serve a public health need.[6,15,17] Through DTCA patients become educated about different disease states, which can assist them in making better treatment decisions and create more knowledgeable patients in the

TABLE 23–2. PhRMA GUIDING PRINCIPLES FOR DTCA[17]

1. DTCAs should follow all FDA standards including the absence of off-label promotion.

2. The company should obtain insight from patients and health care professionals to identify what educational information should be included in DTCA.

3. Prescription medications should be clearly identified as such in the DTCAs.

4. The ad should encourage patients to discuss the risks and benefits of the advertised medication with their prescribers.

5. Health care professionals should be educated about new prescription medications prior to the release of DTCA in order to be able to accurately respond to patient questions.

6. Once unknown safety risks about an advertised product are discovered, companies should edit or remove DTCA while continuing collaboration with the FDA.

7. All new DTCAs should be submitted to the FDA prior to public release. DTCAs that have been significantly changed (including additional indications, new patient populations, additional safety information, or new outcome claims) should also be submitted to the FDA. If companies would like to obtain FDA comments they should submit a feedback request with the DTCA. Timelines for review are 30 days for priority review and greater than 30 days for nonpriority.

8. All printed DTCA should contain the FDA's MedWatch number or Web site to report adverse events. Television DTCA should point patients to print advertisements with the FDA's MedWatch information and/or present the organization's toll-free number.

9. The ad should clearly identify the use of actors as health care professionals and disclose any financial compensation if actual health care professionals are utilized.

10. If a celebrity advocate is used in the DTCA, the claims made by the celebrity should reflect their factual views and experiences while taking the medication.

11. When applicable, the DTCA should also highlight alternatives to treat the condition being advertised such as diet and lifestyle changes.

12. Television DTCA that discuss a particular product should present the major risks and the approved indications.

13. Medication benefit and risk information should be balanced including information about boxed warnings (presented in plain language). Television DTCA should point patients to where they can obtain additional information about product risks and benefits.

14. The disease state should be presented seriously and reverently throughout the DTCA.

15. DTCA that may be inappropriate for children should not be aired or published in mediums where children could witness the advertisement.

16. Information about the disease and health awareness should be presented in DTCA.

17. Patient assistance programs for the uninsured and underinsured population should be mentioned in DTCA when applicable.

health care environment.[1,6,10,11,17,26] A related point is that DTCA can help improve the quality of patient–professional interactions and help patients identify meaningful questions to ask of their health care providers, as well as improve adherence to prescribed treatment.[6,10,15,17] DTCA provides patients with information about treatment options available early on, which can result in lower health care costs.[10] Similarly, DTCA may also increase appropriate care for underdiagnosed diseases.[1,6,10,15,17] It has been asserted that if medication therapy is started sooner because of DTCA in a disease that could eventually lead to surgery if not treated, health care costs can be saved.[10] However, there is limited data to support this claim.[10] Supporters mention that DTCA can lower drug prices due to increased competition between products.[10] DTCA also has been credited with reducing the stigma of certain diseases making them acceptable for discussion (e.g., psychiatric disorders).[6,10,11,15]

OPPOSITION TO DTCA

In contrast, many who oppose DTCA express its potential threat to public health.[15] DTCAs could contain inaccurate or misleading information in addition to inadequate information about adverse effects and risks.[1,15] Sixty-five percent of physicians reported that patients tend to underestimate the risks and overemphasize the benefits of a drug, mostly after viewing a television advertisement.[9] A study analyzing television drug advertisements found that patients remembered the benefits of a drug more easily than the risks.[9] This may be due to the dominance of visual messages over audio when presented jointly and the fact that much of the safety information is presented verbally in television advertisements.[10] Patients may also overemphasize a product's benefits because DTCA is known to exaggerate the happiness achieved with a medication.[10]

Opponents of DTCA state that FDA regulations are too lenient because the pharmaceutical companies are only held responsible for the information presented in DTCA if there is a violation.[10] As a result, some advertisements presented have inappropriate information included. For example, in 1996 only 65% of newspaper and magazine DTCA were reported to be fair balanced.[7] Unfortunately, consumers will remember the information presented in an ad even if there are violations.[10] The PhRMA has released DTCA guidelines that suggest companies should submit DTCA to the FDA for review prior to distribution; however, these guidelines are optional and unenforceable.[10]

The content of DTCA is usually not written in lay person language (i.e., an eighth-grade reading level), making it challenging for consumers to understand the content.[10] Along these lines the use of words such as usually, mild, may, etc., to describe safety information may lead to consumer confusion about the exact meaning of these terms.[10]

There have also been multiple reports of statistical overexaggeration of product benefits in advertisements.[30] Particularly, in DCTA, this paper points out that only two of 67 advertisements in U.S. magazines presented results of the promoted drug verses placebo as absolute rates of clinical outcomes. Other advertisements only presented data in the form of relative risk reduction (RRR); absolute risk reduction (ARR) was not included (see Chapters 5 and 8 for further information about RRR and ARR). Some provided references to clinical studies, but did not provide any data from the studies in the advertisements. One additional advertisement claimed that the promoted drug provided a clinical cure compared to competitors, but did not explain exactly what was defined as a clinical cure. In a study assessing 16 advertisements, only one ad provided adverse effect frequency using quantitative methods, two presented using comparative relationships, and the majority used a qualitative approach.[30] Prevalence of the disease state the product is treating is also rarely reported in advertisements. In a study from 2004, only three of 31 advertisements provided disease state prevalence information.[30]

Due to DTCA, there has been an increase in patients requesting advertised medications during their provider visits.[7] This can lead to the undermining of health care professional authority and hinder the provider–patient relationships.[3,6,10,11] This has been reported in the literature by 30% of patients and 39% of physicians who participated in a national survey.[10] In particular, if a physician refuses to prescribe a medication that the patient is requesting, the patient is more likely to switch physicians.[10] This pressure on prescribers from consumers can increase the risk of inappropriate prescribing.[3,4,6,10,11,15] An FDA study reported about 50% of physicians felt some pressure to prescribe a particular medication after a patient reported seeing a DTCA for the product.[9,26] One study found that during physician visits, 40% of patients requested a medication they saw on a DTCA and about 50% of the requests were granted by the doctor.[10] However, a study conducted in 2006 reported that of the patients who requested a medication due to a DTCA, only about 2% to 7% received a prescription for the product in the end.[10] It has been reported that patients may try to fit the type of patient who is presented in the DTCA, which can also lead to inappropriate prescribing and diagnosis, and ultimately unnecessary side effects.[6,10] A study found that about half of physicians, participating in a focus group discussion, presumed that patients diagnosed themselves accurately based on DTCA.[6] Also, this increase in unnecessary prescribing can lead to an increase in prescription drug spending.[8]

The added time for providers and patients to discuss DTCA during scheduled appointments could take away from other important aspects of the appointment and lead to negative patient outcomes.[11] DTCA can lead to unnecessary physician visits and make patients believe they have a particular disease.[1,8,10] For example, critics blame DTCA for converting menopause from a normal life process into an insufficient hormone disease.[10]

In addition, use of DTCA to advertise me-too drugs can increase health care costs since many patients will request the brand name drug when there may be inexpensive generic options available.[4,10,15] A study found that patients were more likely to switch from lansoprazole to omeprazole in areas that were more exposed to DTCA since omeprazole was advertised via DTCA and lansoprazole was not.[6] The expense of DTCA may also drive up the consumer costs for the product as pharmaceutical companies increase prices to compensate for advertising costs.[5] For example, one study found that the cost of clopidogrel increased by $0.40 (12%) per unit after the launch of the DTCA campaign.[5,6] In a study assessing television DTCA, the high-cost medications had longer air time for the ads (60 seconds) compared to medium cost medications (47.9 seconds).[1]

Critics mention that the safety information required in the DTCA could cause patients to have concerns about the safety of a medication and may lead to issues with patient compliance.[10] However, most of the time DTCA is released to the public before the majority of the safety information is collected (i.e., postmarketing surveillance).[10] For example, rofecoxib (Vioxx®), which was one of the most promoted medications in the United States. ($100 million/year spent on promotion), was not discovered to cause myocardial infarction (80,000 to 140,000 cases) or stroke until after the DTCA campaign.[6,10] This additional safety information led to its voluntary recall in 2004.[6,10] Another example of a highly marketed product whose side effects were not fully discovered until after DTCA was tegaserod (Zelnorm®), which was later withdrawn from the market due to increased risk of cardiovascular-related adverse effects.[18,31]

For the many reasons described above, information included in DTCA (in addition to advertisements intended for health care professionals) should be closely scrutinized for errors, promotional violations, and other misleading information.

SUGGESTIONS FOR IMPROVEMENT

Suggestions for the improvement of DTCA have been reported in the literature. One suggestion would eliminate the need for DTCA altogether. A group of representatives from industry, government, and academia would be tasked to create public service announcements discussing appropriate treatment for conditions that are known to cause morbidity or mortality, have effective and safe treatments available, and are identified as being undertreated and underdiagnosed.[8,10] This solution has not been implemented at this time. The U.S. Institute of Medicine (IOM) proposed enforcing a 2-year delay from the time a product is released to launching DTCA.[6,10] This can ensure that adequate time has passed for postmarketing data to be collected and allow physicians to become educated about the product.[10] However, in 2011 the U.S. Congressional Budget Office stated that the benefits of providing information about new medications outweighed the risks and, therefore, the proposal was not supported.[6] To have the FDA review all DTCA before being released to the public is another recommendation.[10] However, this would only be achievable assuming additional user fees were paid to the FDA by the pharmaceutical industry. There was a proposal for such a program in 2008, but it was not funded by Congress and, therefore, could not be enforced by the FDA.

There have also been debates about the most appropriate DTCA format.[32] A study assessing consumer preferences found that more patients preferred the drug facts box format, which is similar to the nonprescription labeling.[32] In addition, more patients were able to recall risk information when presented in this matter. Other suggestions include listing adverse effects on drug advertisements in bullet form from the highest to the lowest possibility of occurring.[11] However, even with these findings, this format for DTCA has not been mandated.

Requiring quantitative data in the DTCAs, as well as mentioning if a generic alternative is available for the product, have also been described as possible solutions.[10] The latter suggestion may not be well accepted by the pharmaceutical industry, but has been suggested in the literature. Another study suggested requirements to include specific information about the population at risk for the condition being advertised, describing **nonpharmacologic treatment**, and discuss the effectiveness of other therapies in the ads.[21]

With the solutions, suggestions, and continued evolvement, the hope for future DTCAs will be a greater emphasis on using medications appropriately, sustained use of medications, and medication adherence.[2]

EVALUATING DTCA

❸ *The balance of risk and benefit information, inclusion of a brief summary of the risks listed in the labeling, a statement encouraging patients to seek information from their physicians, and references to other sources to find the full prescribing information should be included and considered essential content when validating DTCA.*

In general, DTCA must present only accurate statements, maintain a balance of risk versus benefit information throughout, align with the information presented in the FDA-approved labeling, and only present content that is supported by robust evidence.[17,33] When evaluating DTCA, consider using the process outlined in Table 23–3.[34]

TABLE 23–3. ISSUES TO CONSIDER WHEN EVALUATING DTCA[30,34]

Issues for health care professionals and patients to consider:
- Identify what condition or disease state the advertised product treats.
- Determine the reasoning behind why the patient believes they have the advertised condition.
- Decide if the patient would be considered an appropriate candidate for the drug based on the information.
- Recognize if the patient is permitted to take the medication with their current comorbidities .
- Identify if the patient is taking any other medications that could interact with the advertised medication.
- Determine which adverse effects the patient may be concerned about.
- Decide if the drug could be affected by certain foods, dietary supplements, vitamins, or alcohol.
- Pinpoint any other medications (including generic products) that could treat the patient's current condition.
- Determine if other medications to treat this condition have different or less serious side effects.
- Identify if diet and exercise could help the patient with their condition.
- Locate additional information about the disease state and the drug described in the advertisement.

Continued

● **TABLE 23–3. ISSUES TO CONSIDER WHEN EVALUATING DTCA[30,34]** *(Continued)*

Additional issues for health care professionals to consider:

- Determine if absolute risk reduction (ARR) or number needed to treat (NNT) was used to present results (e.g., "Three out of five patients benefit from Drug X.").
- Assess the appropriateness of the use of confidence intervals.
- Identify if statistical power has been adequately explained in the advertisement if referenced.
- Determine if the literature cited is from the main journal in which the data was published and not a from a supplement or symposia.
- Evaluate the appropriateness of presented graphs and tables.
- Recognize if claims are being supported by emotional reports rather than numerical data.

Case Study 23–1

While using a common commercial search engine, you identify a help-seeking advertisement regarding asthma. Since this advertisement is visible to many members of the public, you decide to evaluate whether it is appropriate or not.

- *What information should the help-seeking advertisement include?*
- *What information should the help-seeking advertisement not include?*
- *What other aspects of the advertisement could you assess?*

The FDA also provides information for patients and health care professionals on how to determine if an advertisement is false or misleading based on the type.[35] FDA guidance for evaluating specific types of advertisements is provided in Table 23–4. The FDA encourages patients to report promotional violations to OPDP by calling 301-796-1200 or mailing

● **TABLE 23–4. FDA GUIDANCE FOR EVALUATING SPECIFIC TYPES OF ADVERTISEMENTS[20,22,28]**

A product claim ad should:

- Identify the product's brand and generic name
- State the product's FDA-approved indication (all claims made in the ad must be backed by clinical experience or evidence)
- Include a statement that the product is only available by prescription
- Contain balanced amounts of drug risk and benefit information
- Clearly state the product is intended for adults or children (this includes the use of pictures, such as children being featured for pediatric medications)
- Include the FDA MedWatch statement about reporting serious adverse effects to the FDA
- Contain a brief summary of the product's risks listed in the FDA-approved labeling

TABLE 23–4. FDA GUIDANCE FOR EVALUATING SPECIFIC TYPES OF ADVERTISEMENTS[20,22,28] (*Continued*)

- Encourage patients to ask their physicians about the medication, signifying that the patient cannot make the decision to prescribe
- Include references to other resources to obtain detailed product information including a Web site or toll-free telephone number

A reminder ad should:

- Include a product's brand and generic name
- Not list the product's indication

A help-seeking ad should:

- Include appropriate images of individuals who may be experiencing the discussed symptoms and images of drug products are not included
- List possible symptoms but does not mention a treatment for these symptoms
- Encourage patients to discuss their symptoms and seek medical advice from their prescribers
- Provide company information and references to a telephone number or Web site for more information

a written complaint directly to the division.[24,36] Health care professionals are encouraged to report promotional violations using the Bad Ad program, described below.

Promotions to Health Care Professionals

❹ *Drug promotion to health care professionals makes up the majority of drug promotions activity in terms of financial expenditure on the part of pharmaceutical industry; this information can be effective in eliciting changes in prescribing behavior.* The following sections describe the scope and response to this issue.

Marketing of prescription medications differs from typical consumer products in that one individual—the prescriber—directly controls, to a large extent, purchasing decisions on behalf of the ultimate consumer.[37] For this reason, in addition to the very high expenditures of the pharmaceutical industry on DTCA, even greater financial resources are dedicated to promotions made directly to health care professionals, or detailing. Of the estimated $57.5 billion spent in pharmaceutical promotions in 2004, approximately 35.5% was spent on detailing along with approximately 27.7% and 3.5% spent on drug samples and professional meetings, respectively.[38] In contrast, only 7% was spent on DTCA. Detailing, like any type of marketing, combines use of scientific knowledge, logic, and reason with appeals to emotions through techniques such as slogans and use of wishful thinking.[37] Detailing may be defined as a one-on-one or group interaction in which a pharmaceutical industry representative, who might or might not have a clinical background, provides drug information and marketing materials to a prescriber or health care professional.[37,39] These activities could involve provision of product samples and continuing education. At its core, detailing is designed to produce a change in prescribing behavior. The extraordinary expenditures on detailing and related activities, as well as cases of illegal and unsupported drug promotion to health care professionals suggest that critically assessing the information delivered in these interactions is of vital importance.

LEGAL ISSUES

The same criteria described earlier for DTCA also apply to formal advertisements intended for health care professionals and information promotions such as detailing.[40] Briefly, the information provided must provide fair balance in addressing safety risks and efficacy benefits, describe factual information, and not be misleading. Additionally, information must be consistent with the FDA-approved product labeling (i.e., the package insert), including indications for which the medication may be used.[41] Off-label information may be provided in scientific exchanges and at the request of a health care professional, but not in the context of promotion. The legality of off-label promotion is an often debated First Amendment issue.[41,42]

FDA advertising rules also apply to industry-sponsored education programs that are, in actuality, promotional activities.[40] For a program to be considered independent and nonpromotional (and, thus, qualify as continuing education), the program must be conducted by a third party that controls the educational content. Additionally, all relevant relationships must be disclosed. PhRMA companies adhere to voluntary standards that prohibit direct speaker honorariums, entertainment (e.g., sporting event tickets), gifts, and noneducational practice-related items (e.g., coffee mugs, pens) at continuing education events and during detailing.[43] All programs must be conducted through an independent continuing education provider.

PROMOTION EFFECTIVENESS

The majority of scientific literature assessing health care professionals' interactions with pharmaceutical industry centers around medical students, physicians, and nurse practitioners, and finds success on the part of industry in achieving their desired changes in attitudes and behaviors.[44-51] Little information is available regarding promotions targeted toward pharmacists. Two studies have attempted to quantify exposure to pharmaceutical promotion during medical training, with high proportions of medical students and residents reporting attending sponsored events and receiving gifts.[44,45] Studies vary in the degree to which medical residents and students value industry-sponsored information; however, survey responders perceive that they do not feel prepared to manage these types of interactions, but that drug promotions would not influence their prescribing habits. One survey of nurse practitioners found that this group does not prefer to receive drug information from pharmaceutical industry sources, but also found that approximately

36% have been offered paybacks in return for changes to prescribing habits.[46] Limited research describes which prescribers are more likely to meet with pharmaceutical industry representatives. One cross-sectional study found that factors of nonacademic affiliation, higher prescription volume, urban practice, small practice size, and specialization in primary care were positive correlations with this risk.[47]

Several studies have assessed effects of detailing and related activities on prescribing patterns. Two studies found increased prescribing and loyalty to brand name prescription medications when physicians were exposed to detailing.[18,48] Similar results have been found in a study assessing effectiveness of industry-sponsored continuing education for physicians,[49] although it should be noted that it was conducted prior to publication of current industry guidelines.[43] One systematic review noted that 17 of 29 assessed articles found increased prescribing of a target medication as a result of one-on-one detailing; the remaining studies found no difference in practice.[50] Similarly, five out of eight articles assessing effectiveness of sponsored education events found the expected changes in practice (i.e., increased prescribing of the target medication). In the inpatient setting, one study found that physicians who request a medication to be added to formulary are more likely to have accepted payment from industry to attend or lead symposia or to have personally met with industry representatives from the company producing the medication.[51]

COMBATING MISINFORMATION

❺ *All health care professionals, including pharmacists, should arm themselves using strategies of information mastery and vigilance for flawed reasoning when interacting with pharmaceutical sales representatives.* Systematic and individual strategies for combating potential misinformation provided by the pharmaceutical industry are discussed in the following sections.

Both approaches are needed to ensure that undesired effects of drug promotions to health care professionals are minimized. This need is illustrated by several cases in which the pharmaceutical industry was fined for inappropriate promotion to health care professionals, including cases brought against the manufacturers of olanzapine (Zyprexa®), gabapentin (Neurontin®), and valdecoxib (Bextra®) for off-label promotion and/or lack of fair balance.[52]

A number of systematic strategies are active or have been proposed to decrease the potentially significant effect of promotions on prescribers and pharmacists at local, institutional, and national levels. Several of these strategies are described below:

- **Academic detailing:** Research has demonstrated the value of structured one-on-one visits between traveling clinicians, or academic detailers, and prescribers in terms of evidence-based prescribing habits and increased use of generic medications.[39] Applications of academic detailing are described later in the chapter.

- Conflict of interest policies: Conflict of interest policies have been used in residency programs, colleges of medicine, and health systems in order to decrease the effect of pharmaceutical promotions.[53,54] Many health systems have very specific policies regarding the allowed interactions with industry representatives. The policy may even be that such meetings are prohibited.
- Education: Several studies have assessed effectiveness of educational sessions focusing on pharmaceutical industry interactions with medical students and residents.[55-57] Study participants have generally expressed improved knowledge of the pharmaceutical industry and a greater ability to critically assess promotions, and identified potential behaviors they will change as a result of the program (e.g., stop seeing industry representatives).
- National initiatives: In the United States, OPDP is responsible for review of submitted promotional materials, monitoring at professional meetings for inappropriate promotion, and review of Internet sites related to prescription medications.[58]
- Representative tracking: Health systems often use industry credentialing programs to enforce institutional policies regarding content, frequency, and length of meetings between clinicians and industry representatives.[59] These programs allow health systems administrators to know when representatives are on campus and with whom they are meeting.

Additionally, several professional organizations provide guidelines regarding information provided by the pharmaceutical industry. The American Society of Health-Systems Pharmacists (ASHP) guides members that a third party should control educational content of all industry-sponsored continuing education.[60] Similarly, the American Medical Association (AMA) recommends physicians select continuing education that is accredited and fair balanced. Promotional continuing education should be clearly denoted as such.[61] Both organizations counsel members to limit interactions with the pharmaceutical industry to professional, scientific exchange of information and to avoid situations in which professional judgment is at risk and impropriety may be perceived.[60,61]

Even in the presence of systematic approaches to preventing misinformation in drug promotions, the need for pharmacists, and other health care professionals, to critically evaluate specific information provided in drug promotions is clear. Considering the volume of medical information emerging every day, the task of analyzing, retaining, and synthesizing this information can be monumental.[62] For this reason, health care professionals must develop skills and confidence in searching the medical literature and practicing evidence-based medicine (i.e., information mastery) using both patient-specific and general approaches (i.e., top down versus bottom up; see Chapter 7). It is recommended that health care professionals preferentially use tertiary drug information resources that are either FDA approved (i.e., the prescribing information) or prepared and published by unbiased sources (e.g., *AHFS® Drug Information*, Micromedex 2.0). If health care professionals do meet with pharmaceutical industry representatives or use other promotional materials, they should be prepared to rigorously assess pharmaceutical promotions in the same way they would any tertiary resource (see Chapter 3). Additionally, health care professionals should evaluate any print pharmaceutical promotions distributed by industry representatives using strategies similar to DTCA, outlined in Tables 23–1 to 23–3.

Many pharmaceutical industry representatives use flawed logic in order to persuade prescribers and pharmacists that their product is the ideal choice for their patients.[37] Errors in reasoning can introduce self-doubt on the part of the health care professional and increase likelihood of a behavior change. It is important to identify when arguments are logical and when they are irrational. In particular, pharmacists who manage pharmacy and therapeutics committee initiatives should be vigilant in their awareness of flawed logic and misleading messages. One of the best methods for combating logical fallacies is reviewing relevant information prior to interacting with an industry representative. See Table 23–5 for examples of misleading strategies that industry representatives might use. See Table 23–6 for general recommendations for interacting with pharmaceutical industry representatives.

TABLE 23–5. EXAMPLE LOGICAL FALLACIES USED IN PHARMACEUTICAL PROMOTION[37]

Fallacy	Description	Example
Appeal to authority	Appeal to knowledge of a known expert with or without conferring with that expert	"I just spoke with the Head of Surgery who says he used Drug X in nearly every case."
Appeal to pity	Appeal to the inner desire to do good without focusing on evidence	"Patients who my other prescribers work with have benefited so much from Drug X. It's really been life-changing for them."
Bandwagon effect	Appeal to popularity with or without confirming if that popularity is true or false	"All the other tertiary medical centers in the city have added Drug X to formulary."
Red herring	Including extraneous, irrelevant details in an argument	"In clinical studies, Drug X had a lower rate of headache [2%] compared to Drug Y [3%]."

TABLE 23–6. RECOMMENDED PRACTICES FOR PHARMACEUTICAL INDUSTRY INTERACTIONS[61]

Conduct visits politely and professionally.
Determine the content of meetings ahead of time.
Clearly communicate expectations for content and duration of meetings with the representative.
Prepare for meetings using unbiased tertiary resources and review of primary literature.
Come prepared with specific questions in mind.
Use active listening skills.
Use clinical thinking to catch potential errors in reasoning.

Case Study 23–2

As part of your work with the pharmacy and therapeutics committee at an academic, tertiary care hospital, you are asked to conduct monthly meetings with pharmaceutical industry representatives. Your goal for these meetings is to stay up-to-date on competitive pricing information.

- *What systems should you ensure are in place prior to scheduling such visits?*
- *What strategies should you use to prepare for visits once you know which representatives will be attending?*
- *What strategies can you use to remain objective during the visits?*

ADVERTISING TO HEALTH CARE PROFESSIONALS

❻ *Health care professionals are encouraged to report advertising violations to the FDA's Bad Ad program.* All health care professionals have a responsibility to report inappropriate drug promotions using the process described below.

Health care professionals, particularly prescribers, are also targets of drug promotion in the form of print advertisements in medical journals.[63,64] One study found that approximately 16% of the pages in one oncology journal were devoted to drug promotion.[63] Advertisements appearing in medical journals are subject to the same standards as other print advertisements discussed earlier in the chapter, as well as ideally be in compliance with a journal's advertising policy. Advertising policies should be robust and available to the reader. Advertisements in these journals should be assessed using the same methods described for DTCA.

The FDA's Bad Ad program encourages prescribers to report misinforming or incorrect prescription drug advertising and promotion to FDA.[33,36] This assists OPDP in identifying and ceasing such advertisements.[33] Advertisements for products such as dietary supplements, medical devices, and nonprescription drugs should not be reported through the Bad Ad program since OPDP does not regulate the promotion of these products. In the past, OPDP obtained information about prescription drug promotion violations through complaints and comments about medication promotion, medical conference observations, review of company submitted promotional materials, and Internet searches.[36] Due to the absence of FDA employees at dinner programs, promotional speaker events, and prescribers' offices, the FDA seeks the help of health care professionals to report promotional violations through this program.[36]

If an ad is found to be in violation, the FDA can take enforcement action and/or continue to monitor additional advertisement activities.[33] Advertising methods that are assessed and can be reported through the Bad Ad program include information presented in printed or written drug promotional materials or by sales representatives, presentations by program speakers, as well as advertisements on radio or television.[33,36]

Common violations identified in drug advertisements include inadequate risk information, overexaggeration of benefits, off-label or unapproved information, and false or deceiving comparisons with other medications.[33,36] For example, ads could say that the medication works in as little as 2 days, but in reality most patients might not see an effect for months.[36] Another example in reference to pharmaceutical representatives is statements that the adverse effects that occurred in clinical trials are not as likely to occur in practice.

Comments to the FDA through the Bad Ad program can be submitted anonymously; once received, they are analyzed by a member of the OPDP team.[33] FDA accepts comments from health care professionals via email: BadAd@FDA.gov, or by phone: 855-RX-BADAD (855-792-2323).

Case Study 23-3

You have been asked to attend a dinner program sponsored by the pharmaceutical industry. The main goal for you attending the program is to learn about a new product to treat rheumatoid arthritis.

- *How do you interpret the information being presented at the program?*
- *What are the common violations that can occur in this setting?*
- *How do you report a violation to the FDA?*

ACADEMIC DETAILING

❼ *Academic detailing programs, often led by pharmacists, are designed to combat pharmaceutical industry detailing by providing evidence-based information in the form of one-on-one or small group interactions between a clinician and prescribers.* The following sections address the design, effectiveness, and roles for pharmacists in academic detailing.

Academic detailing, also known as counterdetailing, prescriber outreach, and prescriber support and education is a proactive approach developed to combat proliferation of potentially biased information provided by pharmaceutical industry sales representatives in prescriber workplaces.[39,65,66] The goal of academic detailing is to provide objective, scientific evidence to prescribers in order to improve patient outcomes. While originally focused on increasing use of generic medications when the practice emerged in the 1980s, today's academic detailing programs have expanded clinical roles including promotion of evidence-based medicine and dissemination of comparative effectiveness research. Although most commonly associated with outpatient settings, academic detailing programs have also been reported in inpatient and long-term care practices.[67,68] Pharmaceutical and academic detailing are similar in that both are designed to change prescribing behavior.[39,65,66,69]

Program Design

The core process of an academic detailing program is outlined in Table 23–7.[66,67] At its heart is a one-on-one, face-to-face interaction between a traveling health care professional (e.g., physician, pharmacist, nurse) and a prescriber.[39,65,66,69] The academic detailer may also have a concurrent academic or clinical appointment.[65,66] While the original format for these interactions was inspired by the success of pharmaceutical detailing, a key difference is that academic detailing is intended to focus purely on evidence-based information without a promotional perspective.[39,65,66,69] Individuals providing academic detailing should have knowledge of clinical and information sciences as well as experience in providing direct patient care.[65] Interactions between the detailer and the prescriber should be nonjudgmental, empathetic, and professional.

The most accepted goal of academic detailing is promotion of rational prescribing.[39,65,66] One somewhat controversial aspect of academic detailing is whether improving cost savings–related outcomes should also be a core function of these initiatives.[65] Programs are occasionally accused of allowing pursuit of cost savings to supersede promotion of evidence-based medicine. While simply encouraging use of generic medications in

TABLE 23–7. CORE FUNCTIONS OF AN ACADEMIC DETAILING PROGRAM[39,66,67]

- Identify a target therapeutic issue based on local trends (e.g., demographics, endemic disease states, prescriber preference, prescribing patterns).
- Identify a target prescriber population based on specific criteria (e.g., level of experience, prescribing patterns).
- Synthesize the available evidence using strategies discussed in Chapters 2 and 7.
- Provide the synthesized evidence in an engaging small group or one-on-one format using a concise message that can be easily implemented into practice.
- Monitor program using identified metrics related to scope (e.g., quantity and quality of visits) and effectiveness (e.g., generic versus brand prescribing, therapeutic area-specific issues).
- Develop relationships with prescribers by increasing communication and face time.

place of branded product is a generally accepted aim, therapeutic substitution of a different medication in the same class is a more divisive issue. Differences in philosophy may vary depending on the organization sponsoring the program; for-profit and government organizations may be more likely than academic groups to acknowledge a cost savings goal.[39,65,66,69]

For-profit, nonprofit, government, and academic organizations are all known to sponsor academic detailing programs.[39,65-71] Many of the most successful programs are collaborations among multiple groups. Large-scale academic detailing has been conducted by several Canadian provinces and at a national level in Australia; several states in the United States are considering or have developed programs modeled after the success of programs in these countries (where large scale academic detailing has a much longer history).[65,66] One of the most well-known academic detailing programs in the United States is the Independent Drug Information Service (iDiS), a division of the Pennsylvania Department of Aging's Pharmaceutical Contract for the Elderly (PACE) program.[70] This program spends approximately $600 million annually to provide medication to over 300,000 elderly patients who are ineligible for Medicaid.[65,70] PACE reports that cost savings generated from improving prescribing of common chronic medications (e.g., antihypertensives, anti-inflammatories) more than cover the costs of this program.[65,66] The content for iDiS visits is developed by an independent group of physicians, the National Resource Center for Academic Detailing (NaRCAD), located at Harvard Medical School and Brigham and Women's Hospital, and then provided by 10 academic detailers in approximately 1000 physician visits annually.

Another example of an American academic detailing collaboration is the South Carolina Medicaid Academic Detailing Program (SCORxE), a collaboration of the South Carolina Department of Health and Human Services and the South Carolina College of Pharmacy.[65,71] This program focuses on providing pharmacist-led academic detailing with prescribers who provide care for rural and urban Medicaid patients who have cancer, human immunodeficiency virus (HIV), or mental health disorders. These disease states were selected based on state law prohibiting legal prescribing restrictions in HIV and mental health. The programming is provided by four full-time pharmacists across at least nine counties.

Nationally, leadership in the area of academic detailing comes from NaRCAD, an Agency for Healthcare Research and Quality (AHRQ)-supported initiative.[72] NaRCAD collaborates with states, including Pennsylvania and South Carolina, and private organizations to determine their specific needs in an academic detailing program, based on local medication use.[65,66,73] Additionally, the service translates important comparative effectiveness research into usable tools, conducts education on academic detailing best practices and implementation, and helps organizations develop an assessment plan for their programs.[73] A final key role of NaRCAD is enlarging the network of organizations providing academic detailing in order to encourage information exchange.

Case Study 23–4

As part of your work in a large health system with a network of physician office clinics, you are asked to develop an academic detailing program designed to improve safety, efficacy, and cost-effectiveness of prescribing in an area of psychiatry.

- *How would you go about determining which class of medications or disease state on which to focus?*
- *How would you develop your clinical materials? Which external organizations could you partner with?*
- *Would you take a one-on-one or group approach to academic detailing? Discuss why you selected the strategy you did.*
- *What metrics could you assess to determine the effectiveness of your program?*

Effectiveness

While theoretical and observational data suggest huge potential for improvement in clinical and economic outcomes from academic detailing programs,[74,75] results from prospective, interventional studies assessing effectiveness of academic detailing programs have been mixed.[65,66,68,76-81] The nationwide academic detailing program in Australia has demonstrated significant cost-effectiveness; however, less public information is available regarding tangible cost savings of such programs in the United States.[75] From a clinical perspective, some individual programs have demonstrated both improved prescribing practices in addition to some cost savings in areas such as control of vasodilator use, adherence to hypertension clinical practice guidelines and evidence-based treatment of gastrointestinal reflux disease (GERD) and related disorders.[76-78] Another study found improved prescribing practices regarding use of antipsychotics in long-term care.[68] Conversely, some studies have had only marginal clinical and economic results.[79,80] One study suggests academic detailing targeted toward resident physicians can be an effective strategy for improving rational prescribing.[81] Most published studies have limited generalizability due to publication in past decades, conduct in a specific HMOs or institution, and interventions performed by a low number of individuals; however, these same limitations could signal good internal validity of individual programs and customizing based on local need, a key principle of academic detailing.[68,76-80] Another concern regarding effectiveness of academic detailing is that the resources dedicated to these programs are much less than the resources dedicated toward pharmaceutical detailing on the part of industry.[65,66,74] A meta-analysis of academic detailing studies found a consistent small benefit in terms of changes in targeted practice behavior, but did not assess pharmacoeconomic outcomes.[82]

Pharmacy Role

With their strong academic background in drug information and drug literature evaluation, pharmacists can be ideally positioned to engage in academic detailing.[39,65,66] Indeed, many of the academic detailing programs described in clinical literature and the media are centered around a team of pharmacists.[65-67,69,76,80,81] Pharmacists with postgraduate training in drug information may be particularly well equipped for these types of positions as a result of their special skills in drug information service management, evidence-based medicine, and communications.[83] Pharmacists seeking to engage in academic detailing should critically assess local demographics and prescribing patterns in order to identify a specific detailing target, network and collaborate with established programs through organizations such as NaRCAD and local key stakeholders, and strive to build strong interpersonal relationships with target prescribers. Finally, as with any novel clinical service, identifying and monitoring key metrics is vital to justify direct and indirect costs of the program. Considering the mixed results of published studies and their remote time of publication, pharmacists participating in academic detailing are encouraged to share more current effectiveness information.

Conclusion

Drug promotion, including DTCA and promotion to health care professionals, represents significant expenditure on the part of the pharmaceutical industry. The controversial issues surrounding DTCA, in particular, continue to raise concerns about the benefits and harms of providing this type of information to patients. Detailing and direct advertisement to health care professionals continues to be an effective method of promotion. The FDA calls on health care professionals to play a key role in reporting drug promotions violations related to advertising, detailing, and continuing education. As drug promotional methods evolve, pharmacists will continue to serve both health care professionals and the public as a valuable source in deciphering and evaluating materials distributed by the pharmaceutical industry. Academic detailing may be one avenue for drug information specialists and others to combat the influence of drug promotions on prescribing.

Self-Assessment Questions

1. Which of the following activities are considered to be drug promotion?
   I. Advertisement to patients
   II. Advertisement to health care professionals
   III. Detailing to health care professionals
   a. I
   b. III
   c. I and II
   d. II and III
   e. I, II, and III

2. World Health Organization (WHO) recommendations support DTCA for which of the following product types:
   I. Nonprescription drugs
   II. Prescription drugs
   III. Vitamins and minerals
   a. I
   b. III
   c. I and II
   d. II and III
   e. I, II, and III

3. Which of the following regulations gave the FDA authority over prescription drug advertising?
   a. The Food and Drug Administration Amendments Act
   b. Kefauver-Harris Amendment
   c. The Food, Drug, and Cosmetic Act
   d. WHO Ethical Criteria for Medicinal Drug Promotion

4. Which type of DTCA includes only disease state information and, therefore, is regulated by the FTC?
   a. Help-seeking ads
   b. Reminder ads
   c. Product claim ads
   d. Television ads

5. Which of the following drugs are not permitted to be advertised using reminder ads?
   a. OTC medications
   b. Pediatric medications

    c. Boxed warning medications

    d. Prescription medications

6. Which of the following components of product claim ads are *not* required by FDA regulations?

    a. Fair balanced risks and benefits

    b. FDA's MedWatch statement

    c. Drug indication

    d. Mechanism of action

7. The PhRMA guiding principles for DTCA are currently enforced by the FDA.

    a. True

    b. False

8. According to the PhRMA guiding principles for DTCA which of the following ads are acceptable?

    a. A printed advertisement for a cholesterol medication that includes information about the patient assistance program sponsored by the company

    b. A television commercial portraying a child playing outside for a medication for an allergy medication indicated for adults

    c. An advertisement for an obesity medication that fails to mention diet and exercise as adjunctive therapy

    d. A television advertisement for an erectile dysfunction medication being aired during Saturday morning cartoons

9. Which of the following actions is the FDA not permitted to take against a drug company for DTCA violations?

    a. Request a corrected advertisement be broadcasted

    b. Seize the company's drug supply

    c. Issue warning letters

    d. Levy fines against the companies

10. Which of the following suggestions for improvement of DTCA was considered by Congress in 2008 but not passed?

    a. FDA reviewing all DTCA ads before released to the public

    b. Group of representatives creating public service announcements

    c. Two-year delay from product release to DTCA

    d. Standardized format for all DTCA

11. A pharmaceutical representative is permitted to discuss off-label use of prescription medications as long as those uses are supported by clinical literature.

    a. True

    b. False

12. All of the following are proposed means to combat potential for biased information discussed in pharmaceutical detailing *except*:
    a. Academic detailing to prescribers based on identified issues
    b. Developing conflict of interest policies outlining permitted interactions
    c. Education to physicians-in-training regarding information mastery
    d. Requiring detailing to be performed by a health care professional

13. The red herring logical fallacy refers to:
    a. Bandwagon effect
    b. Making the discussion personal
    c. Providing distracting, unrelated detail
    d. Referencing local content experts

14. Academic detailing programs ideally are designed to:
    a. Decrease use of brand medications
    b. Promote evidence-based prescribing
    c. Provide cost savings to third-party payers
    d. Punish low-performing physicians

15. Academic detailing programs in the United States have been shown to:
    a. Achieve the desired change in prescribing behavior
    b. Achieve national improvements in economic outcomes
    c. Decrease the rate of evidence-based prescribing
    d. Have similar success to pharmaceutical detailing

REFERENCES

1. Brownfield ED, Bernhardt JM, Phan JL, Williams MV, Parker RM. Direct-to-consumer drug advertisements on network television: an exploration of quantity, frequency, and placement. J Health Commun. 2004 Nov-Dec;9(6):491-7.
2. Bulik BS. Pharmaceutical marketing [Internet]. Chicago (IL): Ad Age; 2011 Oct 17 [cited 2013 April 14]. Available from: http://gaia.adage.com/images/bin/pdf/WPpharmmarketing_revise.pdf
3. Greene JA, Herzberg D. Hidden in plain sight marketing prescription drugs to consumers in the twentieth century. Am J Public Health. 2010 May;100(5):793-803.
4. Hansen RA, Chen SY, Gaynes BN, Maciejewski ML. Relationship of pharmaceutical promotion to antidepressant switching and adherence: a retrospective cohort study. Psychiatr Serv. 2010 Dec;61(12):1232-8.
5. Law MR, Soumerai SB, Adams AS, Majumdar SR. Costs and consequences of direct-to-consumer advertising for clopidogrel in Medicaid. Arch Intern Med. 2009 Nov 23;169(21):1969-74.
6. Mintzes B. Advertising of prescription-only medicines to the public: does evidence of benefit counterbalance harm? Annu Rev Public Health. 2012 Apr;33:259-77.

7. Norris P, Herxheimer A, Lexchin J, Mansfield P. Drug promotion. What we know, what we have yet to learn. Reviews of materials in the WHO/HAI database on drug promotion. EDM Research Series No. 032 [Internet]. World Health Organization and Health Action International, 2005 [cited 2013 Apr 14]. Available from: http://apps.who.int/medicinedocs/pdf/s8109e/s8109e.pdf

8. Ross JS, Kravitz RL. Direct-to-consumer television advertising: time to turn off the tube? J Gen Intern Med. 28(7):862-4.

9. Vastag B. FDA considers tightening regulations for direct-to-consumer advertising. J Natl Cancer Inst. 2005 Dec 21;97(24):1806-7.

10. Ventola CL. Direct-to-consumer pharmaceutical advertising: therapeutic or toxic? P T. 2011 Oct;36(10):669-84.

11. Womack CA. Ethical and epistemic issues in direct-to-consumer drug advertising: where is patient agency? Med Health Care Philos. 2013 May;16(2):275-80.

12. 2012 US pharmaceutical promotion spending [Internet]. Irvine (CA): Cegedim Strategic Data; [updated 2013 Jan; cited 2013 May 29]. Available from: https://www.cegedimstrategicdata.com/Downloads/Documents/White%20Papers/2012_promotional_spending.pdf

13. Othman N, Vitry A, Roughead EE. Quality of pharmaceutical advertisements in medical journals: a systematic review. PLoS One. 2009 Jul 22;4(7):e6350.

14. Palmer E. Top 10 drug advertising spends—Q1 2012 [Internet]. Fierce Pharma; 2012 Aug 9 [cited 2013 Apr 14]. Available from: http://www.fiercepharma.com/special-reports/top-10-drug-advertising-spends-q1-2012

15. Keeping watch over direct-to-consumer ads [Internet]. Silver Spring (MD): U.S. Food and Drug Administration; 2010 May [cited 2013 Apr 21]. Available from: http://www.fda.gov/downloads/ForConsumers/ConsumerUpdates/ucm107180.pdf

16. Ethical criteria for medical drug promotion [Internet]. Geneva: World Health Organization; 1988 [cited 2013 Apr 20]. Available from: http://apps.who.int/medicinedocs/documents/whozip08e/whozip08e.pdf

17. PhRMA guiding principles direct to consumer advertisements about prescription medicines [Internet]. Washington, DC: PhRMA; [updated 2008 Dec; cited 2013 Apr 18]. Available from: http://www.phrma.org/sites/default/files/pdf/phrmaguidingprinciplesdec08final.pdf

18. Dorn SD, Farley JF, Hansen RA, Shah ND, Sandler RS. Direct-to-consumer and physician promotion of tegaserod correlated with physician visits, diagnoses, and prescriptions. Gastroenterology. 2009 Aug;137(2):518-24.

19. Basics of drug ads [Internet]. Silver Spring (MD): U.S. Food and Drug Administration; [updated 2012 Sep 13; cited 2013 Apr 21]. Available from: http://www.fda.gov/Drugs/ResourcesForYou/Consumers/PrescriptionDrugAdvertising/ucm072077.htm

20. Correct help-seeking ad [Internet]. Silver Spring (MD): U.S. Food and Drug Administration; [updated 2012 Sep 13; cited 2013 Apr 21]. Available from: http://www.fda.gov/Drugs/ResourcesForYou/Consumers/PrescriptionDrugAdvertising/ucm082288.htm

21. Frosch DL, Krueger PM, Hornik RC, Cronholm PF, Barg FK. Creating demand for prescription drugs: a content analysis of television direct-to-consumer advertising. Ann Fam Med. 2007 Jan-Feb;5(1):6-13.

22. Reminder ad (correct) [Internet]. Silver Spring (MD): U.S. Food and Drug Administration; [updated 2012 Sep 13; cited 2013 Apr 21]. Available from: http://www.fda.gov/Drugs/ResourcesForYou/Consumers/PrescriptionDrugAdvertising/ucm083573.htm

23. Sumpradit N, Ascione FJ, Bagozzi RP. A cross-media content analysis of motivational themes in direct-to-consumer prescription drug advertising. Clin Ther. 2004 Jan;26(1):135-54.

24. Prescription drug advertising: questions and answers [Internet]. Silver Spring (MD): U.S. Food and Drug Administration; [updated 2012 Sep 13; cited 2013 Apr 21]. Available from: http://www.fda.gov/Drugs/ResourcesForYou/Consumers/PrescriptionDrugAdvertising/UCM076768.htm

25. Kefauver-Harris amendments [Internet]. Silver Spring (MD): U.S. Food and Drug Administration; 2012 Oct 10 [updated 2013 Apr 11; cited 2013 Apr 27]. Available from: http://www.fda.gov/ForConsumers/ConsumerUpdates/ucm322856.htm

26. The impact of direct-to-consumer advertising [Internet]. Silver Spring (MD): U.S. Food and Drug Administration; [updated 2013 Apr 12; cited 2013 Apr 27]. Available from: http://www.fda.gov/Drugs/ResourcesForYou/Consumers/ucm143562.htm

27. CFR-Code of Federal Regulations Title 21: Part 202—prescription drug advertising [Internet]. Silver Spring (MD): U.S. Food and Drug Administration; [updated 2012 Apr 1; cited 2013 Apr 27]. Available from: http://www.accessdata.fda.gov/scripts/cdrh/cfdocs/cfCFR/CFRSearch.cfm?fr=202.1

28. Product claim ad (correct) [Internet]. Silver Spring (MD): U.S. Food and Drug Administration; [updated 2012 Sep 13; cited 2013 Apr 21]. Available from: http://www.fda.gov/Drugs/ResourcesForYou/Consumers/PrescriptionDrugAdvertising/ucm082284.htm

29. Warning letters and notice of violation letters to pharmaceutical companies [Internet]. Silver Spring (MD): U.S. Food and Drug Administration; [updated 2012 Jan 25; cited 2013 Apr 21]. Available from: http://www.fda.gov/Drugs/GuidanceComplianceRegulatoryInformation/EnforcementActivitiesbyFDA/WarningLettersandNoticeofViolationLetterstoPharmaceuticalCompanies/default.htm

30. Lexchin J. Statistics in drug advertising: what they reveal is suggestive what they hide is vital. Int J Clin Pract. 2010 Jul;64(8):1015-8.

31. Public Health Advisory: tegaserod maleate (marketed as Zelnorm) [Internet]. Silver Spring (MD): U.S. Food and Drug Administration; 2007 Mar 30 [updated 2010 June 23; cited 2013 Apr 27]. Available from: http://www.fda.gov/Drugs/DrugSafety/PostmarketDrugSafetyInformationforPatientsandProviders/DrugSafetyInformationforHeathcareProfessionals/PublicHealthAdvisories/ucm051284.htm

32. Aikin KJ, O'Donoghue AC, Swasy JL, Sullivan HW. Randomized trial of risk information formats in direct-to-consumer prescription drug advertisements. Med Decis Making. 2011 Nov-Dec;31(6):E23-33.

33. Reporting misleading Rx drug promotion [Internet]. Silver Spring (MD): U.S. Food and Drug Administration; [cited 2013 Apr 17]. Available from: http://www.fda.gov/downloads/Drugs/GuidanceComplianceRegulatoryInformation/Surveillance/PrescriptionDrugAdvertisingandPromotionalLabeling/UCM209847.pdf

34. Prescription drug advertising: questions to ask yourself [Internet]. Silver Spring (MD): U.S. Food and Drug Administration; [updated 2009 Jun 24; cited 2013 Apr 21]. Available from: http://www.fda.gov/Drugs/ResourcesForYou/Consumers/PrescriptionDrugAdvertising/ucm071915.htm

35. Prescription drug advertising [Internet]. Silver Spring (MD): U.S. Food and Drug Administration; [updated 2012 Sep 20; cited 2013 Apr 26]. Available from: http://www.fda.gov/Drugs/ResourcesForYou/Consumers/PrescriptionDrugAdvertising/default.htm

36. Bad Ad program FDA aims to keep drug promotion truthful [Internet]. Silver Spring (MD): U.S. Food and Drug Administration; 2011 Apr [cited 2013 Apr 26]. Available from: http://www.fda.gov/downloads/ForConsumers/ConsumerUpdates/UCM211935.pdf

37. Shaughnessy AF, Slawson DC, Bennett JH. Separating the wheat from the chaff: Identifying fallacies in pharmaceutical promotion. J Gen Intern Med. 1994;9:563-8.

38. Gagnon MA, Lexchin J. The cost of pushing pills: a new estimate of pharmaceutical promotion expenditures in the United States. PLoS Med. 2008;5(1):29-33.

39. National Resource Center for Academic Detailing. About academic detailing [Internet]. Boston (MA): Brigham and Women's Hospital and Harvard Medical School, Department of Medicine, Division of Pharmacoepidemiology and Pharmacoeconomics; [cited 2013 Apr 26]. Available from: http://www.narcad.org/about/aboutad/.

40. Abood RR. Pharmacy practice and the law. 7th ed. Burlington (MA): Jones & Bartlett Learning; 2014.

41. Greenwood K. The ban on "off-label" pharmaceutical promotion: constitutionally permissible prophylaxis against false or misleading commercial speech? Am J Law Med. 2011;37:278-98.

42. Kesselheim AS, Avorn J. Pharmaceutical promotion to physicians and First Amendment rights. New Engl J Med. 2008;358:1727-32.

43. Pharmaceutical Research and Manufacturers of America. Code on interactions with health care professionals [Internet]. Washington, DC: Pharmaceutical Research and Manufacturers of America; [cited 2013 Apr 29]. Available from: http://www.phrma.org/code-on-interactions-with-healthcare-professionals

44. Sierles FS, Bordkey AC, Cleary LM, et al. Medical students' exposure to and attitudes about drug company interactions. JAMA. 2005;294(9):1034-42.

45. Hodges B. Interactions with the pharmaceutical industry: experiences and attitudes of psychiatry residents, interns, and clerks. CMAJ. 1995;153(5):553-9.

46. Clauson KA, Khanfar NM, Polen HH, Gibson F. Nurse prescribers' interactions with and perceptions of pharmaceutical sales representatives. J Clin Nurs. 2008;18:228-33.

47. Alkhateeb FM, Khanfar NM, Clauson KA. Characteristics of physicians who frequently see pharmaceutical sales representatives. J Hosp Mark Public Relations. 2009;19:2-14.

48. Hansen RA, Chen SY, Gaynes BN, Maciejewski ML. Relationship of pharmaceutical promotion to antidepressant switching and adherence: a retrospective cohort study. Psychiatr Serv. 2010;61(12):1232-8.

49. Bowman MA, Pearle DL. Changes in drug prescribing patterns related to commercial company funding of continuing medical education. J Cont Educ Health Prof. 1988;8:13-20.

50. Spurling GK, Mansfield PR, Montgomery BD, et al. Information from pharmaceutical companies and the quality, quantity, and cost of physicians' prescribing: a systematic review. PLoS Med. 2010;7(10):e1000352.

51. Chren MM, Landefeld CS. Physicians' behavior and their interactions with drug companies. A controlled study of physicians who requested additions to a hospital drug formulary. JAMA. 1994;271:684-9.

52. Lexchin J. Models for financing the regulation of pharmaceutical promotion. Global Health [Internet]. 2012 Jul 11 [cited 2013 Apr 26]; 8:24. Available from: http://www.globalizationandhealth.com/content/8/1/24

53. Epstein AJ, Busch SH, Busch AB, Asch DA, Barry CL. Does exposure to conflict of interest policies in psychiatry residency affect antidepressant prescribing? Med Care. 2013;51(2):199-203.

54. Grande D, Frosch DL, Perkins AW, Kahn BE. Effect of exposure to small pharmaceutical promotional items on treatment preferences. Arch Intern Med. 2009;169(9):887-93.

55. Fugh-Berman AJ, Scialli AR, Bell AM. Why lunch matters: assessing physicians' perceptions about industry relationships. J Cont Ed Health Prof. 2010;30(3):197-204.

56. Shankar PR, Singh KK, Piryani RM. Knowledge, attitude and skills before and after a module on pharmaceutical promotion in a Nepalese medical school. BMC Res Notes [Internet]. 2012;5(8). Available from: http://www.biomedcentral.com/1756-0500/5/8

57. Shankar PR, Singh KK, Piryani RM. Student feedback about the skeptic doctor, a module on pharmaceutical promotion. J Educ Eval Health Prof [Internet]. 2011 Aug 11 [cited 2013 Apr 26]; 8(11). Available from: http://dx.doi.org/10.3352/jeehp.2011.8.11

58. U.S. Food and Drug Administration. Office of Prescription Drug Promotion [Internet]. Silver Spring (MD): U.S. Food and Drug Administration, Center for Drug Evaluation and Research, Office of Prescription Drug Promotion; [updated 2011 Oct 17; cited 2013 Apr 29]. Available from: http://www.fda.gov/Drugs/GuidanceComplianceRegulatoryInformation/Surveillance/DrugMarketingAdvertisingandCommunications/default.htm

59. Reptrax. About Reptrax [Internet]. Flower Mound (TX): IntelliCentrics, Inc.; [cited 2013 Apr 29]. Available from: https://www.reptrax.com/about/reptrax

60. American Society of Health-Systems Pharmacists. ASHP guidelines on pharmacists' relationships with industry [Internet]. Bethesda (MD): American Society of Health-Systems Pharmacists, ASHP Council on Legal and Public Affairs; 1991 Nov 20 [updated 2001; cited 2013 Apr 29]. Available from: http://www.ashp.org/Import/PRACTICEANDPOLICY/PolicyPositionsGuidelinesBestPractices/BrowsebyDocumentType/GuidelinesMain.aspx

61. American Medical Association. AMA's Code of Medical Ethics: 9.011 Continuing medical education [Internet]. Chicago (IL): American Medical Association, Council Ethical and Judicial Affairs; 1993 Dec [updated 1996 Jun; cited 2013 Apr 29]. Available from: http://www.ama-assn.org/ama/pub/physician-resources/medical-ethics/code-medical-ethics.page

62. Slawson DC, Shaughnessy AF, Bennett JH. Becoming a medical information master: feeling good about not knowing everything. J Fam Pract. 1994;38(5):505-9.

63. Yonemori K, Hirakawa A, Ando M, et al. Content analysis of oncology-related pharmaceutical advertising in a peer-reviewed medical journal. PLoS One. 2012;7(8):e44393.

64. Kesselheim AS. Covert pharmaceutical promotion in free medical journals. CMAJ. 2011;183(5):534-5.
65. The Hilltop Institute. Academic detailing: a review of the literature and states' approaches [Internet]. Baltimore (MD): University of Maryland, Baltimore County, The Hilltop Institute; 2009 Jan 18 [cited 2013 Apr 29]. Available from: http://www.hilltopinstitute.org/publication_view.cfm?pubID=270&st=tbl_Publications
66. Reck J. A template for establishing and administering prescriber support and education programs: a collaborative, service-based approach for achieving maximum impact [Internet]. Hallowell (ME): Prescription Policy Choices; 2008 Jul [cited 2013 Apr 26]. Available from: http://www.policychoices.org/reports.shtml
67. Levinson W, Dunn PM. Counter-detailing. JAMA. 1984;251(16):2084.
68. Avorn J, Soumerai SB, Everitt DE, et al. A randomized trial of a program to reduce the use of psychoactive drugs in nursing homes. N Engl J Med. 1992;327:168-73.
69. Greg ME. Confessions of a pharmacy counter-detailer. Drug Topics [Internet]. 2011 Apr 15 [cited 2013 May 23]. Available from: http://drugtopics.modernmedicine.com/drug-topics/news/modernmedicine/modern-medicine-now/confessions-pharmacy-counter-detailer
70. Pennsylvania Department of Aging. PACE, PACENET, and PACE Plus Medicare [Internet]. Harrisburg (PA): Pennsylvania Department of Aging; [cited 2013 Apr 26]. Available from: http://www.aging.state.pa.us/portal/server.pt/community/pace_and_affordable_medications/.
71. SCORxE. What is SCORxE? [Internet]. Columbia (SC): South Carolina College of Pharmacy, SCORxE; [cited 2013 Apr 26]. Available from: http://www.sccp.sc.edu/centers/SCORxE/.
72. National Resource Center for Academic Detailing. About us [Internet]. Boston (MA): Brigham and Women's Hospital and Harvard Medical School, Department of Medicine, Division of Pharmacoepidemiology and Pharmacoeconomics; [cited 2013 Apr 26]. Available from: http://www.narcad.org/about
73. National Resource Center for Academic Detailing. Our services [Internet]. Boston (MA): Brigham and Women's Hospital and Harvard Medical School, Department of Medicine, Division of Pharmacoepidemiology and Pharmacoeconomics; [cited 2013 Apr 26]. Available from: http://www.narcad.org/services
74. Pew Prescription Project. Cost effectiveness of prescriber education ("academic detailing") programs [Internet]. Boston (MA): Pew Prescription Project; 2008 Mar 12 [cited 2013 Apr 26]. Available from: http://www.communitycatalyst.org/.
75. Soumerai SB, Avorn J. Economic and policy analysis of university-based drug "detailing." Med Care. 1986;24(4):313-31.
76. Avorn J, Soumerai SB. Improving drug-therapy decisions through educational outreach. N Engl J Med. 1983;308(24):1457-63.
77. Simon SR, Rodriguez HP, Majumdar SR, Kleinman K, Warner C, Salem-Schatz S, et al. Econcomic analysis of a randomized trial of academic detailing interventions to improve use of antihypertensive medication. J Clin Hypertens (Greenwich). 2007;9(1):15-20.
78. Ofman JJ, Segal R, Russell WL, Cook DJ, Sandhu M, Maue SK, et al. A randomized trial of an acid-peptic disease management program in a managed care environment. Am J Managed Care. 2003;9(6):425-33.

79. Fanzini L, Boom J, Nelson C. Cost-effectiveness analysis of a practice-based immunization education intervention. Ambul Pediatr. 2007;7(2):167-75.
80. Farris KB, Kirking DM, Shimp LA, Opdycke RAC. Design and results of a group counter-detailing DUR education program. Pharm Res. 1996;13(10):1445-52.
81. Wall GC, Smith HL, Craig SR, Yost WJ. Structured pharmaceutical representative interactions and counterdetailing sessions as components of medical resident education. J Pharm Pract. 2013;26:151.
82. O'Brien MA, Rogers S, Jamtvedt G, Oxman AD, Odgaard-Jensen J, Kristoffersen DT, et al. Educational outreach visits: effects on professional practice and health care outcomes. Cochrane Database Syst Rev. 2007;17(4):CD000409.
83. American Society of Health-System Pharmacists. Educational outcomes, goals, and objectives for a drug information PGY2 pharmacy residency [Internet]. Bethesda (MD): American Society of Health-System Pharmacists; 2008 Mar [cited 2013 Apr 26]. Available from: http://www.ashp.org/menu/Accreditation/ResidencyAccreditation.aspx

24

Chapter Twenty-Four

Pharmacy Informatics: Enabling Safe and Efficacious Medication Use

Joshua C. Hollingsworth • Brent I. Fox

Learning Objectives

After completing this chapter, the reader will be able to

- List the activities that occur at each step of the medication use process.
- Define pharmacy informatics and other core informatics terms.
- Discuss the role of pharmacy informatics at each step of the medication use process.
- Describe challenges implementing computerized provider order entry.
- Describe the components of an e-prescribing system.
- Describe the role of the three primary components of a clinical decision support system.
- Describe limitations of health information technology that is used during the transcription step of the medication use process.
- Compare and contrast the health information technology used during dispensing in acute care and community pharmacy settings.
- Define the role of bar code medication administration.
- Describe the role of the three primary components of a clinical surveillance system.
- Describe the changing role of the patient in the United States (U.S.) health care system.
- Explain the importance of interoperability to the future of the U.S. health care system, including the role of the U.S. government.
- Describe the goal and structure of Meaningful Use.
- Define privacy, security, and confidentiality as they relate to protected health information.

Key Concepts

1 The medication use process is a system of interconnected parts that work together to achieve the common goal of safe and effective medication therapy.

2 All pharmacists are impacted by the electronic information systems that make up pharmacy informatics in virtually every aspect of practice.

3 The two broad categories of information used in pharmacy informatics, as well as other clinical informatics domains, are patient-specific information and knowledge-based information.

4 The vision of health care is becoming more patient centered.

5 The current health care system is decentralized and fragmented. Because of this, significant communication gaps exist when multiple health care institutions provide care for the same patient. Substantial evidence suggests that more effective communication would improve patient care and reduce medical errors, such as adverse drug events.

6 The desired result of interoperable systems and electronic health records (EHRs) is to readily provide all health practitioners in all locations, including the pharmacy, with access to information about a patient's care, as needed.

7 The Center for Medicare and Medicaid Services (CMS) created the Meaningful Use program to incentivize the use of certified EHR technology. The Meaningful Use program focuses on (1) improving quality, safety, and efficiency, (2) engaging patients and their families, (3) improving care coordination, as well as public and population health, and (4) maintaining privacy and security of protected health information (PHI). In general, Meaningful Use criteria address the use of specific components of EHRs (like prescribing systems) to achieve specific outcomes, which can be process oriented or patient oriented.

Introduction

Pharmacists of today have a multitude of responsibilities within their scope of practice. Whether verifying and filling prescriptions, compounding medications, advising patients on proper medication use, or collaborating with other practitioners in the care of patients, at the forefront of a pharmacist's responsibilities is a focus on the safe and effective use of medication therapy. Specifically, pharmacists aim to maximize patient safety while minimizing medication misadventures, such as medication errors and adverse drug events, which are covered in Chapters 15 and 16. And, given the sheer amount of information involved and available today, this focus on safety and efficacy can only be reasonably obtained via pharmacists' management of the information and related information systems involved in support of the medication use process. Pharmacists, regardless of practice setting, must be able to input, access, share, evaluate, and utilize information in these systems to support their efforts in patient care.

Medication Use Process

❶ *The medication use process is a system of interconnected parts that work together to achieve the common goal of safe and effective medication therapy.* The interconnected parts include the people, systems, procedures, and policies that manage medications and related information in patient care. It should be noted here that Chapter 14 further covers a portion of the medication use process, specifically in the context of quality improvement. The medication use process is cyclical in nature and begins with the prescribing stage. In this stage, the practitioner assesses whether medication therapy is warranted and, if so, orders therapy accordingly. The health information technology (HIT) utilized at the prescribing stage includes computerized provider order entry (CPOE), electronic prescribing (e-prescribing), and clinical decision support systems (CDSS), including various medication references.

In the next stage of the medication use process, the transcription stage, the ordered medication enters the pharmacy computer system, a pharmacist assesses the appropriateness of the order, and any issues or discrepancies are addressed. HIT tools used at the transcription stage include CPOE and e-prescribing. Various drug information references, often electronic in nature, may be used and may be built into the systems (e.g., drug interaction screening systems). Next is the dispensing stage. Here, the medication is prepared and distributed from the pharmacy, either directly to the patient or to a health care provider. There are many HIT tools utilized in the dispensing stage, including bar code verification, automated dispensing cabinets, syringe fillers, total parenteral nutrition compounders, and other robotics.

Following the dispensing stage is the administration stage in which the medication is reviewed for appropriateness and then given to, or taken by, the patient. Health care providers, caregivers, the patient, and the patient's family may be involved in the administration stage, depending on the setting. HIT tools used here may include point-of-care bar coding, electronic medication administration records (eMARs), and intelligent infusion (smart) pumps. The final stage in the medication use process is monitoring. At the monitoring stage, the patient's response to the medication therapy is assessed, outcomes are documented, and interventions are made as necessary. HIT tools used here include adverse drug event (ADE) surveillance, antibiotic/drug surveillance, and rules engines. The following is a brief description of some of the HIT tools mentioned above[1]:

- **Adverse drug event (ADE) monitoring:** Computer programs that use electronic data and predetermined rules to identify when an ADE may have occurred or is about to occur to a patient within a hospital. This is separate from such programs as MedWatch (see Chapter 15), which is used to report adverse effects to the U.S. Food and Drug Administration (FDA).
- **Automated dispensing cabinets (ADCs):** Automated devices with a range of functions. Core capabilities include medication storage and retrieval for administration to patients, especially in patient care areas, as well as audit trails of cabinet access. Other functions can include medication charging and automated inventory management.
- **Bar code verification:** The use of bar code scanning to ensure that the correct drug, strength, and dosage form were dispensed in the drug selection process and the five rights of medication administration (i.e., right patient, right drug, right dose, right route, right time) are followed at the point of care.
- **Clinical decision support systems (CDSS):** Computer programs that augment clinical decision making by combining referential information with patient-specific information to prevent negative actions and update providers of patient status.
- **Computerized provider order entry (CPOE):** A process allowing medical provider instructions to be electronically entered for the treatment of patients who are under a provider's care.
- **Electronic medication administration record (eMAR):** An electronic version of the traditional medication administration record. It supports patient safety by incorporating clinical decision support and bar-coded medication administration. It also enables real-time documentation and billing of medication administration.
- **Electronic prescribing (e-prescribing):** The electronic process in which a prescription is initially entered in an electronic format and then verified and processed in an electronic format, resulting in a labeled medication product, supportive documentation, and an updated, sharable patient electronic medication profile.
- **Intelligent infusion (smart) pumps:** Infusion pumps containing software designed to help eliminate pump programming errors through the use of standardized drug databases and dosing parameters.
- **Rules engines:** Computer programs, similar to ADE monitoring systems, with built-in, logic rules designed to aid in monitoring specific aspects of patient care. For example, a rule developed in an attempt to prevent hypoglycemia in patients receiving insulin may require documentation of the patient's meal being delivered prior to the patient receiving mealtime insulin.

Pharmacy Informatics

The term informatics simply refers to the use of computers to manage data and information. Informatics exists at the intersection of people, information, and technology.[2] Pharmacy informatics refers to a form of clinical informatics that is applied to the discipline of pharmacy. More specifically, **pharmacy informatics** focuses on the use of information, information systems, and automation technology to ensure safe and effective medication usage. ❷ *All pharmacists are impacted by the electronic information systems that make up pharmacy informatics in virtually every aspect of practice.* For example, patient records, medication administration and usage information, insurance information, as well as laboratory tests and results are just a few of the categories of information that are managed in electronic environments.

❸ *The two broad categories of information used in pharmacy informatics, as well as other clinical informatics domains, are patient-specific information and knowledge-based information.*[3] Patient-specific information, which is created and applied in the process of caring for individual patients, includes medication and medical histories, laboratory test results, radiology interpretations, immunization histories, physical assessments, and other information that is unique to the specific patient. Today, this information is generated and housed in health care facilities, such as pharmacies, hospitals, and clinics. Consumer health informatics, a rapidly growing field, has created an environment in which patients themselves are also generating and managing health-related information in addition to and outside of these traditional settings. Aspects of consumer health informatics can include Internet-based direct-to-consumer advertising (see Chapter 23) and research activities.

Knowledge-based information, on the other hand, forms the scientific basis of health care and includes referential information (about medications, procedures, disease states, etc.), clinical practice guidelines, as well as many other domains of health and medical knowledge.[3] Pharmacists and other healthcare providers make patient care decisions based on a combination of patient-specific and knowledge-based information, a process that can often be a real challenge. Informatics addresses this challenge by using information technology (IT) to manage information, and the medication use process is the context in which pharmacists work to promote safe and effective medication therapy. The following sections describe the role of pharmacists, pharmacy informatics, and other HIT in the medication use process.

Order entry

In the 1999 report *To Err Is Human: Building a Safer Health System*, the Institute of Medicine (IOM) estimated that 44,000 to 98,000 deaths occur each year in U.S. hospitals due to adverse drug events (ADEs). Chapters 15 and 16 provide a closer examination of adverse drug events and the larger topic of medication misadventures; brief statistics are provided here. Nineteen percent of the ADEs were deemed to be due to medication errors, by far the largest category of adverse events noted in the IOM report. The causes of errors and patient injury related to order entry identified in the report included illegible handwritten reports, manual order entry, and the use of nonstandard abbreviations.[4] Further, a study by Bates and associates,[5] which looked at more than 4000 hospital admissions over a 6-month period, found that errors resulting in preventable ADEs occur most often (i.e., 56% of cases) at the prescribing stage of the medication use process. As such, it is imperative that pharmacists identify and prevent ADEs at this early stage in the medication use process. The three HIT tools that can aid in doing so include CPOE, electronic prescribing, and CDSS.

Computerized Provider Order Entry

CPOE, as described earlier, is the process allowing medical provider instructions to be entered electronically for the treatment of patients under a provider's care. Orders entered via a CPOE system are communicated to the medical staff and appropriate departments over a computer network. CPOE eliminates illegible handwriting, decreases medical errors as well as the delay in order completion, improves patient care, and is, therefore, an important component in health care information systems.[6,7] Although features of a CPOE system may vary, ideal features are described here.

Provider orders should be standardized across the organization (see Chapter 12), but may also be individualized based on the provider or the provider's specialty through the use of order sets. Orders should be communicated to all departments and health care providers involved in the patient's care. Patient-centered decision support, including display of the patient's medical history, current test results, and evidence-based guidelines to support treatment options, should be readily available. CPOE systems must support clinical workflows through algorithms that provide clear, concise, and actionable advice and warnings. The order entry process should be simple and allow efficient use by new or infrequent users. Access must be secure, and a permanent record of access needs to be created with an electronic signature (i.e., any legally recognized means of indicating that a person accepts the contents of an electronic message). The CPOE system should be portable, accepting and managing orders from all departments through various devices, including desktop and laptop computers, smartphones, and tablets. Data should be collected for training, planning, and analysis of patient safety events as part of ongoing quality initiatives. Diagnoses should be linked to orders at the time of order entry in order to support drug-condition checking, improve documentation, and support appropriate charges. Like all HIT systems, appropriate backup and downtime procedures should be established and routinized.

Despite having the ability to decrease ADEs, CPOE also potentially introduces new types of errors.[8] Inexperienced providers and staff using CPOE may actually cause slower order entry and person-to-person communication, especially at first. Alerts and warnings that appear too frequently may lead to **alert fatigue**, a situation in which a provider ignores or overrides CDSS messages. Many other types of errors can occur, serving as a strong reminder that all healthcare providers share responsibility to ensure safe use of CPOE and other HIT systems. As such, implementation of CPOE in a complex medical environment can take years and requires ongoing design changes in order to adequately fit unique care settings. Given these issues, as well as providers' resistance to change and the costs involved, adoption of this technology by providers and hospitals in the United States has been slow. However, use of CPOE is expected to increase as more hospitals become aware of the financial benefits of CPOE and as hospitals comply with **Meaningful Use** criteria (see Key Concept #7 and below). A study by RAND Health found that the U.S. health care system could save $70 billion or more annually, as well as reduce ADEs and improve the quality of care, if CPOE and other HIT were widely adopted.[9]

• For wide adoption to be realized, there are certain barriers that must be overcome. In 2004, Poon and colleagues published a report identifying and addressing these barriers.[10] First is provider and organization resistance to change and CPOE adoption. Reasons cited for this resistance vary and include perceptions such as paper methods are faster or more efficient, and that implementation attempts would be costly and unsuccessful. The authors of the report identified four key areas on which to focus to overcome resistance. Strong hospital leadership is a necessary factor of implementation of CPOE. Physician champions (i.e., well-respected physicians) should be identified and involved. Workflow concerns should be addressed and users should be reassured throughout the implementation process. And lastly, organizational expertise, being those providers who are more comfortable with IT or who have had experience with CPOE, should be leveraged.

• The second major barrier identified is the high cost of CPOE implementation and lack of capital. Strategies identified to overcome high costs include realigning the hospital's priorities to focus on patient safety, leveraging external influences such as published literature to increase awareness about patient safety, and measuring CPOE's impact on hospital efficiency. The last major barrier identified was selection of a specific CPOE product from the many options available. As such, the report's authors concluded that the product or company selected should be committed to the CPOE market, willing and able to adapt products to specific hospital workflows, able to provide tools that help evaluate product functionality, as well as able to provide information and references for other CPOE systems implemented by the company.

Electronic Prescribing (e-prescribing)

Although many definitions exist, e-prescribing is commonly defined as ambulatory CPOE. A more precise definition would be a prescription entered by a prescriber directly into an electronic format using agreed-upon standards that is securely transmitted to the pharmacy that the patient chooses. Faxes and printed prescriptions are not e-prescriptions. One of the primary early challenges to nationwide e-prescribing was a network on which to transfer the prescriptions. Surescripts provides the connection network and verification between prescribers, insurance providers, and pharmacies. The National Council for Prescription Drug Programs (NCPDP), which is accredited by the American National Standards Institute, provides the standards for provider identification and telecommunication of pharmacy claims in this process.[11]

Aside from the prescriber, Surescripts, and the pharmacy, there are many other components that make up an e-prescribing system. These components include the computer software, the hardware needed to run the software, the organizations that support transmission and sharing of data, data standardization, authorization of payment, communications to the pharmacy, and the processing of prescriptions within the pharmacy. The e-prescribing software should provide functionality to support accurate, efficient, and safe entry and transmission of prescriptions. The U.S. government provides incentives to health care providers who implement e-prescribing and electronic medical records (EMRs) that meet certain minimal requirements. Such functionality includes generating a complete medication list; support for prescription ordering, printing, and electronic transmission; inclusion of alerts for unsafe conditions (e.g., allergies); providing information on lower cost, therapeutic alternatives; and providing information on formulary and patient eligibility based on the patient's drug plan.[12]

The overall functionality of the e-prescribing software depends on the management of multiple databases. A drug database is necessary and should include decision support functions, such as therapeutic categories, drug–drug and drug–disease interactions, dose range checking, as well as allergy warnings. A pharmacy database, which supports selection of and communication with the patient's specific pharmacy, is needed. A user database, consisting of a list of prescribers and other users along with their authority to prescribe, Drug Enforcement Agency (DEA) number, and other identifiers, is also needed. A patient database, listing patients and all pertinent patient information to support e-prescribing functions, must be included and managed. Other databases that are necessary include medication insurance plans/formularies and medication profile information for individual patients. Depending on the functionality of the e-prescribing software, additional clinical information may also be available, such as laboratory results, patient problems and diagnoses, and information from prior visits.

To fully comprehend the functionality of an e-prescribing system, an understanding of prescribing workflow is necessary. The first step is patient registration and eligibility verification, which generally occurs prior to or at the time the patient arrives for an appointment. Here, the patient's insurance coverage and address are verified, and the patient is put on a readily available selection list within the e-prescribing system for prescribers. The patient's medication history and prescription eligibility, which are generally retrieved from Surescripts, are assessed next. Following this is the medication entry step. Since prescription entry can vary greatly between and within practices, the e-prescribing system should support quickly transitioning between patients, data gathering, and ordering. Portable devices and the ability to quickly log into an immobile device (e.g., desktop computer) are needed to support this type of workflow. Although not yet addressed by federal regulations, delegating the task of medication entry to support staff introduces the potential for errors as reading and translating written prescriptions is often involved in this approach. The next step in the prescribing workflow is prescriber selection of the pharmacy to which the prescriptions should be sent. A common error at this stage is selection of the wrong pharmacy from the searchable database. Once the pharmacy is selected, the prescription is transmitted to the pharmacy using standard NCPDP SCRIPT interface transactions. Although federal law, as of June 1 2010, does allow controlled substances to be prescribed electronically, not all states have authorized such prescribing, particularly for Schedule II controlled substances.[13]

One area that has great potential for improvement with e-prescribing is the renewal authorization process (i.e., authorization by the prescriber for additional refills). Prior to e-prescribing, renewal authorization required multiple telephone calls and was highly interruptive. Now, pharmacies can initiate electronic renewal requests, which can be electronically processed and returned by the prescriber.

Clinical Decision Support Systems

According to the American Medical Association, clinical decision support (CDS) is described as "providing clinicians, patients or individuals with knowledge and person specific or population information, intelligently filtered or presented at appropriate times, to foster better health processes, better individual patient care, and better population health."[14] CDSS are the computing systems that provide CDS. The three basic components of a CDSS include an inference engine, a knowledge base, and a communication mechanism. The inference engine, also known as the reasoning engine, forms the brain of the CDSS, working to link patient-specific information with information in the knowledge base. It evaluates the available information and determines what to present to the user. The knowledge base is composed of varied clinical knowledge, such as treatment guidelines, diagnoses, and drug–drug or drug–disease interactions. The communication mechanism allows entry of patient information and is responsible for communicating relevant information back to the clinician. A CDSS that checks a patient's age and immunization history against vaccination guidelines and then presents recommendations to a provider serves as a useful example.

CDS can be generated in a variety of forms, including alerts, reminders, information displays, CPOE, electronic templates, and guidelines. CDSS have been employed in many clinical care domains and have the ability to support a wide range of complex decisions at various stages in the patient care process. In terms of preventive care, CDSS can provide reminders for vaccinations, cancer screenings, cardiovascular risk reduction, as well as other preventive measures. A study by Shea and associates found a 77% increase in the use of preventive practices when computer reminders were used.[15] There are several CDSS that have been designed to help clinicians diagnose based on the signs and symptoms exhibited by a patient. These systems have the potential to reduce diagnostic errors, and should be linked with an EMR to achieve their full potential.[16] CDSS are used to provide evidence-based treatment at the point of care, often drawing upon evidence-based guidelines, which are covered in Chapter 7.

Medication decision support is a large portion of the knowledge base for any CDSS. Basic support in this area includes drug-allergy checking, basic dosing guidance, formulary decision support, duplicate therapy checking, and drug–drug interaction checking. In the case of formulary decision support, CDSS can prompt prescribers of the preferred medications (according to the hospital's or insurer's formulary) at the point in time in which they are selecting from available medications. This allows prescribers to implement agreed-upon formularies (see Chapter 12) within their practice settings with minimal disruption. More advanced decision support may include dosing suggestions for geriatric patients or patients with renal insufficiency, guidance for medication-related laboratory testing, drug–disease and drug–lab interaction checking, and drug-pregnancy contraindication checking. CDSS are also used for follow-up or corollary orders as well as adverse event monitoring. In fact, a study by Overhage et al. showed a 25% improvement in corollary orders (orders that are routine under certain situations, such as a stool softener when a patient is receiving a narcotic) with the use of CDSS.[17] The main benefits of CDSS use include the ability to decrease adverse drug events, costs, and length of patient stay as well as improve clinical workflow, provide useful information at the point of care, draw attention to possible drug interactions, and provide reminders of warranted follow-up interventions.

CDSS also have their limitations. For instance, developing and maintaining a comprehensive knowledge base is time consuming and resource intensive. CDSS need to communicate with other clinical information systems, such as EMRs, CPOE systems, and pharmacy systems. And excessive alerting can lead to alert fatigue and clinicians ignoring the warnings.

Transcription

Transcription occurs when prescribed medications are transferred, either manually or electronically, to the pharmacy. Once received, pharmacists must interpret the medication order and make an assessment in regard to any drug-related problems. The goal of this process is to transform the order into a dispensable form that can be safely and correctly interpreted at the administration step. Pharmacists may use CDSS, pharmacy computer systems, and evidence-based medicine tools at this stage to perform their cognitive and administrative functions.

Pharmacists have traditionally relied on CDSS within the pharmacy information system to support safe and efficacious decision making regarding the filling of prescriptions. Although the use of CDSS at the prescribing stage helps improve the quality of orders received by the pharmacy, problems still exist with orders originating from CPOE systems and e-prescriptions. For instance, CPOE systems, while reducing certain errors, have been to found to increase other types of errors. A study by Koppel and associates found that a widely used CPOE system actually facilitated 22 types of medication error risks, including pharmacy inventory displays being mistaken for dosage guidelines, fragmented CPOE displays that prevent full view of a patient's medications, and inflexible ordering formats that result in wrong orders.[18] As such, pharmacists must remain diligent in their review of orders prior to dispensing.

One of the main aspects of support provided by pharmacy CDSS software is information pertaining to drug–drug interactions (DDIs). This information is meant to augment and increase pharmacists' ability to detect clinically significant interactions. However, a study by Saverno and associates, which analyzed the ability of pharmacy information systems and associated CDS to detect DDIs at 64 Arizona pharmacies, indicated that many pharmacy CDSS perform suboptimally in terms of identifying well-known, clinically relevant interactions. Specifically, only 28% of the participating pharmacies accurately identified the interactions and noninteractions involved in the study's fictitious patient medication orders.[19] This further reiterates the point that pharmacists must remain diligent when reviewing orders to be dispensed.

Dispensing

Medications are prepared and distributed to patients in the dispensing stage of the medication use process. The actual activities involved at this step vary depending on the setting (i.e., institutional or community pharmacy). However, there are many similarities shared between the two settings, including acquiring medications from a supplier, stocking medications based on needs, as well as safely and accurately preparing and dispensing medications based on the transcribed order. Further, there are many HIT tools utilized at the dispensing stage in both settings. That said, the two settings also have their differences when it comes to dispensing and the HIT tools used in the process.

ACUTE CARE PHARMACY SETTING

Many aspects related to dispensing from an acute care pharmacy (i.e., institutional pharmacy) can be automated by HIT. All automated systems utilized must be able to uniquely identify managed products, receive and interpret medication orders, perform appropriate dose calculations as needed, and report transactions to other automated systems for billing or other purposes. In order for this to occur, all prescription medication packaging must be marked with an assigned, 10-digit National Drug Code (NDC), a requirement by the Food and Drug Administration (FDA). All NDCs consist of three parts: a labeler code, a drug code, and a package code in one of the following configurations: 4-4-2, 5-4-1, or 5-3-2, representing labeler-drug-package. The labeler code is assigned by the FDA and identifies the vendor responsible for the final packaging of the drug. The drug code, which is assigned by the vendor, identifies the drug form and strength of the product. Lastly, the package code, also assigned by the vendor, identifies the packaging level type and size (e.g., unit, box, case, etc.). There is no central repository of NDCs and, although manufacturers are required to report NDCs to the FDA, approval is not required. For automation to work properly, the pharmacy and related automated systems must maintain a current and accurate list of known NDCs. Compounded preparations, on the other hand, require their own unique bar codes produced by the pharmacy.[1]

Carousel cabinets, automated dispensing cabinets, robotic cart filling systems, and sterile compounding devices are some of the other prominent HIT tools used in automated drug distribution systems in acute care pharmacies. Carousel cabinets contain shelves that are attached to a carousel, which rotates shelves for medication selection. Benefits of carousel cabinets include the freeing up of floor space, reduced walking associated with drug distribution, and more accurate accounting of inventory. Automated dispensing cabinets (ADCs) are similar to carousels, except they do not use rotating shelves. ADCs, which may be located either in the pharmacy or on patient-care units, maintain inventory and audit trails as well as perform charging functions. Access to inventory contained in ADCs requires the user to log in, maintaining an audit trail of receiving and dispensing activity. ADCs can be configured with a variety of different drawers so that specified users may only have access to certain drawers or even specific drawer sections. Despite being able to limit access in this way, none of the drawers control the amount of product removed, which can be seen as a limitation. In some situations (such as emergencies), override functions are permitted.[1] Despite the obvious benefit of override access, this practice has also been associated with medication errors, such as obtaining the wrong strength of medication and obtaining a medication after it has been discontinued.[20,21]

While not as common as ADCs, robotic cart filling systems are commonly found in hospital settings as well. They utilize bar coding to locate, obtain, package, and deliver medications. This is done by filling unit-dose carts and most often requires significant repackaging efforts, as the medications must be in containers that can be manipulated by the device. The preparation of sterile products for administration can also be automated. The FDA classifies the devices that automate sterile dose preparations as pharmacy compounding devices.[22] Total parenteral nutrition (TPN) compounders are an example of this type of device. TPN compounders first compute a TPN formulation based on clinical requirements, and then drive a machine to deliver the correct ingredients in the correct amounts and sequence.

COMMUNITY PHARMACY SETTING

In the community pharmacy, pharmacy information management systems (PIMS) serve as the core piece of HIT that supports pharmacy operations, managing all data associated with prescriptions, patients, and prescribers. They contain key databases, such as drug files, DEA and national provider identifier numbers, physician contact information, prescription pricing tables, third-party plan details, and patient profiles. The PIMS software and related databases commonly reside on a server in the pharmacy, but they may be located on a central server, allowing access from multiple sites. In the **software as a service (SaaS)** or **application service provider (ASP)** options, both the data and software are hosted off-site. PIMS may also have integrated workflow systems with multiple workstations assigned specific tasks (e.g., intake, processing, and verifying of prescriptions). Bar code scanning is an integral component of this workflow, which allows the tracking of every prescription through the filling queue. Such workflow systems provide efficiency and are usually found in high-volume pharmacies.[1]

Other HIT utilized in the community pharmacy setting includes automated counting systems and robotics, interactive voice response (IVR) systems (i.e., the automated menu a caller is prompted through using the phone number pad), document scanning, and electronic signature capture. Refill requests are commonly routed into the PIMS filling queue via IVR, which guides patients in entering in their refill information. This practice reduces the number of phone calls that must be made and handled by pharmacy staff and also gives patients the ability to submit refills after hours. The Internet is also being utilized for patient entered refill requests to the same effect. Further, IVR systems, along with text messaging, are being utilized to automate outbound contact with patients, such as prescription pickup reminders and other, informative messages.

Another way new or refill prescriptions can enter the PIMS queue is via e-prescribing. E-prescribing is a feature of almost every PIMS, most of which route prescriptions through the Surescripts network. Faxed and paper prescriptions are scanned during intake, making the then digitized prescription available at the filling and verification steps. The goal of digitization is to reduce the amount of paper handled and provide a faster way to file, index, share, and search for information.[1]

Through the use of counting systems and/or robotic dispensing systems, the majority of a community pharmacy's prescription volume can be automated. Counting systems include countertop devices and stand-alone cabinets, while robotic dispensing fills and labels vials. Bar codes are used in the dispensing process to match the medication with the patient and the prescription as entered in the computer system. This use of bar codes allows multiple checks as an additional layer of safety. Bar code scanning can tie will-call management into the technology-driven workflow and provides another searchable data point.[1] Bar codes on will-call bags are scanned when bags are hung. This information is updated in the pharmacy computer system for quick retrieval when the patient arrives, using light to identify the hanging bag in some instances.

Administration

Depending on the setting, medications may be administered by a health care provider, such as a physician, nurse, or pharmacist; a caregiver; or the patient themselves. The two major HIT tools being used in hospital settings at this stage of the medication use process are bar code medication administration (BCMA) systems and eMARs. BCMA systems are used at the point of care to ensure the five rights of medication administration are followed. While use of these systems has been increasing steadily, there is a major issue that hinders implementation. While most products used in the inpatient care setting have bar codes, there are some products that still require pharmacy to create and attach the bar code. Also, products that are compounded for local use, such as intravenous antibiotics, need special bar codes that are not supported by the basic linear bar coding format. Two-dimensional bar codes can at least partly solve this issue. Alongside BCMA systems, the use of eMARs replaces paper records currently used to document medication administration. eMARs decrease the potential for errors by eliminating the need to handwrite changes in medications and allowing a medication change to be updated in real time in the patient's medical record.[1]

Monitoring

Pharmacists' monitoring activities vary greatly depending on their work setting and available resources. No matter the setting, however, monitoring activities should result in clinical interventions, when necessary. A clinical intervention is the act of interceding with the intent of modifying the medication use process. The broad categories of monitoring activities, and, therefore, clinical interventions, performed by pharmacists include activities that promote safety, activities that promote quality, and activities that promote efficiency and cost-effectiveness. For instance, a pharmacist may intercept a medication ordered for which the patient has an allergy. Or a pharmacist may identify a less expensive, therapeutic alternative to the prescribed medication in order to decrease costs for the patient.[1]

In the hospital setting, clinical surveillance systems are at the core of monitoring efforts. Clinical surveillance refers to active surveillance or watchful waiting that includes a collection and analysis of patient-specific information that is then used to drive decisions. These systems are most often used by pharmacy to monitor information from the pharmacy system (i.e., medication lists), laboratory results, and patient demographics from the admission/discharge/transfer system. Rules are built to identify potential problems. For example, a rule may monitor all patients for orders of naloxone, which is used to treat opioid overdose. Another rule may monitor for all patients receiving ranitidine whose platelet count has decreased to less than 50% of the previous value, suggesting an occurrence of rare thrombocytopenia. Patients meeting these predefined rules are presented to pharmacy staff for follow-up and evaluation.

Once a need is established and a clinical intervention has taken place, the process must be well documented. The purpose of clinical intervention documentation is multifaceted. One primary purpose is to demonstrate the cost and quality impact of programs, such as clinical pharmacy services. Documenting clinical interventions can also be used for staff performance improvement as well as quality improvement activities. Documentation gives insight into what clinical staff members are doing, and, therefore, allows constructive feedback to be provided. Similarly, clinical intervention documentation can be utilized to improve workflow.

There are certain basic elements that a good documentation system should have. The system should be easy to use and fit into the existing workflow as much as possible. It should allow for quick documentation that includes sufficient details. Specifically, the system should have the capability to add or modify interventions, manage drug and prescriber databases, and mirror the organization's security policies. Further, all documentation should be searchable, and the documentation system should provide a complete record of all clinical activities. Ideally, all practitioners providing care to the same patient would document all monitoring and intervention activities in a shared record. The record would then be accessible by all other providers who are also caring for that particular patient. In fact, a primary objective of the Pharmacy eHIT Collaborative, a multiorganizational group focused on the role of pharmacists in the emerging electronic health record landscape, is to ensure that this is the case for the monitoring efforts of pharmacists.[23] Reporting, which is the critical output of the documentation system, should be quick and easy. It should allow real-time selection and inclusion of any combination of documented fields in the system.[1]

Case Study 24–1

You are a student pharmacist completing an inpatient pharmacy administration rotation. Through your rotation experiences, you have observed and interacted with a variety of health information technologies and automation used to manage medications within the institution. Your preceptor gives you the following assignment.

• *Name the commonly encountered technologies used at each step of the medication use process to ensure safe and efficacious medication therapy.*

The Future: Informatics in the U.S. Health Care System

❹ *The vision of health care is becoming more patient centered.* Health care is transitioning from industrial age medicine, which places focus on professional care, is segmented, and is also highly expensive, to a new approach. This new approach, alternatively described as information age health care, encourages lower cost individual care, getting friends and family involved, and using self-help networks as first-line approaches.[24] This transformation has been given the label participatory care, in that the new approach involves patients as highly active, decision-making members of their own care team. **Health 2.0**, being the utilization of health care–related tools provided by Web 2.0, is the Web-oriented extension of this new participatory care approach. Web 2.0 simply refers to those applications of the Internet that are interactive and social, allowing for collaboration and interactivity among patients, caregivers, and providers. Facebook (https://www.facebook.com/) is probably the most prominent example of Web 2.0. Facebook, as is well known, is a social networking portal that allows users to interact and share pictures, videos, and links, among other things. Patientslikeme® (http://www.patientslikeme.com/), being a Health 2.0 social networking portal, is similar to Facebook except that it focuses on allowing people with the same medical condition to communicate with each other about health-related issues.

Other Web 2.0 and Health 2.0 resources include blogs, wiki sites, Twitter (https://twitter.com/), and **personal health records (PHRs)**. With a blog, anyone can post his or her thoughts on any topic at a particular site on the Internet as a blog entry. Readers can then leave related comments directly below the published material. Wiki sites allow the publication of monographs via group participation, and the published material can be updated at any time. The most well-known example of a wiki site is Wikipedia, "the freeencyclopediathatanyonecanedit."[25] AsforHealth2.0, RxWiki (http://www.rxwiki.com/) is a wiki site that provides patients with drug monographs compiled by pharmacists.

Twitter is a Web 2.0 service with the sole focus being the ability to send short messages to groups. Twitter users can follow one or more members as well as be followed by members who want to keep up with the insights of those they find interesting. Examples of some pharmacy applications for this kind of resource include promoting medication adherence, prompting health behaviors, and producing warnings for patients. One of the best ways to learn about Health 2.0 resources (including primary literature, for example) is to search for "Health 2.0 journal" in your preferred search engine.

PHRs are Health 2.0 applications that provide the patient increased opportunity to participate in the collection, maintenance, and sharing of their personal health-related information through a Web-based environment. All the information is patient maintained, and PHRs should be designed as a lifelong resource of patient health information. PHRs are ideally kept in a Web-accessible, electronic format that is secure and private but also universally available to providers treating the patient. Further, the ability to move information from a patient's EMR, which is maintained by a health care organization, to the patient's PHR increases patient involvement in their own health care. Along with this ability, patients should also have the ability to annotate the information coming in from their providers or EMR. It should be noted here that the PHR does not and is not meant to replace the legal record of any provider.[26] In order for PHRs to be interoperable and share data with other systems as described, standards of data communication must be established and utilized. Current agreed upon standards include Continuity of Care Record (CCR) and Extensible Markup Language (XML). Strong levels of data encryption and passwords are also required. Although still evolving, there are dozens of PHRs available today. Two examples include Microsoft's HealthVault (https://www.healthvault.com) and AHIMA's MyPHR (http://www.myphr.com/).

Case Study 24–2

Your preceptor approaches you one morning and tells you about a new committee within the hospital that she has been asked to chair. The committee's role is to explore the emerging Health 2.0 domain and identify potential ways the hospital can become involved. Knowing that you are a tech savvy person, your preceptor asks you to help conduct some of the initial research into the Health 2.0 domain. You are given the following assignment.

- *What are the primary journals that address the Health 2.0 domain?*
- *Suggest a few ways the hospital can use popular Web 2.0 tools for Health 2.0 efforts.*

Interoperable Electronic Health Records

❺ *The current health care system is decentralized and fragmented. Because of this, signifi- cant communication gaps exist when multiple health care institutions provide care for the same patient. Substantial evidence suggests that more effective communication would improve patient care and reduce medical errors, such as adverse drug events.*[4,27] Beyond the clinical improvements, there are also major financial benefits to be had, with greater health information exchange and interoperability potentially saving the U.S. health care system $77.8 billion annually.[28] **Interoperability** is the ability of disparate computer systems to exchange information in a manner that allows the information to be used meaningfully.[29] ❻ *The desired result of interoperable systems and EHRs is to readily provide all health practitioners in all locations, including the pharmacy, with access to information about a patient's care, as needed.* As such, new health information systems (HIS) should focus on ensuring effective communication of data between and within institutions, which includes a focus on data transfer across applications, devices, and geographical locations. Communication standards are necessary to achieve this desired level of meaningful data exchange.

CURRENT STANDARDS

Several health care standards exist today. For instance, the NCPDP developed an e-pre- scribing standard, NCPDP SCRIPT, for the transmission of prescription information, along with relevant medical history information, electronically between prescribers, pharmacies, and payers. As mentioned before, NDCs, created by manufacturers and registered with the FDA, are used as a standard way to signify the drug manufacturer, drug formulation, and packaging type. RxNorm, produced by the National Library of Medicine (NLM), is a standard for supporting semantic interoperability between phar- macy systems and drug terminologies by providing a standardized naming system for generic and branded drugs.[30] Unified Medical Language System (UMLS), also main- tained by the NLM, enables interoperability between computer systems, such as EHRs, by providing a set of files and software that bring together many medical vocabularies and standards.[31] Contained within the UMLS is the Logical Observation Identifiers Names and Codes (LOINC) terminology for laboratory test results and procedures. Another important medical terminology version also contained within UMLS is the Sys- tematized Nomenclature of Medicine-Clinical Terms (SNOMED CT). SNOMED CT maps to diagnosis and billing codes known as the International Classification of Disease- tenth revision (ICD-10). Further, Current Procedural Terminology (CPT®) codes, pro- duced by the American Medical Association (AMA), provide medical nomenclature used to report medical procedures and services performed under private and public health insurance plans.[32]

THE GOVERNMENT'S ROLE IN INTEROPERABILITY

Technical standards are one piece of the interoperability puzzle. Other challenges include finding an organization or group to lead the charge through associated business, administrative, and financial considerations. The U.S. government has been leading these efforts, beginning in 2004 when President George W. Bush targeted computerizing health records in his State of the Union Address. That same year, President Bush established the Office of the National Coordinator for Health Information Technology (ONC) within the Office of the Secretary of Health and Human Services (HHS).[33] The two major goals of the ONC were widespread adoption of EHRs by 2014 and the creation and implementation of an interoperable health information infrastructure.

● In order to increase adoption and Meaningful Use of EHRs by providers and hospitals, CMS has developed a monetary incentive program. ❼ *The Meaningful Use program incentivizes hospitals and physicians to use EHRs to achieve specific outcomes, which may be process oriented or patient oriented. For example, 60% of medication orders should be entered electronically or >50% of patients should have electronic access to their medical information within 36 hours after discharge. The goals of the Meaningful Use program are to (1) improve quality, safety, and efficiency, (2) engage patients and their families, (3) improve care coordination, as well as public and population health, and (4) maintain privacy and security of protected health information (PHI).* It is hoped that the adoption of and compliance with Meaningful Use will result in better clinical outcomes, improved population health, increased health care transparency and efficiency, more robust data for research, and the empowerment of individuals and patients.[34]

● Further, there are specific objectives, broken down into three stages, set by CMS that eligible providers and hospitals must achieve to qualify for the incentive program. Stage 1 focuses on providers capturing patient data and sharing that data with either the patient or other health care providers. Stage 2, which begins in 2014 and focuses on advanced clinical processes, requires that a specified number of core and menu objectives be met. Specifically, all of the 15 core objectives must be met, which includes items such as the use of CPOE and e-prescribing, maintaining active drug and allergy lists, checking for drug–drug and drug–allergy interactions, implementation of CDS, and protection of electronic health information. As for the 10 menu objectives, which include items such as submitting electronic data to immunization registries, drug formulary checking, electronic access to health information for patients, and patient-specific education resources, five must be met.[35] Stage 3, which begins in 2016 and is currently still being formalized, will focus specifically on improved patient outcomes.

Case Study 24–3

You are wrapping up your rotation, and your preceptor comes to you with a final assignment. She has been tasked with representing the Pharmacy Department on the committee that is overseeing the implementation of electronic health records in the institution. She knows very little about EHRs and asks the following questions to get started.

- *What group or organization is overseeing the EHR Meaningful Use program?*
- *Why would a hospital or provider want to start Meaningful Use earlier rather than later?*
- *What are the stages of Meaningful Use?*

Greater Emphasis on Security, Privacy, and Confidentiality of Protected Health Information

As interoperability advances and more patient data are shared across providers and organizations, the issues of security, privacy, and confidentiality of **protected health information (PHI)** inevitability arise. Protected health information includes any information that can be used to identify a person, including information about medical conditions, payment for care, or actual care delivered.[1] Privacy refers to being free from unauthorized intrusions and the protection of PHI. In health care organizations, privacy is accomplished through policies that determine how and what information is gathered, stored, and used, as well as how patients are involved in the process. Security here refers to restricting access to patient health data to everyone except those with authorized access. This is accomplished through the use of electronic tools, such as login identifications and password protection. Confidentiality here refers to the provider-client privilege that, under most circumstances, any health-related information communicated between a provider and a patient is private. PHI can be in any form (e.g., written, oral, or electronic), and examples include patient name, address, Social Security number, e-mail address, or any other part of a medical record that could be used to identify a patient.[1]

As health care providers, pharmacists need to be aware of the existing and emerging regulations that apply to the security, privacy, and confidentiality of PHI. For instance, the Health Breach Notification Rule, passed into law in 2009, requires that covered entities provide notice to patients following a breach in security. Also, the Patient Safety and Quality Improvement Act of 2005 (Patient Safety Act) establishes a framework that allows providers to voluntarily and confidentially report patient safety events to patient safety organizations for aggregation and analysis purposes.[36]

HEALTH INSURANCE PORTABILITY AND ACCOUNTABILITY ACT

Another major piece of legislation with which pharmacists and other providers need to be intimately familiar is the Health Insurance Portability and Accountability Act (HIPAA), passed into law in 1996. The main component of concern here is the HIPAA Privacy Rule, which establishes how medical information should be handled. The major goal of the Privacy Rule is to ensure proper protection of individuals' health information while also allowing the flow of health information needed to provide high-quality health care. As such, the law defines PHI, describes how health care organizations can use and disclose PHI, and outlines the requirements of health organizations to protect PHI from inappropriate disclosure and misuse. For instance, the Privacy Rule specifies that PHI can be transmitted and used for treatment, payment, and operations (TPO) processes (i.e., general health care operational use). And, as it is not intended to prevent providers from discussing the treatment of their patients, the rule specifies that some incidental disclosures of PHI are permitted. That said, reasonable safeguards, such as speaking in a low voice, not discussing patient care in the presence of others, and closing patient charts after use, should be used to limit such incidental disclosures. There are also certain disclosures, permitted by law, which may be made to governmental agencies for such purposes as law enforcement, research, workers' compensation, and organ donation. Further, the HIPAA Privacy Rule requires that health care organizations notify patients of their rights when receiving care and also provides them with a process to exercise those rights. Also, patients should be given the opportunity to agree or object to disclosures of their PHI while under the care of a health care organization.[1,37]

There is also the HIPAA Security Rule, which covers electronic PHI (ePHI). ePHI is simply PHI stored in electronic form. Health care organizations are required by the Security Rule to ensure the integrity, confidentiality, and availability of all ePHI created, received, maintained, or transmitted by the organization. As such, most all organizations have fax, Internet, and e-mail policies that outline appropriate use in order to protect ePHI.[38]

Conclusion

Pharmacy informatics is the scientific discipline found at the intersection of people, data, and technology systems. It is governed by business, technical, and regulatory standards to ensure optimal use of patient-specific and knowledge-based information. Pharmacists rely on informatics to support all of their activities associated with the medication use process. As EHR adoption increases in the United States, pharmacists and other health care providers will continue to see a growing role of informatics in their practice, regardless of the setting.

Self-Assessment Questions

1. Which of the following represents the correct order of the medication use process?
   a. Monitoring, prescribing, transcribing, administration, follow-up
   b. Prescribing, transcribing, dispensing, administration, monitoring
   c. Transcribing, dispensing, administration, monitoring, documentation
   d. Assessment, prescribing, transcribing, administration, monitoring
   e. None of the above

2. Pharmacy informatics includes:
   a. People
   b. Information
   c. Technology
   d. a and b
   e. a, b, and c

3. The two primary types of information used in pharmacy informatics include:
   a. Patient specific and clinical expertise
   b. Clinical expertise and knowledge based
   c. Patient specific and knowledge based
   d. Referential and guidelines
   e. None of the above

4. The primary similarity between CPOE and e-prescriptions is they:
   a. Are easy to implement because they do not disrupt workflow
   b. Both address the dispensing stage of the medication use process

    c. Eliminate illegible prescriptions

    d. Eliminate all errors related to prescribing

    e. c and d

5. The role of Surescripts is to:

    a. Certify controlled substance schedule II prescriptions for authenticity

    b. Provide the communication network for e-prescriptions

    c. Create standards for CPOE transmission

    d. Define Meaningful Use standards

    e. Provide financial support for e-prescription adoption

6. The three components of clinical decision support systems include:

    a. CPOE system, transmission network, transmission standards

    b. Knowledge base, e-prescription network, transmission standards

    c. Communication mechanism, knowledge base, CPOE system

    d. Inference engine, knowledge base, communication mechanism

    e. None of the above

7. The main benefits of CDSS include the ability to decrease:

    a. Adverse drug events

    b. Costs

    c. Length of stay

    d. All of the above

    e. a and b

8. Prescriptions created electronically (by CPOE and e-prescribing) have already undergone clinical review by CDSS when they reach the pharmacists for transcription. Research suggests that:

    a. These prescriptions are ready for dispensing, requiring no additional review

    b. Problems still exist with prescriptions created electronically

    c. Pharmacists must remain diligent when reviewing all prescription orders

    d. Physicians do not rely on the information presented to them by CDSS

    e. b and c

9. The NDC is necessary to support automation of the medication use process. Challenges with use of the NDC include:

    a. There is no single repository of NDCs

    b. The FDA does not actually approve NDCs

    c. NDCs are too long for some automation to read

    d. a and b

    e. All of the above

10. Dispensing automation commonly found in hospitals include:
    a. Carousel cabinets
    b. Automated dispensing cabinets
    c. Robotic cart filling systems
    d. Sterile compounding devices
    e. All of the above

11. The core technology supporting pharmacy operations in the community setting is:
    a. Pharmacy information management system
    b. Robotic vial filling systems
    c. Interactive voice response
    d. Electronic signature capture
    e. Document scanning systems

12. The three categories of data making up clinical surveillance systems are:
    a. Radiology, diagnoses, pharmacy
    b. Patient demographics, pharmacy, laboratory
    c. Laboratory, radiology, patient demographics
    d. Diagnoses, patient demographics, radiology
    e. Diagnoses, pharmacy, nutrition

13. Which of the following is an example of Health 2.0?
    a. Personal health records
    b. PatientsLikeMe.com
    c. Promoting medication adherence through Facebook
    d. Sending health messages through Twitter
    e. All of the above

14. The ultimate, desired result of interoperability is:
    a. The provision of a patient's complete care history to all providers
    b. More accurate and efficient billing for health care services
    c. Streamlined prescription routing from institutional clinics to community pharmacies
    d. Improved clinical decision making though access to knowledge-based information
    e. All of the above

15. Goals of Meaningful Use of EHRs include:
    a. Improve quality of health care
    b. Engage patients in their own care

c. Improve coordination of care

d. Maintain privacy and security of protected health information

e. All of the above

REFERENCES

1. Fox BI, Thrower MR, Felkey BG, eds. Building core competencies in pharmacy informatics. Washington, DC: American Pharmacists Association; 2010.

2. Hersh W. A stimulus to define informatics and health information technology. BMC Med Inform Decis Mak. 2009;9(1):24.

3. Hersh W. Medical Informatics—improving health care through information. JAMA. 2002;288:1955-8.

4. Kohn LT, Corrigan JM, Donaldson MS, eds. To err is human: building a safer health system. Washington, DC: National Academies of Science 2000:1-5.

5. Bates DW, Cullen DJ, Laird N, et al. Incidence of adverse drug events and potential adverse drug events. Implications for prevention. ADE Prevention Study Group. JAMA. 1995;274(1):29-34.

6. Kaushal R, Shojania KG, Bates DW. Effects of computerized physician order entry and clinical decision support systems on medication safety: a systematic review. Arch Intern Med. 2003;163(12);1409-16.

7. Bates DW, Leape LL Cullen DJ, et al. Effect of computerized physician order entry and a team intervention on prevention of serious medication errors. JAMA. 1998;280(5):1311-6.

8. Koppel R, Metlay JP, Cohen A, et al. Role of computerized physician order entry systems in facilitating medication errors. JAMA. 2005;293(10):1197-203.

9. Hillestad R, Bigelow JH. Health information technology. Can HIT lower costs and improve quality? [Internet]. California: RAND Corporation; 2005 [cited 2012 Dec 28]. Available from: http://www.rand.org/pubs/research_briefs/RB9136.html. Accessed on December 28, 2012.

10. Poon EG, Blumenthal D, Jaggi T, et al. Overcoming barriers to adopting and implementing computerized physician order entry systems in U.S. hospitals. Health Aff. 2004;23(4):184-90.

11. National Council for Prescription Drug Programs [Internet]. Scottsdale (AZ): National Council for Prescription Drug Programs; About—Contact Us; [cited 2012 Dec 28]:[about 1 screen]. Available from: http://www.ncpdp.org/About-Us

12. Centers for Medicare and Medicaid Services. Electronic Prescribing (eRx) Incentive Program [Internet]. Baltimore (MD): Centers for Medicare and Medicaid Services; 2013 May 28 [cited 2012 Dec 28]:[about 3 screens]. Available from: http://www.cms.hhs.gov/ ERxIncentive

13. U.S. Department of Justice Drug Enforcement Administration, Office of Diversion Control. Notices—2012 [Internet]. Springfield (VA): Drug Enforcement Administration; 2012 Aug 1 [cited 2012 Dec 28]:[about 3 screens]. Available from: http://www.deadiversion .usdoj.gov/fed_regs/notices/2012/fr0801_4.htm

14. Osheroff JA, Teich JM, Middleton B, et al. A roadmap for national action on clinical decision support. J Am Med Inform Assoc. 2007;14(2):141-5.

15. Shea S, DuMouchel W, Bahamonde L. A meta-analysis of 16 randomized controlled trials to evaluate computer-based clinical reminder systems for preventive care in the ambulatory setting. J Am Med Inform Assoc. 1996;3(6):399-409.

16. Berner ES. Clinical decision support systems: theory and practice. 2nd ed. New York, NY: Springer; 2007.

17. Overhage JM, Tierney WM, Zhou XH, et al. A randomized trial of "corollary orders" to prevent errors of omission. J Am Med Inform Assoc. 1997;4(5):364-75.

18. Koppel R, Metlay JP, Cohen A, et al. Role of computerized physician order entry systems in facilitating medication errors. JAMA. 2005;293(10):1197-1203.

19. Saverno KR, Hines LE, Warholak TL, et al. Ability of pharmacy clinical decision-support software to alert users about clinically important drug–drug interactions. J Am Med Inform Assoc. 2011;18(1):32-37.

20. Oren E, Griffiths LP, Guglielmo BJ. Characteristics of antimicrobial overrides associated with automated dispensing machines. Am J Health Syst Pharm. 2002;59(15);1445-8.

21. Kester K, Baxter J, Freudenthal K. Errors associated with medications removed from automated dispensing machines using override function. Hosp Pharm. 2006;41:53-537.

22. Class II special controls guidance document: pharmacy compounding systems; final guidance for industry and FDA [Internet]. Rockville (MD): U.S. Department of Health and Human Services, Food and Drug Administration, Centers for Devices and Radiological Health; 2001 Mar 12 [cited 2012 Dec 29]:[9 p.]. Available from: http://www.fda.gov/downloads/medicaldevices/deviceregulationandguidance/guidancedocuments/ucm073589.pdf

23. Pharmacy e-Health Information Technology Collaborative Home page [Internet]. Alexandria (VA): Pharmacy e-Health Information Technology Collaborative; c2011 [cited 2012 Dec 29]. Available from: http://www.pharmacyhit.org/.

24. Smith R. Information technology and consumerism will transform health care worldwide. BMJ. 1997;314:1495.

25. Wikipedia: The Free Encyclopedia [Internet]. Wikipedia; [cited 20112 Dec 29]. Available from: http://en.wikipedia.org/wiki/Main_Page

26. AHIMA e-HIM Personal Health Record Work Group. The role of the personal health record in the EHR. J AHIMA. 2005;76(7):64A-D.

27. eHealth Initiative. Migrating toward Meaningful Use: the state of health information Exchange. Washington, DC: eHealth Initiative; August 2009. Available from: http://www.sftvision.com/2009SurveyReportFINAL.pdf

28. Walker J, Pan E, Johnson D, et al. The value of health care information exchange and interoperability [Internet]. Bethesda (MD): Health Affairs; 2005 Jan 19 [cited 2012 Dec 29]:[8p.]. Available from: http://content.healthaffairs.org/content/suppl/2005/02/07/hlthaff.w5.10.DC1

29. The National Alliance for Health Information Technology report to the Office of the National Coordinator for Health Information Technology on defining key health

information technology terms [Internet]. Department of Health and Human Services; 2008 Apr 28 [cited 2012 Dec 29]. 40 p. Available from: http://cdm16064.contentdm.oclc .org/cdm/singleitem/collection/p266901coll4/id/2086/rec/10

30. U.S. National Library of Medicine [Internet]. Bethesda (MD): U.S. National Library of Medicine; 1993 Oct 10 [updated 2013 Jul 3]. RxNorm overview; 2005 May 5 [updated 2013 Mar 5; cited 2012 Dec 29]:[about 14 screens]. Available from: https://www.nlm.nih.gov/ research/umls/rxnorm/overview.html

31. U.S. National Library of Medicine [Internet]. Bethesda (MD): U.S. National Library of Medicine; 1993 Oct 10 [updated 2013 Jul 3]. UMLS quick start guide; 2011 Mar 30 [updated 2012 Jul 27; cited 2012 Dec 29]:[about 2 screens]. Available from: http://www .nlm.nih.gov/research/umls/quickstart.html

32. American Medical Association. About CPT® [Internet]. Chicago (IL): American Medical Association; c1995-2013 [cited 2012 Dec 29]:[about 1 screen]. Available from: http:// www.ama-assn.org/ama/pub/physician-resources/solutions-managing-your-practice/ coding-billing-insurance/cpt/about-cpt.page

33. Bush GW. Executive Order 13335—incentives for the use of health information technology and establishing the position of the National Health Information Technology Coordinator [Internet]. Washington, DC: Federal Register; 2004 Apr 27 [cited 2012 Dec 29]:[3 p.]. Available from: http://www.gpo.gov/fdsys/pkg/FR-2004-04-30/pdf/04-10024.pdf

34. HealthIT.gov. Meaningful use definitions and objectives [Internet]. Washington, DC: The Office of the National Coordinator for Health Information Technology; [cited 2012 Dec 29]:[about 1 screen]. Available from: http://www.healthit.gov/providers-professionals/ meaningful-use-definition-objectives

35. An introduction to the Medicaid EHR Incentive Program for eligible professionals [Internet]. Baltimore (MD): Centers for Medicare and Medicaid Services; [cited 2012 Dec 29]:[94 p.]. Available from: http://www.cms.gov/Regulations-and-Guidance/Legislation/ EHRIncentivePrograms/Downloads/EHR_Medicaid_Guide_Remediated_2012.pdf

36. Summary of selected federal laws and regulations addressing confidentiality, privacy and security [Internet]. Washington, DC: The Office of the National Coordinator for Health Information Technology; 2010 Feb 18 [cited 2012 Dec 29]:[12 p.]. Available from: http:// www.healthit.gov/sites/default/files/federal_privacy_laws_table_2_26_10_final_0.pdf

37. Summary of the HIPAA Privacy Rule [Internet]. Washington, DC: U.S. Department of Health and Human Services; 2005 May [cited 2012 Dec 29]:[25 p.]. Available from: http:// www.hhs.gov/ocr/privacy/hipaa/understanding/summary/privacysummary.pdf

38. HIPAA administrative simplification [Internet]. Washington, DC: U.S. Department of Health and Human Services; 2006 Feb 16 [cited 2012 Dec 29]:[101 p.]. Available from: http://www .hhs.gov/ocr/privacy/hipaa/administrative/privacyrule/adminsimpregtext.pdf

SUGGESTED READINGS

1. Fox BI, Thrower MR, Felkey BG, eds. Building core competencies in pharmacy informatics. Washington, DC: American Pharmacists Association; 2010.

2. The Office of the National Coordinator for Health Information Technology [Internet]. Washington, DC: U.S. Department of Health and Human Services; [updated 2011 Feb 18; cited 2012 Dec 12]. Available from: http://healthit.hhs.gov

3. Journal of the American Medical Informatics Association, http://jamia.bmj.com/.

4. Friedman CP. A 'fundamental theorem' of biomedical informatics. JAMIA. 2009;16:169-70.

5. Pew Internet and American Life Project, http://www.pewinternet.org/.

6. American Society of Health-System Pharmacists. Technology-enabled practice: vision statement by the ASHP Section of Pharmacy Informatics and Technology. Am J Health Syst Pharm. 2009;66:1573-77.

7. Journal of Medical Internet Research, http://www.jmir.org

8. Journal of Participatory Medicine, http://www.jopm.org

9. Journal of Biomedical Informatics, http://www.sciencedirect.com/science/journal/15320464

10. Pharmacy Informatics, http://www.pharmacy-informatics.com

11. Dumitru D, ed. The pharmacy informatics primer. Bethesda (MD): American Society of Health-System Pharmacists; 2009.

Appendices

Appendix 2–1

Drug Consultation Request Form

☐ Completed (Review Pending)	**DRUG CONSULTATION REQUEST FORM**	LOG# _____
☐ Reviewed	DRUG INFORMATION SERVICE	Final QA Check _____
☐ Communicated	NATIONAL INSTITUTES OF HEALTH	

REQUESTER INFORMATION

Date Received _____   Time Received _____ AM / PM *(circle one)*

Name _____   Phone# _____   FAX# _____

Pager# _____   e-mail _____

INTERNAL:	EXTERNAL:	AFFILIATION CATEGORY:
☐ MD ☐ DDS	☐ Pharmacist	☐ Institute _____
☐ RN	☐ Physician	☐ Clinic _____
☐ Pharmacist	☐ General Public	☐ Pt Care Unit _____
☐ Other Professional _____	☐ Other Healthcare Professional _____	☐ Other _____
☐ NIH Patient	☐ Other Professional/Organization _____	
☐ Other _____		

HOW RECEIVED: ☐ Phone   ☐ Voice Mail   ☐ E-Mail   ☐ Mail   ☐ FAX   ☐ In Person   ☐ Referred by :_____

PRIORITY: ☐ Urgent   ☐ High Priority   ☐ Routine   ☐ Low Priority

ORIGINAL QUESTION / REQUEST

CLEAR STATEMENT(S) OF ACTUAL DRUG INFORMATION NEED

PERTINENT PATIENT DATA / BACKGROUND INFORMATION

Name _____   Pt Care Unit/Clinic _____   ☐ Inpatient ☐ Outpatient

Age _____   Race _____   ☐ Male ☐ Female   Height _____ cm _____ ft _____ in   Weight _____ lb _____ kg

Primary Diagnosis _____   Allergies/Intolerances _____

End-Organ Function _____   Special Circumstances _____

CC:

HPI:

PMH:

FH:

SH:

ROS:

Meds:

PE:

Labs:

Diagnostics:

Problem List:

LOG# _____

CLASSIFICATION(S) OF REQUEST

☐ Administration (Routes/Methods)
☐ Adverse Effects/Intolerances
☐ Allergy/Cross Reactivity
☐ Alternative Medicine
☐ Biotechnology/Gene Therapy
☐ Clinical Nutrition/Metabolic Support
☐ Compatibility/Stability/Storage
☐ Contraindications/Precautions
☐ Cost/Pharmacoeconomics
☐ Dose/Schedule
☐ Drug Delivery Devices/Systems/Forms
☐ Drug Interactions (Drug-Drug, Drug-Food)
☐ Drug of choice/Therapeutic Alternatives/Therapeutic Use
☐ Drug Standards/Legal/Regulatory
☐ Drug Use in Special Populations
   (Effects of Age, Organ System Function, Disease,
   Extracorporeal Circulation, etc.)
☐ Excipients/Compounding/Formulations

☐ Investigational Products (Pre-Clinical and Clinical)
☐ Lab Test Interferences (Drug-Lab Interactions)
☐ Monitoring Parameters
☐ Nonprescription Products
☐ Patient Information/Education
☐ Pharmacokinetics (LADME/TDM)
☐ Pharmacology/Mechanisms/Pharmacodynamics
☐ Physicochemical Properties
☐ Poisoning/Toxicology (Environmental/Occupational Exposure,
   Mutagenicity, Carcinogenicity)
☐ Pregnancy/Lactation/Teratogenicity/Fertility
☐ Product Availability/Status
☐ Product Identification (Tablet/Capsule)
☐ Product Identification (Generic, Brand, Orphan,
   Foreign, Chemical Substances, Discontinued Products, etc.)
☐ Product Information
☐ Study Design/Protocol Development/Research Support
☐ Other _____

REQUEST CATEGORY

☐ Patient Care   ☐ Research   ☐ Other _____

RESPONSE (Referenced)

REFERENCES (Numbered)

TRACKING / FOLLOW-UP

Request Received By_____
Response Formulated By_____

Reviewed By_____
Response Communicated By_____
Time Required to Answer_____

☐ Documents/Literature Provided   ☐ Verbal Response   ☐ E-Mail   ☐ Written Response/Consult

OUTCOME / FOLLOW-UP

Appendix 2–2

Examples of Questions for Obtaining Background Information from Requestors[*]

Regardless of the type or classification of the question, the following information should be obtained:

1. The requestor's name
2. The requestor's location and/or page number
3. The requestor's affiliation (institution or practice), if a health care professional
4. The requestor's frame of reference (e.g., title, profession/occupation, rank)
5. The resources the requestor has already consulted
6. If the request is patient-specific or academic
7. The patient's diagnosis and other medications
8. The urgency of the request (negotiate time of response)

The following are examples of questions that can be asked to clarify the initial query and elicit pertinent background information. Please note that this Appendix addresses selected categories of queries and lists only a sampling of questions that can be posed to the requestor (i.e., it is not a comprehensive list).

Availability of Dosage Forms
1. What is the dosage form desired?
2. What administration routes are feasible with this patient?
3. Is this patient alert and oriented?
4. Does the patient have a water or sodium restriction?
5. What other special factors regarding drug administration should be considered?

Identification of Product
1. What is the generic or trade name of the product?
2. Who is the manufacturer? What is the country of origin?
3. What is the suspected use of this product?
4. Under what circumstances was this product found? Who found the product?
5. What is the dosage form, color markings, size, etc.?
6. What was your source of information? Was it reliable?

---

[*]Originally prepared by Craig Kirkwood

General Product Information

1. Why is there a particular concern for this product?
2. Is written patient information required?
3. What type of information do you need?
4. Is this for an inpatient, outpatient, or private patient?

Foreign Drug Identification

1. What is the drug's generic name, trade, manufacturer, and/or country of origin?
2. What is the dosage form, markings, color, strength, or size?
3. What is the suspected use of the drug? How often is the patient taking it? What is the patient's response to the drug? Is the patient male or female?
4. If the medication was found, what were the circumstances/conditions at the time of discovery?
5. Is the patient just visiting, or are they planning on staying?

Investigational Drug Information

1. Why do you need this information? Is the patient in need of the drug or currently enrolled in a protocol?
2. If a drug is to be identified, what is the dosage form, markings, color, strength, or size of the product?
3. Why was the patient receiving the drug? What is the response when the patient was on the drug? What are the patient's pathological conditions?
4. If a drug is desired what approved or accepted therapies have been tried? Was therapy maximized before discontinued?

Method and Rate of Administration

1. What dosage form or preparation is being used (if multiple salts available)?
2. What is the dose ordered? Is the drug a one-time dose or standing orders?
3. What is the clinical status of the patient? For example, could the patient tolerate a fluid push of [ ] mL? Is the patient fluid or sodium restricted? Does the patient have CHF or edema?
4. What possible delivery routes are available?
5. What other medications is the patient receiving currently? Are any by the same route?

Incompatibility and Stability

1. What are the routes for the patient's medications?
2. What are the doses, concentrations, and volumes for all pertinent medications?
3. What are the infusion times/rates expected or desired?
4. What is the base solution or diluent used?
5. Was the product stored and handled appropriately, based on requirements?
6. When was the product compounded/prepared?

Drug Interactions

1. What event(s) suggest that an interaction occurred? Describe.
2. For the drugs in question, what are the doses, volumes, concentrations, rate of administration, administration schedules, and length of therapies?
3. What is the temporal relationship between the drugs in question?
4. Has the patient received this combination or a similar combination in the past?
5. Other than the drugs in question, what other drugs is the patient receiving currently? When were these started?

Drug-Laboratory Test Interference

1. What event(s) suggest an interaction occurred? Describe.
2. For the drug in question, what is the dose, volume, concentration, rate of administration, administration schedule, and length of therapy?
3. What is the temporal relationship between drug administration and laboratory test sampling?
4. What other drugs is the patient receiving?
5. Has clinical chemistry (or the appropriate laboratory) been contacted? Are they aware of any known interference similar to this event?
6. Was this one isolated test or a trend in results?

Pharmacokinetics

1. Which product (e.g., drug, dose, brand) is being used?
2. What is the dose and route of the drug?
3. What is the patient's age, sex, height, and weight?
4. What are the disease being treated and the severity of the illness?
5. What is the patient's hepatic and renal function?
6. What other medications is the patient receiving?
7. What physiologic conditions exist (e.g., pneumonia, severe burns, or obesity)?
8. What are the patient's dietary and ethanol habits?

Therapeutic Levels

1. Is the patient currently receiving the drug? Have samples already been drawn? At what time?
2. What is the disease or underlying pathology being treated? If infectious in nature, what is the organism suspected/cultured?
3. If not stated in the question, what was the source of the sample (blood, urine, saliva; venous or arterial blood)?
4. What was the timing of the samples relative to drug administration? Over what period of time was the drug administered and by what route?
5. What were the previous concentrations for this patient? Was the patient receiving the same dose then?
6. How long has the patient received the drug? Is the patient at steady state?

Therapy Evaluation/Drug of Choice

1. What medications, including doses and routes of administration, is the patient receiving?
2. What are the patient's pathology(ies) and disease(s) severity?
3. What are the patient's specifics: age, weight, height, gender, organ function/dysfunction?
4. Has the patient received the drug previously? Was the response similar?
5. Has the patient been adherent?
6. What alternative therapies has the patient received? Was therapy maximized for each of these before discontinuation? What other therapies are being considered?
7. What monitoring parameters have been followed (serum concentrations/levels, clinical status, other clinical lab results, objective measurements, and subjective assessment)?

Dosage Recommendations

1. What disease is being treated? What is the extent/severity of the illness?
2. What are the medications (all) being prescribed? Has the patient been adherent?
3. Does the patient have any insufficiency of the renal, hepatic, or cardiac system?
4. For drugs with renal elimination, what are the serum creatinine/creatinine clearance, blood urea nitrogen (BUN), and/or urine output? Is the patient receiving peritoneal dialysis or hemodialysis?
5. For drugs with hepatic elimination, what are the liver function tests (LFTs), bilirubin (direct and indirect), and/or albumin?
6. For drugs with serum level monitoring utility, characterize the most recent levels per timing relative to dose and results.
7. Are these lab values recent? Is the patient's condition stable?
8. Does this patient have a known factor that could affect drug metabolism (ethnic background or acetylator status)?

Adverse Events

1. What are the name, dosage, and route for all drugs currently and recently prescribed?
2. What are the patient specifics (age, sex, height, weight, organ dysfunction, and indication for drug use)?
3. What is the temporal relationship with the drug?
4. Has the patient experienced this adverse relationship (or a similar event) with this drug (or similar agent) previously?
5. Was the suspected drug ever administered before? Why was it discontinued then?
6. What were the events/findings that characterize this adverse drug reaction (include onset and duration)?
7. Has any intervention been initiated at this time?
8. Does the patient have any food intolerance?
9. Is there a family history for this ADR and/or drug allergy?

Toxicology Information
1. What is your name, relationship to the patient, and telephone number?
2. What are the patient specifics (age, sex, height, weight, organ dysfunction, and indication for drug use)?
3. Is this a suspected ingestion or exposure?
4. What is the product suspected to have been ingested? What is the strength of the product and the possible quantity ingested (e.g., how much was in the bottle)?
5. How long ago did the ingestion occur?
6. How much is on the patient or surrounding area?
7. How much was removed from the patient's hands and mouth? Was the ingestion in the same room where the product was stored?
8. What has been done for the patient already? Has the poison control center or emergency department been called?
9. Do you have syrup of ipecac available (only if recommended by a poison control center)? Do you know how to give it properly?
10. What is the patient's condition (sensorium, heart rate, respiratory rate, temperature, skin color/turgor, pupils, sweating/salvation, etc.)?
11. Does the patient have any known illnesses?

Teratogenicity/Drugs in Pregnancy
1. What is the drug the patient received and what was the dose? What was the duration of therapy?
2. Is the patient pregnant or planning to become pregnant?
3. When during pregnancy was the exposure (trimester or weeks)?
4. What are the patient specifics (age, height, weight, sex)?
5. Was the patient adherent?
6. For what indication was the drug being prescribed?

Drugs in Breast Milk/Lactation
1. What is the drug the patient received and what was the dose? What was the duration of therapy?
2. How long has the infant been breast-feeding?
3. Has the infant ever received nonmaternal nutrition? Is bottle feeding a plausible alternative?
4. What is the frequency of the breast feeds? What is the milk volume?
5. How old is the infant?
6. Does the mother have hepatic or renal insufficiency?
7. What was the indication for prescribing the drug? Was this initial or alternate therapy?
8. Has the mother breast-fed previously while on the drug?

Appendix 3–1

Performing a PubMed Search

PubMed Search

PubMed is a database which is maintained by the National Library of Medicine and is available to the public at no charge. This database is available online at http://www.ncbi.nlm.nih.gov/PubMed. The information indexed by PubMed includes Medline, OldMedline (articles from the 1950s to the mid-1960s), as well as citations for additional life science journals.

This database is especially helpful when looking for off-label uses of medications. For example, if a prescriber contacts you asking for information about the efficacy of fluoxetine in treatment of anorexia nervosa, it may be appropriate to seek information from the primary literature. A PubMed search might be a good place to start this search. When performing a search using PubMed one can begin with just a key word, for example, fluoxetine. As Figure 1 shows, just using the term fluoxetine yields in 10,310 results. The results can be narrowed by entering a second key word, such as anorexia nervosa, and combining the two terms with the Boolean operator AND.

While the addition of a second search term (see Figure 2) did narrow the results, there are still 88 results that match these two terms. At this time it may be wise to explore the limit options provided by the database. Limits allow the user to restrict the number of results returned for a search. Some databases allow searches to be limited by a variety of factors, including language of publication, year of publication, type of article (e.g., human study, review, case report), or type of journal where publication is found. Since the requestor is seeking efficacy data, it is appropriate to limit these search results to just clinical trials.

By limiting the results to only human clinical trials published in English, 23 citations of possible interest have been identified (Figure 3). It is now necessary to look at the abstracts for these citations (Figure 4) and determine if these are helpful to provide a response to the query. By clicking on the blue hyperlink an abstract is displayed; this abstract summarizes the information in the article, as well as provides complete citation information for that specific article. If the publisher's Web site offers full text of an article, a link is provided at the top of the page to the journal Web site. Some journals charge a fee for access to the full-text article while others do not. Those journals not charging for an article are clearly marked as "free full text." You can then select that icon and go directly to a full-text PDF or html of the desired article.

One additional helpful feature offered by PubMed is the "Related citations" link. The database will first identify the key words or Medical Subject Headings (MeSH) associated with the article selected and then identify secondary words and terms. The database will then compare these terms (both primary and secondary terms) with other articles indexed in PubMed to determine which other articles include similarly ranked terms and, therefore, might be of interest.

The best way to effectively search this database is by experience. However, PubMed offers a tutorial to gain additional experience in how to most effectively conduct literature searches. This interactive tutorial session is available at http://www.nlm.nih.gov/bsd/disted/pubmedtutorial/.

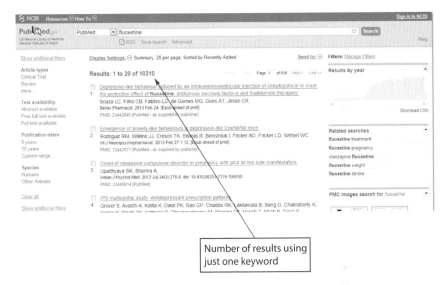

Number of results using just one keyword

Figure 1. Key word search.

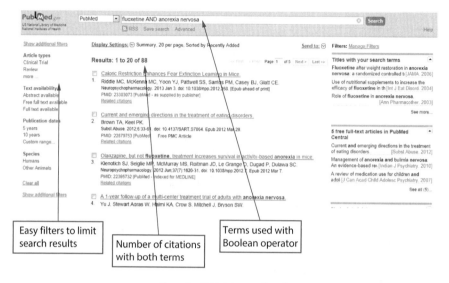

Figure 2. Multiple key word search.

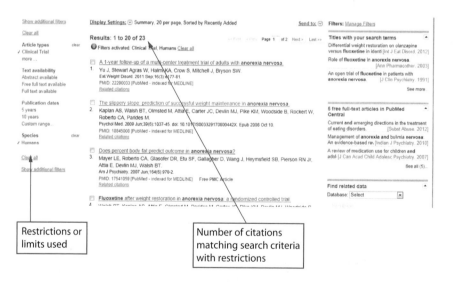

Figure 3. Results of search with restrictions.

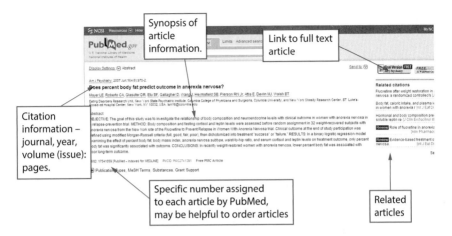

Figure 4. PubMed abstract.

3-2

Appendix 3–2

Selected Primary Literatures Sources

Journal Title	Publisher	ISSN	Areas Covered
American Journal of Health-System Pharmacy: AJHP	American Society of Health-System Pharmacy	1079-2082	Clinical and managerial areas of pharmacy practice in health systems
American Journal of Pharmacy Education	American Association of Colleges of Pharmacy	0002-9459	Scholarship and advancement of pharmacy education
Annals of Internal Medicine	American College of Physicians	0003-4819	Internal medicine, including management of disease states
Annals of Pharmacotherapy	Sage Journals	1060-0280	Safe, effective, and economical use of drugs
Antimicrobial Agents and Chemotherapy	American Society for Microbiology	0066-4804	Information regarding the use of antimicrobial agents
Archives of Internal Medicine	American Medical Association	0003-9926	Focus on the diagnosis and treatment of disease states
Clinical Pharmacokinetics	Adis International Limited	0312-5963	Focus on pharmacokinetic and pharmacodynamic properties of drugs
Clinical Pharmacology and Therapeutics	Nature Publishing Group	0009-9236	The effect of drugs on the human body
Drug Information Journal	Drug Information Association	0092-8615	Technology related to disseminating drug information
Drug Topics	Thomson Healthcare	0012-6616	Focus on issues impacting community pharmacy and on new drug therapies
Drugs	Adis International Limited	0012-6667	Pharmacotherapeutic aspects of both new and established drugs
Formulary	Advanstar Communications Incorporated	1082-801X	Contemporary issues in drug policy management and pharmacotherapy

continued

Journal Title	Publisher	ISSN	Areas Covered
Hospital Pharmacy	Thomas Land Publishers Incorporated	0018-5787	Issues related to pharmacy in institutional settings
JAMA (the Journal of the American Medical Association)	American Medical Association	0098-7484	New research and review information that impacts health care
Journal of Cardiovascular Pharmacology	Lippincott Williams & Wilkins	0160-2446	New information about the treatment of cardiovascular disease.
The Journal of Clinical Pharmacology	Lippincott, Williams & Wilkins	0091-2700	Clinical information about the safety, tolerability, efficacy, therapeutic use, and toxicology of drugs
Journal of Pharmaceutical Sciences	Wiley	0022-3549	Application of physical and analytical chemistry to pharmaceutical sciences
Journal of Pharmacology and Experimental Therapeutics	American Society for Experimental Pharmacology and Therapeutics	0022-3565	Covers interaction between chemicals and biological systems as well as metabolism, distribution, and toxicology.
Journal of Pharmacy and Pharmacology	Pharmaceutical Press	0022-3573	Addresses a variety of practice areas including drug delivery systems, biomaterials and polymers, and implications of human genome on drug therapies.
Journal of the American Pharmacists Association	American Pharmacists Association	1544-3191	News, information, and research in the area of pharmacotherapeutic management
Medical Letter on Drugs and Therapeutics	Medical Letter, Inc.	0025-732X	Provides information on new drug therapies and drugs of choice for disease management
New England Journal of Medicine	Massachusetts Medical Society	0028-646X	Results of recent research considered important to the practice of medicine
Pharmaceutical Research	Plenum Press	0724-8741	Emphasis on drug delivery, drug formulation, pharmacokinetics, pharmacodynamics, and drug disposition
PharmacoEconomics	Adis International Limited	1170-7690	Information regarding the economical use of drug therapies
Pharmacological Reviews	American Society of Pharmacology and Experimental Therapeutics	0031-6997	Current topics of interest including cellular pharmacology, drug metabolism and disposition, renal pharmacology, and neuropharmacology

continued

Journal Title	Publisher	ISSN	Areas Covered
Pharmacotherapy	IOS Press	0277-0008	Published by American College of Clinical Pharmacy and focused on original research in clinical practice
Pharmacy Times	Romaine Pierson Publishing Incorporated	0003-0627	Focus on new drug therapies and patient counseling as it relates to community pharmacy
Therapeutic Drug Monitoring	Lippincott Williams & Wilkins	0163-4356	Fosters exchange of knowledge between fields of pharmacology, pathology, toxicology, and analytical.
U.S. Pharmacist	Jobson Publishing Corporation	0148-4818	Information regarding the practice of community pharmacy

Appendix 4–1

Questions for Assessing Clinical Trials

OVERALL ASSESSMENT

- Was the article published in a reputable, peer-reviewed journal?
- Are the investigator's training/education/practice sites adequate for the study objective?
- Can the funding source bias the study?

TITLE/ABSTRACT

- Was the title unbiased?
- Did the abstract contain information not found within the study?
- Did the abstract provide a clear over view of the purpose, methods, results, and conclusions of the study?

INTRODUCTION

- Did the authors provide sufficient background information to demonstrate the rationale for the study?
- Were the study objectives clearly identified?
- What were the major null hypothesis and alternate hypothesis?

METHODS

- Was an appropriate study design used to answer the question?
- Were reasonable inclusion/exclusion criteria presented to represent an appropriate patient population?
- Was a selection bias present?
- Was subject recruitment described? If so, how were subjects recruited? Was the method appropriate?
- Was IRB approval obtained?
- Was subject informed consent obtained?
- Were the intervention and control regimens appropriate?
- What type of blinding was used? Was this type appropriate?
- Was randomization included? If so, what type was used? Was this appropriate?
- Who generated the allocation sequence, enrolled participants, and assigned participants to groups? Was this appropriate?

- Which ancillary treatments were permitted? Would they have affected the outcome?
- Was a run-in period included? How does this affect the results?
- Did the investigators measure compliance? How was compliance measured? Was compliance adequate?
- Was the primary endpoint appropriate for the study objective?
- Were secondary endpoints measured? If so, were they adequate for what was being studied?
- Were planned subgroup analyses planned? If so, were they appropriate?
- Was the method used to measure the primary endpoint appropriate?
- What type of data best describes the primary endpoint?
- Were data collected appropriately?
- What number of patients was needed for the primary endpoint to detect a difference between groups (power analysis)? Was the necessary sample size calculated? Were there enough patients enrolled to reach this endpoint?
- What were the alpha (α) and beta (β) values? Were these appropriate?
- Were the statistical tests used appropriate?

RESULTS

- Were the numbers of patients screened, enrolled, administered treatment, completing, and withdrawing from the study reported? Were reasons for subject discontinuations reported? Were withdrawals handled appropriately?
- Was the trial adequately powered?
- Were the subject demographics between groups similar at baseline? If not, were the differences likely to have an affect on the outcome data?
- Were data presented clearly?
- Were the results adjusted to take into account confounding variables?
- Was intention-to-treat analysis used? Was this appropriate?
- Were estimated effect size, p-values, and confidence intervals reported?
- Were the results statistically significant? Clinically different?
- Was the null hypothesis accepted or rejected?
- Can the trial results be extrapolated to the population?
- Based on the results, could a Type I or Type II error have occurred?
- Are subgroup analysis presented? Are these appropriate?
- Was ancillary therapy included? Did this affect the study results?
- Were therapy adverse effects included?

CONCLUSIONS/DISCUSSION

- Did the information appear biased, and did the trial results support the conclusions?
- Were trial limitations described?
- Did the investigators explain unexpected results?

- Are the results able to be extrapolated to the population?
- Were the study results clinically meaningful?

REFERENCES

- Were the references listed well represented (e.g., current, well-representing the literature)?
- Is a comprehensive list of published articles related to the trial objective presented?

Appendix 5–1

Beyond the Basics: Questions to Consider for Critique of Primary Literature

RANDOMIZED CONTROLLED TRIAL

- Refer to Chapter 4, Drug Literature Evaluation I: Controlled Clinical Trial Evaluation

PHARMACOECONOMIC ANALYSIS

- Refer to Chapter 6, Pharmacoeconomics

NONINFERIORITY TRIAL

- Is the reference drug's efficacy established using adequate historical data and/or addition of a placebo arm?
- Are the participants and outcome measures for the noninferiority similar compared to previous studies that confirmed the efficacy of the reference drug (e.g., constancy assumption)?
- Is the method used to determine the noninferiority (NI) margin predetermined before the study, both clinically and statistically sound, and the reasoning clearly stated in the article?
- Was a per-protocol analysis used? If so, did they also perform an intention-to-treat analysis?
- Was the sample size modified as the study progressed? If so, was a clear explanation of how the blinded information was handled and by what method these modifications were determined also provided?
- Was this study an attempt to rescue a failed superiority trial?

N-OF-1 TRIAL

- Was assignment of active and control treatment to study periods randomized?
- Was the study blinded?
- Were multiple observation periods used?
- Were study endpoints clearly defined?
- Was the washout period between study periods adequate?

ADAPTIVE CLINICAL TRIAL (ACT)

- Are the methodologies used to make adaptive changes in the trial adequately described?
- What logistical issues exist and have they been adequately addressed?
- Are the adaptive changes based on evidence and good clinical judgment?
- Did extensive adaptation to the protocol occur during the study?
- To what extent is intrusion of bias noted?
- Who has access to the information created from interim analyses?
- If the study was stopped early, is the totality of evidence adequate?

STABILITY STUDY

- Were study methodologies and test conditions clearly defined?
- Were validated assays used?
- Were assays validated using time-zero measurements and an adequate number of test samples taken?

BIOEQUIVALENCY STUDY

- Did the protocol define the characteristics of the subjects?
- Were confounding factors (e.g., smoking, alcohol use) identified and controlled?
- Was a crossover design used?
- Was the study randomized and blinded?

PROGRAMMATIC RESEARCH

- Were one of two options used for subject comparison: (1) comparison of subjects to those not using the program or service, (2) comparison of subjects before or after initiation of the program or service?
- Was the program or service clearly defined?
- Did the authors specify from whose perspective (e.g., patient, provider, physician, third-party payer) the study was undertaken?
- If costs were analyzed, were all costs associated with provision of the program or service included in the analysis, including personnel, inflationary changes, and cost savings had the intervention not occurred?
- Were clinically important outcome parameters used to assess effectiveness of the program or service?

COHORT STUDY

- Was the research question clearly stated?
- Were inclusion and exclusion criteria described in detail?
- Were exposed and unexposed subjects similar in terms of demographic characteristics and susceptibility to disease states?
- Was selection bias obviously present?

- Were confounding factors obviously present?
- Were the same efforts to measure outcomes made in each group?
- Were 95% confidence intervals calculated?
- Were follow-up rates the same for the exposed and unexposed groups?

CASE-CONTROL STUDY

- Was predisposition of disease similar in cases and controls except for exposure to the risk factor?
- Were cases and controls matched?
- Was exposure to the risk factor similar to that which would occur in the general population?
- Did cases and controls undergo similar diagnostic evaluations?
- Were investigators who assessed patients or collected data blinded to the status of the subject as a case or control?
- Did the investigators compare cases with several different control groups?
- Were 95% confidence intervals calculated?

CROSS-SECTIONAL STUDY

- Did investigators ensure accuracy in data collection?
- If a survey or questionnaire was used, was it validated?
- Were the inclusion and exclusion criteria clearly defined and stated?
- Was selection of cases clearly described?

CASE STUDY, CASE REPORT, OR CASE SERIES

- Did the authors recognize the preliminary nature of the results (i.e., recommendations for clinical application of the results should be guarded)?

SURVEY STUDY

- Was the survey instrument valid and reliable? Was a pretest or pilot test conducted on the survey instrument?
- Was the sample size large enough to detect a difference between groups?
- Was the survey objective and carefully planned?
- Were data quantifiable?
- Was the sample representative of the target population?
- Was response rate high enough to reflect results that would be expected of the target population?
- Did the investigators determine whether nonresponders differed from responders?

POSTMARKETING SURVEILLANCE STUDY

- Was a large enough sample studied to reflect current uses of and side effects associated with the new drug therapy?
- Were appropriate methods used to measure clearly defined endpoints?

NARRATIVE (NONSYSTEMATIC) REVIEWS—QUALITATIVE

- Was an extensive search for available studies undertaken?
- Did the authors use a variety of resources to identify studies for inclusion in the review article?
- Was the review article focused on a clearly defined population?
- Did the studies included in the review article use valid research methods?
- Did the author examine reasons for differences in study results and conclusions?
- Were outcomes of the studies clinically important?
- Did the author consider benefits and risks of the drug therapy?

SYSTEMATIC REVIEWS—QUALITATIVE

- Did the authors clearly define the research question?
- Was the review article focused on a clearly defined patient population?
- Was an extensive search for available studies undertaken?
- Did the authors consider using results from both published and unpublished studies in the analysis?
- Did the authors clearly define criteria for study inclusion in the analysis?
- Did the authors list studies that were included in and excluded from the analysis?
- Did the authors provide details concerning methodologies of studies used in the analysis?
  - Were included studies addressing the same clinical question(s)?
  - Did all included studies use appropriate doses, regimens, and routes of administrations for both treatments and comparators?
  - Were all included studies of appropriate duration?
- Were those who selected studies for inclusion in the analysis blinded to the names of the original authors, place of publication of the study, and final study results?

META-ANALYSIS—QUANTITATIVE

- Did the authors clearly define the research question?
- Was the review article focused on a clearly defined patient population?
- Was an extensive search for available studies undertaken?
- Did the authors consider using results from both published and unpublished studies in the analysis?
- Did the authors clearly define criteria for study inclusion in the analysis?
- Did the authors list studies that were included in and excluded from the analysis?
- Did the authors include gray literature in the analysis?
- Did the authors provide details concerning methodologies of studies used in the analysis?
  - Were included studies addressing the same clinical question(s)?
  - Did all included studies use appropriate doses, regimens, and routes of administrations for both treatments and comparators?
  - Were all included studies of appropriate duration?

- Was a funnel plot provided to determine if publication bias was potentially present?
- Were tests of homogeneity performed and results reported?
- Were those who selected studies for inclusion in the analysis blinded to the names of the original authors, place of publication of the study, and final study results?
- Were appropriate statistical tests used and the probability of Type I and Type II errors considered?
- Were 95% confidence intervals calculated?
- Were results presented in a forest plot?

PRACTICE GUIDELINES

- Is there an explicit description of the procedures used to identify, select, and combine evidence?
- Are the recommendations valid?
- Are the guidelines regularly reviewed and updated to incorporate new evidence as it becomes available?
- Was the guideline peer reviewed?
- Can the recommendations be generalized to a larger population?
- Was the source of funding for the development of the guideline provided and could it bias the conclusions?
- If another group of experts were to independently develop a guideline on the same clinical situation, would the recommendations be the same (are the recommendations reliable)?

QUALITY-OF-LIFE STUDIES

- Are HR-QOL instruments validated?
- If a series of HR-QOL measurements are used, does this result in a valid HR-QOL battery?
- Are HR-QOL instruments sensitive to changes in the patients' status as the trial progresses?
- Are important aspects of patients' lives measured, as determined by patients themselves?
- Is timing of HR-QOL measurements to answer the research questions appropriately related to anticipated timing of the clinical effects?
- Were sequences of HR-QOL assessments conducted in the same order for all patients?
- Was mode of data collection (self-report versus trained interviewer) appropriate for type of questions being asked?
  - If mode of data collection was a trained interviewer, could the interview location lead to biased answers?
- Were response rates to questionnaires reported?
- Is there missing data?
  - If missing data exist, is there a specific pattern that suggests author manipulation providing desired results (missing data could have countered author's hypothesis)?
- If a multicenter trial, did all sites evaluate HR-QOL?
- Is the QOL instrument valid for examining the specific disease in question?
- Are both positive and negative findings reported?

- Are adverse drug events and HR-QOL measurements considered separately?
- Is impact of treatment effects included with HR-QOL measurements?
- Is there evidence that culturally defined factors may have impacted patient HR-QOL measurements and/or the assessment of these measurements?
- Does there appear to be a bias on the part of the study researchers?
- Were general measures of QOL evaluated?

DIETARY SUPPLEMENT MEDICAL LITERATURE

- Which plant part was utilized?
- Was a standardized botanical extract utilized?
- Was the study product standardization appropriate?
- Was a specific plant species or specific salt form utilized?
- Was the study dose appropriate?
- Was trial length appropriate to perceive treatment effects or differences?
- Was sample size sufficient to detect a difference between groups if one exists?

Appendix 7–1

Grade Evidence Profile: Antibiotics for Children with Acute Otitis Media

Quality Assessment						Summary of Findings					
						Number of patients		Relative risk (95% CI)	Absolute risk		Quality
Number of studies (Design)	Limitations	Inconsistency	Indirectness	Imprecision	Publication bias	Placebo	Antibiotics		Control risk[a]	Risk difference (95% CI)	
Pain at 24h											
5 (RCT)	No serious limitations	No serious inconsistency	No serious indirectness	No serious imprecision	Undetected	241/605	223/624	RR 0.9 (0.78-1.04)	367/1000	Not significant	⊕⊕⊕⊕ High
Pain at 2-7 d											
10 (RCT)	No serious limitations	No serious inconsistency	No serious indirectness	No serious imprecision	Undetected	303/1366	228/1425	RR 0.72 (0.62-0.83)	257/1000	72 fewer per 1000 (44-98)	⊕⊕⊕⊕ High
Hearing, inferred from the surrogate outcome abnormal tympanometry—1 mo											
4 (RCT)	No serious limitations	No serious inconsistency	Serious indirectness (because of indirectness of outcome)	No serious imprecision	Undetected	168/460	153/467	RR 0.89 (0.75-1.07)	350/1000	Not significant	⊕⊕⊕o Moderate
Hearing, inferred from the surrogate outcome abnormal tympanometry—3 mo											
3 (RCT)	No serious limitations	No serious inconsistency (because of indirectness of outcome)	Serious indirectness	No serious imprecision	Undetected	96/398	96/410	RR 0.97 (0.76-1.24)	234/1000	Not significant	⊕⊕⊕o Moderate
Vomiting, diarrhea, or rash											
5 (RCT)	No serious limitations	Serious inconsistency (because of inconsistency in absolute effects)	No serious indirectness	No serious imprecision	Undetected	83/711	110/690	RR 1.38 (1.09-1.76)	113/1000	43 more per 1000 (10-86)	⊕⊕⊕o Moderate

[a] The control rate is based on the median control group risk across studies.

GRADE = Grading of Recommendations Assessment, Development, and Evaluation; RCT = randomized controlled trials; CI = confidence interval; RR = risk ratio.

Reproduced from Journal of Clinical Epidemiology, Vol 64, Gordon Guyatt, Andrew D. Oxman, Elie A. Akl, Regina Kunz, Gunn Vist, et al. GRADE guidelines: 1. Introduction GRADE evidence profiles and summary of findings tables. Pp. 383-394, Copyright 2011, with permission from Elsevier.

9-1

Question Example

DRUG INFORMATICS CENTER

St. Anywhere Hospital

Name of Inquirer:	Dr. Meghan J. Malone	Date: XX/XX/XX
Address	2184 Fall St. Seneca Falls, NY 13148	Time Received: XX:XX am/pm
		Time Required: 5 hours
		Nature of Request: Therapeutics
Telephone Number:	(315)555-1212	Type of Inquirer: Pharmacist

QUESTION

A young, adult male patient recently arrived from Japan and presented to the physician sparse medical records indicating he is suffering from tsutsugamushi disease. Because of the language difficulties, little is known about the patient, other than he is taking drug X for the illness. Physical examination reveals a patient in some discomfort with elevated temperature, swollen lymph glands, and red rash. All other findings appear to be normal. (*Note:* The person answering this question obtained as much background as possible about the patient.) The physician has little information on the disease and would like to know if that drug X is the most appropriate treatment.

ANSWER

Tsutsugamushi disease is an acute infectious disease seen in harvesters of hemp in Japan.[1] It is caused by *Rickettsia tsutsugamushi*. Common symptoms of the disease include fever, painful swelling of the lymph glands, a small black scab in the genital region, neck or axilla, and large dark-red papules. The disease is known by a number of other names, including akamushi disease, flood fever, inundation fever, island disease, Japanese river fever, and scrub typhus.[2-4] (*Note:* Background information presented.) The standard treatment of the disease includes either drug X or drug Y, although there are several other less effective treatments.[5-7] In the remainder of this paper, a comparison of the two major drugs will be presented. (*Note:* Clear objective for paper is presented.)

A thorough search of the available literature was conducted. Unfortunately, there were few textbooks available on this disease. A search of MEDLINE® (1966 to present) and EMBASE's *Drugs and Pharmacology* (1980 to present) produced a number of articles that were obtained and are reviewed below. (*Note:* This documents the type of search and acts as a lead-in to the remainder of the body of the paper.)

Smith and Jones[8] performed a double-blind, randomized comparison of the effects of drug X and drug Y in patients with tsutsugamushi fever. Patients were required to be between 18 and 70 years old, and could not have any concurrent infection or disorder that would affect the immune response to the disease (e.g., neutropenia, AIDS). Twenty patients received 10 mg of drug X three times a day for 15 days. Eighteen patients received 250 mg of drug Y twice a day for 10 days. The two groups were comparable, except that the patients receiving drug X were an average of 5 years younger ($p < 0.05$). Drug X was shown to produce a cure, both in terms of symptoms and cultures in 85% of patients, whereas drug Y only produced a cure in 55.5% of patients. The difference was statistically significant ($p < 0.01$). No significant adverse effects were seen in either group. Although it appears that drug X was the better agent, it should be noted that drug Y was given at its minimally effective dose, and may have performed better in a somewhat higher dose or longer regimen. (*Note:* Evaluative comments made about article.)

(*Note:* Other articles would be described at this point.)

Based on the literature found, it appears that drug Y is generally accepted as the better agent, except in those patients with severe renal insufficiency. Because this patient does not appear to be suffering from that problem, it is recommended that he receive a 3-week course of drug Y at a dose of 500 mg three times a day. Renal function should be monitored weekly. The patient should receive an additional week of therapy, if the symptoms have not been gone for the final week of therapy. (*Note:* This patient's situation was specifically addressed, rather than just presenting a general conclusion.)

Signature: _____ Date: March 20, 2014

Mia Q. Pharmacist, Pharm.D.

REFERENCES

(Present references here.)

Appendix 9–2

Abstracts

Abstracts are a synopsis (usually 250 words or less) of the most important aspect of an article. They should be clear, concise, and complete enough for readers to have a reasonable understanding of the important portions of the article.[1] Since they are the most commonly read part of an article, they must be accurate and avoid the three most common errors: differences in information presented in the abstract and in the body of the article, information given in the abstract that was not presented in the article, and conclusions presented in the abstract that are not supported by information in the abstract.[2-4]

There are basically three types of abstracts that are seen in the literature. The first two (descriptive and informational) are somewhat traditional; however, they do not convey as much information as structured abstracts. Structured abstracts were originally designed to convey more information, and have been in use since the 1980s. The type of abstract to be used depends on the type of information and the requirements of the particular place the work is being submitted or used.

In addition to writing an abstract, some journals ask that indexing terms be submitted. Whenever possible, Medical Subject Headings (MeSH) from the National Library of Medicine should be used for the indexing terms. Each of the abstracts will be discussed in more detail in the following sections.

DESCRIPTIVE ABSTRACTS

A descriptive abstract, as its name implies, simply describes the information found in an article. Few specific details are given and it is primarily used in a review article. An example of this type of abstract is as follows:

> Lists of references that should be available, depending on location of the drug information service, are presented. These lists are specific to community, hospital, long-term care facility, and academic sites. Included are general references, indexing and abstracting services, and journals. Specialty references that would be useful in specific circumstances are also presented. In addition, the equipment and software necessary to access the computerized resources is shown for the individual references.

INFORMATIONAL ABSTRACTS

Informational abstracts concisely summarize the factual information presented in a study. This type of abstract is more applicable to clinical studies.

Key points to include in an informational abstract:

- Study design (e.g., double-blind, crossover)
- Purpose
- Number of patients and other demographic aspects
- Dosages
- Results
- Conclusions

An example of this type of abstract is as follows:

> A double-blind, randomized comparison of the effects of drug X and drug Y was performed in patients with tsutsugamushi fever, in order to determine whether either drug was superior in efficacy or safety. Twenty patients received 10 mg of drug X three times a day for 15 days. Eighteen patients received 250 mg of drug Y twice a day for 10 days. The two groups were comparable, except that the patients receiving drug X were an average of 5 years younger ($p < 0.05$). Drug X was shown to produce a cure, both in terms of symptoms and cultures in 85% of patients, whereas drug Y only produced a cure in 55.5% of patients. The difference was statistically significant ($p < 0.01$). No significant adverse effects were seen in either group. Drug X was shown to be significantly better than drug Y in the treatment of tsutsugamushi fever.

STRUCTURED ABSTRACTS

Due to perceived deficiencies in abstracts,[5] including lack of sufficient information,[6] a new type of abstract was presented in 1987[7] and later updated in 1990.[8] This structured abstract was designed to present more information about clinical studies and possibly laboratory studies, as compared to the informational abstract presented earlier.[9,10] This type of abstract is not meant for case reports, studies of tissues or animals, opinion articles, and position papers.[7] Abstracts following this standard seem to be gaining in popularity[11] and have been mandated by an influential group of journals (e.g., *The New England Journal of Medicine,*[12] *Annals of Internal Medicine,*[7] *JAMA: Journal of the American Medical Association,*[8] *British Medical Journal,*[13] *Canadian Medical Association Journal,*[14] *Chest*[15]), sometimes in a somewhat modified form, although this type of abstract may not be used in the majority of articles found in popular medical journals.[16] This type of abstract has also been suggested in the pharmacy literature.[17] Although the overall acceptance and approval of this format of abstract appears to be good, there are some who disapprove.[18-20] Also, there is some data suggesting that structured abstracts do not always contain as much information as they should, if the published rules are followed,[21] and that they do not necessarily contain any more useful information than informational abstracts.[22]

It is worth noting that articles with structured abstracts are indexed with a greater number of terms in MEDLINE®, which may make it easier to find such articles in a computer search.[23]

An abstract following this procedure would contain the following subheadings and information:

- *Objective*—The main objective of the study and key secondary objectives.
- *Design*—The basic design of the study (e.g., randomized, double-blind, crossover, placebo-controlled, prospective versus retrospective) and duration of any follow-up.

- *Setting*—The location and level of clinical care available at that location (e.g., tertiary care hospital, ambulatory clinic). Also, if a single or multiple locations were involved.
- *Patients or other participants*—Description of the patients, including illnesses and key sociodemographic features, and how they were selected for the study (including whether it was a random, volunteer, etc. sample); it should also include the number of patients who refused to enroll in the study, proportion of the patients completing the study, and number of patients withdrawn due to adverse effects or other reasons.
- *Intervention(s)*—A brief description of any treatment(s) or intervention(s).
- *Main outcome measure(s)*—The main study outcome measurements, as planned before data collection was begun; if most of the article covers other material (e.g., data or hypotheses not planned to be observed before the study was started), that should be made clear.
- *Results*—The method(s) by which patients were assessed and the main results of the study, including any blinding. Statistical significance (particularly confidence intervals, odds ratios, numerators, and denominators) and levels of significance should be mentioned. Absolute, rather than relative, differences are presented (e.g., "adverse effects were seen in 5% of patients in group A and 10% of patients in group B," rather than "group B had twice as many adverse effects"). The response rate should be provided in survey articles.
- *Conclusion(s)*—The key conclusion(s) directly supported by the evidence presented in the study and their clinical application(s) as well as a statement regarding whether further study is necessary should be included.

An example of this type of abstract is as follows:

Study objective— To compare the safety and efficacy of drug X and drug Y in the treatment of tsutsugamushi fever.

Design—Randomized, double-blind trial

Setting—Tertiary care, military hospital located on Guam

Patients—Sequential sample of 40 young (age 20 to 37), otherwise healthy male patients with tsutsugamushi fever. Patients randomly divided into two equal groups. Two patients were removed from the group receiving drug Y, due to transfer to U.S. mainland hospitals. The two groups were comparable, except that the patients receiving drug X were an average of 5 years younger ($p < 0.05$).

Interventions—Twenty patients received 10 mg of drug X three times a day for 15 days. Eighteen patients received 250 mg of drug Y twice a day for 10 days.

Main outcome measures—Physician and patients' global assessment of disease activity; five-point scale from 0 (no symptoms) to 5 (severe disability). Presence or absence of organism on laboratory specimens.

Results—Drug X was shown to produce a cure, both in terms of symptoms and cultures in 85% of patients, whereas drug Y only produced a cure in 55.5% of patients. The difference was statistically significant ($p < 0.01$). No significant adverse effects were seen in either group.

Conclusions—Drug X was shown to produce significantly higher cure rates than drug Y in the treatment of tsutsugamushi fever, with no difference in adverse effects. Additional trials at different doses and lengths of therapy should be performed.

A method to prepare a structured abstract for a review article differs from the first example.[24] This method would only be applicable in specific situations, where a number of similar studies were evaluated together. It would not be useful in a situation where a number of dissimilar articles dealing with the same topic were discussed (e.g., a review of all therapies for a particular disease). Such an abstract would consist of the following items:

- *Purpose*—The main objective of the review article, including information about the population tested, how they were tested, and the outcome.
- *Data sources*—A brief summary of data sources and the time periods covered.
- *Study selection*—The number of studies covered in the article and how they were selected for inclusion.
- *Data extraction*—A description of the guidelines for abstracting data and how those guidelines were applied.
- *Data synthesis*—The main results of the review and the method to obtain the results are outlined.
- *Conclusions*—Important conclusions, including applications and need for further study.

An example of this type of abstract would be as follows:

Purpose—To evaluate the effect of the antihistamine, drug X, on symptoms of allergic reactions, as determined by physicians' and patients' global symptom assessment.

Data sources—Studies published from January 1980 to December 2013 were identified by computer searches of MEDLINE® and Embase—*Drugs and Pharmacology*—and hand searching of bibliographies of the articles identified via the computer search.

Study selection—Fifty-three studies evaluating the effects of drug X in the treatment of allergies were located.

Data extraction—Descriptive data regarding the population, dosing, effects, and adverse effects were assessed, along with the study's quality.

Results of data analysis—Subjective and objective measures of effectiveness demonstrated that drug X decreased or eliminated allergy symptoms approximately 80% of the time in a variety of patient types (e.g., seasonal allergic rhinitis, perennial allergic rhinitis, anaphylaxis). The only adverse effects seen were dryness of mucous membranes and sedation, seen in approximately 5% and 2% of patients, respectively.

Conclusions—Drug X is an effective agent for the treatment of allergic reactions. It has a low incidence of typical antihistamine adverse effects. Further studies should be performed to verify the effectiveness of Drug X in comparison to other drugs commonly used for anaphylaxis.

A version of a structure abstract has also been proposed for use in describing clinical practice guidelines (see Chapter 7 for more information about such guidelines).[25] The format is as follows:

- *Objective*—Provides the primary objective of the guideline. This must include the health problem, along with the targeted patients, providers, and settings.
- *Options*—This includes the various clinical practice options that were considered when the guideline was formulated.
- *Outcomes*—Presents the significant health and economic outcomes that were considered when the alternative practices were considered.

- *Evidence*—Describes how and when the evidence was gathered, selected for use, and synthesized.
- *Values*—Describes how values were assigned to the potential outcomes, along with who was involved in doing so.
- *Benefits, harms, and costs*—Provides both the type and magnitude of the benefits, harms, and costs that might be expected from using the guideline.
- *Recommendations*—Provides a summary of the key recommendations.
- *Validation*—Describes any external validation of the guidelines that was conducted.
- *Sponsors*—Provides a list of the people who developed, funded, and/or endorsed the guideline.

An example of this type of abstract would be as follows:

- *Objective*—To determine the best initial therapy for allergic rhinitis. This guideline is intended for physicians and pharmacists to determine the best way to start therapy, particularly in the community.
- *Options*—Different nonprescription medications are considered first (antihistamines, decongestants [systemic and local], cromolyn), with the place for prescription intranasal steroids in initial therapy.
- *Outcomes*—The major outcomes evaluated are relief of symptoms, adverse effects, and direct cost to the patient.
- *Evidence*—All randomized, controlled clinical trials published in English found in MEDLINE from 1990 to 2012 were considered. In regard to costs, the average retail cost of the medication and the cost of a physician visit (for prescription medications) were calculated, based on the therapy used in the studies.
- *Values*—A group of three board certified allergy physicians and three pharmacists (Pharm.D. and either Board Certified Pharmacotherapy Specialist or Board Certified Ambulatory Care Pharmacist) were appointed by the American Academy of Allergy, Asthma & Immunology to review and evaluate the studies and pharmacoeconomic data. Patients were not represented.
- *Benefits, harms, and costs*—Use of a second-generation antihistamine (e.g., loratadine, cetirizine) provides the greatest efficacy with the least cost. Decongestants may be of value in the first few days, but are contraindicated in hypertensive patients. All other therapies have less effectiveness or greater cost.
- *Recommendations*—Patients suffering from allergies should begin therapy with a second-generation antihistamine, preferably about a week prior to anticipated allergen exposure. If therapy cannot be started early, pseudoephedrine may be used for up to 3 days as part of initial therapy in patients without hypertension or other contraindication. If this therapy is not sufficient, patients should be evaluated by a physician and prescribed an intranasal steroid spray.
- *Validations*—This recommendation was reviewed by three reviewers in the normal peer-review process established by the American Academy of Allergy, Asthma & Immunology.
- *Sponsors*—Development of this recommendation was funded by the American Academy of Allergy, Asthma & Immunology.

REFERENCES

1. Staub NC. On writing abstracts. Physiologist. 1991;34:276-7.
2. Pitkin RM, Branagan MA. Can the accuracy of abstracts be improved by providing specific instructions? A randomized controlled trial. JAMA. 1998;280:267-9.
3. Pitkin RM, Branagan MA, Burmeister LF. Accuracy of data in abstracts of published research articles. JAMA. 1999;281:1110-1.
4. Winker MA. The need for concrete improvement in abstract quality. JAMA. 1999;281:1129-30.
5. Huth EJ. Structured abstracts for papers reporting clinical trials. Ann Intern Med. 1987;106:626-7.
6. Narine L, Yee DS, Einarson TR, Ilersich AL. Quality of abstracts of original research articles in CMAJ in 1989. CMAJ. 1991;144:449-53.
7. Ad Hoc Working Group for Critical Appraisal of the Medical Literature. A proposal for more informative abstracts of clinical articles. Ann Intern Med. 1987;106:598-604.
8. Haynes RB, Mulrow CD, Huth EJ, Altman DG, Gardner MJ. More informative abstracts revisited. Ann Intern Med. 1990;113:69-76.
9. Rennie D, Glass RM. Structuring abstracts to make them more informative. JAMA. 1991;266:116-17.
10. Haynes RB. Dissent. More informative abstracts: current status and evaluation. J Clin Epidemiol. 1993;46:595-7.
11. Ripple AM, Mork JG, Knecht LS, Humphreys BL. A retrospective cohort study of structured abstracts in MEDLINE, 1992-2006. J Med Libr Assoc. 2011;99(2):160-163.
12. Relman AS. New "Information for Authors"—and readers. NEJM. 1990;323:56.
13. Lock S. Structure abstracts. Now required for all papers reporting clinical trials. BMJ. 1988;297:156.
14. Squires BP. Structured abstracts of original research and review articles. CMAJ. 1990;143:619-22.
15. Soffer A. Abstracts of clinical investigations. A new and standardized format. Chest. 1987;92:389-90.
16. Nakayama T, Hirai N, Yamazaki S, Naito M. Adoption of structured abstracts by general medical journals and format for a structured abstract. J Med Libr Assoc. 2005;93(2):237242.
17. Kane-Gill S, Olsen KM. How to write an abstract suitable for publication. Hosp Pharm. 2004;39:289-92.
18. Spitzer WO. Second thoughts. The structured sonnet. J Clin Epidemiol. 1991;44:729.
19. Heller MB. Dissent. Structured abstracts: a modest dissent. J Clin Epidemiol. 1991;44:739-40.
20. Heller MB. Structured abstracts. [letter] Ann Intern Med. 1990;113:722.
21. Froom P, Froom J. Variance and dissent: Presentation. Deficiencies in structured medical abstracts. J Clin Epidemiol. 1993;46:591-4.
22. Scherer RW, Crawley B. Reporting of randomized clinical trial descriptors and use of structured abstracts. JAMA. 1998;280:269-72.
23. Harbourt AM, Knecht LS, Humphreys BL. Structured abstracts in MEDLINE®, 1989–1991. Bull Med Libr Assoc. 1995:83(2):190-5.
24. Mulrow CD, Thacker SB, Pugh JA. A proposal for more informative abstracts of review articles. Ann Intern Med. 1988;108:613-5.
25. Hayward RSA, Wilson MC, Tunis SR, Bass EB, Rubin HR, Haynes RB. More informative abstracts of articles describing clinical practice guidelines. Ann Intern Med. 1993;118:731-7.

9-3

Appendix 9–3

Bibliography

Although there seems to be a different method to prepare a bibliography for every English class ever given, there is fortunately a standardized method to prepare a bibliography in medical writing. This method is used by the National Library of Medicine and has been incorporated into the *Uniform Requirements for Manuscripts Submitted to Biomedical Journals* and published in *Citing Medicine*[1-3]; it has been used widely since the 1970s in both journals and other medical writing. This method will be presented here.

References in the bibliography are placed in the order they are first cited in the text of a document, and each reference is assigned a consecutive Arabic number. Those cited only in tables or figures are numbered according to the place the table or figure is identified in the text. References are not listed multiple times in the bibliography, if they are cited more than once in the text of the document. Instead, subsequent citations to the same reference use the original reference number. It should also be noted that *Ibid* is not used. The reference number in the text will be the Arabic number in parenthesis or, commonly, superscript. This number is often cited after the sentence that contains the fact being referenced. If there are several references used to prepare a specific sentence, they may be listed at the end of the sentence or throughout the sentence. Also, if the sentence is a lead-in to an abstract, the authors' names are commonly listed followed by the reference number. See the sentences below for examples.

- Drug X has been shown to cause green rash with purple spots.[2,3]
- Drug Y is useful in the treatment of hypertension,[4] congestive heart failure,[5] and arrhythmias.[6]
- Smith and Jones[7] studied the effects of ...
- Brown *et al.*[9] treated ... (please notice on this example, *al.* is followed by a period since it is an abbreviation, whereas *et* is a full Latin word, and there is no need for a comma after the first author's name)
- Brown and associates[9] treated ... (this is used the same way as the previous example, but is preferred by some people over the use of et al.)

Before getting into the method for listing references and examples, it should be mentioned that there are a number of general rules to be followed:

- Citations are often not found in conclusions of documents. The conclusions are based on the information presented, and cited, earlier in the article.
- Avoid using abstracts as references, if at all possible. Sometimes the information is only published as an abstract, so it is necessary to cite the abstract in this situation.

- Avoid using unpublished observations or personal communications as references. In the latter case, it is proper to insert references to written, but not oral, communications in parentheses in the text only and indicate it will not be formally referenced at the end of publication. Permission must be obtained from the author for the use of this material and this should only be used if the material is not available from a public source of information. A note should be made at the end of the publication stating that permission was given.
- If reference is made to an article that has been accepted by a journal, but not yet published, the phrase *Forthcoming* followed by the year of planned publication should be inserted where the volume and page numbers would normally be listed. It is usually necessary to get permission to cite this type of article, since the publisher may have strict confidentiality rules, and verification of acceptance by the journal should be obtained if that is the case.
- The use of the Internet has increased substantially, so it is important to use the correct citation based on the medium used.
- Only place a period at the end of a Web address if a back slash is the last character in the address.
- For items such as wikis, blogs, databases, when they are still open (people can still add something), use a hyphen with three spaces following it for date of publication. If they are closed (people can no longer add something), list the range of dates it was open.

Examples and some general templates of the above-mentioned and other types of references used in a bibliography are provided in the balance of this appendix. Please note that these should provide adequate direction in how to cite most publications. However, if detailed directions and further examples are needed, the reader is referred to *Citing Medicine*, which is available free on the Internet at http://nlm.nih.gov/citingmedicine.[3]

JOURNAL ARTICLES

To cite a journal article, the following information should be given:

- Last name of author(s) and initials each separated by commas, with a period at the end. Please note that some publications will list only three or six authors followed by the phrase *et al.*
- Title of article (do not use quotation marks, capitalize only the initial word of title and proper nouns in English) followed by a period with the exception when punctuation is already at the end of the title—for example, if a title ends with a question mark or exclamation point, use that instead of the period.
- Journal Title (abbreviated as found in the list of journals at http://www.nlm.nih.gov/tsd/serials/lji.html) followed by a period.
- Date of Publication (year, month [three-letter abbreviation], and day of month [if available]) followed by a semicolon.
- Volume number (listing the issue number in parenthesis) followed by a colon.
- Page numbers (If continuous, use first and last pages separated by a hyphen. Keep page numbers concise (e.g., 561-569 should be 561-9). If separate pages, list the pages separated by a comma and a space. If a combination of continuous and separate pages, use both (e.g., 18-29, 33, 40) followed by a period. If an Internet article does not have page numbers, put the

actual number of pages in square brackets, followed by p. (e.g., [20 p.]). If the article is in unpaginated format (e.g., html, xml), precede the number with the word about (e.g., [about 10 screens] or [about 15 p.])

A condensed version of the above information is as follows:

Author(s). Title of article. Journal Title. Date of Publication;Volume Number(Issue Number): Page Number(s).

Journal on the Internet

Author(s). Title of article. Journal Title [Internet]. Date of Publication [Date of Update; Date of Citation];Volume Number(Issue Number):Page Number(s) or [Length of Article]. Available from: Web Address

Example Journal Citations

Standard Journal Article

Smythe M, Hoffman J, Kizy K, Dmuchowski C. Estimating creatinine clearance in elderly patients with low serum creatinine concentrations. *Am J Hosp Pharm*. 1994 Jan 15;51:198-204.

Beck DE, Aceves-Blumenthal C, Carson R, Culley J, Noguchi J, Dawson K, Hotchkiss G. Factors contributing to volunteer practitioner-faculty vitality. *Am J Pharm Ed*. 1993 Apr;57:305-12.

Journal Article on the Internet

Robinson ET. The pharmacists as educator: implications for practice and education. *Am J Pharm Ed* [Internet]. 2004 [cited 2010 Jun 17];68(3):[4 p.]. Available from: http://www.ajpe.org/aj6803/aj680372/aj680372.pdf

Nemecz G. Evening primrose. US Pharmacist [Internet]. 1998 Nov [cited 1998 Dec 10];23: [about 1 p.]. Available from: http://www.uspharmacist.com/NewLook/Docs/1998/Nov1998/EveningPrimrose.htm

Organization as Author

Task Force on Specialty Recognition of Oncology Pharmacy Practice. Executive summary of petition requesting specialty recognition of oncology pharmacy practice. *Am J Hosp Pharm*. 1994 Jan 15;51:219-24.

Personal Authors and Organization as Author

Wiencke K, Louka AS, Spurkland A, Vatn M, The IBSEN Study Group, Schrumpf E. Association of matrix metalloproteinase-1 and -3 promoter polymorphisms with clinical subsets of Norwegian primary sclerosing cholangitis patients. *J Hepatol*. 2004 Aug;41(2):209-14.

No Author Given

N.Y. court rules against Medicaid co-pay. *Drug Topics*. 1994 Mar;138(3):6.

Article Not in English (Note That the Language Is Stated at the End)

Antoni N. Zur kritjk der irrtümlich sogenannten sehnen- und periostreflexe. *Acta Psychiatrica Neurologica*. 1932;VII:9-19. German.

Volume with Supplement

Nayler WG. Pharmacological aspects of calcium antagonism. Short term and long term benefits. *Drugs*. 1993 Apr;46Suppl 2:40-7.

Issue with Supplement

Graves NM. Pharmacokinetics and interactions of antiepileptic drugs. *Am J Hosp Pharm*. 1993 Dec;50(12 Suppl A):S23-9.

Volume with Part

Katchen MS, Lyons TJ, Gillingham KK, Schlegel W. A case of left hypoglossal neurapraxia following G exposure in a centrifuge. *Aviat Space Environ Med*. 1990 Sep;61(Pt 2):837-9.

Issue with Part

Dudley MN. Maximizing patient outcomes of antiinfective therapy. *Pharmacotherapy*. 1993 Mar-Apr;13(2 Pt 2):29S-33S.

Issue with No Volume

Slaga TJ, Gimenez-Conti IB. An animal model for oral cancer. *Monogr J Nat Cancer Instit*. 1992;(13): 55-60.

No Issue or Volume

Payne R. Acute exacerbation of chronic cancer pain: basic assessment and treatments of break-through pain. *Acute Pain Sympt Manage*. 1998:4-5.

Pagination in Roman Numerals

Koretz RL. Clinical nutrition. *Gastroenterol Clin North Am*. 1998 Jun;27(2):xi-xiii.

Expressing Type of Article (As Needed)

Goldwater SH, Chatelain F. Taking time to communicate [letter]. *Am J Hosp Pharm*. 1994 Feb 1;51: 232, 234.

Talley CR. Reducing demand through preventive care [editorial]. *Am J Hosp Pharm*. 1994 Jan 1;51:55.

Saritas A, Cakir Z, Emet M, Uzkeser M, Akoz A, Acemoglu F. Factors affecting the b-type natriuretic peptide levels in stroke patients [abstract]. *Ann Acad Med Singapore*. 2010 May;39(5):385.

Article Containing a Retraction

Brown MD. Retraction. Am Heart J. 1986;111:623. Retraction of: Slutsky RA, Olson LK. *Am Heart J*. 1984;108:543-7.

Article Retracted

Slutsky RA, Olson LK. Intravascular and extravascular pulmonary fluid volumes during chronic experimental left ventricular dysfunction *Am Heart J*. 1984 Sep;108:543-7. Retraction in: *Am Heart J*. 1986 Mar;111:623.

Article with Published Erratum

Reitz MS Jr, Juo HG, Oleske J, Hoxie J, Popovic M, Read-Connole E. On the historical origins of HIV-1 (MN) and (RF) [letter]. *AIDS Res Hum Retroviruses*. 1992 Aug;8:1539-41. Erratum in: *AIDS Res Hum Retroviruses* 1992 Aug;8:1731.

Item (e.g., Table or Figure) in Article

Hohnloser SH, Pajitnev D, Pogue J, Healey JS, Pfeffer MA, Yusuf S, Connolly SJ. Incidence of stroke in paroxysmal versus sustained atrial fibrillation in patients taking oral anticoagulation or combined antiplatelet therapy: an ACTIVE W substudy. *J Am Coll Cardiol*. 2007 Nov 22;50(22):2156-61. Table 4, Incidence of stoke or non-CNS systemic embolism in patients with paroxysmal versus persistent/permanent AF treated with aspirin plus clopidogrel or OAC; p. 2159.

Unpublished Article

Malone PM. Topics in informatics. *Adv Pharm*. Forthcoming 2004.

BOOKS

To cite a book, which can include manuals, brochures, or fact sheets, the following information should be given:

- Last name of author(s) and initials each separated by a comma and followed by a period. Some publications will list only three authors followed by the phrase *et al.*
- Title of book (capitalize only the initial word of title and proper nouns in English) followed by a period with the exception that punctuation is already at the end of the title—for example, if a title ends with a question mark or exclamation point, use that instead of the period
- Edition, other than first followed by period
- Place of publication (city) followed by colon (if the location is not clear with just a city name, the state or country abbreviation may be placed in parenthesis after the city name and before the colon)
- Name of publisher followed by semicolon
- Year of publication followed by period

A condensed version of the above information is as follows:

Author(s). Title of Book. Edition. Place of Publication: Publisher; Date of Publication.

Book on the Internet:

Author(s). Title of Book [Internet]. Place of Publication: Publisher; Date of Publication [Date of Update; Date of Citation]. Available from: Web Address

Example Book Citations

Standard Book

Albright RG. A basic guide to online information systems for health care professionals. Arlington (VA): Information Resource Press; 1988.

Book on the Internet

DiPiro JT, Talbert RL, Yee GC, Matzke GR, Wells BG, Posey LM, editors. Pharmacotherapy: a pathophysiologic approach [Internet]. 7th ed. New York: McGraw-Hill; 2008 [cited 2010 Jun 15]. Available from: http://www.accesspharmacy.com/resourceToc.aspx?resourceID = 406

Lacy CF, Armstrong LL, Goldman MP, et al, editors. Lexi-comp online [Internet]. Hudson (OH): Lexi-
Comp, Inc.; c1978-2010 [cited 2010 Jun 16]. Available from: http://online.lexi.com/crlsql/
servlet/crlonline

Editor(s) as Author

Chisholm-Burns MA, Wells BG, Schwinghammer TL, Malone PM, Kolesar JM, Dipiro JT, editors.
Pharmacotherapy principles and practice. 3rd ed. New York: McGraw-Hill; 2013.

No Specific Editor(s), Compiler, or Author Identified

Drug facts and comparisons 1999. St. Louis: Facts and Comparisons; 1998.

Organization as Author and Publisher

United States Pharmacopeial Convention, Inc. USAN and the USP dictionary of drug names. Rockville: United States Pharmacopeial Convention, Inc.; 1993.

Volumes (Same Author(s)/Editor(s))

United States Pharmacopeial Convention, Inc. USP dispensing information. 22nd ed. Vol. 2, Advice for
the patient: drug information in lay language. Greenwood Village (CO): Micromedex; 2002.

If on the Internet use the following format:

**Author(s). Title of Book. Volume Number, Volume Title [Internet]. Place of Publication:
Publisher; Date of Publication [Date of Update; Date of Citation]. Available from: Web
Address**

Ross IA. Medicinal plants of the world. Vol. 3, Chemical constituents, traditional and modern medicinal uses [Internet]. Totowa (NJ): Humana Press, Inc.; 2005 [cited 2010 Jun 23]. Available from:
http://metis.findlay.edu:2080/xtf-ebc/search?keyword = pharmacy

*Portion of a Book (e.g., Chapter, Table, Figure, or Appendix) with Author(s) Writing Entire
Book*

Bauer LA. Applied clinical pharmacokinetics. 2nd ed. New York: McGraw-Hill; 2008. Chapter 6,
Digoxin; p. 301-55.

If on the Internet, use the following format:

**Author(s). Title of Book [Internet]. Place of Publication: Publisher; Date of Publication
[Date of Update of Book]. Portion Number, Portion Title; [Date of Update of Portion;
Date of Citation]; Page Number(s) or [Length of Portion]. Available from: Web
Address**

Bauer LA. Applied clinical pharmacokinetics [Internet]. 2nd ed. New York: McGraw-Hill; 2008. Chapter 6, Digoxin; [cited 2010 Jun 23]; [about 20 screens]. Available from: http://metis.findlay.
edu:2209/content.aspx?aID = 3519569

Contribution to Book (Portions of Book Written by Different Authors)

Malesker MA, Morrow LE. Fluids and electrolytes. In: Chisholm-Burns MA, Schwinghammer TL, Wells BG, Malone PM, Kolesar JM, Dipiro JT, editors. Pharmacotherapy principles and practice. 2nd ed. New York: McGraw-Hill; 2010. p. 479-94.

If on the Internet, use the following format:

Chapter Author(s). Chapter Title. In: Author(s)/Editor(s). Title of Book [Internet]. Place of Publication: Publisher; Date of Publication [Date of Citation]. Available from: Web address

Malone PM. Professional writing. In: Malone PM, Kier KL, Stanovich JE, editors. Drug information: a guide for pharmacists [Internet]. 4th ed. New York: McGraw-Hill; 2012 [cited 2012 Oct 17]. Available from: http://www.accesspharmacy.com/content.aspx?aid = 55673619

Book on CD-ROM or DVD

Haux R, Kulikowski C. Yearbook 04 of medical informatics – towards clinical bioinformatics [CD-ROM]. Stuttgart (Germany): Schatteuer; 2004.

Video Clip, Videocast, or Podcast Associated with Book

Author(s). Title of Book [Internet]. Place of Publication: Publisher; Date of Publication. [Video or Videocast or Podcast], Title of Video; [Date of Citation]; [Length of Video]. Available from: Web Address

Brunton LL, Parker KL, Murri N, Blumenthal DK, Knollmann BC, editors. Goodman and Gilman's: the pharmacological basis of therapeutics [Internet]. 11th ed. New York: McGraw-Hill; 2006 [Video], Adrenergic neuroeffector junction; [cited 2010 Jun 23]; [5 min.]. Available from: http://metis.findlay.edu:2209/video.aspx?file = anj_01/anj_01

OTHER MATERIAL

Format and Example Citations (in alphabetical order)

Conference Proceedings

Editor(s). Conference Title; Date(s) of Conference; Conference Location. Place of Publication: Publisher; Date of Publication.

Allebeck P, Jansson B, editors. Ethics in medicine. Individual integrity versus demands of society. Karolinska Institute Novel Conference Series. Proceedings of the 3rd International Congress on Ethics in Medicine; 1989 Sep 13-15; Stockholm. New York: Raven Press; 1990.

If on the Internet, use the following format:

Editor(s). Conference Title [Internet]; Date(s) of Conference; Conference Location. Place of Publication: Publisher; [Date of Citation]. [Length of Publication]. Available from: Web Address

Allebeck P, Jansson B, editors. Ethics in medicine. Individual integrity versus demands of society. Karolinska Institute Novel Conference Series. Proceedings of the 3rd International Congress on Ethics in Medicine [Internet]; 1989 Sep 13-15; Stockholm. New York: Raven Press; [cited 2010 Jun 23]. [8 p.] Available from: http://jmp.oxfordjournals.org/cgi/issue_pdf/backmatter_pdf/13/4.pdf

Conference Paper

Author(s) of Conference Paper. Title of Paper. In: Editors of Conference Proceedings. Conference Title; Date(s) of Conference; Conference Location. Place of Publication: Publisher; Date of Publication. Pages.

Keyserlingk E. Ethical guidelines and codes—can they be universally applicable in a multi-cultural world? In: Allebeck P, Jansson B, editors. Ethics in medicine. Individual integrity versus demands of society. Karolinska Institute Novel Conference Series. Proceedings of the 3rd International Congress on Ethics in Medicine; 1989 Sep 13-15; Stockholm. New York: Raven Press; 1990. p. 137-49.

If on the Internet, use the following format:

Author(s) of Conference Paper. Title of Paper. In: Editors of Conference Proceedings. Conference Title [Internet]; Date(s) of Conference; Conference Location. Place of Publication: Publisher; Date of Publication [Date of Citation]. [Length of Paper]. Available from: Web Address

Keyserlingk E. Ethical guidelines and codes—can they be universally applicable in a multi-cultural world? In: Allebeck P, Jansson B, editors. Ethics in medicine. Individual integrity versus demands of society. Karolinska Institute Novel Conference Series. Proceedings of the 3rd International Congress on Ethics in Medicine [Internet]; 1989 Sep 13-15; Stockholm. New York: Raven Press; 1990 [cited 2010 Jun 23]. [about 2 p.]. Available from: http://jmp.oxfordjournals. org/cgi/issue_pdf/backmatter_pdf/13/4.pdf

Dictionary Definition

Dictionary Name. Place of Publication: Publisher; Date of Publication.Word Being Defined; Page Number.

Stedman's medical dictionary. 27th ed. New York: Lippincott Williams & Wilkins; 2000. Asthenia; p. 158.

If on the Internet, use the following format:

Dictionary Name [Internet]. Place of Publication: Publisher; Date of Publication. Term Being Defined; [Date of Citation]. Available from: Web Address

Merriam-Webster Online [Internet]. Springfield (MA): Merriam-Webster, Inc.; c2010. Blood pressure; [cited 2010 Jun 23]. Available from: http://www.merriam-webster.com/dictionary/blood%20 pressure

Dissertation/Thesis

Author(s). Title [dissertation or master's thesis]. Place of Publication: Publisher; Date of Publication.

Wellman CO. Pain perceptions and coping strategies of school-age children and their parents: a descriptive-correlational study [dissertation]. Omaha (NE): Creighton University; 1985.

If on the Internet, use the following format:

Author(s). Title [dissertation or master's thesis on the Internet]. Place of Publication: Publisher; Date of Publication [Date of Update; Date of Citation]. Available from: Web Address

Mil JW. Pharmaceutical care, the future of pharmacy: theory, research, and practice [dissertation on the Internet]. Groningen (The Netherlands): University of Groningen; 2000 Feb 1 [updated 2009 Sep 8; cited 2010 Jun 23]. Available from: http://dissertations.ub.rug.nl/faculties/science/2000/j.w.f.van.mil/?pLanguage = en&pFullItemRecord = ON

Legal Documents

Please consult: The bluebook: a uniform system of citation. 19th ed. Cambridge (MA): Harvard Law Review Association; 2010.

Newspaper Article

Author(s). Title of Article. Newspaper Title (Edition). Date of Publication;Section:Page Number(Column Number).

Fein EB. Rise in fetal tests prompts ethical debate. The New York Times (National Ed.). 1994 Feb 5;Sect. A:1(col. 2).

If on the Internet, use the following format:

Author(s). Title of Article. Newspaper Title [Internet]. Date of Publication [Date of Update; Date of Citation];Section:Page Number or [Length of Article]. Available from: Web Address

Painter K. Your health: feet bear the strain of extra weight. USA Today [Internet]. 2010 Jun 20 [cited 2010 Jun 23];Health and Behavior:[about 2 screens]. Available from: http://www.usatoday.com/news/health/painter/2010-06-21-yourhealth21_ST_N.htm

Package Insert

Package inserts are commonly cited in professional writing; however, the Uniform Requirements do not address the format to use. The following is a common format that is similar to those presented in this appendix.

Medication Name [package insert]. Place of Publication: Publisher; Date of Publication.

Prilosec® (omeprazole) delayed-release capsules [package insert]. Wayne, PA: Astra Merck; 1998 Jun.

If on the Internet, use the following format:

Medication Name [package insert on the Internet]. Place of Publication: Publisher; Date of Publication [Date of Update; Date of Citation]. Available from: Web Address

Omeprazole [package insert on the Internet]. Bethesda (MD): U.S. National Library of Medicine; 2009 Aug [updated 2009 Dec; cited 2010 Jun 23]. Available from: http://dailymed.nlm.nih.gov/dailymed/drugInfo.cfm?id = 14749

Meeting Presentations of Paper and Poster Sessions

Author(s). Title of Paper or Poster. Paper or Poster session presented at: Conference Title; Date(s) of Conference; Conference Location.

Ciaccia V, Hinders C, Malone M, Morales R, Sanchez A. Comparison of evidence based hypertension guideline model to an alternative model. Poster session presented at: The University of Findlay Symposium for Scholarship and Creativity; 2010 Apr 13; Findlay, OH.

Patent

Inventor(s); Assignee (Applicant). Title. Patent Country patent Country Code Patent Number. Date patent issued.

Schwartz B, inventor; New England Medical Center Hospital, Inc., assignee. Method of and solution for treating glaucoma. United States patent US 5,212,168. 1993 May 18.

Personal Communication

In text citation only (e.g. Letter from or Conversation with; unreferenced, see Notes Section) In Notes Section state that permission was given to reference the letter or conversation.

(Letter from Max Jones to Charlie Smith on June 23, 2010; unreferenced, see Notes Section)

Scientific or Technical Report

Author(s). Title. Place of Publication: Publisher; Date of Publication. Report No.: .

Issued by funding/sponsoring agency:

Shekelle P, Morton S, Maglione M (Southern California Evidence-Based Practice Center/RAND, Santa Monica, CA). Ephedra and ephedrine for weight loss and athletic performance enhancement: clinical efficacy and side effects. Vol. 1, Evidence report and evidence tables. Rockville (MD): Agency for Healthcare Research and Quality; 2003 Mar. (Evidence report/technology assessment; no. 78). Report No.: AHRQPUB03E022. Contract No.: AHRQ-290-97-001.

Issued by performing agency:

Shekelle P, Morton S, Maglione M. Ephedra and ephedrine for weight loss and athletic performance enhancement: clinical efficacy and side effects. Vol. 1, Evidence report and evidence tables. Santa Monica: Southern California Evidence-Based Practice Center/RAND; 2003 Mar. (Evidence report/technology assessment; no. 78). Report No.: AHRQPUB03E022. Contract No.: AHRQ-290-97-001. Sponsored by the Agency for Healthcare Research and Quality.

If on the Internet, use the following format:

Author(s). Title [Internet]. Place of Publication: Publisher; Date of Publication [Date of Citation]. Report No.: Available from: Web Address

Qureshi N, Wilson B, Santaguida P, Carroll J, Allanson J, Culebro CR, Brouwers M, Raina P. Collection and use of cancer family history in primary care [Internet]. Rockville (MD): Agency for Healthcare Research and Quality; 2007 Oct [cited 2010 Jun 23]. (Evidence reports/technology assessments no. 159) Report No.: AHRQPUB08E001. Contract No.: 290- 02-0020. Available from: http://www.ncbi.nlm.nih.gov/bookshelf/br.fcgi?book = erta159

OTHER ELECTRONIC MATERIAL (IN ALPHABETICAL ORDER)

Format and Example Citations (in alphabetical order)

Part of a Blog (Only One Author)

Since this is personal communication, as above, it usually is done as an in-text citation only (Posting on given date from author on given blog; unreferenced, see Notes section). In Notes section, state that permission was given to reference the blog post. Otherwise follow the format given below.

Author of Blog. Title of Blog [blog on the Internet]. Place of Publication: Publisher. [Start Date of Blog]. Title of Part; Date of Publication [Date of Citation]; [Length of Part]. Available from: Web Address

Daria. Living with Cancer [blog on the Internet]. Edmonton (AB): Daria. [2008 Aug]. Chemo went well; 2010 Jun 12 [cited 2010 Jun 16]; [about 1 screen]. Available from: http://daria-livingwithcancer.blogspot.com/.

Part of a Blog (Multiple Authors)

Since this is personal communication, as above, it usually is done as an in-text citation only (Posting on given date from author on given blog; unreferenced, see Notes section). In Notes section, state that permission was given to reference the blog post. Otherwise follow the format given below.

Author of Comment. Title of Blog Comment. Date of Publication of Comment [Date of Citation]. In: Author of Blog. Name of Blog [blog on the Internet]. Place of Publication: Publisher. Date of Publication- . [Length of Comment]. Available from: Web Address

Smith J. Dialysis. 2010 Jun 16 [cited 2010 Jun 16]. In: Kidney Coaching Foundation, Inc. KCF Blog and News [blog on the Internet]. Raleigh (NC): Kidney Coaching Foundation, Inc. c2005-2010- . [about 1 paragraph]. Available from: http://www.thekcf.org/bn/

Computer Program on CD-ROM or DVD

Author(s). Title [Medium]. Version. Place of Publication: Publisher; Date of Publication.

A.D.A.M. Animated dissection of anatomy for medicine [CD-ROM]. Version 2.2. for Windows. Marietta (GA): A.D.A.M. Software, Inc.; 1993.

Database on the Internet

Title of Database [Internet]. Place of Publication: Publisher. Date of Publication [Date of Update; Date of Citation]. Available from: Web Address

PubMed [Internet]. Bethesda (MD): National Library of Medicine. 2004 [cited 2004 Aug 18]. Available from: http://www.ncbi.nlm.nih.gov/entrez/query.fcgi

DRUGDEX [Internet]. Greenwood Village (CO): Thomson Reuters Inc. c1974-2010 [cited 2010 Jun 16]. Available from: http://www.micromedex.com/products/drugdex/

Part of a Database on the Internet (e.g., a single drug monograph out of a publication)

Title of Database [Internet]. Place of Publication: Publisher. Date of Publication. Record Identifier, Title of Part; [Date of Update; Date of Citation]; [Length of Part]. Available from: Web Address

MeSH Browser [Internet]. Bethesda (MD): National Library of Medicine. 2004. unique ID: D015201, Phenytoin; [cited 2004 Aug 18]; [about 670 p.]. Available from: http://www.nlm.nih.gov/mesh/MBrowser.html

DRUGDEX [Internet]. Greenwood Village (CO): Thomson Reuters Inc. c1974-2010. Amiodarone; [updated 2010 Apr 23]; [about 8 screens]. Available from: http://www.micromedex.com/products/drugdex/

Electronic Mail

Since this is personal communication, as above, it usually is done as an in-text citation only (Email on given date from sender to recipient; unreferenced, see Notes section). In Notes section, state that permission was given to reference the email. Otherwise follow the format given below.

Author. Title of Email [Internet]. Message to: Recipient(s). Date of Message [Date of Citation]. [Length of Email].

Malone, Patrick. Drug information textbook [Internet]. Message to: John Stanovich; Mark Malesker. 2010 Jun 14 [2010 Jun 16]. [3 paragraphs].

Encyclopedia Entry

Name of Encyclopedia [Internet]. Place of Publication: Publisher; Date of Publication. Name of Entry; [Date of Update; Date of Citation]; [Length of Entry]. Available from: Web Address

Encyclopedia Britannica Online [Internet]. Chicago: Britannica; 2010. Stroke; [cited 2010 Jun 23]; [about 5 screens]. Available from: http://www.britannica.com/EBchecked/topic/569347/stroke

LISTSERV

Since this is personal communication, as above, it usually is done as an in-text citation only (Posting on given date from sender to given LISTSERV; unreferenced, see Notes section). In Notes section, state that permission was given from the sender to reference the email. Otherwise follow the format given below.

Author. Title of Message. In: Name of LISTSERV [Internet]. Place of Publication: Publisher; Date of Message [Date of Citation]. [Length of Message].

Malone PM. CAMIPR – discussion forum for medication information specialists. In: CAMIPR [Internet]. Iowa City: Consortium for the Advancement of Medication Policy and Research; 2010 May 6 [cited 2010 June 18]. [about 1 p.].

Video Clip, Videocast, or Podcast

Title of Homepage [Internet]. Place of Publication: Publisher; Date of Publication of Homepage. [Video or Videocast or Podcast], Title of Video; Date of Publication of Video (if different from Homepage) [Date of Update; Date of Citation]; [Length of Video]. Available from: Web Address

American Society of Health-System Pharmacists [Internet]. Bethesda (MD): ASHP Advantage; c2010. [Podcast], Multidisciplinary approach to identifying patients at risk for VTE; 2010 May 4 [cited 2010 Jun 23]; [45 min.]. Available from: http://www.ashpadvantage.com/podcasts/

Web site Homepage

Author(s). Title of Homepage [Internet]. Place of Publication: Publisher; Date of Publication [Date of Update; Date of Citation]. Available from: Web Address

American Society of Health-System Pharmacists [Internet]. Bethesda (MD): American Society of Health-System Pharmacists; c1997-2004 [updated 2004 Aug 18; cited 2004 Aug 18]. Available from: http://www.ashp.org/

Part of a Web site

Title of Homepage [Internet]. Place of Publication: Publisher; Date of Publication of Homepage. Title of Part; Date of Publication of Part (if different from Homepage) [Date of Update; Date of Citation]; [Length of Part]. Available from: Web Address

American Society of Health-System Pharmacists [Internet]. Bethesda (MD): American Society of Health-System Pharmacists; c1997-2004. Compounding Resource Center; [updated 2004 Aug 18; cited 2004 Aug 18]; [about 1 screen]. Available from: http://www.ashp.org/compounding

Wiki

Since this is personal communication, as above, it usually is done as an in-text citation only (Posting on given date from author on given wiki; unreferenced, see Notes section). In Notes section, state that permission was given from the author to reference the wiki. Otherwise follow the format given below.

Author of Part. Title of Part of Wiki. Date of Posting [Date of Update; Date of Citation]. In: Title of Wiki [Internet]. Place of Publication: Publisher. Start Date of Wiki- . [Length of Part]. Available from: Web Address

If no author for part:

Title of Wiki [Internet]. Place of Publication: Publisher. Start Date of Wiki- . Title of Part of Wiki; [Date of Update; Date of Citation]; [Length of Part]. Available from: Web Address

Wiki Public Health [Internet]. [place unknown]: WikiPH. [date unknown]- . Health care; [updated 2007 Mar 27; cited 2010 Jun 16]; [about 2 screens]. Available from: http://wikiph.org/index.php?title = Health_care

REFERENCES

1. International Committee of Medical Journal Editors. Uniform requirements for manuscripts submitted to biomedical journals [Internet]. Philadelphia (PA): International Committee of Medical Journal Editors; 2009 [cited 2012 May 15]. Available from: http://www.icmje.org

2. International Committee of Medical Journal Editors. Uniform requirements for manuscripts submitted to biomedical journals: sample references [Internet]. Philadelphia (PA): International Committee of Medical Journal Editors; 2003 [updated 2011 July 15; cited 2012 May 15]. Available from: http://www.nlm.nih.gov/bsd/uniform_requirements.html

3. Patrias K. Citing medicine: the NLM style guide for authors, editors, and publishers [Internet]. 2nd ed. Wendling DL, technical editor. Bethesda (MD): National Library of Medicine (US); 2007 [updated 2011 Sep 15; cited 2012 May 15] Available from: http://nlm.nih.gov/citingmedicine

11-1

Code of Ethics for Pharmacists[1]

Pharmacists are health professionals who assist individuals in making the best use of medications. This Code, prepared and supported by pharmacists, is intended to state publicly the principles that form the fundamental basis of the roles and responsibilities of pharmacists. These principles, based on moral obligations and virtues, are established to guide pharmacists in relationships with patients, health professionals, and society.

I. A pharmacist respects the covenantal relationship between the patient and pharmacist.

Considering the patient–pharmacist relationship as a covenant means that a pharmacist has moral obligations in response to the gift of trust received from society. In return for this gift, a pharmacist promises to help individuals achieve optimum benefit from their medications, to be committed to their welfare, and to maintain their trust.

II. A pharmacist promotes the good of every patient in a caring, compassionate, and confidential manner.

A pharmacist places concern for the well-being of the patient at the center of professional practice. In doing so, a pharmacist considers needs stated by the patient as well as those defined by health science. A pharmacist is dedicated to protecting the dignity of the patient. With a caring attitude and a compassionate spirit, a pharmacist focuses on serving the patient in a private and confidential manner.

III. A pharmacist respects the autonomy and dignity of each patient.

A pharmacist promotes the right of self-determination and recognizes individual self-worth by encouraging patients to participate in decisions about their health. A pharmacist communicates with patients in terms that are understandable. In all cases, a pharmacist respects personal and cultural differences among patients.

IV. A pharmacist acts with honesty and integrity in professional relationships.

A pharmacist has a duty to tell the truth and to act with conviction of conscience. A pharmacist avoids discriminatory practices, behavior or work conditions that impair professional judgment, and actions that compromise dedication to the best interests of patients.

V. A pharmacist maintains professional competence.

A pharmacist has a duty to maintain knowledge and abilities as new medications, devices, and technologies become available and as health information advances.

VI. A pharmacist respects the values and abilities of colleagues and other health professionals.

When appropriate, a pharmacist asks for the consultation of colleagues or other health professionals or refers the patient. A pharmacist acknowledges that colleagues and other health professionals may differ in the beliefs and values they apply to the care of the patient.

VII. A pharmacist serves individual, community, and societal needs.

The primary obligation of a pharmacist is to individual patients. However, the obligations of a pharmacist may at times extend beyond the individual to the community and society. In these situations, the pharmacist recognizes the responsibilities that accompany these obligations and acts accordingly.

VIII. A pharmacist seeks justice in the distribution of health resources.

When health resources are allocated, a pharmacist is fair and equitable, balancing the needs of patients and society.

*Adopted by the membership of the American Pharmacists Association October 27, 1994.

REFERENCE

1. American Pharmacists Association. Code of ethics 1994 [Internet]. [updated Oct 27, 1994 Mar 26, 2010]. Available from: http://www.pharmacist.com/code-ethics.

Appendix 12-1

Pharmacy and Therapeutics Committee Procedure

This appendix includes two policy and procedure operational statements. The first is specifically written to centralize the formulary decision process for a multihospital health system: a Formulary Committee. The second, and closely related, operational statement is written as a model to function as the traditional Pharmacy and Therapeutics Committee for a Hospital's Medical Staff. Both operational statements describe the functions of their related committees based on a certain degree of autonomy. Their membership is ultimately chosen by an administrative leader as a means to best isolate the committee from organizational as well as economic influences. The decision process for each operational statement is intended to create predictability and transparency. To implement this set of operational statements, each Executive Committee of the hospitals in a multihospital system would pass the following resolution:

> The Medical Staff of Alpha Hospital agrees to delegate its Pharmacy and Therapeutic Committee responsibilities to ALPHAOMEGA HEALTH based on the policy and procedures for a "Hospital Formulary System" and a "Hospital Pharmacy and Therapeutics Committee."

The two operational statements can also be combined to reflect the traditional functions of a single hospital, medical staff-based pharmacy, and therapeutics committee. Also, there may be other arrangements where the two operational statements could provide the organizational environment for a closed health system, a pharmacy benefits manager, or one of the new organizational structures created by Federal Legislation in 2004 for the new financing of drug coverage in the United States.

POLICY TITLE: HOSPITAL FORMULARY SYSTEM

I. PURPOSE

To maintain a **HOSPITAL FORMULARY** and a Formulary Committee for all ALPHA-OMEGA HEALTH Hospitals as a means to enhance the quality of health care for all patients served by ALPHAOMEGA HEALTH

II. POLICY

A. The Formulary Committee of ALPHAOMEGA HEALTH will periodically evaluate its performance as a means to improve its ability to support the Vision and Mission of ALPHAOMEGA HEALTH.

B. ALPHAOMEGA HEALTH will maintain one Formulary Committee and a Pharmacy and Therapeutics Committee (P&T COMMITTEE) at each ALPHAOMEGA HEALTH Hospital to implement this POLICY in accord with the applicable Medical Staff Bylaws and this POLICY.

C. The Formulary Committee of ALPHAOMEGA HEALTH will maintain a standard format for a **HOSPITAL FORMULARY** that is based on the provisions of this POLICY.

D. The Formulary Committee will develop and continually revise a list of therapeutic products, a **HOSPITAL FORMULARY**, that reflects the current clinical judgment of the Medical Staff of ALPHAOMEGA HEALTH Hospitals regarding the selection of the best therapeutic products for the health care of hospitalized patients. The Formulary Committee will evaluate the various alternative therapeutic products available and develop the **HOSPITAL FORMULARY** based on an evaluation of each therapeutic product's indications, effectiveness, risks, patient safety, and overall impact on health care costs.

E. The Formulary Committee will collaborate with the P&T Committee at each ALPHAOMEGA HEALTH Hospital to monitor compliance with the provisions of the **HOSPITAL FORMULARY**.

F. The Formulary Committee will support the quality improvement functions of ALPHAOMEGA HEALTH where necessary to improve the use of the **HOSPITAL FORMULARY**.

III. PROCEDURE

A. FORMULARY COMMITTEE DEVELOPMENT

1. The Formulary Committee will recommend, when appropriate, amendments to this POLICY AND PROCEDURE to the Chief Medical Officer of ALPHAOMEGA HEALTH. After revisions to any of these proposed amendments by the Chief Medical Officer, in collaboration with the Formulary Committee, the Chief Medical Officer will submit the amendments to the Executive Committee of the Medical Staff at each ALPHAOMEGA HEALTH Hospital for final approval.

2. The Officers of the Formulary Committee will prepare an Annual Membership Report to the Chief Medical Officer of ALPHAOMEGA HEALTH regarding participation of its Members and any recommendations that may be important to maintain the expertise necessary for the affairs of the Formulary Committee.

3. The Officers of the Formulary Committee will prepare an Annual Report and submit it to the Professional Affairs Committee of ALPHAOMEGA HEALTH for approval. As a result of this review, the Professional Affairs Committee may make recommendations to the Formulary Committee for consideration regarding its affairs or to the Chief Medical Officer regarding amendments to this POLICY AND PROCEDURE.

B. FORMULARY COMMITTEE ORGANIZATION

1. REGULAR MEMBERS

a. MEDICAL STAFF MEMBERS

i. There may be up to 16 Medical Staff members nominated annually by the Chief Medical Officer of ALPHAOMEGA HEALTH, each President or Chief of Staff from the Medical Staff of an ALPHAOMEGA HEALTH Hospital, or the Officers of the Formulary Committee. Any Medical Staff nominee must have demonstrated an active interest in evidence-based therapeutics, a willingness to be an active participant in the affairs of the Formulary Committee, and represent as a group, whenever possible, the specialties of Family Practice, Internal Medicine, Pediatrics, Obstetrics and Gynecology, Hematology and Oncology, Cardiology, Infectious Disease, Pulmonology, and General Surgery.

    ii. From any Nominees, 12-16 will be selected by the Chief Medical Officer of ALPHAOMEGA HEALTH on the basis of maintaining a reasonable balance among the following factors: hospital and outpatient-based physicians, primary care and disease focused physicians, physician liaison to the Medical Staff Executive Committee or P&T Committee of each ALPHAOMEGA HEALTH Hospital, and a balanced representation from the Medical Staffs of the ALPHAOMEGA HEALTH Hospitals.

  b. ADMINISTRATION MEMBER—The Chief Medical Officer of ALPHAOMEGA HEALTH, or designee who is a Medical Staff Member of an ALPHAOMEGA HEALTH Hospital, will be a Member of the Formulary Committee.

2. SPECIAL MEMBERS AND SOURCE OF SELECTION

  a. The Chief Medical Officer of ALPHAOMEGA HEALTH will select Special Members as may be needed to provide administrative or technical support for the affairs of the Formulary Committee. The Special Members will include, at a minimum:

    i. any pharmacist recommended by the Pharmacist in charge at a Hospital Pharmacy of ALPHAOMEGA HEALTH and

    ii. at least one Registered Nurse from among the Nursing Staff of an ALPHAOMEGA HEALTH Hospital.

  b. The Chairperson of the Formulary Committee may select one or more Special Members from the personnel of ALPHAOMEGA HEALTH or the Medical Staff of any ALPHAOMEGA HEALTH Hospital on a temporary basis as may be necessary for:

    i. technical support for the activities of the Formulary Committee or any Ad Hoc Subcommittee of the Formulary Committee or

    ii. information for the deliberations of the Formulary Committee regarding a proposal to add or delete an individual therapeutic product listed on the **HOSPITAL FORMULARY**.

3. FORMULARY COMMITTEE OFFICERS

  a. The CHAIRPERSON will be selected by the Chief Medical Officer of ALPHAOMEGA HEALTH from among the Regular Members of the Formulary Committee. The Chairperson will:

    i. manage the affairs of the Formulary Committee in a manner to

      I) support the active, positive involvement of each Regular and Special Member,

      II) acknowledge any conflict of interests,

      III) initiate a replacement appointment of any Officer, Regular Member, or Special Member becoming inactive during a calendar year,

        IV)   appoint temporary Special Members, and

        V)   select the location for Meetings of the Formulary Committee;

    ii. prepare the Annual Membership and Self-Evaluation reports; and

    iii. appoint an Ad Hoc Committee when necessary to study decisions in greater depth or to arrive at consensus recommendations for consideration by the Formulary Committee whose membership will be:

        I)   six or less members from the Medical Staffs of the ALPHAOMEGA HEALTH Hospitals,

        II) at least one member who is a Regular Member of the Formulary Committee, and

        III) the Secretary, or designee, of the Formulary Committee.

  b. The VICE CHAIRPERSON will be selected by the Chief Medical Officer of ALPHAOMEGA HEALTH from the Regular Members of the Formulary Committee. The Vice chairperson will assume the duties of the Chairperson during their absence.

  c. The SECRETARY will be selected by the Chief Medical Officer of ALPHAOMEGA HEALTH from among the Regular or Special Members of the Formulary Committee. The Secretary will assist the Chairperson in managing the affairs of the Formulary Committee by:

    i. preparing the minutes for each meeting of the Formulary Committee or any of its Ad Hoc Committees,

    ii. sending an Agenda to the Members prior to each meeting of the Formulary Committee,

    iii. maintaining a schedule for the annual regular review by the Formulary Committee of all therapeutic products listed on the **HOSPITAL FORMULARY**, and

    iv. coordinating the preparation of any Drug Monograph or any other report necessary for a meeting of the Formulary Committee by a Pharmacist In Charge, or designee, at an ALPHAOMEGA HEALTH Hospital.

4. TERM OF APPOINTMENT

  a. The Regular and Special Members will be appointed or reappointed each January for 1 year.

  b. Each Officer will be appointed or reappointed each January for 1 year.

5. VOTING

  a. Each Regular Member will have one vote, and each Special Member will have not have a vote.

  b. Any two Regular Members present during a Meeting of the Formulary Committee will constitute a quorum.

  c. The Regular Members present at a meeting of the Formulary Committee should recognize that a decision regarding a special issue may not be appropriate if certain Regular or Special Members having expertise related to the issue are not present. Based on attendance or any other pertinent reason, the Regular Members present at a meeting of the Formulary Committee should delay making any permanent decision when the appropriate expertise is not available during a meeting of the Formulary Committee.

d. A simple majority of Regular Members voting will be required for any action of the Formulary Committee. Any abstention on the basis of a conflict of interests will be noted in the minutes for the meeting.

6. LIAISON—A Regular or Special Member may be appointed by the Chief Medical Officer of ALPHAOMEGA HEALTH to report on the affairs of the Formulary Committee during the deliberations of any other Committee of ALPHAOMEGA HEALTH.

7. MEETINGS—Thpe meetings of the Formulary Committee will be:

    a. scheduled once a month for 1 hour or as may be planned by the Members of the Formulary Committee,

    b. attended by Regular and Special Members only, and

    c. convened at a location arranged by the Chairperson.

8. COMMITTEE PROTOCOLS—The Formulary Committee may also arrange for the:

    a. definitions applicable to the resignation and replacement of any Regular Member, Special Member, or Officer during a calendar year;

    b. management of any potential or actual conflict of interests affecting the participation of a Regular or Special Member during a meeting of the Formulary Committee;

    c. use of ALTERNATIVE MEDICATION for the health care of a patient at any ALPHA-OMEGA HEALTH Hospital;

    d. information necessary to request a change in the list of therapeutic products or other information described in the **HOSPITAL FORMULARY**;

    e. contents of a DRUG MONOGRAPH that must be prepared before a therapeutic product not listed on the **HOSPITAL FORMULARY** is administered to a patient or before a therapeutic product is added to the **HOSPITAL FORMULARY**; and

    f. management of any shortage of a therapeutic product listed in the **HOSPITAL FOR-MULARY** by the:

        i. timely notification of the Medical Staff at each ALPHAOMEGA HEALTH Hospital listing the specific dosage forms in limited or unavailable supply,

        ii. development of alternative strategies for a patient's health care using therapeutic products currently available on the **HOSPITAL FORMULARY** when a therapeutic product becomes either not available or in limited supply,

        iii. collaboration with the appropriate expertise within the Medical Staff of ALPHA-OMEGA HEALTH Hospitals when a rationing protocol is necessary for a critical therapeutic product in limited supply, and

        iv. review of any proposal for a rationing protocol by the Ethics Council of ALPHA-OMEGA HEALTH when the Formulary Committee requests assistance before final approval to ensure that the appropriate ethical standards have been considered.

C. **HOSPITAL FORMULARY FORMAT**

1. Any therapeutic product used in the health care of a patient will be eligible for the **HOS-PITAL FORMULARY**. This includes samples, prescription drugs as defined by the Food and Drug Administration, herbal or other alternative therapies administered topically or enterally, nutraceuticals, nonprescription drugs, vaccines, diagnostic or contrast

agents, radioactive agents, respiratory products, parenteral or enteral nutrients, blood products, intravenous solutions, and anesthetic gases. A therapeutic product may not be considered for the **HOSPITAL FORMULARY** if it would normally be considered a medical device, durable medical equipment, or implant.

2. The **HOSPITAL FORMULARY** will list the therapeutic products approved by the Formulary Committee in a format approved by the Formulary Committee. The format for the **HOSPITAL FORMULARY** will reflect the recommendations of nationally recognized organizations and include certain attributes, where appropriate, as described below.

   a. Any restricted use provision will be defined by credentialing categories in use by the Medical Staffs of ALPHAOMEGA HEALTH Hospitals and be implemented when necessary to monitor or limit the use of a **HOSPITAL FORMULARY** therapeutic product known to be associated with:

      i. an increased risk of a substantial adverse patient reaction,

      ii. a highly specific therapeutic indication, or

      iii. an unusual impact on the overall cost of health care.

   b. Specific patient education provisions will be added for any **HOSPITAL FORMULARY** therapeutic product known to require:

      i. special nutritional adjustments,

      ii. prevention of substantial adverse effects or noncompliance, or

      iii. unique requirements for informed consent.

   c. Continuing education provisions will be added when a Medical Staff Member or qualified Hospital employee requires specialized knowledge prior to or during the administration of a given **HOSPITAL FORMULARY** therapeutic product. This is particularly applicable in the professional areas of oncology and cardiology.

   d. Special information may be added to assist the Medical Staff at each ALPHAOMEGA HEALTH HOSPITAL when necessary to improve the:

      i. level of compliance with prescribing only therapeutic products listed on the **HOSPITAL FORMULARY**,

      ii acceptance of rational therapeutic concepts as a basis for planning health care intervention strategies, and

      iii acceptance of therapeutic interchange strategies involving therapeutic products not listed on the **HOSPITAL FORMULARY**.

3. Each therapeutic product listed in the **HOSPITAL FORMULARY** will normally be stocked in each ALPHAOMEGA HEALTH Hospital's Pharmacy. The Formulary Committee may establish an alternative provision for inventory control of a **HOSPITAL FORMULARY** therapeutic product when the alternative provision will not interfere with the health care of an individual patient hospitalized at an ALPHAOMEGA HEALTH Hospital.

D. **HOSPITAL FORMULARY MAINTENANCE**

1. A proposal for a change in a single therapeutic product listed on the **HOSPITAL FORMULARY** will require a specific set of steps before final approval by the Formulary

Committee. These steps are defined below. The Formulary Committee may make a temporary exception to this provision when necessary to improve the quality of health care to patients at an ALPHAOMEGA HEALTH Hospital.

    a. timely submission of a completed Formulary Request form to any pharmacist at an ALPHAOMEGA HEALTH Hospital by a Medical Staff member of an ALPHAOMEGA HEALTH Hospital or other professional employee of ALPHAOMEGA HEALTH,

    b. review of the Formulary Request by a pharmacist in charge, or designee, of an ALPHAOMEGA HEALTH Hospital's Pharmacy to be sure that it has been fully completed,

    c. preparation of a Drug Monograph, as may be arranged by the Secretary of the Formulary Committee if a new therapeutic product has been proposed by the Formulary Request for the **HOSPITAL FORMULARY,**

    d. preliminary review of the Formulary Request and any associated Drug Monograph by representative specialists affected by any proposed change in the **HOSPITAL FORMULARY,**

    e. initial approval or disapproval of the Formulary Request at one meeting of the Formulary Committee, followed by review for comments at each ALPHAOMEGA HEALTH Hospital's P&T Committee, before final approval or disapproval including any amendments to the Formulary Request at a subsequent meeting of the Formulary Committee.

2. The Formulary Committee will annually review all therapeutic products listed on the **HOSPITAL FORMULARY** according to a schedule of therapeutic classes as may be arranged throughout a calendar year by the Secretary of the Formulary Committee. The review of each class of therapeutic products will require a specific set of events before final approval. These steps are defined below.

    a. review of a class of therapeutic products preliminarily by the pharmacists in charge, or designees, of the ALPHAOMEGA HEALTH Hospital Pharmacies prior to a meeting of the Formulary Committee regarding the possible need to:

        i. initiate a Formulary Request for a new addition to the **HOSPITAL FORMULARY,**

        ii. deletion of a therapeutic product because of production defects, nonuse, nonavailability, recall, or replacement by another therapeutic product, or

        iii. a need to change information included in the **HOSPITAL FORMULARY** such as patient education, professional education, therapeutic interchange, or a restricted use provision;

    b. preliminary review of the proposed revisions to the **HOSPITAL FORMULARY** by representative specialists affected by the proposed revisions;

    c. initial approval or disapproval of the therapeutic product class review at one meeting of the Formulary Committee, followed by review for comments at each ALPHAOMEGA HEALTH Hospital's P&T Committee, before final approval or disapproval including amendments to the class review at a subsequent meeting of the Formulary Committee.

3. The Formulary Committee may authorize certain strategies by the ALPHAOMEGA HEALTH Hospital pharmacies that are necessary to offer the most appropriate

therapeutic products for hospitalized patients. The Formulary Committee may authorize these special strategies when supported by its own decision and the support of each ALPHAOMEGA HEALTH Hospital's P&T Committee. Certain specific strategies to be authorized by this POLICY AND PROCEDURE are listed below.

    a. A class review of **HOSPITAL FORMULARY** therapeutic products as described above may also be initiated when there is a Formulary Request for a therapeutic product that substantially affects the inclusion or supplementary information of other therapeutic products currently listed in the **HOSPITAL FORMULARY**.

    b. The pharmacist in charge, or designee, at all ALPHAOMEGA HEALTH Hospital Pharmacies will arrange to prepare a preliminary or full Drug Monograph before any therapeutic product is dispensed that has not previously been ordered for a hospitalized patient at any ALPHAOMEGA HEALTH Hospital.

    c. The Formulary Committee may provide for automatic therapeutic interchange between a therapeutic product that is not listed for another therapeutic product that is listed on the **HOSPITAL FORMULARY** when supported by appropriate scientific evidence and appropriately considered standards of practice.

    d. The Formulary Committee may also select certain therapeutic products for the **HOSPITAL FORMULARY** that will be dispensed for certain indications or any indication even if prescribed with a "Do Not Substitute" designation. The Formulary Committee will use the same process for this designation as defined above for a new change in the **HOSPITAL FORMULARY**.

E. **HOSPITAL FORMULARY COMPLIANCE**

  1. The P&T Committee of each ALPHAOMEGA HEALTH Hospital will be responsible for monitoring each Medical Staff physician's orders for a therapeutic product that is:

    a. not listed or does not have an automatic therapeutic interchange with a therapeutic product listed on the current **HOSPITAL FORMULARY**,

    b. for an indication not permitted by the **HOSPITAL FORMULARY**, or

    c. for an indication having a restricted use provision.

  2. Any ALPHAOMEGA HEALTH Hospital's P&T Committee may establish a Special Formulary as a means to temporarily support the efforts of its Medical Staff in the health care of hospitalized patients having special requirements that are unique to that Hospital. The Special Formulary therapeutic products will be selected using the same process defined above for a change in the **HOSPITAL FORMULARY**. For a Special Formulary, the other Committees of the Hospital's Medical Staff will provide the advice and consent process. For any therapeutic product listed on an ALPHAOMEGA HEALTH Hospital's Special Formulary for 1 year or more, continued use of the Special Formulary status for the therapeutic product will require the approval of the Formulary Committee.

  3. If a P&T Committee votes to not accept a decision of the Formulary Committee, the Chairperson, or designee, of the P&T Committee will be invited to a subsequent meeting of the Formulary Committee. At this Formulary Meeting, the Formulary Committee will attempt to develop a strategy for resolving the conflict between the original decision of

the Formulary Committee and the respective P&T Committee. In the event that a resolution is not achieved, the issue may be appealed by either Committee to the Professional Affairs Committee for a final decision within 3 months of the appeal.

F. **QUALITY IMPROVEMENT**

1. The Formulary Committee will maintain access to the decisions of other hospital's Formulary or P&T Committees as a resource for the basis in managing difficult decisions regarding the **HOSPITAL FORMULARY**. The hospitals chosen should reflect regional as well as national locations.

2. The Formulary Committee will regularly assess the pending availability of new therapeutic products in the future that will likely require the preparation of a Formulary Request and Drug Monograph.

3. The Formulary Committee will regularly monitor the possible evolution of a shortage involving the availability of a therapeutic product listed on the **HOSPITAL FORMULARY**.

4. The Formulary Committee may recommend to each P&T Committee certain quality improvement projects, such as a Drug Use Evaluations for a certain product that would reflect the health care at all ALPHAOMEGA HEALTH Hospitals.

5. The Formulary Committee will monitor all black box warnings or other Advisories issued by the Food and Drug Administration or pharmaceutical manufacturing company. The Formulary Committee will use the monitoring process as a basis to collaborate with each ALPHAOMEGA HEALTH Hospital's P&T Committee as a means to promote patient safety.

6. The Formulary Committee will maintain a newsletter regarding its decisions and distribute it to each member of the Medical Staff of all ALPHAOMEGA HEALTH Hospitals.

7. The Formulary Committee will collaborate with the P&T Committee at each ALPHAOMEGA HEALTH Hospital to develop educational strategies for the ALPHAOMEGA HEALTH professional employees and each Hospital's Medical Staff that builds support for the principles and priorities used to maintain the **HOSPITAL FORMULARY**.

8. The Formulary Committee will offer consultation when requested or directed by the Board of Directors of ALPHAOMEGA HEALTH, its Committees, or any other ALPHAOMEGA HEALTH Committee regarding therapeutic products in the investigation, protocols, standard order sets, or quality assessment of health care.

9. The Formulary Committee will offer a means to coordinate the standardization of POLICY AND PROCEDUREs for the Pharmacy Departments of ALPHAOMEGA HEALTH Hospitals.

POLICY TITLE: HOSPITAL PHARMACY AND THERAPEUTICS COMMITTEE

I. PURPOSE

To maintain a Pharmacy and Therapeutics Committee as a means to enhance the quality of health care for all patients served by the Alpha Medical Center.

II. POLICY

A. The Pharmacy and Therapeutics Committee of Alpha Medical Center will periodically evaluate its performance as a means to improve its ability to support the Vision and Mission of ALPHAOMEGA HEALTH.

B. The Alpha Medical Center will maintain a Pharmacy and Therapeutics Committee (P&T committee) to implement this POLICY in accord with the applicable Medical Staff By-Laws and this POLICY.

C. The P&T Committee may maintain a SPECIAL FORMULARY at the Alpha Medical Center based on the provisions of the Hospital Formulary System POLICY AND PROCEDURE of ALPHAOMEGA HEALTH.

D. The P&T Committee will monitor compliance with the provisions of the **HOSPITAL FORMULARY**.

E. The P&T Committee will support the quality improvement functions of ALPHAOMEGA HEALTH where necessary to improve the use of the **HOSPITAL FORMULARY**.

F. The P&T Committee will review and approve any POLICY AND PROCEDURE of the Alpha Medical Center Pharmacy.

III. PROCEDURE

A. PHARMACY AND THERAPEUTICS COMMITTEE DEVELOPMENT

    1. The P&T Committee will recommend, when appropriate, amendments to this POLICY AND PROCEDURE to the Administrator of Alpha Medical Center. After revisions to any of these proposed amendments by the Administrator, in collaboration with the P&T Committee, the Administrator will submit the amendments to the Executive Committee of the Alpha Medical Center Medical Staff for final approval.

    2. The Officers of the P&T Committee will prepare an Annual Membership Report to the Administrator of the Alpha Medical Center regarding participation of its Members and any recommendations for changes in its membership that may be important to maintain the expertise necessary for the affairs of the P&T Committee.

    3. The Officers of the P&T Committee will prepare an Annual Report and submit it to the Executive Committee of the Alpha Medical Center Medical Staff for approval. As a result of this review, the Executive Committee may make recommendations to the P&T Committee for consideration regarding its affairs or to the Administrator regarding amendments to this POLICY AND PROCEDURE.

B. FORMULARY COMMITTEE ORGANIZATION

    1. REGULAR MEMBERS AND SOURCE OF SELECTION

        a. MEDICAL STAFF MEMBERS

            i There may be up to eight Medical Staff members nominated annually by the Administrator, or designee, of Alpha Medical Center, the President of the Medical Staff of the Alpha Medical Center, or the Officers of the P&T Committee. Any Medical Staff nominee must have demonstrated an active interest in evidence-based therapeutics, a willingness to be an active participant in the affairs of the P&T Committee, and represent as a group, whenever possible, the specialties of

Family Practice, Internal Medicine, Pediatrics, Obstetrics and Gynecology, Hematology and Oncology, Cardiology, Infectious Disease, Pulmonology, and General Surgery.

  ii From any nominees, eight will be selected by the Administrator, or designee, of Alpha Medical Center on the basis of maintaining a reasonable balance among the following factors: hospital and outpatient-based physicians, primary care and disease focused physicians, physician continuity from year to year, and physician liaison to the Medical Staff Executive Committee of the Alpha Medical Center or the Formulary Committee of ALPHAOMEGA HEALTH.

  b. PHARMACY MEMBERS—The Administrator, or designee, of Alpha Medical Center will select two pharmacists that will include the Pharmacist In Charge of the Hospital's Pharmacy.

  c. NURSING SERVICE MEMBER—The Administrator, or designee, of Alpha Medical Center will select one registered nurse from the Nursing Service.

2. SPECIAL MEMBERS AND SOURCE OF SELECTION

  a. The Administrator, or designee, of Alpha Medical Center may select Special Members as needed to provide administrative or technical support for the affairs of the P&T Committee.

  b. The Chairperson of the Formulary Committee may select one or more Special Members from the personnel of the Alpha Medical Center or its Medical Staff on a temporary basis as may be necessary for:

    i. technical support for the activities of the P&T Committee or any Ad Hoc Subcommittee or

    ii. information for the deliberations of the P&T Committee regarding a proposal to add or delete an individual therapeutic product listed on the **HOSPITAL FORMULARY**.

3. P&T COMMITTEE OFFICERS AND SOURCE OF SELECTION

  a. The CHAIRPERSON will be selected by the Administrator, or designee, of the Alpha Medical Center from the physician Regular Members of the P&T Committee. The Chairperson will:

    i. manage the affairs of the P&T Committee in a manner to:

      I) support the active, positive involvement of each Regular and Special Member,

      II) acknowledge any conflict of interests,

      III) initiate a replacement appointment of any Officer, Regular Member, or Special Member becoming inactive during a calendar year,

      IV) appoint temporary Special Members,

      V) select the location for Meetings of the P&T Committee;

    ii. prepare the Annual Membership and Self-Evaluation reports; and

    iii. appoint an Ad Hoc Committee when necessary to study decisions in greater depth or to arrive at consensus recommendations for consideration by the P&T Committee whose membership will be:

  I) six or less members from the Medical Staff of the Alpha Medical Center,

  II) at least one member who is a physician Regular Member of the P&T Committee, and

  III) the Secretary, or designee, of the P&T Committee.

 b. The VICE CHAIRPERSON will be selected by the Administrator of the Alpha Medical Center from among the physician Regular Members of the P&T Committee. The Vice Chairperson will assume the duties of the Chairperson during their absence.

 c. The SECRETARY will be selected by the Administrator of the Alpha Medical Center from among the Regular or Special Members of the P&T Committee. The Secretary will assist the Chairperson in managing the affairs of the P&T Committee by:

  i. preparing the minutes for each meeting of the P&T Committee or any of its Ad Hoc Committees,

  ii. sending an Agenda to the Members prior to each meeting of the P&T Committee,

  iii. maintaining liaison with the other Committees of the Medical Staff,

  iv. maintaining a schedule for the annual Quality Assurance activities of the P&T Committee, and

  v. assisting in the preparation of any Drug Monograph or any other report necessary for a meeting of the Formulary Committee of ALPHAOMEGA HEALTH.

4. TERM OF APPOINTMENT

 a. The Regular and Special Members will be appointed or reappointed each January for 1 year.

 b. Each Officer will be appointed or reappointed each January for 1 year.

5. VOTING

 a. Each Regular Member will have one vote, and each Special Member will have not have a vote.

 b. Any two physician Regular Members present during a Meeting of the Formulary Committee will constitute a quorum.

 c. The Regular Members present at a meeting of the P&T Committee should recognize that a decision regarding a special issue may not be appropriate if certain Regular or Special Members having expertise related to the issue are not present. Based on attendance or any other pertinent reason, the Regular Members present at a meeting of the P&T Committee should delay making any permanent decision when the appropriate expertise is not available during a meeting of the P&T Committee.

 d. A simple majority of Regular Members voting will be required for any action of the P&T Committee. Any abstention on the basis of a conflict of interests will be noted in the Minutes for the meeting.

6. LIAISON—A Regular or Special Member may be appointed by the Administrator to report on the affairs of the P&T Committee during the deliberations of any other Committee of the Alpha Medical Center.

7. MEETINGS—The meetings of the P&T Committee will be:

 a. scheduled once a month for 1 hour or as may be planned by the Members of the P&T Committee,

    b. attended by Regular and Special Members only,

    c. convened at a location arranged by the Chairperson.

  8. COMMITTEE PROTOCOLS—The P&T Committee may also arrange for the:

    a. use of definitions applicable to the resignation and replacement of any Regular Member, Special Member, or Officer during a calendar year as may be established by the Formulary Committee of ALPHAOMEGA HEALTH and

    b. management of any potential or actual conflict of interests affecting the participation of a Regular or Special Member during a meeting of the P&T Committee as may be determined by the Formulary Committee of ALPHAOMEGA HEALTH.

C. HOSPITAL FORMULARY DEVELOPMENT

  1. The P&T Committee will review for comment at each meeting any therapeutic product recommended for addition or deletion to the **HOSPITAL FORMULARY** by the Formulary Committee of ALPHAOMEGA HEALTH.

  2. The P&T Committee will review for comment at each meeting any class review of therapeutic products by the Formulary Committee of ALPHAOMEGA HEALTH and their recommendations for changes in the **HOSPITAL FORMULARY**.

D. HOSPITAL FORMULARY COMPLIANCE

  1. The P&T Committee will monitor each Medical Staff physician's orders for a therapeutic product that is:

    a. not listed or does not have an automatic therapeutic interchange with a therapeutic product listed on the current **HOSPITAL FORMULARY**,

    b. for an indication not permitted by the **HOSPITAL FORMULARY**, or

    c. for an indication having a restricted use provision.

  2. The P&T Committee may establish a Special Formulary for therapeutic products not listed on the **HOSPITAL FORMULARY** as a means to temporarily support the efforts of the Medical Staff for hospitalized patients having special requirements that are unique to Alpha Medical Center. The Special Formulary therapeutic products will be selected using the same process defined by the ALPHAOMEGA HEALTH Formulary Committee for the **HOSPITAL FORMULARY**. For a Special Formulary, the other Committees of the Alpha Medical Center's Medical Staff will provide the advice and consent process. For any therapeutic product listed on Special Formulary for 1 year or more, continued use of the Special Formulary status for the therapeutic product will require the approval of the Formulary Committee.

  3. If the Alpha Medical Center P&T Committee votes to not accept a decision of the Formulary Committee, the Chairperson, or designee, of the P&T Committee will attend a subsequent meeting of the Formulary Committee. At this Formulary Meeting, the Formulary Committee will attempt to develop a strategy for resolving the conflict between the original decision of the Formulary Committee and the P&T Committee of the Alpha Medical Center. In the event that a resolution is not achieved, the issue may be appealed by either the Formulary Committee or the Alpha Medical Center P&T Committee to the Professional Affairs Committee for a final decision within 3 months of the appeal.

E. QUALITY IMPROVEMENT

1. The P&T Committee will regularly review the decisions of the ALPHAOMEGA HEALTH Formulary Committee as a means to evaluate any issues requiring the development of carefully considered implementation requirements at the Alpha Medical Center, such as the shortage of a therapeutic product.

2. The P&T Committee will maintain an annually revised schedule for Drug Use Evaluations as may be established through consultation with other Medical Staff Committees.

3. The P&T Committee or an Ad Hoc Committee will review all Medication Error Reports.

4. The P&T Committee will quarterly review all Adverse Medication Reaction Reports.

5. The P&T Committee will participate in the development of standard order sets as may be requested by a Member, a group of Members, or a Committee of the Medical Staff. Generally, the P&T Committee will not have primary responsibility of a standard order set unless specifically requested by the Executive Committee of the Medical Staff.

6. The P&T Committee will prepare an annual report to the Executive Committee regarding the overall level of prescribing compliance with the **HOSPITAL FORMULARY**.

7. The P&T Committee in collaboration with the Formulary Committee will monitor all black box warnings or other advisories issued by the Food and Drug Administration or pharmaceutical manufacturing company. The Formulary Committee will use the monitoring process as a basis to collaborate with each P&T Committee of ALPHAOMEGA HEALTH as a means to promote patient safety.

8. The P&T Committee will suggest information to the Formulary Committee for inclusion in the **HOSPITAL FORMULARY** newsletter.

9. The P&T Committee may make recommendations to the Medical Staff of Alpha Medical Center regarding the health care of hospitalized patients regarding the use of the **HOSPITAL FORMULARY** based on the outcome of certain studies undertaken by the P&T Committee. These studies will exclude any direct identification of patient names or medical records.

F. PHARMACY DEPARTMENT POLICY AND PROCEDURE

1. The P&T Committee will periodically review and approve the POLICY AND PROCEDURES of the Alpha Medical Center Pharmacy Department.

2. The review and approval will be, whenever possible, coordinated with the operational statements of the other Pharmacy Departments of ALPHAOMEGA HEALTH Hospitals.

Appendix 12–2

Formulary Request Form

PHARMACY AND THERAPEUTICS COMMITTEE
FORMULARY ADDITION REQUEST

NOTE: Both sides of this form must be completed in order for consideration by the **Formulary Committee** at its next regularly scheduled meeting. You may submit additional information based on the outline of this **request** if more space is required. If you are not a member of the committee, you must also complete a Conflict of Interest Statement and attach it to this request.

Generic Name _____ Brand Name _____

Indications - Describe the FDA-approved or potential off-label uses which have prompted this **request.** _____

_____

_____

Dosing - Describe the specific strength and administration form of this product necessary for this **request.** _____

_____

_____

Comparative Efficacy - Describe how this agent relates to other products in terms of effectiveness.

_____

_____

_____

Contraindications and Warnings - Describe any substantial issues related to this product.

_____

_____

_____

Adverse Effects - List any substantial issues related to this product. _____

_____

Expected Outcomes - Describe how this product would substitute or add to the current **Formulary** products. _____

_____

_____

Cost of Therapy - Describe how this product would change the overall cost of medical care.

_____

_____

_____

Impact on Inpatient Care Processes - Describe any special requirements on the hospital for use of this product such as nursing/medical staff education, standards of care, discharge planning, certification, or standard order sets.

_____

_____

_____

Impact on Outpatient Care Processes - Describe any special requirements on ambulatory care for use of this product such as compliance, follow-up, or monitoring.

_____

_____

_____

Other Considerations - Describe any information not applicable to the above categories.

_____

_____

_____

Requested By - Must be a **Formulary Committee Member** or **Hospital Medical Staff Member**.
Printed Name_____

Signature_____

Response - For record keeping by the **Formulary Committee**.
  Received by a **Formulary Committee Member date** _____
  Initial **Formulary Committee** consideration **date** _____
  Final **Formulary Committee** consifderation **date** _____
Action Taken_____
Notification of Medical Staff Member submitting request date_____

Appendix 12–3

P&T Committee Meeting Attributes[1-3]

I. TIMING

    A. Regular—The choice is often between monthly or bimonthly. Overall, a long-term commitment to one schedule that does not vary is ideal. An atypical but practical variation might include monthly meetings except August and December, in order to adjust for times when it is difficult to get quorum because of vacations and holidays. To support a regular meeting cycle, any cancellation on a sudden, unexpected basis must be avoided virtually without exception. Finally, a 2- to 3-year experience with a given schedule would be necessary to permit members an opportunity to work membership commitment into their own schedule.

    B. Monthly work cycle—Virtually all holidays occur in association with the first or last week of any month during the calendar year. Similarly, Mondays and Fridays frequently have distractions caused by these associated weekend demands. Thus, the second or third Tuesday-Wednesday-Thursday of the calendar month are often the best choice for a regular meeting.

    C. Daily work cycle—Given the character of the discussion above, the start of the morning or afternoon would be ideal for a meeting. The afternoon timing could be associated with a light lunch prior to starting the meeting.

II. MEETING ROOM CHARACTER

    A. Location—A location that minimizes the travel barriers encountered by all the members of the committee is best. In a multihospital organization, this choice may not be ideal if a perception of interhospital territoriality would create a perception of bias in the decisions of the committee. There have also been suggestions regarding the use of teleconferencing.[4] As this becomes a more widely accepted professional tool in the future, the barriers of travel time could be eliminated as a means to incorporate a higher degree of expertise within the members of the committee.

    B. Size—The room should have a rectangular table, or tables set up in a U shape if there are too many members for a single table, with chairs on all sides and enough room for additional chairs next to the walls for guests who might be attending a meeting. The room should allow a comfortable fit for a table that is large enough for the usual attendance as well as appropriate audiovisual equipment. Overall, the room or table should not be so large that the usual attendees might feel isolated and thus less engaged in the agenda of any meeting. Similarly, a full turnout would crowd the room, giving greater emphasis to the character of the deliberations.

C. Seating—This can be highly defined as is seen in cases with assigned seats having a name card displayed on the table for each member. The benefits of universal identity of the members would thus be enhanced, especially if they are generally unknown to each other because of the size of an institution or hospital group. More commonly, there could be no fixed seating arrangements for a more informal tradition that could better support collaboration and open discussion. A decision by the chairperson to sit in different locations would further emphasize this approach to a seating tradition. It is also often good for pharmacy personnel to disperse themselves throughout the room to avoid a feeling of us/them in discussions.

REFERENCES

1. Doyle M, Straus D. How to make meetings work: the new interaction method. New York: Berkeley Publishing Group; 1993.
2. Nair KV, Coombs JH, Ascione FJ. Assessing the structure, activities, and functioning of P&T committees: a multisite case study. P&T. 2000;25(10):516-28.
3. Balu S, O'Connor P, Vogenberg FR. Contemporary issues affecting P&T committees. Part 2: beyond managed care. P&T. 2004;29:780-3.
4. Boedeker B. Virtual pharmacy & therapeutics meetings. The Harry S. Truman VA Hospital experience. Columbia (MO): Harry S. Truman Memorial Veteran's Hospital; 1999 Mar [cited 2004 Jan 27]. Available from: http://www.gasnet.org/esia/1999/march/virtual.html

12–4

Appendix 12–4

Example P&T Committee Minutes

ORGANIZATION, INC.

PHARMACY AND THERAPEUTICS COMMITTEE MEETING

January 21, 20XX

SCHEDULED AT 0700

THESE MINUTES ARE PRIVILEGED AND NOT SUBJECT TO DISCLOSURE OR LEGAL DISCOVERY PROCEEDINGS UNDER (STATUTE NUMBER)

I. **Call to Order**. The members or Guests present or members absent are indicated below (legal names, usually with degrees).

The meeting was called to order by the chairperson at 7:00 AM. The physician members present represented a quorum. The minutes for the previous meeting were presented to the members. The section regarding a report of the chairperson from a discussion with the executive committee about ineligible handwriting and unapproved abbreviations was specifically reviewed by the chairperson. The minutes did not describe the executive committee's request that the P&T committee quarterly forward five to eight examples of physician progress notes that reflect these two issues. The executive committee decided to have the president of the medical staff have individual contact with the medical staff members involved. A motion was made to approve the amended minutes and seconded. There being no further discussion, the motion was approved unanimously. After the vote, there was a brief discussion of the impending transition to a total electronic medical record with physician order entry and its ability to reduce transcribing errors. The physician members expressed concern regarding the ease of order entry. No further action was taken.

II Pharmacy and Therapeutics Committee Organizational Affairs

A. Policy and Procedure Amendments—The chairperson submitted a draft revision of the entire policy and procedure for the P&T committee in response to new standards of TJC and previously discussed requirements for the functions of the committee. The committee reviewed the proposed draft and agreed informally to reconsider it at the next meeting after the chairperson has had a chance to meet with the Chief Medical Officer regarding any other amendments that may be necessary.

B. Committee Procedures

1. Conflict of Interest Disclosure—The chairperson gave the Members the forms neces-

sary to declare any potential or actual conflicts of interest according to the procedure established previously by the committee. The chairperson briefly reviewed this process and emphasized that conflicts of interest were only unacceptable when not acknowledged or no action is taken to resolve them during a meeting of the committee.

2. Formulary Request format—no change
3. Alternate Medication Use—no change
4. Drug Monograph—no change

C. Committee Membership—no action; end of year report due December 31st
D. Annual Report—draft Report due January 5th
E. Ad Hoc Committees—none currently
F. Budget—reports due February, May, August, November

III Formulary System

A. Formulary Maintenance
1. Formulary Additions/Deletions
   a. IV lansoprazole (Prevacid®)
   b. fondaparinux (Arixtra®)
   c. escitalopram (Lexapro®)
2. Formulary Class Reviews
   28:04 General anesthetic agents
   72:00 Local anesthetic agent
   86:00 Smooth muscle relaxants
   24:00 Cardiovascular agents
3. Nonformulary Usage Report
4. Review of Standard Order Sets/Guidelines
   TPN order sheet

IV. Drug Use and Quality Improvement

A. Medication Error Report—no report
B. Adverse Medication Reaction Report—no report
C. Drug Usage Evaluation Report—no report
D. Medication Recall—no report

V. Hospital Pharmacy Policies—no report

VI. Current Medication Shortages

12–5

Appendix 12–5

Chairperson Skills

I. Experience

A. KNOWLEDGE OF FORMULARY ISSUES

This occurs ideally as a result of prior experience on the committee for several years. P&T committee meetings are often associated with an individual hospital, group of hospitals, a staff model health maintenance organization, or an insurance-related pharmacy benefit management (PBM) process. A chairperson's experience in each of these areas would be ideal.

B. PROFESSIONAL PRACTICE

It could be suggested that at least 10 years are required for a pharmacist, nurse, administrator, or physician to have a sense of the overall trends evolving within health care. Within a P&T committee, the chairperson would need this background to best respond to the biases that each member might bring to the deliberations. It is beneficial if the members have had mutual experience with the chairperson at a direct patient care level.

C. LEADERSHIP

The chairperson is likely to be the most essential person for the overall success of a P&T committee. This is most directly related to the organization truism that it is nearly impossible to hold a committee responsible for anything except when a committee is acting as the ultimate authority for an organization. Thus, the value of a P&T committee is related to its ability to serve the common interests of the entire organization affected by its actions. If the costs of the P&T committee members' time are considered, the committee's activities are the result of a very expensive effort. To best utilize this expertise, a chairperson must be skilled at mobilizing these resources in a manner that bests supports the overall efforts of the organization to which it is attached. A previously demonstrated ability to create this role for a committee is the most valuable attribute for use in choosing a committee's chairperson.

II. Meeting Strategies

A. PUNCTUALITY

Given the busy schedules of the members, it is necessary to start and end on time. To open a meeting, it is best to lay out the agenda including any new additions and briefly discuss any items that will require a special discussion. Within 2 to 3 minutes, the chairperson and each member should have an understanding of the scope of the meeting ahead.

B. FAIRNESS

Often the health care process vacillates unpredictably between deductive and inductive reasoning processes. External observers are often baffled by this interplay. Related to this, it is suggested that a strict use of the *Robert's Rules of Order* for a meeting agenda may not facilitate the spontaneity for a committee's members that usually underlies their involvement in the character of health care. It is the responsibility of the chairperson to guide this process and seek out the opinions that the members have for a given issue. Also, if the knowledge necessary to make the best judgment for a given issue does not exist for a decision on the issue, it is important that the chairperson be able to facilitate a consensus that develops a means to rectify the deficiency.

C. INVOLVEMENT

Some members may not normally wish to participate spontaneously during a meeting. It is up to the chairperson to ask these members a specific question that would allow them a meaningful opportunity to participate in a given discussion. Occasionally, the chairperson might ask each member present about their opinion for a final decision being faced by the committee. This strategy should begin at one place around the table moving to each member present clockwise around the meeting room.

12–6

Appendix 12–6

Conflict-of-Interest Declaration

FORMULARY ADDITION REQUEST CONFLICT OF INTEREST STATEMENT

NOTE: This must be submitted along with the actual **Request** form if the person submitting the **Request** is not a member of the Formulary Committee. A copy of the Formulary Committee's Policy on Conflict of Interest Management is attached.

Generic Name _____ Trade Name _____

Substantial Involvement with a Competing Organization - ☐ Yes ☐ No

Please describe if:

1) A member of a health insurance company or another health system Pharmacy and Therapeutics Committee.
2) Another health system medical staff officer.
3) A member of a group practice primarily affiliated with another health system.

Substantial Involvement with a Company which Manufactures the Product or Competes with the Product's Company - ☐ Yes ☐ No

Please describe if:

1) Receiving financial income or support in the last 12 months of more than $100 for research, attendance at a **company** supported seminar, travel to an out-of-town meeting, or participation in a **company** sponsored speaker's bureau.
2) Receiving pharmaceutical products from the **company in** the last 12 months for personal or family use, gifts for family or personal use, or samples for use other than as a courtesy for patients.
3) Maintaining in the last 12 months a substantial ownership of stock (>10% of outstanding shares) in the **company** having >30% of its revenue from sales to **this organization**, its affiliated organizations, or another local health system.

Substantial Inside Information - ☐ Yes ☐ No

Please describe if there are other outside relationships for which involvement in this **request** may be actually or potentially perceived as affecting the decision of the committee such as:

1) Having a substantial position of authority in another organization which might affect a member of the committee for employment or medical staff privileges.

2) Disclosing information about this **request** to another organization directly or indirectly which might give **this organization**, the other organization, or the requester an unfair advantage.

3) Receiving substantial assistance from the company or its representative that manufactures the requested product in the preparation of this **Formulary Addition Request**.

Appendix 13–1

Format for Drug Monograph

INSTITUTION NAME HEADING

Generic Name: Can include other common, nonofficial names, e.g., TPA for alteplase.

Trade Brand Name: If more than one, indicate company that each is from.

Manufacturer (or source of supply): Include Web site address.

Therapeutic Category: For example, Thromobolytic Agent for alteplase

Classification: Note—other classifications, such as the VA Class, can also be used.
- AHFS Number and Classification: If not in the book yet, see the list in the front of the *AHFS Drug Information* book and determine the most appropriate classification.
- FDA Classification: Include specific FDA Web site URL concerning approval.
- Status: Prescription, Nonprescription, and/or Controlled Substance Schedule (if applicable).

Similar agents: A list of common treatments used for the same indication(s).

Summary: Includes a short summary of advantages and disadvantages of the drug, particularly in relation to other drugs or treatments used for each major indication, and any other significant information. Must include indications allowed in the institution.

Recommendations: Indicate whether or not the drug should be added to the drug formulary of an institution, including specifying the indications that it is approved for use in the institution, assuming they would have patients that would be treated for illnesses where this drug might be used. Also indicate specific formulary status for the drug (i.e., uncontrolled, monitored, restricted, conditional—see ASHP guidelines) and whether the drug will replace any other product that might already be on the formulary. In addition, include any information on how the drug is to be placed in any clinical guidelines. For third-party payer monographs, information will need to be included on the payment tier.

Page one of the drug monograph consists of the above information

Pharmacological Data:
- Mechanism of Action (usually brief)
- Bacterial Spectrum (if applicable)

Therapeutic Indications:
- FDA-Approved Indications (see package insert)—Clearly state which indications are FDA approved.
- Potential Unlabeled Uses (list only if they are considered to be acceptable medical practice, although it is allowable to mention others that are early in investigation with a statement that the drug should not be used for them or that they require more study)—Clearly indicate they are not FDA approved.
- How the drug, and similar drugs, fit into clinical guidelines.
- Clinical Comparison (abstract at least two studies; see Appendix 9–2 for more guidelines. Include human efficacy studies and, where available, studies comparing the product to standard therapy. Note: If there are other supportive studies for an indication, they can be covered briefly, if you desire, along with the major study covered in detail. Be sure to note any deficiencies in the studies). Also, pharmacogenomic information may need to be included here and elsewhere.

Bioavailability/Pharmacokinetics:
A table summarizing the following, in comparison to the gold standard, can be very useful.
- Absorption
- Distribution
- Metabolism
- Excretion

Dosage Forms:
- Forms and Strengths—Compare to other agents (consider a table), since new products often have a limited number of dosage forms/routes as compared to established products. Purity and composition information should be included for herbal and alternative medications
- Explain any special information needed for preparation and storage, in comparison to other products. Sometimes a product will be so difficult to prepare or have such a limited shelf-life after preparation that it is not worth stocking

Dosage Range:
- Adults
- Children
- Elderly
- Renal or Hepatic Failure
- Special Administration Requirements
- Any anticipated problems in supplies (i.e., shortages) or restrictions in distribution (e.g., prescriber certification required)

Known Adverse Effects/Toxicities:
- Frequency and Type (A table comparing the drug to others can be a clear and concise way of expressing this information.)

- Prevention of Toxicity
- Risk and Benefit Data

Special Precautions: Usually includes pregnancy and lactation.

Contraindications: List of contraindications

Drug Interactions:

A simple one- or two-sentence statement for each—usually separate various interactions into separate short paragraphs and compare to other drugs.
- Drug–Drug
- Drug–Food
- Drug–Laboratory

Patient Safety Information:

Includes medication error information and product safety information from outside sources (e.g., ISMP, MedWatch, FDA Patient Safety News, United States Pharmacopeia Patient Safety Program)

Patient Monitoring Guidelines:

Include effectiveness, adverse effects, compliance and other appropriate items

Patient Information:

- Name and description of the medication
- Dosage form
- Route of administration
- Duration of therapy
- Special directions and precautions
- Side effects
- Techniques for self-monitoring
- Proper storage
- Refill information
- What to do if dose is missed

Cost Comparison:

Use AWP and institutional prices, and make sure there is a comparison with any similar products at equivalent doses—a pharmacoeconomic analysis (see Chapter 6) is the best method of comparing drugs in this section; remember to include any required concomitant therapy. Providing a spreadsheet file with information to consider different patient circumstances that can change may be helpful.

Date Presented to pharmacy and therapeutics committee, and name and title of the person preparing the document

References:

Follow guidelines as described in Appendix 9–3.

13-2

Appendix 13-2

Example Drug Monograph

Note: This example is based on fictional products and is condensed. It shows examples of most sections in a real drug monograph, but often does not go into all of the details (e.g., a table of adverse effects is seen, but only a couple items are listed, whereas a full drug monograph would list at least all common and/or serious reactions).

St. Anywhere Medical Center (St. AMC)
Pharmacy & Therapeutics Committee
Drug Evaluation Monograph

Generic Name:	artiblood
Brand Name:	MegaBlood
Manufacturer:	MegaPharmics
Therapeutic Category:	Blood substitute
Classification:	AHFS 16:00 Blood Derivatives
	FDA Classification: 1A
	Status: Prescription Only
Similar Agents:	fakered

Summary:

Artiblood is a new perfluorocarbon that has many similarities to the only other product in its class, fakered. Both products have the ability to temporarily replace the oxygen-carrying function of red blood cells in patients in whom use of whole blood or packed red blood cells is impossible due to medical or religious reasons. In general, artiblood was found to be more efficacious than fakered; however, it also has been shown to produce a greater number of adverse effects. The adverse effects are mostly gastrointestinal in nature; however, the increased INR can be a problem in some patients. Artiblood is not metabolized in the body, whereas fakered is approximately 50% metabolized to inactive components. These differences are generally not clinically significant, since the dose of either product is unlikely to need adjustment. Fakered is available in several different volume bags, allowing the dose to be matched more closely to the anticipated patient need. While the cost of fakered appears to be lower, a pharmacoeconomic analysis shows that artiblood would produce the greatest cost savings for the institution.

Recommendations:

It is recommended that artiblood be added to the Drug Formulary for use restricted to those who cannot use natural blood replacement products because of religious reasons or because suitable blood types are not available, including for use in cardiac catheterization procedures. It is not approved for use as a volume expander, except when in conjunction with the previous indications.

Pharmacological Data:

Artiblood is a type of perfluorocarbon, similar to fakered. These products have the unique ability to freely bind with or give up oxygen, depending on the partial pressures of the gas where the product is located (i.e., in the lungs there is an abundance of oxygen, so the product adsorbs oxygen; in the tissues there is a relative deficiency of oxygen, so the product gives up the gas).[1,2] The products do not have direct immunologic properties, nor do they have the ability to aid in blood clotting, although there may be some effect on blood clotting (either interference by coating platelets or precipitation of the clotting pathway mechanism).[3]

In addition to oxygen-carrying capabilities, the products have some plasma volume expansion properties. Artiblood has a similar effect to Dextran 40,[1] whereas fakered's properties are relatively insignificant.[4] Maximum plasma volume expansion occurs within several minutes of administration and lasts for approximately 1 day in normal patients. This results in increased central venous pressure, cardiac output, stroke volume, blood pressure, urinary output, capillary perfusion, and pulse pressure. Microcirculation is improved.

Therapeutic Indications:

Indications:

Artiblood is FDA approved for the short-term replacement of the oxygen-carrying capabilities of blood in patients who cannot use normal whole blood.[1] In addition, the product has been used successfully in cardiac catheter procedures, although this use is not FDA approved.[5] There is some early research into the use of the product as a plasma expansion product, but there is not enough information to support this use.[6]

Fakered is approved only for use in cardiac catheterization,[2] although it is commonly used as a blood replacement product in patients who cannot or will not use whole blood products.[7]

Evidence-Based Clinical Guidelines:

A search of the literature was performed to identify evidence-based clinical guidelines. This included Medline, Embase Drugs and Pharmacology, the National Guideline Clearinghouse Web site, the American College of Cardiology Web site, and approximately a dozen Internet search engines; however, no applicable guidelines were identified.

Clinical Studies:

Max and Sugar[6] conducted a comparison trial of artiblood (500 mL/day administered once daily to over 1 hour to 80 patients) and fakered (750 mL administered once over 90 minutes to 82 patients) in patients (18–80 years of age) suffering from massive blood loss (>1 L), who could not use whole blood due to religious beliefs (e.g., Jehovah's Witnesses). In the artiblood group, all patients were undergoing open-heart surgery, as were 78 of the patients in fakered group. The remainder of the fakered group consisted of gunshot patients. Patients with renal insufficiency (creatinine clearance < 50 mL/min) or diagnosed with liver dysfunction were eliminated from consideration. Both groups were similar, except that the artiblood group had more smokers, which may have had an effect on oxygen requirements. Withdrawals from the artiblood group were for the following reasons: death due to failure of heart-lung machine (one patient), noncompliance with protocol (10 patients), worsening symptoms (three patients), and side effects (one patient—vomiting). The authors noted that protocol compliance problems were due to inappropriate staff education and were not related to the drug itself. In the fakered group, withdrawals were due to side effects one patient, diarrhea; one patient, nausea; one patient, abdominal cramps) and noncompliance with protocol (two patients). The patients were assessed on the following items: oxygen and carbon dioxide content of the blood (samples drawn immediately before and after administration, and every 4 hours for 24 hours), coagulation profile of patient (drawn within 2 hours before and after administration), effect on normal blood chemistry profiles (SMA-20) (drawn within 2 hours before and after administration), and time to discontinuation of supplemental oxygen to the patient. Adverse effects were also noted. Results were analyzed using appropriate statistical methods. Artiblood was found to increase the oxygen-carrying capabilities of the blood in comparison to fakered ($p < 0.01$), although fakered did significantly improve oxygen-carrying capabilities over baseline ($p < 0.05$). While fakered had minimal effect on blood chemistry and coagulation profile, it was noted that INRs were increased in patients receiving artiblood ($p < 0.001$). Other adverse effects, mostly gastrointestinal in nature, were more common with fakered, although the symptoms typically disappeared within 2 hours of administration. Other measured characteristics seemed similar between the two groups. The authors concluded that artiblood was the superior agent, due to increased oxygen-carrying capabilities. The authors downplayed adverse effects, although the effects on INRs do appear worrisome.

[Other studies would be covered here for all likely uses within an institution.]

There were no studies found that demonstrated any effects of genome on either artiblood or fakered therapy.

Bioavailability/Pharmacokinetics[16–18]:

Absorption:

Absorption is not applicable, since these agents are administered by IV infusion.

Distribution:

Artiblood is found in the blood stream, with little being distributed to the tissues. Approximately 5% of fakered is found in the liver, with the rest being in the bloodstream.

Metabolism:

Artiblood is not metabolized in the body, whereas approximately 50% of fakered is broken down to inactive components and is excreted in the bile.

Elimination:

Artiblood has a half-life of 5 to 15 hours. It is excreted unchanged in the urine. The longer half-life is seen in patients with renal insufficiency. Since the drug is usually given as a single dose, renal insufficiency does not pose a significant problem. Fakered has a half-life of 4 to 7 hours in normal patients. Significant renal or hepatic impairment may double the half-life.

Dosage Forms:

Large Volume Parenteral:

- Artiblood—500 mL IV bags
- Fakered—500, 750, and 1000 mL IV bags

No other forms or strengths available. This product will have limited availability for the next 6 months due to the ability of the manufacturer to produce an adequate amount to satisfy demands.

No problems in availability are expected after that point. Due to the restrictions on indicated uses in the institution, this is not expected to cause any difficulties and, therefore, no specific procedures are being mandated to address a possible shortage.

Dosage Range:

The normal dose of artiblood for blood replacement is 500 mL, which may be repeated once after 4 hours. Doses may be cut in half for patients weighing less than 50 kg. No dosage adjustments are necessary in renal or hepatic impairment. The product has not been tested in patients younger than 12 years of age and is not recommended in that population. No dosage adjustment is necessary in the elderly.[1]

Fakered is given in doses of 500 mL to 1 L, with a maximum daily dose of 1.5 L. The dose is adjusted based on clinical response of the patient. The product can be used in patients as young as 6 years of age; however, the initial dose is 250 mL.[2]

Known Adverse Effects/Toxicities:

The two agents are compared in the following table:

Adverse Effect	Artiblood (% of patients)	Fakered (% of patients)
Gastrointestinal		
Nausea	20	7
...	...	...

Special Precautions:

Neither drug has been studied long term; therefore, the effects are not known.

Both products are considered Pregnancy Category C. Tests in pregnant animals have shown adverse effects and no adequate, well-controlled studies have been conducted in humans. There is no information available on the excretion of the drug in human milk. Overall, when considering use in pregnant or lactating women, the physician must consider the benefits versus the risks.

Safety and effectiveness of artiblood in children have not been established, although fakered may be used in children at least 6 years old.

Contraindications:

Both agents are contraindicated in patients with hypersensitivities to the drug or any component of the dosage form.

Drug Interactions:

Drug–Drug Interactions:

Heparin—Effects of heparin or low-molecular weight heparins may be significantly increased by either artificial blood replacement agent, although the effect by artiblood tends to be greater. There is no effect on either artiblood or fakered, although the heparin may improve circulation of the products to underperfused tissues. (Other interactions for both drugs would be listed and compared.)

Drug–Food Interactions:

None are known or expected, since these agents are given intravenously and do not undergo entero-hepatic recirculation.

Drug–Laboratory Test Interactions:

INR—INRs can be increased by both agents, although the effect is more noticeable with artiblood. (Other interactions for both drugs would be listed and compared.)

Patient Safety:

This product has a good patient safety profile, with relatively minor adverse effects (e.g., nausea). Since the product has no coagulation or immunologic activity, health care providers must be aware that it is only used for temporary help in oxygen-carrying capabilities. Other specific safety concerns include:

- Patients on warfarin must have a baseline INR and one each day for the 2 days following administration.
- The product has been on the market less than 6 months and information is limited.
- Product must be refrigerated until approximately 30 minutes prior to infusion.

Patient Monitoring Guidelines:

Monitor patient for objective evidence of effectiveness (e.g., oxygen content of blood and clinical effects). Obtain baseline INR and normal chemistry values, and monitor regularly. Monitor for adverse effects.

Patient Information:

In a patient receiving the product due to trauma, it is likely that he or she will not be able to be given information. In that case, provide the information to the next of kin or guardian. Inform patients that the product is an intravenous product that does not contain any blood products. The patient or family should know that he or she may receive this product once or more during the first day after surgery. The patient or family should be informed that the drug has few noticeable adverse effects other than some gastrointestinal upset; however, the physician or pharmacist should be consulted if anything unusual occurs. The patient or family should know that some blood tests will be regularly performed to exclude the possibility of adverse effects. The nurse will keep the drug refrigerated until approximately 30 minutes before infusion. Warnings about missed doses are irrelevant.

Cost Comparison:

General pricing information:

	AWP	Daily Dose*	St. AMC	Daily Dose*
Artiblood 500 mL	$2500/bag	$2500	$2310/bag	$2310
Fakered 500 mL	$1000/bag	$1000	$800/bag	$800
Fakered 750 mL	$1500/bag	$1500	$1200/bag	$1200
Fakered 1000 mL	$2000/bag	$2000	$1600/bag	$1600

*Assume used one bag of each strength.

Pharmacoeconomic Analysis:

- *Problem Definition*—The objective of this analysis is to determine which artificial blood product should be included on the St. AMC drug formulary.
- *Perspective*—This will be from the perspective of the institution.

- *Specific treatment alternatives and outcomes*—There are two drugs to be compared: artiblood and fakered. It will be assumed that natural blood products are not an alternative, since the ability to use natural products would preclude consideration of the artificial products. The outcomes to be measured are hospital costs.
- *Pharmacoeconomic model*—A cost-benefit analysis will be performed. A cost-utility analysis would be desirable, but insufficient information is available. Note: No published pharmacoeconomic analysis is available. The following is based on information obtained from the literature concerning efficacy, adverse effects, monitoring, etc., and uses St. AMC costs, since outside prices would be irrelevant.

	Cost per Patient	Benefit-to-Cost Ratio	Net Benefit
Cost of artiblood (including administration, monitoring, adverse reactions, etc.)	$5120	$7430/$5120 = 1.45:1	$7430 − $5120 = $2310
Benefits of artiblood (money save by early patient discharge from ICU)	$7430		
Cost of fakered (including administration, monitoring, adverse reactions, etc.)	$4000	$4500/$4000 = 1.125:1	$4500 − $4000 = $500
Benefits of fakered (money saved by early patient discharge from ICU)	$4500		

[**Note to reader**: The above information is a summary of information, including averages, decision analysis, and sensitivity analysis that would be used in a pharmacoeconomic evaluation. While the details could be presented here, that may be distracting and confusing to some readers—a decision must be made as to whether all of the details will be presented. See Chapter 6 for details on how to prepare a pharmacoeconomic analysis of a drug being evaluated by the P&T committee.]

Presented by John Q. Doe, PharmD, to the Pharmacy and Therapeutics committee on February 30, 20XX.

REFERENCES

References would be listed in the order in which they are cited in the text—see Appendix 9–3 in Chapter 9 for format and details.

Appendix 14–1

Tools Used in Quality Assurance

FLOW CHARTS

Flow charts illustrate the steps of a process and how the steps are related to each other. It can be used to describe the process, increase a team's knowledge of the entire process, identify weaknesses or breakdown points in the current process, or design a new process. An example of a flow chart outlining how adverse drug reactions might be addressed within an organization is provided below.

Flowchart: suspected adverse drug reactions

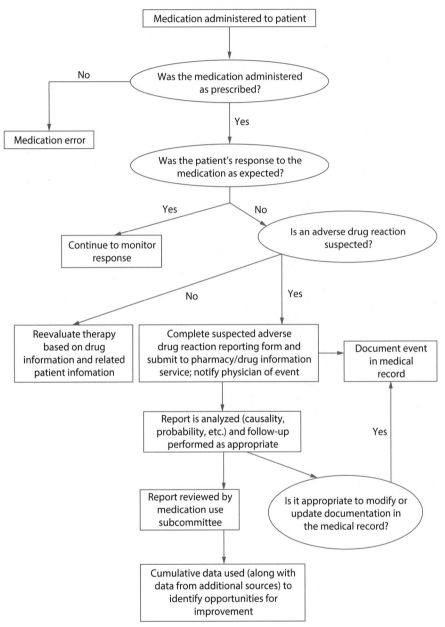

PARETO CHART

Pareto charts are vertical bar graphs with the data presented so that the bars are arranged from left to right on the horizontal axis in their order of decreasing frequency. This arrangement helps identify which problems to address in what order. By addressing the data represented in the tallest bars (e.g., the most frequently occurring problems or contributing factors) efforts can be focused on areas where the most gain can be realized. Pareto charts are commonly used to identify issues to address, delineate potential causes of a problem, and monitor improvements in processes. An example of a Pareto chart is provided below. This example illustrates frequently occurring factors contributing to improper dose medication errors. By focusing on transcription errors as a contributing factor on which to focus quality improvement efforts, the quality improvement team will generally gain more than by tackling the smaller bars.

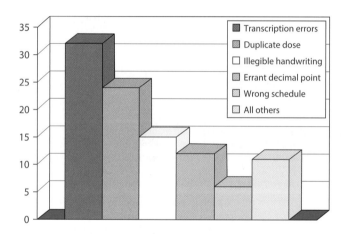

FISHBONE OR CAUSE-AND-EFFECT DIAGRAM

Fishbone or cause-and-effect diagrams represent the relationship between an outcome (represented at the head of the fish) and the possible causes of the outcome (represented as the bones of the fish). The bones of the fish should represent causes and not symptoms of the issue. Fishbone diagrams are commonly used to identify components of a process to address, delineate potential causes of a problem, or identify practitioner groups that participate in producing an outcome and should be represented in the group addressing quality issues in the process(es). An example of a Fishbone chart is provided below.

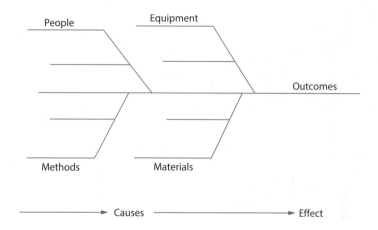

CONTROL CHARTS

Control charts are run charts or line graphs with defined allowable limits of variation. Data are plotted on the graph as they become available with new data points connected to older data by a continuous line. The *x*-axis is usually a measure of time. The control limits help identify which variations in data are important. Control limits are statistically determined based on average ranges and sample size. Fluctuation in data points above and below the average is expected and is referred to as common variation or common cause as long as they remain between the control limits. Data points above the upper control limit or below the lower control limit are referred to as special variation or special cause. Special cause variation indicates that something different is going on outside the normal operation of the process. Also, a series of data points above or below average may indicate a trend in performance that may need to be addressed. As variability in a process is reduced by quality improvement efforts, control limits should be recalculated (and narrowed) based on ongoing data. An example of a control chart is provided below. Calls from pharmacists to prescribers in response to questions or issues related to new medication orders are represented over a 6-month period. Data from the month of July indicates a significant increase in the number of calls made. A quality improvement team evaluating this data would then attempt to identify what contributed to this increase. A potential cause in many institutions might be the influx of new medical housestaff into the organization each July. One potential intervention to reduce this special cause is to improve the orientation of new practitioners to the medication use process within the organization.

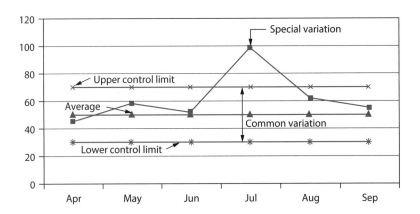

Appendix 14–2

Example of Criteria and Request for Approval

MEDICATION USE EVALUATION CRITERIA

Antiemetic Use in the Prophylaxis of Chemotherapy-Induced Nausea and Vomiting

Request for Approval by Medication Use Evaluation Committee

Purpose of evaluation: The purpose of this Medication Use Evaluation (MUE) is to evaluate the use of antiemetic therapy in the prevention of chemotherapy-induced nausea and vomiting. This agent was selected for evaluation based on its essential role in the management of this patient population, potential inappropriate use, and increased cost relative to other antiemetic agents. This class of medications has not been evaluated within the organization for at least 5 years.

Criteria: A multidisciplinary group including physicians, clinical nurse specialists, staff nurses from the oncology unit, and pharmacists developed the attached criteria. They are submitted for approval by the MUE Committee.

Data Collection: Data will be collected on all patients with orders for this agent written throughout a period of approximately 30 days beginning in mid-January 20XX. A minimum of 50 cases will be reviewed. Pharmacists and clinical nurse specialists will collect data concurrently from the medical record. Patients will be identified by means of the clinical information system.

Results: Results will be presented to this Committee. Information will also be shared with the Cancer Care Committee and Health system Performance Improvement Council. Prescriber-specific results will be confidentially provided to Medical Staff Support for use in the reappointment/recredentialing process.

14-3

Appendix 14-3

Example of MUE Results

MEDICATION USE EVALUATION

Summary of Overall Results

Antiemetic: January-February 20XX

Background: This topic was selected based on high use, potential misuse, and high cost of these agents. Criteria for this evaluation were approved at the MUE Committee's December 20XX meeting. Please refer to attached criteria for additional information.

Total Patients Evaluated (All Indications for Use) = 52

Element	Standard	Results		Compliance
Prescribing				
Indication for use	95%	OVERALL RESULTS		
		Treatment/prevention of nausea/ vomiting (N/F) associated with chemotherapy		100% (52/52)
		Highly emetogenic chemotherapy		46/46
		Anticipatory N/V associated with chemotherapy		6/6
Dispensing/Administering				
Dosing	95%	OVERALL RESULTS		71% (37/52)
		Highly emetogenic chemotherapy		31/46
		Anticipatory N/V associated with chemotherapy		6/6
Monitoring				
Adverse drug reaction(s)	< 10-25% (varies with ADR)	OVERALL RESULTS: Headache: 1 patient Constipation: 1 patient		4% (2/52)

continued

Element	Standard	Results	Compliance
Outcome			
Prevention of nausea and emesis	95%	OVERALL RESULTS	92% (46/50)*
		Highly emetogenic chemotherapy	41/44
		Anticipatory N/V associated with chemotherapy	5/6
Chemotherapy course not interrupted	95%	OVERALL RESULTS (ALL INDICATIONS)	100% (52/52)

*Includes only patients in whom outcome was documented. Outcome was not assessed in two patients who were discharged immediately following administration of chemotherapy.

Summary of Results

Prescribing: Criteria for indication for use were met in all cases.

Dispensing/Administering: Criteria for dosing was met in 37 of 52 cases with all cases involving anticipatory nausea and vomiting meeting criteria.

In 15 cases, patients receiving the antiemetic prior to highly emetogenic chemotherapy received doses not included in the approved criteria. Five of these patients received doses based on an investigational protocol. This dose is now under consideration by the FDA for approval and preliminary results (available only in abstract form) were recently presented at the American Society of Clinical Oncology meeting. Results with the new dosing regimen have been comparable to those with the currently approved doses.

In seven cases not meeting dosing criteria, patients received a single dose prior to chemotherapy consistent with the criteria. However, an additional dose was administered 24 hours after the first dose. These orders were written by two prescribers.

Two cases did not meet dosing criteria because the dose was not adjusted based on renal dysfunction. In both cases, the estimated creatinine clearance was between 20 and 25 mL/min and nephrotoxic drugs were not being administered concurrently. In both cases, the estimated creatinine clearance increased to 30 mL/min or more by day two of the admission (probably due to rehydration of the patient). Neither patient experienced adverse effects.

One dose was not administered within the appropriate timeframe. In this case, the antiemetic dose was administered just 5 minutes prior to the initiation of chemotherapy administration. The nurse administering the antiemetic documented its administration on the way to the patient's room. When she arrived, the patient was not in the room. The dose was administered after he was located, approximately 25 minutes later. The nurse did not correct the actual administration time until after the chemotherapy was administered by a second nurse.

Recommendations:

1. Add new dosing regimen to dosing criteria.
2. Send letters to prescribers giving extra dose.
3. Renal dosing was not significantly outside guidelines. Mention findings in the report to be published in the quality improvement newsletter but do not take prescriber-specific action.

4. The dose administered late was reported via an incident report, no further action by this group is required at this time.

Monitoring: The rate of adverse drug reactions was less than that reported in the literature. This might be reflective of underreporting and underdocumenting of adverse drug events.

Recommendations:

1. The Adverse Drug Event Task Force is currently implementing a new process to improve reporting and documentation. No specific action by this group is required at this time.

Outcome: Ninety-two percent of patients did not experience nausea or vomiting. Outcome was assessable in 50 patients; two patients were discharged immediately following the administration of chemotherapy.

The patient who received his antiemetic dose just 5 minutes prior to chemotherapy experienced moderate nausea and no vomiting. Otherwise, the occurrence of nausea and vomiting was not related to problems with administration or dosing.

Recommendations:

1. 92% success rate is acceptable based on literature, no action is necessary.

General Recommendations:

1. After approval, implement recommendations presented above.
2. Publish results in the Quality Improvement Newsletter following review by the Cancer Care Committee and the Quality Improvement Committee.
3. Perform a follow-up evaluation focusing on dosing issues.
4. Initiate planned assessment of this agent's use in postoperative nausea and vomiting as soon as possible.

14–4

Appendix 14–4

Evaluation Form for Drug Information Response

Request #	Date of Request			
Response by (circle one):	DI Staff	Resident	Student	
Caller (circle type):	MD	RPh	Nurse	Other:

Assessment of Search and Response to Request

	Yes	No	NA	Standard %*
1. Is requestor's demographic information complete?				100%
2. Background information is:				100%
A. Thorough				
B. Appropriate to request				
3. Is the question clearly stated?				100%
4. Search strategy/references:				100%
A. Appropriate references were used				
B. Search was sufficiently comprehensive				
C. Is search strategy clearly documented				
5. Response was:				100%
A. Appropriate for the situation				
B. Sufficient to answer the question				
C. Provided in a timely manner				
D. Integrated with available patient data				
E. Supported by appropriate materials supplied to requestor				
6. If complete response could not be provided within timeframe requested, was requestor advised as to the status of their request and the anticipated delivery of the final response?				100%

* If performance falls below 90% in any category during any month, the service director will coordinate an assessment of the process and report findings and actions will be reported to the P&T committee.

Comments:

Reviewed By: _____

15-1

Appendix 15-1

Kramer Questionnaire*

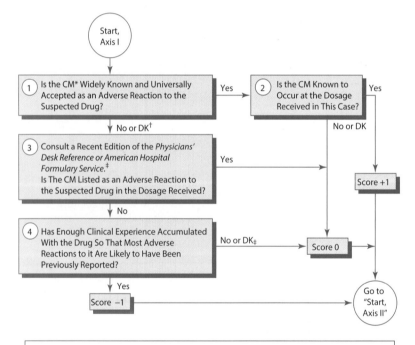

*Abbreviation CM indicates clinical manifestation, the abnormal sign, symptom, or laboratory test, or cluster of abnormal signs, symptoms, and tests, that is being considered as a possible adverse drug reaction.

† Abbreviation DK indicates do not know. This answer should be given when no data are available for the question being answered or when the quality of the data does not allow a firm "Yes" or "No" response.

‡ When these are not available, an equivalent reference source may be used.

Figure 1. Axis I. Previous general experience with drug.

*Kramer MS, Leventhal JM, Hutchinson TA, Feinstein AR. An algorithm for the operational assessment of adverse drug reaction: I. background, descriptions, and instructions for use. JAMA. 1979; 242(7):623-32.

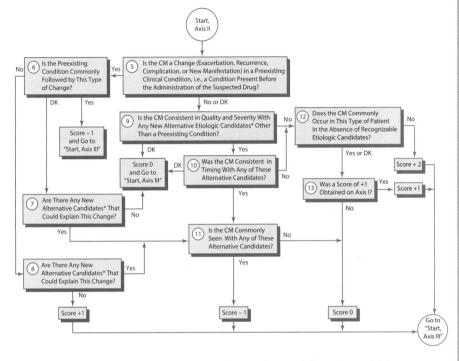

Figure 2. Axis II. Alternative etiologic candidates. For explanation of abbreviations, see Axis I.

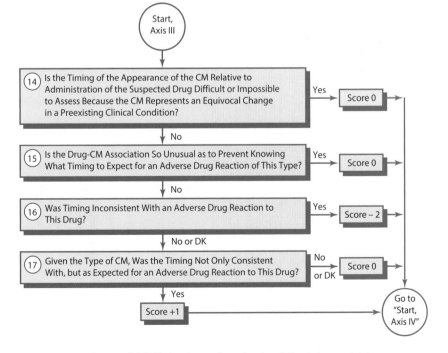

Figure 3. Axis III. Timing of events. For explanation of abbreviations, see Axis I.

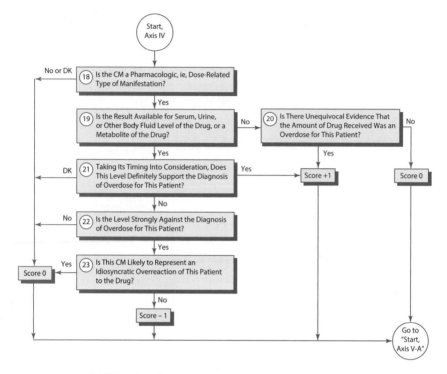

Figure 4. Axis IV. Drug levels and evidence of overdose. For explanation of abbreviations, see Axis I.

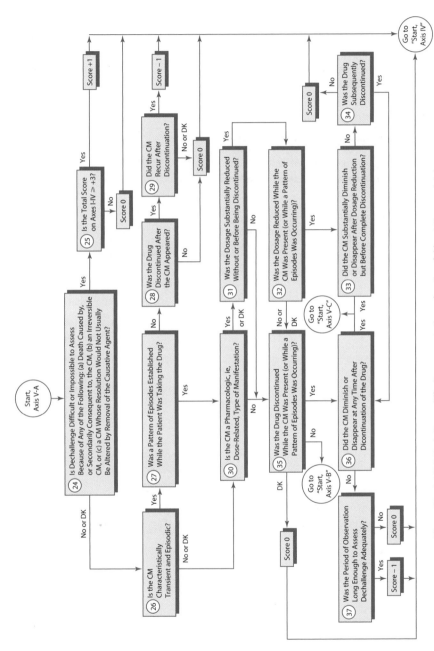

Figure 5A. Axis V-A. Dechallenge: difficult assessments. For explanation of abbreviations, see Axis I.

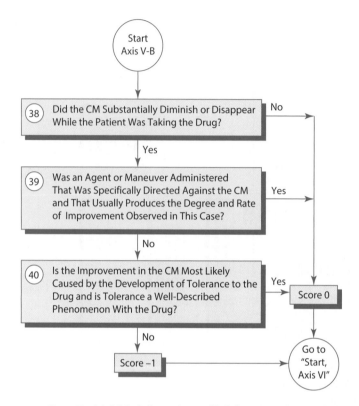

Figure 5B. Axis V-B. Dechallenge: absence of dechallenge. For explanation of abbreviation, see Axis I.

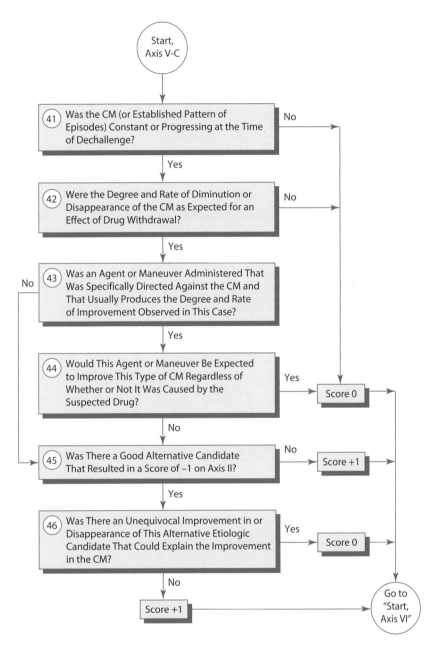

Figure 5C. Axis V-C. Dechallenge: improvement after dechallenge. For explanation of abbreviation, see Axis I.

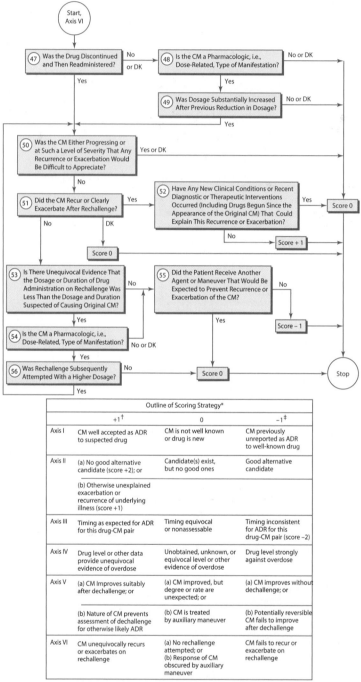

	+1[†]	0	−1[‡]
Axis I	CM well accepted as ADR to suspected drug	CM is not well known or drug is new	CM previously unreported as ADR to well-known drug
Axis II	(a) No good alternative candidate (score +2); or	Candidate(s) exist, but no good ones	Good alternative candidate
	(b) Otherwise unexplained exacerbation or recurrence of underlying illness (score +1)		
Axis III	Timing as expected for ADR for this drug-CM pair	Timing equivocal or nonassessable	Timing inconsistent for ADR for this drug-CM pair (score −2)
Axis IV	Drug level or other data provide unequivocal evidence of overdose	Unobtained, unknown, or equivocal level or other evidence of overdose	Drug level strongly against overdose
Axis V	(a) CM Improves suitably after dechallenge; or	(a) CM improved, but degree or rate are unexpected; or	(a) CM improves without dechallenge; or
	(b) Nature of CM prevents assessment of dechallenge for otherwise likely ADR	(b) CM is treated by auxiliary maneuver	(b) Potentially reversible CM fails to improve after dechallenge
Axis VI	CM unequivocally recurs or exacerbates on rechallenge	(a) No rechallenge attempted; or (b) Response of CM obscured by auxiliary maneuver	CM fails to recur or exacerbate on rechallenge

Outline of Scoring Strategy*

* CM indicates clinical manifestation; ADR = adverse drug reaction.
† Except where noted as +2.
‡ Except where noted as −2.

Figure 6. Axis VI. Rechallenge. For explanation of abbreviation, see Axis I.

15-2

Appendix 15–2

Naranjo Algorithm*

To assess the adverse drug reaction, please answer the following questionnaire and give the pertinent score.

	Yes	No	Don't Know	Score
1. Are there previous conclusive reports on this reaction?	+1	0	0	
2. Did the adverse event appear after the suspected drug was administered?	+2	−1	0	
3. Did the adverse reaction improve when the drug was discontinued or a specific antagonist was administered?	+1	0	0	
4. Did the adverse reaction reappear when the drug was readministered?	+2	−1	0	
5. Are there alternative causes (other than the drug) that could on their own have caused the reaction?	−1	+2	0	
6. Did the reaction reappear when a placebo was given?	−1	+1	0	
7. Was the drug detected in the blood (or other fluids) in concentrations known to be toxic?	+1	0	0	
8. Was the reaction more severe when the dose was increased, or less severe when the dose was decreased?	+1	0	0	
9. Did the patient have a similar reaction to the same or similar drugs in any previous exposure?	+1	0	0	
10. Was the adverse event confirmed by any objective evidence?	+1	0	0	
			Total Score	_____

Score Interpretation

___Definite: ≥ 9

___Probable: 5 to 8

___Possible: 1 to 4

___Doubtful: ≤ 0

---

*Naranjo CA, Busto U, Sellers EM, Sandor P, Ruiz I, Roberts EA, et al. A method of estimating the probability of adverse drug reactions. Clin Pharmacol Ther. 1981;30(2):239-45.

15–3

Appendix 15–3

Jones Algorithm*

START HERE:**

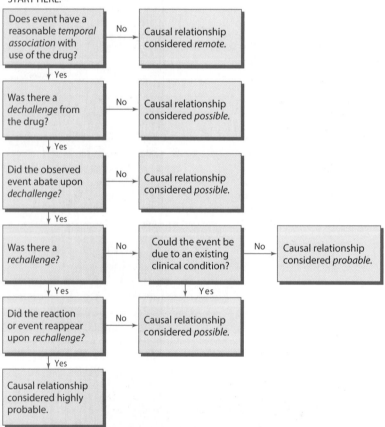

**Each drug is carried through independently; if > 1 drug was dechallenged or rechallenged simultaneously causality for all is ≤ possible.

QUESTIONS:

1. Did the reaction follow a reasonable temporal sequence?
2. Did the patient improve after stopping the drug?
3. Did the reaction reappear on repeated exposure (rechallenge)?
4. Could the reaction be reasonably explained by the known characteristics of the patient's clinical *state*?

---

*Jones JK. Adverse drug reactions in the community health setting: approaches to recognizing, counseling, and reporting. Clin Comm Health. 1982;5(2):58-67.

MedWatch Form

Reset Form

U.S. Department of Health and Human Services

Form Approved: OMB No. 0910-0291, Expires: 6/30/2015
See PRA statement on reverse.

MedWatch

The FDA Safety Information and Adverse Event Reporting Program

For VOLUNTARY reporting of adverse events, product problems and product use errors

Page 1 of 3

FDA USE ONLY

Triage unit sequence #

A. PATIENT INFORMATION

1. Patient Identifier	2. Age at Time of Event or Date of Birth:	3. Sex	4. Weight
In confidence		☐ Female ☐ Male	lb or kg

B. ADVERSE EVENT, PRODUCT PROBLEM OR ERROR

Check all that apply:

1. ☐ Adverse Event ☐ Product Problem *(e.g., defects/malfunctions)*
   ☐ Product Use Error ☐ Problem with Different Manufacturer of Same Medicine

2. Outcomes Attributed to Adverse Event *(Check all that apply)*
   - ☐ Death: _____ *(mm/dd/yyyy)*
   - ☐ Life-threatening
   - ☐ Hospitalization - initial or prolonged
   - ☐ Required Intervention to Prevent Permanent Impairment/Damage (Devices)
   - ☐ Disability or Permanent Damage
   - ☐ Congenital Anomaly/Birth Defect
   - ☐ Other Serious (Important Medical Events)

3. Date of Event *(mm/dd/yyyy)*

4. Date of this Report *(mm/dd/yyyy)*

5. Describe Event, Problem or Product Use Error

(Continue on page 3)

6. Relevant Tests/Laboratory Data, Including Dates

(Continue on page 3)

7. Other Relevant History, Including Preexisting Medical Conditions *(e.g., allergies, race, pregnancy, smoking and alcohol use, liver/kidney problems, etc.)*

(Continue on page 3)

C. PRODUCT AVAILABILITY

Product Available for Evaluation? *(Do not send product to FDA)*

☐ Yes ☐ No ☐ Returned to Manufacturer on: _____ *(mm/dd/yyyy)*

D. SUSPECT PRODUCT(S)

1. Name, Strength, Manufacturer *(from product label)*
   #1 Name:
   Strength:
   Manufacturer:
   #2 Name:
   Strength:
   Manufacturer:

2. Dose or Amount | Frequency | Route
   #1
   #2

3. Dates of Use *(If unknown, give duration) from/to (or best estimate)*
   #1
   #2

4. Diagnosis or Reason for Use *(Indication)*
   #1
   #2

5. Event Abated After Use Stopped or Dose Reduced?
   #1 ☐ Yes ☐ No ☐ Doesn't Apply
   #2 ☐ Yes ☐ No ☐ Doesn't Apply

6. Lot #
   #1
   #2

7. Expiration Date
   #1
   #2

8. Event Reappeared After Reintroduction?
   #1 ☐ Yes ☐ No ☐ Doesn't Apply
   #2 ☐ Yes ☐ No ☐ Doesn't Apply

9. NDC # or Unique ID

E. SUSPECT MEDICAL DEVICE

1. Brand Name

2. Common Device Name

2b. Procode

3. Manufacturer Name, City and State

4. Model # | Lot #

   Catalog # | Expiration Date *(mm/dd/yyyy)*

   Serial # | Unique Identifier (UDI) #

5. Operator of Device
   ☐ Health Professional
   ☐ Lay User/Patient
   ☐ Other:

6. If Implanted, Give Date *(mm/dd/yyyy)*

7. If Explanted, Give Date *(mm/dd/yyyy)*

8. Is this a Single-use Device that was Reprocessed and Reused on a Patient?
   ☐ Yes ☐ No

9. If Yes to Item No. 8, Enter Name and Address of Reprocessor

F. OTHER (CONCOMITANT) MEDICAL PRODUCTS

Product names and therapy dates *(exclude treatment of event)*

(Continue on page 3)

G. REPORTER *(See confidentiality section on back)*

1. Name and Address
   Name:
   Address:
   City: State: ZIP:
   Phone # E-mail

2. Health Professional? ☐ Yes ☐ No

3. Occupation

4. Also Reported to:
   ☐ Manufacturer
   ☐ User Facility
   ☐ Distributor/Importer

5. If you do NOT want your identity disclosed to the manufacturer, place an "X" in this box: ☐

FORM FDA 3500 (2/13) Submission of a report does not constitute an admission that medical personnel or the product caused or contributed to the event.

PLEASE TYPE OR USE BLACK INK

Delete Page

ADVICE ABOUT VOLUNTARY REPORTING
Detailed instructions available at: http://www.fda.gov/medwatch/report/consumer/instruct.htm

Report adverse events, product problems or product use errors with:

- Medications *(drugs or biologics)*
- Medical devices *(including in-vitro diagnostics)*
- Combination products *(medication & medical devices)*
- Human cells, tissues, and cellular and tissue-based products
- Special nutritional products *(dietary supplements, medical foods, infant formulas)*
- Cosmetics
- Food *(including beverages and ingredients added to foods)*

Report product problems - quality, performance or safety concerns such as:

- Suspected counterfeit product
- Suspected contamination
- Questionable stability
- Defective components
- Poor packaging or labeling
- Therapeutic failures (product didn't work)

Report SERIOUS adverse events. An event is serious when the patient outcome is:

- Death
- Life-threatening
- Hospitalization - initial or prolonged
- Disability or permanent damage
- Congenital anomaly/birth defect
- Required intervention to prevent permanent impairment or damage (devices)
- Other serious (important medical events)

Report even if:

- You're not certain the product caused the event
- You don't have all the details

How to report:

- Just fill in the sections that apply to your report
- Use section D for all products except medical devices
- Attach additional pages if needed
- Use a separate form for each patient
- Report either to FDA or the manufacturer *(or both)*

Other methods of reporting:

- 1-800-FDA-0178 - To FAX report
- 1-800-FDA-1088 - To report by phone
- www.fda.gov/medwatch/report.htm - To report online

If your report involves a serious adverse event with a device and it occurred in a facility outside a doctor's office, that facility may be legally required to report to FDA and/or the manufacturer. Please notify the person in that facility who would handle such reporting.

If your report involves a serious adverse event with a vaccine, call 1-800-822-7967 to report.

Confidentiality: The patient's identity is held in strict confidence by FDA and protected to the fullest extent of the law. FDA will not disclose the reporter's identity in response to a request from the public, pursuant to the Freedom of Information Act. The reporter's identity, including the identity of a self-reporter, may be shared with the manufacturer unless requested otherwise.

-Fold Here-

-Fold Here-

The information in this box applies only to requirements of the Paperwork Reduction Act of 1995

The burden time for this collection of information has been estimated to average 36 minutes per response, including the time to review instructions, search existing data sources, gather and maintain the data needed, and complete and review the collection of information. Send comments regarding this burden estimate or any other aspect of this collection of information, including suggestions for reducing this burden to:

Department of Health and Human Services *Food and Drug Administration* *Office of Chief Information Officer* *Paperwork Reduction Act (PRA) Staff* *PRAStaff@fda.hhs.gov*	*Please DO NOT* *RETURN this form* *to the PRA Staff e-mail* *to the left.*	*OMB statement:* *"An agency may not conduct or sponsor, and a person is not required to respond to, a collection of information unless it displays a currently valid OMB control number."*

U.S. DEPARTMENT OF HEALTH AND HUMAN SERVICES
Food and Drug Administration

FORM FDA 3500 (2/13) (Back)   Please Use Address Provided Below -- Fold in Thirds, Tape and Mail

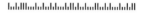

DEPARTMENT OF
HEALTH & HUMAN SERVICES

Public Health Service
Food and Drug Administration
Rockville, MD 20857

Official Business
Penalty for Private Use $300

NO POSTAGE
NECESSARY
IF MAILED
IN THE
UNITED STATES
OR APO/FPO

BUSINESS REPLY MAIL
FIRST CLASS MAIL PERMIT NO. 946 ROCKVILLE MD

POSTAGE WILL BE PAID BY FOOD AND DRUG ADMINISTRATION

MEDWATCH
The FDA Safety Information and Adverse Event Reporting Program
Food and Drug Administration
5600 Fishers Lane
Rockville, MD 20852-9787

Reset Form | Delete Page

U.S. Department of Health and Human Services

MEDWATCH
The FDA Safety Information and
Adverse Event Reporting Program

(CONTINUATION PAGE)

For VOLUNTARY reporting of
adverse events and product problems

Page 3 of 3__

B.5. **Describe Event or Problem** *(continued)*

Back to Form

B.6. **Relevant Tests/Laboratory Data, Including Dates** *(continued)*

Back to Form

B.7. **Other Relevant History, Including Preexisting Medical Conditions** *(e.g., allergies, race, pregnancy, smoking and alcohol use, hepatic/renal dysfunction, etc.) (continued)*

Back to Form

F. **Concomitant Medical Products and Therapy Dates** *(Exclude treatment of event) (continued)*

Back to Form

Appendix 17–1

Investigational New Drug Application

Next Page	Export Data	Import Data	Reset Form

DEPARTMENT OF HEALTH AND HUMAN SERVICES Food and Drug Administration **INVESTIGATIONAL NEW DRUG APPLICATION (IND)** *(Title 21, Code of Federal Regulations (CFR) Part 312)*	Form Approved: OMB No. 0910-0014 Expiration Date: April 30, 2015 *See PRA Statement on page 3.* NOTE: No drug/biologic may be shipped or clinical investigation begun until an IND for that investigation is in effect (21 CFR 312.40)

1. Name of Sponsor	2. Date of Submission *(mm/dd/yyyy)*

3. Sponsor Address	4. Telephone Number *(Include country code if applicable and area code)*

Address 1 *(Street address, P.O. box, company name c/o)*

Address 2 *(Apartment, suite, unit, building, floor, etc.)*

City	State/Province/Region

Country	ZIP or Postal Code

5. Name(s) of Drug *(Include all available names: Trade, Generic, Chemical, or Code)*	6. IND Number *(If previously assigned)*

Continuation Page for #5

7. (Proposed) Indication for Use

Is this indication for a rare disease (prevalence <200,000 in U.S.)? ☐ Yes ☐ No

Does this product have an FDA Orphan Designation for this indication? ☐ Yes ☐ No

If yes, provide the Orphan Designation number for this indication:

Continuation Page for #7

8. Phase(s) of Clinical Investigation to be conducted ☐ Phase 1 ☐ Phase 2 ☐ Phase 3 ☐ Other *(Specify)*: _____

9. List numbers of all Investigational New Drug Applications (21 CFR Part 312), New Drug Applications (21 CFR Part 314), Drug Master Files (21 CFR Part 314.420), and Biologics License Applications (21 CFR Part 601) referred to in this application.

10. IND submission should be consecutively numbered. The initial IND should be numbered "Serial number: 0000." The next submission (e.g., amendment, report, or correspondence) should be numbered "Serial Number: 0001." Subsequent submissions should be numbered consecutively in the order in which they are submitted.. | Serial Number

11. This submission contains the following *(Select all that apply)*

☐ Initial Investigational New Drug Application (IND) ☐ Response to Clinical Hold ☐ Response To FDA Request For Information
☐ Request For Reactivation Or Reinstatement ☐ Annual Report ☐ General Correspondence
☐ Development Safety Update Report (DSUR) ☐ Other *(Specify)*: _____

Protocol Amendment(s)	Information Amendment(s)	Request for	IND Safety Report(s)
☐ New Protocol	☐ Chemistry/Microbiology	☐ Meeting	☐ Initial Written Report
☐ Change in Protocol	☐ Pharmacology/Toxicology	☐ Proprietary Name Review	☐ Follow-up to a Written Report
☐ New Investigator	☐ Clinical ☐ Statistics	☐ Special Protocol Assessment	
☐ PMR/PMC Protocol	☐ Clinical Pharmacology	☐ Formal Dispute Resolution	

12. Select the following only if applicable. *(Justification statement must be submitted with application for any items selected below. Refer to the cited CFR section for further information.)*

Expanded Access Use, 21 CFR 312.300

☐ Emergency Research Exception From Informed Consent Requirements, 21 CFR 312.23 (f)
☐ Charge Request, 21 CFR 312.8

☐ Individual Patient, Non-Emergency 21 CFR 312.310
☐ Individual Patient, Emergency 21 CFR 312.310(d)

☐ Intermediate Size Patient Population, 21 CFR 312.315
☐ Treatment IND or Protocol, 21 CFR 312.320

For FDA Use Only		
CBER/DCC Receipt Stamp	DDR Receipt Stamp	Division Assignment
		IND Number Assigned

FORM FDA 1571 (1/13) | Page 1 of | PSC Publishing Services (301) 443-6740 EF

Previous Page   Next Page

13. Contents of Application – This application contains the following items *(Select all that apply)*

☐ 1. Form FDA 1571 *(21 CFR 312.23(a)(1))*

☐ 2. Table of Contents *(21 CFR 312.23(a)(2))*

☐ 3. Introductory statement *(21 CFR 312.23(a)(3))*

☐ 4. General Investigational plan *(21 CFR 312.23(a)(3))*

☐ 5. Investigator's brochure *(21 CFR 312.23(a)(5))*

☐ 6. Protocol(s) *(21 CFR 312.23(a)(6))*

　☐ a. Study protocol(s) *(21 CFR 312.23(a)(6))*

　☐ b. Investigator data *(21 CFR 312.23(a)(6)(iii)(b))* or completed Form(s) FDA 1572

　☐ c. Facilities data *(21 CFR 312.23(a)(6)(iii)(b))* or completed Form(s) FDA 1572

6. Protocol(s) *(Continued)*

　☐ d. Institutional Review Board data (21 CFR 312.23(a)(6)(iii) (b)) or completed Form(s) FDA 1572

☐ 7. Chemistry, manufacturing, and control data *(21 CFR 312.23(a)(7))*

　☐ Environmental assessment or claim for exclusion *(21 CFR 312.23(a)(7)(iv)(e))*

☐ 8. Pharmacology and toxicology data (21 CFR 312.23(a)(8))

☐ 9. Previous human experience *(21 CFR 312.23(a)(9))*

☐ 10. Additional information *(21 CFR 312.23(a)(10))*

☐ 11. Biosimilar User Fee Cover Sheet *(Form FDA 3792)*

☐ 12. Clinical Trials Certification of Compliance *(Form FDA 3674)*

14. Is any part of the clinical study to be conducted by a contract research organization?　☐ Yes　☐ No

If Yes, will any sponsor obligations be transferred to the contract research organization?　☐ Yes　☐ No

If Yes, provide a statement containing the name and address of the contract research organization, identification of the clinical study, and a listing of the obligations transferred *(use continuation page)*.

Continuation Page for #14

15. Name and Title of the person responsible for monitoring the conduct and progress of the clinical investigations

16. Name(s) and Title(s) of the person(s) responsible for review and evaluation of information relevant to the safety of the drug

I agree not to begin clinical investigations until 30 days after FDA's receipt of the IND unless I receive earlier notification by FDA that the studies may begin. I also agree not to begin or continue clinical investigations covered by the IND if those studies are placed on clinical hold or financial hold. I agree that an Institutional Review Board (IRB) that complies with the requirements set forth in 21 CFR Part 56 will be responsible for initial and continuing review and approval of each of the studies in the proposed clinical investigation. I agree to conduct the investigation in accordance with all other applicable regulatory requirements.

17. Name of Sponsor or Sponsor's Authorized Representative

18. Telephone Number *(Include country code if applicable and area code)*

19. Facsimile (FAX) Number *(Include country code if applicable and area code)*

20. Address

Address 1 *(Street address, P.O. box, company name c/o)*

Address 2 *(Apartment, suite, unit, building, floor, etc.)*

City　State/Province/Region

Country　ZIP or Postal Code

21. Email Address

22. Date of Sponsor's Signature *(mm/dd/yyyy)*

23. Name of Countersigner

24. Address of Countersigner

Address 1 *(Street address, P.O. box, company name c/o)*

Address 2 *(Apartment, suite, unit, building, floor, etc.)*

City　State/Province/Region

Country　ZIP or Postal Code

WARNING : A willfully false statement is a criminal offense (U.S.C. Title 18, Sec. 1001).

25. Signature of Sponsor or Sponsor's Authorized Representative　Sign

26. Signature of Countersigner　Sign

Appendix 17–2

Statement of Investigator

1. NAME AND ADDRESS OF INVESTIGATOR

Name of Principal Investigator

Address 1	Address 2		
City	State/Province/Region	Country	ZIP or Postal Code

2. EDUCATION, TRAINING, AND EXPERIENCE THAT QUALIFY THE INVESTIGATOR AS AN EXPERT IN THE CLINICAL INVESTIGATION OF THE DRUG FOR THE USE UNDER INVESTIGATION. ONE OF THE FOLLOWING IS PROVIDED *(Select **one** of the following.)*

☐ Curriculum Vitae   ☐ Other Statement of Qualifications

3. NAME AND ADDRESS OF ANY MEDICAL SCHOOL, HOSPITAL, OR OTHER RESEARCH FACILITY WHERE THE CLINICAL INVESTIGATION(S) WILL BE CONDUCTED

CONTINUATION PAGE for Item 3

Name of Medical School, Hospital, or Other Research Facility

Address 1	Address 2		
City	State/Province/Region	Country	ZIP or Postal Code

4. NAME AND ADDRESS OF ANY CLINICAL LABORATORY FACILITIES TO BE USED IN THE STUDY

CONTINUATION PAGE for Item 4

Name of Clinical Laboratory Facility

Address 1	Address 2		
City	State/Province/Region	Country	ZIP or Postal Code

5. NAME AND ADDRESS OF THE INSTITUTIONAL REVIEW BOARD (IRB) THAT IS RESPONSIBLE FOR REVIEW AND APPROVAL OF THE STUDY(IES)

CONTINUATION PAGE for Item 5

Name of IRB

Address 1	Address 2		
City	State/Province/Region	Country	ZIP or Postal Code

6. NAMES OF SUBINVESTIGATORS *(If not applicable, enter "None")*

CONTINUATION PAGE – for Item 6

7. NAME AND CODE NUMBER, IF ANY, OF THE PROTOCOL(S) IN THE IND FOR THE STUDY(IES) TO BE CONDUCTED BY THE INVESTIGATOR

8. PROVIDE THE FOLLOWING CLINICAL PROTOCOL INFORMATION. *(Select **one** of the following.)*

☐ For Phase 1 investigations, a general outline of the planned investigation including the estimated duration of the study and the maximum number of subjects that will be involved.

☐ For Phase 2 or 3 investigations, an outline of the study protocol including an approximation of the number of subjects to be treated with the drug and the number to be employed as controls, if any; the clinical uses to be investigated; characteristics of subjects by age, sex, and condition; the kind of clinical observations and laboratory tests to be conducted; the estimated duration of the study; and copies or a description of case report forms to be used.

9. COMMITMENTS

I agree to conduct the study(ies) in accordance with the relevant, current protocol(s) and will only make changes in a protocol after notifying the sponsor, except when necessary to protect the safety, rights, or welfare of subjects.

I agree to personally conduct or supervise the described investigation(s).

I agree to inform any patients, or any persons used as controls, that the drugs are being used for investigational purposes and I will ensure that the requirements relating to obtaining informed consent in 21 CFR Part 50 and institutional review board (IRB) review and approval in 21 CFR Part 56 are met.

I agree to report to the sponsor adverse experiences that occur in the course of the investigation(s) in accordance with 21 CFR 312.64. I have read and understand the information in the investigator's brochure, including the potential risks and side effects of the drug.

I agree to ensure that all associates, colleagues, and employees assisting in the conduct of the study(ies) are informed about their obligations in meeting the above commitments.

I agree to maintain adequate and accurate records in accordance with 21 CFR 312.62 and to make those records available for inspection in accordance with 21 CFR 312.68.

I will ensure that an IRB that complies with the requirements of 21 CFR Part 56 will be responsible for the initial and continuing review and approval of the clinical investigation. I also agree to promptly report to the IRB all changes in the research activity and all unanticipated problems involving risks to human subjects or others. Additionally, I will not make any changes in the research without IRB approval, except where necessary to eliminate apparent immediate hazards to human subjects.

I agree to comply with all other requirements regarding the obligations of clinical investigators and all other pertinent requirements in 21 CFR Part 312.

INSTRUCTIONS FOR COMPLETING FORM FDA 1572
STATEMENT OF INVESTIGATOR

1. Complete all sections. Provide a separate page if additional space is needed.

2. Provide curriculum vitae or other statement of qualifications as described in Section 2.

3. Provide protocol outline as described in Section 8.

4. Sign and date below.

5. FORWARD THE COMPLETED FORM AND OTHER DOCUMENTS BEING PROVIDED TO THE SPONSOR. The sponsor will incorporate this information along with other technical data into an Investigational New Drug Application (IND). INVESTIGATORS SHOULD NOT SEND THIS FORM DIRECTLY TO THE FOOD AND DRUG ADMINISTRATION.

10. DATE *(mm/dd/yyyy)*	11. SIGNATURE OF INVESTIGATOR Sign

(**WARNING**: A willfully false statement is a criminal offense. U.S.C. Title 18, Sec. 1001.)

The information below applies only to requirements of the Paperwork Reduction Act of 1995.

The burden time for this collection of information is estimated to average 100 hours per response, including the time to review instructions, search existing data sources, gather and maintain the data needed and complete and review the collection of information. Send comments regarding this burden estimate or any other aspect of this information collection, including suggestions for reducing this burden to the address to the right:

Department of Health and Human Services
Food and Drug Administration
Office of Chief Information Officer
Paperwork Reduction Act (PRA) Staff
PRAStaff@fda.hhs.gov

"An agency may not conduct or sponsor, and a person is not required to respond to, a collection of information unless it displays a currently valid OMB number."

DO NOT SEND YOUR COMPLETED FORM TO THIS PRA STAFF EMAIL ADDRESS.

FORM FDA 1572 (7/13)   PREVIOUS EDITION IS OBSOLETE.   Page 2 of

Appendix 17–3

Protocol Medication Economic Analysis

Date:
Protocol title:
Study chairperson:

Hospital Cost Analysis

Drug	Hospital Cost per Cycle*	Number of Cycles	Total Cost per Patient	Number of Patients	Total Protocol Cost	Annual Cost
Primary Therapy						
Supportive Care						

*When applicable, doses calculated on 1.7 m^2 or 70 kg at initial dose level and costs include infusion fluids, administration sets, and tubing.

Patient Charge Analysis

Drug	Patient Charge per Cycle*	Number of Cycles	Total Charge per Patient	Number of Patients	Total Patient Billing
Primary Therapy					
Supportive Care					

*When applicable, charges include infusion fluids, administration sets, and tubing.

Reimbursement Risk

Drug	FDA Labeled	Compendium

Comments

Summary

_____

_____

17-4

Appendix 17–4

Investigational Drug Accountability Record

Form approved
OMB No. 0925-0240
Expires: 6/30/91

National Institutes of Health
National Cancer Institute

Investigational Drug Accountability Record

PAGE NO. _____

CONTROL RECORD ☐

SATELLITE RECORD ☐

Name of Institution	Protocol No. (NCI)

Drug Name, Dose Form and Strength

Protocol Title	Dispensing Area

Investigation

Line No.	Date	Patient's Initials	Patient's I.D. Number	Dose	Quantity Dispensed or Received	Balance Forward / Balance	Manufacturer and Lot No.	Recorder's Initials
1.								
2.								
3.								
4.								
5.								
6.								
7.								
8.								
9.								
10.								
11.								
12.								
13.								
14.								
15.								
16.								
17.								
18.								
19.								
20.								
21.								
22.								
23.								
24.								

NIH-2564
9-85

Appendix 18–1

Policy Example: High-Alert Medications

I. PURPOSE:

This policy outlines the process for the safe use of high-alert medications.

II. DEFINITIONS:

When used in this policy these terms have the following meanings:
- A. High-alert medications: Medications that have a higher risk of causing harm when an error occurs.
- B. Independent double verification (IDV):
  1. Is performed by two staff members (as appropriate to the task, e.g., blood administration, breast milk retrieval) in the same proximity but separately, without prompting by another, as an independent cognitive task.
  2. Both professionals will dialog to confirm what was checked independently prior to administration.
  3. IDV of a medication also includes the following steps in addition to the two steps above:
     a. Performed by two professionals (e.g., nurse/pharmacist,/physician [within the approved LPN scope of practice]) in the same proximity but separately, without prompting by another, as an independent cognitive task.
     b. Each professional must check: the actual prescriber's order, drug, calculation, concentration, and other information specific to the medication.
     c. Each professional performing the verification performs all calculations independently without knowledge of any prior calculations and documents the verification in the medical record.

III. POLICY:

It is the policy of the health system that:
- A. All systems and data repositories relating to medication use (medication error reports, adverse drug event reports, etc.) shall be systematically evaluated on an ongoing basis to identify those medications in the hospital formulary determined to be high-alert medications.
- B. Medications being added to the hospital formulary shall be evaluated for their high-alert potential.

C. Medications identified as high-alert shall be targeted for specific error reduction interventions.

D. The following three principles shall be followed to safeguard the use of high-alert medications:

1. Reduce or eliminate the possibility of error (e.g., limit the number of high-alert medications on the hospital formulary; remove high-alert medications from the clinical areas).

2. Make errors visible by detecting serious events before they reach the patient (e.g., follow the five rights and when appropriate utilize the independent double verification process).

3. Minimize the consequences of errors (e.g., stock high-alert medications in smaller volume units of use minimizing the error effect if the medication was administered in error).

E. Engineering safety controls shall be used as appropriate.

IV. PROCEDURE:

A. The Pharmacy and Therapeutics Committee will approve all medications added to the formulary.

B. The following processes for safeguarding high-alert medication use have been implemented:

1. Build in system redundancies (e.g., unit dose drug distribution).

2. Use fail-safes (e.g., pumps with locking mechanisms).

3. Reduce options (e.g., limit concentration available).

4. Utilize engineering safety controls (e.g., oral syringes that will not fit IV tubing, computer systems that force the order of standardized products).

5. Externalize or centralize error-prone processes (e.g., centralize IV solution preparations).

6. Use differentiation (e.g., identify and isolate look-alike and sound-alike products, use generic names).

7. Store medications appropriately (e.g., separate potentially dangerous drugs with similar names or similar packaging).

8. Screen new products (e.g., inspect all new drugs and drug delivery devices for poor labeling and/or packaging).

9. Standardize and simplify order communication (e.g., only approved abbreviations will be used, all verbal orders will be read back verbatim to the ordering physician).

10. Limit access (e.g., high-alert medications will be securely stored).

11. Use of constraints (e.g., pharmacy will screen all medication orders, automatic stop orders or duration limits).

12. Standardize or automate dosing procedures (e.g., use of standard dosing charts rather than calculating doses based on weight or renal function when appropriate).

C. When initiating any high-alert medication by any route, and for those high-alert medications administered via pump, and with all subsequent bag/syringe changes and with dose changes requiring pump adjustment, the following must occur:

1. Independent double verification, each professional will independently:

a. Review/verify the physician order in the medical record (i.e., on the physician's order sheet or in the clinical information system).

    b. Verify the correct medication, dose (all required dosage calculations must be done independently by each nurse), frequency/rate/titration, and route against the order.

      1) Note: After the initial IDV, ongoing titration in Level I areas is exempt from the IDV process for each continuing adjustment.

      2) Some medications require IDV of pump settings at change of shift (e.g., insulin).

      3) Additional information regarding medication-specific IDV requirements is available in the IDV Policy and Procedure.

  2. The nurse administering the medication will:

    a. Identify the patient using two acceptable identifiers.

    b. Verify the correct connection/patient access when administering the medication via an intravenous drip, trace the flow of the medication from the bag > to the pump > to the patient access, prior to hanging the medication.

    c. Document the verification.

D. When an infusion device with prebuilt infusion parameters is used and pre-set infusion parameters are not available for a high-alert medication (e.g., when the medication is new and not yet added to the library), independent double verification of the medication parameters programmed into the pump must occur prior to initiation of the infusion.

V. DOCUMENTATION:

As appropriate in the medical record or clinical information system.

VI. REFERENCES:

  A. Institute for Safe Medication Practices (ISMP); *ISMP's list of high-alert medications.* 2008.

  B. Patient Care Policy and Procedure #0282, *Independent Double Verification.*

  C. Patient Care Policy and Procedure #0500, *Verbal Orders.*

  D. Patient Care Policy and Procedure #0700, *Abbreviations.*

  E. Patient Care Policy and Procedure #0282, *IDV.*

  F. Patient Care Policy and Procedure #5010, *Anticoagulant Safety.*

  G. Patient Care Policy and Procedure #5020, *Chemotherapy: Oncology/Hematology.*

  H. Patient Care Policy and Procedure #5070, *Electrolyte Infusions.*

  I. Patient Care Policy and Procedure #5117, *Insulin Intravenous Infusions.*

  J. Patient Care Policy and Procedure #5130, *Medication Administration.*

  K. Patient Care Policy and Procedure #5131, *Medfusion Syringe Infusion Pump.*

  L. Patient Care Policy and Procedure #5140, *Medication Use Analysis/Error Prevention.*

  M. Patient Care Policy and Procedure #5150, *Moderate/Deep Sedation/Analgesia.*

VII. ATTACHMENTS:

High-Alert Medications/Classes, one page.

Source: Used by permission from Orlando Health, Orlando, FL. www.orlandohealth.com.

High-Alert Medications/Classes	Safeguards, Etc.
Chemotherapy agents (all routes, includes antineoplastic, biological, immunological agents used for malignant oncology and hematology diagnoses)	Chemotherapy Policy and Procedure outlines requirements for independent double verification(IDV) of order, laboratory parameters, body surface area, medication, dose, route, frequency, etc.
	Chemotherapy order form (or electronic equivalent) required
	Only attending physicians with chemotherapy privileges may write orders
	No verbal or telephone orders allowed (except to clarify as outlined in policy)
	Only Chemo-verified RN's may administer (exceptions are made for some oral agents, refer to the Chemotherapy Policy and Procedure for details)
IV Electrolytes (i.e., potassium chloride and phosphate, concentrated sodium chloride, magnesium sulfate, calcium chloride, and calcium gluconate)	Independent double verification required (IDV not required for 1000 mL pre-mixed IV solutions)
	No concentrated products outside Pharmacy (*Rare exceptions exist, but only with specific safeguards*)
	Electrolyte policy provides specific administration parameters and limits
	Electrolyte replacement protocol includes dosing and monitoring parameters
	Standard concentrations/premixes
Intravenous/subcutaneous anticoagulants (i.e., heparin, lepirudin, enoxaparin, argatroban, bivalirudin—excluding flushes)	Independent double verification required
	Weight-based protocol for heparin. The prescriber must designate the specific protocol (e.g., Cardiac, Noncardiac) to be implemented
	Duplication warning in Clinical Information System
	Standardized order review requirements for enoxaparin and fondaparinux
	Standardized laboratory assessments for heparin, enoxaparin, and fondaparinux for treatment of deep vein thrombosis/pulmonary embolism
	Premixed heparin solutions in standard concentrations
Neuromuscular blocking agents	IDV required
	Availability limited to specific units and access limited on these units (e.g., emergency department, operating room, intensive care unit)
	Special labeling of packages
	Standard concentrations established
Insulin	IDV required (Note: verification of the insulin product is not required when insulin is supplied directly from pharmacy in patient-specific units of use (e.g., prefilled syringes versus vials)
	Floor stock limited to specific agents and Pharmacy removes unused patient-specific vials from patient care units daily
	Resources include the Insulin Infusion Policy and the IV push insulin parameters defined within policy
	Sliding scale order sets create a consistent process

continued

High-Alert Medications/Classes	Safeguards, Etc.
Anesthetic agents used outside the OR (e.g., propofol, ketamine, methohexital, etomidate, dexmedetomidine)	IDV required
	Guidelines for use and administration of propofol
	These agents have been added to the Moderate-Deep Sedation Policy with defined safeguards for use
Warfarin	IDV required
	Standard administration time to allow access to International Normalized Ratio (INR) results prior to daily dosing
	Laboratory monitoring standards and standardized order review processes
	Critical value—clinical laboratory calls with INR results >5
	Automated dispensing cabinet (ADC) inquiry—nurse is asked if he/she knows the patient's current INR as warfarin is being taken from ADC for administration to the patient
	Pharmacy monitoring of at-risk patients

18-2

Appendix 18–2

Policy Example: Medication Shortages and Backorders

I. PURPOSE:

The purpose of this policy is to outline an appropriate response to current or impending medication shortages in order to provide patients appropriate alternative therapy. In addition, the policy will ensure proper communications among the health system facilities to develop a unified action plan in addressing medication shortages.

II. DEFINITIONS:

When used in this policy these terms have the following meanings:
  A. Shortage: A drug product shortage is a supply issue that affects how the pharmacy prepares or dispenses a drug product or influences patient care when prescribers must use an alternative agent.
  B. Backorder: A short-term and/or long-term unavailability of drug products.

III. POLICY:

  A. It is the policy of the health system that medication shortages and/or backorders shall be handled in an efficient, consistent, and timely manner.
  B. Pharmacy Services shall gather information and work collaboratively to assess alternatives, develop communication plans, and ensure safety when handling medication shortages or backorders.

IV. PROCEDURE:

  A. The individual aware of the shortage or backorder will notify the Corporate Pharmacy Contracting Coordinator as soon as it has been identified.
  B. On identification of a medication shortage the Corporate Pharmacy Contracting Coordinator or designee will activate the communications with the pharmacy buyers to obtain an accurate inventory count and site-based utilization data.
  C. The pharmacy buyers will also proceed with the following steps:

1. Sending a completed Medication Shortage Form (Attachment A) to the site-based Pharmacy Management Team and the Corporate Pharmacy Contracting Coordinator. The entire form must be completed to the extent possible. Any information not readily available may be left blank.

2. Conduct an accurate and complete inventory inclusive of medication supply in satellite pharmacies, automated dispensing cabinets, storage, main pharmacy, code carts, medication kits, and other procedural areas.

3. During severe shortages (less than 2-week supply) the decentralized medication stock (ADM, satellite pharmacy, etc.) will be quarantined to the main pharmacy with the approval of the Pharmacy Manager or designee. The Pharmacy Manager or designee must communicate this decision with the pharmacy staff.

4. Maximize purchasing according to allocation at each site.

5. Transfer and balance the utilization of the remaining supply with facilities in greatest need and inform site-based Pharmacy Management Team.

D. For severe and acute shortages a group (Backorder Action Team) will convene under the direction of the Corporate Pharmacy Contracting Coordinator. The group will be responsible for developing a detailed backorder/shortage action plan for alternatives, communications, and a monitoring of the backorder for updates. The group may be inclusive of, but not limited to, the Drug Information Coordinator, Pharmacy Managers, Operations Coordinators, Clinical Coordinators, and when applicable Clinical Specialist, Pyxis® System Specialist, Pharmacy Information Systems Coordinator, Pharmacy Buyer, Pharmacy Educator, and Risk Management.

E. The Drug Information Coordinator will assist with developing a list of alternatives and a plan for substitution in the event the medication supply becomes depleted. This plan must be forwarded to the site-based Pharmacy Manager or designee. Therapeutic substitutions must receive the approval of the Pharmacy and Therapeutics Committee Chair or designee prior to implementation.

F. The organizational backorder/shortage action plan should include the following information: current supply and utilization, how long will current supplies last, anticipated duration of the shortage/backorder, plan to conserve current supply (assessment of medical necessity [patient prioritization]), development of therapeutic alternatives, and dosing when all supplies are depleted.

G. With a clear operational assessment of impact and a clinical impact on patient care, the group will develop a communication plan when appropriate (for pharmacists, nurses, physicians, respiratory therapists, or other health care professionals as needed). The Pharmacy Manager or designee will implement the communication plan for each site, respectively.

1. Plans to address a corporate shortage will include notification of at least the following groups and individuals:

a. Chief Nursing Officer, Clinical Unit Educators, and Nurse Managers

b. Chief of Staff, Chief Medical Officers, and Medical Department Chairpersons. Notices to the Clinical Information System and faxes can be facilitated via Medical Staff Support and Information Services.

   c. Managers of other departments impacted by the shortage/backorder (such as the clinical laboratory, respiratory therapy, radiology, infection control, and others).

   d. Information Services should be notified if clinical information systems are impacted (e.g., if an alternative medication must be added to the system, if an interchange must be implemented, etc.)

  2. Committees with oversight for the clinical area should also be notified as appropriate, such as the Corporate Code Blue Committee, Critical Care Committee, Surgical Issues, and others.

  3. Plans may be site specific as appropriate.

V. DOCUMENTATION:

None.

VI. REFERENCE:

ASHP Guidelines on Managing Drug Product Shortages. Am J Health-Syst Pharm. 2009;66:1399-1406.

VII. ATTACHMENTS:

  A. Medication Shortage/Backorder Form, one page
  B. Decision Flow Diagram

Source: Used by permission from Orlando Health, Orlando, FL. www.orlandohealth.com.

Medication Shortage/Backorder Form

Pharmacy: _____

Drug Name: Generic: _____

Brand: _____

Drug formulation(s) and/or strength(s) affected: _____

_____

Therapeutic interchanges affected: _____

Backorder or Discontinuation. If backorder, anticipated duration/resupply date: _____

Current Supply: _____

Current Usage: _____

How much additional supply can be obtained: _____

Cost concerns related to obtaining product from outside sources: _____

Reason for shortage/backorder (if known):

    ☐ Raw and bulk material unavailability
    ☐ Manufacturing difficulties
    ☐ Voluntary recalls
    ☐ Manufacturer production decisions (e.g., discontinuation of product)
    ☐ Orphan drug products
    ☐ Restricted drug distribution
    ☐ Industry consolidations
    ☐ Market shifts
    ☐ Unexpected increases in demand
    ☐ Nontraditional distributors (e.g., international)
    ☐ Natural disasters
    ☐ Other: _____

Other comments: _____

Threat to Patient Care and Cost Assessments:
Assessment by Pharmacy Contracting Coordinator:
    ☐ Alternative sources (other wholesalers, direct purchases, etc.):
Assessment by Drug Information Coordinator:
    ☐ Alternative therapies: _____
    ☐ Medical necessity: _____

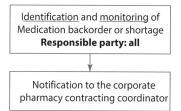

Identification and monitoring of
Medication backorder or shortage
Responsible party: all

↓

Notification to the corporate
pharmacy contracting coordinator

↓

Corporate Contracting Coordinator will inform ALL Pharmacy Buyers

↓

Pharmacy Buyers will proceed with following steps once notified:
- Conduct an accurate and complete inventory (ADM, main pharmacy, satellite, code carts etc.)
- Complete Medication Shortage Form (Attachment A) and send to Pharmacy Management Team and Corporate Contracting Coordinator
- Quarantine decentralized supply when applicable for severe shortages (with approval from Pharmacy Manager or designee)
- Maximize purchasing according to allocation
  Transfer supplies to sites in greatest needs (inform Pharmacy Manager)

↓

The health system is experiencing
severe or acute shortage

↓

Corporate Contracting Coordinator:
- Pursue alternative sources for securing additional supply

Corporate Pharmacy Contracting Coordinator or Site-based Pharmacy Manager:
- Convenes a call or a meeting with the Backorder Action Team to develop a backorder/shortage action plan
- Backorder Action Team to develop a communication plan for the health care team as appropriate
- Pharmacy Manager or designee must implement plan at their individual sites
- Plan must be revised and redistributed as the situation evolves

Drug Information Coordinator
- Develop a list of alternatives and a plan for therapeutic substitution when necessary
- Receive endorsement/approval from Pharmacotherapy Committee Chair or designee
- Pharmacy Manager or designee must implement plan at their individual sites

22-1

Appendix 22–1

Response Letter Drug A—Incidence of Yellow Stripes

DRUG A—Adverse Event—Yellow Stripes

Dear Dr. Smith,

Thank you for your inquiry. The following information is provided in response to your question regarding the use of DRUG A® and the incidence of yellow stripes appearing on the skin.

Please note that the information provided is not intended to advocate the use of our product in any manner other than as described in the enclosed full prescribing information.

INDICATION(S)

DRUG A® is indicated for the relief of moderate to severe hiccups in patients 18 years of age or older.[1]

PRESCRIBING INFORMATION

Please refer to the following sections of the enclosed Full Prescribing Information that are relevant to your inquiry: ADVERSE REACTIONS, WARNINGS, PRECAUTIONS.[1]

LITERATURE SEARCH RESULTS

A literature search of MEDLINE databases (and other resources) pertaining to the incidence of yellow stripes appearing on the skin associated with the use of DRUG A® was conducted through May 2010.

CLINICAL STUDIES

In phase III efficacy and safety studies of DRUG A® for the relief of moderate to severe hiccups, yellow stripes appearing on patients skin was reported in 7% of patients (see Table: Incidence of Yellow Stripes Appearing on Skin).[2]

TABLE 1 INCIDENCE OF YELLOW STRIPES APPEARING ON SKIN[2]

Adverse Event	DRUG A®	Placebo
Yellow stripes on skin	7%	7%

In a 12-month long-term safety study, the incidence of yellow stripes appearing on the skin was evaluated. DRUG A® users reported yellow stripes on their skin with an incidence rate of 9% (see Table: Incidence of Yellow Stripes Appearing on Skin—Long-Term Study).[3]

TABLE 2 INCIDENCE OF YELLOW STRIPES APPEARING ON SKIN—LONG-TERM STUDY[3]

Adverse Event	DRUG A®	Placebo
Yellow stripes on skin	9%	8%

Multiple case reports were identified reporting yellow stripes appearing on patient's skin.

In a report by Jones and associates,[4] a 90-year-old woman suffering from severe hiccups reporting yellow stripes appearing on the skin within 4 days of starting treatment. She was treated with DRUG FIX-IT® and her yellow stripes resolved immediately.

In a report by Jones and associates,[5] a 20-year-old man suffering from moderate hiccups reported yellow stripes on his skin within 2 minutes of starting treatment. The patient did not seek treatment, continued taking DRUG A®, and the yellow stripes resolved.

ADVERSE EVENT REPORTING

Please see the enclosed Prescribing Information for the complete safety and drug interaction information on our product. In order to monitor the safety of our products, we encourage clinicians to report adverse events by calling 1-800-555-9999 from 9 am to 9 pm Mountain Time, Monday through Sunday. Adverse events may also be reported to the FDA MedWatch program by phone (1-800-FDA-1088), fax (1-800-FDA-0178), or e-mail (www.fda.gov/medwatch). To view a description of ongoing clinical trials for our products, please visit www.clinicaltrials.gov.

REFERENCES

1. DRUG A® [package insert]. Awesome Drugs R Us, Inc. Any Town, USA; 2010.
2. Jones Z, et al. Efficacy and safety of DRUG A® in the treatment of hiccups. JAHA. 2009;6542:735-746.
3. Jones Y, et al. Long-term safety of the use of DRUG A® in severe hiccups. JAHA. 2009; 6543:887-896.
4. Jones A, et al. 90-year old woman with yellow stripes. Hiccup Central. 2009;78(4):232-235.
5. Jones B, et al. 20-year old male with resolved yellow stripes. Hiccup Central. 2010;83(3):196-199.

Glossary

A priori   In clinical trial design, this distinguishes something that is done before the study is started. Determining specific study criteria prior to study initiation.

Absolute risk reduction   The difference in the percentage of subjects developing the adverse event in the control group versus subjects in the intervention group. Also refers to the number of subjects spared the adverse event by taking the intervention compared to the control.

Abstracting service   A database that provides abstracts and citations for journal articles.

Abstracts   A synopsis (usually of 250 words or less) of the most important aspect(s) of an article.

Academia   Pertaining to a college, school, or other educational institution.

Academic detailing   A process by which a health care educator visits a physician to provide a 15- to 20-minute educational intervention on a specific topic. Information provided is based on the physician's prescribing patterns and evidence-based medicine to improve prescribing.

Accountable care organization   A collaborative group of hospitals, doctors, and other providers of health care who coordinate their patient care efforts for Medicare patients. An emphasis is placed on minimizing duplication of effort and preventing medical errors, in particular, for the chronically ill.

Action-guides   A term coined by Beauchamp and Childress to refer to a hierarchical approach to analysis of an ethical issue when forming particular judgments about the issue.

Active control   A standard therapy or procedure (but not a placebo) used in a study to determine the difference in effect produced by the study intervention.

Adaptive clinical trial   A trial design, also known as group sequential design, that allows adaptation of various components such as inclusion/exclusion criteria, dosing, efficacy outcomes, and duration of trial based on continuously emerging knowledge throughout the study.

Adjunctive therapy   A therapy (e.g., medication, exercise, diet) that all subjects within a study receive. Since all subjects are receiving, it is not considered a study bias since the effect of this therapy occurs among all subjects within the study.

Adverse drug event (ADE)   An ADE is defined as an injury from a medicine or lack of intended medicine. An ADE refers to all adverse drug reactions (ADRs), including allergic or idiosyncratic reactions, as well as medication errors that result in harm to a patient.

Adverse drug event (ADE) monitoring   Computer programs that use electronic data and predetermined rules to identify when an ADE may have occurred or is about to occur.

Adverse drug event (ADE) trigger tool   It is an augmented chart review method that uses automated systems to identify alerts or triggers to efficiently identify patients with potential ADEs. The triggers are cues that a patient may have experienced an error and/or adverse event. When these triggers are identified, it is suspected that the patient may have experienced a medication error. The patient's chart is reviewed for evidence of error and/or level of harm and data are collected and collated to determine potential common causes.

Adverse drug reaction (ADR)   Defined broadly, any unexpected, unintended, undesired, or excessive response to a medicine. The Food and Drug Administration's (FDA) definition of ADRs is: "any adverse event associated with the use of a drug in humans, whether or not considered drug related, including the following: adverse event occurring in the course of the use of a drug product in professional practice; an adverse event occurring from drug overdose, whether accidental or intentional; an adverse event occurring from drug abuse; an adverse event occurring from drug withdrawal; and any significant failure of expected pharmacologic action." Adverse drug reactions also include drug interactions. Defined by the World Health Organization (WHO) as "any response that is noxious, unintended, or undesired, which occurs at doses normally used in humans for prophylaxis, diagnosis, therapy of disease or modification of physiological function." Several other definitions are available; many of those are discussed in Chapter 15.

Agenda for Change   An initiative adopted by the JCAHO in 1986 intended to improve standards by focusing on key functions of quality of care, to monitor the performance of health care organizations using indicators, improve the relevance and quality of the survey process, and enhance the accuracy and value of JCAHO accreditation.

Aggregate indicators   Provide a summary of the frequency, or timeliness, of a process by aggregating numerous cases.

Aggregator   A piece of software that is used to automatically collect information from RSS and Weblog sites, which allows the user to look at material from many of those sites at one time and in one place.

Alert fatigue   A situation in which clinical decision support system (CDSS) alerts and warnings appear too frequently resulting in a provider ignoring or overriding these messages.

Alert fatigue   A situation in which clinical decision support system (CDSS) alerts and warnings appear too frequently resulting in a provider ignoring or overriding these messages.

Alpha (level of significance)   The probability of a false positive result in a study. Criterion for rejecting the null hypothesis. It is the upper bound of the Type I error rate. The value (usually 0.05) that is set prior to the beginning of a study and in which the p-value is compared at the end of the study to determine if statistical difference is present in the outcome being measured. A p-value less than alpha (e.g., 0.001 < 0.05) is interpreted as a statistical difference was determined between the intervention and control groups of a study. Also is the amount of error the researchers are willing to accept that a false-positive result is identified between the study intervention and control groups (e.g., alpha of 0.05 is up to a 5% chance of a false-positive result).

Alternative hypothesis   Sometimes referred to as the research hypothesis. The hypothesis that states there is some difference or relationship between the therapy under investigation and the control.

Alternative medicine   An approach to health care outside conventional medicine. Alternative medicine refers to using a nonmainstream approach in place of conventional medicine.

American Hospital Formulary System (AHFS) classification   A classification that can be found in the *AHFS Drug Information* reference book, published by the American Society of Health-Systems Pharmacists. It groups agents by use and/or drug class into specific numbered categories (e.g., 24:32.04 Angiotensin-Converting Enzyme Inhibitors).

Analysis   Analysis is the critical assessment of the nature, merit, and significance of individual elements, ideas, or factors. Functionally, it involves separating the information into its isolated parts so that each can be critically assessed. Analysis requires thoughtful review and evaluation of the quality and overall weight of available evidence.

Analytic research   Quantitative research conducted in a controlled environment to determine cause-and-effect relationships.

Ancillary therapy   A therapy (e.g., medication, exercise, diet) that is disproportional in use among the subjects in the groups within a study and has an effect on the outcome being measured; this can lead to a difference in effect between the groups, which can bias the study results.

Antibiotic use review (AUR)   Retrospective evaluation of antibiotic use. Usually quantitative and limited to identifying patterns of use.

Application service provider (ASP)   See Software as a Service (SaaS).

Appraisal of Guidelines for Research and Evaluation (AGREE) II instrument   A structured instrument to assess the quality of guidelines, provide a methodological strategy for the development of guidelines, and inform what information and how information ought to be reported in guidelines.

Article proposal   A letter asking the publisher whether they would be interested in possibly publishing something on a particular topic written by the person(s) who are inquiring.

Aspect of care   A term used in quality assurance programs to indicate the title that describes the area being evaluated.

Assay sensitivity   The process of ensuring that a drug truly has a notable effect by utilizing high-quality clinical trials of the drug against placebo.

Assumption of the risk   A defense in the law of torts, which bars a plaintiff from recovery against a negligent party if the defendant can demonstrate that the plaintiff voluntarily and knowingly assumed the risks at issue inherent to the dangerous activity in which he or she was participating at the time of his or her injury.

Attributable risk   The difference in the rate of a condition when comparing an exposed population to an unexposed population. This is primarily used in cohort studies and is considered an epidemiological term.

Automated dispensing cabinets (ADCs)   Automated devices with a range of functions. Core capabilities include medication storage and retrieval for administration to patients, especially in patient care areas, as well as audit trails of cabinet access. Other functions can include medication charging and automated inventory management.

Autonomy   Autonomy is the personal rule that is free from both controlling interferences by others and from personal limitations that prevent meaningful choice. Autonomous individuals act intentionally, with understanding, and without controlling influences.

Avatar   A movable three-dimensional image used to represent some body in cyberspace.

Bar code verification   The use of bar code scanning to ensure that the correct drug, strength, and dosage form were dispensed in the drug selection process and the five basic patient rights (i.e., right patient, right drug, right dose, right route, right time) are followed at the point of care.

Beneficence   A basic principle of consequentialist theory that expresses the duty to promote good.

Berkson's bias A type of selection bias noted in case-control studies and is produced when the probability of hospitalization of cases and controls differs. This probability can be increased based on the specific exposure being studied and increases the chance of hospital admission.

Beta The probability of a false-negative result in a study.

Bias An intentional or unintentional systematic error in the way a study is designed, conducted, analyzed, or reported.

Bibliography A list of references, usually seen at the end of a piece of professional writing.

Biocreep (also known as placebo creep) The phenomenon that results in the reference drug becoming no better than placebo in NI trials. This occurs when a somewhat inferior test drug is chosen as the reference drug for a future generation of NI trials. After multiple generations of this occurring, the final result is a future reference drug that is no better than placebo.

Bioequivalence studies Research that evaluates whether products are similar in rate and extent of absorption.

Biologics license applications (BLA) A biologics license application is a submission that contains specific information on the manufacturing processes, chemistry, pharmacology, clinical pharmacology, and the medical effects of the biologic product. It is a request for permission to introduce, or deliver for introduction, a biologic product into interstate commerce.

Black letter rules Principles of law that are known generally to all and are free from doubt and ambiguity. Also known as hornbook law, since they are in a format that would probably be enunciated in a hornbook.

Blinding A study technique used in research to reduce bias by having the study subjects and/or investigators not know which group the study subjects are assigned.

Blog See Weblog.

Body area network (BAN) A multidevice, interconnected computer system carried on a person. Sometimes referred to as a wearable computer.

Boolean operators (logical operators) Words used to combine search terms (i.e., AND, OR, NOT) when using computerized databases.

Case law The aggregate of reported cases; the law pertaining to a particular subject as formed by adjudged cases.

Case report A descriptive record of a single individual (case report) in which the possibility of an association between an observed effect and a specific intervention or exposure is described (often an unexpected complication of treatment or procedure) based on detailed clinical evaluation and history of the individual.

Case series A grouping of records (case studies) that documents a practitioner's experiences, thoughts, or observations related to the care of multiple patients with similar medical situations.

Case study A record of descriptive research that documents a practitioner's experiences, thoughts, or observations related to the care of a single patient. Not useful to test a hypothesis but can serve to generate pilot information to design future controlled trials.

Case-control study A retrospective trial design (often using medical charts or cases) strictly based on the observation of a group of people that have experienced a similar outcome. The study is used to determine the possible exposure these patients have had, which would lead to this known outcome.

Categorical variable A variable measured on a nominal or ordinal scale.

CD-ROM   See Compact disc-read only memory.

Civil liability   Negligent acts and/or omissions, other than breach of contract, normally independent of moral obligations for which a remedy can be provided in a court of law. This form of liability is imposed under civil laws and processes, not criminal law. For example, a person injured in someone's home can bring suit under civil liability law.

Clinical decision support systems (CDSS)   Computer programs that augment clinical decision making by combining referential information with patient-specific information to prevent negative actions and update providers of patient status.

Clinical investigation   Any experiment in which a drug is administered or dispensed to one or more human subjects. An experiment is any use of a drug (except for the use of a marketed drug) in the course of medical practice. Although there are many other definitions, this is the FDA's definition and would seem the appropriate one to use given the nature of this topic. Please note that the FDA does not regulate the practice of medicine and prescribers are (as far as the agency is concerned) free to use any marketed drug for off-label use.

Clinical practice guidelines   Recommendations for optimizing patient care that are developed by systematically reviewing the evidence and assessing the benefits and harms of health care interventions.

Clinical response letters   Written correspondence that contains company-approved content in response to an unsolicited request for medical information.

Clinical Safety Officer (CSO)   Also known as the regulatory management officer (RMO). This will be the sponsor's Food and Drug Administration contact person. Generally, the CSO/RMO assigned to a drug's investigational new drug application will also be assigned to the new drug application.

Clinical significance   The clinical importance of data generated in a study, irrespective of statistical results. Usually refers to the application of study results into clinical practice. Also, can be called clinical meaningfulness.

Clinically significant   A result large enough to cause an effect on an efficacy outcome measure that noticeably changes a patient's condition.

Closed formulary   A drug formulary that restricts the drugs available within an institution or available under a third-party plan.

Coauthor   Any individual who writes a portion of an article, chapter, book, etc. This includes individuals other than the primary author, whose name is normally listed first on a publication.

Cohort study   A prospective trial design strictly based on the observation of a group of people who experience a known exposure over time. The study is used to determine outcomes to this exposure.

Commercial IND   An IND for which the sponsor is usually either a corporate entity or one of the institutes of the National Institutes of Health (NIH). In addition, CDER may designate other INDs as commercial, if it is clear the sponsor intends the product to be commercialized at a later date.

Community rule   See Locality rule.

Compact disc-read only memory (CD-ROM)   A storage and retrieval system for large quantities of computerized data. Modern computers usually cannot only read the data on these disks, but usually can write new data to disks designed to accept that new data.

Comparative negligence   The allocation of responsibility for damages incurred between the plaintiff and the defendant, based on the relative negligence of the two.

Complementary and alternative medicine An approach to health care outside conventional medicine. Complementary medicine refers to using a non-mainstream approach *together with* conventional medicine. Alternative medicine refers to using a non-mainstream approach *in place of* conventional medicine.

Compliance A measure of how well instructions are followed. In a study, compliance refers to how well a patient follows instructions for medication administration and how well the investigator follows the study protocol.

Computer network An interconnection of computers and computer-related devices (e.g., printers, modems) that allows the devices to interchange data, electronic mail, programs, and other files. In addition, a network allows sharing of peripheral devices, such as printers, modems, fax boards, etc. Normally, this interconnection is via a dedicated wiring system (other than telephone/ modem communication); however, wireless connections are becoming common.

Computer-based clinical decision support systems software that is designed to assist clinical decision making which utilizes both patient-specific information and clinical knowledge to make assessments or recommendations in clinical practice.

Computerized provider order entry (CPOE) A process allowing medical provider instructions to be electronically entered for the treatment of patients who are under a provider's care.

Concurrent indicator An indicator used in any quality assurance program that determines whether quality is acceptable while an action is being taken or care is being given.

Concurrent negligence The wrongful acts or omissions of two or more persons acting independently, but causing the same injury.

Confidence interval Range calculated for a study result in which the true value for the population exists; the percentage association with the range (e.g., 95%) indicates the confidence in which the true population value is within the range. For instance, the investigators are 95% confident that the mean blood pressure lowering effect of the medication for the population is between –8 to –12 mmHg for the 95% confidence interval of (–8 to –12 mmHg).

Confidentiality A moral rule, related to the principle of autonomy, which specifically addresses the individual client's right to give or refuse consent relative to release of privileged information.

Conflict of interest A situation in which the interests of an investigator conflicts with the study purpose, design, and/or result interpretation. An investigator may be a stock holder of and/or speaker for a pharmaceutical company; the study may be designed to produce favorable results and/or be interpreted or promoted with a bias to use the study intervention.

Confounder A known or unknown variable that has the potential to mask actual associations or falsely demonstrate a nonexisting but apparent association between the defined related variable (exposure) and outcome(s) being studied. The real issue occurs when the confounder is unevenly distributed between the exposure and nonexposure study groups, leading to confusion interpreting the results. Unevenly distributed confounders are common in cohort studies since this imbalance is the product of not using a randomization schedule that evenly distributes the confounder between the groups.

Consent A moral rule related to the principle of autonomy which states that the client has a right to be informed and to freely choose a course of action.

Consequential damages Also called special damages; damages claimed and/or awarded in a lawsuit which were caused as a direct foreseeable result of wrongdoing. Consequential damages occur with injury or harm that does not ensue directly and immediately from the act of a party, but only from some of the results of such act, and that is compensable by a monetary award after a judgment has been rendered in a lawsuit.

Consequentialist theories   An ethical theory which holds that the rightness or wrongness of decisions or actions is determined by the total of good that is achieved or harm that is prevented.

Constancy assumption   A determination made that past studies being used to determine the non-inferiority (NI) margin in an NI trial are similar in design and conduct compared to the NI trial regarding features that could alter the effect size of the reference drug compared to placebo.

Consumer health information (CHI)   Information actively sought by the patient in response to their need for more information about their health. Information is not individualized for a specific patient but rather general health information.

Content filter   A term used to limit a search to specific things, such as specific drugs or disease states.

Continuous indicators   Provide a simple count, or time estimate, related to a process (e.g., average turnaround time on medication orders).

Continuous quality improvement (CQI)   The term given to the methodologies used in the process of Total Quality Management. Efforts to improve quality are part of each participant's responsibilities on an ongoing basis.

Continuous variable   A variable measured on an interval or ratio scale.

Contract research organization (CRO)   An individual or organization that assumes one or more of the obligations of the sponsor through an independent contractual agreement.

Control group   The group of test animals or humans that receive a placebo (a dosage that does not contain active medicine) or active (a dosage that does contain active medicine) treatment. For most preclinical and clinical trials, the FDA will require that this group receive placebo (commonly referred to as the placebo control). However, some studies may have an active control, which generally consists of an available (standard of care) treatment modality. An active control may, with the concurrence of the FDA, be used in studies where it would be considered unethical to use a placebo. A historical control is one in which a group of previous patients is compared to a matched set of patients receiving the new therapy. A historical control might be used in cases where the disease is consistently fatal (i.e., acquired immunodeficiency syndrome [AIDS]). (Refer to Chapter 4 for additional information on control groups).

Controlled clinical trial   Research design that prospectively and directly compares plus measures and quantifies differences in outcomes between an intervention and control. This is the best study design to determine a cause-and-effect relationship between an item under investigation and an outcome.

Controls   A treatment (placebo, active, historical) used for comparison in a study to measure a difference in effect against an investigational agent. The investigator usually wishes to determine superiority of a new treatment over the control in terms of efficacy and safety.

Copayment   Payment made by an individual who has health insurance at the time the service is received to offset the cost of care. Copayments may vary depending on the service rendered.

Cost-benefit analysis (CBA)   A study where monetary value is given for both costs and benefits associated with a drug or service. The results are expressed as a ratio (benefit-to-cost), and the ratio is used to determine the economic value of the drug or service.

Cost-benefit study   A study where monetary value is given for both costs and benefits associated with a drug or service. The results are expressed as a ratio (benefit to cost), and the ratio is used to determine the economic value of the drug or service.

Cost-consequence analysis (CCA)   An informal variant of a cost-effectiveness analysis (CEA). The costs and various outcomes are listed but no evaluations are conducted.

Cost-effectiveness analysis (CEA)   A study where the cost of a drug or service is compared to its therapeutic impact. Cost-effectiveness studies determine the relative efficiency of various drugs or services in achieving desired therapeutic outcomes.

Cost-effectiveness ratio (CER)   The CER is the ratio of resources used per unit of clinical benefit, and implies that this calculation has been made in relation to doing nothing or no treatment.

Cost-effectiveness study   A study where the cost of a drug or service is compared to its therapeutic impact. Cost-effectiveness studies determine the relative efficiency of various drugs or services in achieving desired therapeutic outcomes.

Cost-minimization study   A study that compares costs of drugs or services that have been determined to have equivalent therapeutic outcomes.

Cost-utility analysis (CUA)   A study that relates therapeutic outcomes to both costs of drugs or services and patient preferences, and measures cost per unit of utility. Utility is the amount of satisfaction obtained from a drug or service.

Cost-utility study   A study that relates therapeutic outcomes to both costs of drugs or services and patient preferences and measures cost per unit of utility. Utility is the amount of satisfaction obtained from a drug or service.

Covenant   An ethical covenant in medical ethics suggests an implicit contract between the client and the health care provider that broadly describes the relationship involved whenever a health care service is provided, including the provision of information. Within this contract the service recipient has a right to competently provided service, as well as respectful treatment. The service recipient also has an obligation to provide needed information to the provider in a respectful manner.

Coverage error   It is a bias in a statistic that occurs when the target population you want to survey does not coincide with the sample population that is actually surveyed. This can be an issue when observing a sample of the population instead of the entire population.

Coverage rules   Criteria for specific drugs determined by the health plan in conjunction with the pharmacy and therapeutics committee that is used to determine if a prescription is covered. Criteria are based on evidence-based medicine.

CQI   See Continuous quality improvement.

Criteria   Definitions of safe and effective use of medications used to assess components of the medication use process that are endorsed by the organization within which they are to be applied. Criteria summarize an organization's definition of appropriate or acceptable use of the medication.

Crossover study   A study where each subject receives all study treatments, and endpoints during the various treatments are compared.

Cross-sectional   Data that is measured one time.

Cross-sectional study   A trial design involving data collection only once on members of the study population that represents a snapshot in time. These members are not required to be studied all at once, but each member can be studied at a different time. The key is that the data collected represents a specific period in time.

Cybermedicine   A concept broader than telemedicine that includes the marketing, relationship creation, advice, prescribing, and selling pharmaceuticals and devices in cyberspace.

Dechallenge   In relation to adverse drug reactions, this occurs when the drug is taken away and the patient is monitored to determine whether the adverse drug reaction (ADR) abates or decreases in intensity.

Decision analysis   A tool that can help visualize a pharmacoeconomic analysis. It is the application of an analytical method for systematically comparing different decision options. Decision analysis graphically displays choices and performs the calculations needed to compare these options.

Deep pocket   Practical consideration that involves the naming of additional codefendants in personal injury lawsuits to provide assurance to the plaintiff that there will be sufficient assets to pay the judgment.

Degrees of freedom   The number of data points that are free to vary.

Delta   The amount of difference that the investigators wish to detect between intervention and control groups in a study.

Deontological theory   An ethical theory that seeks to establish what is a right or wrong decision or action on the basis of prioritizing specific recognized ethical rules or principles.

Descriptive research   Quantitative research that describes naturally occurring events.

Descriptive statistics   Statistics that describe data such as medians, modes, and standard deviations.

Diagnostic review bias   It occurs when the reference test results are not definitive and the study test results affect or influence how the final diagnosis is established.

DIC   See Drug information center.

Dichotomous variable   A variable that has two mutually exclusive categories.

Digital video disk (DVD)   Also known as digital versatile disk. A disk that physically resembles a CD-ROM, but allows the storage of much larger amounts of data. It requires a special reading/writing device in a computer, although this device may also be combined with that used for CD-ROMs. DVDs have been used to a large extent to store and replay movies; however, it is being used on computers to store large amounts of computer data, particularly large multimedia files.

Direct medical costs   One of four categories of costs in pharmacoeconomic studies. These are the medically related inputs used directly in providing the treatment.

Direct nonmedical costs   One of four categories of costs in pharmacoeconomic studies. These are costs directly associated with treatment, but are not medical in nature. Examples include travel, food, and lodging to get to a place of treatment.

DIS   See Drug information service.

Discount rate   A term from finance which approximates the cost of capital by taking into account both the projected inflation rate and the interest rates of borrowed money, and then estimates the time value of money.

Drug class review   A drug evaluation monograph comparing all products in a particular class of drugs. It is used to determine what products will be available for use.

Drug evaluation monograph   A structured document covering all aspects of a particular drug product or class of drugs. It compares similar agents and is used to determine which products will be available for use.

Drug formularies   See Formulary.

Drug formulary system   See Formulary system.

Drug informatics   The electronic management of drug information.

Drug information   Facts or advice on drugs (including chemicals that has medicinal, performance-enhancing or intoxicating effects) regarding a specific patient or a group of patients.

Drug information center (DIC)   A physical location where pharmacists have the resources (e.g., books, journals, computer systems, etc.) to provide drug information. This area is generally staffed by a pharmacist specializing in drug information, but may be used by a variety of the pharmacy staff or other individuals.

Drug information service   A professional service providing drug information. This service is normally located in a drug information center.

Drug interaction   The Food and Drug Administration defines this as "a pharmacologic response that cannot be explained by the action of a simple drug, but is due to two or more drugs acting simultaneously."

Drug master file (DMF)   A submission to the FDA that may be used to provide confidential detailed information about facilities, processes, or articles used in the manufacturing, processing, packaging, and storing of one or more human drugs.

Drug product   The final dosage form prepared from the drug substance.

Drug promotion   Information provided by the pharmaceutical industry through advertising, detailing, and other printed material intended to increase sales of a medication.

Drug regimen review (DRR)   The monthly evaluation of nursing home charts by pharmacists.

Drug substance   Bulk compound from which the drug product is prepared. An active ingredient that is intended to furnish pharmacological activity or other direct effect in the diagnosis, cure, mitigation, treatment, or prevention of disease or to affect the structure or any function of the human body.

Drug use evaluation (DUE)   Concurrent evaluation of prescribing and outcome only. Multidisciplinary involvement.

Drug use review (DUR)   A program related to outpatient pharmacy services designed to educate physicians and pharmacists in identifying and reducing the frequency and patterns of fraud, abuse, gross overuse, or inappropriate or medically unnecessary care. DUR is typically retrospective in nature and utilizes claims data as its primary source of information.

Due care   See Reasonable care.

Duty   A moral or legal obligation.

Editorial   A commentary usually written by an expert that describes study strengths and limitations plus the application of the study results to practice. This is published in the same journal issue as the study, but not all studies have an accompanying editorial.

Electronic mail (e-mail)   Brief messages sent from one computer to another, similar in use to interoffice memos. This serves as a quick, informal method of written communication. Also, e-mail may be used to send other items, such as word processing files, graphics, video, etc., to others.

Electronic medication administration record (eMAR)   An electronic version of the traditional medication administration record. It supports patient safety by incorporating clinical decision support and bar-coded medication administration. It also enables real-time documentation and billing of medication administration.

Electronic prescribing (e-prescribing)   Prescription entered by a prescriber directly into an electronic format using agreed-upon standards, which is securely transmitted to the pharmacy that the patient chooses. Faxes and printed prescriptions are not e-prescriptions.

E-mail   See Electronic mail.

Endpoint   A parameter measured in a clinical study. The primary endpoint is the major variable analyzed and reflects the main objective of the study. Secondary endpoints are additional variables of interest monitored during clinical studies.

Endpoint, Primary   See Primary endpoint.

Endpoint, Secondary   See Secondary endpoint.

Error, Type I   See Type I error.

Error, Type II   See Type II error.

Ethical theories   Integrated bodies of principles and rules that may include mediating rules that govern cases of conflicts.

Ethics   The philosophical inquiry of the moral dimensions of human conduct. An ethical issue involves judgments between right and wrong human conduct or praiseworthy and blameworthy human characters.

Ethics (defined by AACP)   Philosophical inquiry into the moral dimensions of human conduct.

Ethics (defined by Beauchamp and Childress)   A generic term for several ways of examining the moral life.

Evidence-based medicine (EBM)   A philosophy of practice and an approach to decision making in the clinical care of patients that involves making individual patient care decisions based on the best currently available evidence.

Exclusion criteria   Characteristics of subjects defined prior to starting the study that are used as parameters to disqualify subjects from enrolling in the study (e.g., patients with cancer, lactating females, patients receiving corticosteroid therapy).

Exculpatory clause   An exculpatory clause is part of an agreement which relieves one party from liability. It is a provision in a contract which stipulates (1) one party is relieved of any blame or liability arising from the other party's wrongdoing, or (2) one party (usually the one that drafted the agreement) is freed of all liability arising out of performance of that contract. An exculpatory clause will not be enforced when the party protected by the clause intentionally causes harm or engages in acts of reckless, wanton, or gross negligence or when found to be unreasonable under the particular circumstances (e.g., a restaurant checks a person's coat but the ticket states they are not responsible for loss or damage).

Exploratory research   Research of a qualitative nature in which the investigators examines an unknown area to generate hypotheses.

Extemporaneous compounding   The practice of compounding prescriptions from a list of several ingredients—usually performed by a pharmacist.

External validity   Quality of the study design that allows the result to be applied to practice. Study results are meaningful to practitioners and can be used for patient care.

Failure mode and effects analysis (FMEA)   FMEA is a structured proactive method of evaluating a process to identify the gaps—how the process might fail. The process includes identification of the likelihood of each of the failures along with its relative impact to the patient. This provides a prioritization of action plans to drive improvement and reduce the likelihood of failure.

Fair balance   A quality of drug promotions where similar attention is given to safety risks (e.g., contraindications, precautions/warnings, adverse effects) and efficacy benefits.

False negatives   Individuals with the disease who were incorrectly identified as being disease free by the test.

False positives   Individuals without the disease who were incorrectly identified as having the disease by the test.

Fellowship   A directed, highly individualized postgraduate training program designed to prepare the participant to function as an independent investigator. The purpose of fellowship training programs is to develop competency and expertise in the scientific research process, including hypothesis generation and development, study design, protocol development, grantsmanship, study coordination, data collection, analysis and interpretation, technical skills development, presentation of results, and manuscript preparation and publication. A fellowship candidate is expected to possess appropriate practice skills relevant to the knowledge area of the fellowship. Such skills may be obtained through prior practice experience or completion of a residency program.

Fidelity   A principle of moral duty in deontological theory that addresses the responsibility to be trustworthy and keep promises.

File transfer protocol (FTP)   A method to transfer files from one computer to another.

Follow-up study   A study where subjects exposed to a factor and those not exposed to the factor are followed forward in time and compared to determine the factor's influence on disease state development. Also called a cohort study.

Food and Drug Administration (FDA)   The agency of the U.S. government that is responsible for ensuring the safety and efficacy of all drugs on the market.

Forest plot   A preferred method to display the results from a meta-analysis and includes the 95% confidence intervals for the primary efficacy outcome for each study included in the meta-analysis with the overall resulting 95% confidence interval for the meta-analysis.

Formulary   A continually revised list of medications that are readily available for use within an institution or from a third-party payer (e.g., insurance company, government) that reflects the current clinical judgment of the medical staff or the payer. Restrictions on this list may be placed that indicate certain drugs will not be reimbursed by insurance, or will only be reimbursed if several other alternative are tried first.

Formulary decision supports (FDS)   Program (often software) used to enhance compliance with formulary by guiding the prescriber to preferred formulary drugs over those considered nonformulary.

Formulary system   A method used to develop a drug formulary. It is sometimes even thought of as a philosophy.

Funnel plot   A scatter plot of treatment effect versus sample size of studies included in a meta-analysis. They are used to assist in detecting potential publication bias which is a form of selection bias based on the magnitude, direction, or statistical significance of the study results.

Galley proofs   A copy of a written work as it is to be published. The purpose of this document is to allow the author(s) to make a final check to ensure everything is correct before actual publication.

Gantt chart   Project management tool used to plan and monitor elements of a project.

Gender bias   Showing favoritism or discrimination toward a selected gender.

Good clinical practice (GCP)   A standard for the design, conduct, monitoring, analyses, and reporting of clinical trials that provides assurance that the results are credible and accurate, and that the rights of study subjects are protected.

Grading of Recommendation, Assessment, Development, and Evaluation (GRADE) system A standardized system for grading the quality of the evidence and the strength of recommendations in clinical practice guidelines.

Gray literature Documents provided in limited numbers outside the formal channels of publication and distribution. The concern with these documents in that they may include inaccurate information (not completely correct information), misinformation (incorrect information), and disinformation (false information deliberately provided in order to influence opinions) that can confound study results.

Health 2.0 The utilization of health care related tools provided by Web 2.0.

Health applications (apps) Software for devices designed to manage various aspects of health for the specific user.

Health Insurance Portability and Accountability Act of 1996 Commonly referred to as HIPAA, this act includes privacy restrictions for electronic health records.

Health literacy It is the capability of patients to read or hear health information, understand it, and then act on health information.

Health maintenance organization (HMO) Form of health insurance whereby the member prepays a premium for the HMO's health services, which generally include inpatient and outpatient care.

Health Plan Employer Data and Information Set (HEDIS) A set of performance measures used to compare managed health care plans.

Health product information Identified by Project Destiny as a service area where as pharmacists augment patient's health care by providing information to patients based on information from prescription history, patient profiles, and purchases.

Health-related quality of life (HR-QOL) Term used to represent the value assigned to quality and quantity of life that can be modified by various factors such as impairments and perceptions that are caused by disease, injury, treatment, or medical policy.

Heterogeneity Noted in meta-analyses, this describes a situation where there are differences in the way the studies being included in the meta-analysis were conducted. Ideally, all studies included should be identical in design and the way they are conducted (same doses used, same inclusion/exclusion criteria, same outcome measurements, same duration, etc.). There can be different degrees of heterogeneity; however, if there are significant variations in true effects underlying the studies, then the meta-analysis results are in question.

HIPAA See Health Insurance Portability and Accountability Act of 1996.

Hippocratic Oath A central ethical tradition of Western medicine that is committed to producing good for one's patient and protecting that patient from harm. There is a special emphasis placed on the responsibility of the medical professional to the specific patient.

Historical data Data used in research that were collected prior to the decision to conduct the study (e.g., medical records, insurance information, Medicaid databases).

Historical evidence of sensitivity to drug effects (HESDE) In noninferiority trials this concept applies to appropriately designed and conducted past trials using the reference drug and regularly exhibiting the reference drug to be superior to placebo.

HMO See Health maintenance organization.

Homogeneity   As used with meta-analyses, homogeneity measures the differences or similarities between the several studies included in the meta-analysis. Ideally, all studies included should be identical in design and the way they are conducted (same doses used, same inclusion/exclusion criteria, same outcome measurements, same duration, etc.).

Homogenicity tests   Tests used when conducting a meta-analysis to determine the similarity of studies whose results were combined for the analysis.

Homoscedasticity   In correlation and regression, the variability around the best fit line of the linear relationship is constant across all data points.

http—hypertext transfer protocol   A method by which information is encoded and transmitted on the World Wide Web.

https   A secure form of http, used to transmit confidential information, such as credit card numbers.

Hyperlink   Also called a link; it is a word, group of words, or image that can be clicked on to jump (link) to another place within the same document or to an entirely different document. When you move the cursor over a link in a Web site, the arrow will turn into a little hand. Hyperlinks are the most essential ingredient of all hypertext systems, including the Internet.

Hypothesis   The researchers' assumptions regarding probable study results. The research hypothesis or alternative hypothesis (H_A) is the expectations of the researchers in terms of study results. The null hypothesis (H_0) is the no difference hypothesis, which assumes equality amongst study treatments. The null hypothesis is the basis for all statistical tests and must be rejected in order to accept the research hypothesis.

In vitro   Experiments conducted using components of an organism that have been isolated from their usual biological surroundings. These types of experiments are also referred to as "test tube experiments."

In vivo   Experiments conducted in living organisms in their intact state.

Incidence rate   Measures the probability that a healthy person will develop a disease within a specified period of time. It is the number of new cases of disease in the population over a specific time period.

Inclusion criteria   Characteristics of subjects defined prior to starting the study that are used as parameters to enroll participants in the study (e.g., males and females between 50 and 75 years of age with a prior myocardial infarction).

Incremental cost-effectiveness ratio (ICER)   Is the ratio of the change in costs to incremental benefits of a therapeutic intervention or treatment.

Independent data monitoring committee   A group of experts that are independent of the ongoing clinical study they are monitoring. This group looks at the blinded data being generated by the study to determine if changes or adjustments should be made about how the study is being conducted.

Indexing service   A searchable database of biomedical journal citations.

Indicator drug   A drug that, when prescribed, may offer evidence that an adverse effect to a drug may have occurred. Pharmacists can then investigate further to determine whether there really was an adverse effect. Examples are found in Chapter 17.

Indicators   Measures or screens for quality and can focus on structure, process, or outcomes.

Indirect medical costs   One of four categories of costs in pharmacoeconomic studies. Indirect costs involve costs that result from the loss of productivity due to illness or death.

Inference engine   Also known as the reasoning engine, this forms the brain of the clinical decision support system, working to link patient-specific information with information in the knowledge base. It evaluates the available information and determines what to present to the user.

Inferential statistics   Statistics (i.e., parametric and nonparametric tests) that determine the statistical importance of differences between groups and allow conclusions to be drawn from the data.

Informatics specialist   An individual that has advanced medication information skills with a keen understanding of computer and information technology.

Information therapy   Evidence-based patient education and/or medical information presented at an appropriate time to most effectively assist the patient in making a specific health decision or change in their behavior.

Informed consent   The document signed by a subject, or the subject's representative, entering into a trial that informs him or her of his or her rights as a research subject, plus potential benefits and risks of the trial. This document indicates that the person is willing to participate in the study.

Inherent drug risks   Are unique to the drug and usually identified in the package insert, but do not include probable or common side effects.

Injunction   A judicial remedy issues in order to prohibit a party from doing or continuing to do a certain activity.

Institutional Review Board (IRB)   A group of individuals from various disciplines (e.g., lay people, physicians, pharmacists, nurses, clergy) who evaluate protocols for clinical studies to assess risks to the research participants and benefits to society. Approval of a local IRB (i.e., an IRB located in the community in which the study is to be conducted) is necessary prior to initiation of a clinical study involving patients.

Intangible costs   One of four categories of costs in pharmacoeconomic studies. Includes such items as the costs of pain, suffering, anxiety, or fatigue that occur because of an illness or the treatment of an illness.

Intelligent infusion (smart) pumps   Infusion pumps containing software designed to help eliminate pump programming errors.

Intention-to-treat (ITT)   A study design technique used to include results of all subjects in the final analysis even when the subject does not complete the entire study.

Intention-to-treat analysis   Analysis of all subject results randomized in a clinical trial regardless of whether they completed or dropped out of the study.

Interim analysis   Evaluation of data at specified time points before scheduled termination or completion of a study.

Internal validity   Internal validity refers to the extent to which the study results reflect what actually happened in the study (i.e., appropriate and sound study methods).

Internet   A worldwide computer network.

Interoperability   The ability of disparate computer systems to exchange information in a manner that allows the information to be used meaningfully.

Interval data   Data in which each measurement has an equal distance between points, but an arbitrary zero (e.g., temperature in Fahrenheit).

Interval scale   A scale of measurement that has rank ordered data with meaningful distance between two ranks, but no natural zero.

Interventional study   A study where the investigator introduces a factor and examines the factor's influence on certain variables or outcomes.

Intranet   A computer network with restricted access, as within a health-system.

Inverse variance test   A statistical test commonly used to combine continuous data in meta-analyses.

Investigational device exemption (IDE)   An approved IDE means that the IRB (and FDA for significant risk devices) has approved the sponsor's study application and all requirements under 21CFR812 are met. It allows the use of a device in a clinical investigation to collect safety and effectiveness data.

Investigational new drug   A drug, antibiotic, or biological that is used in a clinical investigation. The label of an investigational drug must bear the statement: "Caution: New Drug-Limited by Federal (or United States) law to investigational use."

Investigational new drug application (IND)   A submission to the FDA containing chemical information, preclinical data, and a detailed description of the planned clinical trials. Thirty days after submission of this document to the FDA by the sponsor, clinical trials may be initiated in humans (unless a clinical hold is placed by the FDA). When the FDA allows the studies to proceed, this document allows unapproved drugs to be shipped in interstate commerce.

Investigator   The individual responsible for initiating the clinical trial at the study site. This individual must treat the patients, ensure that the protocol is followed, evaluate responses and adverse reactions, solve problems as they arise, and ensure proper conduct of the study.

JCAHO   Joint Commission on Accreditation of Healthcare Organizations. See The Joint Commission.

Joint and several liability   Refers to the sharing of liabilities among a group of people collectively and also individually. If the defendants are "jointly and severally" liable, the injured party may sue some or all of the defendants together, or each one separately, and may collect equal or unequal amounts from each.

Just Culture   Just Culture is a term coined by David Marx, which is a structured accountability model that supports patient safety and a learning culture. It is intended to balance recognition and understanding of system contribution to errors with an understanding of human error concepts in order to facilitate an accountability process that is valued by leadership and staff. When applied consistently and fairly it is also a proactive approach to identifying gaps in system processes.

Justice   A concept that relates to fairness and tendering what is due, resource allocation, and providing that to which the individual is entitled.

Key opinion leaders   Health care professionals considered to be experts in their area by their peers. Key opinion leaders are often highly regarded for their expertise in publications, speaking engagements, and influential value in the medical community.

Kurtosis   Refers to how flat or peaked the curve appears. A curve with a flat or board top is referred to as platykurtic while a peaked distribution is described as leptokurtic.

Language bias   Occurs when only specific articles are included in a review or study that are published in a specific language such as the review author's native language. The issue is that potentially important articles are eliminated from the review.

Law   Involves written rules set by the whole society, or its representatives, that address the responsibilities of that society's members.

Learned intermediary   A doctrine of products liability law and personal injury law; the manufacturer of a prescription drug fulfills its duty to warn of potentially harmful effects of the drug by informing the prescribing physician and is not also obligated to warn the user. The prescribing physician acts as a learned intermediary between the manufacturer and the consumer and has the primary responsibility of warning patients of the hazards of prescribed pharmaceutical products. This doctrine is an exception to the rule that one who markets goods must warn foreseeable ultimate users of dangers inherent in their products.

Letter-to-the-editor   Comments from readers of a study or other article published in a journal. These are published in a latter issue of the same journal and usually have a reply from the original study/article author(s). Occasionally, short reports of a case or small study may be reported this way.

Level of evidence   A scale used to categorize the overall quality of a specific clinical trial. The reliability of the results can be inferred from the category given a trial.

Life table methods   In the context of cohort study life tables, data are collected by following patients throughout their lives or a specific duration of their life and then compiled into tables for such uses as survival or mortality analyses comparing exposed to nonexposed situations.

Listserver   A service offered by some e-mail systems that allows a member of the listserver to send an e-mail message to one particular Internet address where it will be sent to all members of the listserver. This acts as a dynamic distribution list for e-mail messages.

Local area network (LAN)   A group of computers connected in a way that they may share data, programs, and/or equipment over a small geographic area (e.g., building, department).

Locality rule   Legal doctrine created in the latter part of the nineteenth century that stated that the local defendant practitioner would have his or her standard of performance evaluated in light of the performance of other peers in the same or similar communities. Also known as community rule.

Logical operator   A term such as AND, OR, NOT, NEAR, or WITH that can be used in searching a computer database.

Logit   See Log-odds.

Log-odds   A linear transformation of probability. That is, probability is bounded between 0 and 1, log-odds transform probability to a continuous scale ranging from $-\infty$ to $+\infty$. The log-odds become the dependent variable in logistic regression.

Longitudinal   Data that is measured repeatedly over time.

Macro   Level of decision-making sets policy for the health system, as a standard established for an entire profession, or through government as law/regulation for the society as a whole.

Mail service drug program   Program that provides free home delivery for up to a 90 day supply of maintenance prescription drugs.

Mainframe computer   A large centralized computer that is used via computer terminals or other devices. This term is becoming blurred as smaller computer systems gain greater capabilities.

Managed care organization (MCO)   Health care provider who contracts with participating providers to provide a variety of services to enrolled members.

Mantel-Haenszel test   Statistical test commonly used to combine categorical data in meta-analyses.

Marginal (or incremental) cost-utility ratio   It is the gain in a benefit from an increase, or loss from a decrease, in a good or service, such as the quality-adjusted life years (QALY). It is calculated to estimate the added cost for an added benefit, not calculated when the added benefit comes at a lower cost.

Marginal cost-effectiveness ratio   The additional cost of one unit expansion of a single intervention.

Matching   A statistical technique which is used to evaluate the effect of a treatment by comparing the treated and nontreated units in an observational study such as case-control studies. The goal is to identify a nontreated patient with similar observable characteristics for every treated patient (cases and controls are similar), so treatment effect can be measured more accurately.

Material issue of fact   Genuine issue of material fact is a legal term often used as the basis for a motion for summary judgment. A summary judgment is proper if there is no genuine issue of material fact and the movant is entitled to a judgment as a matter of law. Such a motion will be granted if the party making the motion proves there is no genuine issue of material fact to be decided. When the moving party makes a *prima facie* showing that no genuine issue of material fact exists, the burden shifts to the nonmoving party to rebut the showing by presenting substantial evidence creating a genuine issue

MCO   See Managed care organization.

Mean (arithmetic mean)   The most common measure of central tendency for data measured on an interval or ratio scale and is best described as the average numerical value for the data set. Calculated as the sum of the observations divided by the number of observations. The arithmetic average of a set of numbers.

Meaningful Use   A set of standards defined by the CMS as the use of certified EHR technology to (1) improve quality, safety, and efficiency, (2) engage patients and their families, (3) improve care coordination, as well as public and population health, and (4) maintain privacy and security of PHI.

Measurement error   Occurs when the collection of data is influenced by the interviewer or when the survey item itself is unclear from the respondent's point of view.

Measures of association   Calculation and interpretation of nominal study results using relative risk (RR), relative risk reduction (RRR), absolute risk reduction (ARR), and numbers needed to treat (NNT).

Median   The absolute middle value of a set of number.

Medical executive committee   A committee that acts as the administrative body of a medical staff in an institution. It is responsible for overseeing all aspects of care within the institution. This committee may be known by other names at specific institutions.

Medical Literature Analysis and Retrieval System (MedLARS)   The computerized information retrieval system at the National Library of Medicine.

Medical Subject Headings (MeSH terms)   A thesaurus of official indexing terms used when searching some of the databases of the National Library of Medicine (e.g., MEDLINE, TOXLINE).

Medication error   Any preventable event that may cause or lead to inappropriate medication use or patient harm while the medication is in the control of the health care professional, patient, or consumer. Such events may be related to professional practice, health care products, procedures, and systems, including prescribing; order communication; product labeling, packaging, and nomenclature; compounding; dispensing; distribution; administration; education; monitoring; and use.

Medication guides Information for drug and biological products that the FDA determines pose a serious and significant public health concern requiring the distribution of FDA-approved patient medication information that is necessary to patients' safe and effective use of the drug products.

Medication information Facts or advice on medicines regarding a specific patient or a group of patients.

Medication misadventure Any iatrogenic hazard or incident associated with medications that is an inherent risk when medication therapy is indicated; is created through either omission or commission by the administration of a medicine or medicines during which a patient may be harmed, with effects ranging from mild discomfort to fatality; may be attributable to error (human or system, or both), immunologic response, or idiosyncratic response; is always unexpected or undesirable to the patient and the health professional; and whose outcome may or may not be independent of the preexisting pathology or disease process It includes adverse drug events (ADEs), adverse drug reactions (ADRs), and medication errors.

Medication therapy management Medication therapy management is a distinct service or group of services that optimizes drug therapy with the intent of improved therapeutic outcomes for individual patients.

Medication tier status An indication, usually designated by the payer for prescriptions, as to whether a medication is a preferred agent within its class (i.e., first tier), second choice (second tier), third choice (third tier), or not covered. Each "tier" is generally associated with decreasing payment from the payer and increasing patient responsibility for the cost of the drug, with "not covered" (or nonformulary) being entirely the patient's responsibility to pay.

Medication usage patterns Trends and patterns of drug use. Often influenced by reimbursement decisions and formularies of insurance companies, Medicare and Medicaid, direct-to-consumer advertising, etc.

Medication use evaluation (MUE) A part of the overall performance improvement program within institutional settings that provides in-depth assessment of the medication use process including prescribing, dispensing, administering, monitoring, and outcome. Multidisciplinary involvement.

MedLARS See Medical Literature Analysis and Retrieval System.

MedWatch The FDA Medical Products Reporting Program that monitors clinically significant adverse drug events and problems with medical products. Information is found at http://www.fda.gov/medwatch.

Meso Level of decision making variably described as occurring at the institutional/organizational level or at community/regional levels of health care.

Meta-analysis A study design where results of previously conducted similar clinical trials are combined, statistically analyzed, and new data are created for interpretation. Meta-analyses are especially useful when previous studies are inconclusive or controversial. They are also useful where sample size of multiple similar studies are too small to detect a statistically significant difference, but combining them will provide adequate sample size to meet a set power.

Micro Level of health care related decision making, which involves decisions made at the individual professional–patient level of health care.

Middle technical style A writing style used by professionals addressing professionals in other fields. It tends to be formal and avoids use of the first person (e.g., I, us). Technical jargon is avoided in this writing style.

Mode   The most frequently occurring value or category in the set of data. A data set can have more than one mode.

Modified systematic approach   A seven-step approach to answering drug information requests that includes (1) secure demographics of requestor, (2) obtain background information, (3) determine and categorize ultimate question, (4) develop strategy and conduct search, (5) perform evaluation, analysis, and synthesis, (6) formulate and provide response, and (7) conduct follow-up and documentation.

Morbidity   Detrimental consequences (other than death) related to a treatment, exposure, or disease state.

MTM   See Medication therapy management.

MUE   See Medication use evaluation.

Multicollinearity   Two or more variables have extremely high correlations (e.g., >0.90) indicating that they are redundant or that they are measuring the same construct.

Narrative review   See Nonsystematic review.

Narrow therapeutic index   Used to describe a drug with small differences in dose or blood concentration that may lead to dose and blood concentration dependent serious therapeutic failures or adverse drug reactions.

National Committee for Quality Assurance (NCQA)   An organization dedicated to assessing and reporting on the quality of managed care plans; it surveys and accredits managed care organizations much like JCAHO accredits hospitals.

National Patient Safety Goals (NPSGs)   Program established and updated by The Joint Commission to assist health care organizations to address safety concerns related to patient safety.

NCQA   See National Committee for Quality Assurance.

Negative formulary   A drug formulary that starts out with every marketed drug product and specifically eliminates products that are considered inferior, unnecessary, unsafe, too expensive, and so forth.

Negligence   Failure to exercise that degree of care that a person of ordinary prudence or a reasonable person would exercise under the same circumstances. Elements of a negligence case include (1) duty breached, (2) damages, (3) direct causation, and (4) defenses absent.

Negligent misrepresentation   Occurs when the defendant carelessly makes a representation or statement without reasonable basis to believe it to be true. The burden of proof that is required passes to the person who made the statement who must prove that the statement was either not one of fact but opinion and that he or she had reasonable ground to believe and did believe that the facts represented were true.

Network meta-analysis   Also referred to as a multiple treatment comparison meta-analysis or mixed treatment meta-analysis, it is a network of randomized controlled trials which is developed where all these trials have one intervention in common. This network allows an indirect estimate for comparison of interventions A and B when head-to-head trials do not exist.

New drug application (NDA)   The application to the FDA requesting approval to market a new drug for human use. The NDA contains data supporting the safety and efficacy of the drug for its intended use.

New molecular entity (NME)   A compound that can be patented and has not been previously marketed in the United States in any form.

NNT   See Number needed to treat.

N-of-1 Study   A controlled study conducted in a single subject where periods of exposure to a treatment are compared to periods of exposure to a placebo or alternative therapy, such as standard of care, to determine the effects of the treatment on various variables and outcomes in the subject.

Nominal data   Data that are categorical (e.g., yes/no; male/female).

Nominal scale   A scale of measurement that places data into mutually exclusive categories without reference to rank order.

Noninferiority   Any difference shown in a noninferiority design trial between two treatments is small enough to conclude the test drug has an effect not too much smaller (no worse) than the active control or reference drug.

Noninferiority margin   A prespecified amount of effect used to show the test drug's treatment effect is not worse than the reference drug by more than this specific degree.

Noninherent drug risks   Are created by the particular drug in combination with some extrinsic factor that the pharmacist should reasonably know about.

Nonmaleficence   A basic principle of consequentialist theory which encompasses the duty to do no harm.

Nonparametric statistics   Statistical tests used to analyze data that is not normally distributed such as nominal and ordinal data.

Nonparametric tests   Statistical tests that do not assume a conditional normal distribution.

Nonpharmacologic treatment   Treatment options focusing on a holistic approach to patient care (e.g., nutrition and exercise-related interventions).

Nonpublic unsolicited requests   A nonpublic unsolicited request is an unsolicited request that is directed privately to a firm using a one-on-one communication approach.

Nonresponse bias   A type of bias called nonresponse bias where the answers of respondents differ from the potential answers of those who did not answer the survey. This is the result of a nonresponse error associated with the survey.

Nonresponse error   Occurs when a significant number of subjects in a sample do not respond to the survey. The potential result of this is a type of bias called nonresponse bias where the answers of respondents differ from the potential answers of those who did not answer.

Nonsystematic review   A review article that summarizes previously conducted research, but does not provide a description of the systematic methods used to identify the research included in the article. Also called a narrative review.

NPSG   See National Patient Safety Goals.

Null hypothesis   The hypothesis that states there is no difference or relationship in the data. Statement of no difference in outcome between the intervention and control; created before the beginning of a study. This statement is either rejected or failed-to-be-rejected (i.e., accepted) at the end of the study based upon the p-value compared to the alpha value.

Number needed to treat   A measure used to determine the effectiveness of an intervention. This measure states the average number of patients who need to be treated with the intervention to prevent one additional negative outcome such as a myocardial infarction. The higher the value, the less effective is the intervention.

OBRA '90   See Omnibus Reconciliation Act of 1990.

Observational study   A study where the investigator analyzes naturally occurring events.

Observer bias   Tendency for observer/investigator to consciously or unconsciously distort what they see and record as the effect in a clinical trial situation. In other words, seeing what they expect to see.

Odds ratio   A measure of association between an exposure and an outcome. This ratio represents the chances that an outcome will occur given a particular exposure compared to the chances of the outcome occurring in the absence of that exposure.

Off-label information   Information that originates from sources (e.g., clinical studies, case reports) outside of the FDA-approved prescription drug labeling.

Omission negligence   Consulting the correct source, but failure to locate the correct answer(s) when providing information.

Omnibus Reconciliation Act of 1990 (OBRA '90)   A statute (Public Law 101-508) focused on drug benefits provided under Medicaid. The statute requires pharmacists to conduct drug utilization review (DUR) including prescription screening, patient counseling, and documentation of interventions.

Omnibus test   A statistical test of an overall difference. That is, the test indicates if at least one difference or relationship is statistically significant.

One-tailed test   A hypothesis that makes claim to the direction of the difference or relationship.

Online   The process of connecting to a remote computer via modem or network.

Open formulary   A formulary that allows any marketed drug to be ordered in an institution or under a third-party plan. Can be considered an oxymoron.

Ordinal data   See Ordinal scale.

Ordinal scale   A scale of measurement that has rank order, but makes no reference to the distance between ranks.

Ordinary care   See Reasonable care.

ORYX™   A JCAHO initiative to mandate the use of performance measurement tools to monitor outcomes and integrate these data into the accreditation process.

Outcome indicators   Quality assurance indicators that review whether the final desired result was obtained from whatever action was being reviewed.

Outcomes   A change in a patient's health status (e.g., recovery, death, disability, disease, discomfort, and dissatisfaction) that can be attributed to the care provided.

Outcomes research   A systematic investigation which seeks to provide evidence about which interventions are best for certain types of patients and under certain circumstances. An attempt to identify, measure, and evaluate the end results of health care services. It may include not only clinical and economic consequences, but also outcomes, such as patient health status and satisfaction with their health care.

Overview   A general term for a summary of the literature. It includes nonsystematic (narrative), systematic (qualitative), and quantitative (meta analyses) reviews.

p value   The probability of obtaining a test statistic as large or larger than the one actually obtained, conditional on the null hypothesis being true. It is the remaining area under a given probability distribution.

P&T committee   See Pharmacy and therapeutics committee.

Pair-wise meta-analysis   Traditional method to compile a meta-analysis by synthesizing the results of different trials to obtain an overall estimate of the treatment effect (one intervention relative to the control). The key is that all trials have the same intervention. All trials used are comparing treatment A to treatment B.

Parallel forms   A technique to test reliability of responses to questions in a survey by the responders. The technique usually consists of alternatively worded survey items placed throughout the survey. The parallel concept applies in that a question is asked in a positive manner in one place and in a negative manner in another place of the survey instrument. The answers to these alternate questions undergo a correlation analysis to determine the relatedness of the respondents alternate answers.

Parallel study   A study where two or more groups receive different treatments and the outcomes are compared.

Parameter   A measurement that describes part of the population.

Parameter negligence   Failure to consult the correct source in providing information.

Parametric statistics   Statistical tests used to analyze data with a normal (e.g., bell-shaped) distribution. Commonly used to analyze ratio and interval data.

Parametric tests   Statistical tests that assume a conditional normal distribution.

Parenteral admixtures   Solutions containing drug products for intravenous administration.

Patient education   Delivers written or verbal drug information through a planned activity initiated by a health care provider with the goal of changing patient behavior, improve adherence, and ultimately improve health.

Patient pocket formulary   Pocket-sized drug formulary listing top therapeutic drug classes, preferred products within those classes, cost index for the products, and other pertinent information.

Patient Safety Organizations (PSO)   The Patient Safety and Quality Improvement Act of 2005 (Patient Safety Act) authorized the creation of a nationwide network of Patient Safety Organizations (PSOs) to improve safety and quality through the collection and analysis of data on patient events.

Patient-centered medical home (PCMH)   Team-based healthcare delivery led by a physician or other primary care provider, but including multiple other types of providers, including pharmacists, to optimize patient outcomes.

PBM   See Pharmacy benefit management companies.

Peer review   A quality assurance program that centers on the evaluation of specific individuals by other similar professionals. Also, the process where a group of experts review a manuscript for accuracy and appropriateness for publication in a biomedical journal.

Per protocol analysis   Assessment of the study results in only those subjects completing the entire study duration.

Performance indicators   Items used to measure quality as part of the check function of quality improvement. The indicators typically focus on the process or outcomes of a care system, although they can also focus on structure.

Per-protocol   A study design technique to analyze the study results of only those subjects who completed the entire duration of the study.

Personal health records (PHRs)   Health 2.0 applications that provide the patient increased opportunity to participate in the collection, maintenance, and sharing of their personal health-related information through a Web-based environment.

Perspective   A pharmacoeconomic term that describes whose costs (such as the insurer, or the patient) are relevant based on the purpose of the study.

Pharmaceutical care   The responsible provision of drug therapy for the purpose of achieving definite outcomes that improve a patient's quality of life.

Pharmacoeconomics   The description and analysis of the costs of drug therapy to health care systems and society—it identifies, measures, and compares the costs and consequences of pharmaceutical products and services.

Pharmacoepidemiologic studies   A type of study that combines clinical pharmacology and epidemiology design concepts to study the use of and the effects of drugs in large numbers of people.

Pharmacovigilance   The process of preventing and detecting adverse effects from medications.

Pharmacy and therapeutics (P&T) committee   A group in an institution or company that oversees any and/or all aspects of drug therapy for that institution or company. In hospitals, it is usually a subcommittee of the medical staff. May be known by a variety of similar names, such as pharmacy and formulary committee, drug and therapeutics committee (DTC), or formulary committee.

Pharmacy benefit design   Contract that specifies the level of coverage and types of pharmaceutical services available to the health plan member.

Pharmacy benefit management (PBM) companies   Organizations that manage pharmaceutical benefits for managed care organizations, medical providers, or employers.

Pharmacy informatics   Focuses on the use of information, information systems, and automation technology to ensure safe and effective medication usage.

Pharmacy network   Select pharmacies and pharmacy chains where members of a health plan have to go to get their prescriptions filled, usually at a lower cost.

Placebo   A pharmaceutical preparation that does not contain a pharmacologically active ingredient, but is otherwise identical to the active drug preparation in terms of appearance, taste, and smell.

Placebo creep (also known as biocreep)   The phenomenon that results in the reference drug becoming no better than placebo in noninferiority trials. This occurs when a somewhat inferior test drug is chosen as the reference drug for a future generation of NI trials. After multiple generations of this occurring, the final result is a future reference drug that is no better than placebo.

Placebo effect   A phenomenon where the patient has a perceived or actual improvement in their medical condition after receiving placebo treatment.

Poison information   A specialized area of drug information. By definition, it is the provision of information on the toxic effects of an extensive range of chemicals, as well as, plan and animal exposures.

Poison information center   A place that specializes in research, management, and dissemination of toxicity information. A physician usually directs it, although a pharmacist directs many on a day-to-day basis. Often, pharmacists and nurses provide staffing of these centers.

Policy   A broad, general statement that takes into consideration and describes the goals and purposes of a policy and procedure document.

Popular technical style   A writing style used by professionals addressing lay people. This is less formal than writing addressed to professionals.

Population   Every individual in the entire universe with the characteristics or disease states under investigation. Since entire populations are generally very large, a sample representative of the population is usually selected for an investigation.

Positive formulary   A drug formulary that starts out with no drug products and specifically adds products, after appropriate evaluation, that are needed by the institution or company.

Post hoc   In clinical trial design, this distinguishes something that is done after the study is completed.

Postgraduate year one (PGY1) residency   An organized, directed, accredited program that builds on knowledge, skills, attitudes, and abilities gained from an accredited professional pharmacy degree program. The first-year residency program enhances general competencies in managing medication use systems and supports optimal medication therapy outcomes for patients with a broad range of disease states.

Postgraduate year two (PGY2) residency   An organized, directed, accredited program that builds on the competencies established in postgraduate year one of residency training. The second-year residency program is focused on a specific area of practice. The PGY-2 program increases the resident's depth of knowledge, skills, attitudes, and abilities to raise the resident's level of expertise in medication therapy management and clinical leadership in the area of focus. In those practice areas where board certification exists, graduates are prepared to pursue such certification.

Postmarketing surveillance   The process of continually monitoring and reviewing suspected adverse reactions associated with medications once they reach the market and are available to the public. Legislation mandates this activity for pharmaceutical manufacturers and the U.S. Food and Drug Administration (FDA), but health care providers can also participate by reporting adverse drug events, adverse drug reactions, and medication errors to the FDA and other regulatory bodies.

Postmarketing surveillance study   A study designed to examine drug use and frequency of side effects following approval by the Food and Drug Administration (FDA).

Power   The ability of a study to detect a difference between a study intervention and control if a difference exists. Usual minimum target value is 80%; power increases by increasing sample size, which also decreases the probability of a Type II or beta error.

Power analysis   A statistical procedure conducted by the investigators to determine a sample size for the trial.

Preferred drug product   Specific drug product within a specific therapeutic class selected as the most appropriate to treat a specific disease or condition as determined by the pharmacy and therapeutics committee.

Preferred therapeutic class   Specific drug class selected as the most appropriate to treat a specific disease or condition as determined by the pharmacy and therapeutics committee.

Prescribability   The ability of a drug to be prescribed for the first time.

Prevalence   Measures the number of people in the population who have the disease at a given time.

Prima facie   A fact presumed to be true unless it is disproved. That is, evidence that is sufficient to raise a presumption of fact or to establish the fact in question unless rebutted.

Primary author   The author listed first on a publication. Sometimes referred to as the *first author*.

Primary endpoint   An outcome measured by the study investigators that quantifies the difference in effect between the intervention and control of the clinical trial. The results of this outcome measurement are used to answer the primary study objective. This outcome is also used by the study investigators to determine other study methods (e.g., sample size, statistical tests, duration, dose, patient type to enroll).

Primary literature   Original research published in biomedical journals.

Principles   In ethical analysis, a principle is relatively broad and fundamental in scope, and guides ethical decision-making or actions.

Prior authorization   Authorization from the health plan or pharmacy benefit manager in conjunction with the pharmacy and therapeutics committee for specified medications or specified quantities of medications. Request is reviewed against preestablished criteria which are based on evidence-based medicine.

Privacy   A rule within the principle of autonomy, more generally relating to the right of the individual to control his or her own affairs without interference from or knowledge of outside parties.

Probabilistic sensitivity analysis   A sensitivity analysis that allows one to determine how the results of an analysis would change when these best guesses or assumptions are varied over a relevant range of values. In cost-effectiveness analysis, probability distributions are created for each factor about which there is uncertainty. By simulating the results of random samplings from these distributions, it enables judgments to be formed about the decisions in relation to each factor.

Procedures   Specific actions to be taken.

Process   Refers to the set of activities that occur between the patient and the provider, encompassing the services and products that are provided to patients and the manner in which the services are provided.

Process change   Making a change to routine process. It may be through changes in policy or procedures, implementation of new services, acquisition of new equipment, changes in staffing, generation of regular notifications, or other methods. It is used to correct practice when quality assurance/drug usage evaluation/medication usage evaluation shows a deficiency.

Process indicators   Quality assurance indicators based on the presence or absence of policies and procedures. These assume that if policies and procedures are appropriate they will be effective and be properly performed.

Process mapping   A workflow diagram that provides a clear and consistent understanding of the steps and/or parallel processes required to accomplish a task. This is a process undertaken in many industries as an approach to developing standardized work as part of process improvement. It generally identifies variations within a process that may contribute to excess waste or risk.

Product label   The information affixed to the product and used to identify the contents.

Product labeling   Product information including prescribing information.

Professional ethics   Rules of conduct or standards by which a particular group in society regulates its actions and sets standards for its members.

Professional writing   Any written communication prepared in the fulfillment of the practice of a profession.

Programmatic research   Research focused on the impact and economic value of programs and services provided by pharmacists in community and institutional settings.

Project management   A discipline or science that is goal oriented, organized, detailed, and has built-in accountability.

Prospective indicator   An indicator used in any quality assurance program that determines whether quality is acceptable before an action is taken or care is given.

Prospective study   A study where data are collected forward in time from date of study initiation.

Protected Health Information (PHI)   A term under the HIPAA Privacy Rule which refers to individually identifiable health information that can be linked to a particular person. Specifically, this information can relate to the individual's past, present, or future physical or mental health or condition, the provision of health care to the individual, or past, present, or future payment for the provision of health care to the individual. Common identifiers of health information include names, social security numbers, addresses, and birth dates.

Protopathic bias   When a treatment for the first symptoms of a disease or other outcome appears to cause the outcome. In this case, the first symptoms of the outcome of interest are the reason for the treatment under study and not the outcome itself. For instance, early symptoms of pancreatic cancer can be the symptoms of diabetes since beta cells are being destroyed by the cancer.

Proximate cause   Cause which immediately precedes and produces the effect, as distinguished from the remote or intervening cause.

Public unsolicited requests   An unsolicited request made in a public form, whether directed to a firm specifically or a forum at large.

Publication bias   To selectively pick publications and not include all publications available on the topic for the article.

Pure technical style   A writing style used by professionals addressing other professionals in the same field. It tends to be formal and avoids use of the first person (e.g., I, us). Technical jargon can be used in this writing style.

Push technology   A method by which information is actively sent to users' computers with little, if any, effort required by the user. The information may be displayed as a screen saver or the computer may in some way let the user know that the information is available to be displayed (e.g., pop up notification).

p-value   A statistical value calculated based on the study results. When this number is less than the α-value, it is interpreted as the probability of rejecting a true null hypothesis or the probability of chance being the reason that a difference in the results between the two groups was calculated.

QR (Quick Response)   Codes A type of two-dimensional bar code that provides more information than is possible with a standard UPC barcode. It is increasingly common to find these codes on advertisements or items available for purchase, where the code can be scanned by an application on a smartphone to provide referral to a Web site where further information may be found on something of interest.

Qualitative systematic review   See Meta-analysis or Systematic review.

Quality   A degree or grade of excellence that can be applied to goods, services, processes or even people.

Quality assessment and assurance committee   A committee found in long-term care facilities to evaluate quality of care, including drug usage evaluation.

Quality assurance   A process used to ensure that something is done or made well enough. It is usually retrospective and focuses only on a particular component within a process, not the entire process.

Quality measure   When this term is used in health care, it is used to indicate methods of quantifying the type of care a patient received (indicators may include details about processes and organization structure, overall patient outcomes, and even patients' perceptions of the quality of the care received).

Quality of life   This is an evaluation of a patient's living situation based on the patient's environment, family life, financial situation, education, and health. It is used in quality assurance programs when developing indicators. In some cases, quality-of-life aspects will take precedence over the absolute best treatment. For example, a quick cure to a disease state may not be as desirable when it costs so much that a family is bankrupted in the process.

Quality-adjusted life years (QALY)   A QALY is a health-utility measure combining quality and quantity of life, as determined by some valuations process.

Quantitative systematic review   See Meta-analysis or Systematic review.

Quantity limits   Set quantity of drug that can be prescribed, which is set by the health plan in conjunction with the pharmacy and therapeutics committee and is usually based on FDA-prescribing guidelines.

Random error   See Sample error.

Randomization   A process used in a study in which all subjects enrolled in the study have an equal opportunity to be in any of the study groups. This is used to reduce bias, enable the groups to be as similar as possible at baseline, and is required to validate certain statistical tests.

Randomized clinical trial   See Controlled clinical trial.

Range   The difference between the highest data value and the lowest data value.

Rate-based indicators   Usually measure the proportion of activities, or patients, that conform to a desired standard (e.g., the proportion of stat orders that are dispensed within 15 minutes).

Ratio data   Rank ordered data in which each measurement has a meaningful equal distance between points and also an absolute/natural zero (e.g., temperature in Kelvin).

Ratio scale   A scale of measurement that has rank ordered data with meaningful distance between ranks and a natural zero.

Reasonable care   Also called due care or ordinary care; conduct that an ordinarily prudent or reasonable person would normally exercise in a particular situation to avoid harm to another, taking the circumstances into account. The concept of due care is used as a test of liability for negligence and usually made on a case-by-case basis where each juror has to determine what a reasonable man or woman would do.

Reasoning engine   See Inference engine.

Rechallenge   In relation to adverse drug reactions, this occurs when the drug is discontinued and, after the adverse drug reactions (ADR) abates, the patient is given the same medication in an attempt to elicit the response again.

Referee   An expert in a particular area who reviews a written document to determine whether it is appropriate for publication.

Refereed publication   A publication in which the editors have experts in the appropriate field review items submitted for possible publication to determine whether those items are of suitable quality.

Regulatory project manager (RPM)   This is the sponsor's primary FDA contact person. Each application that is submitted is assigned a regulatory project manager (RPM). Contact information for the RPM is provided in the letter sent to the applicant acknowledging receipt of the application. If the RPM is changed during the course of the review, the applicant is notified by the new RPM.

Relative risk   The risk of developing a disease or adverse event in those participants exposed to a specific variable compared to those not exposed to that variable.

REMS   See Risk evaluation and mitigation strategy.

Research hypothesis   (also known as the alternative hypothesis) It is a difference between the therapy under investigation and the control.

Residual value   The difference between the model predicted dependent variable and the actual dependent variable value.

Respondeat superior   Refers to the proposition that the employer is responsible for the negligent acts of its agents or employees.

Response bias   See Measurement error.

Restatement (Second) of Torts   "An attempt by the American Law Institute to present an orderly statement of the general common law of the United States, including in that term not only the law developed solely by judicial decision, but also the law that has grown from the application by the courts of statutes..." It takes into account other factors, such as the modern trend of the law according to influential jurisdictions and well thought out opinions.

Retrospective indicator   An indicator used in any quality assurance program that determines whether quality was acceptable after an action was taken or care was given.

Retrospective study   A study that analyzes historical data (e.g., previously collected data such as medical records or insurance information).

Risk Evaluation and Mitigation Strategy (REMS)   A risk management plan required by the FDA that goes beyond requirements in the drug prescribing information to manage serious risks associated with a drug.

Risk minimization action plans (RiskMAPs)   A strategic safety program designed to meet specific goals and objectives in minimizing known risks of a product while preserving its benefits.

RiskMAPs   See Risk minimization action plans.

Robustness   The ability of the statistical test to produce correct test statistics and parameter estimates in the presence of assumption violations.

Root cause analysis (RCA)   In response to a sentinel or serious event, the expectation of The Joint Commission is that the organization will conduct a timely, thorough, and credible analysis to determine root causes of the event, develop and implement an action plan to reduce the risk of recurrence, and monitor the effectiveness of the plan and its implementation.

RSS   This acronym has multiple meanings, but is usually defined as Really Simple Syndication. It is a method by which an aggregator program collects information from Web sites and Weblogs (blog), which is then displayed as a collation. This allows individuals to monitor new or additional information on the Internet without having to use a browser to go to multiple Web sites.

Rule   In ethical analysis, a rule guides ethical decision making or actions, but is relatively specific in context and restricted in scope.

Rules engines   Computer programs, similar to ADE monitoring systems, with built-in, logic rules designed to aid in monitoring specific aspects of patient care.

Run-in phase   A short duration of patient assessment but prior to being enrolling in the study. Various reasons exist for this phase and include assessment of medication compliance, meet an inclusion criteria (e.g., LDL-C less than 130 mg/dL), and allow for medication washout.

Sample   A group of subjects, taken from the population, who are enrolled in a study; these individuals should represent the population in order for the study results to be extrapolated to the population.

Sample frame   A term describing the population that will actually be drawn from to make up the sample.

Sample precision   A measure of how close an estimator is expected to be to the true value of a parameter.

Sample size   The number of subjects in a study.

Sampling bias   See sampling error.

Sampling error   In statistics, this is incurred when the statistical characteristics of a population are estimated from a subset or sample of that population. The statistics on that sample such as means and variances differ from the parameters of the entire population because not all members of the entire population are used (also known as sample error).

Secondary endpoint   An outcome measured by the study investigators that quantifies the difference in effect between the intervention and control of the clinical trial, but not considered the focus of the study. The results of this outcome measurement are used to answer secondary study objectives. For example, a study compares a statin to placebo to determine if the statin can reduce the risk of having a stroke (primary endpoint); change in LDL-C levels are also compared between the two groups (secondary endpoint).

Secondary literature   Resources that index and/or abstract literature from biomedical journals.

Selection bias   Study subjects who meet the study inclusion/exclusion criteria but are not randomized into either the intervention or control (i.e., excluded from the study).

Selection bias   An error in selection method to obtain individuals or groups to take part in a scientific study.

SEM   See Standard error of the mean.

Sensitivity   The probability that a diseased individual will have a positive test result. It is the true positive rate of the test. The ability of a test to correctly identify those with the disease.

Sensitivity analysis   Tests that are undertaken to determine the influence of various criteria or conditions on study results. Sensitivity analyses are commonly used in meta-analyses and pharmacoeconomic research.

Sentinel event   The Joint Commission defines a sentinel event as an unexpected occurrence involving death or serious physical or psychological injury, or the risk thereof. Serious injury specifically includes loss of limb or function. The phrase "or the risk thereof" includes any process variation for which a recurrence would carry a significant chance of a serious adverse outcome. Such events are called *sentinel* because they signal the need for immediate investigation and response.

Sentinel indicators   Reflect the occurrence of a serious event that requires further investigation (e.g., adverse drug-related event, death).

Skewness   The measure of symmetry of a curve.

Smartphone   A cellular device that has Internet capabilities and supports various software functions.

Social media   Form of electronic communication allowing interactions with users to share information, messages, and other various forms of content.

Software as a service (SaaS)   (also known as application service provider [ASP]) A computing model in which an organization's data and software are hosted by an off-site vendor who is responsible for maintaining data storage as well as the equipment on which it is stored.

Special Protocol Assessment   Is a statement from the U.S. Food and Drug Administration that an uninitiated or ongoing Phase III trial's design, clinical endpoints, and statistical analyses are adequate for FDA approval.

Specificity   The probability an individual without a disease will have a negative test result.

Sponsor   An organization (or individual) that takes responsibility for and initiates a clinical investigation. The sponsor may be an individual or pharmaceutical company, government agency, academic institution, private organization, or other organization.

Sponsor-investigator   An individual who both initiates and conducts a clinical investigation (i.e., submits the IND and directly supervises administration of the drug as well as other investigator responsibilities).

Stability study   A study designed to determine the stability of drugs in various preparations.

Stakeholder   Any individual who affects or is affected by the problem or issue addressed by the policy.

Standard   A term used in quality assurance program that indicates how often an indicator must be complied with. The level of compliance will be set at either 0% (i.e., never done) or 100% (i.e., always done). A threshold, which allows compliance of between 0% and 100%, has sometimes been used instead of a standard.

Standard deviation   (1) A measurement of the range of data values (i.e., variability) around the mean. (2) The measure of the average amount by which each observation in a series of data points differs from the mean. In other words, how far away is each data point from the mean (dispersion or variability) or the average deviation from the mean.

Standard error of the mean (SEM)   An estimate of the true mean of the population from the mean of the sample. Mathematically, SEM is calculated as the standard deviation divided by the square root of the sample size. Ninety-five percent of the time, true mean of the population lies within +2 standard errors of the sample mean. Describes the precision of the mean of a sample of data that is being used to estimate some unknown or "true" value of the mean of the target population. The standard error of the mean (SEM) increases as the variability of the data increases, and decreases as the sample size increases.

Standard gamble   One method used in measuring health preferences. Each subject is offered two alternatives. Alternative one is treatment with two possible outcomes: either the return to normal health or immediate death. Alternative two is the certain outcome of a chronic disease state for life. The probability of dying is varied until the subject is indifferent between alternative one and alternative two. Used to assess his or her quality-adjusted life years (QALY) estimate.

Statistic   A measurement that describes part of a sample.

Statistical significance   The impact of a study in terms of the outcome of statistical tests conducted on the data. A study is said to be statistically significant when statistical tests demonstrate a difference between treatment groups.

Statute   Written law enacted by a legislature other than that of a municipality.

Step therapy   Prescribing guidelines set by the health plan in conjunction with the pharmacy and therapeutics committee that specify which drugs should be prescribed first before more expensive drugs will be covered. Guidelines are based on evidence-based medicine.

Stratification   An advanced type of randomization to produce study groups as similar as possible; considers baseline demographic information of the subjects selected for the study.

Strict liability   Also called absolute liability; the legal responsibility for damages, or injury, even if the person was not at fault or negligent. Strict liability has been applied to certain activities, such as holding employers absolutely liable for the torts of their employees, but it is most commonly associated with claims for injuries resulting from defectively manufactured or designed products. A successful plaintiff need only show that the product was in fact defective in design or manufacture, rendering it unreasonably dangerous and the cause of injury.

Structure   Refers to the characteristics of providers, the tools and resources at their disposal, and the physical or organizational settings in which they work.

Structure indicators   Quality assurance indicators based on the presence or absence of items, such as staffing patterns, available space, equipment, resources, or administrative organization.

Study objective   A brief statement of the goals and purpose of a research study.

Subgroup analysis   Evaluation of study results within a subset of subjects enrolled in the study according to specific demographic (e.g., age, gender, disease state).

Subject   An individual who participates in a clinical investigation (either as the recipient of the investigational drug or as a member of the control group).

Summary judgment   A party moving (applying) for summary judgment is attempting to avoid the time and expense of a trial when the outcome is obvious. A party may also move for summary judgment in order to eliminate the risk of losing at trial, and possibly avoid having to go through discovery (i.e., by moving at the outset of discovery), by demonstrating to the judge, via sworn statements and documentary evidence, that there are no material factual issues remaining to be tried. If there is nothing for the fact finder to decide, then the moving party asks rhetorically, why have a trial? A dispute over a material fact on which the outcome of a legal case may rely, and which, therefore, must be decided by a judge or jury; a dispute which precludes summary judgment.

Surrogate endpoint   A study measurement (e.g., laboratory value or physical assessment) that serves as a substitute marker for an actual clinical outcome. It is an effect that can be easily measured to correlate an outcome that is more difficult and/or time-consuming to measure (e.g., lowering LDL-C levels [measured effect] should result in reducing cardiovascular events [predicted outcome] such as myocardial infarction, stroke, or death).

Survey research   Research where responses to questions asked of subjects are analyzed to determine the incidence, distribution, and relationships of sociological and psychological variables.

Switchability   The ability to exchange one drug for another.

Symposium   A meeting focused on a particular topic.

Synthesis   Synthesis is the careful, systematic, and orderly process of integrating varied and diverse elements, ideas, or factors into a coherent response. This process relies not only on the type and quality of the data gathered, but also on how the data are organized, viewed, and evaluated. Synthesis, as it relates to pharmacotherapy, involves the careful integration of critical information about the patient, disease, and medication along with pertinent background information to arrive at a judgment or conclusion.

Systematic review   A summary of previously conducted studies where the research to be included in the review is systematically identified; however, the results are not statistically combined as would occur with a quantitative systematic review or meta-analysis. Also called a qualitative systematic review.

Target drug program   A program that evaluates the use of a medication or group of medications on an ongoing basis. Within these programs, interventions are usually made at the time of discovery based on established criteria or guidelines.

Target population   The entire group a researcher is interested in because this is the population that the findings of the survey are meant to generalize and the researcher wishes to make inferences and draw conclusions.

Telemedicine   It is defined as the use of telecommunications and interactive video technology to provide health care services to patients who are at a distance.

Telnet   A program for microcomputers that causes the computer to mimic a dumb terminal, so that it can run programs on other computers (usually minicomputers or mainframes) over the Internet or other computer networks.

Ten major considerations   A tool containing 10 items identified to evaluate a clinical trial article that if any single item is considered a limitation, the reliability of the entire article is questionable and the results deemed possibly unreliable.

Teratogenicity   Toxicity of drugs to the unborn fetus.

Tertiary literature/resources   Textbooks and drug compendia (includes full-text computer databases) that consists of established knowledge.

The Joint Commission (TJC)   Organization that accredits health care organizations and programs in the United States.

Third-party payer   Organization that pays for or underwrites coverage for health care expenses for another entity.

Third-party plan   A method of reimbursement for medical care in which neither the care provider nor the patient is charged. Third-party payers include insurance, health maintenance organizations, and government entities.

Threshold   A term used in quality assurance program that indicates how often an indicator must be complied with. Unlike standards, thresholds can be set at any level of compliance from 0% to 100%.

Tiered copayment benefit   A pharmacy benefit design that encourages patients to use generic and formulary drugs, by requiring the patient to pay progressively higher copayments for brand name and nonformulary drugs.

Time trade-off   A method for measuring health preferences. The subject is offered two alternatives. Alternative one is a certain disease state for a specific length of time t, the life expectancy for a person with the disease, then death. Alternative two is being healthy for time x, which is less than t. Time x is varied until the respondent is indifferent between the two alternatives. The proportion of the number of years of life a person is willing to give up ($t - x$) to have his or her remaining years (x) of life in a healthy state is used to assess his or her quality-adjusted life years (QALY) estimate.

TJC See The Joint Commission.

Tort liability Civil wrongs recognized by law as grounds for a lawsuit.

Total quality management (TQM) A management concept dealing with the implementation of continuous quality improvement.

TQM See Total quality management.

Treatment effect A mean difference in the outcome measure over time between two drugs (i.e., drug minus placebo or test drug minus reference drug)

Treatment order effect A situation where the order in which patients receive the treatment in a trial (generally a crossover design) affects the results of that trial.

Trohoc study See Case-control study.

True experiment A study where researchers apply a treatment and determine its effects on subjects.

True negatives Individuals without the disease who were correctly identified as being disease free by the test.

True positives Individuals with the disease who were correctly identified as diseased by the test.

Two-tailed test A hypothesis that does not claim a direction of the difference or relationship.

Type I error The probability of a false positive result. The probability of a type I error is equal to alpha and occurs when the null hypothesis is rejected when it is in fact true. Falsely rejecting the null hypothesis when, in fact, the null hypothesis is true.

Type II error The probability of a false negative result. The probability of a type II error is equal to beta and occurs when the null hypothesis is accepted when it is in fact false. Failing to reject the null hypothesis when, in fact, the null hypothesis is false.

Unexpected drug reaction The Food and Drug Administration defines this as "one that is not listed in the current labeling for the drug as having been reported or associated with the use of the drug. This includes an ADR that may be symptomatically or pathophysiologically related to an ADR listed in the labeling but may differ from the labeled ADR because of greater severity or specificity (e.g., abnormal liver function versus hepatic necrosis)."

Uniform resource locator—URL An Internet address (e.g., http://druginfo.creighton.edu).

Unsolicited requests Requests initiated by persons or entities that are completely independent of the relevant firm.

USENET news A large number of discussion groups that are replicated in numerous places on the Internet. Users can read items posted on a topic and can contribute their own items to be posted.

Validity The truthfulness of study results. Internal validity refers to the extent to which the study results reflect what actually happened in the study (i.e., appropriate and sound study methods). External validity is the degree to which the study results can be applied to patients routinely encountered in clinical practice.

Validity filter A type of term or limit used to narrow a search to only the highest quality studies, such randomized controlled trial or double-blind.

Validity, External   See External validity.

Validity, Internal   See Internal validity.

Value   Has been assigned many definitions, but within health care, it usually reflects the ratio of quality and costs (value = quality/cost).

Variables   Factors (characteristics that are being observed or measured) that are the focus of a study. The independent variable (e.g., treatment) causes change in the dependent variable (e.g., outcome).

Variance   A measurement of the range of data values (i.e., variability) about the mean. Variance is the square of the standard deviation.

Veracity   This term addresses the obligation to truth telling or honesty.

Vicarious liability   Also called imputed liability or imputed negligence; the doctrine that attaches responsibility on one person for the failure of another, with whom the person has a special relationship (such as parent and child, employer and employee, husband and wife, or owner of vehicle and driver), to exercise such care as a reasonably prudent person would use under similar circumstances. Ordinarily, the independent negligence of one person is not imputable to another person.

Virtual private network (VPN)   A method to connect computers over a distance, for example, over the Internet, which allows secure transmission of confidential data.

Warranty   An assurance by one party to a contract of the existence of a fact upon which the other party may rely, intended to relieve the promisee of any duty to ascertain the fact for himself or herself. Amounts to a promise to indemnify the promisee for any loss if the fact warranted proves untrue. Warranties may be express (made overtly) or implied (by implication).

Web 2.0   Simply refers to those applications of the Internet that are interactive and social, allowing for collaboration and interactivity among patients, caregivers, and providers. Web 2.0 is not new software but a different strategy to use the Web. The Web goes beyond being a search engine and a source of information to include a platform to create, share, and collaborate in developing new knowledge. Social networking is the phenomenon of online communities in which people share interests and/or activities with one another and is an outgrowth of Web 2.0.

Web browser   A computer program used to access information on the World Wide Web. The most popular programs are Microsoft Internet Explorer, Google Chrome, and Mozilla Firefox.

Web portal   A Web site that acts as an interface to the Internet for users. Many Internet search engines are considered to be Web portals. A variation on this, the enterprise portal, can also be used by an institution to help guide employees to necessary information within the institution or out on the Internet.

Weblog   (also known as blog) This is a public Web site where a person maintains a journal that is open to viewers.

Web site   A group of Web pages that will provide information to the person requesting that information. These pages are generally grouped under one main Internet address (URL).

Wide area network (WAN)   A group of computers connected in a way that they may share data, programs, and/or equipment over a distance (e.g., connection between computers owned by an institution that are scattered in clinics around a city).

Wikis   Web sites which allows its users to add, modify, or delete its content via a Web browser usually using a simplified markup language or a rich-text editor. Wikis are powered by wiki software,

are created collaboratively, and can be community Web sites and intranets, for example. Some permit control over different functions (levels of access). For example, editing rights may permit changing, adding, or removing material. Others may permit access without enforcing access control.

World Wide Web (WWW)   Computers connected to the Internet that provide a graphical interface to a variety of information that is available as text, pictures, sounds, databases, and other electronic files. Generally accessed using a Web browser, such as Internet Explorer.

XHTML—extensible HTML   A combination of HTML and Extensible Markup Language.

XML—Extensible Markup Language   A superset of HTML that provides information on the content of a Web page, presentation of the information (how it looks), and semantics (what it means). This is designed to make it easier to find more relevant information using search engines.

z-score   The distance a data point is from its variable's mean in standard deviation units.

Answers for Case Studies

Chapter 3

CASE STUDY 3–1

Common side effects would be included in all major compendia (e.g., Micromedex® 2.0, Clinical Pharmacology, or Facts & Comparisons) which would be a good initial search. In addition, some of the adverse effect specific resources (e.g., Meyler's Side Effects of Drugs) would be appropriate to consult for less common side effects.

CASE STUDY 3–2

- There are a variety of resources that could be consulted for this information including the text Drugs in Pregnancy and Lactation or some of the major compendia (possibly, Micromedex® 2.0 or Clinical Pharmacology).
- The resources classify levofloxacin as an agent with unknown safety, but likely to be safe.
- In order to best answer this question, the requestor should determine if the disease state has other treatment options which have more data available and if the infant is receiving any formula supplementation.

CASE STUDY 3–3

- The student might start a search for general information in a toxicology text such as Goldfrank's Toxicologic Emergencies. That could be followed with a search in Micromedex® 2.0 to find some general toxicology information; specifically the POISONDEX component of that resource would provide comprehensive information on this topic.
- The student would do best to search using the generic name of the medication, in this case using chlorpheniramine.

CASE STUDY 3–4

In a case you are not familiar with a term, a general Internet search might be a good start to help streamline your search. An Internet search shows that AMDUCA stands for Animal Medicinal Drug Use Clarification Act of 1994. Knowing that the term refers to a specific piece of legislation, you would be prompted to consider searching the American Veterinarian Medical Association Web page or Food and Drug Administration Web page.

CASE STUDY 3–5

- Since this would be an off-label use, there may be less data in the tertiary resources. In this case it is likely more efficient to do a search in the secondary resources. Medline is a good place to start.
- Initially conducting a search with no restrictions/limits ensures that valuable information is not missed.
- If the initial search yields a significant number of results, then a restriction to human clinical trials would be beneficial. When conducting this search it is important to realize that the term female sexual arousal disorder has changed over time, so maybe a more general search for female sexual dysfunctions will give more responses. In addition, searching for the specific drug sildenafil will yield useful data, but expanding the search using the class of drugs will provide more data.

CASE STUDY 3–6

Since the patient specifically provided you the news venue, going directly to the NBC Web page would be an excellent start. Since content changes quickly on news pages, possibly a general Internet search might be needed if the story was run a while back.

CASE STUDY 3–7

- Tertiary resources could provide a good overview on how a treatment might work in a large patient population, appropriate dosing, as well as provide a quick summary of safety data. The disadvantage is the lag time from when the information is updated until it is published, so recently discovered safety or efficacy information might not be included in that type of resource.
- Primary literature would provide very timely information, but in a case like this the volume of primary literature can be overwhelming and make it difficult to navigate.

Chapter 4

CASE STUDY 4–1

1. Yes, any study enrolling human subjects requires IRB approval. This is especially true since this clinical trial is evaluating an investigational agent and subjects may be at risk while partaking in this research. The IRB approval is needed to protect the enrolled subjects.
2. Placebo being selected as the control for this controlled clinical trial is appropriate. The purpose of this study is to measure and quantify the weight changes produced by lorcaserin. In addition, this study was designed to determine a cause-and-effect relationship with lorcaserin (cause = lorcaserin; effect = body weight changes).
3. This indicates that 68% (one standard deviation from the mean) of the body weight loss in the subjects of this trial treated with lorcaserin were measured to be between 3.4 and 8.2 kg.
4. Since all subjects were to follow the same diet and exercise program, this would be classified as adjunctive therapy. The diet should not interfere with measuring a difference in weight changes between lorcaserin and placebo since both groups are following the same diet and exercise regimens.

5. The probability of rejecting a true H_0 is $< 0.1\%$. Since this p-value is less than the stated α-value, H_0 would be rejected and H_1 accepted. The probability of a Type I error is less than 0.1%. In addition, the probability of chance being the reason a difference was calculated between lorcaserin and placebo would be less than 0.1%.

6. Weight loss has been associated with lowering the risk of diabetes and cardiovascular disease. However, this study did not directly measure the number of subjects developing diabetes or reduction in the incidence of cardiovascular events (e.g., myocardial infarction). Lorcaserin did lower body weight, but these results cannot be used to claim this agent reduces the risk in developing diabetes or cardiovascular events. The primary endpoint results would be considered a surrogate endpoint for the reduction of diabetes and cardiovascular events.

CASE STUDY 4–2

1. Double-blinding is the most appropriate blinding type. The primary and secondary endpoints are subjective in nature. Thus, neither the subjects nor the investigators should know who were randomized to which group. Reduction in pain will, most likely, not be reported by individuals knowing they are taking placebo. In addition, the probability is highly likely that changes in pain scores reported by both subjects and investigators would be biased if the therapy is known.

2. Ordinal. This type of data is classified as ranked or scaled. Subjects rated their pain during this trial using a scale. Rating pain on a scale is not dichotomous (e.g., yes/no data) and does not have equal intervals (as does continuous data).

3. Mode and median are the appropriate measures of central tendency to present ordinal data. The mode is the most frequently occurring observation of the data set. The median is the point in which 50% (or middle) of the data in the set are above and 50% of the data are below.

4. A power analysis is conducted by the investigators to determine a sample size for the trial. Power is the ability of the study to detect a difference between the intervention and control if a difference exists. An appropriate study power is at least 80%. This trial had a power of 90%. Study power increases with increasing sample size (and reduces the probability of a Type II error). A trial with 90% power requires a larger sample size than 80% power.

5. According to the results of this study, duloxetine appears to be efficacious in reducing this pain type compared to placebo. However, other pain agents were not assessed in this clinical trial. Thus, the claim that duloxetine is more efficacious than other agents and duloxetine should be used as initial therapy cannot be supported with this controlled clinical trial.

CASE STUDY 4–3

1. RRR = 21%
   RRR = 1 − RR. RR = (212/9120)/(265/9081) = 0.023/0.029 OR 2.3%/2.9% = 0.79
   RRR = 1 − 0.79 = 21%
   The apixaban reduced the baseline risk of a stroke or systemic embolism by 21% over warfarin. This result indicates that apixaban reduces stroke or systemic embolism greater than adjusted-dose warfarin.

2. ARR = 0.6%
   ARR = (265/9081) − (212/9120) = 0.029 − 0.023 OR 2.9% − 2.3% = 0.6%
   A total of 0.6% (or 55) patients were spared a stroke or systemic embolism by receiving apixaban versus adjusted-dose warfarin. This result indicates that apixaban reduces stroke or systemic embolism risk versus adjusted-dose warfarin.

3. NNT = 167
   NNT = 1/ARR = 1/([265/9081] − [212/9120]) = 1/0.006 = 167

A total of 167 patients need to be treated with apixaban for a median of 1.8 years to prevent one stroke or systemic embolism that would otherwise occur with adjusted-dose warfarin.

4. The hazard ratio (HR) for stroke or systemic embolism in this patient sample is 0.79 and the investigators are 95% confident that the true HR in the general population lies between 0.66 and 0.95. The value of equality (one) is not contained in this range, indicating the risk of stroke and systemic embolism is lower with apixaban versus adjusted-dose warfarin. Also, the result is statistical significance and potentially clinical significance.

5. This family member is an overall healthy male with minimal risk factors for stroke, other than his atrial fibrillation. He is well controlled on adjusted-dose warfarin, appears to be pleased with therapy, and is at low/moderate risk for bleeding adverse events. Unless he specifically desires to change therapy due to reasons other than those surrounding efficacy of warfarin (i.e., bleeding risk or adherence issues), continuing with his warfarin therapy is acceptable. Evaluating the primary endpoint result and all the measures of association calculations, the magnitude of difference between these two treatments may not warrant changing his stabilized and effective warfarin therapy in which no bleeding episodes have occurred.

Chapter 5

CASE STUDY 5-1

- Null hypothesis: The test drug (alginate/antacid) fails to exhibit noninferiority to the reference drug (omeprazole) or at the very least the results are inconclusive for noninferiority versus inferiority.

  Alternative hypothesis: The test drug (alginate/antacid) is noninferior to the reference drug (omeprazole).

- How the noninferiority (NI) margin was determined. Did the investigators set the NI margin prior to the study being conducted? Did the investigators confirm omeprazole's efficacy against placebo which is referred to as assay sensitivity? Were historical trials and this NI study identical as possible regarding important characteristics (referred to as constancy assumption)?

- Yes, both intention-to-treat (ITT) and per-protocol (PP) analyses were used. Comparison between the two would have shown any concerns that the ITT approach diluted the results to show noninferiority. Smaller observed treatment effects can result with an ITT analysis since patients did not necessarily complete the duration of the trial and experience the maximum effect of alginate/antacid. Using just an ITT analysis with an NI trial design can significantly increase the risk of falsely claiming noninferiority. The FDA recommends performing both ITT and PP analyses and checking to see if there are significant differences between the results. An explanation by the authors as to why there was a significant difference is expected.

- See Figure 5-1. For this noninferiority trial design, the conclusion would be that alginate/antacid is noninferior to omeprazole regarding short-term symptomatic efficacy in moderate GERD in a general practice setting.

- See Figure 5-1. For this noninferiority trial design, the result would be inconclusive regarding noninferiority for alginate/antacid compared to omeprazole since the 95% CI crosses over the NI margin instead of being located completely on one side noninferior or the other side inferior of the NI margin.

- Performing a superiority analysis after noninferiority has been established is acceptable and appropriate. It is generally not acceptable or appropriate to seek the conclusion of noninferiority from a failed superiority trial.

CASE STUDY 5-2

- Null hypothesis: The test drug (linagliptin) fails to exhibit noninferiority to the reference drug (glimepiride) or at the very least the results are inconclusive for noninferiority versus inferiority. Alternative hypothesis: The test drug (linagliptin) is noninferior to the reference drug (glimepiride).
- In this case, there was no mention of NI margin. This situation dictates utilization of the p-value that resulted from the noninferiority statistical testing. The set alpha is 0.05. They reported a p-value of 0.03. The resulting p-value is less than the set alpha and, therefore, the null hypothesis is rejected in favor of the alternative hypothesis. For this study, the alternative hypothesis stated that the test drug (linagliptin) is noninferior to the reference drug (glimepiride).
- A modified intention-to-treat (mITT) analysis was used. Each patient that was placed in the evaluation group had received one dose of treatment, had a baseline HbA_{1c} measurement, and had at least one on-treatment HbA_{1c} measurement. The issue with mITT analyses involves the potential for smaller observed treatment effects since patients did not necessarily complete the duration of the trial and experience the maximum effect of linagliptin. This effect can dilute the results to show a false noninferiority between the two treatments. This is why the FDA recommends performing both ITT and per-protocol (PP) analyses to see if there are significant differences in results between the two analyses. An explanation from the authors as to why there was a significant difference is expected.
- A result showing a p-value greater than the set alpha would prevent us from rejecting the null hypothesis that states: failure to show noninferiority.
- Performing a superiority analysis after noninferiority has been established is acceptable and appropriate. It is generally not acceptable or appropriate to seek the conclusion of noninferiority from a failed superiority trial.

CASE STUDY 5-3

- Observation studies provide no guarantee that the two groups have similar characteristics with the exception of being in the same observational cohort study. The women consuming four or more cups of coffee may be made up of healthier subjects than the group of women that consumed less than one cup of coffee per day.
- Other factors (some not even known at this time) not controlled by this observational study may be playing an important protective role in those women that had an associated reduction in endometrial cancer risk. Potential confounding factors include health of immune system, genetic familial effects, and exposure to other factors that may be causing the cancer. There are many other confounding factors that can be identified.
- The outcome should be measured the same way and at the same frequency for both groups. Adequate follow-up should be determined.
- No cause-effect relationship can be determined with an observational study such as this cohort study.

CASE STUDY 5-4

- The quality of the meta-analysis depends on the quality of the individual studies used to develop the meta-analysis in addition to the homogeneity of the studies as a whole.
- Publication bias is a form of selection bias where publication of studies is based on the magnitude, direction, or statistical significance of the results. It is documented that researchers are more likely to publish studies that demonstrate positive effects of drugs.

  The investigators utilized a technique called funnel plot to identify the potential existence of publication bias. A funnel plot is a scatter plot of treatment effect versus study size. If this plot shows an inverted symmetrical funnel, publication bias is probably not present. An asymmetrical funnel plot indicates the possibility that publication bias is present (see Figure 5–6).

- Factors that suggest a lack of high homogeneity or in other words high heterogeneity between studies: difference in primary outcome measure used, differences in participant attrition, difference in study design, differences in intervention duration, and wide variations in the vasoactive ingredient (polyphenol) between trials.

- The authors used a forest plot to provide the results of this meta-analysis because the reader can easily visualize the similarities and differences noted between studies and a confidence interval is included which provides additional information about the variability of the results for individual studies.

- Based on the findings reported here, although there is a statistically significant difference between chocolate and control, these findings are probably not clinically significant. Therefore, the authors should conclude that chocolate does not effectively reduce blood pressure in hypertensive patients.

- Proprietary content of active ingredients prevents you from being able to confirm whether any of the other products contain the same amount, or more or less than the product that provided this evidence. Also, specific plant parts utilized in a study are important to consider. If a trial evaluated the use of a herb's root, but the product for which a practitioner is searching for information about contains the herb's leaves and flowers, the results cannot be extrapolated. Unfortunately, not knowing the amount or exact part of the pelargonium plant used for the study prevents us from using this evidence for making evidence based clinical decisions for our patients.

- The majority of dietary supplement trials are conducted in Europe and Asia. Appropriateness of generalizability of results to a practitioner's own patient population must always be considered, just as with standard drug trials.

- Probably not with this trial although it might take longer than 7 days to completely alleviate the symptoms of acute bronchitis so this would need to be taken into consideration. In this study, we saw clear clinical improvement in the patients receiving pelargonium.

- Small subject population is a common flaw with dietary supplement trials. This study utilized a reasonable number of patients to have some comfort with external validity. Also, the number of patients were adequate to meet power and show a difference between treatment groups. In addition, adverse reactions or drug interactions can be overlooked in smaller groups versus a larger one. This could be a reason why no adverse drug effects were noted.

Chapter 7

CASE STUDY 7–1

Establish transparency.   Transparency should be planned from the beginning. Explicit details should be recorded throughout development. This information as well as funding information will need to be made publicly available.

This first step is similar to selecting topics for a medication use evaluation program. There are specific disease conditions that possess the maximum potential for benefit from guideline development and implementation. These disease conditions share common characteristics such as high prevalence, high frequency/severity, availability of high-quality evidence supporting reduction in morbidity and mortality with treatment, feasibility of guideline implementation, potential cost-effectiveness, evidence that current practice is not optimal, evidence of practice variation, and the availability of personnel, expertise, and resources to implement a practice guideline if one is developed.

Manage conflict of interest.   Before the development group is selected, individuals being considered for membership will need to declare in writing all potential conflicts of interest. Conflicts of interest not only include financial conflicts of interest, but also intellectual conflicts which may occur as a result of previous research published by the individual, institutional conflicts of interest, and patient–public activities.

Establish a multidisciplinary guideline development group.   Developing a clinical practice guideline should be considered a multidisciplinary process involving groups that have a stake in the development and implementation of the guideline. Patient involvement is especially important in helping to formulate and prioritize the questions to be addressed by the guideline. Anyone with expertise in guideline development would be valuable to the panel.

CASE STUDY 7–2

Conduct a systematic search for evidence.   Several key steps are involved in conducting a systematic search for evidence. An appropriate topic for guideline development must be selected, the clinical questions to be addressed must be defined, and the study screening selection criteria should be determined before the systematic search is conducted. Once the systematic search for evidence has been done, individual studies should be appraised and then the body of evidence should be synthesized.

Selecting a topic for guideline development is similar to selecting topics for a medication use evaluation program. There are specific disease conditions that possess the maximum potential for benefit from guideline development and implementation. These disease conditions share common characteristics such as high prevalence, high frequency/severity, availability of high-quality evidence supporting reduction in morbidity and mortality with treatment, feasibility of guideline implementation, potential cost-effectiveness, evidence that current practice is not optimal, evidence of practice variation, and the availability of personnel, expertise, and resources to implement a practice guideline if one is developed.

Defining the clinical questions to be addressed is critical to be successful in searching for the necessary evidence and providing useful valid conclusions. Many guideline development groups use the PICO format for framing the question. The "P" stands for patients who are being considered for the question. Which treatment intervention to be considered is represented by the "I," and the "C" stands for comparison or main alternatives that should be compared to the intervention. Finally, the "O" stands for what outcome is most important to the patient such as mortality, morbidity, treatment complications, rates of relapse, physical function, quality of life, and costs.

The study screening selection criteria includes the types of published or unpublished research to be considered so that appropriate literature searches may be performed. The panel needs to decide if they will accept evidence from previous guidelines, meta-analyses, systematic reviews, randomized, controlled trials, observational studies, diagnostic studies, economic studies, and qualitative studies. This process may be revisited at various stages of guideline development depending on the results of the original search.

Typically, a search is first conducted to identify previously completed guidelines and systematic reviews that involve related questions. The actual retrieval process should include a search of available bibliographic resources. Next a search of any specialized databases related to the subject of the guideline should be performed. Citations listed in published bibliographies, textbooks, and identified literature should be reviewed to identify other evidence not produced from database searches. Search terms can be identified from the clinical questions developed earlier by the panel.

Several different methods exist for evaluating studies identified in the literature. The primary purpose of appraising individual studies is to identify issues with trial design or any potential biases that would affect internal or external validity. Some issues to consider include basic trial design, sample size, statistical power, selection bias, inclusion/exclusion criteria, choice of control group, randomization methods, comparability of groups, definition of exposure or intervention, definition of outcome measures, accuracy and appropriateness of outcome measures, attrition rates, data collection methods,

methods of statistical analysis confounding variables, unique study population characteristics, and adequacy of blinding.

Evidence represented by selected studies should be summarized in a format that allows the panel to begin developing conclusions. Best formats facilitate consideration of the characteristics and quality of individual studies, consistency of the results between studies, overall size of the evidence database, and size of treatment effects for benefits and harms.

CASE STUDY 7–3

Establish evidence foundations for and rating strength of recommendations.   Recommendations in a guideline must be worded carefully and clearly communicate that the expected outcomes will be achieved if the recommendations are followed. These recommendations should be written to stand alone since users may not read the full guideline document. Confusion exists for the end user because a variety of grading systems are currently used by different guideline development groups. For each guideline that is used, practitioners are required to read the grading scheme description so they will correctly interpret the strength of the recommendations, quality of the evidence, and the balance between benefits and harms of the interventions considered. To minimize this confusion and potential for misinterpretation, a standardized system such as the Grades of Recommendation Assessment Development and Evaluation (GRADE) should be used by the panel to grade recommendations in the practice guideline being developed.

Articulate recommendations.   A standardized form should be used to detail exactly what the recommendation is and when it should be done. Strong recommendations should be phrased so that compliance with the recommendation(s) can be evaluated.

Conduct an external review.   Once a draft of the guideline has been created, it should undergo external review. All relevant stakeholders should be involved in the external review. Based on feedback from the external review, revisions may be required for the guideline to meet its intended goals. As with many steps in the guideline development process, one of the keys in this step is documentation. The decisions and actions taken in response to the recommendations from external review should be carefully documented. It is particularly important if there are critical recommendations that the guideline panel decides to reject that the reason for that decision is documented. At the time of external review or immediately following it prior to publication of the final guideline, a draft should be made available to the general public for comment.

Establish a plan for updating the guideline.   It is important that a plan for updating the guideline be established. The publication date and dates of systematic reviews used in the guideline should be clear. A plan to regularly review the literature to identify new technology or new evidence that may affect the guideline should be made, and a review interval to update the guideline should be established by the panel. The duration of the interval is dependent on the topic and knowledge of ongoing studies. A plan should also be made for an expiring guideline.

CASE STUDY 7–4

The seven categories of guideline implementation barriers that limit or restrict complete prescriber adherence include lack of awareness, lack of familiarization, lack of agreement, lack of self-efficacy (disbelief they could perform the behavior or activity recommended by the guideline), lack of outcome expectancy (disbelief that expected outcome would occur by following guideline), inertia of present practice (lack of motivation to change current practice), and a host of external barriers such as patient resistance, patient embarrassment, lack of reminder system, cost to patient, and lack of time.

Chapter 8

CASE STUDY 8–1

1. The population of interest is postmenopausal women.
2. Random sampling was used from the convenience of the endocrinologist's office.
3. Yes. Patients were randomized to treatment group, and a placebo group was included.
4. The DV is calcium absorption. It is measured on a continuous (ratio) scale.
5. The IV is treatment group. The IV is ordinal in that the treatment groups can be rank ordered by dose size. The IV has four levels—placebo, 500 IU, 2500 IU, and 5000 IU. The size of the vitamin D dose is what is manipulated by the researcher.
6. Yes, baseline calcium absorption and 25OHD measurements could be potential covariates.
7. No, because the DV is continuous, the normal distribution should be attempted initially.
8. No. Both variables are continuous, so they should be presented as mean, standard deviation.
9. Data transformation is never wholly incorrect, so it could be done. However, because the data has severe positive skewness, a natural log transformation works better. With that said, a more appropriate option would be to use the gamma, inverse Gaussian, exponential, log-normal, Weibull, or Gompertz distributions, as described in Table 8–1.

CASE STUDY 8–2

1. No. Although patients are randomized to groups, there is no placebo or control group. That is, both groups receive some form of treatment.
2. This study uses a parallel-group design with 1:1 randomization. Participants are randomly assigned to one, and only one, treatment group.
3. No. The researchers did not specify that they were interested in EACA having less bleeding than TXA. They only stated they were interested in differences between EACA and TXA. This hypothesis could be answered with either more or less bleeding. Therefore, a two-tailed hypothesis would be most appropriate.
4. Differences.
5. Twice. Once at pre-op baseline and another 2 days post-op.
6. No. The authors collected baseline hemoglobin at baseline they intended to use as a covariate. The only option is to test for group differences using a continuous covariate is ANCOVA.
7. Yes. With a continuous DV, linear regression can handle any number of covariates measured on any scale. Because this study has covariates in addition to the IV, a multivariable linear regression is most appropriate.
8. Yes. The patients are nested within doctors who are nested within hospitals. Forgetting about clustering can lead to inaccurate standard errors and bias in the statistical inference.

Chapter 9

CASE STUDY 9–1

- Since the topic is known and the boss informed you that you are the sole author, it is possible to skip some of the first steps listed in this chapter. Also, it is known where it will be published—in the policy and procedure section of the institutional intranet. So, the first thing to do is probably review the format of policies and procedures in the institution, to determine what needs to written. As a part of this, determine that it needs to be written in the middle technical style, since it is being aimed at a variety of health care practitioners (e.g., pharmacist, physician, nurse). Then, it is necessary to do research into the topic.

- First, organize the material. This can be done in conjunction with preparation of an outline of the order in which the material needs to be covered. That outline can done on a word processor and serve as the template for the document. In many cases, the way the institution lays out its policy and procedure documents can serve as a good part of the outline. Then proceed to write the material. At this stage, simply make sure everything necessary is recorded in the document. The document can be written in order of the topics, or each individual section may be written separately, in whatever order is easiest. Also, remember to cite material as the document is written. Besides being appropriate to give credit, it is also useful for the future when someone may have to come back to revise the document after several years and may not otherwise be able to tell the origin of some of the information.

- Some would say to just present it to the pharmacy and therapeutics committee, but there are a couple of things that need to be done first. To start, the author should reread and edit the document. Then, get others who have expertise in the area to read and edit the document. These others should include one or more representatives from each group affected by the document (e.g., pharmacist, physician, nurse). An effort must be made to make sure the document is in a logical order, covers all aspects of the topic, and is understandable. Then incorporate any necessary revisions. This process may need to be done several times (e.g., some chapters in this book went through a dozen versions before being submitted to the publisher).

CASE STUDY 9-2

First, clarify who the Web site is addressing—the audience. It will be different for patients versus other health care practitioners. Sometimes it will be both groups. Then, in relationship to the above, determine what information or features need to be on the Web site. Then determine what equipment (e.g., computer hardware and software) and budget are available to prepare the Web site.

CASE STUDY 9-3

First, be sure to prepare slides on something that is compatible with the program used at the meeting. Then determine what information needs to be on the slides. Generally, assume that each slide should be shown for a minute or two. Each slide should be kept simple, with a maximum of five bullet points and five words per bullet point, so that attendees can concentrate on the message. Also, remember that the speaker is not to read directly from the slides, but use them just as a jumping off spot for the presentation and to organize thoughts.

Chapter 10

CASE STUDY 10-1

- Factors that favor finding the pharmacist liable for negligence:
  - Pharmacist is a specialist (e.g., BCPS).

- ° Anticoagulation clinical pharmacist.
  - ° Reasonable pharmacist should know that an INR of 5.2 in a patient on warfarin places the patient at increased bleeding risk.
  - ° Reasonable pharmacist would question the use of the two medications together and document the same. For example, enoxaparin may be used for bridging anticoagulation when initiating warfarin but the INR of 5.2 would not indicate warfarin initiation.
- No. While combing these two drugs may increase the risk of serious or life-threatening bleeding complications, enoxaparin and warfarin may be used together to treat acute deep vein thrombosis with or without pulmonary embolism. However, where the pharmacist possesses special knowledge of the patient's condition, there is a responsibility of the patient to clarify the order.
  - ° If there is any protocol or guideline used at the clinic which was not followed.
  - ° If there was no follow up or documentation of the rationale for the combo.
- Yes. The courts would hold a specialist to a higher standard. The fact that the pharmacist is the anticoagulation clinic pharmacist and is board certified places this individual into a higher liability category.

  If there was a collaborative practice agreement it would be seen as a voluntary undertaking to provide expanded services to the physician and patient.
- All three would be liable—the pharmacist, physician, and clinic under the theory of respondeat superior for actions of employee.

CASE STUDY 10-2

- The pharmacist fell below the standard of care. A health system pharmacist has access to the patient's renal function tests. Dispensing metformin without checking renal function falls below the standard. Not following a pharmacy department policy which requires both checking and documentation of the patient's creatinine clearance prior to dispensing metformin also falls below the standard of care.

  Looking at the elements of negligence: (1) duty was breached; (2) damages resulted; (3) the damages would seem to be directly caused by the breach of the duty; and (4) defenses to not checking the renal function or following the policy are absent.

CASE STUDY 10-3

- Several activities occurring in this case violate the copyright law.
  - ° Mere listing of all drugs which should not be crushed—derived from published references.
  - ° Not classroom use.
- Permission must be obtained to use material that is paraphrased, abridged, or condensed. However, a new table created from data that is copyrighted sources would probably not require permission in this case.
- Unless the reference was government materials, permission must be obtained. In looking at fair use, a four-pronged test is used—(1) nature and character of use, (2) nature of the work, (3) the proportional amount copied, and, most importantly, (4) the effect on the market for the copied work.
- You take several direct sentences without providing source reference. One of the references is out of print.

  One factor in copying infringement is the amount copied. Even though only several sentences were copied, there is no minimal amount or threshold quantity standard where fair use would be presumed.

  The fact that some of the material is out of print does not mean the material is in the public domain. Out of print does not necessarily mean out of copyright. The rights revert to the author, and the underlying copyright remains unaffected.

CASE STUDY 10-4

- HIPAA prohibits:
  - The pharmacist sharing PHI and diagnosis in an area where it was easily overheard by others.
  - PHI faxed to a fax machine in an unsecured area where many people have access.
- Safeguards:
  - Private area
  - FAX machine should be in a private area.
  - Reasonable steps should be taken. Examples of such steps include: confirming with the intended recipient that the receiving fax machine is located in a secure area or the intended recipient is waiting by the fax machine; pre-programming and testing fax numbers for frequent recipients of DI faxes to avoid errors associated with misdialing; double-checking the recipient's fax number prior to transmission; using a fax cover sheet with an erroneous transmission statement and advising to notify the sender immediately and arrange for return or destruction of the fax; promptly checking all fax confirmation sheets to determine that faxed material was received at the intended fax number.

Chapter 11

CASE STUDY 11-1

- Assessment of whether this drug information request constitutes a potential ethical dilemma:
  1. What does it mean to you if confronting an ethical dilemma for such judgments of right or wrong to be ultimate/fundamental?
  2. How do you interpret what it means for an ethical issue to be universal, in your own words?
  3. Who are the various parties whose welfare could be impacted by the resolution to this situation, if indeed it does constitute an ethical dilemma?
- Background information to obtain to clarify this information request:
  1. What are facts of this case that you will want to learn more about before reaching a determination of whether it is indeed an ethical dilemma? (For example: What is the clinical condition of the patient in question? and, What standards or patient care commitments has your institution established for addressing patient pain issues?)
  2. Considering who is affected is really a continuation of item #3 above defining an ethical dilemma. However, it may help you further to consider specific people involved in the case at hand—the patient himself; the supervising physician; the various other staff and trainees who must try to meet this patient's needs under the circumstances at hand, and may learn to address future patients' needs based on their experience; family members of the patient who will observe their loved ones' suffering; the future patients who will be treated in similar or different ways based on the accumulating experience from this case.
  3. What cultural perspectives might be at work for the prescribing physician (imagine for instance an older practitioner, or one trained in a particular perspective relative to standards of pain control). Likewise, what is the culture in the case environment relative to lines of authority, or freedom to question authority, or approaches to patient rights?

- Given that a specific patient's welfare must be addressed, this case certainly involves a micro level of ethical decision making; however, as is often the case with ethical dilemmas, it might be argued that there are also meso level decision-making issues to be considered: What standards is the organization held to in meeting the pain control needs of its patients? What policies are there established within the organization regarding supervision/accountability of practitioners charged with patient care relative to specified standards ?
- Refer to the listing of rules and principles provided in the chapter—Which if any seem to have relevance to this case?
- Remember that rules often apply best to more narrow cases, and may be reasonably limited in some circumstances to meet the demands of more fundamental ethical principles. Decisions about competing principles will often rely on the decision makers' priorities relative to primacy of anticipated good/bad consequences of the action (for the individual only? how about for society?) versus for instance certain core beliefs about fundamental rights (e.g., deontological principle prioritizing "respect for persons").
- What kinds of standards, policies, or procedures might be useful to this nurse specialist, both to aid in her ethical decision making and to provide support in her dealings with the prescriber and other involved staff as well as the patient/family?

Refer to the article *Ethical dilemmas: Controversies in pain management* by Janet Brown to read the analysis of a similar case.[1]

REFERENCE

1. Brown J. Ethical dilemmas: controversies in pain management. Adv Nurse Pract. 1997:69-72.

CASE STUDY 11–2

- First recognize and understand the meaning of these characteristics as they apply to this specific case—however, final determination of whether they apply will require the reader to first address other steps of analysis below.
- There are a number of important factual questions that Dr. Rich is honor bound to address before deciding on any ethical dimensions of this case:
  1. Examples: What is the drug in question? How available is it, other than relative to cost? Will use for the patient at hand impact availability for other patients with more clear-cut and pressing indications for use?
  2. What is the level of evidence supporting or refuting the agent's efficacy and safety when used for the requested purpose?
     - At a macro level of decision making, cost effectiveness is often deemed another appropriate factor to consider in recommendations for use at a population level.
     - However, policies on unlabeled use quite often also include "special circumstances" where a prescriber may be allowed to prescribe a specific therapy in a particular case with coverage provided, based on the available evidence supporting such use in similar cases.
  3. What policies/procedures exist on appropriate action to address: when other alternatives are available to treat the medical condition, the seriousness of case brought up for "waiver" status, and general societal norms regarding prescriber/patient choice in desperate cases are other factors for meso or macro level decision makers to determine.
- Certainly the professional must address this dilemma at a meso level. His or her decision making may be improved if he or she also thinks about what his or her responsibility is to the individual patients who will undoubtedly be impacted by the decision, as well as overall macro (system or societal) level consequences of policies established by this and similar organizations.

- How do you think the principles of Respect for Autonomy or Fidelity might apply to this case? How do you think Justice Theory might speak in favor of restrictions; for instance, in availability of scarce drugs for fully indicated therapies versus use for less-proven therapies?
- Please imagine a specific product and case in order to personally decide how you would prioritize the various pertinent rules and principles in order to make a decision in such a case as this. Do you think that you would be justified in simply acting on the orders from your job supervisor, regardless of the factual circumstances and possible ethical issues of the case?
- Organizational strategies that might best prepare this pharmacist to most effectively respond to ethical dilemmas:

1. What organization policies or standards do you think should be established in managed care organizations to support ethical decision making pertinent to cases such as this one?
2. Do you think there are laws or regulations that should be in place at the governmental level to guide managed care organizations in providing ethical service to their insured populations? If so, what measures do you think could be useful?

Chapter 12

CASE STUDY 12-1

- See Appendix 12–6 for an example of routine agenda items. Review the minutes from the previous meeting. Add agenda items based on the meeting minutes such as follow-up information or new agenda items that came from discussion. Verify agenda with Director of Pharmacy and P&T Committee Chair.
- You would need to know some background on the formulary application, who requested it and for what application. You would need to be familiar with similar agents within category (if applicable) for comparable indications, dosing, cost, etc. It is not unreasonable to have several communications with the person requesting the new medication or other specialists who may have insight into formulary justification.

  The summary page should include the following: generic name, trade name, indications, clinical pharmacology, pharmacokinetics, adverse reactions, drug interactions, dosing, product availability and storage, drug safety/REMS, pricing, conclusion, and references.
- Intranet communication, e-mails, newsletters, personal communication, dissemination through appropriate meetings.

CASE STUDY 12-2

- Nonformulary request form
- All proton pump inhibitors (esomeprazole, lansoprazole, dexlansoprazole, omeprazole, pantoprazole, rabeprazole) are generally considered therapeutically equivalent. While there are many examples of published interchange protocols (both inpatient and outpatient), there may be a given patient who may have a better tolerability and response for one product over another.
- Most inpatient hospitals have preprinted orders for preapproved therapeutic interchanges. This form has been approved by the P&T committee. The pharmacist has been granted the responsibility to automatically fill the order with the equivalent dose of pantoprazole. Once the form is

completed it becomes part of the medical record (electronic or paper). If an interchange is chosen for a medication that is not on the preapproved therapeutic interchange list, then a new order must be written for the alternative agent.
- You can tell the physician the process for filling out the formulary request form.

CASE STUDY 12–3

- Physicians, pharmacists, nurses, students, and administrators affiliated with the health system.
- Newsletters, announcements at meetings, intranet communication, e-mail messages, personal communication, or even posting alerts in specific areas of the hospital.
- Current inventory, expected length of shortage, alternative agents available.
- In the case of furosemide, other loop diuretics are available alternatives. You may find it necessary to restrict the remaining inventory to specific hospital units or for a specific diagnosis. You may emphasize that during the shortage oral furosemide should be used whenever possible. It would be wise to produce a comparative chart for equivalent dosing and route of administration for alternative loop diuretics (bumetanide, furosemide, or torsemide). This comparison chart can be sent along with the message regarding the shortage.

Chapter 13

CASE STUDY 13–1

- Steps to add this drug to the formulary:
  - Review nonformulary utilization and indications for use.
  - Review utilization of similar agents in the therapeutic class (if applicable) that are on the formulary.
  - Seek input from the appropriate specialists who would have knowledge of the product or recommendations for formulary status.
  - Review available literature to evaluate clinical evidence.
  - Consider discussions with pharmacists at other hospitals.
  - Determine financial implications of product addition by reviewing cost information with purchasing agent and contract information from the wholesaler and manufacturer.
  - Prepare a drug monograph.
- Essential elements of a medication monograph:
  - Generic name (Trade name)
  - Approval rating
  - Therapeutic class
  - Sound/Look-alike
  - Indications/place in therapy
  - Adverse effects
  - Drug interactions
  - Recommended monitoring
  - Dosing
  - Product availability and storage

- ° Drug safety/REMS
- ° Comparative pricing information/pharmacoeconomic analysis
- ° Formulary implications/Conclusion/Recommendation
- ° References
- Sources of information to develop a complete, evidence-based, medication monograph:
  - ° Current published clinical studies and abstracts
  - ° Nonpublished data or data awaiting publication (contact manufacturer)
  - ° Current package labeling
  - ° Obtaining a formulary kit from the manufacturer may be helpful for double-checking information, but this should not be the primary reference source for your monograph
  - ° Check current evidence-based clinical guidelines

CASE STUDY 13–2

- Each of the following would be necessary, with comparison to other similar products. Essentially, it will be a quick comparison of the major similarities and differences, which can be fit on a single page.
  - ° Generic name and trade name
  - ° Indications
  - ° Clinical pharmacology
  - ° Pharmacokinetics
  - ° Adverse reactions
  - ° Drug interactions
  - ° Dosing
  - ° Product availability and storage
  - ° Drug safety/REMS
  - ° Evidence-based clinical guidelines
  - ° Recommendation

- The following information should be included:
  - ° All of the previous mentioned items
  - ° Defined tier status for copayments
  - ° Restrictions—such as prior approvals
  - ° REMS

- Different types of formulary status recommendations:
  - ° Added for uncontrolled use by the entire medical staff.
  - ° Added for monitored use—No restrictions placed on use, but the drug will be monitored via a quality assurance study (e.g., drug usage evaluation and medication usage evaluation) to determine appropriateness of use. This is a tie-in to the institution's quality assurance/drug usage evaluation process. Note: This category does not mean that the patient is monitored, since that is necessary for every drug. It means that the quality and appropriateness of how the drug is used are monitored.
  - ° Added with restrictions—The drug is added to the drug formulary, but there are restrictions on who may prescribe it and/or how it may be used (e.g., specific indications, certain physicians or physician groups, and certain policies to be followed).
  - ° Conditional—Available for use by the entire medical staff for a finite period of time.
  - ° Not added/deleted from formulary. The product can be ordered as a nonformulary product, but will not be routinely stocked in the pharmacy. Nonformulary products may take up to 24 hours or longer to obtain.

Chapter 14 _____

CASE STUDY 14–1

Possible responses include:
- Staff do not know that the medication should be infused over 60 minutes.
- The medication label does not provide infusion-time directions to the nurse administering the medication.
- Nurses are not using the smart features of the infusion pumps that would default to the appropriate infusion rate for a 60-minute infusion.
- Staff are rushed and opt to infuse medications more rapidly in order to get everything done.

CASE STUDY 14–2

Possible responses include:
- Physicians (surgeons, medicine/family medicine, infectious disease specialists)
- Nurses from the perioperative areas, inpatient units, and home care areas
- Pharmacists
- Discharge planners/case managers who help plan for discharge and arrange home care

CASE STUDY 14–3

Existing guidelines or standards for warfarin use to assist in drafting criteria for MUE can be found using any of the following:
- Search the medical literature.
- Ask practitioners with experience/expertise in this area.
- Professional organizations (pharmacy, nursing, medical).
- Identify any prior evaluations of this topic with the organization.
- Post an inquiry on professional listservs.

Chapter 15 _____

CASE STUDY 15–1

- There was no dechallenge in this case; the patient has been taking the product continuously for about 6 weeks.
- Although there was not a formal dechallenge and rechallenge, the patient reports taking the product again after her symptoms abate. Her symptoms reappear each time.
- Yes. The patient's symptoms are always preceded by administration of the drug, and they disappear soon afterward.
- Yes, the patient's symptoms are consistent with the known pharmacology of *ZygoControl Weight Loss*. The product contains synephrine, which has stimulant effects. The pharmacology of synephrine is similar to its isomer, phenylephrine.
- Using clinical judgment, you can determine that the product is likely responsible for the side effects described. This is supported by the fact that the symptoms occurred after ingestion of the

product, the symptoms recurred following rechallenge, and the symptoms are consistent with the known pharmacology of the ingredients contained in the product. You could also complete one of the algorithms discussed above in order to assess the likelihood that this reaction was caused by *ZygoControl Weight Loss.*

CASE STUDY 15-2

- There are several options for reporting the reaction to the FDA. You can report this ADR to the MedWatch program by phone, or by filling out Form 3500 and submitting it through mail, fax, or the Internet. Because this ADR involved a nonprescription natural supplement product, you also have the option of reporting the reaction through a third-party system such as Natural Medicines Watch, or directly to the product's manufacturer or distributor. These entities will forward your ADR report to the FDA.
- You patient can report the ADR either by completing MedWatch Form 3500B, or contacting one of the FDA's Consumer Complaint Coordinators.

Chapter 16

CASE STUDY 16-1

- Advantages and disadvantages of including multiple cases in the root cause analysis process:
  - Combining cases of similar types provides a larger volume of information from which to extract potential causes common to many events. For example, reviewing one case and making major system changes may in fact miss the most common factor that is causing the events. The power of multiple cases increases the chance that the frequent causative reasons are identified, which can then be addressed.
  - One disadvantage is that each case that is included in an aggregate root cause analysis (RCA) requires adequate investigation in order to understand the causes and, therefore, takes more time. All the cases are then reviewed in aggregate to determine those most common causes.

CASE STUDY 16-2

- Questions you would like to ask the pharmacist involved in the error as part of an interview:
  - It is important to ask staff to provide a description of the situation as they remember it, without leading questions. It is also very important to interview staff early to prevent unintentional alterations to the story based on fading memory or hearing other discussions related to the event.
  - Ask the pharmacist to describe what happened and what they remember.
  - Ask the pharmacist what they do if/when they realize an error has occurred. What resources are they aware of to identify what patient they may have entered the orders on in error—many computer systems have a searching function that enables a report that identifies all patients on a given drug?
  - Ask other pharmacists what their process is when interrupted to ensure they are entering orders on the correct patient.

- Classification of error as human-error only, system-error only or combination:
- It depends on the information that is gathered during interviews and observation of the usual process. If there exists the opportunity to devise a no-interruption zone for order entry (in which telephone calls are received by other staff), then this is a system opportunity. It is a human error in that it was not an intentional action and the system set up the pharmacist to potentially fail. It is likely considered a combination of both human error and system contributing cause.

CASE STUDY 16–3

- System issues that contributed to the error:
  - ○ The nurse had more patients than the recommended nurse:patient ratio.
  - ○ The drug label had the volume first and the drug listed second, yet the infusion pump requires programming the drug first and the volume second, setting up the nurse to program it incorrectly.
- Your reaction as manager of the unit:
  - ○ Were the actions as intended? Did the nurse intentionally program the pump incorrectly? No.
  - ○ Was the person under the influence of unauthorized substances? No.
  - ○ Did he or she knowingly violate a safe operating procedure? There was not a required double check and pump programming was taught to all staff upon institution of the new pumps. She did not make a conscious choice to skip steps within the process or subvert the process.
  - ○ Do they pass the substitution test described above? When this was discussed with several other nurses, two of the three noted that they had made a similar error and/or caught a similar error. This appears to be a skill-based error in which the nurse has done it many times and this time there was a slip. Would others have made the same decisions and, if so, less likely to be culpable? If not, were there deficiencies in training or experience? The training must be carefully considered. Providing didactic information without practice or competency testing is not the most appropriate method of teaching staff. Adequate practice is needed to develop good habits and skill-based actions.
  - ○ Does the individual have a history of unsafe acts? This is the first error of this type that has been identified for this nurse. If not, again less likely to be culpable.
- Identifying potential system fixes:
  - ○ The label design should match the entry in the pump if at all possible. Rearranging or increasing the visibility of the required information for programming is another option.
  - ○ Providing adequate staffing ratios to decrease the risk of competing priorities with multiple patients is appropriate.
- What other system fixes can you think of?

CASE STUDY 16–4

- Identifying system or process issues:
  - ○ The epidural medication was brought into the patient's room before there was an order, at the request of the anesthesiologists. They wanted to have everything ready when the patient and team decided it was time for the epidural. This increases the risk of inadvertent administration due to availability.
  - ○ The nurse had not placed an identification band on the patient, which is required for use of the medication bar-code scanning process. Part of this was because of the lack of immediate availability of labels in the patient's room or on admission, requiring the nurse to go searching for the identification band. A contributing factor was found to be a prior tolerance of not using the bar-code scanning on this unit.
  - ○ The nurse did not use the bar-code scanning technology to verify the medication prior to administration. This would have detected the error prior to administration to the patient if used correctly. This was partly due to the lack of patient identification band and a unit tolerance

to inconsistent use of this technology. This unit experienced a difficult implementation with this process that was ineffective at times, leading nurses to skip the process.

  ○ The nurse picked up the wrong medication, didn't closely read the label, and prepared the incorrect medication. Contributing factors to this human error include the similar bag size and look of the two medications, a rushed nature, and a low suspicion of risk—never having experienced an error or problem in the treatment of a laboring mother in this manner. This nurse was fatigued due to her work schedule and distracted, both of which increase the risk of a human error.

• Read the related article cited below to identify additional information about the case. Lead a discussion related to system errors and their impact on health care professional's behaviors and the potential impact to patients.

Smetzer J, Baker C, Byrne FD, Cohen MR. Shaping systems for better behavioral choices: lessons learned from a fatal medication error. Jt Comm J Qual Patient Saf. 2010 Apr;36(4):152-63.

  a. Discuss challenges with implementation of new technology.
  b. Discuss challenges in culture and prioritization of safety principles.
  c. Discuss confirmation bias and look-alike packaging.

Chapter 17

CASE STUDY 17–1

• Yes, the product is going to be used in a different patient population and be infused using a different route of administration. In both cases the risk profile is higher for the new usage and as such submission of a new IND is going to be required.

The company may select to work with Dr. Smith's data to further develop the product, develop an appropriate protocol, and submit the IND to the FDA.

Alternatively, the company may select to simply support Dr. Smith as he develops a protocol and IND for submission. In that case the company will provide Dr. Smith with a letter of cross reference for his use in supporting his IND application.

CASE STUDY 17–2

• A well-researched comparison of the risks of liver metastases as compared to the risks of cirrhosis will be needed to justify further development of this product using this route of administration. In addition, submission of an REMS will be crucial.

• Appropriate components of the REMS:
  ○ Letters to health care providers
  ○ Patient medication guide
  ○ Patient registry to track enrollment of patients receiving the drug via this route of administration
  ○ Patient monitoring of liver function tests

CASE STUDY 17–3

• The IRB is likely to determine that not only must this risk be included in the consent form, but that if the purpose of the new studies is to obtain further information about this risk, that must be explained to the subjects as part of the consent form.

- Children are considered a special population in clinical research. 45CFR46 specifies criteria for the evaluation of risk as compared to benefit when research is conducted in children. In this case it is likely that an IRB would still consider this study to be approvable since the product holds the promise of potential benefit to the patient in addition to the known risks. In children prior to the age of legal majority (as defined by state law), their guardians are responsible for making health care decisions for them. In some situations the agreement of one guardian is sufficient; however, if the IRB has determined that there is risk to the child and no direct benefit to them, the agreement of both guardians is required. In addition, the agreement of the child (referred to as assent) is also required.
- The point at which a child reaches the age of majority they must provide their own consent to participate in the study.

Chapter 18

CASE STUDY 18-1

- Steps used to approach this assignment:
  - Collect information on the background related to this formulary decision.
  - If unfamiliar with the role and development of an automatic therapeutic interchange, engage in background readings to help understand this type of policy, including the strengths and limitations.
  - Determine what the standard format/template will be for policies.
  - Conduct a systematic search to determine comparative dosing, safety profiles, and cost considerations.
  - Review the information gathered in your search and consider this information in the context of the needs of the health system.
  - Solicit input from colleagues in similar institutions or professional organizations for sample policies.
  - Prepare a draft policy that is specific, yet succinct, and well referenced.
  - An automatic therapeutic interchange should include specific guidance on how nonformulary agents will be converted to the formulary agents and should include all potential medications, all usual prescribed regimens (i.e., drug, dose, route, frequency) with an equally specific regimen for the formulary agent.
  - Convene a group of stakeholders and solicit input on the policy.
- A variety of resources can be used in this process. As discussed in Chapter 3, an appropriate search should begin with tertiary references and should progress to secondary resources and eventually to primary literature in this scenario. The safety and efficacy of the HMG-CoA reductase inhibitors is well documented in the tertiary literature and resources such as Micromedex®, AHFS® Drug Information, and textbooks (e.g., *Pharmacotherapy Principles and Practice*) are a good starting point for understanding a comparison of the agents with respect to clinical efficacy, safety profile, and dosing and administration considerations, in addition to other parameters. Following a thorough search of the tertiary literature, in this case, it is appropriate to conduct a literature search in a secondary database (e.g., PubMed®) to identify primary literature that supports a conversion from one agent to another. Adequate clinical trials should be collected and evaluated to assess the appropriateness of such a therapeutic interchange policy. Ideally, comparative head-to-head studies would be available to draw conclusion about comparative efficacy and safety. Finally, cost should be obtained directly from the pharmacy department regarding institution-specific pricing to develop a cost comparison for the conversion to the formulary agent.

- Once the information is collected from tertiary and primary resources, a thorough evaluation should be conducted. This will involve a critical assessment of the literature in the context of the needs of the organization.
- Stakeholder and identify key stakeholders for this policy are defined as follows:
  - A stakeholder is an individual who has a vested interest in the matter and policy in question.
  - For the policy on an HMG-CoA reductase inhibitor automatic therapeutic interchange, the key stakeholders would be physicians in the specialties of cardiology, internal medicine, and family medicine. This policy would affect the pharmacy department and clinical pharmacists practicing in these specialties as well.
  - Once a draft policy is developed, it should be presented to key stakeholders for review and input prior to its presentation for approval by a pharmacy and therapeutics committee or medical director. This can be accomplished in several ways. Perhaps a formal meeting of the stakeholders could be convened (e.g., expert panel) or individual discussions and dissemination of the draft could be handled by the pharmacist responsible for drafting the policy.

Chapter 19

CASE STUDY 19-1

- Drug information questions that TH has either requested or implied:
  - What is meant by the term "not on formulary?"
  - What *is* covered on this patient's prescription formulary?
  - What other options (pharmacologic [Rx and OTC] or nonpharmacologic are there besides what the patient has determined to be an expensive prescription drug?
- Sue might begin to answer each of these questions as follows:
  - "Not on formulary" means that a medication is not listed in a prescription drug plan as being paid for nor provided at a discounted rate through a prescription insurance plan.
  - Prescription formulary coverage information may be determined in a variety of ways, including visiting http://medicare.gov for Medicare recipients, typing prescription insurance provider + formulary + the calendar year you desire (e.g., 2014) in an Internet search engine, searching select drug information databases such as Epocrates® or Lexicomp®, or within e-prescribing platform formulary decision support systems.
  - Alternative treatments for heartburn may be researched within current treatment guidelines. Accurate, reputable treatment guidelines may be quickly found in sources such as National Guidelines Clearinghouse (NCG), the Iowa Drug Information Service, PubMed®, as well as through links from the Web sites of the American Society of Health-System Pharmacists (ASHP) at http://www.ashp.org/bestpractices or from the American Pharmacists Association™.
- Reputable databases with information geared specifically toward the patient, and with materials that have been reviewed and placed at eighth-grade reading level or below include Clinical Pharmacology, Facts and Comparisons Online, Lexicomp, and Micromedex.
- Clinical Pharmacology®, Facts and Comparisons Online®, and Lexicomp®, each contain patient-oriented materials in both English and Spanish. In addition, the Lexicomp® database includes medication leaflets in up to 19 additional languages, and Micromedex®'s Patient Connect Suite includes medication information in up to 15 languages geared toward the patient (although the reading level for the additional languages in LexiComp® and Micromedex® is not specified).

CASE STUDY 19-2

- In general, the most important thing to advise the consumer is to avoid flushing medication and avoid pouring them down the drain (according to the SMARxT DISPOAL™ Campaign). Consumers should be encouraged to take advantage of medication take-back collection days. If none are available, methods for safe personal disposal of medications can be found on the Institute for Safe Medical Practice Web site (http://www.ismp.org) as well as the Pharmacist's Letter Web site (http://www.pharmacistsletter.com). A very small number of drugs may be flushed (due to the potential risk of inappropriate exposure), and these are listed online at http://www.fda.gov/downloads/Drugs/ResourcesForYou/Consumers/BuyingUsingMedicineSafely/EnsuringSafeUseofMedicine/SafeDisposalofMedicines/UCM337803.pdf as well as in Table 19-1 of this chapter.
- While multiple governmental initiatives exist to promote the safe and appropriate disposal of unused, unwanted, and expired medications (e.g., The White House Office of National Drug Control Policy and that of the U.S. Fish and Wildlife Service's SMARxT DISPOSAL campaign), these are not enforceable laws on the consumer.

CASE STUDY 19-3

- Examples of such quality indicators include, but are not limited to, efficiency (resource use), structure, process, intermediate outcomes, long-term outcomes, and patient centeredness. Newer measures may include those focused on medication-related patient safety (e.g., detecting/preventing medication errors and adverse drug reactions).
- Yes it is, and it falls under the quality measure related to patient centeredness.
- Yes; The U.S. Department of Health and Human Services, as part of the Accountable Care Organization model has specified and published 33 required quality measure that are evaluated in order to determine payment structure for patient care networks (including ambulatory care settings).

Chapter 20

CASE STUDY 20-1

- As a pharmacist in a busy pharmacy, it is important to triage the problems in front of you. In this situation, you have multiple things going on and you are the only pharmacist on duty. It is up to you to decide what takes priority. This patient may be making decisions about her health based solely on information found online. If the patient follows through on her plan to stop taking the antidepressant, she will be at risk of being harmed. This should make her your top priority.

  The patient in this particular case is actually seeking input from you in her attempt to have a dialogue about quitting her antidepressant. You would be negligent in your duties if you did not choose to counsel the patient on the pros and cons of obtaining health information online, danger of stopping an antidepressant abruptly, and risk of recurrence of her depression. As a pharmacist, you have a professional obligation to engage with your patients and provide them with the education and tools to obtain the best health care possible. Patients are increasingly using alternative sources beyond health care providers for advice and/or counseling, which makes it vital that pharmacists initiate even difficult conversations.

- First, the patient should be encouraged to continue to take an active role in her own health care. Patient empowerment has many positives for health outcomes. On the flipside, it is important to make the patient aware that when taking her health care into her own hands there can be negative consequences as well. It is crucial that she involve a health care practitioner if she decides to change her therapy in anyway.

Second, agree with your patient that there are a lot of good places to find health information out there but that it is really important they identify quality Web sites to obtain that information. Even then, every individual is different and the information they find on these Web sites may not necessarily be patient specific or applicable to his or her situation. For example, the patient in this case is making a decision to discontinue her antidepressant based on other patients' opinions of the medication. These other patients quite possibly have an entirely different health situation. Encourage the patient to take these concerns to her primary care practitioner so that they may have a discussion on whether or not what she found online is relevant to her situation. Seems like it is missing a space between the period and the T in third. Third, you review suggestions for determining a quality health information Web site, thereby ensuring she is obtaining information from reputable sources and bringing information to discuss with her health care practitioner that has value. In this specific case, you are extremely busy and unable to meet now so you should arrange a time to call the patient or make an appointment for her to come back in to discuss her plans.

Our role is to support the patient and their beliefs. Show respect and the desire to collaborate with them and you will gain their trust. Trivialize what they bring to you and insist that the health care practitioner is the expert and the one who knows best and you may damage the relationship beyond repair.

- Safety first. If the patient has made up her mind that there is no stopping her from discontinuing her antidepressant immediately, advising her how to do so safely becomes your number one priority. First, direct the patient to see her primary care practitioner as soon as possible. Together they can work out a plan of action to taper her off the medication and possibly get her started on something she feels more comfortable taking. The practitioner may also establish a plan in order to monitor the patient for signs of relapse into depression.

If you sense the patient will not consult her physician, it is important to counsel her on possible withdrawal symptoms she may experience as well as the consequences of quitting her medication all at once without tapering. Also arrange a follow up time after your initial discussion to evaluate the control of her depression and how well she tolerated stopping the medication. At follow-up, if the patient is suicidal or at imminent risk of harming herself or someone else it is imperative you seek immediate assistance.

CASE STUDY 20-2

- The first question that should come to mind as a pharmacist is whether or not the patient has discussed the use of this particular app with his physician. Although the tracking of health data to assist in the management of a disease state can be extremely helpful for the patient, it can become dangerous when an app is making clinical recommendations about treating a condition without the supervision of a health care professional.

Second, it is important to confirm the patient is not currently in a health crisis. Although the patient sings the app's praises because of the positive difference he feels in terms of his disease state since downloading it, you want to verify that his blood glucose levels truly are well controlled. Depending on the situation, some disease states may be easier than others to evaluate at the pharmacy. Most of the time the patient will need to be redirected back to their physician in order to be sure that the app has been helping not hurting. At that time, it's a perfect opportunity for the patient and physician to discuss the mobile software and whether or not it will be a part of their treatment plan going forward.

Finally, you should ask more questions about the particular app in question. Was it developed by a credible source? Are clinical recommendations based on evidence? Is the app capable of tailoring a recommendation to a specific patient? The answers to these questions and others may help you better guide the patient in whether the app is a reliable one or in some cases FDA approved as a medical device to use in managing a disease state.

- In this particular scenario, it seems the patient has not just dipped his toes into the mobile health arena but has jumped head first. The app he describes using puts him, the patient, in a position to be very reliant on a device to make therapeutic decisions his physician would normally make. While it seems the application does factor in patient-specific data when making its decisions, without the supervision of a clinician this is risky territory.

  The single best piece of advice you can give a patient who is interested or has been using mobile health apps is to always check with a health care professional before making any changes to their prescribed medication regimen. Use of mobile health software by a patient wanting to get more involved in their health should never be discouraged; in fact, the benefits seen in patients who use apps to keep track of health and fitness progress, find health information, and stay connected with others in their health situation are infinite. The danger lies when patients start using apps as a sole resource to diagnose, manage their disease state, adjust their medication regimens, etc. Smartphone applications with these types of capabilities should be used in conjunction with a physician. In some cases, they may be medically prescribed.

CASE STUDY 20-3

In general, there are five key areas that are important to consider when evaluating a new mobile health application: credibility, accuracy, whether or not it is evidence based, ease-of-use, and health literacy. There are several questions under each key area that are important to ask yourself as a reviewer of an app.

- Credibility of application
  Are credentials of the app suitable?
  Are authors/publishers clearly listed?
  Are there advertisements?
  Is the organization that developed the app reputable?
  Are there disclaimers of content?
- Accuracy of information
  Is it peer reviewed?
  Is the information current and/or frequently updated?
  Are recent and reputable guidelines used to support recommendations made?
  Are references cited?
- Evidence-based medicine
  Are recommendations evidence based?
  Do recommendations target a specific audience or are they general in nature?
  Are opinion statements clearly marked?
  Are users directed to a health care professional before making changes to health care routine?
- Ease-of-use
  Does the app fit to the screen?
  Is the setup of the app well designed and organized?
  Is the app easily navigated?
  Does the app have a search function?
  Is there a main menu that helps clearly lay content out?
- Health literacy
  Is medical jargon used easy for the lay reader to understand?
  Is font and setup of app easy-to-read?
  Does app gear information for the consumer?

Unfortunately, even after thoroughly reviewing a mobile health app using the five key areas there still may be some questions as to whether or not it is an app that is capable of making therapeutic decisions for a patient. In these instances, it may be best to suggest contacting the developer of the software to better determine how their particular app arrives at therapeutic decisions.

Chapter 21 _____

CASE STUDY 21–1

Answers for Case Studies
1. d
2. d

Chapter 22 _____

CASE STUDY 22–1

1. Awesome Drugs R Us, Inc. should prepare standard operating procedures (SOPs) to make their employees aware of the regulations governing their job functions.
2. Awesome Drugs R Us, Inc. should include, at a minimum, Title 21 of the Code of Federal Regulations and pertinent Food and Drug Administration (FDA) Guidance documents in education materials on external regulations for their staff.
3. The medical affairs department at Awesome Drugs R Us, Inc. is responsible for all company sponsored clinical trial programs related to investigation Drug A®. The medical affairs staff are also responsible for corresponding with field staff and key opinion leaders in addition to reviewing promotional and marketing materials in anticipate of launch of Drug A®. If approved, medical affairs will be responsible for reviewing Drug A® product labeling and marketing dossiers.
4. Other departments Awesome Drugs R Us, Inc. should consider developing include medical information, medical science liaisons, and field based outcomes liaisons. Responsibilities of each include:

Medical Information:
- responds to inquiries, provides training, and drafts materials for internal and external audiences
- reviews promotional materials to ensure fair-balance of risk and benefit information
- develops portions of formulary dossier
- responds to escalated medical information requests, some may be off-label requests

Medical science liaisons (MSLs):
- supports scientific affairs and medical information staff out in the field
- maintains close relationships with key opinion leaders
- engage in clinical conversations
- cover a large geographic area while supporting a single product

Field-based outcomes liaisons (FBOLs):
- demonstrates the value of Drug A® to managed care organizations, pharmacy benefit managers and others in decision making or purchasing positions
- creates tools to help clinicians evaluate the value of Drug A® such as a risk stratification tool

CASE STUDY 22–2

- Medical education is the department which would review grants for education programming for Drug A®.
- Medical information and medical affairs will be involved in approving marketing materials for Drug A®. They will work closely with legal and regulatory staff.

CASE STUDY 22–3

- Awesome Drugs R Us, Inc. should draft a standard response letter discussing the similarities and differences between Drug A® and STRIPES™ in terms of mechanism of action, side effects, and other characteristics, in anticipation of inquiries regarding product comparisons to STRIPES™ and other investigational compounds.
- Awesome Drugs R Us, Inc. should anticipate questions on yellow stripes and anything related to that adverse event (AE) based to their similar indication to STRIPES™.

CASE STUDY 22–4

- Awesome Drugs R Us, Inc. will document patient reports of yellow stripes on Form FDA 3500A.
- Awesome Drugs R Us, Inc. is not required to share reports of yellow stripes with any additional agency or organization. Awesome Drugs R Us, Inc. has chosen to voluntarily inform the Institute for Safe Medication Practices and has alerted a patient advocacy group for those suffering from mild to moderate hiccups of the increased incidence of yellow stripes and how to report the adverse effect.

CASE STUDY 22–5

- FDA communicates safety information to patients in many ways beyond updating the prescribing information (package insert). Some of the ways FDA communicates safety information includes:
  - Drug Safety Communications
  - Medication Guides
  - Patient Package Inserts
  - Communication Plans
  - Elements to Assure Safe Use

CASE STUDY 22–6

- The manufacturer of SPOTS™ should consider voluntarily submitted a proposed Risk Evaluation and Mitigation Strategy (REMS) with their New Drug Application based on the known risks associated with Drug A® and STRIPES®.

CASE STUDY 22–7

- Pharmacists cannot dispense single ingredient albuterol CFC MDIs after December 31, 2008. Information to support this answer is found on FDA's Web site (www.fda.gov) by searching for "albuterol CFC phase out". One helpful resource is titled "Making the Switch: Prepare your patients for the phase-out of CFC-propelled albuterol inhalers". This article was also featured in the November 2008 issue of *Pharmacy Today*, the official publication of the American Pharmacists Association.

- Yes, the pharmacist may automatically switch patients from an albuterol CFC to and HFA inhaler. Information to support this answer may be found in the online article mentioned above. The article states, "Any of the three HFA propelled products containing the active moiety albuterol (ProAir HFA Inhalation Aerosol, Proventil HFA Inhalation Aerosol, and Ventolin HFA Inhalation Aerosol) are acceptable replacements for CFC propelled products containing albuterol, even though they are not generically equivalent to CFC-propelled products."
- Counseling points are provided in the article mentioned above regarding the differences patients may notice when switching from CFC to HFA albuterol inhalers. The patient should be counseled using this information, which states, "Notably, the force of the spray of an HFA-propelled inhaler may feel softer than that of a CFC-propelled inhaler. Patients should be reassured of the drug's effectiveness, even though the spray may taste different or not feel as strong as that from a CFC inhaler."
- The FDA also provides a response to pricing concerns in the article mentioned above. Regarding pricing, the FDA notes, "Because no generic products are available, patients may also have concerns about the higher cost of HFA propelled albuterol inhalers. Some drug companies have patient assistance programs that make medicines available to patients at no cost or at a lower cost. In addition, some patients may be able to get help paying for medicines from CMS [Centers for Medicare & Medicaid Services]."

  The FDA does not have statutory authority to investigate or control the prices charged for marketed drugs. Prices are established by manufacturers, distributors, and retailers. FDA does not stipulate what drugs insurance companies may cover or to what extent the drug may be covered. The Federal Trade Commission (FTC) enforces a variety of federal antitrust and consumer protection laws. The FTC accepts complaints on their Web site on the prices of marketed drugs. Please ponder the last part of this question; there is no right or wrong answer.
- Evaluating both sides of an argument helps develop empathy and understanding for opposite points of view. Express your concern for the mother's fears. Listen carefully for what help she needs. Share appropriate information about the Montreal Protocol, as required by the Clean Air Act, and the United States agreement as a signatory country to follow its terms, including the elimination of the use of CFCs.

Chapter 23

CASE STUDY 23-1

- A help-seeking advertisement should include a list of possible symptoms for a particular disease and appropriate images of individuals who may be experiencing the discussed symptoms. The advertisement should encourage patients to discuss their symptoms and seek medical advice from their physicians. In addition, the advertisement should provide company information and references to a telephone number or Web site for more information.
- The help-seeking advertisement should not include images or references to drug products to treat listed symptoms.
- Additional evaluation of the advertisement can be completed using the PhRMA *Guiding Principles*. Accuracy of the disease state information being presented should be assessed. In addition, the seriousness and respectfulness of the disease state should be maintained throughout the advertisement. Help-seeking advertisements that may be inappropriate for children should not be presented in mediums where children have access to the advertisement.

CASE STUDY 23-2

- It is very important to have a clear conflict of interest policy in place. This policy and procedure should guide who may meet with the pharmaceutical industry, how often individuals should meet with industry representatives, what topics are discussed, and what types of information and/or items may be exchanged. It is also wise to have a system in place to track and document these visits. Finally, it is also beneficial to complete a training session or course regarding best practices for industry interactions.
- Prior to the visit, it is recommended to determine what medications will be discussed, either by directly asking the representative or by reviewing their portfolio. Key evidence-based information from resources such as the prescription drug labeling will be used. It is also helpful to conduct a primary literature search and ensure you are up-to-date with current clinical literature regarding the medications.
- Be polite and professional but also use active listening skills to detect use flawed logic (e.g., appeal to authority, red herring).

CASE STUDY 23-3

- Health care professionals should critically analyze all information presented at these programs for accuracy, reliability, and potential violations.
- Common violations likely to occur in this setting include inadequate risk information, overexaggeration of benefits, presenting off-label or unapproved information, making false or deceiving comparisons with other medications.
- Health care professionals can report advertising violations to the FDA through the Bad Ad program via email: BadAd@FDA.gov or by phone: 855-RX-BADAD (855-792-2323).

CASE STUDY 23-4

- Some type of needs assessment should be done prior to launching an academic detailing programing. Possible sources of data include review of prescribing practices, patient demographics, financial data, and survey of health care professionals and/or patients.
- Materials used in academic detailing should be developed using an evidence-based approach; they should draw from tertiary resources and primarily literature. One organization that may provide validated materials is NaRCAD. Academic institutions may also serve as valuable partners.
- The advantage of a one-on-one approach is that it may facilitate a more meaningful discussion as well as allow for privacy of the prescriber. However, a group approach has the advantage of potentially reaching a larger audience. Either approach could be considered depending on the scope and goals of the program.
- Metrics should be specific to the intervention targets and actionable. For example, if a program was designed to promote evidence-based use of antihypertensives, prescribing patterns could be monitored with the goal of observing increased adherence to an institutional guideline. If increasing use of generic medications was a goal, prescription data could also be monitored to ensure effectiveness. Finally, humanistic data may also be collected in the form of prescriber and/or patient survey.

Chapter 24

CASE STUDY 24–1

- Commonly encountered technologies used:
    - Prescribing—computerized provider order entry, clinical decision support systems, electronic prescribing
    - Transcribing—clinical decision support systems
    - Dispensing—automated dispensing cabinets, carousel cabinets, robotic cart filling systems, sterile compounding devices
    - Administration—bar code medication administration systems, electronic medication administration records, intelligent infusion pumps
    - Monitoring—clinical surveillance systems, clinical documentation systems

CASE STUDY 24–2

- *Journal of Medical Internet Research, Journal of Participatory Medicine.*
- Initially, Web 2.0 tools, such as Facebook, can be used to provide general information about services offered, showcase the expertise of staff, and provide basic health and medical information. As the institution's comfort with the technology grows, Facebook can be used for online question and answer sessions, to host videos of highly advanced procedures, and to provide patient perspectives on their experiences at the facility.

    Twitter can also be used to send the latest news about significant additions to the medical staff, inform followers about upcoming clinical education classes, and highlight the acquisition of high tech tools for patient care. As resources become available and as patients express interest, Twitter may also be used for targeted messaging to remind patients of activities that encourage healthy behaviors. Ultimately, the information that is shared on Facebook, Twitter, or any other medium should address the needs of the institution's patients while maintaining privacy and confidentiality. The best way to find out what information patients want to receive or access electronically is to ask them.

CASE STUDY 24–3

- What group or organization is overseeing the EHR Meaningful Use program?
    - Centers for Medicare & Medicaid Services (CMS)
- Why would a hospital or provider want to start Meaningful Use earlier rather than later?
    - To receive the monetary incentives offered by CMS and because implementation is expected to result in better clinical outcomes, improved population health, increased health care transparency and efficiency, more robust data for research, and the empowerment of individuals and patients.
- What are the stages of Meaningful Use?
    - Answer is fine as is (i.e., There are three stages of Meaningful Use, focused on (1) capturing patient data and sharing that data with either the patient or other health care providers, (2) advanced clinical processes, and (3) improved patient outcomes.)
- The Office of the National Coordinator for Health Information Technology
- The Centers for Medicare and Medicaid Services
- There are three stages of Meaningful Use, focused on (1) capturing patient data and sharing that data with either the patient or other health care providers, (2) advanced clinical processes, and (3) improved patient outcomes.

Answers for Self-Assessment Questions

Chapter 1

1. c	6. e	11. a
2. e	7. a	12. e
3. b	8. b	13. e
4. c	9. d	14. a
5. e	10. c	15. a

Chapter 3

1. a	6. c	11. d
2. c	7. d	12. d
3. c	8. c	13. b
4. a	9. e	14. b
5. b	10. e	15. e

Chapter 4

1. e	6. b	11. a
2. b	7. a	12. e
3. a	8. d	13. b
4. d	9. c	14. d
5. c	10. e	15. c

Chapter 5

1. c	6. d	11. b
2. a	7. c	12. a
3. b	8. c	13. d
4. d	9. c	14. a
5. c	10. b	15. d

Chapter 6

1. d	6. d	11. b
2. c	7. a	12. a
3. c	8. d	13. b
4. c	9. a	14. a
5. b	10. c	15. c

Chapter 7

1. e	6. c	11. e
2. c	7. b	12. e
3. d	8. d	13. c
4. d	9. b	14. a
5. e	10. e	15. b

Chapter 8

1. a	6. e	11. b
2. e	7. c	12. d
3. a	8. b	13. a
4. c	9. b	14. e
5. d	10. a	15. a

Chapter 9

1. e	6. b	11. b
2. b	7. b	12. b
3. b	8. a	13. b
4. e	9. a	14. d
5. b	10. a	15. b

Chapter 10

1. a	6. b	11. c
2. e	7. e	12. d
3. b	8. e	13. b
4. b	9. a	14. e
5. d	10. e	15. e

Chapter 11

1. a, c, and d	6. b, c, and d	11. b
2. a	7. a	12. d
3. a, b, c, d (There could be relevance of any of these rules/principles.)	8. a	13. c
	9. b, c, and d	14. d
4. b	10. a, b, and d	15. a, b, c, and d
5. d		

Chapter 12

1. a	6. d	11. d
2. a	7. d	12. d
3. d	8. a	13. b
4. c	9. a	14. a
5. a	10. a	15. a

Chapter 13

1. a	6. d	11. d
2. a	7. e	12. a
3. b	8. b	13. a
4. a	9. a	14. a
5. a	10. d	15. a

Chapter 14

1. d	6. e	11. c
2. d	7. a	12. c
3. a	8. e	13. e
4. d	9. c	14. e
5. e	10. d	15. e

Chapter 15

1. d	6. a	11. e
2. c	7. d	12. c
3. c	8. c	13. e
4. d	9. a	14. e
5. b	10. e	15. a

Chapter 16

1. b	6. b	11. a
2. c	7. a	12. e
3. c	8. c	13. b
4. d	9. e	14. a
5. c	10. b	15. c

Chapter 17

1. a	6. c	11. d
2. b	7. b	12. b
3. c	8. d	13. e
4. a	9. a	14. d
5. c	10. c	15. c

Chapter 18

1. c	6. b	11. c
2. d	7. e	12. b
3. a	8. b	13. a
4. d	9. e	14. e
5. a	10. e	15. c

Chapter 19

1. b	6. b	11. b
2. c	7. d	12. c
3. d	8. b	13. b
4. b	9. e	14. d
5. d	10. a	15. a

Chapter 20

1. e	6. e	11. d
2. e	7. b	12. c
3. d	8. e	13. c
4. e	9. d	14. e
5. e	10. b	15. d

Chapter 21

1. d	6. e	11. d
2. d	7. d	12. c
3. c	8. d	13. d
4. a	9. d	14. e
5. d	10. d	15. a

Chapter 22

1. b	6. d	11. c
2. a	7. a	12. b
3. a	8. d	13. a
4. c	9. b	14. b
5. d	10. c	15. d

Chapter 23

1. e	6. d	11. b
2. a	7. b	12. d
3. b	8. a	13. c
4. a	9. d	14. b
5. c	10. a	15. a

Chapter 24

1. b	6. d	11. a
2. e	7. d	12. b
3. c	8. e	13. e
4. c	9. d	14. a
5. b	10. e	15. e

Index

Canadian Coordinating Office of Health
Technology Assessment, 302*t*
Cancer
ALLCure drug, 844
anticancer agents, in various stages of drug
development, 14
breast cancer
Kaplan-Meir method and, 443-445,
443*f*, 444*f*
Oncoplatin vs.Oncotaxel, 297-300, 299*t*
oprelvekin (Neumega®), 47-50
cervical, 215
chemotherapy
BSC *versus* Oncoplatin and Oncotaxel
(case study), 297-301, 298*t*, 299*t*
chemotherapy-induced peripheral
neuropathy, 169-170
double checks, 818
error, 803
regime library, medical informatics, 20
thrombocytopenia with, 48, 50
VP-CAP comparison, 287
clinical trials
Internet recruitment, 121
placebos, 123
endometrial, 220
European Organization for Research and
Treatment of Cancer, 247
Functional Assessment of Cancer
Therapy, 247
Functional Living Index-Cancer, 247
lung cancer studies, 215*f*, 221*f*, 222, 223,
372, 403
medical informatics and, 20
National Cancer Institute, 86, 857
*National Comprehensive Cancer Network's
Drugs and Biologics Compendium*, 529, 855
non-small cell lung cancer, 287
off-label drug use and, 529-530
placebos and, 123
SCORxE, 1033
screenings, CDSS, 1054
testicular, 468
uterine, 223
venous thrombosis, 129
*Cancer Epidemiology, Biomarkers, and
Prevention*, 220
Cancer Today, 89
CANCERLIT, 86
CAP. *See* Cyclophosphamide, doxorubicin, and
cisplatin
CAPE. *See* Center for the Advancement of
Pharmaceutical Education
Captopril, 129
Carbamazepine, 201, 202, 766
Care. *See also* Health care; Managed care
pharmacy; Quality improvement
continuum of, 8, 814, 885
due care, 506, 509, 518, 537
reasonable care, 507-508, 513

Career and leadership opportunities. *See* Drug
information specialists
CareNotes System, 913
*Casarett & Doull's Toxicology: The Basic Science
of Poisons*, 64*t*, 77
Case history studies. *See* Case-control studies
Case reports, 190*t*, 226-227
Case series, 190*t*, 226-227
Case studies
ADRs, 749-750, 764
BSC *versus* Oncoplatin and Oncotaxel,
297-301, 298*t*, 299*t*
cohort study design, 220
controlled clinical trials, 159-160, 168-170
drug evaluation monographs, 693
drug information education and training, 964
drug information in ambulatory care, 910-911,
919, 922-923
drug information resources, 68, 75-76, 78, 81,
88-89, 92-93, 95
drug promotion, 1024, 1030, 1031, 1034
ethical issues, 582-592
evidence-based clinical practice guidelines,
320, 325, 334, 340
investigational drugs, 844, 848, 851-852
legal aspects of DI practice, 507, 508-509,
540, 548
medication errors, 797, 802, 806, 819-820
meta-analyses, 244-245
natural products, 256-257
pharmaceutical industry, 980-981, 984, 985,
992, 993, 999-1000
pharmacy informatics, 1060, 1061, 1064
professional writing, 477, 485, 493
P&T committees, 624-625, 639, 649-650
quality improvement, 717, 724, 726
response-recommendations for drug
information queries, 46-57
as study design type
described, 226-227
N-of-1 trials compared to, 202*t*, 226
purpose, 190*t*
TXA-EACA comparison, 399-400
vitamin D-calcium absorption, 376-377
Case Studies in Pharmacy Ethics, 593
Case-control studies (case-referent studies, case
history studies, retrospective studies),
190*t*, 221-224, 221*t*, 224*t*
Cases. *See* Court cases
Catalog of Teratogenic Agents, 64*t*, 75
Categorical distribution, 368*t*
Categorical variables, 356
Causality, of ADRs, 745-751
Cause-and-effect relationships
ADRs, 745, 751
controlled clinical trials, 117, 121, 188,
190*t*, 213
observational study designs, 188, 213
survey research, 188, 227
CBA. *See* Cost-benefit analysis

Comparative Effectiveness Plus tool, IDIS, 87.
    See also Iowa Drug Information Service
Comparative negligence, 518
Compendia, major, 63*t*, 64*t*, 82
Compendium of Pharmaceuticals and
    Specialties, 73
Compendium of Veterinary Products (CVP),
    64*t*, 79
Complementary and alternative medicine (CAM)
    Clinical Pharmacology database, 912
    in drug evaluation monograph, 673
    growing use of, 16-17
    National Center for Complementary and
        Alternative Medicine, 94*t*
    Natural Medicines Comprehensive
        Database, 914
    resources on, 17, 94*t*
Compliance. *See* Adherence
Composite endpoints, 129-130, 148, 166
Compounding, veterinary, 79-80
Computer Software Act of 1980, 543
Computer technology. *See* Informatics;
    Information technology
Computer-based clinical decision support
    systems (CDSSs). *See also* Pharmacy
    informatics
    clinical practice guidelines implementation
        through, 339
    medical records, 12
    pharmacy informatics, 1047, 1048, 1050,
        1053-1054, 1055
Computerized provider order entry (CPOE), 3,
    20, 646, 786, 814, 816, 1048, 1050-1051
Conclusion section
    clinical trials, 110*t*, 149-150
    professional writing projects, 473-474
Concurrent cohort study. *See* Prospective
    cohort study
Concurrent data collection, for MUE, 729
Concurrent negligence, 518
CONDOR trial, 115-116, 118, 126, 130-131, 133,
    141, 143, 166. *See also* Controlled clinical
    trials
Conference on Guideline Standardization
    (COGS), 470
Confidence intervals (CIs)
    controlled clinical trials, 154-156
    NI trials, 193
    statistical significance and, 389-391, 389*f*, 390*f*
Confidentiality principle, 581, 586*f*
Conflict of interest
    ACPE accreditation standards, 957
    in clinical practice guideline development,
        316, 317*t*, 319
    commercial support of educational
        activities, 552
    in document submission, 475
    in formulary management, 632
    IRBs and, 851
    policies, drug promotions, 1028

in published research, 113, 164
referees, 476
Wikipedia entries, 531-532
Confounders, 122, 128, 207*t*, 217, 218-219, 355
Consensus-based clinical practice guidelines,
    245-246. *See also* Evidence-based clinical
    practice guidelines
Consent
    ethics inquiry and, 581, 586*f*
    informed consent
        of clinical trial subjects, 124-125
        off-label use and, 527-530, 528*t*
Consequential damages, 516
Consequentialist theory, 574-575, 579, 580, 581,
    585, 586, 589
Consolidated Standards of Reporting Trials
    (CONSORT), 109, 199, 469
Constancy assumptions, 196-197
Constraints, for writing newsletters and Web
    sites, 478-479
Consumer Assessment of Healthcare
    Providers and Systems program
    (CAHPS), 712
Consumer health information (CHI). *See also*
    Community pharmacy practice
    on Internet, 93-94, 94*t*
    local libraries, 93
    patient education *versus*, 933-934
    social media for, 10-11, 934, 935*t*-936*t*,
        937-939
Consumer "privacy bill of rights," Obama
    administration, 550
Consumer Reports, 935*t*
Content, of newsletters and Web sites, 483
Contingency tables, 372, 372*f*, 401, 402, 403, 415
Continuing medical education (CME)
    ACCME, 504, 551-552
    described, 336, 504, 551, 977
Continuous attribute, 706*t*
Continuous quality improvement (CQI), 312,
    340, 706*t*, 709, 719-720. *See also* Quality
    improvement
Continuous variables, 356
Continuum, of care, 8, 814, 885
Contraceptives, 127, 512, 525, 596, 597, 692, 992
Contract drug information centers
    (fee-for-service), 19-20
Contract research organization (CRO), 832
CONTRAST study. *See* Evaluation of Corlopam
    in Patients at Risk for Renal Failure-A
    Safety and Efficacy Trial
Control groups
    controlled clinical trials, 121-124
    historical controls, 122, 123, 832
    investigational drugs, 832
Control limits, for MUE, 704, 714, 727-728,
    727*f*, 730
Controlled clinical trials, 105-186. *See also*
    Randomized controlled trials; Study
    designs